Textbook of Clinical Otolaryngology

Abdulsalam Al-Qahtani
Hassan Haidar • Aisha Larem
Editors

Textbook of Clinical Otolaryngology

Springer

Editors
Abdulsalam Al-Qahtani
Hamad Medical Corporation
Doha, Qatar

Hassan Haidar
Hamad Medical Corporation
Doha, Qatar

Aisha Larem
Hamad Medical Corporation
Doha, Qatar

ISBN 978-3-030-54087-6 ISBN 978-3-030-54088-3 (eBook)
https://doi.org/10.1007/978-3-030-54088-3

This Springer imprint is published by the registered company Springer Nature Switzerland AG
The registered company address is: Gewerbestrasse 11, 6330 Cham, Switzerland

Dedicated
To my parents
To my wife Fatima
To my children Alreem, Faisal, Noof
To my family and friends
who have always been my strength and moral support

Abdulsalam Al-Qahtani

Preface

During my two decades as an otolaryngologist, I came across several broad otolaryngology textbooks. I felt that there was a lack of brief textbooks appropriate for otolaryngology practitioners and physicians taking written and oral board examinations, re-certification, and in-service exams. So, we decided to fill this void and wrote a condensed book to suit the purpose, covering most of the ORL-HNS topics. The book consists of many recent advances in head and neck, fascioplastic, otology, laryngology, rhinology, audiology, and pediatrics subspecialties. It covers issues related to allergy, sleep medicine, trauma, and the basics of otolaryngology systemic diseases.

The book is a joint effort of Hamad Medical Corporation researchers and some of the world's prominent authors. I want to thank each of them for their contributions to this book and for making my long-standing dream of publishing a textbook a reality.

I hope that this book will fulfill its primary objective in adding to the otolaryngology specialty information pool and helping the trainees to prepare well for their board review.

Doha, Qatar — Abdulsalam Al-Qahtani

Preface

Attractively designed and effectively presented, this textbook is the happy culmination of our keen and long-drawn focus on clinical otolaryngology. It serves as an essential guide to help users recognize, diagnose, and manage a range of common and important ear, nose, and throat conditions. Lucid presentation was of particular importance when approaching each subject, as we intended to facilitate the easy recall and reproduction of concepts by students and practitioners. This rapid reference is a must-have book for all otolaryngologists, audiologists, and speech therapists.

We intended this book for our departments, residents and fellows, our colleagues, and the patients who will ultimately benefit from advances in our field. We hope our readers can build upon the achievements described in this book. I owe my own achievements to my parents, my wife Fatima, my children Hawraa and Ali, and all my friends. I cannot thank them enough.

Doha, Qatar

Hassan Haidar

Preface

Otolaryngology, head and neck surgery, is a fascinating specialty concerned with the medical and surgical treatment of conditions involving ear, nose, throat, and neck. Its expertise ranges from managing possible life-threatening tumors or infections to providing improved quality of life by treating dizziness and hearing and speech pathologies.

Authoring the *Textbook of Clinical Otolaryngology* was inspired by my passion for teaching and training. Thus, this book, which is intended primarily for otolaryngology trainees, will provide the knowledge they require to progress in the field. The book covers most of the specialty's common and advanced topics. It will give the reader gradual, easy-to-locate, and practical information on diagnosis, testing, disease processes, and up-to-date strategies for treatment and management. The book hopefully will be of interest to otolaryngologists and all the medical and surgical specialties and related disciplines.

The book is structured to combine conventional with contemporary thoughts, theory with practical tips, and international standards with national or regional norms. The chapters are blended and organized to flow naturally, but each is adequately self-contained. The materials were chosen from books, magazines, research papers, and the Internet to represent my viewpoints and experiences.

I feel privileged to be on the editorial board, along with my colleagues Dr. Al-Qahtani and Dr. Haidar. I am also grateful to the many senior professors, colleagues, trainees, friends, and loved ones who have given so generously their time, resources, and support in contributing to this book.

I dedicate this work to my beloved country, Qatar. I owe my achievements to my mom Amna, my family, and friends, while I am not able to thank them enough.

I would be happy to hear from the readers of this book.

Doha, Qatar — Aisha Larem

Contents

Part VII Pediatrics

Part VIII Facial Plastics

Part I

Audiology

General Audiology

1

Ma'in Ali Al Shawabkeh, Hassan Haidar,
and Khaled Abdulhadi

1.1 Introduction

Audiological tests are essential in clinical practice as they can guide the management and determine the treatment option for patients. These tests should always be taken as a battery of tests and not relying on a single test, as this will help to give a whole picture of the patient.

1.2 Definitions

- *Sound*: It is the energy that travels in waves within a medium (like air). A sound wave is composed of compression (more dense) and rarefaction (less dense) waves. Two important terms related to sound are intensity and frequency.
- *Frequency*: It is the number of waves per second. Hertz (Hz) is the unit used for measurement of frequency. It is related to the pitch of the sound. The higher the frequency is, the more pitch the sound will be. Sound in nature is complex, which means it is composed of more than one frequency. Pure tone sound, that is, sound composed from single frequency, is rarely found in nature but usually used in audiometer for hearing assessment. Humans are capable of hearing sounds between 20 and 20,000 Hz [1].
- *Noise*: It is a complex aperiodic sound; it can be a white noise if it composed of all the frequencies, a narrow-band noise if it is composed of certain frequencies (above and below specific frequency), or speech noise if it is composed of speech frequencies (i.e., 300–3000 Hz).
- *Intensity*: It is the strength of the sound and consists of the amount of energy produced in an area per time. It correlates to the loudness of the sound. Decibel is the unit used to measure the intensity or loudness of sounds. The normal conversation usually is about 60 dB, and the quiet countryside is about 30 dB. One hundred and ten decibel can cause discomfort in the ear, and 130 dB can cause pain in the ears [2].
- *Decibel*: It is a relative measure of the intensity of sound. It represents a logarithmic expression of two intensities ratios.
- *Sound pressure level (SPL)*: It is related to the intensity of the sound and considered an absolute pressure reference level for the decibel. Zero dB SPL = 0.0002 dyn/cm^2.
- *Hearing level (HL)*: It is the most common reference used in audiometers. Zero dB HL means that normal human ears will perceive

M. A. Al Shawabkeh · K. Abdelhadi
ENT Department, Hamad Medical Corporation, Doha, Qatar
e-mail: Khadi@hmc.org.qa

H. Haidar (✉)
ENT Department, Hamad Medical Corporation, Doha, Qatar

Hamad Medical Corporation, Doha, Qatar

A. Al-Qahtani et al. (eds.), *Textbook of Clinical Otolaryngology*,
https://doi.org/10.1007/978-3-030-54088-3_1

the sound at any given frequency in 50% of the times.

- *Sensation level (SL)*: Here, the reference is the threshold for an individual. Zero SL means that an individual can hear the sound at a given frequency in 50% of the times.
- *Recruitment*: It is the abnormal growth of loudness. It indicates a cochlear hearing loss. Patients with this condition are poor candidates for hearing aid.
- *Most comfortable level*: It is the intensity of the sound that is more comfortable to the patient.
- *Loudness discomfort level*: It is the intensity of the sound that will produce discomfort to the patient.
- *Dynamic range*: It is the range between the loudness discomfort level and the most comfortable level. Patients with recruitment will have a reduced dynamic range.

1.3 Assessment of Hearing

1.3.1 Clinical Tests

1.3.1.1 Tuning Fork Tests

There are different forks with each having specific frequencies. There are 128, 256, 512, 1024, 2048, and 4096 Hz. Five hundred twelve Hertz tuning fork is the most suitable one used for hearing assessment, because the one with low frequency will give a bone vibration sensation that means it is felt rather than heard, while the one with high frequencies will give a short decay time [3].

Weber test: It is the test of lateralization; the tuning fork is put on the middle of the forehead after being activated, and then assess where the patient will hear the sound better.

- Normal hearing: there will be no lateralization of the sound (in the center).
- Unilateral Conductive hearing loss (CHL): he will lateralize the sound to the diseased ear.
- Unilateral Sensorineural hearing loss (SNHL): the patient lateralizes the sound to the normal ear.

Table 1.1 Interpretation of negative and positive Rinne tests' results of the different types of tuning forks

256 Hz	512 Hz	1024 Hz	Degree of air-bone gap (AB gap) (dB)
Negative Rinne	Positive Rinne	Positive Rinne	20–30
Negative Rinne	Negative Rinne	Positive Rinne	30–45
Negative Rinne	Negative Rinne	Negative Rinne	45–60

Rinne test: In this test, the tuning fork (after being activated) is put on the mastoid process for a given ear (it will assess the bone conduction (BC)) and then 2 cm lateral to the external auditory canal of that ear (it will assess the air conduction (AC)), and the patient is asked which sound heard better.

- Normal hearing: It will give a positive Rinne, which means AC is better than BC.
- CHL: It will give a negative Rinne, which means BC is better than AC.
- SNHL: It will give a positive Rinne. Look at Table 1.1, which gives an interpretation of negative and positive Rinne tests' results of the different types of tuning forks.

For other tuning forks clinical tests, look at Table 1.2.

1.3.2 Audiometric Tests

1.3.2.1 Pure Tone Audiometry

The audiometer is a device used for hearing assessment. It can measure the threshold for air conduction and bone conduction. In AC, 250, 500, 1000, 2000, 4000, and 8000 Hz are used, while in BC, 8000 Hz is not measured. Pure tone average (PTA) is the average threshold of AC. Table 1.3 shows the different symbols used in an audiogram.

Hearing assessment can show:

(a) Normal hearing: if all threshold within the normal level.

Table 1.2 Other tuning forks clinical tests

Test	How to perform the test	Normal hearing	CHL	SNHL
Bing test	The tuning fork is put on the mastoid process of the ear, and the examiner closes and opens the patient's ear canal by his finger	Positive Bing, which means the patient will hear the sound louder when the ear is occluded	Negative Bing; there will be no change in the appreciation of the sound while the ear is opened or closed	Positive Bing
Schwabach test	The tuning fork is put on the mastoid process of the patient till the sound will stop, then the examiner will put that fork to his mastoid process	Normal Schwabach; The patient will stop hearing the sound same as the examiner (given that the examiner has a normal hearing)	Prolonged Schwabach; the patient will hear the sound for a more extended period than the examiner	Diminished Schwabach; the patient will stop hearing the sound before the examiner
Absolute bone conduction	The tuning fork is put on the patient's mastoid process and then on the examiner's mastoid process. The external auditory canal of the patient and the examiner should be occluded	Both the patient and the examiner will hear the sound for the same period	Both the patient and the examiner will hear the sound for the same period	The patient will hear the sound for a shorter period

Note: In Gelle test, the tuning fork is put on the patient's mastoid process, and then a different amount of pressure level is applied to the tympanic membrane (TM). Patients with normal TM and ossicles will notice a decrease of sound while the pressure is increased, while patients with ossicular discontinuity or fixation will appreciate no change in sound. It was used before to detect patients with otosclerosis

Table 1.3 Different symbols used in an audiogram

Interpretation	Right ear	Left ear
Unmasked AC	○	X
Masked AC	△	□
Unmasked BC	<	>
Masked BC	[	]
No response	↙	↘
Soundfield	S	S

(b) CHL: if BC within normal threshold but AC shows some hearing loss.
(c) SNHL: Both AC and BC show the same degree of hearing loss.
(d) Mixed: Both AC and BC show a hearing loss, but AC has more severe hearing loss than BC.

Look at Fig. 1.1 that represents a different type of audiograms.

Note

- Maximal CHL is 60 dB, and it is found in cases of an intact TM with ossicular discontinuity.
- Low-frequency SNHL: found in endolymphatic hydrops.
- High-frequency SNHL: found in presbycusis and ototoxicity.
- Carhart notch: found in otosclerosis.
- 4 kHz Notch: found in noise-induced hearing loss.
- Cookie Bit (U-shaped): found in hereditary hearing loss.

Masking

Interaural attenuation is the amount of sound needed to make it cross to the contralateral ear (non-tested ear); because of that, the tested sound should not exceed that level to prevent

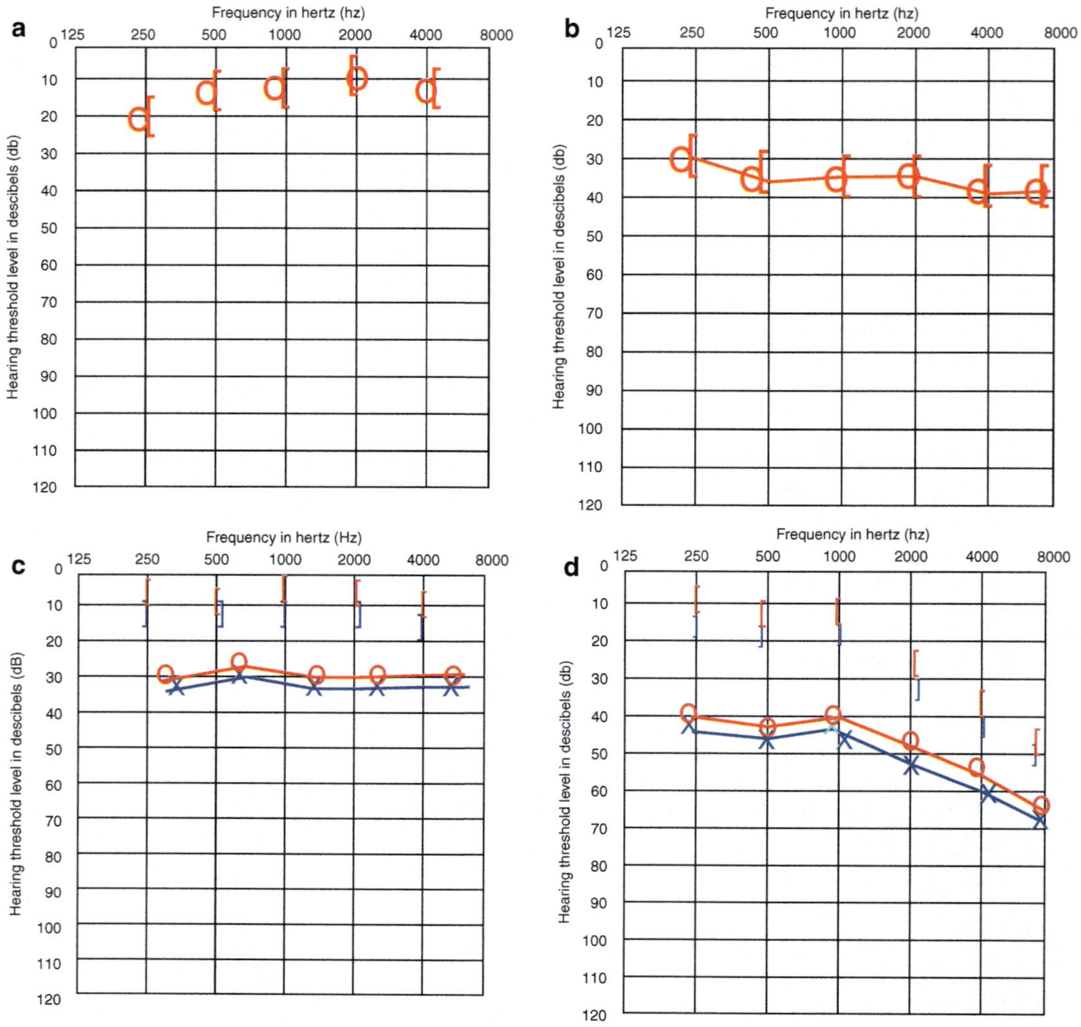

Fig. 1.1 Different types of audiograms. (**a**) Normal hearing in the right ear, (**b**) mild SNHL in the right ear, (**c**) bilateral CHL, (**d**) bilateral mixed hearing loss

crossover, otherwise masking is needed. In AC testing, the interaural attenuation for stimuli delivered via headphones ranges from 35 to 50 dB, and it is 60 to 65 dB for the stimuli delivered via the earphones. In BC testing, it is 0 dB [4].

To prevent crossover, masking should be used in the non-test ear. Masking is a narrow-band noise for pure tone audiometry or wideband noise for speech audiometry. Masking should be used while doing AC test in cases where the AC in the tested ear is more than 40 dB the BC in the non-tested ear for the headphones, or AC in the tested ear is more than 70 dB the BC in the non-tested ear for the insert earphones. Masking also should be used in the BC test if the AB gap in the tested ear is more than 10 dB.

While testing a dead ear, sound can cross to the non-test ear giving *a shadow curve*.

For degree of hearing loss, look at Table 1.4.

1.3.2.2 Speech Audiometry

Here the stimulus is the spoken words; it can be either Speech Reception Threshold (SRT) or Word Recognition Score (WRS) (Speech Discrimination Score):

Table 1.4 Degree of hearing loss

0–25 dB HL	Normal
26–40 dB HL	Mild
41–55 dB HL	Moderate
56–70 dB HL	Moderately severe
71–90 dB HL	Severe
Above 91	Profound

Table 1.5 The interpretation of WRS results

WRS (%)	Interpretation
90–100	Normal
76–88	Slight difficulty
60–74	Moderated difficulty
40–58	Poor
40	Very poor

Note: In normal individuals, as the intensity of the sound at which PB words are presented increases, the score will increase until it reaches 100%. In SNHL of cochlear origin, it will reach a plateau at which the WRS score will not increase. However, in SNHL of retrocochlear origin, as sound's intensity increases, WRS will not maintain that plateau and then it will fall down; this condition is called *RollOver Phenomenon*. Look at Fig. 1.2

(a) SRT: the stimulus is spondee words (i.e., two-syllable words that have the same stress on each syllable as in "eardrum"). The threshold is the lowest intensity at which the patient repeats the words in 50% of the time. SRT should be within 10 dB of the measured PTA.

(b) WRS: the stimulus is phonetically balanced (PB) words, which are presented to the patient at 30–40 dB above SL. The patient will hear 50 words. The result is the percentage of the words that the patient will repeat correctly. The interpretation of the results is shown in Table 1.5.

1.3.2.3 Immittance/Impedance Test

Tympanometry

This device is composed of a probe inserted in the tested ear canal. It has three channels, the first will deliver a 226 Hz tone, this tone will go to TM and then either get reflected or absorbed, the second channel will collect the reflected sound, and the last channel will make changes of the pressure inside the ear canal. A compliant TM will reflect less sound than a stiff TM. This test is an objective one, and it can measure ear canal volume of the tested ear and the compliance of its TM at different pressure levels, which will be shown on a chart called tympanogram. A normal test will show a type A graph; in adults, the peak compliance will be 0.3–1.4 (mean 0.8), the peak will be at average 0 mm H_2O pressure (between −50 mm H_2O till +50 mm H_2O is considered normal), and ear canal volume is 0.6–1.5 mL (mean 1.1). In pediatrics, the peak compliance will be 0.2–0.9 (mean 0.5), the peak will be at average 0 mm H_2O pressure (between −50 mm H_2O till +150 mm H_2O is considered normal), and ear canal volume is 0.4–1.0 mL (mean 0.7). There are five types of tympanogram graphs:

1. Type A: is the normal one and discussed above.
2. Type B: a flat one, and it can indicate either:
   (a) Fluid behind the TM: the volume of the ear canal will be normal.
   (b) TM perforation: the volume of the ear canal will be high.
   (c) A plugged probe by either poor fitting or wax: the volume of the ear canal will be low.
3. Type C: the peak will be at negative pressure, and this will indicate Eustachian tube dysfunction.
4. Type As: The peak will be shallow, and this can indicate wither:
   (a) Otosclerosis.
   (b) Tympanosclerosis.
   (c) Malleus fixation.
5. Type Ad: The peak will be high, and this indicates either:
   (a) Flaccid TM.
   (b) Ossicular discontinuity.

Look at Fig. 1.3 which shows different types of tympanograms.

Acoustic Reflex

In the case where there is an exposure to a high-intensity sound, there will be a reflective contraction of the bilateral stapedial muscle making the TM stiffer; this is a protective mechanism of the ear against high-intensity sounds. This reflex is

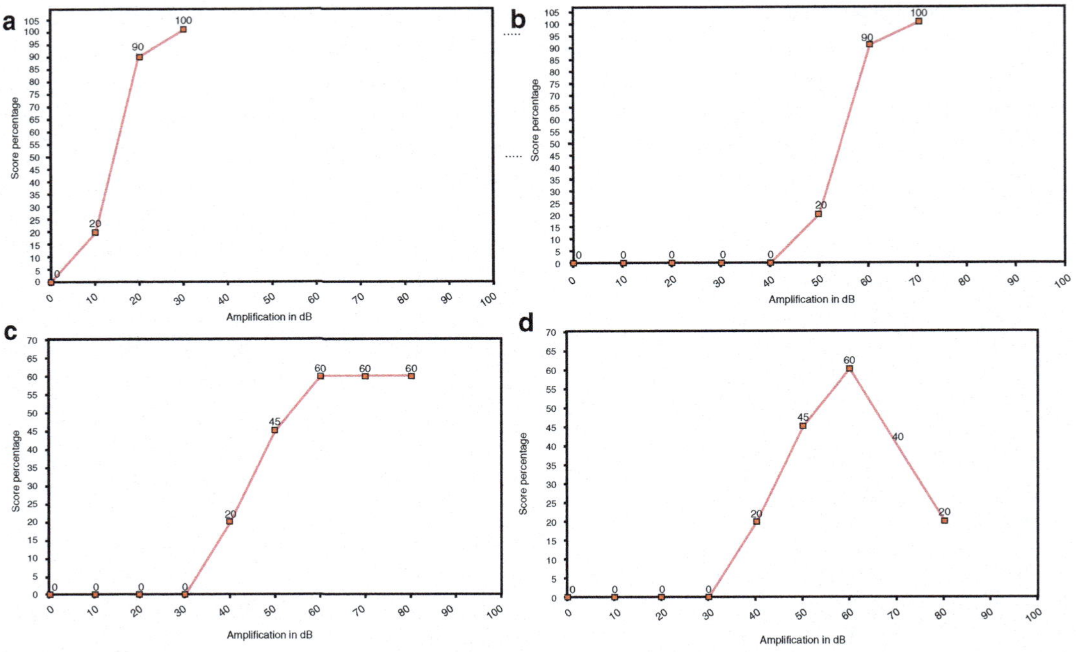

Fig. 1.2 (**a**) Normal speech audiogram. (**b**) Speech audiogram for a patient with CHL. (**c**) Speech audiogram for a patient with a cochlear lesion notice that WRS has reached a plateau and maintained at that level. (**d**) Speech audiogram for a patient with retrocochlear lesion, notice how WRS did not maintain at that plateau, and it fell down; this condition is called Roll Over

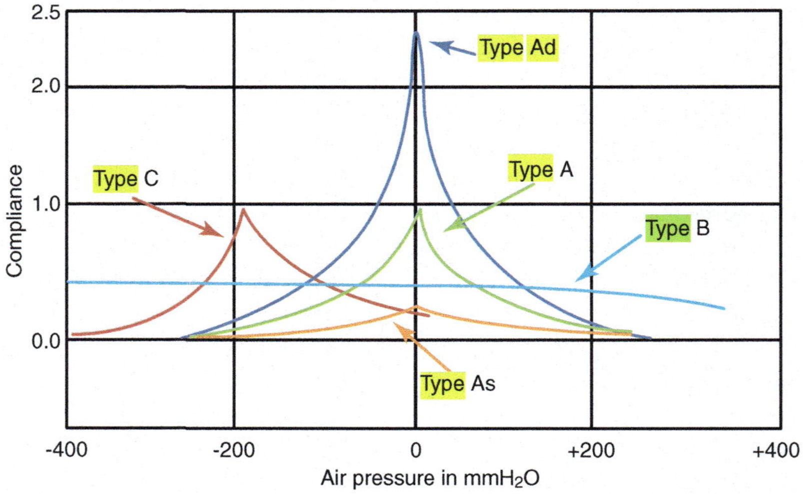

Fig. 1.3 Different types of tympanogram: Type A: normal tympanic compliance, Type As: increased stiffness of the tympano-ossicular system indicative of ossicular fixation, Type Ad: hypermobile drum indicative of ossicular discontinuity. Type B: suggestive of a glue ear. Type C: negative pressure in the middle ear space (nasal congestion, or ear infection). (Adapted from Mansour S., Magnan J., Nicolas K., and Haider H. (2018). Middle ear disease)

called Acoustic reflex. It will occur if the sound's intensity is 70–100 dB SL. The Arc of this reflex is like the following:

- The sound will pass to the cochlea, and then it will go to the ipsilateral cochlear nucleus via CN VIII. From there, it will go to the trapezoid body. Then the signal will pass from the trapezoid body to the bilateral superior olives. After that, it will go to the facial nuclei, and then it stimulates the stapedial muscle via CN VII.
- The acoustic reflex is an objective study. It is measured by introducing a sound at different frequencies (500, 1000, and 2000 Hz) in any of the ears, and the change of compliance for both ears will be detected via a probe.

Acoustic Reflex Interpretation

1. In the case of unilateral SNHL: if hearing loss is more than 60 dB in one ear, then acoustic reflex will be absent in both ears if the signal was introduced in that ear. However, there will be bilateral acoustic reflex if the signal was presented in the normal ear.
2. In the case of unilateral CHL: the reflex will be absent in both ears if the sound is introduced in the ear with the CHL. However, if the sound is introduced in the normal ear, the reflex will be only in that ear and absent in the other ear (as ossicles cannot transmit the stapes signal to the TM).
3. In the case of unilateral facial nerve palsy: If the signal is introduced in the ipsilateral ear with the facial palsy, then acoustic reflex will be absent in that ear but present in the other ear. If the signal is introduced in the other ear, bilateral acoustic reflex will happen. Acoustic reflex can be valuable in cases of facial palsy, as the return of that reflux can indicate the return of the facial nerve function, and that will show a favorable prognosis.
4. In the case of brainstem injury: Acoustic reflex will happen only in the stimulated ear, that is, there will be no crossover of the signal.

Stapedial reflex decay: It happens in CN VIII lesion. In that condition, if the signal is introduced to the diseased ear 10 dB above the acoustic reflex threshold and it is sustained for 10 s, the reflex amplitude will go down to 50%.

Other uses of acoustic reflex are in testing infants and young children and detecting malingering.

1.4 Special Tests of Hearing

1.4.1 Otoacoustic Emissions (OAE)

The normal outer hair cells will emit low-intensity sounds, either spontaneously (which is called spontaneous OAE and presents in 40–60% of the normal ears) or acoustic stimulation (called evoked OAE). The spontaneous OAE is present in 40–60% of normal. The evoked OAE can be:

1. *Stimulus Frequency OAE*: It is generated after a stimulus with a particular frequency (low-tone).
2. *Transiently Evoked OAE (TEOAE)*: It is generated after a broadband tone stimulus (click), which is presented at 80–85 dB SPL. It is indicated in cases of neonatal screening as its presence will suggest a hearing threshold of at least 20–40 dB.
3. *Distortion Product OAE (DPOAE)*: It is generated after applying two stimuli with two different pure-tone frequencies. DPOAE can test hearing at higher frequencies (1000–8000 Hz). It is indicated in neonatal screening, noise-induced hearing loss, and ototoxicity [5].

OAE is absent in cases of cochlear SNHL >30 dB, and middle ear diseases.

OAE is an objective study and can be used in:

1. Neonatal screening.
2. Monitoring Ototoxicity.
3. Noise-induced hearing loss.
4. Distinguishing cochlear from retrocochlear hearing loss.

5. Detecting Auditory Neuropathy; a condition where the patients have abnormal ABR but normal OAE.

1.4.2 Auditory Brainstem Response (ABR)

Other names for this test are Brainstem Auditory Evoked Response or potential (BAEP) and Brainstem Evoked Response Audiometry (BERA).

Auditory stimulation will generate an electrical response in the VIII cranial nerve and the brainstem. ABR is a test that can detect this electoral response. It is composed of three electrodes, a positive electrode put on the high forehead, a negative electrode put on the ipsilateral mastoid, and a common electrode put on the contralateral mastoid. ABR utilizes a stimulus that will generate a stimulus that travels all through the auditory pathway. The stimulus can be a broadband frequency spectrum (click ABR) or frequency specific 500, 1000, 2000, and 4000 Hz (tone burst ABR). The response will be collected as waves; each wave will indicate a specific anatomical site from which it was generated as the following:

- Wave I: Distal part of CN VIII.
- Wave II: proximal part of CN VIII.
- Wave III: Cochlear nucleus.
- Wave IV: superior olivary complex.
- Wave V: Lateral lemniscus.
- Waves VI and VII: inferior colliculus.

1.4.2.1 Parameters Used in ABR

1. Absolute latencies, look at Table 1.6.
2. Interpeak intervals (interwave latencies):
   - Normal values for interpeak I–III intervals is 2 m s, III–V is 2 m s, and I–V is 4 m s.
3. Interaural wave V latency:
   - It is abnormal if more than 0.4 m s.

Table 1.6 ABR absolute latencies

Wave	Latency (m s)
Wave I	1.5
Wave II	2.5
Wave III	3.5
Wave IV	4.5
Wave V	5.5
Wave VI	6.5

1.4.2.2 ABR Interpretation

1. Wave I is absent or delayed: cochlear lesion.
2. Wave V is absent or delayed: upper brainstem lesion.
3. I–III inter-peak latency prolongation: lower brainstem lesion.
4. III–V inter-peak latency prolongation: upper brainstem lesion.
5. I–V inter-peak latency prolongation: whole brainstem lesion.

1.4.2.3 ABR Interpretation According to the Type of Hearing Loss

1. Normal hearing: all the parameters are within normal values.
2. CHL: delayed absolute latencies, especially for wave I.
3. Sensory hearing loss: Delayed absolute latencies. Wave I is absent. Interpeak latencies are within normal limits. Waves have poor morphology.
4. Neural hearing loss: Delayed absolute latencies except for wave I, which is within normal limits. Interpeak latencies are delayed. Waves have poor morphology.

ABR threshold testing: by utilizing Click stimuli: 1000–4000 Hz. Trace Wave V starting at an 80 dB, and then continue down until wave V is no longer seen (30–20 dB).

1.4.2.4 Factors Affecting ABR

1. Age: In infants, the absolute latency of wave III and V is longer than adults [6].
2. Gender: females have shorter latencies for the waves III and V [7].
3. Some pharmacological medications like phenytoin, lidocaine, and alcohol can affect ABR. However, sedatives, general anesthetics, and neuromuscular blocking agents do not affect ABR.
4. Body temperature: the decreased temperature will increase the latencies [8].

1.4.2.5 Application of ABR

1. Auditory threshold testing.
2. Identifying the hearing loss.
3. Classification of type of deafness (conductive or sensorineural).
4. Neonatal hearing screening.
5. Identification of retrocochlear pathology.
6. Neurosurgical interoperative monitoring.

1.4.3 Electrocochleography (ECoG)

An electrode is inserted at the promontory through the TM; it will measure the electrical potential that arises from CN VIII and the cochlea. These potentials are:

1. Cochlear microphonic (CM): it is the alternating current that arises from the outer hair cells.
2. Summating potential (SP): it is the direct current that arises from the stria vascularis and the hair cells.
3. Compound action potential (AP): it is the summation potential of many nerve fibers.

Clinical Applications of ECoG

1. Diagnosis and monitoring patients with Meniere's disease: the SP/AP ratio will be above 30%.
2. Intraoperative monitoring of peripheral auditory pathway.
3. Auditory neuropathy detection.
4. Differentiates cochlea from retrocochlear lesions.
5. Detecting hearing threshold for infants and young children.

1.4.4 Other Tests Like

(a) *Alternate binaural loudness balance test*: It is a test to detect recruitment. In this test, a tone is applied to the deaf and normal ears in an alternating way. The intensity of the sound in the deaf will start at 20 dB above its threshold, and then it will be increased by 20 dB until the loudness will match the normal ear. The initial difference between the deaf ear and normal ear will be maintained throughout the test in the conductive and neural deafness. However, in cochlear lesion, recruitment may be seen.

(b) *Short Increment Sensitivity Index (SISI)*: In this test, a continuous tone will be presented to the patient at 20 dB above the threshold and continues for 2 min, and every 5 s, there will be an increase in the intensity of the sound by 1 dB. Patients should indicate when this increase in sound's intensity will happen. Interpretation: in the cochlear lesion, SISI score will be 70–100%, while in neural hearing loss, SISI score will be between 0% and 20%, and in CHL, SISI score will be less than 15%. The main concept of this test is based on the fact that patients with cochlear hearing loss will have an increased ability to distinguish smaller changes in sound's intensities.

(c) *Threshold Tone Decay Test*: In this test, a tone with 4000 Hz frequency is presented to the patient continuously for about 60 s. The intensity of that tone will be 5 dB above the patient's hearing threshold. The patient should be able to hear the sound continuously till the end of the 60 s. If he is not able to do that, then the sound intensity will be increased by 5 dB, and the test will be repeated similarly until the patient will be able to hear the sound for the whole period. The result is expressed of dB decay. If the decay is more than 25 dB, then this indicates a retrocochlear lesion.

Take-Home Messages

- Audiological tests should always be taken as a battery of tests and not relying on a single test as this will help to give a whole picture of the patient.
- Tuning forks can be used in different clinical hearing assessment tests like Weber, Rinne, Bing, Absolute bone conduction, Schwabach, and Gelle tests. It

is essential to know how to interpret the results of these tests, especially the results of Weber and Rinne tests.

- Pure tone audiometry and speech audiometry are audiometric tests used commonly in clinical practice. Hearing level is the most common reference used in audiometers.
- Masking, which is a narrow-band noise for pure-tone audiometry or wideband noise for speech audiometry applied to the non-tested ear, will prevent the crossover of the signal from the tested ear to the other ear; it is used in some instances.
- Tympanometry and acoustic reflex are Immittance/Impedance tests. There are five types of tympanogram graphs: A, As, Ad, B, and C.
- Patients with recruitment, which is an abnormal growth of loudness, have a reduced dynamic range, and they are poor candidates for hearing aid.
- OAE spontaneous or evoked. The evoked OAE is either Transiently Evoked OAE or Distortion Product OAE. OAE is an objective test that can be used in neonatal screening, monitoring ototoxicity, noise-induced hearing loss, distinguishing cochlear from retrocochlear hearing loss, and detecting Auditory Neuropathy.
- Other nomenclatures for ABR are Brainstem auditory evoked response or potential (BAEP) and brainstem evoked response audiometry (BERA). It is an objective study that measures the electrical response in the VIII cranial nerve and the brainstem after a signal stimulation. It can be used for testing the auditory threshold, identifying hearing loss, classification of the type of deafness (conductive or sensorineural), neonatal hearing screening, identification of retrocochlear pathology, and during neurosurgical interoperative monitoring.
- Electrocochleography has a clinical application in diagnosis and monitoring patients with Meniere's disease, where the SP/AP ratio will be above 30%.
- Alternate binaural loudness balance test, Short Increment Sensitivity Index (SISI), and Threshold Tone Decay Test are other audiological tests sometimes used in clinical practice.

References

1. Purves D, Augustine GJ, Fitzpatrick D, et al., editors. Neuroscience. 2nd ed. Sunderland, MA: Sinauer Associates; 2001. The Audible Spectrum.
2. Hearing loss and deafness: normal hearing and impaired hearing. InformedHealth.org [Internet]. Cologne, Germany: Institute for Quality and Efficiency in Health Care (IQWiG); 2006. 2008 May 15 [Updated 2017 Nov 30].
3. Wahid NWB, Attia M. Weber Test. [Updated 2020 Feb 14]. In: StatPearls [Internet]. Treasure Island, FL: StatPearls Publishing; 2020. Available from: https://www.ncbi.nlm.nih.gov/books/NBK526135/
4. Flint P, Haughey B, Lund V, Niparko J, Robbins K, Regan Thomas J, Lesperance M. Cummings otolaryngology. 6th ed. Philadelphia: Elsevier; 2014.
5. Abdala C, Visser-Dumont L. Distortion product otoacoustic emissions: a tool for hearing assessment and scientific study. Volta Rev. 2001;103(4):281–302.
6. Sharma M, Bist SS, Kumar S. Age-related maturation of wave V latency of auditory brainstem response in children. J Audiol Otol. 2016;20(2):97–101. https://doi.org/10.7874/jao.2016.20.2.97.
7. López-Escámez JA, Salguero G, Salinero J. Age and sex differences in latencies of waves I, III and V in auditory brainstem response of normal hearing subjects. Acta Otorhinolaryngol Belg. 1999;53(2):109–15.
8. Gold S, Cahani M, Sohmer H, Horowitz M, Shahar A. Effects of body temperature elevation on auditory nerve-brain-stem evoked responses and EEGs in rats. Electroencephalogr Clin Neurophysiol. 1985;60(2):146–53.

Part II

Otology/Neurology

Temporal Bone Imaging

2

Karen Nicolas and Ahmed Elsotouhy

Abbreviations

CBCT	Cone-beam CT
CPA	Cerebellopontine angle
CSF	Cerebrospinal fluid
CSOM	Chronic suppurative otits media
CT	Computed Tomography
EAC	External auditory canal
IAC	Inner auditory canal
IAC	Internal auditory canal
LSCC	Lateral semicircular canal
LVA	Large vestibular aqueduct
MDCT	Multidetector-CT
ME	Middle Ear
MRI	Magnetic Resonance Imaging
OW	Oval window
PSCC	Posterior semicircular canal
RW	Round window
SSCC	Superior semicircular canal
TB	Temporal Bone
TM	Tympanic membrane

Key Points

- The main CT Imaging modalities as MDCT and CBCT are described with advantages and inconvenients. MRI is described with its general imaging characteristics, main sequences for temporal bone imaging, and dedicated sequences for special pathologies. MRI-Contraindications are briefly reviewed.
- CT-Anatomy and MRI-Anatomy are demonstrated on several slices through the main anatomic regions of the temporal bone by both techniques.
- A systematic reading structure is proposed, that approaches the temporal bone from outside to inside, and determines for each anatomic site the essential structures to evaluate. Key images, the most adapted reconstruction plane, and pathologic manifestations at each anatomic site are described and illustrated.
- The temporal bone surfaces and surroundings are often involved by spread of temporal bone pathologies: especially infectious pathologies, as necrotizing otitis externa and chronic suppurative otitis media (CSOM) with or without cholesteatoma tend to extend beyond. Also the tegmen is a predestinated site of weakness in patients with

K. Nicolas (✉)
MEIH Hospital Mount Lebanon and Lebanese University, Beirut, Lebanon

A. Elsotouhy
Neuroradiology Department, Hamad Medical Corporation, Doha, Qatar

A. Al-Qahtani et al. (eds.), *Textbook of Clinical Otolaryngology*,
https://doi.org/10.1007/978-3-030-54088-3_2

poor mastoid development or lysis and pathologic communications through the tegmen are described. Further entities are tumors involving the IAC or glomus tumors that have been illustrated.

- Postoperative imaging findings are briefly illustrated for ossicular reconstructions and stapes prosthesis. The important role of MRI diffusion-weighted imaging for residual/recurrent cholesteatoma is pointed out, also for associated complications to be aware of, during surgical revision. Follow-up after intervention for vestibular schwannoma is a long-term survey that needs reproducible exact measurements of slow growing residues.

2.1 Introduction

Imaging technology has greatly improved over the last two decades; high-resolution CT has been overcome by multidetector CT techniques and more recently complemented by Cone-beam CT (CBCT) with its lesser radiation and higher resolution for some middle ear structures.

MR imaging has been developed to thinner slices and 3D imaging, with specific sequences for otologic and neurotologic pathologies.

Thus, imaging nowadays is one of the basic diagnostic mainstays of temporal bone pathology to orient surgical indications and elucidate possible anatomical abnormalities. In consequence, the preoperative and postoperative counseling of the patients is rendered more informative and enlightened.

Principal imaging methods, basic anatomy, and essential imaging keys are presented.

It remains that adequate communication between the clinician and the radiologist is a prerequisite to select the best imaging protocol. Finally, the postoperative feedback from the clinician to the radiologist constitutes the main source of improvement of diagnostic expertise.

2.2 Temporal Bone Imaging Techniques

2.2.1 MDCT (Multidetector-CT)

2.2.1.1 CT Acquisition and Processing

Acquisition of a data volume of the temporal bone is actually done by slice thicknesses of 0.5–0.6 mm or less, that permit standard reformation of thin slices on each ear alone in the axial (Fig. 2.1) and coronal plane (Fig. 2.2). The standard axial plane is reached when the whole LSCC is visible on one slice (Fig. 2.1d).

Most common supplementary reformations are

- *"Axial stapes" plane*: to evaluate the whole stapes and footplate on one image (Fig. 2.3) [1].
- *Poeschl plane*: to evaluate the bony coverage of the SSCC (Fig. 2.4), if doubtful on the coronal plan.
- *Sagittal plane*: to assess relation from malleus head and anterosuperior wall of the tympanic cavity.

Injection of iodine contrast is almost never required, except for suspected vascular lesions.

- Advantages of MDCT: short examination time, modality almost everywhere available, providing an overall view on the two temporal bones, the nasopharynx, most parts of the sinuses, and the base of skull.
- Inconvenients of MDCT: Considerable radiation exposure, especially in children, and important metallic artifacts from several prosthesis or cochlear implants.

2.2.2 CBCT (Cone-Beam CT)

It is a recent imaging method based on a cone of radiation turning around the patient (instead of the X-ray fan beam rotating spirally around the patient). Preliminary results of institutions that use already CBCT in their daily practice confirm its utility [2] and further implementation as a second and complementary imaging method is predictable.

2.2.2.1 Advantages

- Radiation is less (several former studies estimated the difference at least 3–10 times less

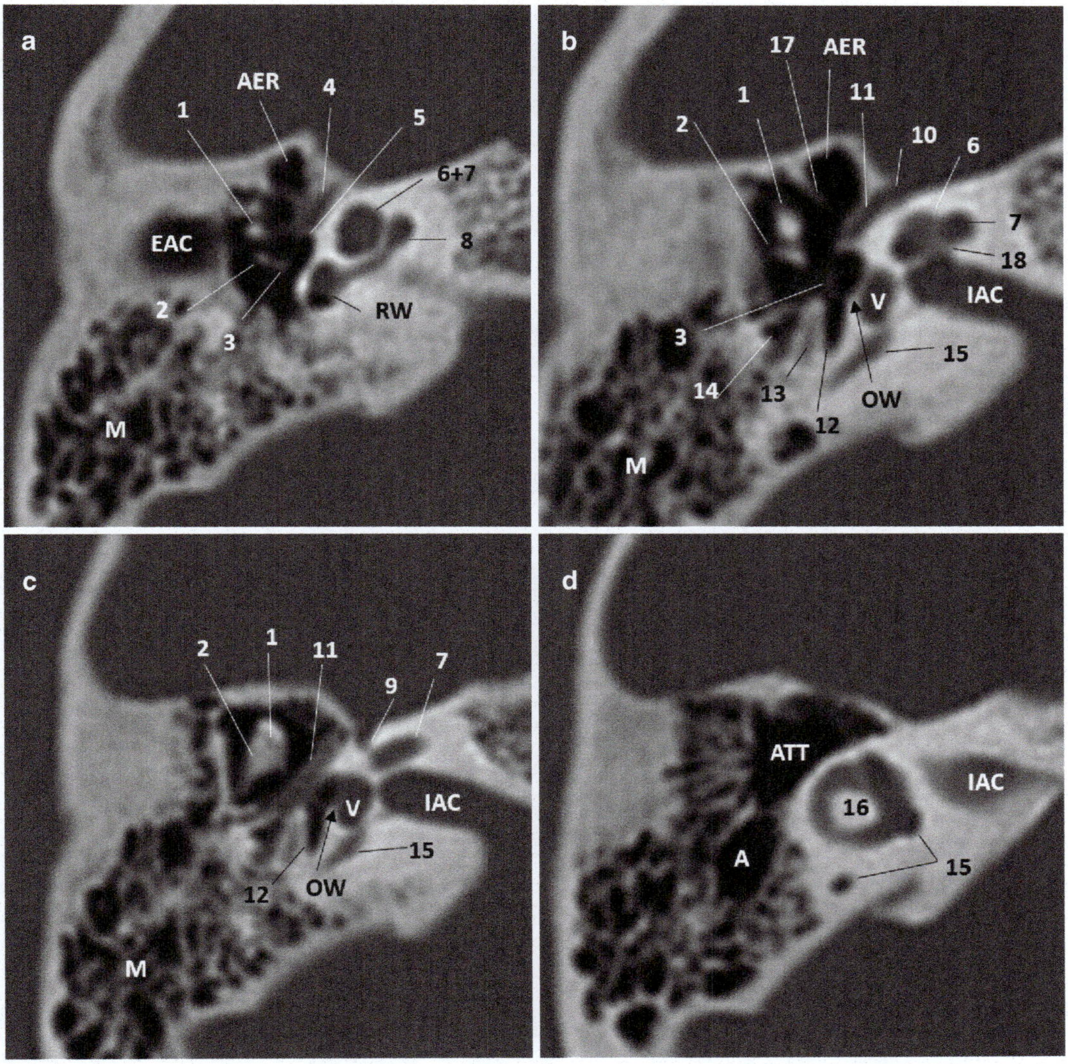

Fig. 2.1 Main anatomic structures on consecutive axial CT cuts from **a** to **d** of the middle ear from caudal to cranial. (1) Malleus, (2) Incus, (3) Stapes, (4) Tensor tympani muscle, (5) Cochleariform process, (6) Last turn cochlea, (7) Mid turn cochlea, (8) Basal turn cochlea, (9) Labyrinthine portion N VII, (10) Geniculate ganglion, (11) Tympanic portion of N VII, (12) Sinus tympani, (13) Stapedial muscle, (14) Facial recess, (15) PSCC, (16) LSCC (standard plan), (17) Cog, (18) Modiolus. *AER* anterior epitympanic recess, *EAC* external auditory canal, *M* mastoid, *RW* round window, *IAC* internal auditory canal, *V* Vestibule, *OW* oval window, *A* antrum, *ATT* attic

for CBCT versus MDCT [3, 4]), but exact evaluation of radiation dose is much difficult, probably underestimation of the CBCT dose because of its beam geometry that cannot be fully evaluated by the standard dose evaluation of MSCT [5–7].

- Strikingly higher spatial resolution for interfaces with high difference of density (air-bone or air-tissue-contrast) has been shown, especially in cadaveric specimen [8, 9] with excellent visibility of ossicular chain and articulations [10], also cochlear anatomy and the facial nerve.
- Much less metallic artifacts than MDCT [8, 11] predestinating CBCT for prosthesis and cochlear implant controls [12].

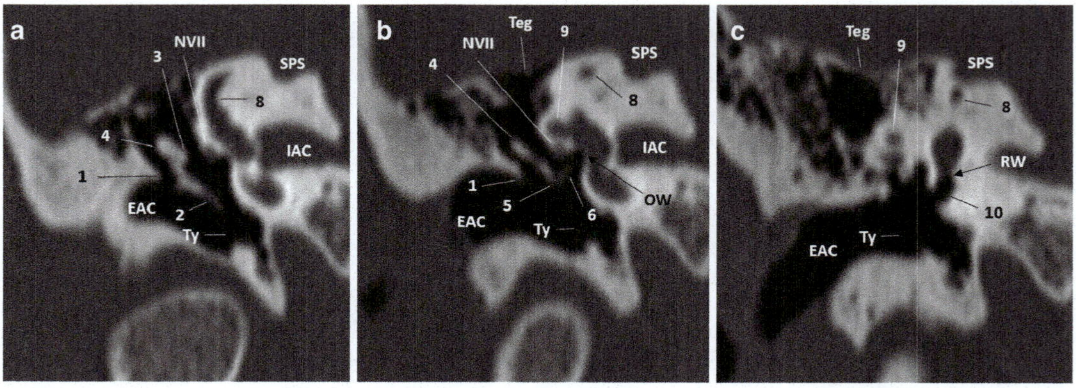

Fig. 2.2 Anatomy on coronal CT slices from **a** to **c** from anterior to posterior: (1) Scutum, (2) Malleus handle, (3) Malleus neck, (4) Incus body, (5) Incudo-stapedial joint, (6) Stapes, N VII facial nerve, (8) SSCC, (9) LSCC, (10) Recess towards the round window. *EAC* external auditory canal, *Ty* tympanic membrane, *IAC* internal auditory canal, *SPS* superior petrosal sinus, *OW* oval window, *RW* round window, *Teg* tegmen

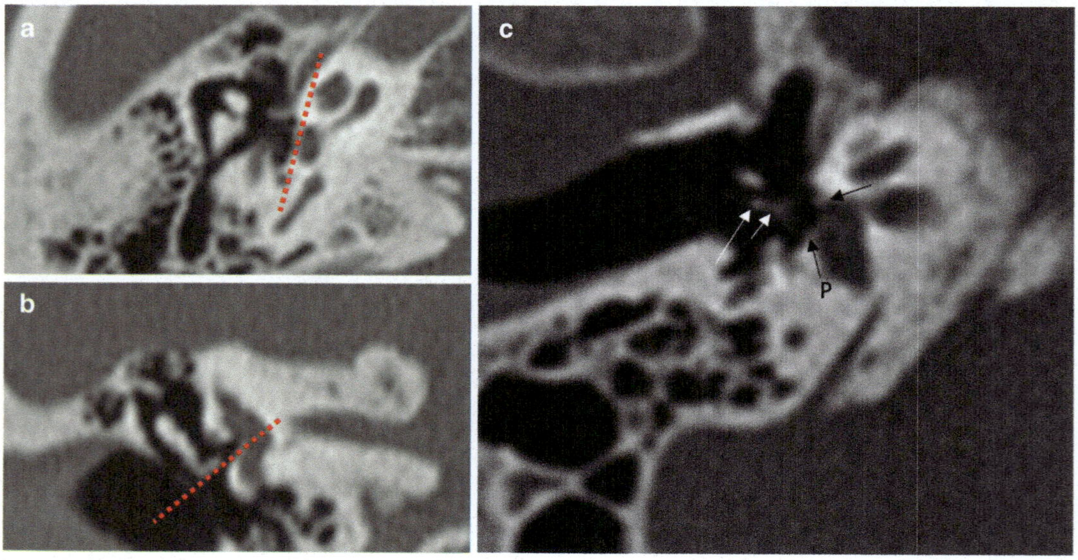

Fig. 2.3 Axial stapes plan: (**a**) on axial CT, the red reference parallel to the footplate for reconstruction → obtain (**b**): Second red reference line along the stapes axis (red dotted line) → obtain (**c**): axial stapes plan with the whole stapes on one slice. Thin footplate (P) between the two black arrows

2.2.2.2 Inconvenients

- Although CBCT has high specificity for otosclerosis, its sensitivity for inactive, sclerotic foci was found to be very low [13]. Others stated that more fenestral lesions were found by MSCT than by CBCT, whereas retrofenestral lesions were equally diagnosed by both techniques [14].
- Lack of soft-tissue contrast resolution limits the use of CBCT in general diagnostic imaging of the temporal bone [10].
- Small field of view enables only one side examination per acquisition.

2.2.3 MR Imaging

2.2.3.1 General MR Imaging Characteristics

- 1.5 Tesla MRI, most available and providing a good standard image quality and evaluation of any anatomic region of head and neck.

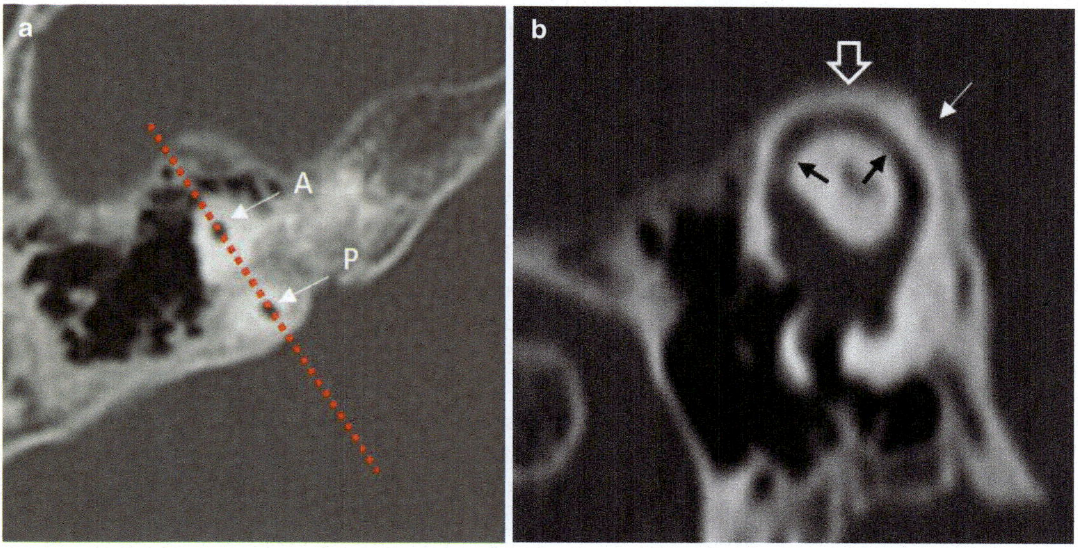

Fig. 2.4 (**a**) Poeschl Plan: axial CT through the upper TB, above the level of axial CT slices of Fig. 2.1d. Red reference line through the anterior (A) and posterior (P) limb of the SSCC for reconstruction → obtain (**b**) the whole SSCC on one slice (small black arrows), the bony coverage (empty arrow) can be assessed. Superior petrosal sinus (white arrow)

- 3.0 Tesla MR using a higher magnetic field strength and providing overall higher imaging quality and newer sequences (see Sect. 2.2.3.2).
- MR is a nonirradiating imaging method using radiofrequency pulses and gradients [15] providing a highly superior soft-tissue characterization in comparison to CT.
- Terminology: different shades of gray on the image are described as follows:
  – white as *high signal intensity*.
  – gray as *intermediate signal intensity*.
  – black as *low signal intensity*.
- Standard sequences are T1-, T2-weighted, or Flair (fluid attenuated) sequences.
  – *T1w*: liquid (as CSF) is hypointense, fat is hyperintense.
  – *T2w*: liquid (as CSF) is hyperintense, fat is also hyperintense.
  – *Flair*: CSF is hypointense, inflammatory or proliferative tissues are hyperintense.
- Gadolinium contrast administration (intravenous) is used to search for pathologic hyperintense contrast uptake on *T1w sequences with fat suppression* (the normally hyperintense fat signal becomes hypointense and permits better discrimination of the contrast uptake) in case of
  – Suspected vascular tumors in the middle ear cavity or around the jugular foramen,
  – Labyrinthitis, acute mastoiditis, lesions in the internal auditory canal (IAC)/cerebellopontine angle (CPA)

2.2.3.2 Dedicated Sequences for Temporal Bone Imaging

High-Resolution 3D T2-Weighted Sequence (3D Drive/CISS/FIESTA/etc.)

This is the essential sequence for middle and inner ear imaging because of high spatial resolution due to inframillimetric slice thickness. It shows

- High contrast between the hypointense vestibulocochlear and facial nerve bundles along their trajectory through the IAC and the hyperintense CSF in the IAC
- The normally hyperintense fluid signal of the membranous labyrinth or pathologic loss of signal
- Different signal intensities for different fluid or solid middle ear pathologies.

Diffusion-Weighted Imaging (DWI)

Diffusion imaging is based on the random Brownian motion of water molecules in a voxel of tissue. If their free motion becomes reduced, a restricted diffusion appears. The *B* value indicates the degree of diffusion weighting applied, starting by B0 and raising up to mostly B1000 s/mm^2. The ADC value (apparent diffusion coefficient) is calculated as B0–B1000, appearing black in case of a positive restriction, white in absence of restriction.

In the middle ear cleft, cholesteatoma was found to be the almost unique pathologic condition that exhibits diffusion restriction. DWI technics are continuously improving. Numerous studies [16, 17] confirmed the advantages of non-echoplanar DWI techniques over previous echoplanar techniques for the detection of cholesteatoma (minimal detection size actually of 2 mm).

3D Flair Imaging 4 h Delayed After Gadolinium Injection for 3 T MRI

This imaging technique has been proposed already since 2009 [18] and continuously improved [19] and implicated in daily imaging routines with 3 T MRT. Recently [20], the combined analysis of vestibular endolymphatic hydrops and perilymphatic enhancement of the cochlea gave combined sensitivity of 79.5% and specificity of 93.6% for Menière's disease.

2.2.3.3 Contraindications

- Foreign metallic bodies in the eye represent an absolute contraindication.
- Cochlear implants represented for longtime an absolute contraindication for MRI, but implants with easier access to MRI have been very recently FDA approved and will be subject of further innovations.
- Prosthesis made of nonmagnetic metals and alloys, including titanium, platinum, and tantalum, showed no potential for movement and were safe by 1.5 Tesla MRI and all above [21].

  Exception: Stainless steel prostheses (mainly used in the years 1960s and 1970s) have been shown to move in several experiments, and their MRI safety may be compromised [22].

2.3 Cross-Sectional Anatomy of the Temporal Bone

2.3.1 Cross-Sectional CT-Anatomy

The temporal bone (TB) is embryologically composed by the fusion of four different bones that are the petrous bone, squamous bone, tympanal bone and styloid bone. The fusion lines of these different parts persist in form of visible sutures on rather all CT-Scans, not to be confused with fracture lines!

Basic sectional views on the most important anatomical structures on the axial, coronal view, the axial stapes plan [1] and the Poeschl plan are shown in the following figures (Figs. 2.1, 2.2, 2.3, and 2.4) [23].

2.3.2 Cross-Sectional MR-Anatomy

Only 3D high-resolution T2-weighted images (Drive, CISS, FIESTA, etc.) with inframillimetric slice thickness show the trajectory of the seventh and eighth cranial nerves inside the IAC in detail (Fig. 2.5). At the "Bill's bar" at the fundus of the IAC, the facial nerve runs in the anterosuperior segment, the cochlear nerve in the anteroinferior segment, and the superior and inferior vestibular nerves in the posterior segments (mnemonic: 7up & Coke Down) (Fig. 2.5c). The different turns of the cochlear and the semicircular canals are well individualized on T2w images due to their liquid components (Fig. 2.6).

2.4 Systematic Reading of Temporal Bone Structures Imaging and Most Frequent Pathologies

In general, CT is the first imaging method of investigation of the outer ear and the middle ear structures. The osseous labyrinth is well seen by CT as by MRI, whereas MRI is the leading imaging method for the content of the membranous labyrinth, the IAC, and all condensation images of the mastoid and tympanic cavity, that are clinically doubtful for complicated infectious disease or cholesteatoma.

A systematic evaluation of the temporal bone can be done along the following steps

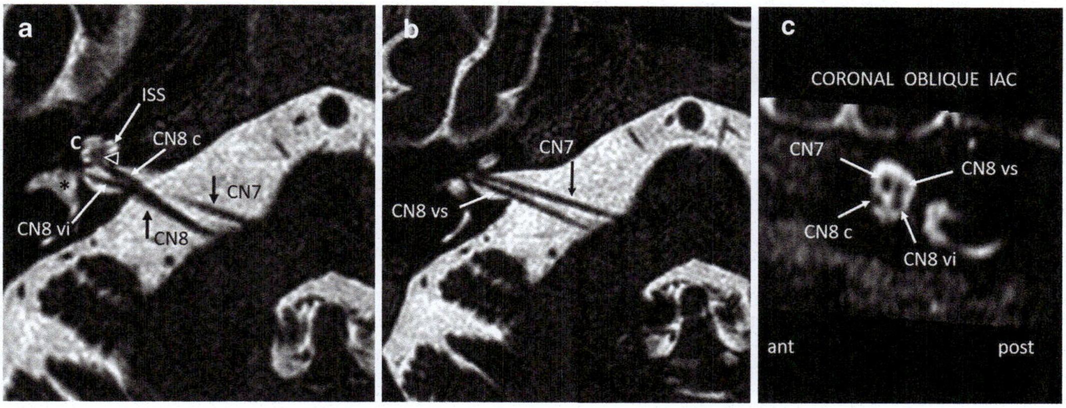

Fig. 2.5 (**a**) Transversal 3D HR T2w Drive image at inferior part of the IAC, (**b**) at upper part of the IAC, (**c**) coronal oblique reformation perpendicular to the lateral end of IAC. Different nerves: CN7 facial, CN8 vestibulocochlear bundle, CN8vi vestibularis inferior, CN8vs vestibularis superior, CN8c cochlear. Interscalar septum (ISS), vestibule (asterisk), cochlea (C), modiolus (empty triangle)

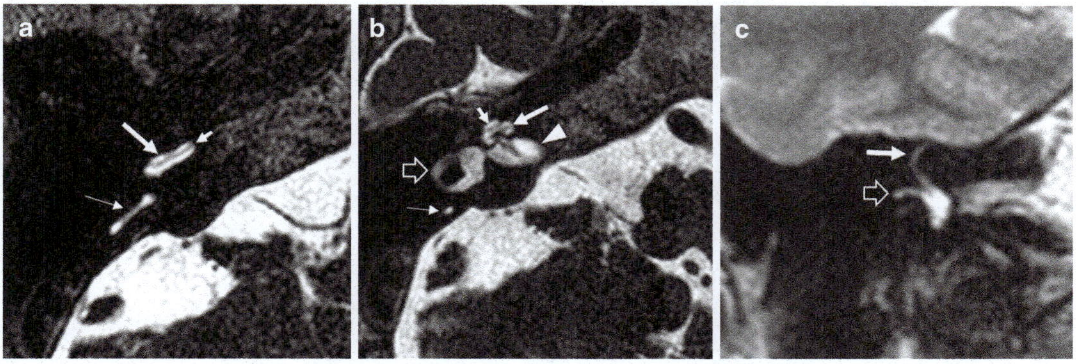

Fig. 2.6 (**a**) Transversal MRI 3D HR T2w Drive image inferior to the IAC: basal cochlear turn (thick long arrow), ISS interscalar septum (short arrow), inferior limb of the PSCC (thin arrow). (**b**) Slightly cranial to (**a**) at level of IAC: mid cochlear turn (thick long arrow), last cochlear turn (small arrow), LSCC (empty arrow), PSCC (thin arrow), IAC (arrowhead). (**c**) Coronal MRI T2w: lateral limb of SSCC (white arrow) and LSCC (empty arrow)

progressing from the outer to the inner ear structures, mentioning for each structure main pathologies and their aspects.

2.4.1 External Auditory Canal (EAC)

- Osseous borders: discontinuity by *persistent foramen of Huschke*, traumatic, or erosive (*infectious or tumoral* origin)
- Scutum (to analyze in the coronal plan!): It is the upper medial bony limit of the tympanic bone, on which the pars flaccida of the ear drum inserts: intact (Fig. 2.2) or amputated (Fig. 2.9a), amputation may indicate an *acquired cholesteatoma.*
- Skin: focally or generally thickened, to refer to the clinical context and inspection as in *external necrotizing otitis* (Sect. 2.5.1.2).

2.4.1.1 *EAC Stenosis or Atresia*

EAC atresia can be completely or incompletely atretic. A number of key points should be looked for [24]:

- Width of the middle ear cavity (should be >3 mm to be suitable for surgical indication [25])
- Stapes malformations: present or not; often associated with a lack of oval window formation.
- VII course identification (Fig. 2.7).
- Look for congenital cholesteatoma behind the atresia plate.

2.4.2 Tympanic Membrane (TM)

Exclusive role of CT

- Tympanic membrane retraction towards the cavity [26]:
  - If close contact to the incudostapedial chain, focal lysis of the joint can be observed (Fig. 2.8a).
  - If retracted on the middle attic wall, it can be very close to the tympanic facial nerve canal (Fig. 2.16a).
- *Perforation:* size and site, central or marginal (Fig. 2.8b).
- Thickening or *myringosclerosis* (Fig. 2.8c).

2.4.3 Tympanic Cavity

The tympanic cavity has a complex anatomy, with numerous osseous limits to analyze and ways of communication with the nasopharynx by the Eustachian tube, with the mastoid by the

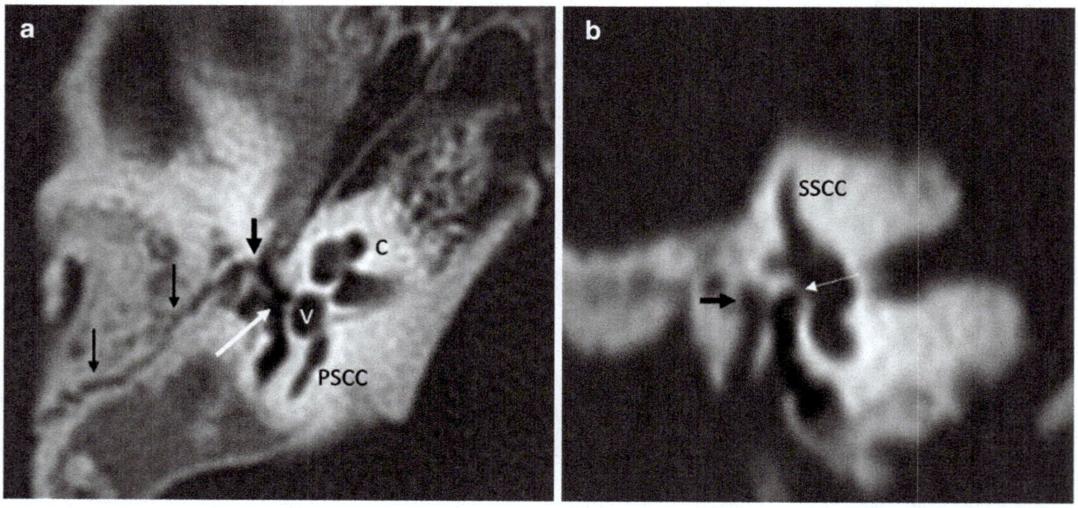

Fig. 2.7 (**a**) Axial CT: Complete atresia of EAC, tympanic bone absent, petrosquamous suture (black arrows). Small cavity (short black arrow) with rudimentary ossicular chain, stapes present (white arrow). Normal inner ear structures (C cochlea, V vestibule, PSCC). (**b**) Coronal CT: horizontal portion of VII (black arrow) advanced at level of the oval window (white arrow)

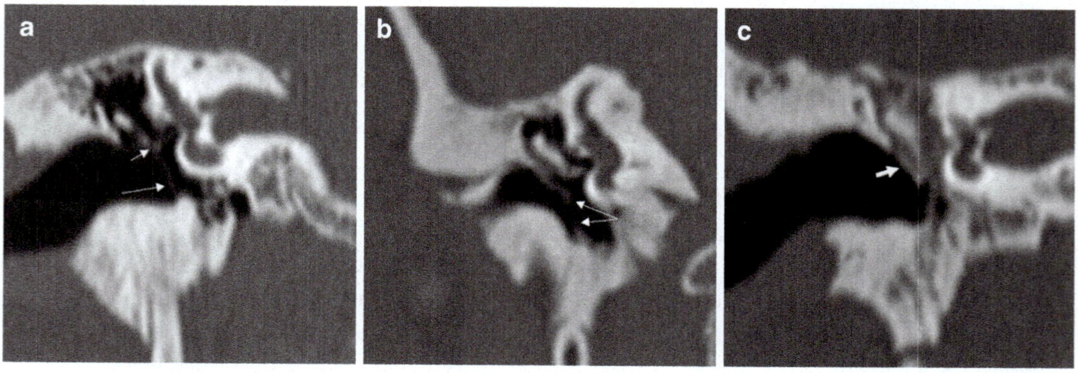

Fig. 2.8 Coronal CT: (**a**) thin TM (arrows) retracted on incudostapedial joint with focal lysis (small arrow). (**b**) Perforation (between arrows) of the thickened TM. (**c**) Myringosclerosis (arrow)

aditus ad antrum, and with the otic capsule via the oval and round windows (Figs. 2.1 and 2.2).

The most frequent pathologies are infectious or inflammatory diseases that concern the tympanic cavity and contents and may extend to all adjacent structures.

Major role of CT

- Aeration/condensations (special look for the different recesses as AER, sinus tympani).
- Bony walls (intact/dehiscent/lytic) especially the tegmen (coronal plan, Fig. 2.2b).
- Tegmen slope (sagittal plan [27]).

2.4.3.1 *Cholesteatoma*

Most often, cholesteatoma is a clinically established diagnosis.

Role of CT: Typical bony erosions are best demonstrated by CT (amputation of the scutum, or the cog), and/or typical rounded or irregular lobulated condensation images in the tympanic cavity (Fig. 2.9a) with adjacent ossicular chain lysis (Fig. 2.9a,b). Bony walls look smoothened in contact with a complete condensation of the lumen of antrum and/or tympanic cavity and disappearance of visible trabeculations (Fig. 2.9c). Erosion of the bony limit of the LSCC is another sign of bony lysis, important to be known before surgery.

Role of MR: Diffusion images have shown sensitivities from 0.86 to 0.93 and specificities from 0.88 to 0.97 for detection of cholesteatoma in large meta-analysis in 2013 and 2017 [28, 29]. Sensitivities range around 90–100% to detect cholesteatoma as small as 2 mm [30].

Especially if the condensations concern the AER, a hidden space for otoscopic evaluation, CT may show condensations and the disappearance of the cog (Fig. 2.10a).

MR permits to confirm the small cholesteatomatous process in the AER (Fig. 2.10b–d).

2.4.4 Ossicular Chain

Exclusive role of CT

- Topography of the ossicles.
- *Post-traumatic discontinuity*, most often incudostapedial (Fig. 2.11a), less frequently incudomallear (Fig. 2.11b), rarely stapedial fractures (axial stapedial plan! (Fig. 2.11c)).
- *Fixity of the ossicular chain* can be congenital, as the malleus bar, that is fixing the malleus to the anterior attic wall (Fig. 2.12a), or due to a malformative attachment of the ossicular chain, as a hypoplastic incus that is retracted to the Fallopian canal (Fig. 2.12b), or a malformed hypoplastic stapes inserting on a very dense footplate (Fig. 2.12c).
- Fixity can also be acquired, as a result of postinflammatory reaction inside the tympanic cavity, as by tympanosclerosis that can involve

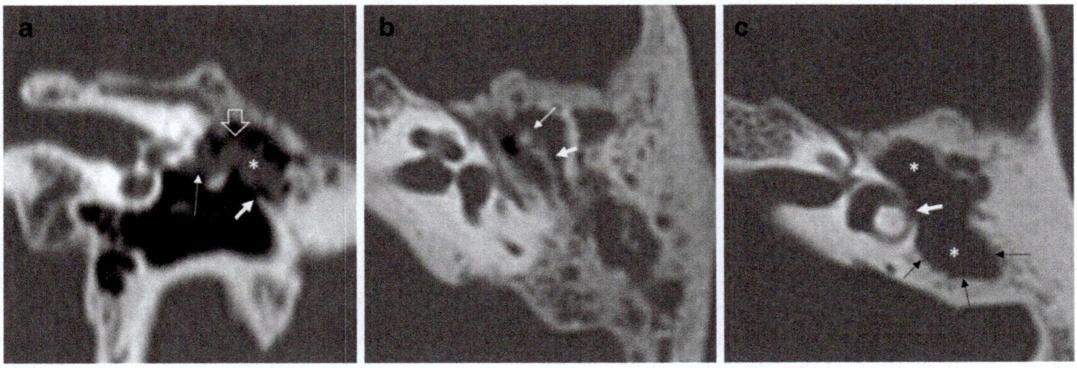

Fig. 2.9 (**a**) Coronal CT: amputation of scutum (short white arrow), irregular attical lobulated soft-tissue mass (asterisk) in contact with the VII (long arrow), advanced lysis of ossicles (empty arrow). (**b**) Axial CT: partial lysis of malleus head (thin arrow) and advanced lyses of incus (thick arrow). (**c**) Complete condensation of the atticoantral spaces (double asterisks) with smoothening of the borders (black arrows), erosion of LSCC (white arrow)

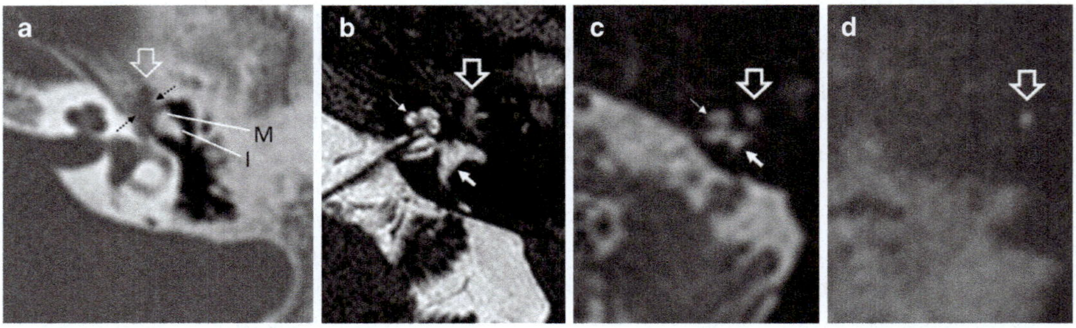

Fig. 2.10 Small cholesteatoma invading the AER. (**a**) Axial CT: soft-tissue mass in the AER (empty arrow), associated to probable lyses of the cog (should be an osseous ridge between dotted arrows). *M* malleus head, *I* incus. (**b**) Axial MRI HR T2 Drive, (**c**) Diff w B0 image: (**d**) Diff w B1000 image: AER (empty arrow) cochlea (slim arrow), vestibule (thick arrow), positive restriction only in the AER in (**d**), very specific for cholesteatoma

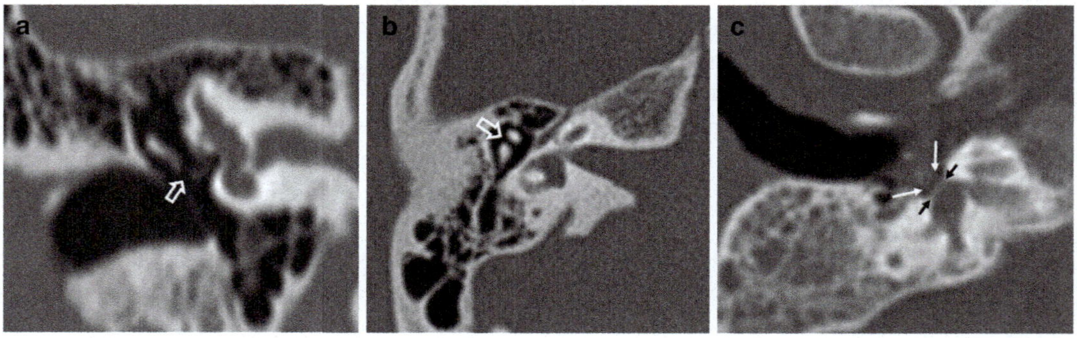

Fig. 2.11 (**a**) Coronal CT: discontinuity of incudostapedial joint (empty arrow), (**b**) axial CT: discontinuity of incudomalleal joint (empty arrow). (**c**) Axial CT reconstruction in stapes plan: discontinuity between distal crura of the stapes (white arrows) and footplate (between black arrows)

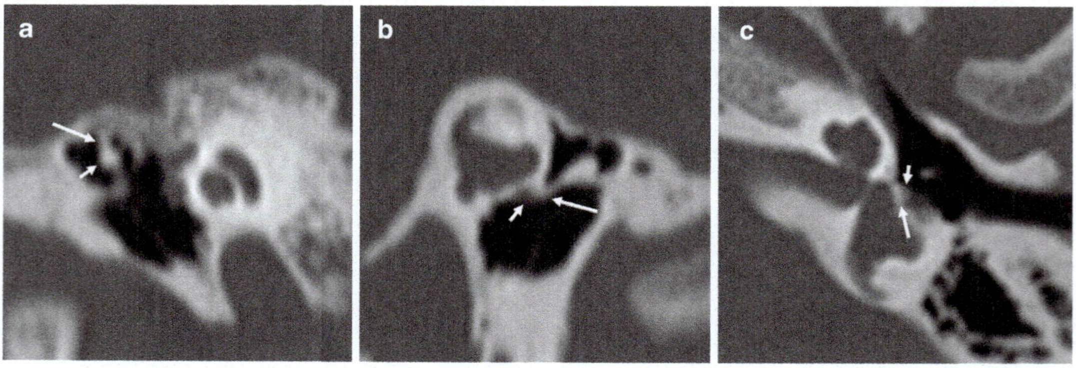

Fig. 2.12 Ossicular chain fixities: (**a**) coronal CT: large bony attachment (long arrow) of malleus head (short arrow) to the tegmen. (**b**) Coronal CT: hypoplastic long process of the incus (long arrow) attached on the Fallopian canal (short arrow). (**c**) Axial CT: hypoplastic stapes with very short crura (short arrow) inserting on a thick and very dense footplate (long arrow)

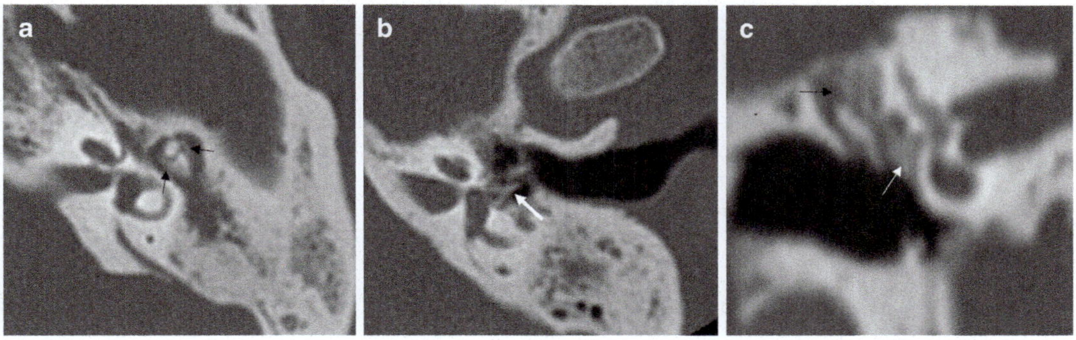

Fig. 2.13 Tympanosclerosis: axial CTs: (**a**) typical periarticular calcifications (arrows) of incudomallear joint, (**b**) important thickening and hyperdensity of stapes superstructure (arrow). (**c**) Coronal CT with diffuse calcified condensations of oval window niche (white arrow) and inner attic (black arrow)

the malleolar complex alone, the stapedial complex alone, or the whole cavity with malleus and stapedial fixity [31] (Fig. 2.13).

2.4.5 Oval Window

- Oval window niche (normal height or reduced).
- *Hypoplasia* of the oval window.
- Footplate: normal thickness, or thickening (to evaluate on axial stapes plan! (Fig. 2.3), especially in pathologies like *otosclerosis, stapedial ankyloses, or tympanosclerosis* [31].
- Fissula antefenestram situated immediately anteriorly to the anterior wall of the oval window is the most common site for *otosclerosis* (Fig. 2.14a).

Major role of CT: high specificity and sensitivity (over 90%) [32] for typical foci of otosclerosis in the fissula antefenestram, for pericochlear extension (Fig. 2.14b) with or without contact to the cochlear endosteum, calcifications of cochlear turns as sign of advanced stage. Classification systems in use according to Veillon [33], or Symons and Fannings [34] especially for more advanced stages.

2.4.6 Round Window

Major role of CT: The round window represents the contact face between the middle ear cavity and the scala tympani of the cochlea. Otosclerosis of the round window is not rare, observed in up to 13% of patients with otosclerosis. A radiologic classification of RW invasion and their audiological impacts has been established [35].

- Round window membrane partially or completely thickened (Fig. 2.14d).
- Round window recess accessible or obliterated (Fig. 2.14e).
- Round window hypoplastic (Fig. 2.14f).

2.4.7 Facial Nerve

The facial nerve has a complex trajectory from its origin at the lateral pons, its cisternal portion traversing the CPA, labyrinthine portion until the geniculate ganglion, the horizontal tympanic portion along the medial attic wall until the second genu, and the vertical mastoid portion through the mastoid until the stylomastoid foramen (Fig. 2.15). Need for axial and coronal images to assess the whole trajectory.

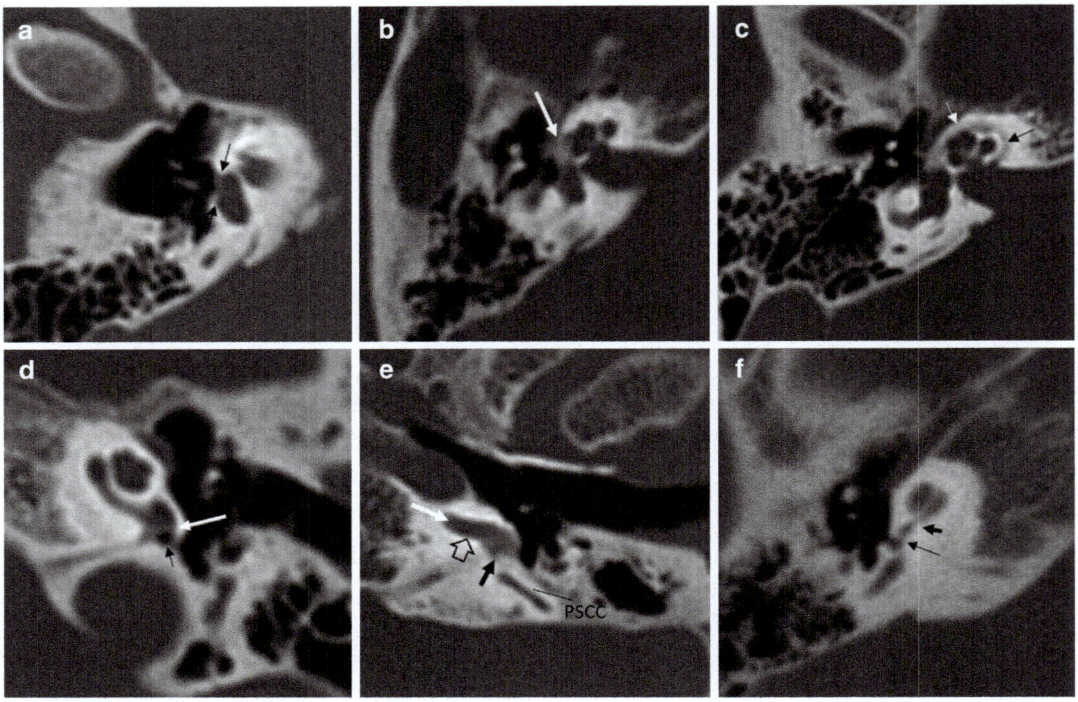

Fig. 2.14 Axial CT (**a**) axial stapes plan: global thickening of the footplate (between black arrows). (**b**) Large otosclerotic focus of the fissula antefenestram (arrow), already in close contact with the cochlear endosteum. (**c**) Extended pericochlear otosclerosis, partially in close contact with the endosteum (white arrow), some foci stay at distance of the endosteum (black arrow). (**d**, **e**) Axial CTs of round window otosclerosis, in (**d**) thickened round window membrane (white arrow), round window recess aerated (thin black arrow). (**e**) Typical otospongiotic focus obliterating the whole round window recess (black arrow): RW4. Scala tympani (empty arrow), spiral ligament (long white arrow). (**f**) Hypoplastic round window (long arrow), stenotic proximal basal turn (short arrow)

- TM can be retracted on the VII canal (Fig. 2.16a).
- Second portion with normal position in the canal, or overhang, coming in contact with the ossicular chain or not (Fig. 2.16b).
- Bony canal integrity of the second and third portions or erosion (Fig. 2.16c).
- An enlarged angle between the first and second portions is observed in cases with X linked deafness or cochlear hypoplasia type IV, strongly associated with Gusher syndrome (Fig. 2.21c) [36].

2.4.7.1 *Facial Nerve Paralysis*

Role of CT: maybe the exam of first approach, to eliminate any gross pathology along the temporal facial nerve trajectory.

MRI is the method of choice: essentially with injected T1 sequences to analyze the facial nerve trajectory from the brainstem to the fundus of the internal auditory canal and to visualize soft-tissue lesions along the lateral course of the nerve.

- A normal facial nerve faintly enhances in the geniculate ganglion, tympanic, and mastoid segments.
- In *Bell's palsy*, there is enhancement of the cisternal and labyrinthine segments, and greater degree of enhancement in, geniculate ganglion, tympanic, and mastoid segments.
- *VII schwannoma*, the most frequent tumoral pathology of this nerve, shows strong contrast enhancement.
- *Hemangiomas* of the facial nerve typically occur at the geniculate ganglion and show also avid contrast enhancement. [37].

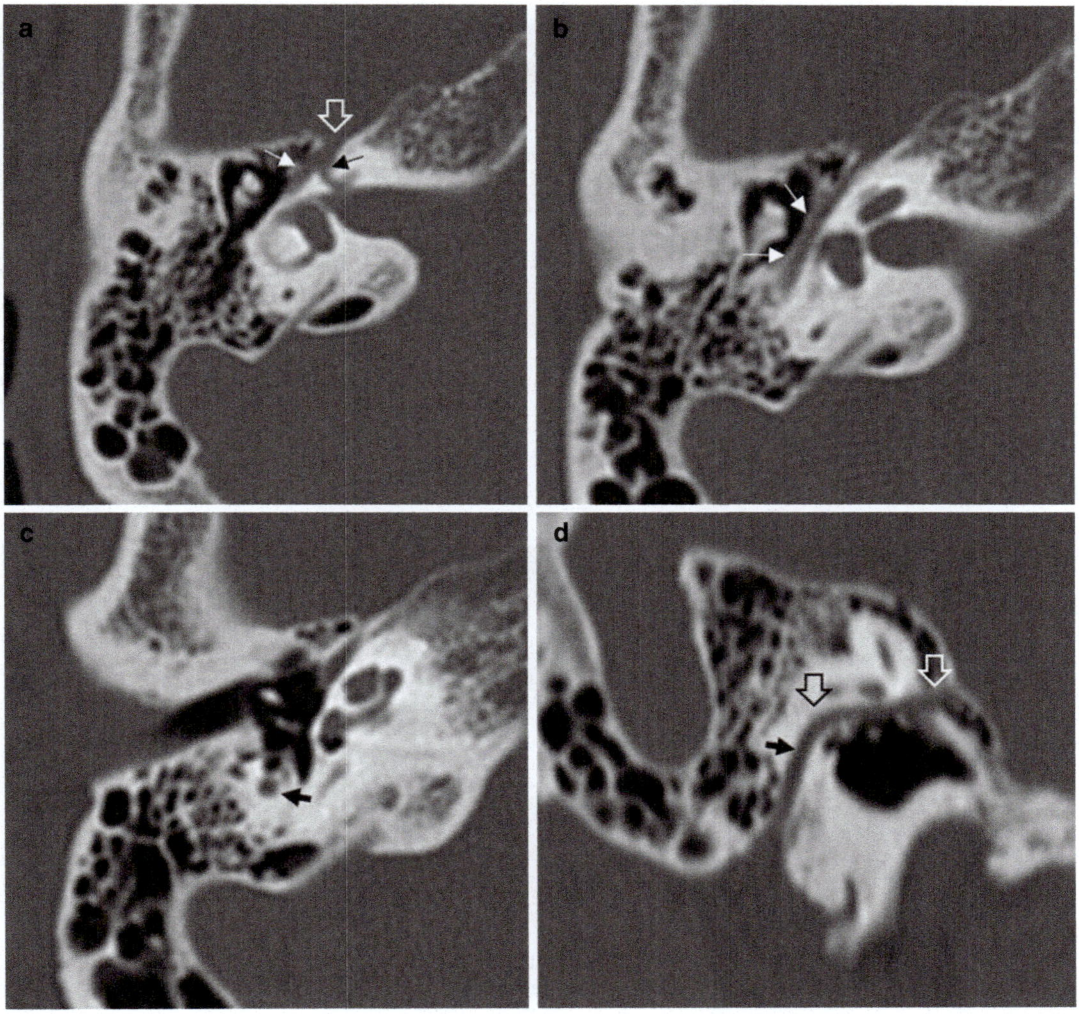

Fig. 2.15 Facial nerve trajectory on axial CT from cranial to caudal (**a**–**c**) and (**d**) oblique reconstruction along the tympanic and mastoid segments: (**a**) First labyrinthine segment (black arrow), geniculate ganglion (empty arrow), proximal tympanic segment (white arrow), *note here the normal small angle between the first and second portion of the facial nerve*. (**b**) Tympanic segment (arrows), (**c**) mastoid segment (arrow), (**d**) third mastoid segment (black arrow), second genu (black empty arrow), geniculate ganglion (empty white arrow)

2.4.8 Mastoid and Sigmoid Sinus

The pneumatization status of the mastoid (Fig. 2.17) as well pneumatized, diploic, or sclerotic informs about a predisposing condition for infectious and inflammatory pathologies.

The aeration status characterizes the absence or presence of condensations and their distribution in the middle ear cleft: one axial key image through the long axis of the incudomallear chain shows AER, Attic, and Antrum on the same slide (Fig. 2.17a) that are indicative of infection or inflammatory process [38].

- Trabeculations are preserved or lytic.
- Sigmoid sinus is normal or anteriorly positioned.
- Jugular bulb situation position is normal or high.
- Shape of tegmen slope (on coronal and sagittal images).

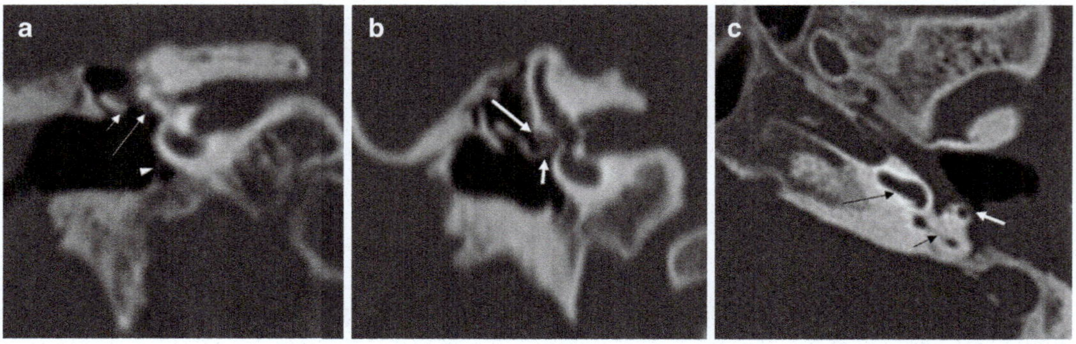

Fig. 2.16 Coronal CT (**a**, **b**): (**a**) TM retraction on the incus (small arrow), and tympanic VII (long arrow), inferior retracted TM (arrowhead). (**b**) Prominent VII (long arrow), in close contact to stapes superstructure (short arrow). (**c**) Erosion of the mastoid segment of the VII (white arrow) inferior to the second genu, in contact with large condensations in mastoidectomy cavity. Basal cochlear turn (long black arrow), PSCC (short black arrow)

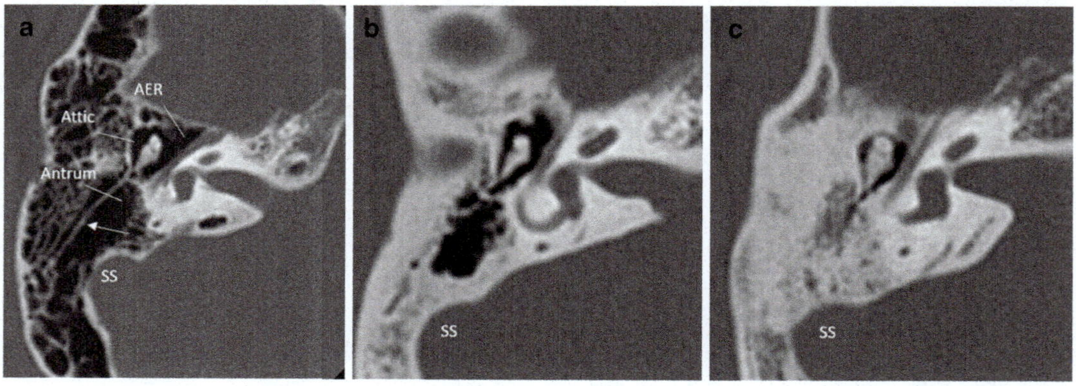

Fig. 2.17 Mastoid-pneumatization status: (**a**) well pneumatized, see the AER, Attic, and Antrum on the same slide, additional finding a Koerner septum (arrow). (**b**) Diploic, (**c**) sclerotic. *SS* sigmoid sinus

2.4.9 Petrous Apex

The internal auditory canal bisects the petrous apex into a large anterior portion that typically contains bone marrow and a smaller posterior portion that is derived from the otic capsule.

Role of CT

- Evaluation of the development of the petrous apex: Sclerotic or pneumatized or filled with condensation images.
- Expansile lesion, preserved limits, or destructive (Fig. 2.18).

Role of MRI: In case of expansile bone erosion, MR may identify the content. *Cholesterol granuloma* is the most common lesion arising in the petrous apex. Classically, it occurs in a pneumatized petrous apex and a long-standing history of ME cleft dysventilation syndrome. MRI is specific for the diagnosis with hyperintense signal on T1 and T2, no contrast enhancement. A hypointense rim on T2-weighted images may be present, which is due to hemosiderin or a preserved rim of bone [39].

In asymmetric petrous apex pneumatization with a unilaterally nonpneumatized apex, its spongiotic signal intensity similar to the clivus on different MRI sequences is also relatively high on

T2- *and* T1-weighted images and should not be mistaken for cholesterol granuloma (Fig. 2.19). The pneumatized side is most often devoid of signal due to the aeration, or shows condensation.

Other lesions are *cholesteatoma*, *cephalocele*, *petrous apicitis* (*Gradenigo syndrome*), or *petrous carotid aneurysm*. Benign and malignant tumors, other vascular lesions, fibrous dysplasia-can affect the petrous apex.

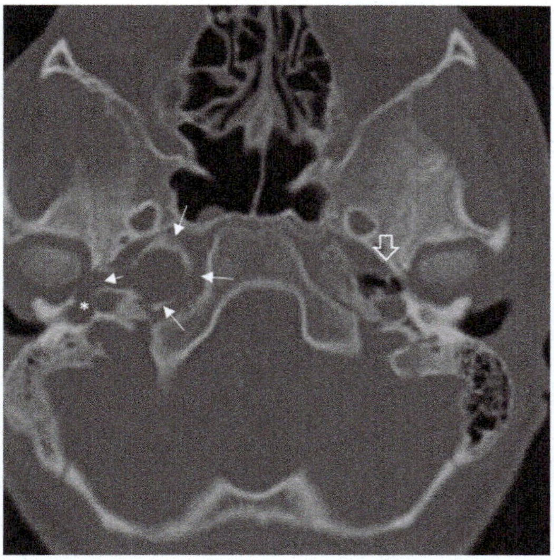

Fig. 2.18 Axial CT showing an expansile soft-tissue lesion in the petrous apex (thin arrows), surrounded by a thickened cortical bone, and continuous extension (short arrow) into the tympanic cavity (asterisk). Normal left petrous apex with some aerated cells (empty arrow)

2.4.10 Cochlea

Normal development with a spiral structure of 2½ to 2¾ turns and visibility of the osseous spiral lamina separating scala tympani from scala vestibuli on CT and MRI. The modiolus should also be recognized (Fig. 2.1b).

2.4.10.1 *Cochlear Anomalies*

Jackler et al. [40] made the first classification of *inner ear malformations*. Since 2002, Sennaroglu proposed an adapted classification [41] from the complete aplasia of the membranous labyrinth (Michel deformity) and common vestibulo-cochlear cavity to different types of incomplete partition.

They are important to distinguish, because their therapeutical approach is different (Fig. 2.20) [42].

CT and MRI have similar value to detect morphologic anomalies of the osseous labyrinth.

Four additional types of *cochlear hypoplasia* are

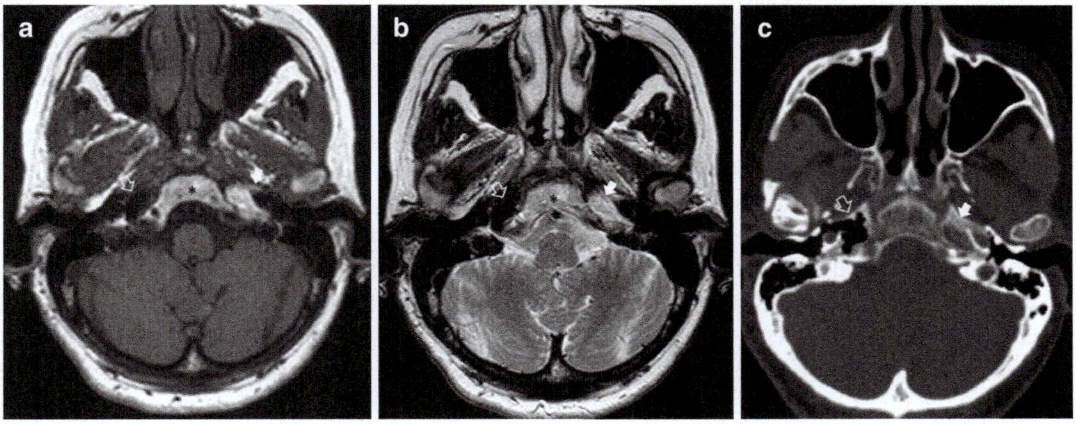

Fig. 2.19 (**a**) Axial T1w and (**b**) axial T2w MR images show high density of the left petrous apex (plain arrows), with equal density to the bone marrow of the clivus (asterisk). Well pneumatized right petrous apex devoid of signal (empty arrows). (**c**) Axial CT: well pneumatized right petrous apex (empty arrow), nonpneumatized spongiotic petrous apex on the left (plain arrow)

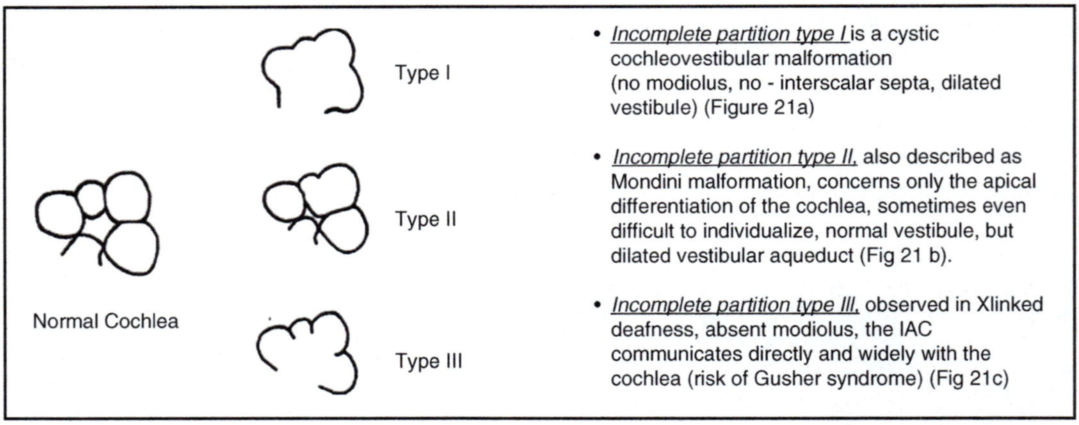

Fig. 2.20 Representation of different types of congenital cochlear malformations with incomplete partition according to Sennaroglu [42]

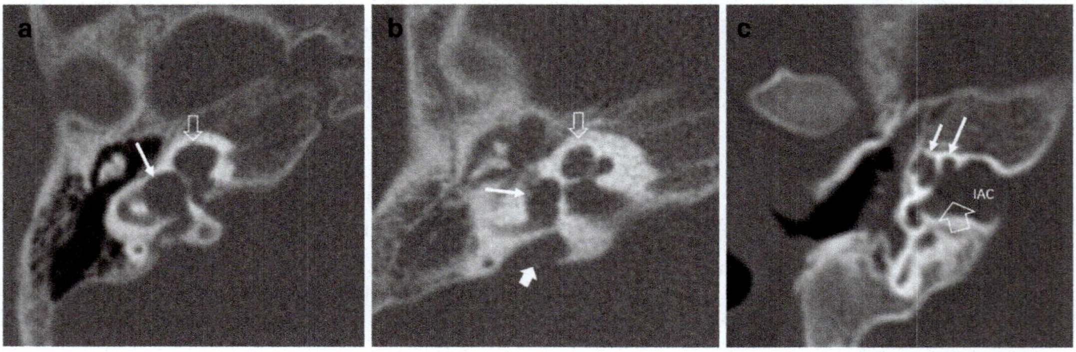

Fig. 2.21 Incomplete partition (**a**) type I: cystic cochleovestibular malformation, cochlea: empty arrow, vestibule: arrow, (**b**) type II (Mondini): apical incomplete partition (empty arrow), almost normal vestibule (white arrow), LVA (plain arrow). (**c**) Type III (x-linked deafness): large IAC, communicating widely (empty arrow) with the basal turn of the cochlea (long arrow), no modiolus! Mid and apical turns of cochlea (short arrow)

- *Type I* budlike, hypoplastic cochlear bud (Fig. 2.26b).
- *Type II* cystic hypoplastic cochlea without modiolus but with enlarged vestibular aqueduct.
- *Type III* cochlea with less than two turns, vestibule and SCC are hypoplastic.
- *Type IV* cochlea with smaller external dimensions, normal basal turn, and hypoplastic mid and apical turn. Enlarged angle of cisternal and tympanic portion of the VII (also risk of gusher syndrome) (Fig. 2.22) [36].

2.4.10.2 *Labyrinthitis*

CT confirms the end stage of labyrinthine calcifications of scala tympani or scala vestibule or both (Fig. 2.23a).

MRI: Acute labyrinthitis can be seen on MR images as diffuse contrast enhancement of the membranous labyrinth. Later, MRI may show diffuse loss of liquid signal on T2w images due to fibrosis that may not be visible on CT (Fig. 2.23).

2.4.10.3 *Imaging Workup for Cochlear Implant*

As shown in Figs. 2.21, 2.22, and 2.23, CT and MRI of the temporal bones allow excellent depiction of inner ear malformations and are routinely used in the evaluation of pediatric sensorineural hearing loss [43]. However, 80% of congenital SNHL are of membranous origin and will not reveal pathologic findings on imaging [44].

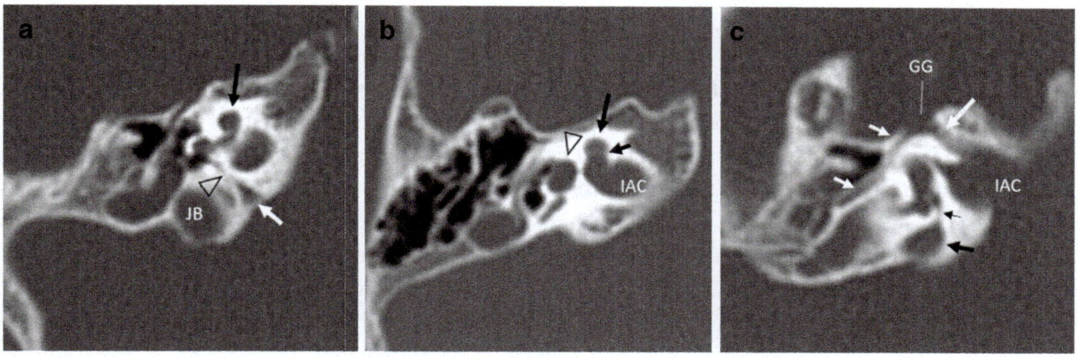

Fig. 2.22 Reconstructed CT images of cochlear hypoplasia type II: (**a**) hypoplastic mid and apical cochlear turns (black arrow). Normal aspect of the cochlear duct, with triangular opening to the posterior fossa (white arrow) anterior to the jugular bulb (JB), very thin aqueduct (arrowhead) until insertion to the basal turn of the cochlear. (**b**) Absent modiolus (short arrow), direct communication between IAC and the hypoplastic cochlea (long arrow), normal sized vestibule (empty triangle). (**c**) Large IAC, enlarged angle at the geniculate ganglion (GG) between the enlarged labyrinthine portion (long white arrow) and tympanic portion (small white arrows) of the VII. Typical LVA (thick black arrow), the proximal isthmic portion is thin (always)

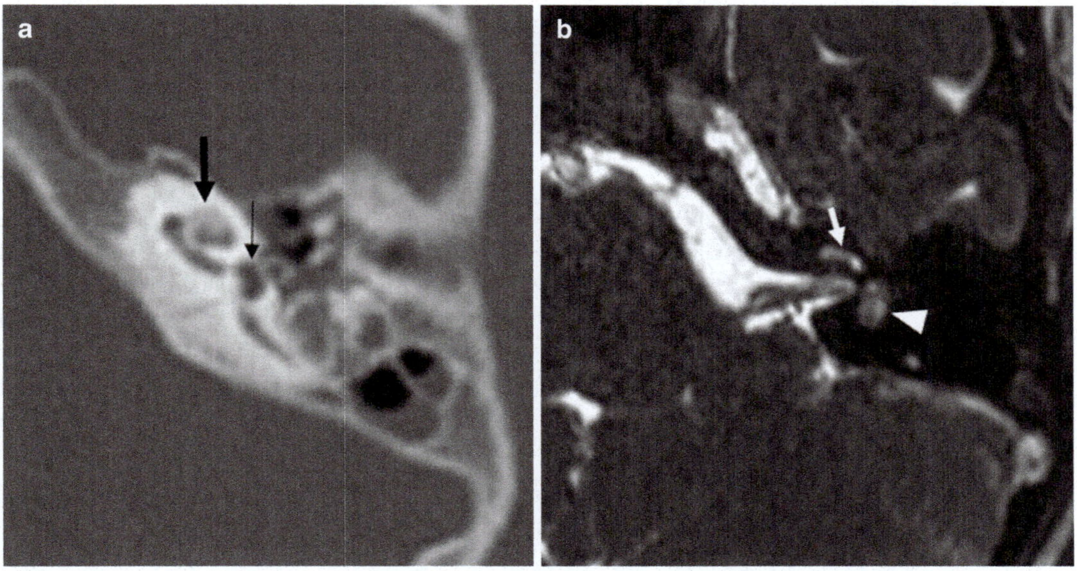

Fig. 2.23 (**a**) Axial CT: calcification of the mid and apical turns of the cochlea (thick arrow). Still normal hypodensity of the vestibule (thin arrow). (**b**) Axial CISS MRI: obscuration of fluid signal intensity in cochlear midturn (arrow), and almost complete absence of liquid signal in the vestibule (arrowhead)

CT may be the exam of first intention that will show an osseous malformation in about 20%.

MRI becomes essential in the workup before cochlear implant, because of its high credibility about

- Patency or obliteration of the cochlear turns.
- Presence of a normally sized cochlear nerve or its absence (Fig. 2.27).
- Absence of lesions of the auditory pathways or the auditory cortex and absence of unexpected associated pathologies which could eventually compromise the long-term safety or function of the cochlear implant.

2.4.11 Cochlear Aqueduct

The cochlear aqueduct has a very thin petrous part arising from the basal turn of the cochlea, to enlarge and widen with a triangular shape at its opening in the subarachnoid space anterior to the jugular foramen (close to the pars nervosa). Only very rare cases of pathologic widening of the whole aqueduct have been reported [45] (Fig. 2.22a).

2.4.12 Vestibule

- Morphology and size of the vestibule can be involved in vestibulocochlear malformations as for example in the incomplete partition type I (Fig. 2.21a).
- Calcifications (rarely in otosclerosis) can appear during ossifying labyrinthitis.

MRI is very sensitive to assess the loss of fluid signal intensity inside the vestibule, corresponding to inflammatory tissue, or fibrosis before calcification (Fig. 2.23b).

The role of 3 Tesla MRI in Menière's disease with delayed acquisition after Gadolinium has already been described in Sect. 2.2.3.2.

2.4.13 Vestibular Aqueduct

Originating from the medial wall of the vestibule, it surrounds the endolymphatic duct. Its proximal part is thin, widening distally, ending in the endolymphatic sac in the posterior fossa. It should not be wider than the superior limb of the PSCC. The Cincinnati criteria [46] consider the vestibular aqueduct as dilated when the mid section of the vestibular aqueduct diameter is greater than 1.0 mm or posterior outside diameter greater than 2.0 mm. LVA (large vestibular aqueduct) is associated to several cochlear or vestibular malformations (Fig. 2.21b), but can also be an isolated finding, and it was found in SNHL of children in 32–39% [46].

2.4.14 Semicircular Canals

- *Anomalies in size or shape* of one or more of the three canals. Complete absence of the posterior labyrinth (Fig. 2.24a) is a rare malformation that is often associated with Charge syndrome [47]. In these cases, arrest of the development must have happened in the 6th gestational week [40]. During the development until the 22nd week, the SSCC forms first, followed by the PSCC and latest the LSCC. However, anomalies of the PSCC (Fig. 2.24b) can be found with a normal LSCC. Anomalies of semicircular canals are the most frequent anomalies found in children with profound hearing loss [48].
- Anomalies of dimension of the canal island are not rare, most often the bony island inside the LSCC is too small (Fig. 2.24c), if inferior to 2.6 mm [49].

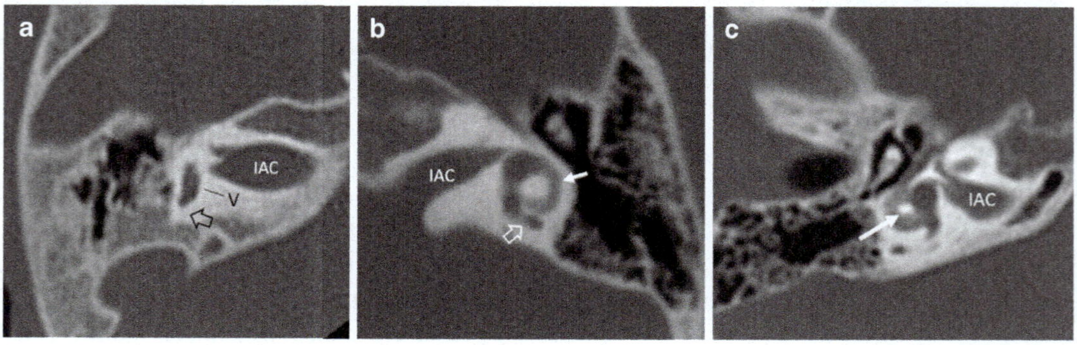

Fig. 2.24 Axial CT-cuts with anomalies of the posterior labyrinth: (**a**) complete absence of the posterior labyrinth (empty arrow) (**b**) very short PSCC (empty arrow), normal LSCC (plain arrow) (**c**) very small bony island of 2 mm inside the LSCC (white arrow). *V* vestibule, *IAC* internal auditory canal

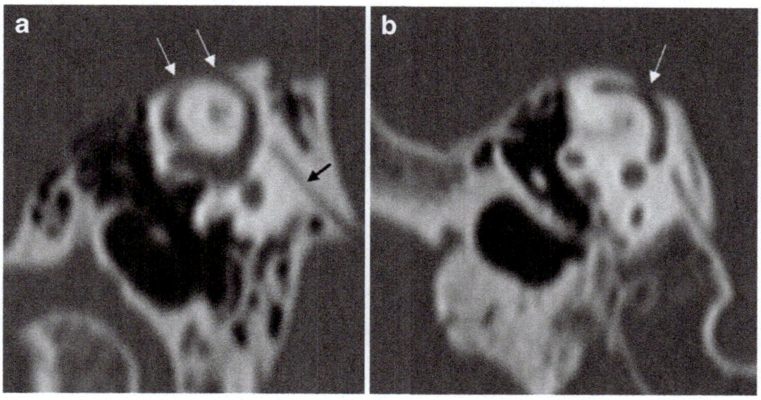

Fig. 2.25 CT Poeschl plan: (**a**) axial CT: dehiscence of the bony cover of the SSCC between the white arrows. Notice also the linear appearance of the vestibular aqueduct in this plan (black arrow). (**b**) Dehiscence of the SSCC with the superior petrosal sinus (arrow)

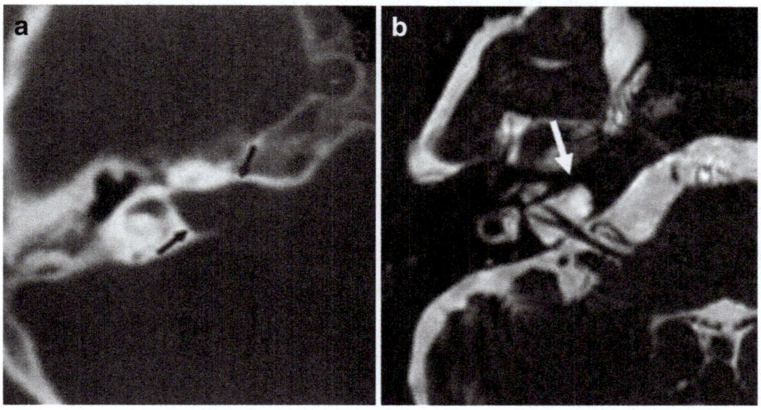

Fig. 2.26 (**a**) Axial CT: enlarged IAC (between arrows), (**b**) axial MR T2w image showing dural ectasia inside the IAC (white arrow)

- Calcification of parts of the lumen, especially after labyrinthitis [50].
- Dehiscence of the bony coverage especially of the SSCC, evaluation on reconstructed images along the Poeschl plan (demonstrated in Fig. 2.4) [51] (Fig. 2.25).

2.4.15 Inner Auditory Canal (IAC)

Normal variants in configuration are funnel shaped, cylindrical, or bud-shaped (Fig. 2.26) [52]. The IAC is considered as stenotic if the diameter is inferior to 2 mm (Fig. 2.27a).

MRI is essential to confirm the presence of the cochlear nerve in case of stenotic IAC (Fig. 2.27b, c) especially before cochlear implant planning (see Sect. 2.4.10).

2.5 Temporal Bone Surfaces: Topographic Pathologies

2.5.1 Lateral Surface

2.5.1.1 *Anomalies of the Auricle*

Usually an indicator of congenital aural dysplasia and not routinely included in the cross-sectional

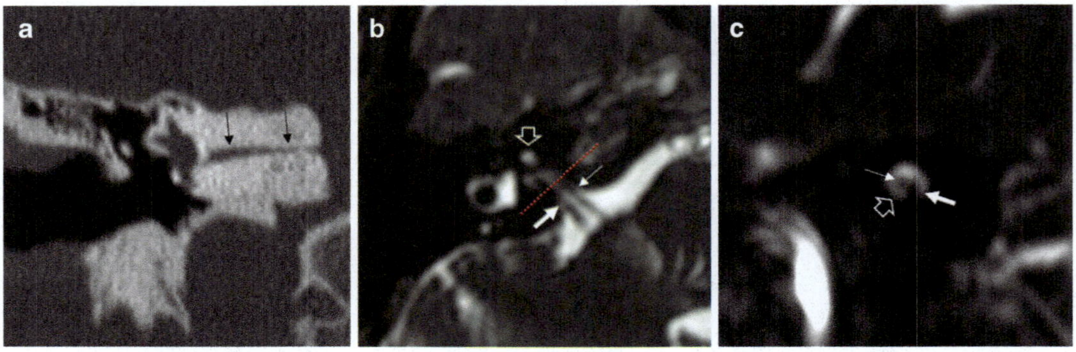

Fig. 2.27 (**a**) Coronal CT: severely stenotic IAC (arrows). (**b**) Axial HR T2w MRI: posteriorly the vestibular nerve (thick arrow) and anteriorly the facial nerve (thin arrow) inside the canal. Rudimentary cochlea type I hypoplasia (empty arrow). Red reference line for sagittal oblique reconstruction in (**c**): only the vestibular nerves (thick arrow) and the VII (thin arrow) are present, absence of the cochlear nerve (empty arrow)

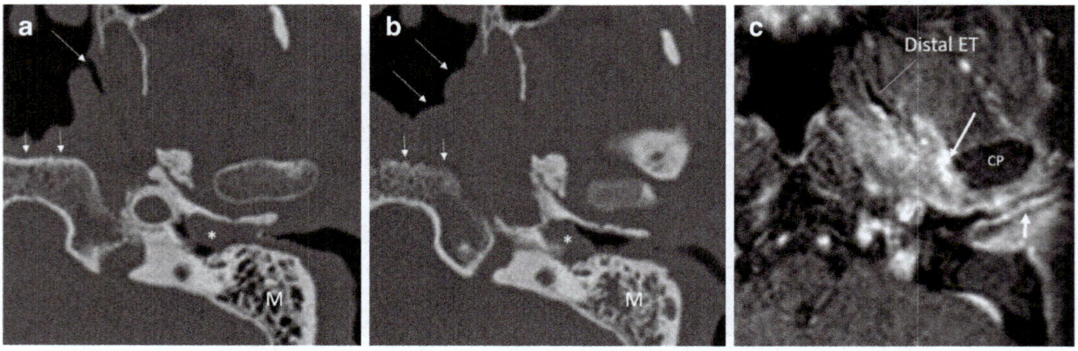

Fig. 2.28 Patient with painful external necrotizing otitis. (**a**) Initial axial CT: condensations confined to EAC (asterisk), intact clivus (white arrows), well aerated mastoid (M). (**b**) Six months later, persistent pain: condensations progressed into the ME cleft (asterisk), lysis of the anterior cortex of the clivus (short arrows). Swelling of nasopharyngeal walls (long arrows). (**c**) T1 w SPIR post Gd MR with important contrast uptake along the EAC (short arrow), inside the temporomandibular joint (long arrow) around the condyloid process (CP) and surrounding the proximal Eustachian tube (ET) that is a virtual lumen in the posterior continuity with the distal ET

imaging unless for special requests in tumor or plastic surgery.

Role of MR permits detailed analyses of the auricle and evaluation of eventual intraosseous extension of skin tumors after i.v. injection of gadolinium.

2.5.1.2 *External Necrotizing Otitis*

CT is often the first approach and may show in the beginning of the process only soft-tissue thickening in the EAC in spite of heavy otalgia (Fig. 2.28a).

Pathways of Infection Spread

- Anteriorly through the fissures of Santorini to the fatty tissue of the temporomandibular joint (Fig. 2.28b, c) that becomes thickened, to the masticator space, to the parotid.
- Anteromedially to the para-nasopharyngeal fatty tissue with obliteration of the normal fat planes.
- Further medially to the preclival fatty tissue and spreading over the midline to the contralateral side with lysis of the clivus cortex as sign of osteomyelitis of the skull base (Fig. 2.28b). This is a sign of advanced disease, often complicated by superior involvement of the skull base and inferior cranial nerves, especially IX, X, and X [53].
- Administration of i.v. iodine contrast is not helpful, because the uptake of inflammatory tissues does not show on CT.

MR, in contrary, is highly superior to evaluate the exact anatomical location and extent of soft-tissue infiltration/infection especially with T1 w post Gadolinium (fat sat) [54] (Fig. 2.28c).

2.5.1.3 *Subperiosteal Abscess*

In the context of acute otomastoïditis, one extra-temporal complication along the lateral mastoid surface (Fig. 2.29) is the subperiosteal abscess that concerns most often children.

CT is the first imaging method of choice, usually indicated when intracerebral complications are suspected, showing the lack of trabeculations in the mastoid/antrum, and often small erosions of the bony walls of the mastoid. It should be done with i.v. contrast administration to show subperiosteal collection lateral to the mastoid.

2.5.2 Posterior Surface

2.5.2.1 *Extratemporal Intracranial Complications of CSOM*

CT: Extratemporal spread of infection from the mastoid posteriorly may cause epidural collections in close proximity to the sigmoid sinus (Fig. 2.29a), or even intracerebral abscess formations. Contrast injection is needed!

MR: Sigmoid sinus thrombosis can occur (Fig. 2.29b), best confirmed on MR venography (Fig. 2.29c), that is an imaging technique based on the flow void volume on T2, *without need of intravenous contrast injection*.

2.5.2.2 Endolymphatic Sac

The normal endolymphatic sac is often very small. MR is the only method to visualize the endolymphatic sac.

- *Endolymphatic sac tumors* are very rare.

CT: soft-tissue masses with prominent intratumoral calcifications and permeative bone erosions along the posterior surface of the petrous bone [55].

MR: heterogeneous signal intensity on both T1- and T2-weighted images [56].

2.5.2.3 IAC Meatus and the Cerebellopontine Angle

MR is the method of choice: large differential diagnosis in case of tumors of the IAC/CPA angle (most frequently *vestibular schwannoma* in 60–90%, and *meningioma*, rarely *epidermoid* or *hemangioma* [57, 58].

MR: Inside the IAC, vestibular schwannoma appears iso (35%) or slightly hypointense (65%) to brain tissue on T1w images, strongly enhancing after Gd administration (Fig. 2.30 [59].

2.5.3 Superior Surface

2.5.3.1 Tegmen Tympani

It is the lateral aspect of the superior surface, part of the floor of the middle cranial fossa.

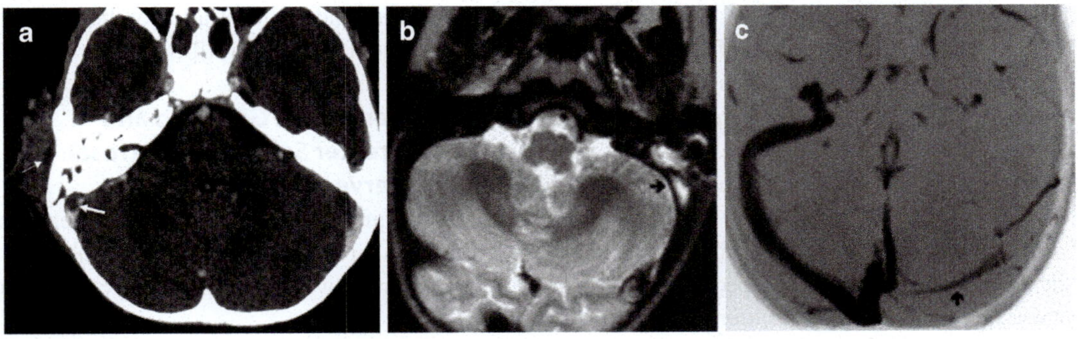

Fig. 2.29 (**a**) Axial CT in a young child after i.v. contrast showing a lateral subperiosteal collection (thin arrow) and also posterior extradural collection, that is insinuating in the sigmoid sinus (SS, thick arrow). (**b** and **c**) Another adult patient with left otomastoïditis complicated by SS - thrombosis: (**b**) hyperintense aspect of thrombotic clot in the SS (arrow), (**c**) typical image of left SS - thrombosis (arrow) on MR venography

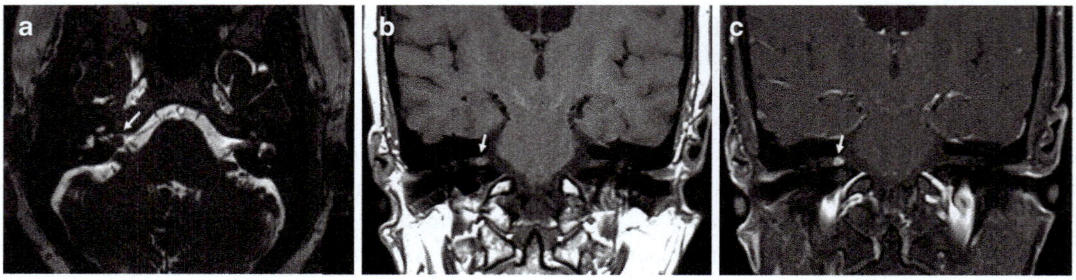

Fig. 2.30 Vestibular intracanalicular schwannoma: (**a**) Axial CISS and (**b**) coronal T1 WI MRI before and (**c**) after i.v. contrast administration: (**a**) small right intracanalicular lesion as lack of fluid signal in the IAC (arrow), (**b**) spontaneously isodense on T1w MR to brain tissue (arrow), (**c**) homogenously enhancing postcontrast (arrow)

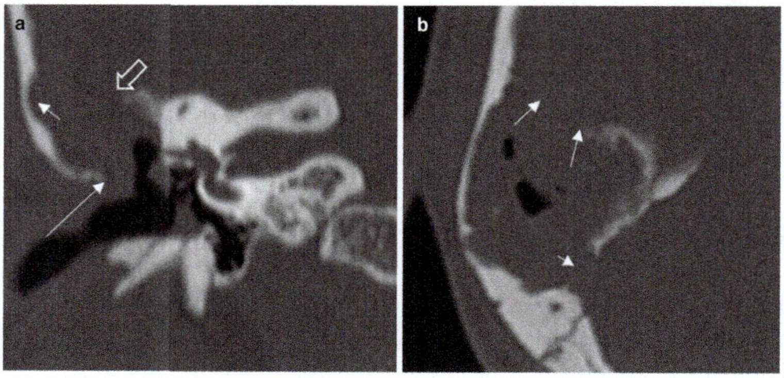

Fig. 2.31 (**a**) Coronal CT: large amputation of the scutum (long arrow) and huge soft-tissue mass (cholesteatoma) occupying the whole attic, and extending into the middle cranial fossa through a large tegmen defect, causing scalloping of the lateral skull (short small arrow). (**b**) Axial CT showing the huge mass at the level of the lytic tegmen, almost complete lysis of the anterior limit (long arrows) and posterior limit (short arrow)

CT: Extension of an ME cholesteatoma through a lytic or dehiscent tegmen into the middle cranial fossa can be already obvious by CT (Fig. 2.31).

MR: In case of discontinuity of the tegmen and nonspecific soft-tissue densities in the middle ear cleft, MRI can show *meningoencephalocele* herniating into the ME (Fig. 2.32) that may be spontaneous, or coexist with a cholesteatomatous process inside the ME cleft.

Also CSF leak through a tegmen defect causing otoliquorrhea can be suspected on CT but needs the diagnostic contribution of MR for the eventual underlying conditions. Proof of this communication can be done by intrathecal injection of contrast and demonstration of the contrast inside the middle ear cleft [60].

2.5.3.2 Geniculate Ganglion and Greater Superficial Petrosal Nerve

- Most frequent pathologies of these nervous structures are *schwannomas or hemangiomas*, both are well demonstrated by *MR with Gd*.

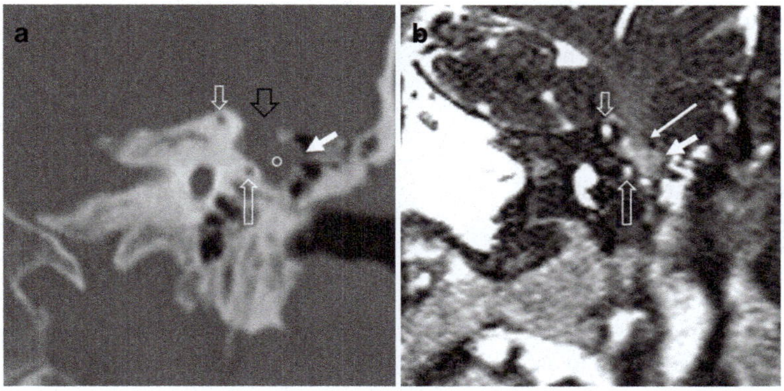

Fig. 2.32 (**a**) Coronal CT: tegmen discontinuity (empty black arrow), obliteration of the attic with convex borders (thick arrow). Density measurement of this condensation (circle) is 1 UH, corresponding to liquid! (**b**) Coronal HR T2w MR showing continuity of cerebral tissue (long arrow) into the superior attic and moderately hyperintense fluid signal in the underlying sac (thick arrow), representing meningoencephalocele. For (**a** and **b**): *SSCC* short empty arrow, *LSCC* long empty arrow

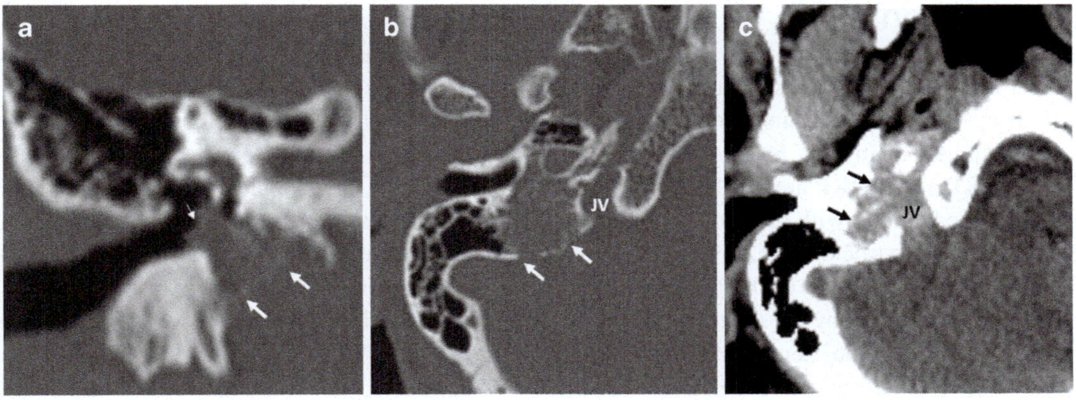

Fig. 2.33 Coronal CT: (**a**) hypotympanic soft-tissue mass (small arrow), diffuse infiltration of the posteroinferior mastoid (thick arrows) (**b**) axial CT diffuse infiltration of the inferior mastoid (arrows). *JV* jugular vein. (**c**) Axial post-contrast CT, diffuse enhancement of the jugulotympanic glomus tumor (arrows)

2.5.4 Inferior Surface

- Posterior boundary of the mandibular fossa
  - Thickening of soft tissue, erosions as sign of eventual spread of infectious diseases
- Jugular foramen, foramen of the carotid artery, numerous cranial nerves passing through the pars nervosa (Nerfs IX, X, XI), and their pathologies

2.5.4.1 *Glomus Tumor*

CT: shows almost always a bulging soft-tissue mass in the hypotympanum typically with important contrast uptake, associated to erosive lesions of the mastoid adjacent to the jugular bulb (Fig. 2.33).

MRI: permits to precise the extension from the glomus of the tympanic nerve to the nerfs of the jugular foramen and extension at the base of skull [61].

2.6 Input of Postoperative Imaging/Follow-Up

Tympanostomies and tympanoplasties do not require scanographic evaluation unless complications. Tympanoplasty leads often to an opaque TM that does not permit otoscopic analysis of the underlying structures. CT permits to reveal retrotympanic processes as developing cholesteatoma (Fig. 2.34a).

2.6.1 Ossicular Reconstruction (Incus Interposition, PORP/TORP)

Incus interposition appears with typical ossicular density but modified in form and position, establishing a continuity between TM and stapes. **PORP and TORP** are synthetic prostheses that engage laterally with the TM, medially with the stapes superstructure (PORP, Fig. 2.34b) or directly with the footplate (TORP). Displacement can be demonstrated by CT (Fig. 2.34c).

CBCT: some studies demonstrated a good visibility of the TORP and analysis of its distal positioning on the footplate with the help of three-dimensional CBCT reformatting [62].

2.6.2 Stapes Prosthesis

CT: Some prostheses are very dense on CT, causing streak artifacts, that should not be mistaken for fibrotic bands (Fig. 2.35a). Metallic artifacts yield to a 0.5 mm overestimation of size and intravestibular length of metallic prosthesis with conventional CT scan [63].

Other types of prosthesis appear with much lower density and do not produce artifacts (Fig. 2.35b).

The prosthesis may have lost the contact with the long incus process (empty loop sign, Fig. 2.35b). The tip of the prosthesis may be deviated on the footplate or show a deep insertion into the vestibule (Fig. 2.35b). Recurrence of the otosclerotic process around the footplate or fibrous bands that cause relapse of fixity can be seen by CT [64, 65].

Also CT can demonstrate pneumolabyrinth as a stapedotomy complication [66].

MR: can give precision about intravestibular pathologies:

- Granuloma development with inflammatory labyrinthitis, typically with intermediate T1, hypointense T2w images, and contrast enhancement post Gd.
- Intra labyrinthine hemorrhage (hyperintense in T1 and T2).
- Suppurative labyrinthitis with intense Gd enhancement [67].

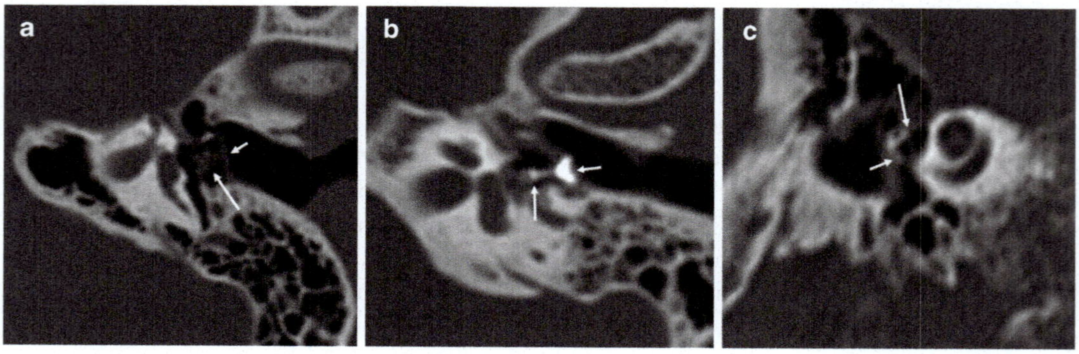

Fig. 2.34 CT of (**a**) Tympanoplasty as a thick linear structure (short arrow), hiding mesotympanic cholesteatoma formation (long arrow). (**b**) PORP with satisfactory contact with the TM (short arrow), medially with the stapes head (arrow). (**c**) Displaced PORP, only partially in contact with the TM (short arrow), its distal tip is disconnected (long arrow)

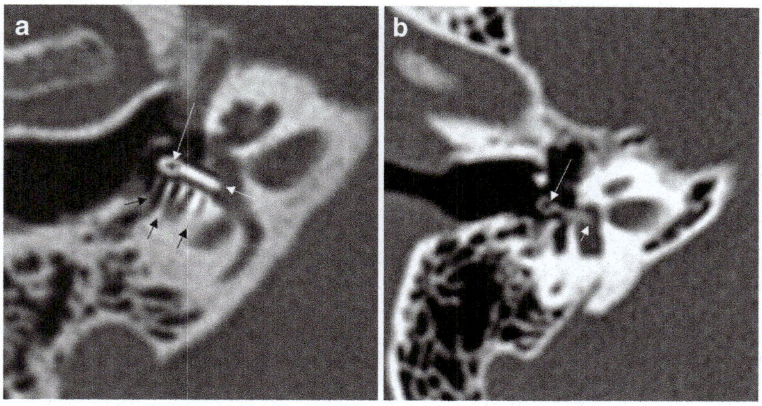

Fig. 2.35 CT reconstructed in the axial stapes plan of two different types of stapes prosthesis: (**a**) prosthesis of titanium, the ring (long arrow) shows a black center due to high density artifact (it is not empty). Multiple streak artifacts (small black arrows). Tip of prosthesis (white short arrow) enters about 1/3 of transversal diameter into the vestibule. (**b**) Another type of prosthesis is less dense, showing a real empty loop (long arrow). The distal tip is far advanced into the vestibule, about 2/3 of the transversal diameter

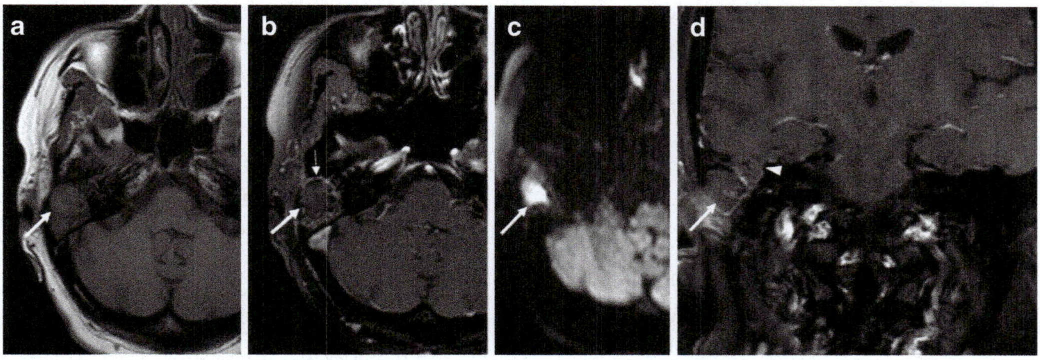

Fig. 2.36 (**a**) ax T1w MR: large atticoantral isointense lesion (arrow), (**b**) ax T1w MR with Gd, no contrast uptake (thick arrow) but thin surrounding rim enhancement (small arrow). (**c**) DW B1000 image: strong restriction (arrow) confirming cholesteatoma. (**d**) On coronal T1wMR: associated meningoencephalocele (arrowhead), medial to the cholesteatoma (arrow)

2.6.3 Recurrent/Residual Cholesteatoma

CT has a high negative predictive value in a well-aerated middle ear cleft with no evidence of abnormal soft tissue [68]. Recurrent cholesteatoma is suspected, when soft-tissue formations are associated to new bone erosions on comparative studies, although the attenuation characteristics are nonspecific.

MR: As diffusion-weighted images have a high predictive value for residual/recurrent cholesteatoma (see Sects. 2.2.3.2 and 2.4.3), non-EPI DWI MR may help to classify patients into groups with indication for second look surgery versus follow up [69, 70].

However, the MR exploration must always include conventional sequences to avoid false-positive interpretations from eventual fat grafts or hemorrhage [71], and to search for associated anomalies that are important to consider during surgery, as associated meningoencephalocele (Fig. 2.36).

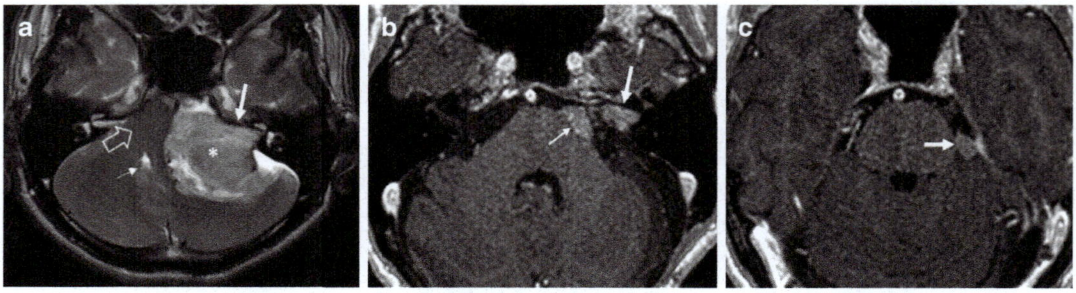

Fig. 2.37 Axial MR T1w after Gd: (**a**) initially huge vestibular schwannoma occupying the whole IAC (white thick arrow) and CPA angle (asterisk) with important mass effect on the pons (empty arrow) and forth ventricle (small arrow). (**b**) Postoperative residual tissues left in the IAC (thick arrow), in close contact with the pons (small arrow) and (**c**) in the upper posterior angle of the cerebellopontine cisterna (arrow) 2 years after subtotal resection with facial nerve preservation

2.6.4 Vestibular Schwannoma

MRI is routinely performed after resection as base line exploration, to assess residual or recurrent tumor, as well as for suspected complications, as there are fat graft necrosis, CSF leakage, infection, cerebral infarction, venous sinus thrombosis, hemorrhage, cerebellar atrophy, and endolymphatic fluid loss [72]

- Almost every first control by MRI shows residual enhancement in the surgical bed.
  - If the enhancement is linear, it is mainly corresponding to scar and/or granulation tissue and can persist for 1 year or longer.
  - If the enhancement is nodular, it is almost always residual tissue [73] (Fig. 2.37). Very exact reproducible measurements are necessary over time to evaluate disease progression for these slow growing processes.

2.7 Conclusion

Temporal bone imaging is considered nowadays the main diagnostic tool to enrich the clinical and therapeutical approaches. It orients surgical indications and helps to anticipate eventual abnormalities or complications that may modify the surgical outcome. Several imaging tools are available for most dedicated imaging, and this chapter emphasizes the utility of CT versus MR imaging depending on the clinical evaluation and course of the disease. CT and MRI are complementary methods, both can be often necessary to elucidate several pathologies. Constant feedback between otologist and radiologist is a key to improve our experience regard to ear disease management.

Take-Home Messages

- CT is the first imaging modality for middle ear pathologies with conductive hearing loss, especially in otosclerosis, tympanosclerosis, chronic suppurative otitis media, cholesteatoma, SSCC dehiscence, or congenital malformations.
- In the postoperative follow-up, CT demonstrates especially prosthesis status (preferably by CBCT when available) and follow-up of otosclerosis progress.
- MRI better differentiates doubtful middle ear condensations that are suspicious for cholesteatoma, recurrence of cholesteatoma, and extension beyond the limits of the temporal bone of any infectious or tumoral process.
- MRI is the key imaging method to analyze the content of IAC and of CPA. It is part of the systematic workup before cochlear implant.
- CT and MRI are often complementary methods. A constant collaboration between otologist and radiologist is essential to improve imaging diagnosis for better ear disease management.

References

1. Gentric JC, Rousset JR, Garetier M, Ben Salem D, Meriot P. High-resolution computed tomography of isolated congenital anomalies of the stapes: a pictural review using oblique multiplanar reformation in the "axial stapes" plane. J Neuroradiol. 2012;39(1):58–64.
2. Lemmerling M, de Foer B. Temporal bone imaging. New York: Springer; 2014.
3. Daly MJ, Siewerdsen JH, Moseley DJ, et al. Intraoperative cone-beam CT for guidance of head and neck surgery: assessment of dose and image quality using a C-arm prototype. Med Phys. 2006;33:3767–80.
4. Loubele M, Bogaerts R, Van Dijck E, et al. Comparison between effective radiation dose of CBCT and MSCT scanners for dentomaxillofacial applications. Eur J Radiol. 2009;71:461Y8.
5. Miracle AC, Mukherji SK. Conebeam CT of the head and neck, Part 1: Physical principles. AJNR Am J Neuroradiol. 2009;30(6):1088–95.
6. Mori S, Endo M, Nishizawa K, et al. Enlarged longitudinal dose profiles in cone-beam CT and the need for modified dosimetry. Med Phys. 2005;32:1061–9.
7. Kyriakou Y, Deak P, Langner O, et al. Concepts for dose determination in flat-detector CT. Phys Med Biol. 2008;53:3551–66. Epub 2008 Jun 13.
8. Gupta R, Bartling SH, Basu SK, et al. Experimental flat-panel high-spatial resolution volume CT of the temporal bone. AJNR Am J Neuroradiol. 2004;25:1417–24.
9. Dahmani-Caussea M, Marxa M, Deguinea O, Frayssea B, Lepageb B, Escudé B. Morphologic examination of the temporal bone by cone beam computed tomography: comparison with multislice helical computed tomography. Eur Ann Otorhinolaryngol Head Neck Dis. 2011;128(5):230–5.
10. Miracle AC, Mukherji SK. Conebeam CT of the head and neck, Part 2: Clinical applications. AJNR Am J Neuroradiol. 2009;30:1285–92.
11. Aschendorff A, Kubalek R, Hochmuth A, et al. Imaging procedures in cochlear implant patients: evaluation of different radiological techniques. Acta Otolaryngol Suppl. 2004;552:46–9.
12. Ruivo J, Mermuys K, Bacher K, Kuhweide R, Offeciers E, Casselman JW. Cone beam computed tomography, a low-dose imaging technique in the postoperative assessment of cochlear implantation. Otol Neurotol. 2009;30(3):299–303. https://doi.org/10.1097/mao.0b013e31819679f9.
13. Révész P, Liktor B, Liktor B, Sziklai I, Gerlinger I, Karosi T. Comparative analysis of preoperative diagnostic values of HRCT and CBCT in patients with histologically diagnosed otosclerotic stapes footplates. Eur Arch Oto-Rhino-Laryngol. 2016;273(1):63–72. 10p.
14. Redfors YD, Gröndahl HG, Hellgren J, Lindfors N, Nilsson I, Möller C. Otosclerosis: anatomy and pathology in the temporal bone assessed by multi-slice and cone-beam CT. Otol Neurotol. 2012;33:922–7.
15. Mangrum W, Christianson K, Duncan S, et al. Duke review of MRI principles. Philadelphia, PA: Mosby; 2012.
16. Dremmen MH, Hofman PA, Hof JR, Stokroos RJ, Postma AA. The diagnostic accuracy of non-echo-planar diffusion weighted imaging in the detection of residual and/or recurrent cholesteatoma of the temporal bone. AJNR Am J Neuroradiol. 2012;33:439–44.
17. Dudau C, Draper A, Gkagkanasiou M, Charles-Edwards G, Pai I, Connor S. Cholesteatoma: multishot echo-planar *vs* non echo-planar diffusion-weighted MRI for the prediction of middle ear and mastoid cholesteatoma. BJR Open. 2019;1:20180015.
18. Naganawa S, Satake H, Iwano S, Fukatsu H, Sone M, Nakashima T. Imaging endolymphatic hydrops at 3 tesla using 3DFLAIR with intratympanic Gd-DTPA administration. Magn Reson Med Sci. 2008;7(2):85–91.
19. Venkatasamy A, Veillon F, Fleury A, Eliezer M, Abu Eid M, Romain B, Vuong H, Rohmer D, Charpiot A, Sick H, Riehm S. Imaging of the saccule for the diagnosis of endolymphatic hydrops in Meniere disease, using a three-dimensional T2-weighted steady state free precession sequence: accurate, fast, and without contrast material intravenous injection. Eur Radiol Exp. 2017;1:14.
20. Bernaerts B, Vanspauwen R, Blaivie C, van Dinther J, Zarowski A, Wuyts F, Vanden Bossche S, Offeciers E, Casselman JW, De Foer B. The value of four stage vestibular hydrops grading and asymmetric perilymphatic enhancement in the diagnosis of Menière's disease on MRI. Neuroradiology. 2019;61: 421–9.
21. Fritsch M. MRI scanners and stapes prosthesis. Otol Neurotol. 2007;28:733–8.
22. Syms MJ. Safety of magnetic resonance imaging of stapes prostheses. Laryngoscope. 2005;115:381–90.
23. Mansour S, Magnan J, Nicolas K, Haidar H. Middle ear diseases. New York: Springer; 2018. p. 471–73.
24. Patil AR, Bhalla A, Gupta P, et al. HRCT evaluation of microtia: a retrospective study. Indian J Radiol Imaging. 2012;22(3):188–94.
25. Gassner EM, Mallouhi A, Jaschke WR. Preoperative evaluation of external auditory canal atresia on high-resolution CT. AJR Am J Roentgenol. 2004;182(5):1305–12.
26. Mansour S, Magnan J, Haidar H, Nicolas K. Tympanic membrane retraction pocket, overview and advances in diagnosis and management. New York: Springer; 2015.
27. Mansour S, Magnan J, Haidar H, Nicolas K, Louryan S. Comprehensive and clinical anatomy of the middle ear. 2nd ed. New York: Springer; 2019. p 44.
28. Li P, Linos E, Gurgel R, Fischbein N, Blevins N. Evaluating the utility of non–echo-planar diffusion-weighted imaging in the preoperative evaluation of cholesteatoma: a meta-analysis. Laryngoscope. 2013;123:1247–50.
29. Lingam R, Bassett P. A meta-analysis on the diagnostic performance of non-echoplanar diffusion-weighted

imaging in detecting middle ear cholesteatoma: 10 years on. Otol Neurotol. 2017;38:521–8.
30. Jindal M, Riskalla A, Jiang D, Connor S, O'Connor AF. A systematic review of diffusion-weighted magnetic resonance imaging in the assessment of postoperative cholesteatoma. Otol Neurotol. 2011;32:1243–49.
31. Mansour S, Magnan J, Nicolas K, Haidar H. Middle ear diseases. New York: Springer; 2018 chapter tympanosclerosis pages 169-181 and/or chapter otosclerosis pages 1-33.
32. Lagleyre S, Sorrentino T, Calmels MN, Shin YJ, Escudé B, Deguine O, Fraysse B. Reliability of high-resolution CT scan in diagnosis of otosclerosis. Otol Neurotol. 2009;30(8):1152–9.
33. Veillon F, Stierle JL, Dussaix J, et al. Otosclerosis imaging: matching clinical and imaging data. J Radiol. 2006;87:1756–64.
34. Marshall AH, Fanning N, Symons S, Shipp D, Chen JM, Nedzelski JM. Cochlear implantation in cochlear otosclerosis. Laryngoscope. 2005;115:1728–33.
35. Mansour S, Nicolas K, Ahmad HH. Round window otosclerosis: radiologic classification and clinical correlations. Otol Neurotol. 2011;32(3):384–92.
36. Sennaroglu L, Bajin MD, Pamuk E, Tahir E. Cochlear hypoplasia type four with anteriorly displaced facial nerve canal. Otol Neurotol. 2016;37:407–9.
37. Gupta S, Mends F, Hagiwara M, Fatterpekar G, Roehm PC. Imaging the facial nerve: a contemporary review. Radiol Res Pract. 2013;2013:248039. 14 pages.
38. Mansour S, Magnan J, Nicolas K, Haidar H. Middle ear diseases. New York: Springer; 2018. p. 296–300.
39. Razek AA, Huang BY, et al. Lesions of the petrous apex: classification and findings at CT and MR imaging. Radio Graphics. 2012;32:151–73.
40. Jackler RK, Luxford WM, House WF. Congenital malformations of the inner ear: a classification based on embryogenesis. Laryngoscope. 1987;97:2–14.
41. Sennaroglu L, Saatci I. A new classification for cochleovestibular malformations. Laryngoscope. 2002;112:230–41.
42. Sennaroglu L. Cochlear implantation in inner ear malformations – a review article. Cochlear Implants Int. 2009;11(1):4–41.
43. Joshi V, Navlekar SK, Kishore G, Reddy K, Kumar E. CT and MR imaging of the inner ear and brain in children with congenital sensorineural hearing loss. Radiographics. 2012;32:683–98.
44. Sennaroğlu L, Bajin M. Classification and current management of inner ear malformations. Balkan Med J. 2017;34:397–411.
45. Mukherji SK, Baggett HC, Alley J, Carrasco VH. Enlarged cochlear aqueduct. AJNR Am J Neuroradiol. 1998;19:330–2.
46. Vijayasekaran S, Halsted MJ, Boston M, Meinzen-Derr J, Bardo DME, Greinwald J, Benton C. When is the vestibular aqueduct enlarged? A statistical analysis of the normative distribution of vestibular aqueduct size. Am J Neuroradiol. 2007;28(6):1133–8.
47. Morimoto AK, Wiggins RH III, Hudgins PA, Hedlund GL, Hamilton B, Mukherji SK, Telian SA, Harnsberger HR. Absent semicircular canals in CHARGE syndrome: radiologic spectrum of findings. AJNR Am J Neuroradiol. 2006;27(8):1663–71.
48. Wu WJ, He XB, Tan LH, Hu P, Peng AO, Xiao ZA, Yang S, Wang T, Qing J, Chen X, Li JK, Peng T, Dong YP, Liu XZ, Xie DH. Imaging assessment of profound sensorineural deafness with inner ear anatomical abnormalities. J Otol. 2015;10:29–38.
49. Purcell D, Fischbein N, Patel A, Johnson J, Lalwani A. Two temporal bone computed tomography measurements increase recognition of malformations and predict sensorineural hearing loss. Laryngoscope. 2006;116:1439–46.
50. Lemmerling M, Vanzieleghem B, Dhooge I, Van Cauwenberge P, Kunnen M. CT and MRI of the semicircular canals in the normal and diseased temporal bone. Eur Radiol. 2001;11:1210–9.
51. Minor LB, Solomon D, Zinreich JS, Zee DS. Sound- and/or pressure-induced vertigo due to bone dehiscence of the superior semicircular canal. Arch Otolaryngol Head Neck Surg. 1998;124:249–58.
52. Marques S, Ajzen S, D'Ippolito G, Alonso L, Isotani S, Lederman H. Morphometric analysis of the internal auditory canal by computed tomography imaging. Iran J Radiol. 2012;9(2):71–8.
53. Mani N, Sudhoff H, Rajagopal S, Moffat D, Axon P. Cranial nerve involvement in malignant external otitis: implications for clinical outcome. Laryngoscope. 2007;117:907–10.
54. van Kroonenburgh A, van der Meer WL, Bothof RJP, van Tilburg M, van Tongeren J, Postma AA. Advanced imaging techniques in skull base osteomyelitis due to malignant otitis externa. Curr Radiol Rep. 2018;6:3.
55. Kumar M, Ramakrishnaiah R, Muhhamad Y, Van Hemert R, Angtuaco E. Endolymphatic sac tumor. Radiol Case Rep. 2011;6(3).
56. Sun YH, Wen W, Wu JH, Song JM, Guan H, Wang KX, Xu MQ. Endolymphatic sac tumor: case report and review of the literature. Diagn Pathol. 2012;7:36.
57. Casselman J, Lu CH, De Foer B, Delanote J. Schwannomas of the cochleo-vestibular nerve (Schwannomes du nerf vestibulo-cochléaire). In: Veillon F, editor. Imagerie de l'oreille et de l'os temporal. Tome 4, chapitre 26. Paris: Lavoisier; 2013. p. 921–57.
58. Bonfort G, Veillon F, Debry C, Kehrli P, Chibbaro S. VIIIth nerve cavernous hemangioma mimicking a stage 1 acoustic schwannoma. Neurochirurgie. 2015;61:352–5.
59. Mulkens TH, Parizel PM, Martin JJ, et al. Acoustic schwannoma: MR findings in 84 tumors. AJR Am J Roentgenol. 1993;160(2):395–8.
60. Schubiger O, Valvanis A, Stuckmann G, Antonuccci F. Temporal bone fractures and their complications: examination with high resolution CT. Neuroradiology. 1986;28:93–9.

61. Mravic M, LaChaud G, Nguyen A, Scott M, Dry S, James A. Clinical and histopathological diagnosis of glomus tumor: an institutional experience of 138 cases. Int J Surg Pathol. 2015;23(3):181–8.
62. Komori M, Yanagihara N, Hyodo J, Miuchi S. Position of TORP on the stapes footplate assessed with cone beam computed tomography. Otol Neurotol. 2012;33:1353–6.
63. Warren FM, Riggs S, Wiggins RH III. Computed tomographic imaging of stapes implants. Otol Neurotol. 2008;29:586–92.
64. Ali HI, Khater NH. Otosclerosis and complications of stapedectomy: CT and MRI correlation Alexandria. J Med. 2018;54:197–201.
65. Kösling K, Plontke SK, Bartel S. Imaging of otosclerosis. Fortschr Röntgenstr. 2020; https://doi.org/10.1055/a-1131-7980.
66. Ziade G, Barake R, El Natout T, El Natout M-A. Late pneumolabyrinth after stapedectomy. Eur Ann Otorhinolaryngol Head Neck Dis. 2016;133(5):361–3.
67. Rangheard AS, Marsot-Dupuch K, Mark A, Meyer B, Tubiana JM. Postoperative complications in otospongiosis: usefulness of MR imaging. AJNR Am J Neuroradiol. 2001;22:1171–8.
68. Barath K, Huber AM, Stämpfli P, Varga Z, Kollias S. Neuroradiology of cholesteatomas. AJNR Am J Neuroradiol. 2010;32:221–9.
69. Keeler JA, Kaylie DM. Cholesteatoma: is a second stage necessary? Laryngoscope. 2016;126:1499–500.
70. Steens S, Venderink W, Kunst D, Meijer A, Mylanus E. Repeated postoperative follow-up diffusion-weighted magnetic resonance imaging to detect residual or recurrent cholesteatoma. Otol Neurotol. 2016;37:356–61.
71. Juliano AF, Ginat DT, Moonis G. Imaging review of the temporal bone: Part II. Traumatic, postoperative, and noninflammatory nonneoplastic conditions. Radiology. 2015;276:655–72.
72. Ginat DT, Martuza RL. Postoperative imaging of vestibular schwannomas. Neurosurg Focus. 2012;33:E18.
73. Carlson ML, Van Abel KM, Driscoll CL, et al. Magnetic resonance imaging surveillance following vestibular schwannoma resection. Laryngoscope. 2012;122:378–88.

The External Ear

3

Aisha Larem, Adham Aljariri, and Zaid Altamimi

3.1 Introduction

The ear consists of three parts: the external, middle, and internal ear. All three parts play an essential rule in the hearing function of the ear. The auricle concentrate (collects and localizes) the sound waves from different directions and directs them to the ear canal, then into to the middle, and then into the cochlea. The external ear is the outermost part of the ear, and it is subdivided into auricle (Pinna) and the external auditory canal (EAC). The external ear is subjected to different types of disorders with a higher risk for trauma, infections, and foreign body impaction than the other parts of the ear [1]. In this chapter, the pathologies of the auricle and the EAC are discussed and divided into congenital, acquired, and inflammatory. A brief overview of the embryology, anatomy, and physiology of the external ear is discussed below.

A. Larem (✉) · A. Aljariri · Z. Altamimi
Hamad Medical Corporation, Doha, Qatar
e-mail: alarem@hamad.qa; AAljariri@hamad.qa; ZAITamimi@hamad.qa

3.1.1 Embryology

The ear is originating from the three embryonic layers, ectoderm, mesoderm, and endoderm. The auricle develops from the fusion of six mesodermal hillocks which arises from the first and the second branchial arches [1]. The external ear canal is derived from the first branchial groove (cleft). EAC ends at the tympanic membrane (TM), a structure developed from the three embryonic layers. Different congenital anomalies can affect the external ear, and it includes microtia, anotia, canal atresia, prominent auricles (Bat ears), pits, or sinuses.

3.1.2 Anatomy

The auricle is the visible portion of the external ear. The auricular cartilage is composed of elastic cartilage; the auricle sensory innervation is by the greater auricular, the lesser occipital nerves (branches of the cervical plexus), auriculotemporal nerve (branch of the mandibular nerve), and branches of the facial and vagus cranial nerves. The sensory nerve innervation of the auricle is demonstrated in Fig. 3.1. The external auditory canal is approximately 24 mm in length. The outer one-third (8 mm) is formed by cartilage, and the medial two-thirds are formed by bone.

A. Al-Qahtani et al. (eds.), *Textbook of Clinical Otolaryngology*,
https://doi.org/10.1007/978-3-030-54088-3_3

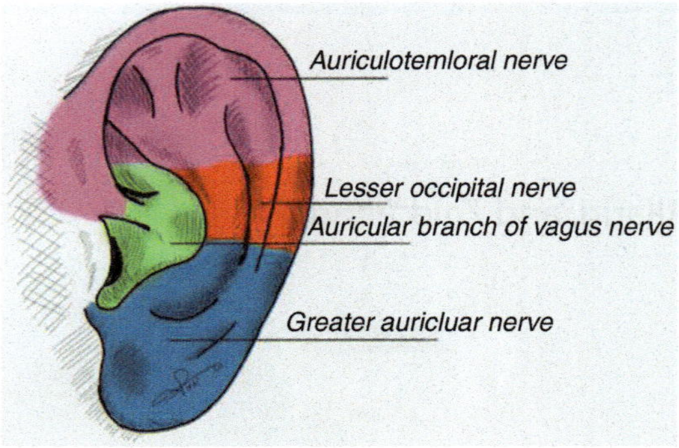

Fig. 3.1 Schematic drawing to the auricle with sensory nerve supply

EAC is lined with stratified squamous epithelium that contains hair follicles, sebaceous glands, and special cerumen gland that secret cerumen. The sloughed epithelium along with any impacted material in the EAC is sloughed out in a centrifugal manner to expel externally.

3.1.3 Physiology

The auricle and the external auditory canal work to concentrate the sounds from surroundings and lead to rising specific resonant frequencies, concha gives resonant to the 5300 Hz and the external auditory canal to 3000 Hz. The external ear also plays a role in sound localization by interaural time difference (difference in time of sound arrival between ears) and interaural amplitude difference (amplitude difference in sound perceiving between the two ears) [1].

3.2 Auricle

3.2.1 Congenital Anomalies of the Auricle

The embryogenesis of the outer/middle ear is different from inner ear, and for this reason, the external ear malformations are frequently associated with the middle ear rather than inner ear malformations.

3.2.1.1 Prominent Ear (Bat Ear)

It occurs due to underdeveloped antihelical fold with/without an overdeveloped conchal bowl. The auricle will be in an abnormal position from the side of the head which is more than 2 cm and at an angle of more than 30° [2].

It has no major functional impairment but can induce psychological distress and emotional trauma for the child (social stigmatization), especially during the school age.

The main treatment is through surgical correction by otoplasty. Surgery usually performed before a child starts school at 4–6 years old. Different techniques have been described including Mustarde, Fritsch, Farrior, and Furnas techniques. Surgical complications such as telephone ear deformity, inadequate correction (asymmetry), hematoma, infection, keloid, suture extrusion, and chondritis can occur. Other management option includes ear splinting at the neonatal period before the age of 3 months [3].

3.2.1.2 Periauricular Pits, Sinuses, and Cysts

Pits are small depressions at the anterior ascending limb of the helix and can be isolated or associated with other extracutaneous manifestations. Preauricular pits do not require management unless they become repeatedly infected or discharging squamous material where surgical excision becomes indicated.

Cysts in the preauricular area may drain desquamated debris if they have sinus or pus if they got infected. Figure 3.2a shows an infected periauricular sinus. Surgical excision is the treatment of choice in case of recurrent infections. Complete excision is essential to prevent recurrence which can be achieved by dissecting out the tract with the guidance of lacrimal probes or methylene blue dye down to the underlying temporalis fascia if needed. It is important to know that this anomaly is different from the branchial cleft cyst anomalies. Figure 3.2b shows intraoperative periauricular sinus identification and excision.

3.2.1.3 Skin Tags

Commonly found in preauricular area, single or multiple, and in some cases contain cartilage.

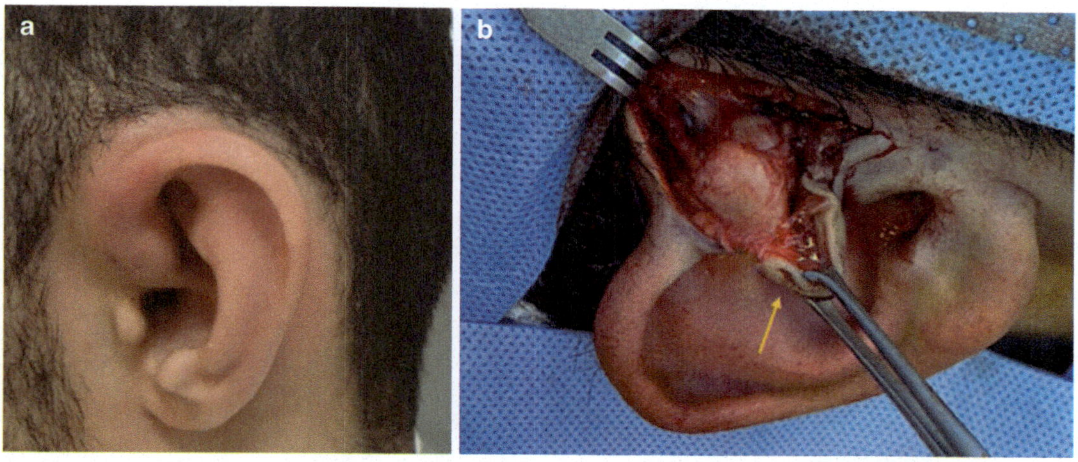

Fig. 3.2 (**a**) Infected periauricular sinus, (**b**) Intraoperative images of periauricular sinus excision (yellow arrow) on the sinus

Audiological evaluation is recommended when they are present. It can be removed surgically with primary wound closure. Figure 3.3 shows a left ear tag.

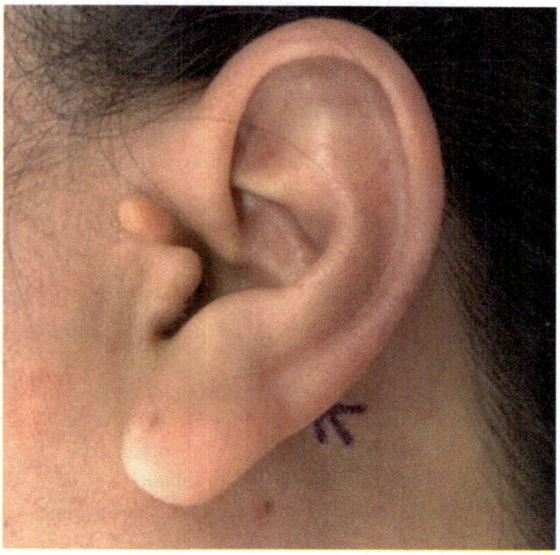

Fig. 3.3 Left ear tag

3.2.1.4 Microtia

Microtia is a malformation of the auricle, which results in a small, deformed auricle (see Fig. 3.4). In case of a complete absence of the auricle, the malformation is called anotia. The incidence of microtia and anotia is 1 to 3 per 10,000 births [4]. It is often associated with atresia. It is found more commonly in males, and more than 75% of cases are unilateral with predominance to the right side. It occurs sporadically or in association with other malformations or syndromes such as Treacher–Collins syndrome, hemifacial microsomia, and Goldenhar syndrome. Prenatal exposure to isotretinoin, thalidomide, and alcohol can increase the risk of microtia [4].

The affected child needs audiological evaluation and may warrant radiologic evaluation for EAC, middle ear, and inner ear [4]. The developmental abnormalities of the auricle can be classified into four grades of severity as shown in Table 3.1 [5].

The management of microtia is achieved by surgical reconstruction or prosthesis for cosmetic reasons. Different surgical reconstruction techniques can be used which often require several stages, and these techniques include Brent and Nagata. The reconstruction is done by utilizing costal cartilage autograft which offers suitable integrity and enough tissue. The surgical intervention is usually performed at the age between 5 and 6 years old (preschool), and it is considered as the first step surgery in case it is associated with aural atresia to ensure a field without scars or compromised blood supply to avoid failure and necrosis of the implanted auricular framework.

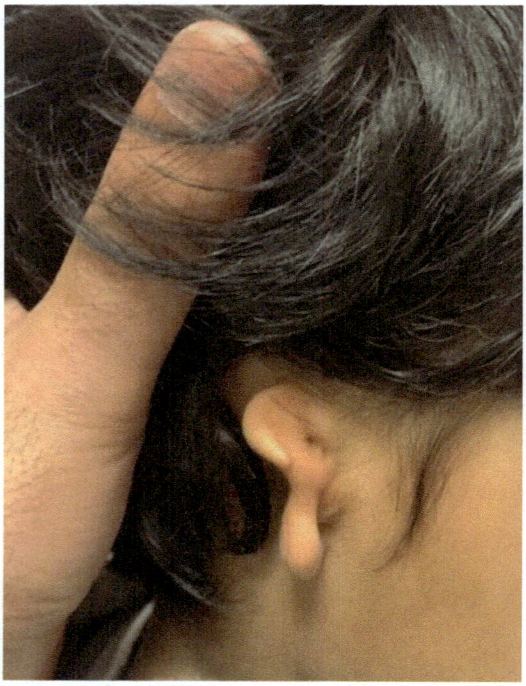

Fig. 3.4 A lateral view demonstrating right ear microtia

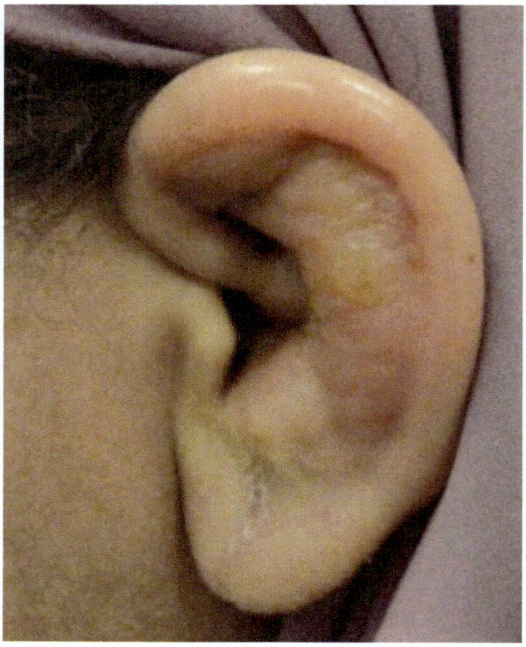

Fig. 3.5 Left auricular perichondritis sparing ear lobule

Table 3.1 Developmental abnormalities of the auricle

Grade	Malformations
I	Abnormal auricle with all identifiable subunits
II	Smaller than grade I auricle with severely underdeveloped or absent subunits, lower half of ear often more developed than upper half
III	"Peanut ear" small piece of disorganized cartilage with a malformed lobule
IV	Anotia (complete absence of the auricle and lobule)

3.2.2 Acquired and Inflammatory Conditions of the Auricle

3.2.2.1 Keloids and Hypertrophic Scars

These are an excessive growth of tissues due to an abnormal response to tissue injury and scar formation. Hypertrophic scars are limited within injury borders, while keloids grow beyond the wound boundaries. Patients with darker skin, genetic predisposition, and wounds closed under tension are prone to develop this abnormal scarring.

Options of treatment include surgical excision with intralesional steroid injection, silicone sheeting, pressure bandages, laser, and cryotherapy. Keloids have a high chance of recurrence, while hypertrophic scar tends to regress with time.

3.2.2.2 Chondritis/Perichondritis

An inflammatory condition involves the perichondrium (Perichondritis) and/or the auricular cartilage (chondritis). It can be secondary to infections, trauma, or as a manifestation of rheumatologic disease as in relapsing polychondritis. The most common pathogen is *Pseudomonas aeruginosa*. It presents as painful erythematous swelling sparing the pinna (see Fig. 3.5). Relapsing polychondritis can affect larynx, trachea, and nose as well as present with recurrent progressive attacks of perichondritis with elevated ESR thought to be due to autoimmune disorder [6].

Treatment by topical and oral antibiotics is generally sufficient in mild cases, and rarely surgical debridement is needed. Corticosteroids therapy is recommended if presumed relapsing polychondritis.

3.2.2.3 Bacterial Infections

It includes impetigo, erysipelas, furunculosis and carbunculosis, and auricular abscess depending on the depth and the layer of the soft-tissue infection.

Impetigo and Erysipelas

Impetigo is a superficial skin infection of the epidermis caused by *Staphylococcus aureus* that leads to a honey-colored crust that is contagious. It is treated with topical antibiotics.

Erysipelas, where the bacterial infection is deeper in the skin (dermal infection), presents with diffuse erythema and swelling of the auricle that spreads along a well-demarcated border. It is caused by B-hemolytic streptococcus, and it may be associated with systemic symptoms as fever [7]. It is treated with appropriate topical and systemic antibiotics. Cellulitis of external ear results from spreading otitis externa or penetrating injury to the canal, and treatment is by systemic antibiotics.

Furunculosis and Carbunculosis

Furunculosis and carbunculosis arise from hair follicles infection of the lateral ear canal. The pathogen is typically *Staphylococcus aureus*. It presents with localized firm or fluctuant painful mass and erythema of the lateral EAC (see Fig. 3.6). Treatment includes appropriate antibiotics and may need incision and drainage if collection is formed [7].

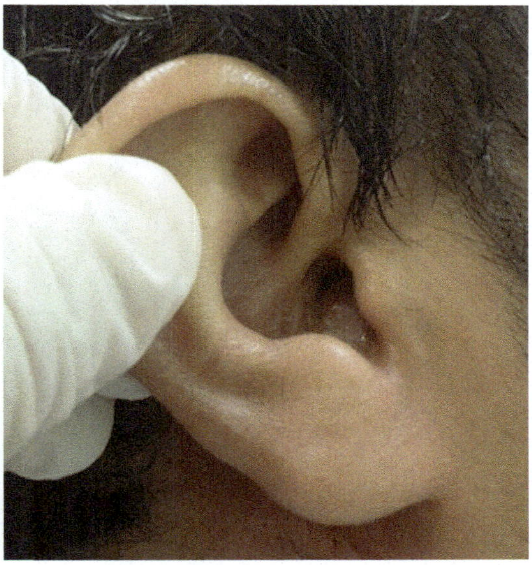

Fig. 3.6 Furuncle in right EAC

Auricular Abscess

Auricular abscess presents with pain, erythema, and fluctuation over the affected area. It can arise secondary to trauma, hematoma, insect bite, or ear piercing. Treatment is by incision and drainage and systemic antibiotics.

3.2.2.4 Ramsey Hunt Syndrome (Herpes Zoster Oticus)

It represents a reactivation of latent viral infection affecting geniculate ganglia of the facial nerve, caused by the Varicella Zoster virus. It can affect other cranial nerves.

The clinical manifestations include facial paralysis, severe ear pain, and unilateral vesicular eruption spread along dermatomes affecting external auditory canal and concha, and cranial nerve VIII involvement causes vertigo and hearing loss. It also includes residual facial weakness after an acute attack in 30–50% of the patient [8]. Treatment includes antiviral therapy, systemic steroids, and supportive care with eye protection.

3.2.2.5 Traumatic Injuries

Hematoma

It usually arises from blunt traumas (sports-related injury), but it can be induced by any minor trauma. Auricular hematoma presents as a painless swelling of the auricle with fading of auricular features (see Fig. 3.7). The separation of the cartilage from its blood supply in the perichondrium can lead to ischemia, then necrosis, and subsequently to cauliflower deformity.

Hematoma requires to be evacuated by aspiration followed by the application of a splint or bolster. In case of recurrence, a proper incision and drainage with splinting should be done to prevent cauliflower ear deformity. Antibiotics (fluoroquinolone) can be administered to avoid infections.

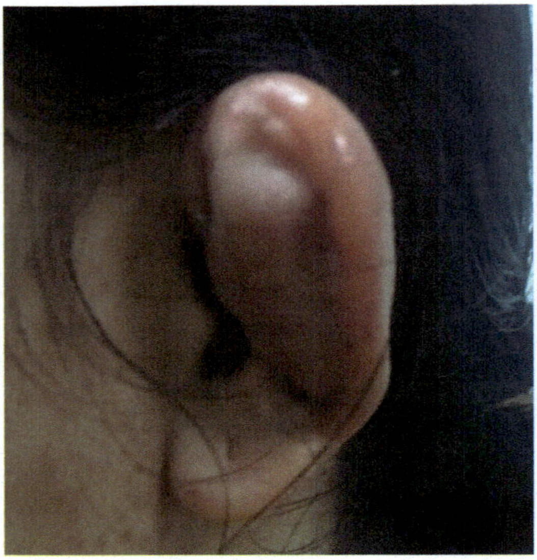

Fig. 3.7 Auricular hematoma

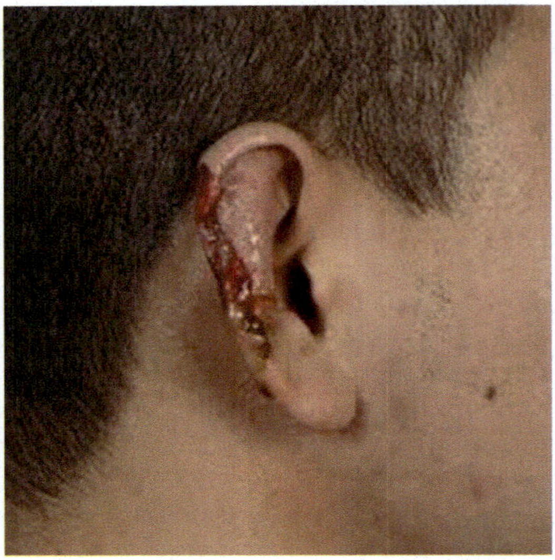

Fig. 3.8 Traumatic helical rim defect of right auricle

Auricular Pseudocysts

It is endochondral cyst-like degeneration with no epithelial or endothelial lining of the anterior surface of the auricle also termed idiopathic pseudocystic chondromalacia. It is believed to result from recurrent minor trauma. It occurs mainly in young adults as a painless mass and can be confused with auricular hematomas. It may require treatment which includes aspiration followed by intralesional steroid injection with a high chance of recurrence or surgical intervention with incision and drainage, curettage, and obliteration with a sclerozing agent.

Laceration and Avulsion

Lacerations can be superficial involving skin only or deep extending into the cartilage, and in both cases, there is a risk of chondritis. Surgical reconstruction is required; most of the lacerations without a significant tissue loss can be closed primarily after irrigation with conservative debridement, supportive management with tetanus shot, and appropriate antibiotics coverage should be given. In the case of exposed cartilage, it can be covered with wedge excision, local flaps, or burial in a postauricular pocket for later reconstruction. In case of helical rim defect (Fig. 3.8), a small defect may be closed primarily if less than 2 cm, while in larger one (more than 2 cm), a chondrocutaneous advancement flap can be used [9].

Avulsions can be partial or complete, and in partial with a well-preserved pedicle, it can be treated by reattachment of the affected part, while complete avulsion requires urgent replantation with microvascular anastomosis, which is difficult and challenging to repair.

3.2.2.6 Other

The auricle may be affected by other disorders such as frostbite, seborrheic dermatitis, allergic contact dermatitis (Fig. 3.9), gout (tophi), chondrodermatitis nodularis chronica helicis, and psoriasis.

3.3 External Auditory Canal (EAC)

3.3.1 Congenital Anomalies of the External Auditory Canal

3.3.1.1 Aural Atresia

Aural atresia is uncommon condition occurring in 1 in 10,000–20,000 patients [10]. It has a high association with microtia. Although in most of the time it is a non-syndromic, it can be seen in syndromes as Treacher Collins, Crouzon, Nager,

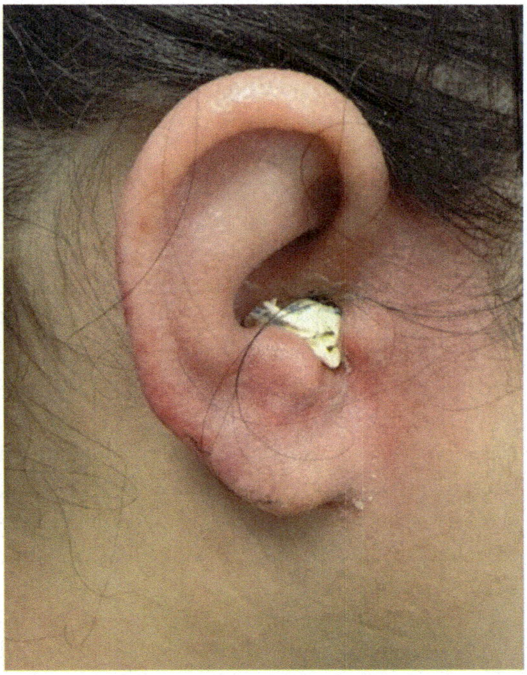

Fig. 3.9 Allergic contact dermatitis in the auricle against bismuth iodoform paraffin paste (BIPP) pack post tympanoplasty

Goldenhar, Klippel–Feil, and Pierre Robin. It can be bilateral in one-third of the cases [10]. Fusion of malleus and incus is the most common middle ear anomaly, and footplate is usually normal. The facial nerve is typically displaced more anterior, superior, and lateral than in the normal anatomy [11].

The management in unilateral atresia does not require immediate intervention if the contralateral ear hearing is normal, but in bilateral atresia, an early amplification is essential in infants with bilateral significant hearing loss. The non-surgical rehabilitative option is achieved by bone conduction hearing aids such as bone-anchored hearing aid (BAHA). The surgical repair can be performed at age 6–7 years old after microtia repair if present, and patient with a major malformation (poor mastoid pneumatization, abnormal or absent oval window/footplate, abnormal facial nerve course, and abnormalities of the inner ear) is a poor candidate for surgical repair. There are three surgical approaches for repair of aural atresia that include the mastoid, the anterior, and the modified anterior approaches. The most frequent complications of the surgical reconstruction are canal stenosis and failure to achieve an adequate hearing level [12].

3.3.2 Acquired and Inflammatory Conditions of the External Auditory Canal

3.3.2.1 Cerumen Impaction

Cerumen is a desquamated epithelium mixed with sebum and watery secretions produced from sebaceous glands and modified apocrine sweat glands, respectively. The predisposing factors to develop cerumen impaction include the use of hearing aids, cotton buds, earplugs, the presence of a narrow EAC, and genetic predisposition in some cases. It is considered as one of the most common complaints in the ENT clinics, where the patients present with ear fullness, ear discomfort, tinnitus, autophony, decreased hearing, and itching.

Cerumen removal is the most performed procedure in ENT clinics and is done through suction, low-pressure irrigation, or using a hook. Cerumen-softening ear drops are also helpful.

3.3.2.2 Foreign Bodies (FB)

It is one of the common presentations to the ENT clinic especially in children less than 6 years old. It can be classified into living and no-living foreign bodies. It is more common in the right ears due to the dominance of right-handedness.

It can be extracted in the office if the patient is cooperative by crocodile forceps, hook, irrigation, or suction. To avoid injury in non-cooperative patients, it is advised to be done under general anesthesia. Living FBs (such as insects) must be killed before removal. Batteries must be removed as soon as possible to avoid chemical burns to the EAC and the drum. Irrigation in the case of seeds is not recommended as it may cause an increase in their size. It is always recommended for young children to examine the ears and the nose after the FB removal to rule out other FBs.

3.3.2.3 External Ear Canal Infections

The EAC may give rise to acute or chronic infections, which can result from bacterial or fungal infections.

Otitis Externa

It is an inflammatory condition of the EAC usually caused by an acute bacterial infection (*for fungal otitis externa, see Sect. "Otomycosis"*). It is caused by a break in the protective barrier (skin) of EAC through direct injury (while cleaning the EAC) or obstruction (e.g., hearing aid, foreign body, cerumen impaction) or change in media to a more alkalotic EAC (swimming). The most common isolated pathogens include *Pseudomonas aeruginosa* and *Staphylococcus aureus* [2]. Clinical manifestations include severe pain, itching, and otorrhea, and physical examination reveals tragal tenderness, canal edema, discharge, erythema, and stenosis. Investigation including swab culture is generally not indicated except for treatment failure.

Treatment of otitis externa depends on ear toileting, topical therapy of antibiotics with steroids, and dry ear precautions. Caution is needed to avoid ototoxic antimicrobials such as aminoglycosides in the case of tympanic membrane perforation. Systemic antibiotics typically are not required unless concurrent otitis media, persistent or severe symptoms, cellulitis, or systemic illness [2].

Chronic infections tend to be related to chronic ear skin conditions, irritation by a foreign body, or manifestation of systemic diseases (e.g., Psoriasis). Chronic otitis externa needs to be treated depending on the etiology, in contact dermatitis avoid the offending agent, and in systemic disease treat the underlying condition [2].

Otomycosis

Otomycosis is a fungal infection of the skin of EAC. The high-risk group includes immunocompromised patients, hearing aid users, and the overuse of topical antibiotics. The most common pathogens include *Aspergillus niger* (most common) and *Candida albicans* [2]. Patients primarily complain of pruritus, ear fullness, and reduce hearing. The clinical examination reveals a white, black, or dotted gray membrane with an appearance of "tissue-paper". Treatment includes frequent ear toileting and using acidifying agents or anti-fungal drops along with dry ear precautions.

Malignant Otitis Externa (MOE)

Malignant otitis externa or necrotizing otitis externa is a progressive infection of the external auditory canal (EAC), the adjacent soft tissues, and the skull base. MOE is usually a disease of the immunocompromised and elderly diabetic patients, though it can occur in immunocompetent patients on very rare occasions [2]. *Pseudomonas aeruginosa* is the most common causative pathogen. Other species of bacteria, such as *Staphylococcus aureus*, and fungal species, including *Aspergillus* and *Candida*, have been reported [2].

The patient commonly presents with longstanding otalgia, described as a severe deep dull pain, and otorrhea, with a finding of granulation tissue at the bony cartilaginous junction of the EAC. Without proper treatment, the infection can spread and involve the cranial nerves, the facial nerve being the most common cranial nerve involved. Other complications include sinus thrombosis, sepsis, intracranial infections, and death.

Diagnosis is mainly based on the patient's history, clinical examination, microbiology, and radiological findings. Consider biopsy and culture of EAC, and check for elevated ESR. CT scan helps in detecting bony erosion, and MRI has a superior role in bone marrow edema, soft-tissue abnormalities, and intracranial extension detection (see Fig. 3.10). Technettium-99m bone scan detects early bone changes and areas of osteoblastic activity, and it is helpful in detecting early disease, while follow-up is monitored better with Gallium-67 citrate and Indium-111 labeled leukocyte, though cost and false-positive results limit their use.

Medical management with administration of prolonged systemic and topical antibiotics, regular EAC toileting, and strict blood sugar control is the cornerstone in the treatment of malignant otitis externa. Surgical debridement has a limited role due to complex access to the

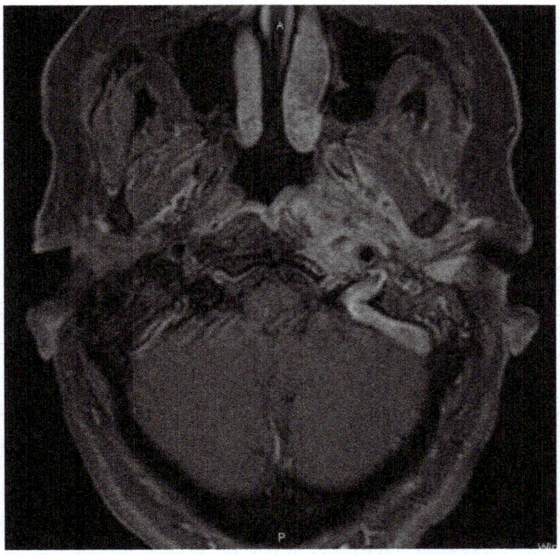

Fig. 3.10 MRI T1 axial image at the level of ear canal showing a significant postcontrast enhancement on the left temporal bone and skull base as compared to right side suggestive of an extensive malignant otitis externa

skull base. Hyperbaric oxygen is used as adjuvant therapy [2].

Myringitis

It is an inflammatory condition of the tympanic membrane (TM) that can be primary or secondary to a middle ear or EAC infection. Granular myringitis is a chronic inflammatory condition of the epidermal layer of the TM. Bullous myringitis occurs when some serous/hemorrhagic bullae formed on the epithelial surface of the TM. It is caused by different pathogens including *Streptococcus pneumonia*, Mycoplasma (bullous myringitis), and viral pathogens (influenza or herpes) [2].

The patient presents with acute severe otalgia, serosanguinous otorrhea, and hearing loss. The physical examination shows bullae on congested inflamed TM (see Fig. 3.11). The audiogram can show sensorineural hearing loss or mixed hearing loss in 65% [2].

Decompression of the bulla provides relief to the pain, topical antibiotic/steroid drop is the treatment of choice along with proper analgesia, and oral macrolides or quinolones may be added to eradicate mycoplasma. Granulation tissue may be treated with surgical removal, chemical cauterization, or vinegar irrigations [13].

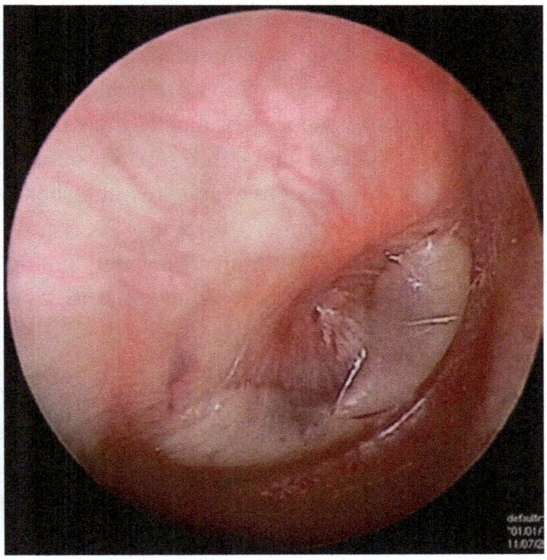

Fig. 3.11 Bullous myringitis

3.3.2.4 Keratosis Obturans and External Auditory Canal Cholesteatoma

Both of keratosis obturans and external auditory canal cholesteatoma are marked by abnormal accumulation of keratin within the medial portion of EAC.

Keratosis Obturans

It represents an abnormal accumulation of dense plug of keratin within the EAC without bony erosion. It is usually a bilateral disorder and affects young adults, and it is associated with bronchiectasis and chronic sinusitis. It presents with severe ear pain and otorrhea secondary to otitis externa, and also presents with conductive hearing loss with a widening of the EAC causing automastoidectomy [14]. It can be diagnosed with a temporal CT scan showing significantly diffuse widening of EAC without boney erosion.

Treatment involves careful, slow, and complete removal of keratin plugs with softening ear drops. It is usually an office-based procedure, and antibiotics/steroid drops are used if the infection exists [14].

External Canal Cholesteatoma

It is a rare condition of cholesteatoma in EAC causing ulceration and erosion of the underlying bone of the inferior posterior part of the canal. It is usually unilateral and affects older patients with focal bony erosion which distinguishes it from keratosis obturans (see Table 3.2). It presents with severe ear pain, otorrhea, and conductive hearing loss and may erode the middle ear or attic. CT scan shows a soft-tissue filling EAC with focal bony erosion.

Treatment is with regular cleaning of the canal from debris, with medications to eradicate otitis externa, and surgery may be required in refractory cases to remove cholesteatoma matrix and necrotic bone with canaloplasty [2].

Table 3.2 The differences between keratosis obturans and external auditory canal cholesteatoma

	Keratosis obturans	External auditory canal cholesteatoma
Age	Young adult	Elderly
Pain	Acute severe pain	Chronic dull pain
Lateralization	Bilateral	Unilateral
Osteonecrosis	Absent	Present
EAC bony erosion	Circumferentially	Focally
Otorrhea	Rare	Frequent

3.3.2.5 Benign Neoplasms

The EAC may give rise to both benign and malignant neoplasms. Benign processes include exostosis, osteoma, and other lesions.

Exostosis

Multiple acquired benign bony outgrowths (hyperostosis) at the EAC periosteum usually in patients have repeated exposure to cold water; therefore, it is called "surfer's ear". Exostosis growths arise from the medial aspect of bony EAC near tympanic annulus, along tympanomastoid and tympanosquamous suture lines. Most of the time it is asymptomatic and appears as narrowing of EAC by multiple, bilateral smooth broad-based sessile masses (see Fig. 3.12).

Treatment is usually unnecessary unless they are large and intervene with hearing or causing repeated ear infections due to cerumen and epithelial debris retaining or to allow a proper hearing aid fitting [15]. All cases being considered for surgery must have a hearing test and CT temporal bone to identify the anatomical landmarks around the bony lesions. Surgical approaches include transcanal or postauricular approach, being aware that facial nerve can be at risk of injury during drilling of the posteroinferior aspect of the bony canal; therefore, intraoperative facial nerve monitor is recommended.

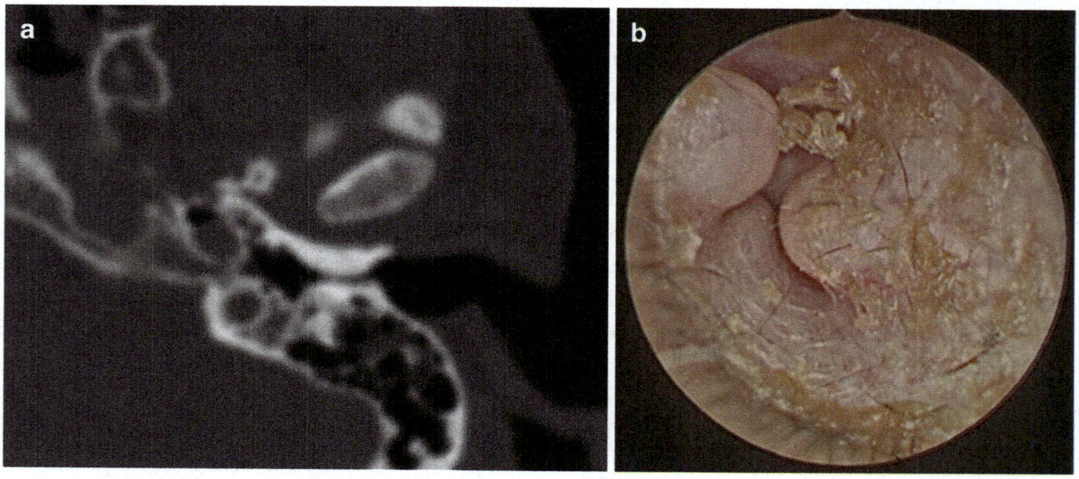

Fig. 3.12 (**a**) Axial CT scan of left ear exostosis, (**b**) Endoscopic view of exostosis

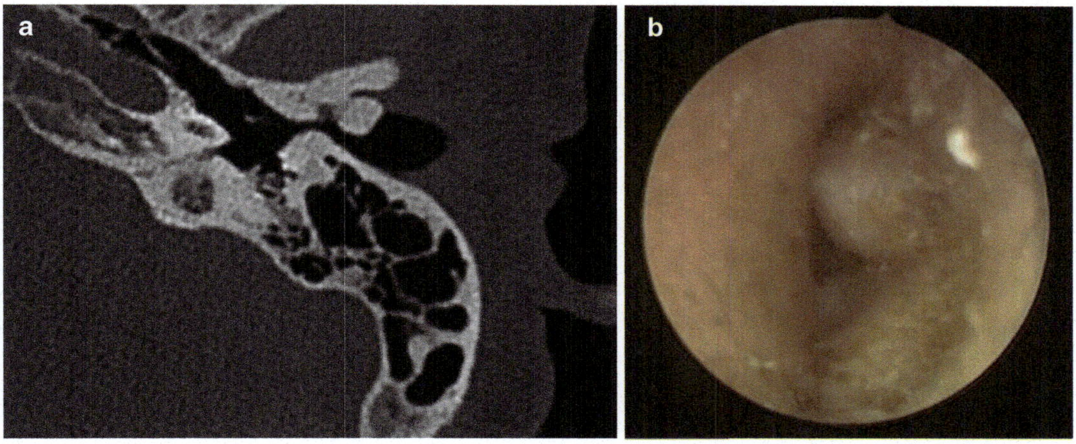

Fig. 3.13 (**a**) Axial CT scan of left ear Osteoma, (**b**) Endoscopic view of Osteoma

Table 3.3 The differences between exostosis and osteoma

	Exostosis	Osteoma
Number of lesion	Multiple	Single
Predisposing factor	Repeated exposure to cold water	Not related to specific exposure
Site	On suture lines of EAC (more medial)	On tympanosquamous suture near bony cartilaginous junction (more lateral)
Lateralization	Bilateral	Unilateral

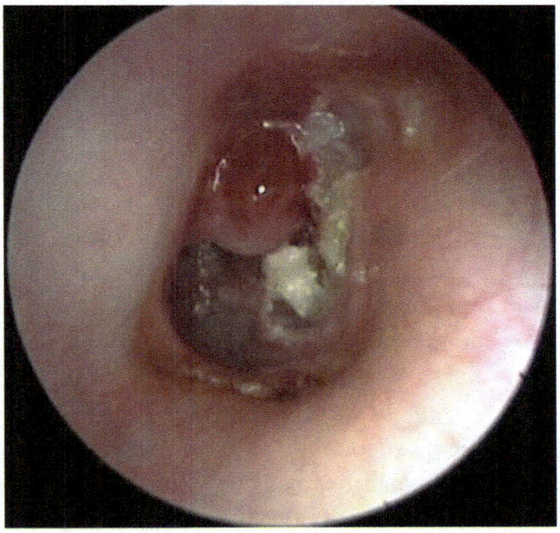

Fig. 3.14 Ear polyp covering the attic area with keratin debris hiding an underlying cholesteatoma

Osteoma

It is a solitary benign bony growth unlike exostosis, mostly at the bony cartilaginous junction, located more laterally in comparison to exostosis. Most of the time it is asymptomatic and appears as narrowing of EAC by single, unilateral pedunculated mass (see Fig. 3.13). See Table 3.3 to check the differences between exostosis and osteoma.

It is usually not treated unless they increase in size causing decrease hearing, recurrent infection, impaction of cerumen, and ear secretions [15].

Aural Polyp

It is a soft-tissue mass that arises in the EAC due to underlying inflammation process, and it can be associated with ventilation tubes, foreign bodies, chronic ear infections, middle ear disease, cholesteatoma, and malignant tumor (see Fig. 3.14). The treatment includes silver nitrate cauterization and topical steroid/antibiotic drops. Excisional biopsy is indicated if unclear etiology or non-resolution polyp, but the surgeon should be aware of the polyp attachments to deeper structures (ossicles, the facial nerve) or its origin if it is coming from intracranial defect (meningoencephalocele, encephalocele); therefore, it should be investigated with radiologic studies (CT and/or MRI) to define the anatomic site of origin.

3.3.2.6 Malignant Neoplasms

Primary cancers of the auricle and EAC include more commonly cutaneous carcinomas (basal cell carcinoma, squamous cell carcinoma, and melanoma) and rarely ceruminous gland tumors (ceruminous adenoma, ceruminous adenocarcinoma, pleomorphic adenoma, and adenoid cystic carcinoma). Basal cell carcinoma is the most common cutaneous carcinoma in the auricle and preauricular area, while squamous cell carcinoma is the most common cutaneous carcinoma in the EAC.

Take-Home Messages

- Prominent Ear (Bat Ear) surgical corrections are usually performed in preschool age (4–6 years old) to avoid social stigmatization.
- Prenatal exposure to isotretinoin, thalidomide, and alcohol can increase the risk of microtia.
- The surgical repair of aural atresia can be performed at age 6–7 years old as a second step after microtia repair if present to ensure a field without scars or compromised blood supply to avoid failure of the auricular reconstruction.
- *Pseudomonas aeruginosa* is considered the most common pathogen in auricular perichondritis, bacterial otitis externa, and malignant otitis externa.
- Keratosis obturans affects mainly young adults, and it is associated with bronchiectasis and chronic sinusitis.
- Radiologic studies by CT and MRI should be performed for aural polyps in case of suspicion of an attachment to deeper structures (ossicles, the facial nerve), or if it is coming from intracranial defect (meningoencephalocele, encephalocele).

References

1. Francis HW. Anatomy of the temporal bone, external ear, and middle ear, Chap. 127. In: Francis HW, editor. Cummings otolaryngology, head and neck surgery. 6th ed. Philadelphia: Elsevier; 2015. p. 1977–8.
2. Farkas LG. Anthropometry of normal and anomalous ears. Clin Plast Surg. 1978;5:401–12.
3. Yotsuyanagi T. Nonsurgical correction of congenital auricular deformities in children older than early neonates. Plast Reconstr Surg. 2004;114(1):190–1.
4. Harris J, Källén B, Robert E. The epidemiology of anotia and microtia. J Med Genet. 1996;33:809.
5. Kountakis SE, Helidonis E, Jahrsdoerfer RA. Microtia grade as an indicator of middle ear development in aural atresia. Arch Otolaryngol Head Neck Surg. 1995;121(8):885–6.
6. Sharma A, Gnanapandithan K, Sharma K, Sharma S. Relapsing polychondritis: a review. Clin Rheumatol. 2013;32(11):1575–83.
7. Brant JA, Ruckenstein MJ. Infections of the external ear, Chap. 137. In: Francis HW, editor. Cummings otolaryngology, head and neck surgery. 6th ed. Philadelphia: Elsevier; 2015. p. 2115–22.
8. Sweeney CJ, Gilden DH. Ramsay Hunt syndrome. J Neurol Neurosurg Psychiatry. 2001;71:149–54.
9. Krunic AL, Weitzul S, Taylor RS. Chondrocutaneous advancement flap for reconstruction of helical rim defects in dermatologic surgery. Australas J Dermatol. 2006;47(4):296–9. Review.
10. Jahrsdoerfer RA. Congenital atresia of the ear. Laryngoscope. 1978;88(Suppl 13):1–46.
11. Schuknecht HF. Congenital aural atresia. Laryngoscope. 1989;99:908–17.
12. De la Cruz A, Teufert KB. Congenital aural atresia surgery: long-term results. Otolaryngol Head Neck Surg. 2003;129(1):121–7.
13. Neilson L, Hussain S. Management of granular myringitis: a systematic review. J Laryngol Otol. 2007;25:1–8.
14. Persaud RAP, Hajioff D, Thevasagayam MS, et al. Keratosis obturans and external ear canal cholesteatoma: how and why we should distinguish between these conditions. Clin Otolaryngol Allied Sci. 2004;29:577–81.
15. Kemink JL, Graham MD. Osteomas and exostoses of the external auditory canal - medical and surgical management. J Otolaryngol. 1982;11(2):101–6.

Otitis Media with Effusion (OME)

4

Amr A. Elhakeem, Ma'in Ali Al Shawabkeh,
and Hassan Haidar

4.1 Introduction

There are different nomenclatures of Otitis Media with Effusion (OME)-like serous otitis media, exudative otitis media, nonsuppurative otitis media, and seromucous otitis media. It is an inflammatory condition of the middle ear where middle ear fluid forms behind an intact tympanic membrane (TM). It is called chronic OME if the fluid persists for more than 3 months. Usually, OME is related to acute otitis media (AOM). However, it can happen without a previous episode of AOM. Nowadays, OME is considered the most common cause of hearing impairment in children.

4.2 Epidemiology

Ninety percent of children have at least one episode of otitis media with effusion by the age of 4. The prevalence among children below 4 years is 10–17%, and it declines to 2–4% for those between 6 and 8 years. It is more common in winter, and males have a slight increase in risk [1].

4.3 Pathogenesis

Two theories can explain OME:

1. Ex vacuo theory: Eustachian tube (ET) obstruction secondary to adenoid hypertrophy or mucosal edema can lead to negative pressure in the middle ear leading to passive transduction of fluid.
2. Inflammatory theory: Gas deficiency can cause hypoxia in the middle ear, which can initiate a mucosal inflammation leading to an active exudation in the middle ear [2].

4.4 **Risk Factors** (Look at Table 4.1)

1. Age: the incidence of OME decreases as age increases, which is due to the maturation of ET and the immune system.
2. ET anatomy: Children have a more horizontal ET, which can make the entry of bacteria easier to the middle ear.
3. Craniofacial abnormalities: there is an increased incidence of OME in patients with cleft lip and palate, as it is believed those conditions can lead to the immaturity of the cartilaginous part of ET.
4. Adenoid: adenoid hypertrophy can lead to ET obstruction and can act as a reservoir for bacteria that increases the incidence of OME.

A. A. Elhakeem (✉) · M. A. Al Shawabkeh
ENT Department, Hamad Medical Corporation, Doha, Qatar
e-mail: aelhakeem@hamad.qa

H. Haidar
Hamad Medical Corporation, Doha, Qatar

A. Al-Qahtani et al. (eds.), *Textbook of Clinical Otolaryngology*,
https://doi.org/10.1007/978-3-030-54088-3_4

Table 4.1 Risk factors of OME

Age
ET anatomy (Horizontal)
Craniofacial abnormalities (cleft lip and palate)
Adenoid hypertrophy
Daycare attendance
Passive smoking
Recurrent middle ear infection
Bacterial biofilms
Allergic rhinitis
Gastroesophageal reflux
Genetic predisposition

5. Daycare attendance.
6. Smoking exposure (passive smoking).
7. Recurrent middle ear infection: bacterial endotoxin initiates OME. *Haemophilus influenzae* and *Moraxella catarrhalis* were found in more frequency as compared to AOM where *Streptococcus pneumoniae* predominates.
8. Biofilms: it plays a vital role in the pathogenesis of OME [3].
9. Allergic rhinitis: it can lead to ET edema and can reduce the immune system function of the upper respiratory tract system.
10. Gastroesophageal reflux: middle ear fluid shows and elevated Pepsin/pepsinogen [4].
11. Genetic predisposition: Having a sibling in whom a ventilation tube was placed is an essential factor in developing OME. Studies involving twins and triplets show genetic susceptibility to OME [5].

4.5 Clinical Features

4.5.1 Symptoms

Acute symptoms are typically absent in OME. Hearing loss is the most common complaint in symptomatic patients; it is conducive with a hearing level of approximately 25 dB [6]. This can affect binaural processing, sound localization, and speech perception. This effect is more pronounced in patients with underlying hearing disabilities [7]. Other symptoms like ear fullness, sleep disturbance, and otalgia can be seen in OME.

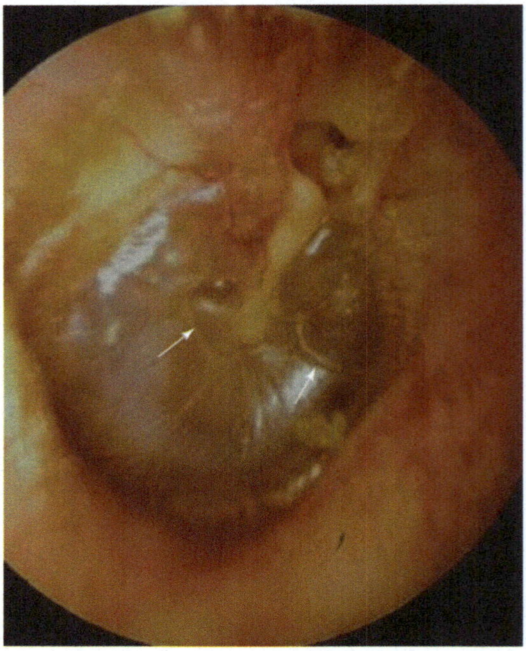

Fig. 4.1 Right ear otomicroscopy: retrotympanic air-fluid level (arrows). (Adapted from Mansour S., Magnan J., Nicolas K., and Haider H. (2018). Middle ear disease)

4.5.2 Otoscopic Findings

1. Air-fluid level, which is the most specific feature. However, it is not the most frequent one (Figs. 4.1 and 4.2).
2. Amber-colored TM (Fig. 4.3).
3. TM can be dull, retracted, and yellow, especially in "Glue ear" where the effusion is thick and looks like glue (Fig. 4.4).
4. In retracted TM, the handle of malleus looks shorter and horizontal with a prominent short process.

4.5.3 Pneumatic Otoscopy

It will show restricted mobility of TM when positive pressure is applied. In clinical practice, this test is not easy to be performed in children [8].

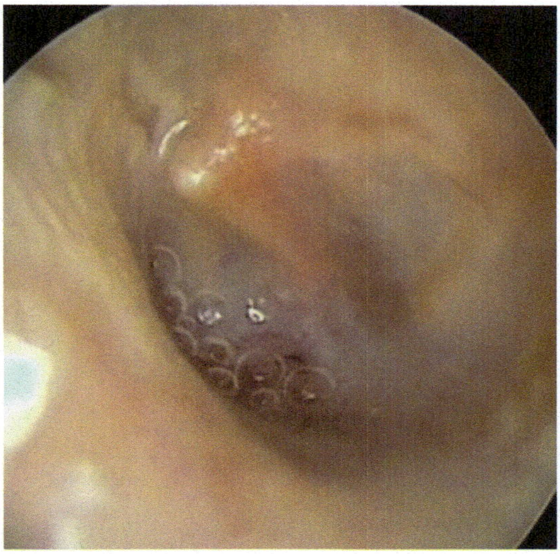

Fig. 4.2 Left ear with serous effusion. After Valsalva maneuver, air bubbles appeared anteriorly. (Adapted from Mansour S., Magnan J., Nicolas K., and Haider H. (2018). Middle ear disease)

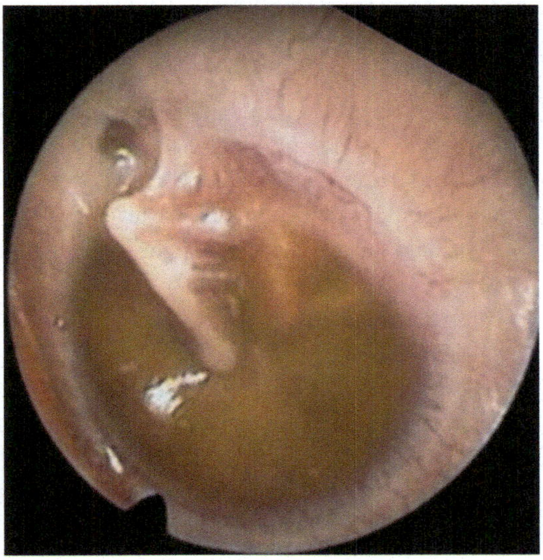

Fig. 4.3 Left ear with abundant serous effusion. (Adapted from Mansour S., Magnan J., Nicolas K., and Haider H. (2018). Middle ear disease)

4.5.4 Tympanometry

It is the most useful test in diagnosing OME. It is a cost-effective and an objective test. Type B (Flat curved) tympanometry is considered pathognomonic for OME (see Fig. 4.5).

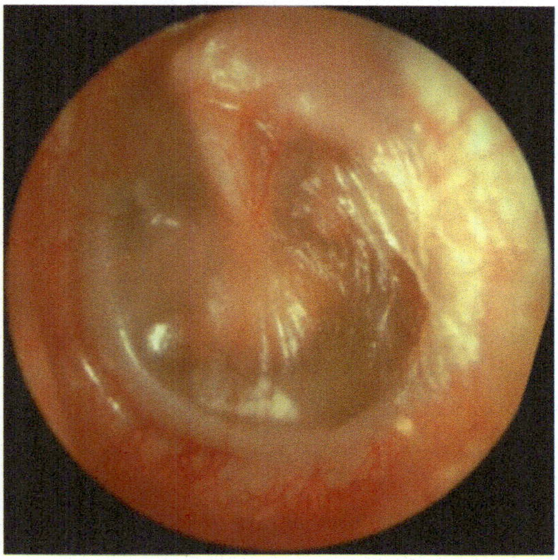

Fig. 4.4 Left ear with mucoid effusion and retracted drum. (Adapted from Mansour S., Magnan J., Nicolas K., and Haider H. (2018). Middle ear disease)

4.5.5 Hearing Assessment

It is recommended in children who have risk factors of speech or learning disorders, or those who have persistent OME for more than 3 months.

Important notes while evaluating patients with OME:

1. The presence of acute signs of infection along with fluid in the middle ear is characteristic of AOM. So, ear pain with bulging of TM excludes OME.
2. In cases of unilateral OME in adults, it is essential to do flexible nasopharyngoscopy to rule out nasopharyngeal mass (see Fig. 4.6).
3. In refractory cases of OME, conditions like nasopharyngeal mass, adenoid hypertrophy, ET congenital defect, IgG subclass deficiencies, and ciliary dyskinesia should be kept in mind.

4.6 The Clinical Course of OME

Eighty-five percent of cases will resolve spontaneously. Thirty to 40% of cases will have recur-

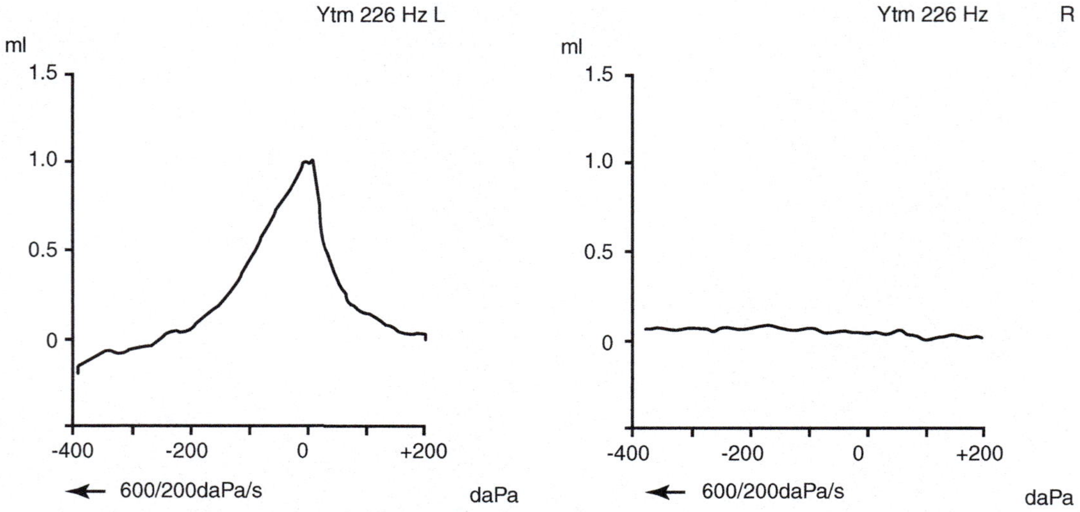

Fig. 4.5 Patient with a normal left ear and a right glue ear; Tympanometry showing curve type A in the left ear and type B in the right ear

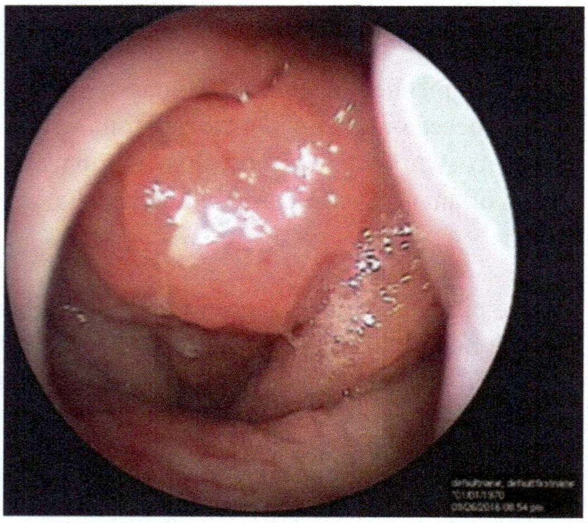

Fig. 4.6 Nasopharyngeal mass compressing the left torus tubarius. (Adapted from Mansour S., Magnan J., Nicolas K., and Haider H. (2018). Middle ear disease)

rent episodes. If effusion persists, then the following pathologies can happen:

1. Tympanosclerosis.
2. Atelectasis, retraction pocket, or adhesive otitis media.
3. Cholesteatoma.

In cases of ventilation tube insertion, if tubes persisted for more than 36 months, then TM perforation can occur.

4.7 Treatment

1. Medical treatment:

   The use of the topical nasal steroid has shown to speed the clearance of OME and prevents recurrences. However, oral steroids, antibiotics, antihistamine, nasal decongestants, and mucolytics did not show any benefit in OME [9].
2. Surgical treatment:

   The benefit of myringotomy and tympanostomy tubes' (TT) insertion is to improve hearing and decrease rates of recurrent otitis media. TT is inserted in the anteroinferior quadrant of TM; posterior positioning of TT is associated with earlier extrusion.

4.7.1 Indication of TT Insertion

1. Patient with OME has symptoms like poor school performance, balance disturbance, or behavioral issues [10].
2. Patient with bilateral OME of less than 3 months and documented hearing loss, especially when hearing loss is more than 30 dB.
3. Changes to TM-like retraction may mandate TT insertion [10].

Note: Children with chronic OME who do not receive TT insertion should be re-evaluated at 3- and 6-month interval until resolution of the effusion [11].

4.7.2 TT Types

1. Short-term tube: Armstrong, Shepard, and Teflon Reuter Bobbin. They last between 6 and 24 months.
2. Long-term tubes: Modified Goode T-tubes, butterfly, Triune, and Paparella II. These tubes can last for years (Fig. 4.7).

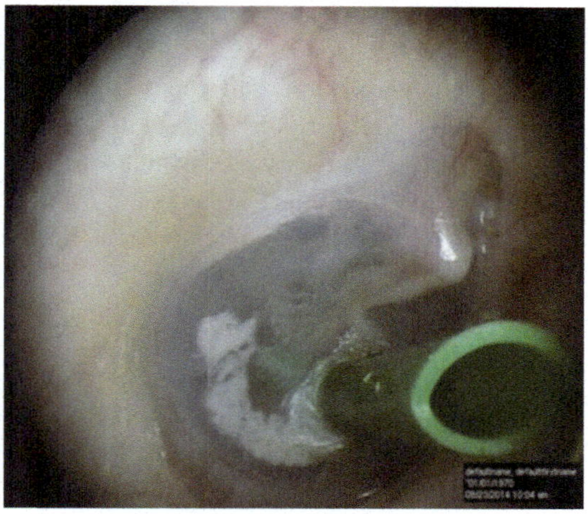

Fig. 4.7 Right ear with T-tube for more than 2 years. (Adapted from Mansour S., Magnan J., Nicolas K., and Haider H. (2018). Middle ear disease)

4.7.3 Role of Adenoidectomy

Adenoidectomy is offered in children who present with nasal obstruction or recurrent rhinorrhea. Moreover, it is considered in cases where the second trial of TT placement is warranted.

4.7.4 The Complications of TT (See Table 4.2)

Short-Term Complications

1. Otorrhea: it is the most common complication. In cases of uncomplicated otorrhea, then topical ear drops can be used.
2. Occlusion of the tube.
3. Premature extrusion.
4. Development of granulation tissue.
5. Intrusion in the middle ear (Fig. 4.8).

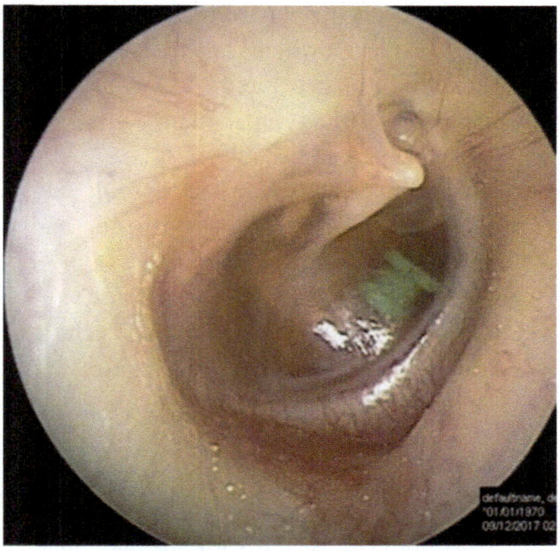

Fig. 4.8 Right ear with the intrusion of the grommet into the ME and recurrence of effusion. (Adapted from Mansour S., Magnan J., Nicolas K., and Haider H. (2018). Middle ear disease)

Table 4.2 Complications of TT

Short-term complication	Long-term complication
Otorrhea	Myringosclerosis
Premature extrusion	Failure of spontaneous tube extrusion
Development of granulation tissue	TM perforation
Intrusion in the middle ear	Development of cholesteatoma

Long-Term Complications

1. Myringosclerosis, which is usually related to TM.
2. Failure of spontaneous tube extrusion.
3. TM perforation; it is more likely if TT remain for more than 36 months.
4. Development of cholesteatoma.

Take-Home Messages

- Ninety percent of children will have middle ear effusion by the age of 4, but the majority will resolve spontaneously.
- Ex vacuo theory and inflammatory theory are the two leading theories that explain the pathogenesis of OME.
- Risk factors of OME are young age, horizontal ET anatomy, craniofacial abnormalities, adenoid hypertrophy, daycare attendance, passive smoking, recurrent middle ear infection, bacterial biofilms, allergic rhinitis, gastroesophageal reflux, and genetic predisposition.
- Acute symptoms are usually absent in OME, and conductive hearing loss is the main complaint in a symptomatic patient. Otoscopic findings can show air-fluid level, which is the most specific feature, Amber-colored TM, or retracted and dull TM. Tympanometry shows a flat curve (type B).
- The use of topical nasal steroids can speed the clearance of the effusion and prevent recurrences.
- TT insertion is indicated in specific situations like children with poor school performance, balance disturbance, or behavioral issues or those with documented hearing loss.
- TT placement can cause some complications: some are short-term like otorrhea, premature extrusion, development of granulation tissue, and intrusion in the middle ear, but others are long-term like myringosclerosis, failure of spontaneous tube extrusion, TM perforation, and development of cholesteatoma.

References

1. Tos M. Epidemiology and natural history of secretory otitis. Am J Otol. 1984;5:459.
2. Mansour S, Magnan J, Nicolas K, Haider H. Middle ear disease. Cham: Springer; 2018. p. 115–42.
3. Ehrlich GD, Veeh R, Wang X, et al. Mucosal biofilm formation on middle-ear mucosa in the chinchilla model of otitis media. JAMA. 2002;287(13):1710–5. https://doi.org/10.1001/jama.287.13.1710. Preliminary Communication April 3, 2002.
4. Miura MS, Mascaro M, Rosenfeld RM. Association between otitis media and gastroesophageal reflux: a systematic review. Otolaryngol Head Neck Surg. 2012;146:345.
5. Casselbrant ML, Mandel EM, Fall PA, et al. The heritability of otitis media: a twin and triplet study. JAMA. 1999;282:2125–30.
6. Fria TJ, Cantekin EI, Eichler JA. Hearing acuity of children with otitis media with effusion. Arch Otolaryngol. 1985;111:10.
7. Roberts JE, Burchinal MR, Zeisel SA. Otitis media in early childhood in relation to children's school-age language and academic skills. Pediatrics. 2002;110:696.
8. Shaikh N, Hoberman A, Rockette HE, Kurs-Lasky M. Development of an algorithm for the diagnosis of otitis media. Acad Pediatr. 2012;12:214.
9. Simpson SA, Lewis R, van der Voort J, Butler CC. Oral or topical nasal steroids for hearing loss associated with otitis media with effusion in children. Cochrane Database Syst Rev. 2011;5:CD001935.
10. Rosenfeld RM, Schwartz SR, Pynnonen MA, Tunkel DE, Hussey HM, Fichera JS, Grimes AM, Hackell JM, Farrison MF, Haskell H, Haynes DS, Kim TW, Lafrenierre DC, Netterville JL, Pipan ME, Raol NP, Schellhase KG. Clinical practice guidelines: tympanostomy tubes in children. Otolaryngol Head Neck Surg. 2013;149(s1):1–35.
11. Teele DW, Klein JO, Rosner BA. Epidemiology of otitis media in children. Ann Otol Rhinol Laryngol Suppl. 1980;89:5.

5 Chronic Suppurative Otitis Media (CSOM)

Salah Mansour, Ma'in Ali Al Shawabkeh, Karen Nicolas, and Hassan Haidar

5.1 Introduction

Chronic suppurative otitis media (CSOM) is a chronic inflammation of the middle ear and mastoid which presents with otorrhea and tympanic membrane perforation (TM). Basic features are otorrhea, a sign of active disease, TM perforation, and inflammatory middle ear mucosa.

TM perforation Can Be

1. *Central perforation:* in which the annulus is preserved. TM perforation can be anterior, posterior, inferior, or subtotal. Historically, this presentation was called tubotympanic disease. *Safe ear* is a new nomenclature for a mucosal disease without cholesteatomatous pathology [1] (Fig. 5.1).
2. *Marginal perforation:* a posterior perforation with loss of the annulus or attic perforation with Pars Flaccida defect. Historically, it was named atticoantral disease. *Unsafe ear*, a new nomenclature, is usually associated with cholesteatoma [1] (Fig. 5.2).

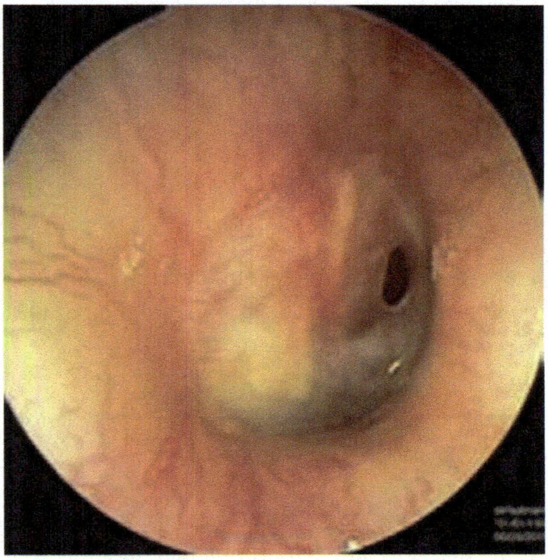

Fig. 5.1 Small anterior perforation of the right ear. (Adapted from cholesteatoma Mansour S., Magnan J., Nicolas K., and Haider H. (2018). Middle ear disease)

5.2 Epidemiology

CSOM is more common in developing countries and less prevalent in developed countries where it is mostly related to tympanostomy tube insertion. Male and female are equally affected [2]. Acute otitis media is a major risk factor for the develop-

S. Mansour (✉)
Centre Medical Westmount Square, Otology, Westmount, QC, Canada

M. A. Al Shawabkeh
ENT Department, Hamad Medical Corporation, Doha, Qatar

K. Nicolas
Radiology Department, Bsalim Hospital, Beirut, Lebanon

H. Haidar
Hamad Medical Corporation, Doha, Qatar

A. Al-Qahtani et al. (eds.), *Textbook of Clinical Otolaryngology*,
https://doi.org/10.1007/978-3-030-54088-3_5

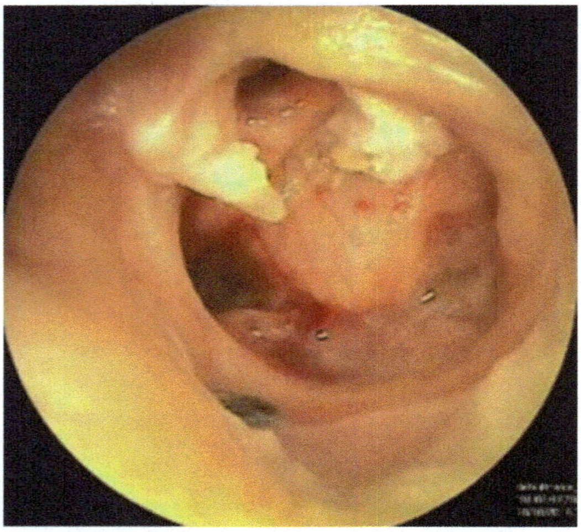

Fig. 5.2 Unsafe CSOM with subtotal and posterosuperior marginal perforation of the left tympanic membrane with keratin debris migrating medially over the incudostapedial joint. (Adapted from Mansour S., Magnan J., Nicolas K., and Haider H. (2018). Middle ear disease)

ment of CSOM. There is still enormous financial burden associated to acute otitis media, CSOM, and sequelae.

5.3 Etiology

CSOM is a multifactorial disease that results from the host and environmental factors. Risk factors are the same as for acute otitis media. Figure 5.3 shows specific factors for CSOM.

Associated Features to CSOM

1. Eustachian tube (ET) dysfunction: Cleft palate, Down's syndrome, patulous ET.
2. Mucosa immune system disorders.
3. Systemic immune deficiency like HIV and hypogammaglobulinemia.
4. Poor mastoid pneumatization.

Healing failure of TM perforation can lead to CSOM. Many factors lie behind this failure:

1. Persistent infection in the middle ear.
2. ET obstruction.
3. Large size perforation.
4. Mucositis, granulation tissue formation, and polyps.

During otitis media, a large number of inflammatory cells and mucosa hyperplasia can lead to hypoxia. ET edema and obstruction can increase hypoxia. Hypoxia leads to overproduction of oxygen radicals, which result in cell damage. The cascade of events presents the following:

- **Inflammation → hypoxia → edema of the mucosa → ulcerations → reparative reaction → granulations → polyps → ossicular lysis** [3]

5.4 Molecular Biology of CSOM

Bacteria endotoxins can stimulate macrophage to produce *TNF-alpha and IL-1* mediators. Immune cells can also produce IL-1 and TNF-alpha. These mediators can damage the host cells and have the potential to enhance the chronicity of otitis media development. Also, *IL-8* plays a role in the chronicity of CSOM [4]. Other cytokines such *IL-6 and INF-gamma* have been found in higher levels in the middle ear mucosa of CSOM [3, 5].

It is crucial to know that IgG and IgA are the most important immunoglobulins in the defense mechanism against mucosal infection (like in CSOM) due to their adherence to the bacterial wall, that is, coating [6]. However, *Pseudomonas aeruginosa*, the main agent of CSOM, lacks effective coating, and that can explain why it is difficult to eradicate this microorganism from the middle ear [7].

5.5 Microbiology of CSOM

1. *Pseudomonas aeruginosa* is the most common microorganism prevalent in CSOM. They are resistant to macrolides, extended-spectrum penicillin, and the first and second-generation cephalosporins, a condition that complicates treatment plans, especially in children.
2. *Staphylococcus aureus* is the second most common organism. Klebsiella and Proteus are other microorganisms isolated in CSOM. Polymicrobial infections are seen in 5–10% of cases Fig. 5.4.

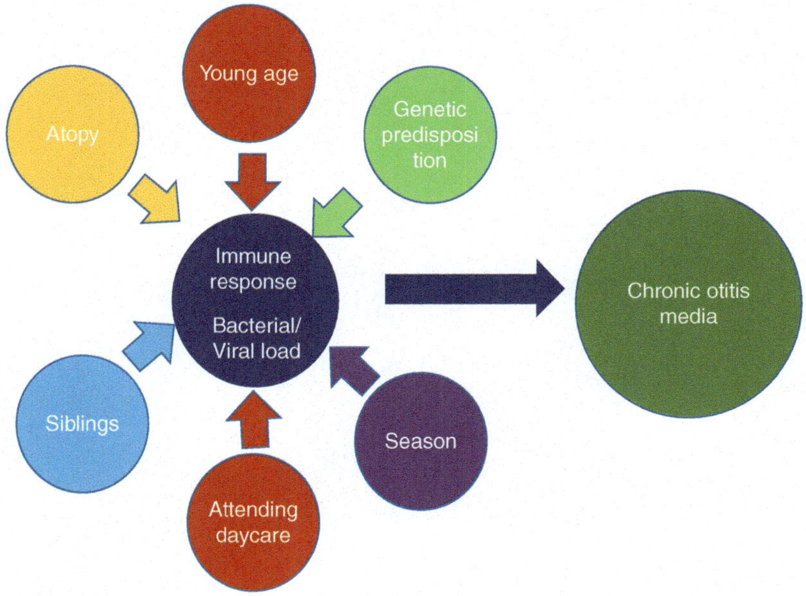

Fig. 5.3 Risks factors for chronic otitis media. (Adapted from Mansour S., Magnan J., Nicolas K., and Haider H. (2018). Middle ear disease)

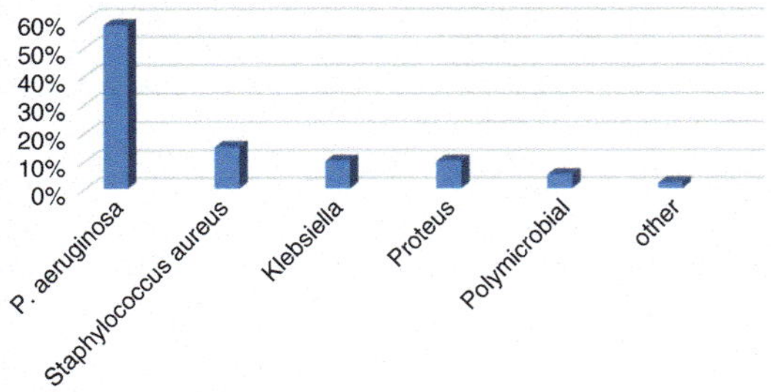

Fig. 5.4 Percentage of different pathogens in CSOM

Biofilms formation is commonly seen in CSOM; they are microorganisms that adhere to each other and are embedded in a self-produced matrix that can act as a self-protector, hence its resistance to antibiotics.

Cases of superimposed fungal infections are encountered in excessive usage of antibiotic ear drops.

5.6 Histopathology of CSOM

Changes observed in the mucosa of the middle ear in CSOM are:

1. Chronic inflammatory infiltrates associated with mucosal edema.
2. Middle ear epithelium metaplasia to respiratory type.
3. Increased number of ciliated cells, goblet cells, increased muco-ciliary clearance, and secretions.
4. Inflammatory granulation tissue and oral polyp during the early stages of healing.
5. Fibrosis and tympanosclerosis in late stage which is a special form of the healing process.

5.7 Ossicular Chain Erosion in CSOM (Fig. 5.5)

Ossicular erosion is much more common in unsafe CSOM than in safe CSOM.

1. The long duration of the inflammatory process is the most harmful factor for the ossicles [8].
2. Incudal necrosis is the most common ossicular pathology seen [8].
3. The stapes lysis is uncommon in a safe ear [8].
4. The malleus is the most resilient middle ear ossicles. In cases of subtotal perforation, the malleus is medialized due to the unopposed action of tensor tympani [8].

Note: TM perforation can lead to a decrease of the sound pressure difference between the external ear and middle ear, leading to hearing loss (HL). HL is dependent on the size of perforation,

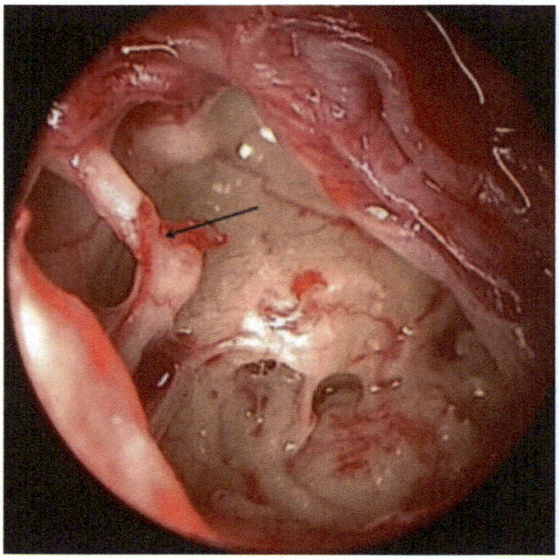

Fig. 5.5 Right chronic ear showing erosion of the lenticular process of the incus with a residual fibrous band (black arrow) connecting incus and stapes [3]

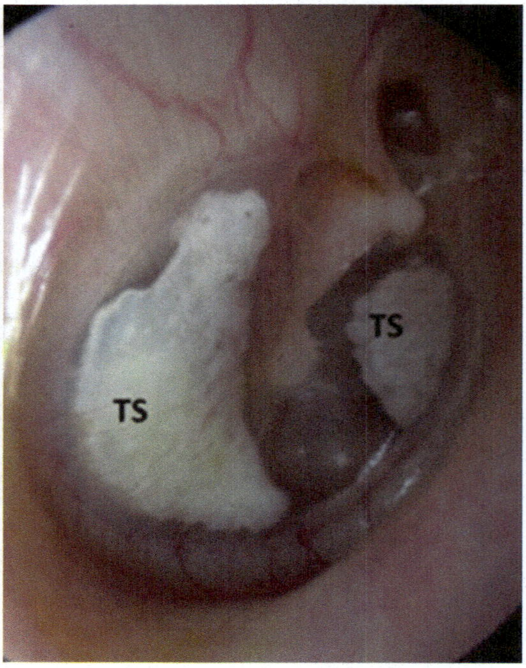

Fig. 5.6 Tympanosclerosis (TS) limited to the tympanic membrane in the right ear

not its location. Also, in the presence of a perforation, HL varies inversely with the volume of the air in the middle ear and mastoid [9].

5.8 Tympanosclerosis in CSOM

Long-standing inflammatory infiltrate may end up with abnormal healing process leaving mostly tympanosclerosis which is a hyaline calcareous deposits found on the tympanic membrane (myringosclerosis) (Fig. 5.6) or the tympanic cavity, ossicular chain, ligaments, or the mastoid with a secondary conductive hearing loss (CHL) (Fig. 5.7) [3].

5.9 Cholesterol Granuloma

The etiology of this entity is still unclear, but it is believed to arise from the same factors leading to CSOM. Negative middle ear pressure can lead to hemorrhage into the ears, the membrane of erythrocytes ruptures releasing the cholesterol inside the ears, and that will act as a nidus for crystal formation and subsequent inflammatory reaction. This can explain the microscopic appearance of cholesterol granuloma as cholesterol crystals surrounded by multinucleated giant cells. Inflammation can lead to the growth of that lesion in size.

Cholesterol granuloma can occur in any part of a pneumatized temporal bone. However, the petrous apex is the most common location. It can be asymptomatic, but in some patients, it can cause mass effect manifested by hearing loss, vertigo, tinnitus, and facial twitching. CT scan can demonstrate an isodense, smooth border mass that does not enhance with contrast. MRI can show a hyperintense mass in both T1 and T2, but it does not enhance with contrast due to its avascularity. In fact, it has a unique feature of hyperintensity on T1 due to its composition of protein, crystal, and hemorrhage, and this feature can distinguish it from cholesteatoma.

Treatment is based on its location and patients' hearing status. Considering the fact that recurrence of cholesterol granuloma after surgical excision is not uncommon, then conservative treatment is advised in asymptomatic patients, and they are followed by serial MRI and CT. Drainage and ventilation are the primary goals of surgical management (see Fig. 5.8).

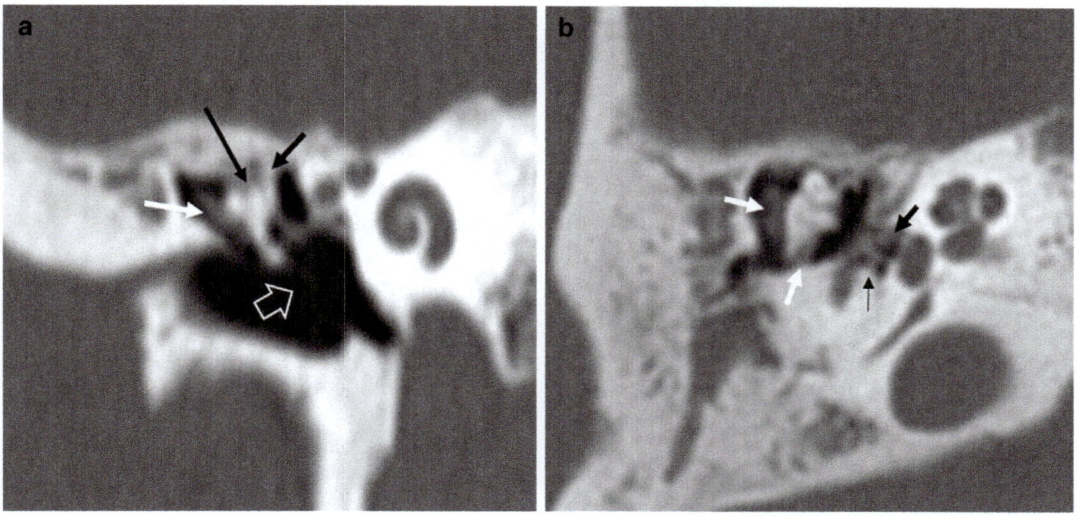

Fig. 5.7 (**a**) Reformatted coronal CT image showing a large tympanic perforation (empty arrow), a large calcified medial attical band (short black arrow), that attaches the malleus head (long black arrow) to the tegmen. Thickened fibrous band along the incus (white arrow). (**b**) Axial CT cut at the level of the attic: thickened bands around the incus (white arrows). Dense and thickened stapes crura (thick black arrow). Thickened stapes tendon (thin black arrow)

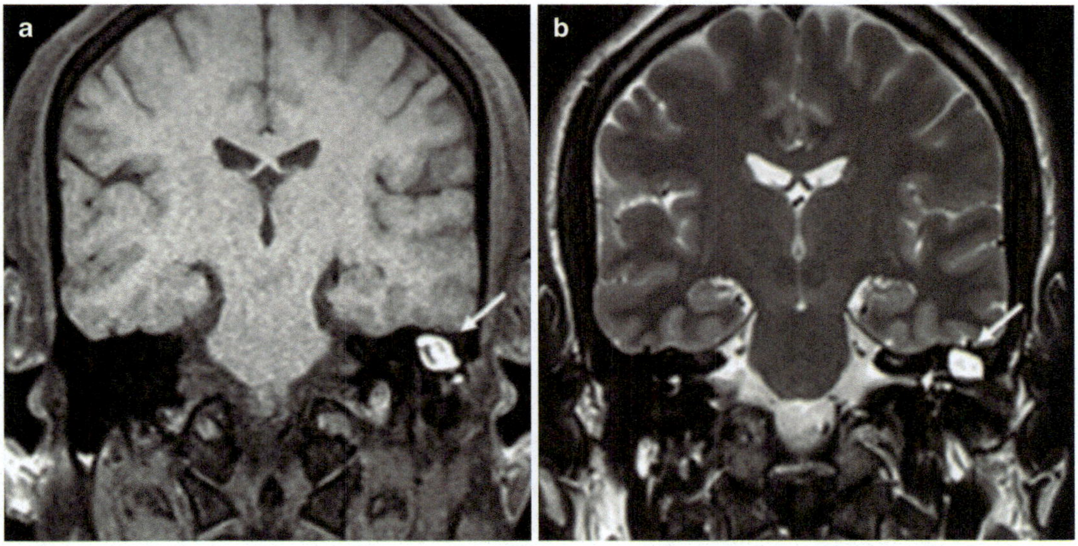

Fig. 5.8 Cholesterol granuloma: *hyper T1, hyper T2* of a left ear. (**a**) Coronal T1-weighted image showing a round mass predominantly hyperintense (arrow), containing some central hypointense structures and (**b**) coronal T2-weighted image showing the same hyperintense aspect of the mass lesion (arrow)

5.10 Clinical Features

The two classic symptoms are otorrhea and hearing loss.

1. Otorrhea: moderate to profuse, continuous or intermittent, serous or mucoid, and sometimes purulent.
2. Hearing Loss (HL): it can be conductive hearing loss (CHL), caused by TM perforation and/or ossicular erosion. HL caused by TM perforation only is larger at low frequencies and decreases with increasing frequencies; it is not related to the location of the perforation [8] and varies inversely to middle ear and mastoid air volume.

5.10.1 Otoscopy

1. **TM perforation**: can vary in size and location (central or marginal). Note: multiple TM perforations associated with pale granulation tissue and facial palsy can indicate tuberculosis.
2. **Status of the mucosa of the middle ear**: Swollen and edematous. Aural polyps may be present.
3. **Ossicular status**: the most common abnormality is the disruption of the incudostapedial joint, necrosis of incus long process, and medialization and shortening of the handle of malleus.
4. **Secondary otitis externa**.
5. **ET** function assessment through nasal mucosa evaluation is highly valuable for the diagnosis and prognosis.

5.10.2 Audiology

Hearing assessment by using 512-tuning fork and audiogram. Depending on the mucosal edema and granulation tissue, TM perforation can lead to CHL between 5 and 40 dB. CSOM can cause sensorineural hearing loss (SNHL) due to the effect of toxins and inflammatory mediators on the inner ear hair cells, mostly on the basal turn. This explains why CSOM patients may be associated with high-frequency SNHL [10].

5.11 Imaging Studies

For patients with CSOM, high-resolution temporal bone CT scan may provide additional information, especially when clinical findings are in favor of a safe ear but with complex clinical presentations as in:

- A long-standing disease with recurrent episodes of active inflammation.
- Cases unresponsive to medical treatment.
- Suspicion of complications.

Preoperative clinico-radiological correlations may orient the surgical strategy.

1. When TM perforation is central and CT shows that **A**ER, **A**ttic and **A**ntrum (AAA spaces) are well aerated: simple condition—*safe ear.*
2. When TM perforation is central, but CT shows extended condensations of AAA spaces or condensation of the AER alone, with the scutum, tegmen, cog, and other bony frontiers of the cavity are intact (image of lysis of the long process of the incus could be associated): this is a presentation of the extensive inflammatory process—*safe ear* [3] Fig. 5.9
3. When TM perforation (not typically central) with condensation images in the ME cavity is associated to any sign of bony lesion (scutum, tegmen, cog, and bony limits of the mastoid

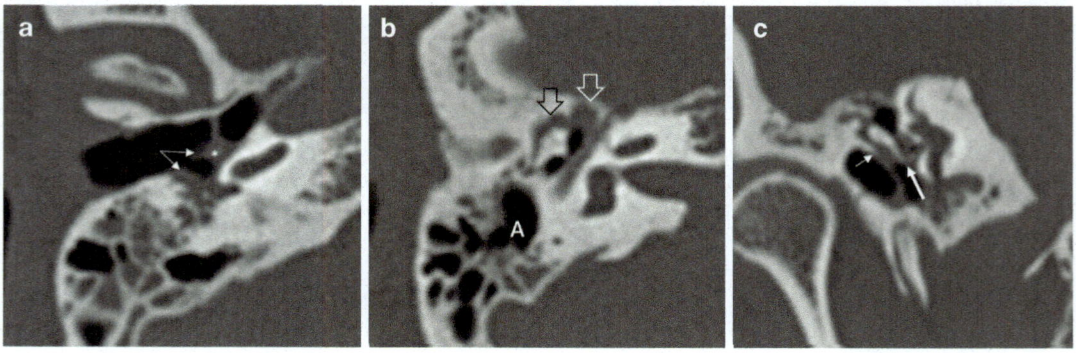

Fig. 5.9 (**a**) Axial CT image showing central perforation (between two small arrows). Condensation images in the ME cavity (asterisk). (**b**) Axial CT showing condensation of the entire attic (external attic: black empty arrow, AER: empty white arrow) *A* antrum. (**c**) Lyses of the incudostapedial joint (long arrow). The scutum is intact! (short arrow). There is extended inflammation, but it is still a **safe ear**

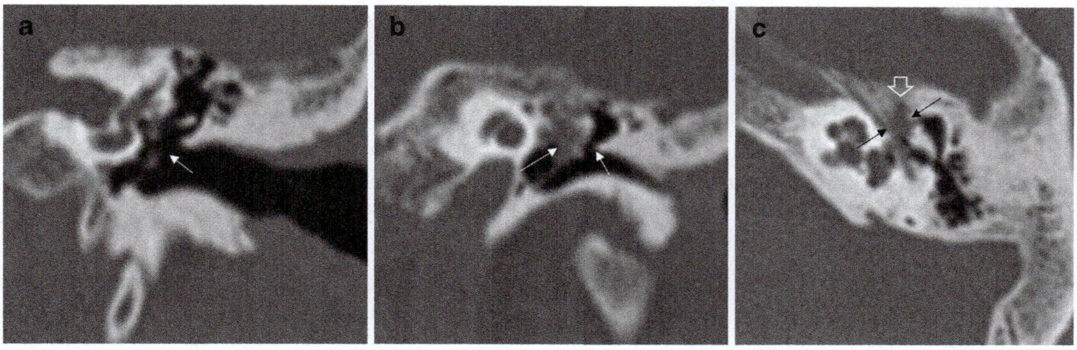

Fig. 5.10 CT of an 88-year-old man with chronic otorrhea and otalgia. (**a**) Coronal CT showing posterosuperior tympanic perforation. (**b**) Coronal CT showing intact scutum (short arrow). Condensation images (long arrow) along the ossicular chain start to erode the malleus. (**c**) Axial CT showing complete condensation of the AER with bone lysis of the anterior bony border (empty arrow) and absence of the cog (should be seen between the black arrows). These are signs in favor of cholesteatoma: unsafe ear

cavity), these features are in favor of an *unsafe ear*—cholesteatoma [3] (Fig. 5.10).

In this context, any lyses of the ossicular chain, incus, and especially of malleus or stapes are in favor of such unsafe ear [3].

5.12 Complications and Sequelae

Nowadays, complications of CSOM are decreasing because of early and better control of the infectious process; nevertheless, they remain of serious concern since they still are life-threatening in unfavorable socioeconomic regions [3] (see Chap. 6).

Complications are due to hematogenic or contiguous spread of the infection [3] and could be:

1. Intratemporal: labyrinthine fistula, VII palsy, Mastoid abscess, petrositis, and labyrinthitis.
2. Extratemporal:
   (a) Intracranial such lateral sinus thrombophlebitis, meningitis, and intracerebral access.
   (b) Extracranial such as subperiosteal abscess or Bezold's.

5.13 Treatment of CSOM

5.13.1 Medical Treatment

The main goal of medical treatment is to obtain dry ear as early as possible before surgical treatment. Medical treatment depends on the following steps:

1. Aural toilet: regular in-office toilet clearance and placement of ear wick in case of edematous external skin canal.
2. Ototopical ear drops: Including:
   (a) Quinolones: they have a low incidence of ototoxicity and vestibulotoxicity.
   (b) Aminoglycosides: they have significant potential of inducing ototoxicity and vestibulotoxicity despite the protective edematous mucosa of the round window membrane in CSOM.
   (c) Neomycin and polymyxin B: fewer than 20% of gram-negative remain sensitive to neomycin, while polymyxin B is still effective.
3. Control of granulation tissue: as these tissues can block the antibiotics from reaching the infected site. Steroid may help in the resolution of the granulation tissues.

In case of failure of topical treatment to treat CSOM, then **systemic oral antibiotics** should be used. The best option is ciprofloxacin, but it should not be given to children below 12 years. Erythromycin or Bactrim are alternatives in these cases. All systemic aminoglycosides should be avoided.

Generally speaking, the topical ear drops should be continued for 6 weeks, while systemic antibiotics should not be used for more than 2 weeks. Systemic corticotherapy for a few days, followed by tapering doses for another few days, enhances the therapeutic control of the active inflammatory process.

5.13.2 Surgery for CSOM

All surgical procedures must be done in respect of basic principles of ME mechanics in relation to the mechanisms of acoustic sound gain [3, 11].

Middle ear mechanics: Sound is transmitted from external auditory canal (EAC) to the cochlea by three mechanisms:

1. ***Ossicular coupling***: it is the transmission of sound pressure from the TM to the oval window through the ossicular chains. Due to the air–fluid interface, the sound will be reflected, causing a 30-dB sound loss, but the coupling effect will overcome this loss by three mechanisms [11]:
   (a) The hydraulic lever effect: due to the Area Ratio 21:1. It is the compression of sound energy and increase of force on the oval window due to the difference of surface area between the TM and the oval window leading to an increase in gain of 26 dB.
   (b) Malleoincudal lever effect: results from the difference in length between the manubrium of malleus and the long process of incus (ratio of 1.3:1). Gain of 2 dB.
   (c) Catenary lever effect: results from stretching of the TM from the annulus to the manubrium of malleus. Gain of 2 dB.
2. ***Acoustic coupling***: Difference of sound pressure on the oval and round window because they are not in the same anatomic localization. Acoustic coupling role is minor in the normal ear with intact TM and ossicles. The acoustic coupling can explain why patients with normal TM and ossicular discontinuity will have more significant HL (60 dB) than those with ossicular discontinuity with perforated TM (40–50 dB), as TM will restrict sound pressure difference transmission to oval and round windows (Figs 5.11, 5.12, and 5.13) [3].

Another consideration in middle ear mechanics is *Phase difference*; a sound stimulus to the inner ear is detected as a net

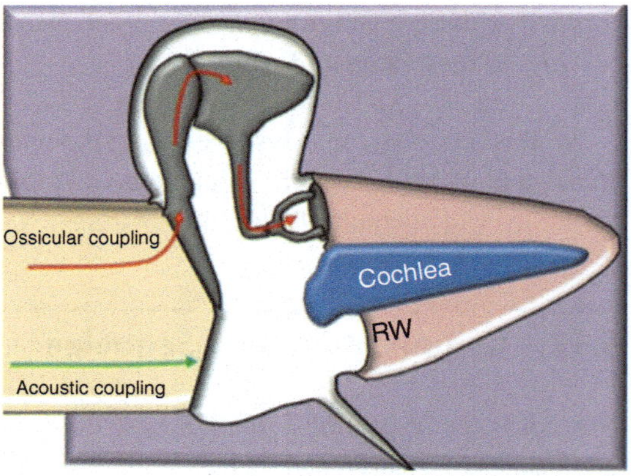

Fig. 5.11 Middle ear mechanics in a normal ear

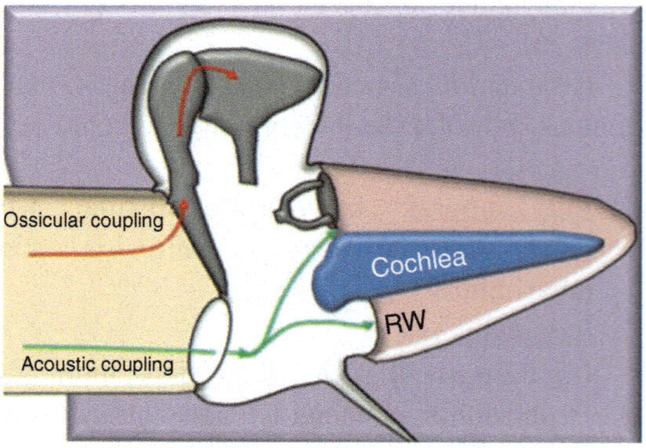

Fig. 5.12 Middle ear mechanics in ear with tympanic membrane perforation and ossicular chain discontinuity. Acoustic coupling with sound pressure difference on the oval window and round window is the main mechanism for transmitting sound energy into the cochlea

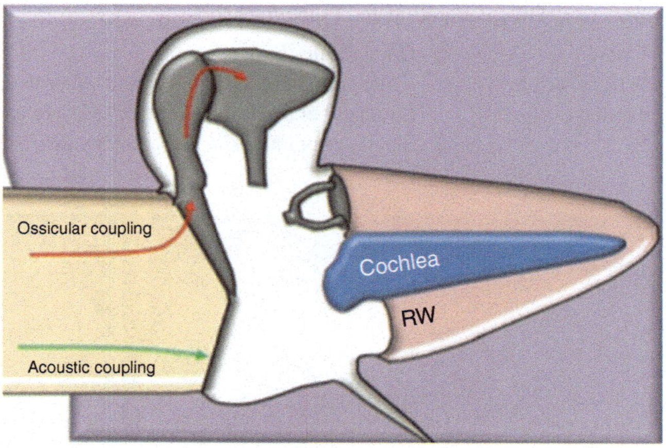

Fig. 5.13 Middle ear mechanics in ear with intact tympanic membrane and ossicular chain discontinuity. Sound energy will not reach the cochlea neither through ossicular coupling nor through acoustic coupling, which will result in a maximal conductive hearing loss

difference in sound pressures between the round and oval windows. This difference is lost if tympano-ossicular mechanisms are absent (as in tympanoplasty types IV and V); in this situation, an unshielded round window will have negative acoustic consequences.

3. **Middle ear aeration** is another essential factor in sound transmission. It contributes to a normal stapes-cochlear impedance and plays an important role in normal ossicular coupling. The minimum amount of air required to maintain ossicular coupling within 10 dB of normal hearing has been estimated to be 0.5 ml [3].

Consideration in pediatric patients: It is preferable to avoid tympanoplasty in pediatric patients below 5 years, and delay it till he or she is 6–9 years old, as there are higher chances of failure due to recurrent otitis media and poor ET dysfunction. Adenoidectomy with or without tonsillectomy could be considered in obstructive cases. ET catheterization is considered. However, confirmed and sustained clinical results remain doubtful since the main issue is the mucosa disease.

Surgical ear reconstruction success may be disappointing to some patients: the hearing benefit after surgery depends not only on the magnitude of the closure of the air-bone gap but also on the level of cochlear function of the operated ear, the hearing level of the contralateral ear, and the symmetry of hearing levels between the two ears.

5.13.2.1 Surgical Techniques in Tympanoplasty (Middle Ear Reconstruction)

The purpose is to reconstruct the TM, reconstruct the ossicular chain (mechanics), and ensure an adequate middle ear aeration.

Tympanic Membrane Repair (Myringoplasty)

Surgical approaches: The choice of myringoplasty depends on the perforation size, the anatomy of EAC, and the surgeon's preference. The main three approaches are:

1. Transcanal: least invasive, used for small perforation or medium-sized perforation, but the whole perforation, especially the anterior rim, should be accessible and the EAC anatomy is favorable.
2. Endaural: It is most useful if limited atticotomy is performed with tympanoplasty.
3. Postauricular: offers better visualization of the anterior rim of the TM.

Canaloplasty can be used when there is bulging of anterior wall of the EAC, narrow EAC, or anterior perforation.

Graft selection: See Table 5.1 for different graft materials in tympanoplasty (Fig. 5.14):

Graft Placement

1. Underlay: Graft put underneath or medial to the perforation.

Table 5.1 Different graft materials in tympanoplasty

Fascia	Good results, easy to handle.
Perichondrium	Same properties, easy to manipulate for beginners.
Cartilage	Stronger but needs to be thinned. May be used for revision procedures.
Fat	Small perforation, simple pathology (dry ear), inlay, outpatient procedure.

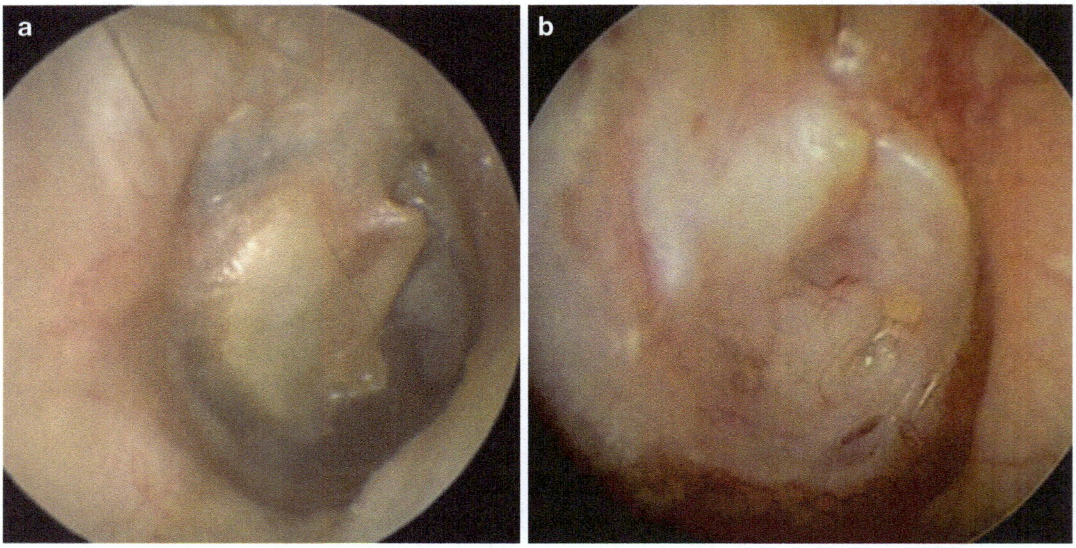

Fig. 5.14 (**a**) Two years after right ear cartilage tympanoplasty for posterior perforation. (**b**) One year after right ear cartilage tympanoplasty for subtotal perforation showing the good vascularization of the graft. The major advantage of cartilage graft is that it retains its rigid quality and resists to reperforation or retraction [3]

2. Overlay technique: Graft put lateral to the fibrous layer of the TM. However, it should be medial to the manubrium to prevent lateralization of the graft. Complete and total removal of the squamous epithelium from the lateral surface of the TM must be insured to avoid iatrogenic cholesteatoma.

The success of any technique depends on the surgeon's expertise rather than on the technique itself.

The advantages and disadvantages of each technique are summarized in Table 5.2.

Table 5.2 The advantages and disadvantages of each technique (underlay/overlay)

	Overlay	Underlay
Advantages	• Excellent exposure • High graft uptake • Applicable to all cases	• Less lateralization • Simpler technique
Disadvantages	• Requires precision • Longer healing time • Blunting, Pearls	• Poor visualization • Difficult with small EAC

TM Repair Outcome

The success rate of myringoplasty is 90%. Myringoplasty failure can be due to:

1. Reperforation: early reperforation is caused by a faulty technique like inappropriate approach selection, small graft, and inappropriate placement of the graft, allowing it to fall into the middle ear space. Late reperforation is often due to infection, graft atrophy, and ET dysfunction.
2. Graft lateralization: happens more in the overlay technique. It can lead to insufficient sound conduction.

3. Atelectasis: ET dysfunction is the leading cause. Other causes are thin graft, not reinforcing the graft by other materials like cartilage, or not ventilating the ear in the primary surgery.
4. Postoperative myringitis: it is a granular reaction of the lateral surface of the TM graft. The patient will complain of slight pain, ear fullness, or otorrhea. It can be an autoimmune response, reaction to the packing materials, or postoperative infection. Treatment options are topical antibiotics, debridement, or silver nitrate cautery. Tympanoplasty can be considered if these options failed.

Ossicular Chain Reconstruction (Ossiculoplasty)

It can be achieved by an allograft (bone or cartilage) or by a synthetic prosthesis. Generally, the prosthesis is divided into:

- Partial ossicular replacement prosthesis (PORP), which is used in cases of absent incus but stapes is present, and
- Total ossicular replacement prosthesis (TORP), which is used in cases of absent incus and stapes superstructure.

Biomechanics of Ossiculoplasty

There are number of factors to be considered in reconstructing the middle ear ossicles:

1. Biological factors: which include:
   (a) *Biocompatibility of the prosthesis*: a biocompatible prosthesis is an inert one that remains stable in a biologic environment without inducing foreign body reaction. Titanium and hydroxyapatite are the most widely used and the most successful implants nowadays, as they have excellent mechanical properties, low extrusion rates, and good hearing results. Titanium prosthesis is more user-friendly. An interface cartilage graft should be used between the prosthesis and TM to minimize extrusion.
   (b) *Middle ear environment:* Fibrotic middle ear mucosa and denuded mucosa during surgery are detrimental to hearing results compared with that of normal middle ear mucosa. The presence of a stapes superstructure is crucial for a favorable hearing result. The presence of malleus is theoretically important for a favorable hearing outcome as well: the malleus is thought to provide better hearing results if incorporated in the reconstruction by preserving the catenary lever.
   (c) *Healing process* which varies with personal immunity conditions.
2. Mechanical factors: The primary goal of ossicular reconstruction is to reach a maximum of coupling the stapes footplate to the TM in order to re-establish the hydraulic lever effect.
   (a) *Prosthesis Axis*: the angle between the stapes and a prosthesis should be less than 45° for optimal sound transmission [12].
   (b) *Tension*: A prosthesis that is too long would stiffen the ME tympano-ossicular system resulting in a reduction of motion and an impaired closure of the air-bone gap [13].
   (c) *Coupling*: Coupling refers to how well prosthesis adheres to the footplate or TM, and the degree of coupling will determine whether or not there is slippage at the end of the prosthesis. Tilting and/or dislocation of the prosthesis are the major causes of poor postoperative hearing results. Apart from biological reasons, prosthesis displacement is the most common cause of the postoperative unsatisfactory hearing results.

Strategies and Techniques in Ossiculoplasty

In cases where the malleus handle is much medialized, resection of the tensor tympani ligament is accomplished to free and positioner the manubrium adequately for better reconstruction. The malleus must be preserved for better stability [3]. Look at Fig. 5.15 for ossiculoplasty strategies and Figs. 5.16, 5.17, 5.18, and 5.19 for further demonstration.

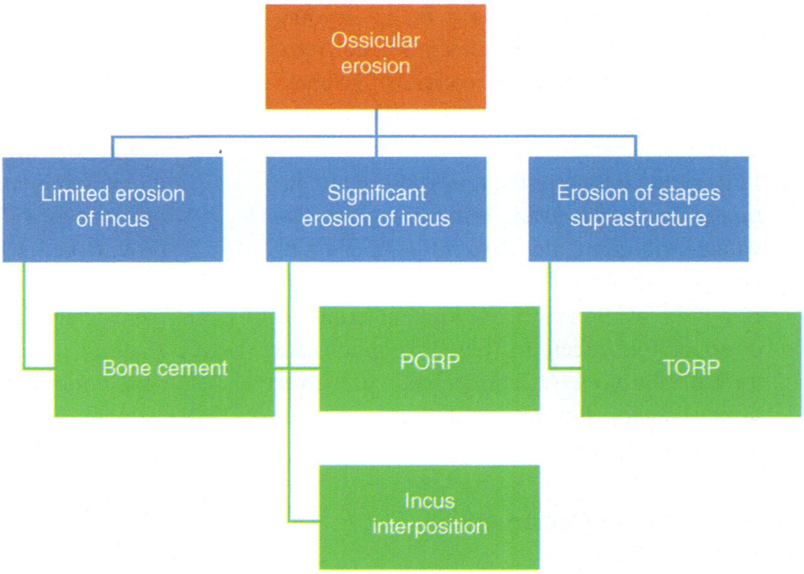

Fig. 5.15 Ossiculoplasty strategies and techniques

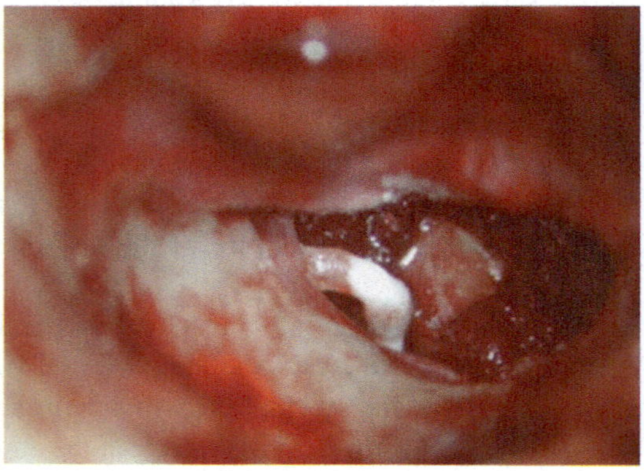

Fig. 5.16 Right ear intraoperative view showing reconstruction of the incudostapedial joint with bone cement

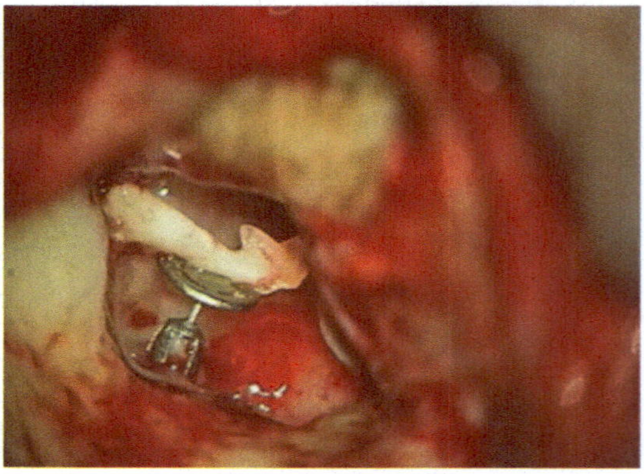

Fig. 5.18 Ossiculoplasty in the left ear using PORP

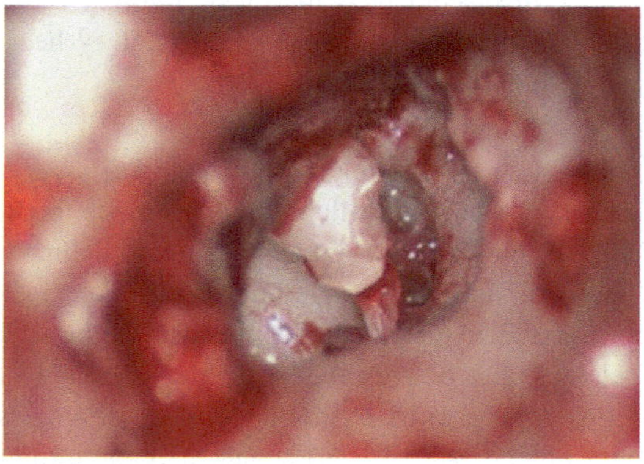

Fig. 5.17 Ossiculoplasty in the left ear using incus interposition

The Outcome of Ossiculoplasty

Postoperative hearing outcomes are considered successful if the postoperative air-bone gap is within 20 dB. Ossiculoplasty may fail for one of three fundamental reasons: a problem with the prosthesis, postoperative adhesions, and recurrent disease.

When only myringoplasty is needed, 80–90% of patients will have an air-bone gap of 20 dB or less. When ossicular reconstruction is necessary, long-term closure of the air-bone gap to less than 20 dB is achieved in 80% of cases in cases where the stapes is intact, and only in about 65% of cases where the stapes superstructure is missing [14].

Critical to the success of the CSOM surgery is the ability of the ME to maintain adequate aeration to ensure good ME mechanics.

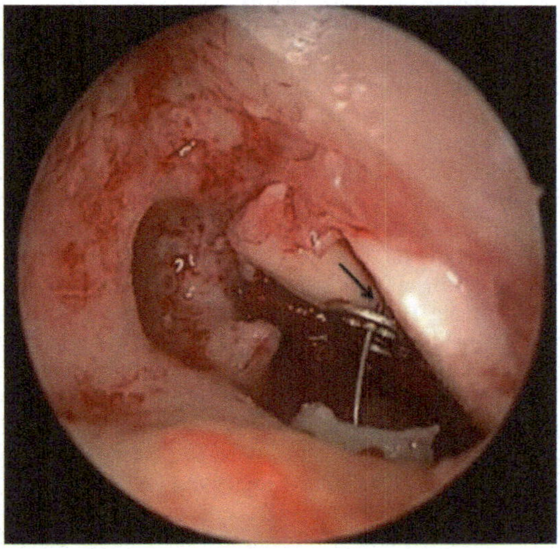

Fig. 5.19 Right ear ossiculoplasty using TORP and cartilage shoe. After finishing middle ear reconstruction and packing the ear canal, a 30° scope is placed in the mastoid attic to look into the middle ear cavity; the TORP is in proper position and is stable. Notice the pin (black arrow) on the headplate of the TORP which is kept intentionally so the TORP will incorporate in the TM cartilage

Complications of Middle Ear Reconstruction

1. Infection.
2. Postauricular incisional site hematomas.
3. Taste disturbance.
4. Ear numbness of the pinna and lobule.
5. CHL due to lateralization of the graft and failure of middle ear spaces aeration (40 dB loss secondary to ME dysventilation and granulation formations.).
6. SNHL, which is a serious complication, can occur due to excessive manipulation of the ossicular chain.
7. Vertigo (rule out fistula).

Complications of Mastoidectomy or Tympano-Mastoidectomy

When mastoidectomy is indicated, according to imaging inputs and surgical strategy review, this surgery may leave, in addition to the above-cited complications, a cerebrospinal fluid (CSF) leak if the dura is violated during the dissection. Moreover, meningoencephaloceles can occur secondary to a large tegmen defect.

CT imaging provides information about the status of the prosthesis and eventual displacement (Fig. 5.20).

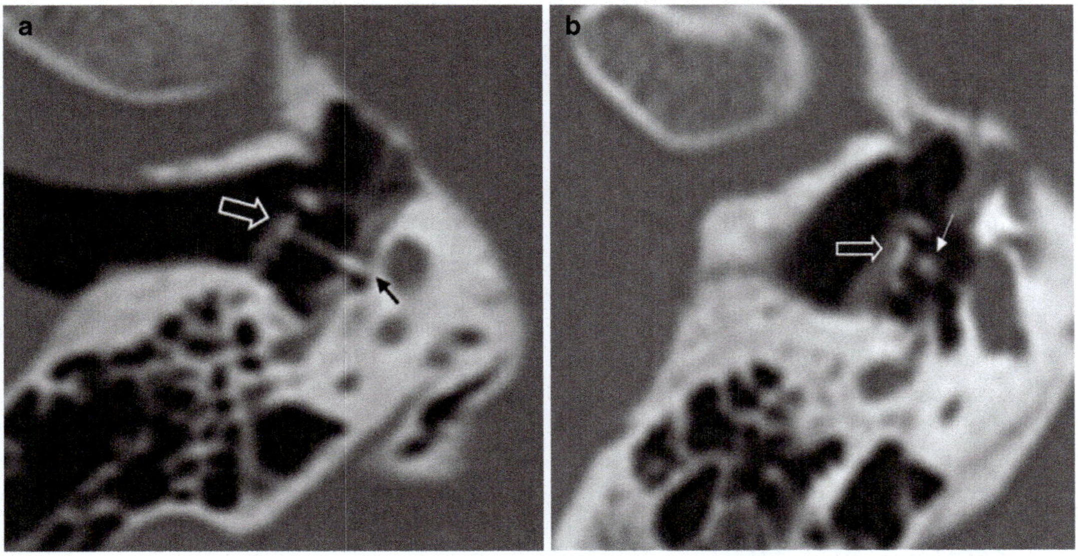

Fig. 5.20 (**a**) Axial CT image along the TORP, that is in close contact with the tympanic membrane (empty arrow), inserting medially on the posterior border of the footplate (arrow): displacement. (**b**) Axial CT image showing a PORP with thickening of the tympanic membrane in contact with the prosthesis (empty arrow), the medial part inserting on the stapes head (arrow)

5.14 Some Unusual Clinical Presentations of CSOM

Tuberculous Otitis Media: The typical feature of the disease is profuse, painless otorrhea not responding to topical and systemic antimicrobial therapies in combined with aural toilet. Examination shows multiple TM perforations and pale exuberant granulations. Complications like facial palsy and SNHL are significantly higher than CSOM without cholesteatoma.

Immunodeficiency: The idiopathic hypogammaglobulinemia is characterized by a deficiency in the IgG fraction of serum globulin, which often presents with otitis media at an early age. Chronic ear disease is sometimes observed in Job's syndrome (lazy leucocyte syndrome).

Wegener's Granulomatosis: Middle ear infection, either as a primary or secondary involvement of the disease, has been described.

Histiocytosis X (Langerhans Cell Histiocytosis): Histiocytosis X involvement of the middle ear is rare and manifests as recurrent otitis with aural polyps.

Take-Home Messages

- In most cases, chronic suppurative otitis media (CSOM) is the result of an initial episode of acute otitis media, and this is why it is of high importance to give AOM the proper care and follow-up in children of 2–3 years old to prevent hearing loss; health workers should ask for all procedures visualizing the eardrum be standardized and validated.
- Clinical evaluation must distinguish between CSOM from other forms of chronic otitis media.
- Imaging is a helpful tool in unresponsive cases to a medical treatment enabling the extent of inflammatory disease in the middle ear cleft so as to differentiate safe from unsafe ear.
- Despite the decrease of morbidity of CSOM, it remains a real burden and residual hearing loss, especially in countries with a lack of public health regimen.

References

1. Mawson S, Ludman H. Disease of the ear: a textbook of otology. 4th ed. London: Edward Arnold Publication; 1979.
2. Matanda RN, Muyunga KC, Sabue MJ, Creten W, Van de Heyning P. Chronic suppurative otitis media and related complications at the University Clinic of Kinshasa. B-ENT. 2005;1:57–62.
3. Mansour S, Magnan J, Nicolas K, Haider H. Middle ear disease. Cham: Springer; 2018. p. 311–81.
4. Elmorsy S, Shabana YK, Raouf AA, Naggar ME, Bedir T, Taher S, Fath-Aallah M. The role of IL-8 in different types of otitis media and bacteriological correlation. J Int Adv Otol. 2010;6:269–73.
5. Si Y, Zhang ZG, Chen SJ, Zheng YQ, Chen YB, Liu Y, Jiang H, Feng LQ, Huang X. Attenuated TLRs in middle ear mucosa contributes to susceptibility of chronic suppurative otitis media. Hum Immunol. 2014;75:771–6.
6. Stanford LE, Raisanen S. Opsonization of middle ear bacteria during chronic suppurative and secretory otitis media. Acta Otolaryngol. 1992;112(1):96–101.
7. Stanford LE, Raisanen S. Secretory IgA- and IgG-coated bacteria in chronically discharging ears. J Laryngol Otol. 1991;105(7):515–7.
8. Haidar H, Sheikh R, Larem A, Elsaadi A, Abdulkarim H, et al. Ossicular chain erosion in chronic suppurative otitis media. Otolaryngol (Sunnyvale). 2015;5:203.
9. Mehta RP, Rosowski JJ, Voss SE, O'Neil E, Merchant SN. Determinants of hearing loss in perforations of the tympanic membrane. Otol Neurotol. 2006;27(2):136–43.
10. Cureoglu S, Schachern PA, Paparella MM, Lindgren BR. Cochlear changes in chronic otitis media. Laryngoscope. 2004;114:622–6.
11. Mansour S, Magnan J, Haidar H, Nicolas K, Louryan S. Comprehensive and clinical anatomy of the middle ear. Cham: Springer; 2013. https://doi.org/10.1007/978-3-642-36967-4.
12. Vlaming MS, Feenstra L. Studies on the mechanics of the reconstructed human middle ear. Clin Otolaryngol Allied Sci. 1986;11(6):411–22.
13. Morris DP, Bance M, Van Wijhe RG. How do cartilage and other material overlay over a prosthesis affect its vibration transmission properties in ossiculoplasty? Otolaryngol Head Neck Surg. 2004;131(4):423–8.
14. Altamimi Z, Haidar H, Larem A, et al. Innovation in otology: stability of ossicular reconstruction. J Bioeng Biomed Sci. 2016;6(5 Suppl).

Cholesteatoma

6

Salah Mansour, Ma'in Ali Al Shawabkeh, Karen Nicolas, and Hassan Haidar

6.1 Introduction

Cholesteatoma is an abnormal growth of the keratinizing squamous epithelium in the middle ear. It could be congenital or acquired. Cholesteatoma is a destructive and expanding lesion that may lead to fatal complications if left untreated.

6.2 Epidemiology

Its annual incidence is 9.2/100,000 in adults and 0.3/100,000 in children with male predominance [1].

It is higher in Caucasian and rare in African. It peaks in the second and third decades [2]. The mean age for congenital cholesteatoma is 6 years.

S. Mansour (✉)
Centre Medical Westmount Square, Otology, Westmount, QC, Canada

M. A. Al Shawabkeh
ENT Department, Hamad Medical Corporation, Doha, Qatar

K. Nicolas
Radiology Department, Bsalim Hospital, Beirut, Lebanon

H. Haidar
Hamad Medical Corporation, Doha, Qatar

6.3 Types of Cholesteatoma

6.3.1 Congenital Cholesteatoma

It is more common in males (3:1). Its location is more common in the superior anterior part of the middle ear facing the Eustachian tube opening (2/3 of the cases). The second most common is the superior posterior part near the incudostapedial joint (Fig. 6.1).

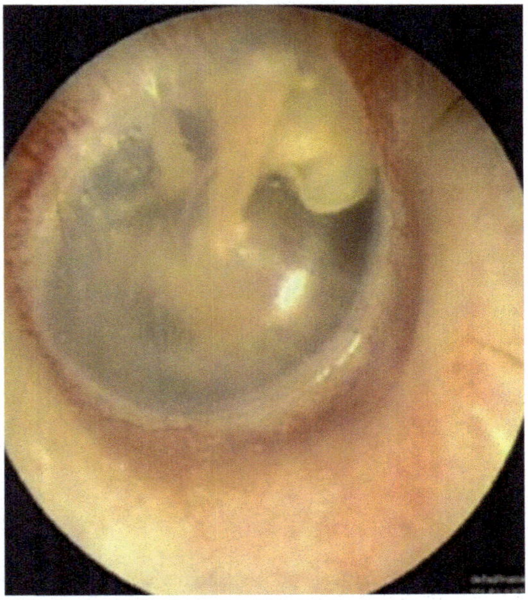

Fig. 6.1 Small congenital cholesteatoma in the anterosuperior quadrant of a right ear. (Adapted from Mansour S., Magnan J., Nicolas K., and Haider H. (2018). Middle ear disease)

A. Al-Qahtani et al. (eds.), *Textbook of Clinical Otolaryngology*,
https://doi.org/10.1007/978-3-030-54088-3_6

Levenson criteria for the diagnosis of congenital cholesteatoma are as follows:

(a) White mass behind an intact tympanic membrane (TM).
(b) No prior history of otorrhea.
(c) No prior history of TM perforation.
(d) No prior history of otologic procedures.
Prior history of otitis media does not rule out congenital cholesteatoma.

6.3.2 Acquired Cholesteatoma

Acquired cholesteatoma has two types:

- ***Primary acquired*:** It is the most frequent type and arises from the progression of tympanic membrane retraction pocket. It can be a retraction from the pars flaccida (more common in adults), from pars tensa (more common in children), or combined (Figs. 6.2 and 6.3).
- ***Secondary acquired*:** It arises from the migration of epithelial membrane through a marginal perforation of the TM, or due to trapped skin through micro-perforation secondary to trauma or surgery.

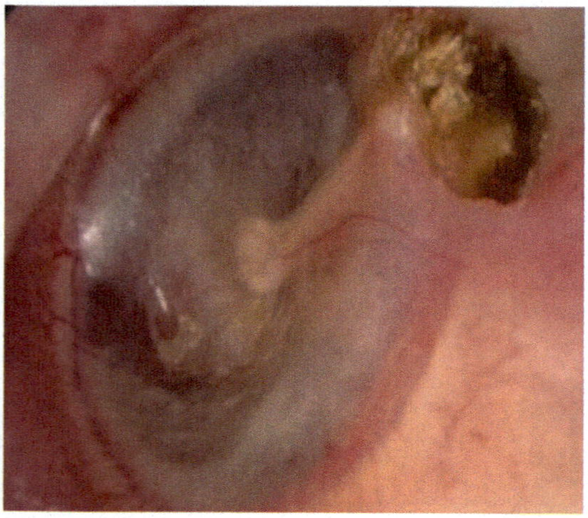

Fig. 6.2 Left attical cholesteatoma. (Adapted from Mansour S., Magnan J., Nicolas K., and Haider H. (2018). Middle ear disease)

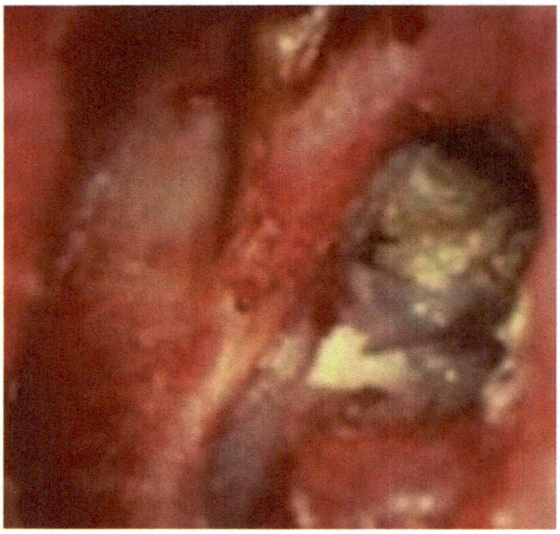

Fig. 6.3 Left ear mesotympanic and retrotympanic cholesteatoma. (Adapted from Mansour S., Magnan J., Nicolas K., and Haider H. (2018). Middle ear disease)

6.4 Histopathology of Cholesteatoma

Light microscopy shows a cyst with three components:

1. Amorphous center composed of squamous keratin debris.
2. Matrix, a stimulated proliferative skin (Keratinizing squamous epithelium).
3. Perimatrix which is granulation tissues and inflammatory cells. It is the site of the inflammatory process.

6.5 Pathogenesis of Cholesteatoma

6.5.1 Theories for Congenital Cholesteatoma

1. Epidermal rest theory: cell rests of non-keratinizing squamous epithelium localized near Eustachian tube ostium, having the potential to become a cholesteatoma.

2. Inclusion theory: migration of cells originatimg from the external auditory canal skin to the middle ear secondary to non-evident injury to the TM [3].

6.5.2 Theories for Acquired Cholesteatoma

1. Invagination theory: the precursors of cholesteatoma are retraction pockets secondary to dysventilation syndrome of the middle ear compartments. Two histological features present in cholesteatoma but not found in retraction pockets: **epithelial hyperplasia and skin migration**.
2. Migration theory: squamous epithelium of the TM or the ear canal skin migrates through the perforated eardrum into the middle ear.
3. Squamous metaplasia theory: this theory stipulated that under chronic inflammation, middle ear mucosa changes into a squamous epithelium. But this theory lacks histological or experimental proof, so such a hypothesis is not accepted anymore.
4. Basal cell hyperplasia (Papillary) theory: a keratin-filled microcysts or buds arise from the basal layer of flaccida epithelium that invade the subepithelial tissue and fuse together to form a cholesteatoma [4].

Recent advances in the pathogenesis of cholesteatoma postulate that the cholesteatoma is a result of the defective healing process, in which the normal maturation end-stage of the wound-healing process will not be achieved (non-stop wound healing process). Moreover, the pathogenesis of this condition does not rely only on the middle ear pathological conditions but also on the immunological status of the bottom of the skin ear canal [5].

6.6 Molecular Biology of Cholesteatoma

1. Histochemical studies found quantitative and qualitative modifications of ***Langerhans' cells***; these cells emit long dendritic expansions, which create a true network between the neighboring cells: keratinocytes and lymphocytes. This close contact between these cells is essential for the immune reaction production [6].
2. There are *paracrine and autocrine interactions* between keratinocytes of the matrix and fibroblasts of the perimatrix that regulate homeostasis and tissue regeneration within a cholesteatoma [4].
3. The fundamental difference between the healing process in a normal skin and in cholesteatoma is that in cholesteatoma, there is a loss of the growth inhibition by "cell to cell contact". Two factors are involved in that:

   (a) The cholesteatoma develops beyond its normal anatomical site for a "skin".
   (b) The inflammatory process produces a self-maintained immunological cycle, which enhances the epithelial growth.

4. The loss of balance between apoptotic and antiapoptotic markers, the increased antiapoptotic activity in cholesteatoma favors its continuing expansion [6, 7].
5. The presence of antibiotic-resistant bacterial Biofilms in cholesteatomas may also explain their aggressiveness [8].

6.7 Cholesteatoma Origin and Growth Pathways [6]

Posterior epitympanic cholesteatoma: It is the most common pattern of spread for cholesteatoma originating from Prussak's space. The cholesteatoma spreads into the superior incudal space lateral to the body of the incus, and from there, it can potentially enter the mastoid through the aditus ad antrum (Fig. 6.4).

Mesotympanic cholesteatoma: the second most common type is mesotympanic cholesteatoma which spreads through the *posterior pouch of von Troeltsch*, following the embryological course of both saccus posticus and saccus superior. It grows medially along the lenticular process and stapes superstructure. Then it may grow upward through the posterior tympanic isthmus

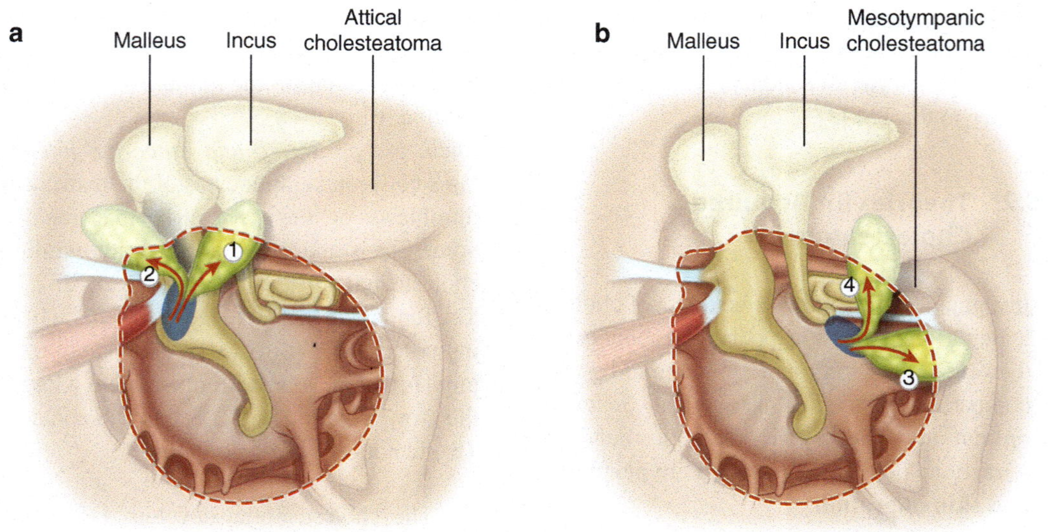

Fig. 6.4 Cholesteatoma origin and spread. (**a**) An attical cholesteatoma usually spreads posteriorly (1) as posterior attical cholesteatoma and rarely anteriorly as anterior attical cholesteatoma (2) and (**b**) mesotympanic cholesteatoma growth pattern into the facial recess and sinus tympani (retrotympanum). (Adapted from Mansour S., Magnan J., Nicolas K., and Haider H. (2018). Middle ear disease)

toward the posterior epitympanum to the mastoid antrum or backward into the sinus tympani (Fig. 6.4).

Anterior epitympanic cholesteatoma: it spreads through the superior malleal fold following the embryologic saccus anticus to enter the epitympanic recess (AER). It may remain there for a time where the geniculate ganglion will be at risk, or progress into the supratubal recess and the protympanum (Fig. 6.4).

Unclassified cholesteatoma: this pattern occurs when cholesteatomas grow beyond multiple middle ear compartments, or when arise from both pars flaccida and pars tensa retraction pockets (PFRP&PTRP).

6.8 Clinical Manifestations

6.8.1 Symptoms

1. Otorrhea: it is a chronic scanty painless foul-smelling discharge.
2. Hearing loss: ossicular erosion is the most common finding (70%), causing conductive hearing loss (CHL) [9]. However, patients may have normal hearing due to the conductive mass effect of cholesteatoma itself.
3. Vertigo: due to the bony erosion of the semicircular canal. Fistula test or Valsalva may reveal the labyrinthine insult. (Tullio phenomenon is dizziness upon exposure to sound, which can happen in conditions like superior canal dehiscence, perilymphatic fistula, and Meniere's disease.)
4. Facial palsy: it may be the first clinical manifestation especially for cholesteatoma in the anterior epitympanic recess (AER).

6.8.2 Otomicroscopy

Otomicroscopy might show marginal TM perforation, erosion of the scutum and/or the ossicles, a retraction pocket, granulation tissue, or a polyp. Caution should be taken if removal of the polyp is decided as it might be attached to the facial nerve or the ossicles.

6.8.3 Audiological Testing

Audiogram usually shows CHL. Speech reception thresholds are normal. Patients may have sensorineural hearing loss, which indicates a labyrinth insult.

6.9 CT Imaging in Cholesteatoma

Cholesteatoma does not have a specific density on CT, because it can demonstrate the same soft-tissue appearance as inflammatory processes, granulation or fibrous tissues, mucosal edema, or even fluid.

CT can show the following:

1. A rounded soft-tissue mass, which is a cardinal sign in the early stages.
2. Erosion of the **scutum**, which is suggestive of pars flaccida cholesteatoma (Fig. 6.5).
3. Erosion of the ossicles: The incus is the most vulnerable of the ossicles. Malleus head and stapes may be lytic in relation to the disease extension and are more suspicious of the cholesteatoma process.
4. Erosion of the **COG** is a sign of an invading cholesteatoma of the AER (Fig. 6.6). The Cog is always preserved in non-cholesteatomatous inflammatory processes. Invasion of the AER with a lysis of the Cog is important to look for, because of the silent progress of the cholesteatoma could make a facial palsy its first clinical sign.
5. Erosion of the **semicircular canals** (labyrinthine Fistula) (Fig. 6.7).
6. Erosion of the **fallopian canal**: integrity of the VII canal is not always easy to confirm by CT. CT can alert the surgeon about abnormal trajectory of the VII (Fig. 6.8).
7. Erosion of the **tegmen** (Fig. 6.8).
8. Extension of cholesteatoma into the mastoid: CT can be strongly indicate an extension of cholesteatoma to the mastoid when filled with condensations with irregular borders, or when the antrum is entirely filled with condensations that have smooth rounded borders (Fig. 6.7).
9. Posterior wall of the external auditory canal lysis: it has an impact on surgical option selection.

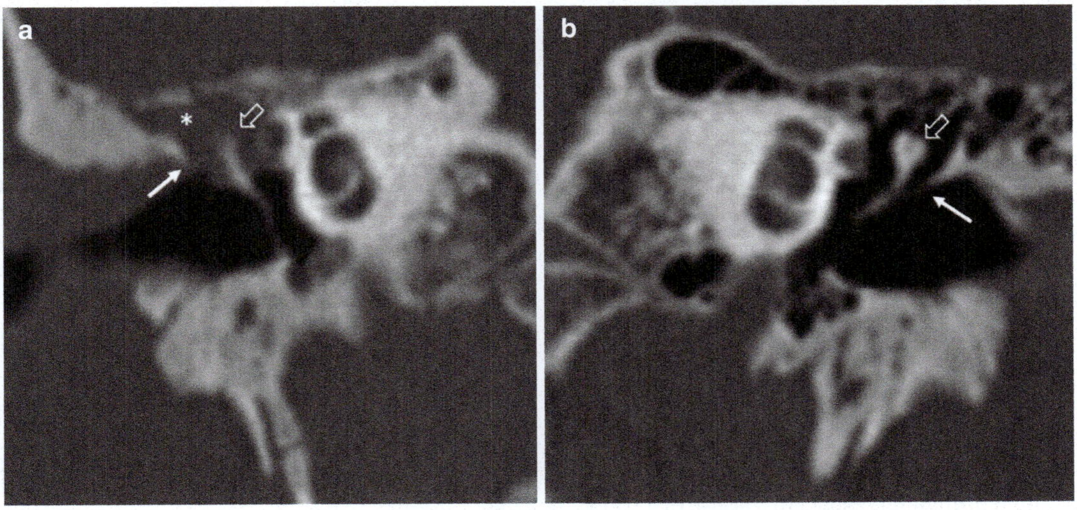

Fig. 6.5 Coronal reformatted CT images: (**a**) Right ear with amputation of the scutum (arrow), Prussak's space cholesteatoma extended to the attic (asterisk), lyses of the malleus head (empty arrow). (**b**) Left normal ear with triangular-shaped scutum (arrow), normal aspect of the malleus head (empty arrow)

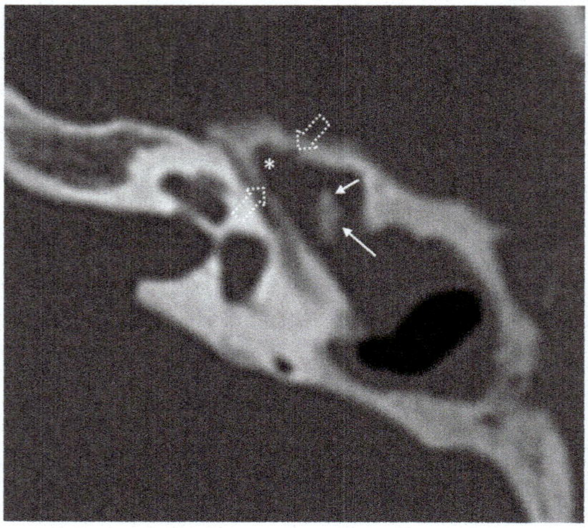

Fig. 6.6 Large atticoantral cholesteatoma also invading the anterior epitympanic recess (asterisk), complete absence of the cog (should be seen between the empty arrows). Lytic ossicular chain: short arrow—lytic malleus head, long arrow—lytic incus

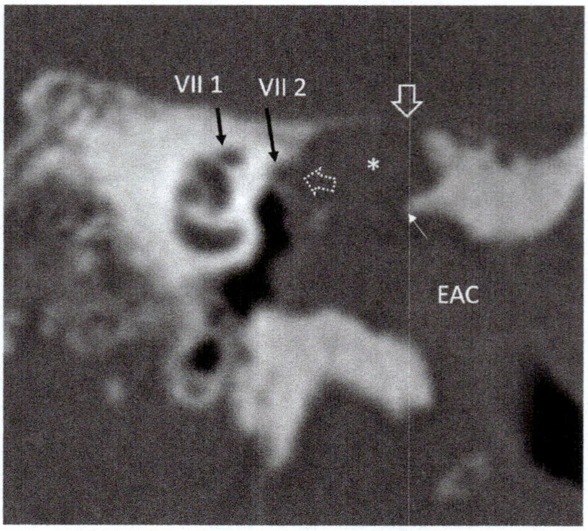

Fig. 6.8 Left coronal CT image, showing a huge cholesteatoma in the attic (asterisk), with lyses of the tegmen (empty arrow), lyses of the facial nerve canal (tympanic portion, dotted empty arrow), and lyses of the scutum (thin arrow). *EAC* external auditory canal

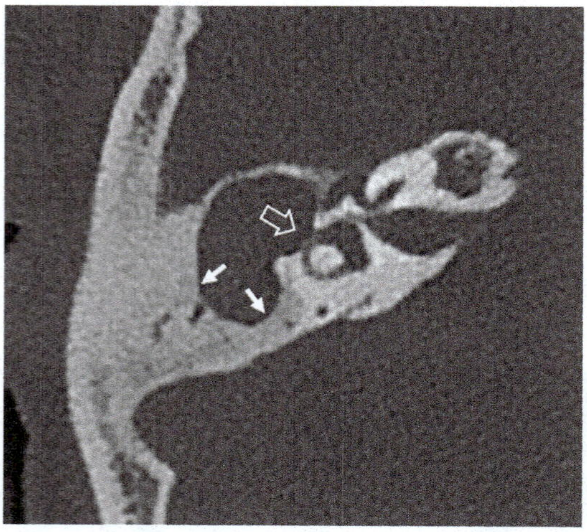

Fig. 6.7 Right side cholesteatoma with labyrinthine fistula secondary to erosion of the anterior limb of the lateral semicircular canal (empty arrow). See also smooth borders of the antrum (arrows) in favor of cholesteatoma

6.10 MRI in Cholesteatoma

MRI permits an almost specific diagnosis of cholesteatoma in the middle ear cleft with diffusion-weighted imaging, especially non-EPI-DWI (see Fig. 6.9), with differentiation from other soft tissues (Table 6.1). It is generally not indicated for the primary diagnosis of cholesteatoma, but rather used in the follow-up with patients postoperatively before second-look indication. In addition, MRI can be considered as a complementary imaging tool when the clinical presentation or CT films suspect complications (see below).

6.11 Management of Cholesteatoma

There is no medical management yet available for cholesteatoma. Surgery of cholesteatoma implies the following:

1. Total eradication of cholesteatoma to obtain a dry and safe ear.
2. Maintain the best condition for wound healing and preserve normal anatomy of the ear.
3. Maintain the best functional status of hearing.

The surgical procedures can be divided into major groups

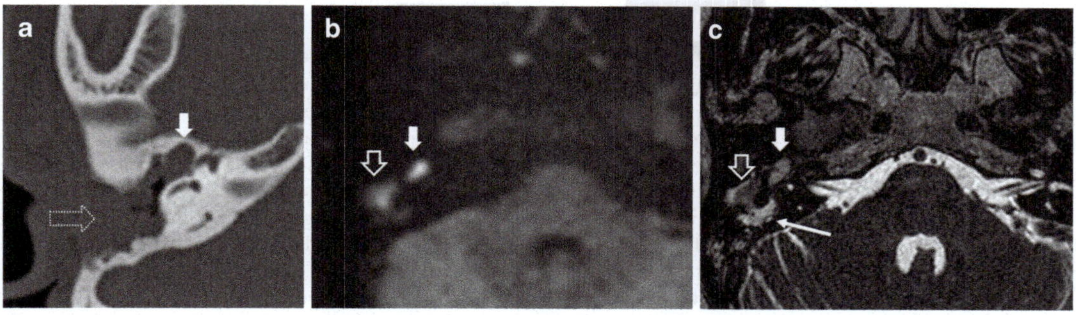

Fig. 6.9 Recurrent cholesteatoma of the right ear: (**a**) axial CT showing non-specific condensations in the cavity of mastoidectomy (open arrow), and oval-shaped condensation of the AER (white arrow). (**b**) Axial diffusion image at B 1000 shows two foci of pathologic restriction corresponding to cholesteatoma in the cavity of mastoidectomy (empty arrow) and in the AER (plain arrow). (**c**) Axial T2 HR Drive image showing the hypointense cholesteatoma in the cavity of mastoidectomy (empty arrow), surrounded by hyperintense effusion (long arrow). Second focus of cholesteatoma in the AER (plain arrow), of intermediate non-specific intensity in this sequence

Table 6.1 Differential diagnosis by MRI [6]

	T1	T2	Diffusion	Gado
Cholesteatoma	Hypointense	Hyperintense	Restriction	No early uptake
Cholesterol granuloma	Hyperintense	Hyperintense	No restriction	No uptake
Granulation tissue	Hypo/intermediate	Hyperintense	No restriction	Uptake
Scar tissue	Hypointense	Hypointense	No restriction	Uptake

1. A closed technique: like canal wall up (CWU) procedure, canal wall down (CWD) with a reconstruction of the ear canal, or CWD with mastoid obliteration.
2. An open technique: CWD, atticotomy without reconstruction or obliteration.

6.11.1 Surgical Procedures

See Table 6.2.

6.11.2 Endoscopy in Cholesteatoma

Otoendoscopy offers better visualization of a disease hidden in areas like sinus tympani, anterior epitympanic recess, and retrotympanum. It permits, better than the microscope, to rule out peroperative residual. In many cases, micro-endoscopic surgery prevails to ensure adequate surgical procedure.

Wet Ear Cavity is the most common reason for revision surgery after CWD mastoidectomy (troublesome mastoid cavity). It is due to the following [10]:

1. Incomplete eradication of the mastoid air-cells disease or inadequate lowering of the facial ridge (85%).
2. A very large cavity or/and inadequate meatoplasty (10%).
3. Recurrent or residual cholesteatoma (5%).

6.11.3 Hearing Rehabilitation in Cholesteatoma Surgery

1. Ossiculoplasty done either by autologous ossicular graft or by prosthesis (partial or total ossicular replacement prosthesis). In extended cases, it is recommended to control the disease process first and do the ossicular reconstruction later. Safe ear prevails on hearing restauration.
2. Bone anchored hearing aid (BAHA) can provide a viable option to improve hearing outcome.

Table 6.2 Comparison between CWU and CWD procedures

	Canal wall down (CWD) procedure	Canal wall up procedure
Indications	1. Cholesteatoma of an only hearing ear. 2. Major erosion of the posterior bony canal wall. 3. History of vertigo due to a labyrinthine fistula. 4. Poor Eustachian tube function. 5. Sclerotic mastoid with limited access to the epitympanum. 6. Patient non-compliant for follow-up.	Indicated in most cases of cholesteatoma, especially for cases with a large pneumatized mastoid and in children *Contraindications* 1. Only hearing ear. 2. A long-standing ear disease after multiple previous procedures and persistent extended pathology. 3. Extensive lysis of the bony ear canal.
Advantages	1. The relatively short duration of the surgery. 2. Attic and the facial recess are well exteriorized; easier surgical in toto removal of the extended disease. 3. Any postoperative cholesteatoma regrowth can readily be seen and removed as an office procedure.	1. More rapid healing. 2. Better quality of life for the patient and normal ear contours. 3. Better fit of hearing aids when needed.
Disadvantages	1. Hearing reconstruction is less successful. 2. Open cavity: the mastoid bowl maintenance can be a lifelong problem. Unpleasant appearance of the meatoplasty. 3. Secondary reconstruction would be less successful. 4. Difficulty fitting of hearing aid because of meatoplasty.	1. Long duration of the surgical procedure in extended pathologies. 2. Unsatisfactory exposure and high rate of residual disease. 3. Staging and multiple surgical looks. It may require a second look after 12 months in adults and 6–9 months in children.

Table 6.3 Complications of chronic otitis media with cholesteatoma (Fig. 6.10)

	Extratemporal	
Intratemporal	Intracranial	Extracranial
Labyrinthine fistula	Lateral sinus thrombosis	Sub-periosteal abscess
Facial paralysis	Meningitis	Bezold's abscess
Petrositis	Extradural abscess	
Labyrinthitis	Subdural abscess	
	Cerebral abscess	

6.11.4 Follow-Up

The rate of recurrence and residual disease is higher in children (30%) than in adults. It is important to ensure as long as possible the follow-up with the patient postoperatively. For children, follow-up should continue until adulthood and longer. MRI imaging can be considered as the first-line follow-up imaging tool to search for disease recurrence.

Otologist should consider the following choices during patients' follow-up, especially in children:

1. Second-look surgery should be offered when complete surgical removal of cholesteatoma was uncertain to the surgeon and the patient has a positive MRI image. (It is to note that MRI is a difficult tool in children because it requires general anesthesia.).
2. When the surgeon was sure of complete removal of cholesteatoma, and when an unequivocal normal microscopic examination is observed in the first 6 months, then MRI can be a substitute for second-look surgery.

6.12 Complications of Chronic Otitis Media with Cholesteatoma [6]

Possible intra- and extratemporal complications are enumerated in Table 6.3 and illustrated by Fig. 6.10.

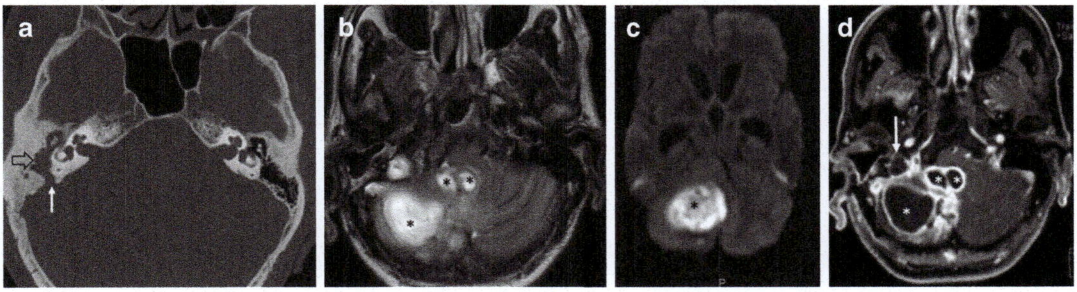

Fig. 6.10 (**a**) Axial HRCT, (**b**) Axial T2-WI MRI, (**c**) Axial DWI MRI, and (**d**) Axial Contrast enhanced tT1-WI MRI. (**a**) Showing CT features of right sided otomastoiditis/cholesteatoma (black empty arrow) with focal bony erosion along the posterior wall (white arrow). (**b**) Multiple right cerebellar abscesses, hyperintense in Flair (asterisk) that show diffusion restriction in **c**, and a typical ring enhancement after Gadolinium in **d**, also subdural empyema (arrow)

Take-Home Messages

- Despite advances in diagnosis and surgery, deficiencies exist worldwide with access to health care facilities, meaning cholesteatoma remains a serious and challenging entity to manage when found within the pediatric or adult population.
- Proper diagnosis and management of each type of cholesteatoma must be achieved through a strict methodology and long-life follow-up.

References

1. Aquino JE, Cruz Filho NA, de Aquino JN. Epidemiology of middle ear and mastoid cholesteatomas: study of 1146 cases. Braz J Otorhinolaryngol. 2011;77(3):341–7.
2. Potsic WP, Korman SB, Samadi DS, Wetmore RF. Congenital cholesteatoma: 20 year experience at the Children's Hospital of Philadelphia. Arch Otolaryngol Head Neck Surg. 2002;126(1): 409–14.
3. Bennett M, Warren F, Jackson GC, Kaylie D. Congenital cholesteatoma: theories, facts, and 53 patients. Otolaryngol Clin N Am. 2006;39(6): 1081–94.
4. Kuo C-L. Etiopathogenesis of acquired cholesteatoma: prominent theories and recent advances in biomolecular research. Laryngoscope. 2015;125(1):234–40.
5. Albino AP, Kimmelman CP, Parisier SC. Cholesteatoma: a molecular and cellular puzzle. Am J Otol. 1998;19(1):7–19.
6. Mansour S, Magnan J, Nicolas K, Haider H. Middle ear disease. Cham: Springer; 2018. p. 311–81.
7. Olszewska E, Chodynicki S, Chyczewski L. Apoptosis in the pathogenesis of cholesteatoma in adults. Eur Arch Otorhinolaryngol. 2006;263(5):409–13.
8. Chole RA, Faddis BT. Evidence for microbial biofilms in cholesteatomas. Arch Otolaryngol Head Neck Surg. 2002;128(10):1129–33.
9. Haidar H, Sheikh R, Larem A, Elsaadi A, Abdulkarim H, et al. Ossicular chain erosion in chronic suppurative otitis media. Otolaryngol (Sunnyvale). 2015;5:203.
10. Li S, Meng J, Zhang F, Li X, Qin Z. Revision surgery for canal wall down mastoidectomy: intraoperative findings and results. Acta Otolaryngol. 2016;136(1):18–22.

Complications of Otitis Media

7

Waqar Aslam and Abdulsalam Al-Qahtani

7.1 Introduction

The term Otitis media (OM) refers to an inflammatory process within the middle ear cleft caused by bacteria and/or viruses. Otitis media can be either acute or chronic. There is no absolute time period, but in general, disease that persists for more than 3 months should be considered as chronic.

Acute otitis media (AOM), in general, is a childhood disease that manifests as a rapid onset of fever and otalgia with a peak incidence around the age of 6–11 months.

Although a rare entity in adults, its incidence is widely quoted as 0.25% per year in adults.

Most commonly involved bacteria are *Streptococcus pneumoniae*, *Haemophilus influenzae*, and *Moraxella catarrhalis*. Mainly *H. Influenzae* is the dominating pathogen, while *S. pneumoniae* is less involved due to vaccination.

Otitis media (OM) comprises a wide spectrum of diseases summarized in Table 7.1.

Table 7.1 Classification of otitis media

Acute otitis media		
	Suppurative	
	Non-suppurative	
	Recurrent	
Chronic otitis media		
	Suppurative	
		Tubotympanic
		Cholesteatoma
	Non-suppurative	
		Otitis media with effusion

7.2 Complications of Acute Otitis Media

Acute otitis media (AOM) is the most common reason for antibiotic prescription in pediatrics population. It is a clinical diagnosis with erythema and bulging of the tympanic membrane with fever and ear pain (Fig. 7.1). Treatment modalities range from observation, analgesia, to antibiotics therapy. Although dramatically decreased, complications of acute otitis media are still a concern. With the resulting morbidity, complications of acute otitis media can be divided into temporal (extracranial) and intracranial [1–4].

7.2.1 Extracranial Complications

- *Tympanic Membrane perforation*
  - Commonest complication of AOM, due to bloody or purulent discharge, usually in the

W. Aslam (✉) · A. Al-Qahtani
Hamad Medical Corporation, Doha, Qatar
e-mail: WKhan1@hamad.qa;
waa4005@qatar-med.cornell.edu

A. Al-Qahtani et al. (eds.), *Textbook of Clinical Otolaryngology*,
https://doi.org/10.1007/978-3-030-54088-3_7

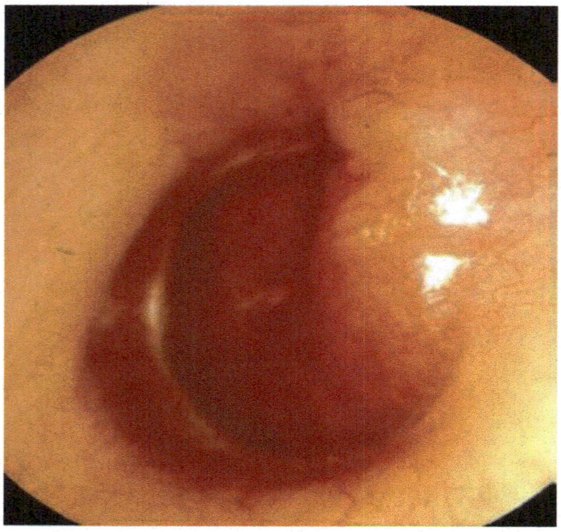

Fig. 7.1 Left ear acute otitis media with bulging of the hyperemic tympanic membrane

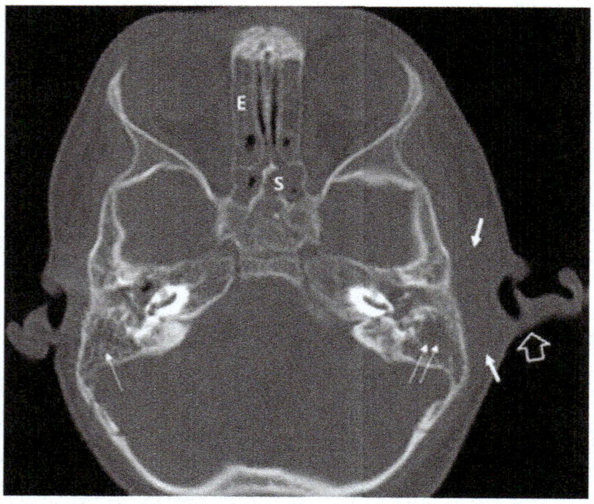

Fig. 7.2 Axial non-contrast CT image of a 2-year-old boy with acute otitis media on both sides. Opacified mastoid air cells with preserved bony septae on the right side (single arrow). On the left side, the mastoid bony septae are resorbed (double arrow): sign of coalescent mastoiditis. Associated post-auricular soft-tissue swelling (between the white arrows) with protrusion of the pinna (empty arrow), with intact mastoid cortex. Note opacified ethmoidal (E) and sphenoidal (S) sinuses

posterior half of pars tensa. Perforation normally heals spontaneously in most of the cases, while in some, it may persist with or without chronic otitis media (COM) [5].

- *Mastoiditis*
  - More in pediatrics population and develops in case of failure of resolution of acute otitis media. Patients present with pain, erythema, tenderness, and auricular protrusion. It can develop concomitantly with the acute infection or after it is subsided. The incidence is higher in areas where antibiotics are not the first line of treatment of AOM. Coalescent mastoiditis may develop about 2–4 weeks in unresolved infections. Etiology is thought to be due to hyperemia and edema associated with infection, poor ciliary clearance with accumulation of inflammatory debris, and poor aeration of the middle ear. Coalescent mastoiditis may be treated medically by antibiotics alone or surgically by mastoidectomy (for eradication of all diseased bone cells) with ventilation tube placement [1].
  - *Types of Acute Mastoiditis*
  - Based on pathological staging, the acute mastoiditis is subdivided into:

    Acute mastoiditis with periostitis, also called incipient mastoiditis, is due to the presence of purulent stuff in the mastoid cavity only.

    Acute coalescent mastoiditis also known as "acute mastoid osteitis" is the acute form of destruction of the thin bony mastoid air cells septae. It may lead to the formation of abscess cavities and further spreads of pus into surrounding areas (Fig. 7.2).

    Masked mastoiditis, also called subacute mastoiditis, refers to a low-grade, subacute, but persistent infection of the middle ear and mastoid with destruction of the mastoid bony septae. It mainly occurs in patients with persistent otitis media with effusion or in those with recurrent episodes of AOM with inadequate antibiotics therapy.
- *Petrositis*
  - It includes petrous apex involvement, Gradenigo's triad of abducens palsy, facial pain, and suppurative otitis media. Although it may not be typically present, it is diagnosed with CT scan or MRI with contrast. It is treated with high-dose systemic antibiotics and variety of mastoidectomy depending on the case [2, 5].

- *Facial palsy*
  - Uncommon these days (incidence 0.005%) due to introduction of antibiotics. It develops due to either dehiscence of tympanic segment in bony fallopian canal, physiologic canaliculi between the middle ear and the fallopian canal, or due to vascular connections between the fallopian canal and the mastoid air cells, leading to intrafallopian inflammatory edema and consequent ischemia and neuropraxia. Patients may develop total or partial paralysis of the facial nerve. Recovery without intervention is usually good. It is treated with systemic antibiotics. Surgical intervention varies from ventilation tube placement to mastoidectomy, depending on the case. Recovery is usually within 4 months. Pediatric patients recover better. Complete paralysis requires more time to recover [1, 5].
- *Labyrinthitis*
  - Can be either serous or suppurative. The infection can spread directly through dehiscent oval window membrane, congenital anomalies, or through membrane of the round window. Usually presents as nausea, vomiting, diaphoresis, hearing loss, tinnitus, and vertigo. Diagnosis is usually clinical in patients with AOM. Treatment is with antibiotics without surgical intervention. The brain usually compensates the vertigo, tinnitus abates with time, but hearing is lost after infection resolution [1, 2, 5].
- *Abscess formation*
  - *Post-auricular abscess*: more common in pediatrics population. It results as an extension of mastoiditis directly through subperiosteal space or by phlebitis of mastoid veins. Subsequent soft-tissue infection causes necrosis and abscess formation (Fig. 7.3). The auricle will be displaced downward and laterally. It is treated with antibiotics, incision, and drainage with or without mastoidectomy depending on the situation [1].

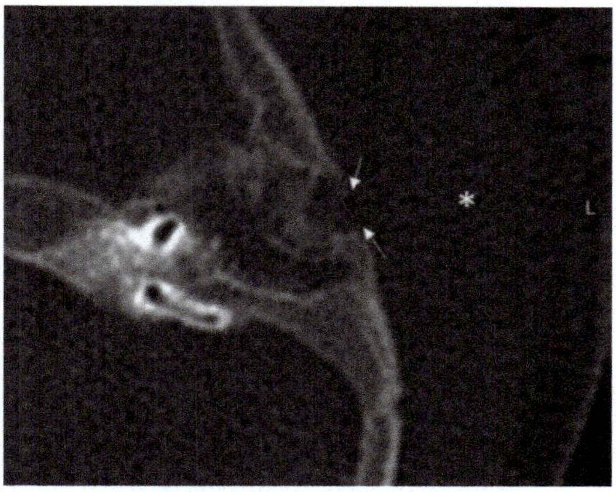

Fig. 7.3 Axial non-contrast CT image of a 1½-year child, with acute otitis media and post-auricular swelling. Destruction of the mastoid cortex (between the two arrows) and soft-tissue thickening (asterisk): subperiosteal abscess

  - *Bezold's abscess*: it's a localized infection in the upper part of the neck deep to sternocleidomastoid muscle. It can develop through direct extension or by hematogenous route. It is more common in older children whose mastoid pneumatization extends into the mastoid tip. It is usually diagnosed by a CT scan. It is treated by incision and drainage of abscess and elimination of mastoid pathology [1].

7.2.2 Intracranial Complications

- *Meningitis*
  - Most common cause of bacterial meningitis. It occurs through direct extension or spread either hematogenously or through the inner ear route. It usually presents with classic meningitis symptoms. MRI head should be done beside other investigational modality for meningitis, to rule out other intracranial pathology or abscess formation. Early diagnosis, initiation of antibiotics, and myringotomy are crucial for its management. Cortical mastoidectomy with ventilation tube insertion can be reserved for patients not responding to medication [6].

- *Extradural abscess*
  - Second most common intracranial complication in which pus collects and localizes between bone and dura. More common with chronic otitis media. Infection spreads and localizes through bone erosion. Treatment is by incision and drainage [5].
- *Subdural empyema*
  - Rare complication of acute otitis media where the pus is localized between dura and arachnoid membranes. The infection spreads through thrombophlebitis. The patient will have focal neurological signs, with signs of meningeal irritation. The condition is treated medically with drainage of pus through burr holes or craniotomy may be required, though medical treatment alone is sufficient.
- *Sigmoid sinus thrombosis*
  - It occurs due to bone erosion in mastoid over the sigmoid sinus. The infection spreads through sinus causing infected thrombus that may extend proximally to the internal jugular vein and superior vena cava reaching systemic circulation causing septicemia. In case otitis media is the only source of infection, myringotomy with antibiotics alone will be sufficient. However, if mastoid is involved, then mastoidectomy is needed to eradicate diseased cells. The role of anticoagulants is not clear [5].
- *Focal otitic encephalitis*
  - Focal inflammatory focus with edema of the brain parenchyma without abscess formation. It is treated with antibiotics [1].
- *Brain abscess*
  - Occurs in the temporal lobe or cerebellum. The treatment includes incision and drainage of the abscess, with eradication of ear infection with prolonged course of antibiotics with or without surgery [2].
- *Otitic hydrocephalus*
  - Increase intracranial pressure in the presence of otitis media in the absence of other central causes such as meningitis or brain abscess. Mechanism is thought to be by decreased venous drainage or abnormal metabolism of CSF by inflamed meninges with resultant brain edema and signs of increased intracranial pressure (ICP) and papilledema. Symptoms include headache with ear pain on the affected side. Diagnosis is confirmed with imaging modalities of the brain, that is, CT scan or brain MRI. Treatment is medically to decrease ICP and eradication of ear infection [1, 7].

7.3 Complications of Chronic Otitis Media

Chronic otitis media (COM) is chronic inflammation of the middle ear and mastoid cavity, which presents with recurrent ear discharges or otorrhea through a tympanic membrane perforation for 2–6 weeks. It can be further classified into suppurative and non-suppurative, with or without cholesteatoma.

7.3.1 Extracranial Complications

- *Labyrinthine fistula*
  - Most common complication of chronic otitis media and can occur in COM with or without cholesteatoma. Lateral semicircular canal being most commonly involved. Mechanism thought to be by direct contact with granulations tissue or cholesteatoma. Many fistulae show spontaneous closure after eradication of cholesteatoma or infection [5].
- *Labyrinthitis*
  - Can occur in COM as well and can be serous as a sterile reaction to bacterial toxin or suppurative due to bacterial infection. Treatment includes antibiotics and steroids, to decrease host inflammatory response as thought to be responsible for hearing loss [5].
- *Mastoiditis*
  - Disease spectrum ranging from mastoid effusion to coalescent mastoiditis. It can occur in both acute and chronic otitis media. Symptomatic coalescent mastoiditis is a rare complication of both AOM and COM. It can be a serious complication to the patient due

to proximity to the posterior cranial fossa, lateral sinuses, facial nerve canal, semicircular canals, and the petrous tip of the temporal bone. Mastoiditis associated with chronic suppurative otitis media (CSOM) may result in bony erosion with temporal lobe abscess and can cause septic thrombosis of the lateral sinus. Clinically, mastoiditis may present with fever, posterior ear pain, and/or local erythema over the mastoid bone, edema of the pinna, or a posteriorly and downward displaced auricle. In coalescent mastoiditis, CT scan demonstrates characteristic loss of the trabecular bone [8].

- *Facial nerve palsy*
  - Can result from both CSOM with or without cholesteatoma and can occur by involvement of the dehiscent facial nerve or through direct bony erosion. Treatment of facial paralysis in CSOM, with or without cholesteatoma, requires surgical intervention [8, 9].
- *Petrositis*
  - Inflammation may extend to petrous apex causing retro-orbital pain, abducens palsy along with otorrhea, a triad known as Gradenigo syndrome. It occurs due to inflammatory changes or lesions involving petrous apex. Chronic petrositis can complicate chronic otitis media with bone remodeling caused by inflammatory changes. It is considered a serious complication due to the close proximity of the petrous apex to intracranial structures and internal carotid artery [5].
- *Tympanosclerosis*
  - Abnormal hyalinization and calcium deposit in the tympanic membrane and middle ear (Fig. 7.4). It can be associated with resolved infection, trauma, or site of tympanostomy tube placement. It appears as white patches on the TM and is more associated with chronic otitis media [1, 5].

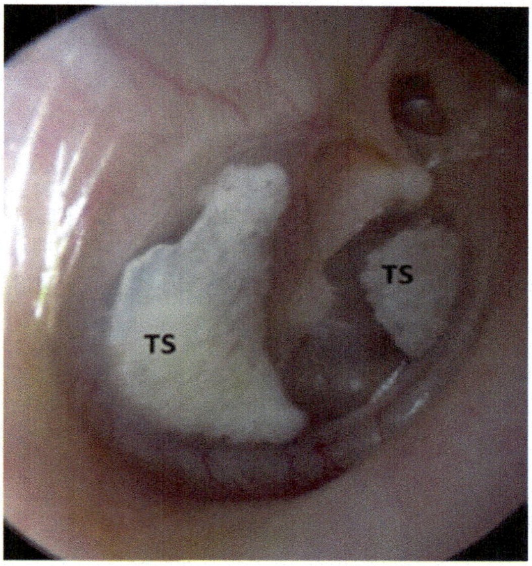

Fig. 7.4 Right ear tympanosclerosis

7.3.2 Intracranial Complications

- They are potentially life-threatening requiring immediate intervention, including suppurative thrombophlebitis of the lateral and/or cavernous sinuses, meningitis, and intracranial abscesses. The incidence has decreased dramatically in the era of antibiotics, with one large review estimating an overall rate of 0.1–2.0%. Signs of intracranial involvement are severe and include systemic symptoms of fever, seizure, headache, nausea, and vomiting, including focal neurological and otological symptoms. Patients who present with such complications should be evaluated and treated promptly. Empiric intravenous antibiotics should be started to cover the typical pathogens including most common offending organisms [2, 5]

Take-Home Messages

- A sound history and good clinical assessment can help early diagnosis of impending complications of acute and chronic otitis media.
- Despite early and prompt use of antibiotics, complications of acute and chronic otitis media can still develop.
- If untreated, the extracranial and intracranial complications can both be fatal.

References

1. Flint PW, Haughey BH, Thomas Robbins K, Lund VJ, Regan Thomas J, Niparko JK, Richardson MA, Lesperance MM. Cummings otolaryngology - head and neck surgery, 3-Volume Set. Expert Consult: Online and Print. 5th ed. Philadelphia: Mosby; 2010.
2. Lustig LR, Limb CJ, Baden R, LaSalvia MT. Chronic otitis media, cholesteatoma, and mastoiditis in adults, Up to date.
3. McCaig LF, Besser RE, Hughes JM. Trends in antimicrobial prescribing rates for children and adolescents. JAMA. 2002;287:3096.
4. Grijalva CG, Nuorti JP, Griffin MR. Antibiotic prescription rates for acute respiratory tract infections in US ambulatory settings. JAMA. 2009;302:758.
5. Brown S. Scott-Brown's otolaryngology, head and neck surgery. 7th ed. London: Hodder Arnold; 2008.
6. Lalwani AK. Current diagnosis and treatment, otolaryngology, head and neck surgery. New York: McGraw-Hill; 2012.
7. Sadoghi M, Dabirmoghaddam P. Otitic hydrocephalus: case report and literature review. Am J Otolaryngol. 2007;28:187.
8. Smith JA, Danner CJ. Complications of chronic otitis media and cholesteatoma. Otolaryngol Clin N Am. 2006;39:1237.
9. Yetiser S, Tosun F, Kazkayasi M. Facial nerve paralysis due to chronic otitis media. Otol Neurotol. 2002;23:580.

Otosclerosis

8

Salah Mansour, Ma'in Ali Al Shawabkeh,
Karen Nicolas, and Hassan Haidar

8.1 Introduction

Otosclerosis is a progressive temporal bone dysplasia that affects the human otic capsule selectively. It causes stapes fixation and is the most common cause of conductive hearing loss in adults with an intact tympanic membrane.

8.2 Epidemiology

It can be divided into clinical and histological [1]. Histological osteosclerosis is a situation when patients have the disease without causing symptoms. Clinical otosclerosis is more common in females (2/1). Family history is found in half of the patients [2, 3]. It is more common in white races and Indian [2, 3] and has a lower rate in Africans. Moreover, it has a tendency to progress during pregnancy [4].

8.3 Pathogenesis

The otic capsule bone normally has two main features that distinguish it from other bones: a very low remodeling rate [5] and the presence of immature cartilage called *Globuli Interossei* [6, 7].

Several factors are involved in the pathogenesis of otosclerosis, which can affect the physiological inhibition of bone turnover in the otic capsule leading to otic dysplasia known as otosclerosis:

1. Genetic inheritance: Mode of inheritance is autosomal dominant with incomplete penetrance [8].
2. Viral infection: It is believed that the persistence of measles infection in the otic capsule is one of the etiological factors of otosclerosis [9].
3. Hormonal effect: Pregnancy may lead to the progression of otosclerosis [4].
4. Autoimmunity: An elevated level of collagen II autoantibody was found in patients with otosclerosis [10].

Electronic Supplementary Material The online version of this chapter (https://doi.org/10.1007/978-3-030-54088-3_8) contains supplementary material, which is available to authorized users.

S. Mansour (✉)
Otology, Centre Medical Westmount Square, Westmount, QC, Canada

M. A. Al Shawabkeh
ENT Department, Hamad Medical Corporation, Doha, Qatar

K. Nicolas
Radiology Department, Bsalim Hospital, Beirut, Lebanon

H. Haidar
Hamad Medical Corporation, Doha, Qatar

A. Al-Qahtani et al. (eds.), *Textbook of Clinical Otolaryngology*,
https://doi.org/10.1007/978-3-030-54088-3_8

8.4 Histology

Classically, otosclerosis has two histological phases: the active phase (spongiosis) manifested by *bone resorption* and a stabilized phase (sclerosis) manifested by *bone deposition* [11, 12] (see Fig. 8.1). Otosclerosis can form in four stages:

1. Stage 1: The resorptive or active stage: bone osteoclasts resorb the endochondral bone.
2. Stage 2: The production of dysplastic immature basophilic bone.
3. Stage 3: The remodeling phase in which the basophilic bone becomes less vascular and replaced by more mature acidophilic bone with the laminated matrix.
4. Stage 4: The mature or otosclerotic stage; a new dense, compact bone with the formation of a woven pattern [11, 12].

The most common site of involvement is the oval window, followed by the round window and the pericochlear area [13].

8.5 Sites of Predilection

Two types of otosclerosis are described based on the location as follows (see Fig. 8.2):

1. **Fenestral involvement** of the oval window and round window niche. Oval window involvement is more commonly found in the *fissula ante-fenestram* in front of the vestibule. Round window otosclerosis is observed in 13% of patients with conductive hearing loss (CHL) and stapedial otosclerosis [7].
2. **Retrofenestral** is the involvement of the pericochlear otic capsule. Usually, it is associated with fenestral otosclerosis. Pure cochlear otosclerosis can cause sensorineural hearing loss (SNHL) without CHL. The earlier the involvement occurs, the more severe the symptoms will be [13, 14].

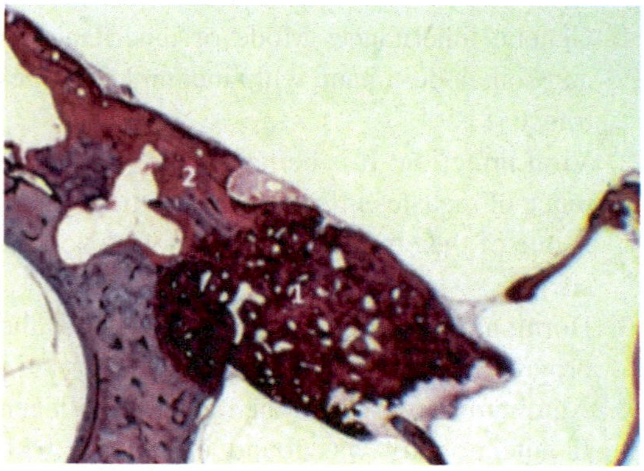

Fig. 8.1 Axial cut of right temporal bone at the level of fissula ante-fenestram showing the two phases of otosclerosis at the same time, active phase (1) and stabilized phase (2) [7]

8.6 Clinical Manifestations

1. **Hearing loss**: progressive CHL in a patient with a normal otoscopy without a history of head trauma or ear infection may indicate otosclerosis. In 10% of the cases, patients complain of mixed hearing loss due to the involvement of the cochlea. Seventy to 80% of cases show bilateral involvement. *Paracusis of Willis* is a phenomenon reported by patients with otosclerosis in which they hear better in a noisy environment [15].
2. **Tinnitus**: Roaring or hissing, but it can be of pulsatile quality due to the hypervascularity in otosclerotic areas [16].
3. **Dizziness**: It is seen in 25–30% of the cases. It can be due to otolithic dysfunction. Vertigo can also be due to endolymphatic hydrops or Meniere's disease, revealed by vestibular evoked myogenic potential (VEMP), and that becomes an important issue to be kept in mind while considering a surgical treatment for such patients [17, 18].

8.7 Clinical Evaluation

1. Otoscopy: shows normal TM. Rarely Schwartze's sign can be seen.
2. Tuning fork: in the early stages, Rinne is negative at 256 Hz only. As the disease progresses, 512 and 1024 Hz forks, Rinne will be negative.
3. Audiological testing:
   (a) <u>Pure tone audiogram</u>: At the start of clinical otosclerosis, a progressive low-frequency

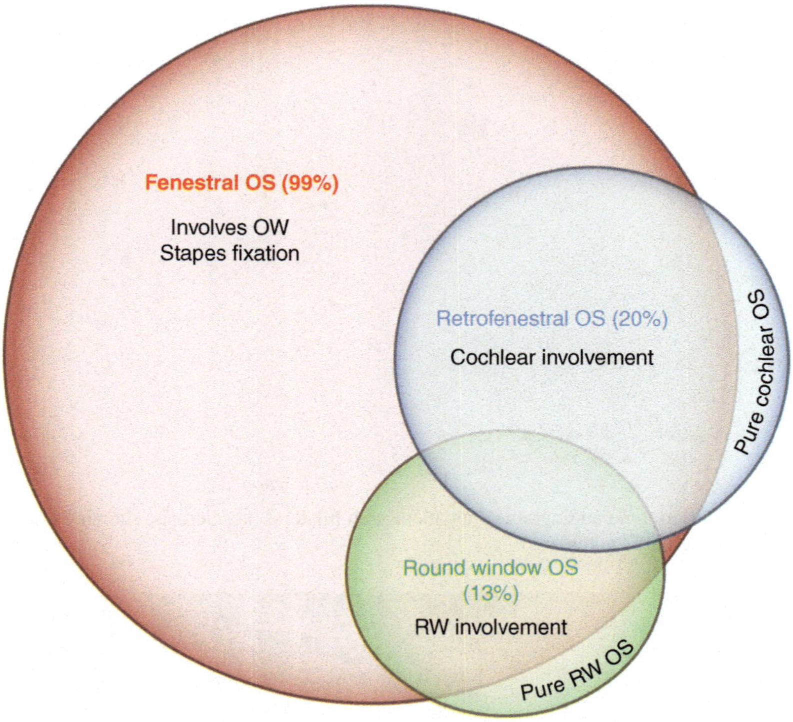

Fig. 8.2 Types of otosclerosis

conductive hearing loss is shown and then high-frequency CHL will occur, changing the audiogram to a flat pattern. If there is no cochlear involvement, then the hearing loss will be conductive with a maximum air-bone gap up to 40 or 50 dB. In the cochlear type, there will be mixed hearing loss in the mid frequencies giving cookie bite appearance [19]. Stapes fixation can give Carhart's notch with an elevation of bone conduction threshold 5 dB at 500 Hz, 10 dB at 1000 Hz, 15 dB at 2000 Hz, and 5 dB at 4000 Hz. Word recognition and speech discrimination scores usually are normal unless there is significant SNHL (see Fig. 8.3).

(b) Tympanogram shows type A or type As.

(c) Stapedial reflex: if the stapes is not yet firmly fixed, it will show an on/off phenomenon. If stapes is fixed, then the stapedial reflex will be absent [20].

8.8 Imaging: High-Resolution CT Scan

CT is considered the gold standard for imaging of otosclerosis [21]: high sensitivity of 91% and 99% specificity. Evaluation of the following is as follows:

1. Oval window: A hypodense area in the fissula ante-fenestram is diagnostic of otosclerosis, footplate thickness being normal, moderately thickened, or even obliterative (above 0.8–0.9 mm) (Fig. 8.4).
2. Round window otosclerosis: A classification system of CT findings of round window otosclerosis (RW1–RW5) correlates with the extent of the pathology in relation to a preoperative and postoperative hearing results [7, 21]: RW1–RW2 do not have an impact on postoperative air-bone gap closure, and RW4–RW5 contraindicate stapedectomy (Fig. 8.5).

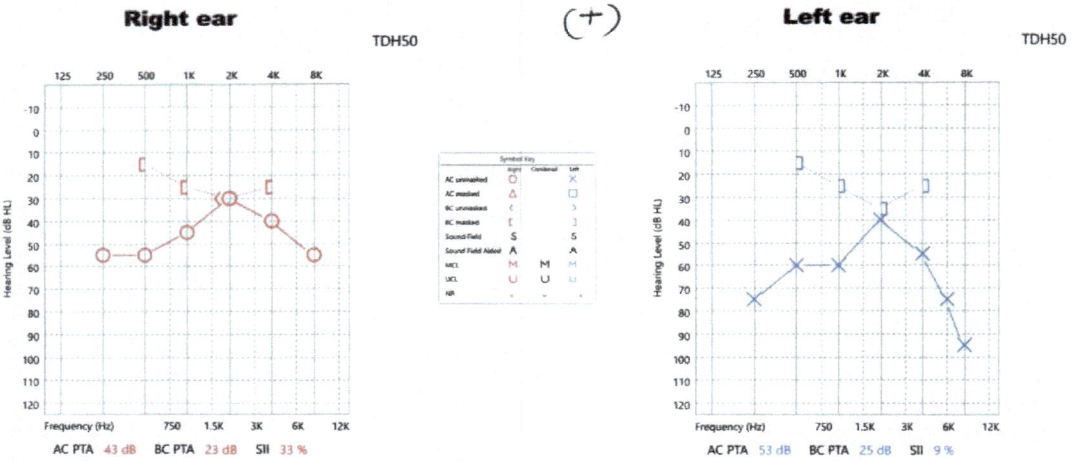

Fig. 8.3 Pure tone audiogram of a patient with bilateral otosclerosis, showing bilateral conductive hearing loss with bilateral Carhart's notch

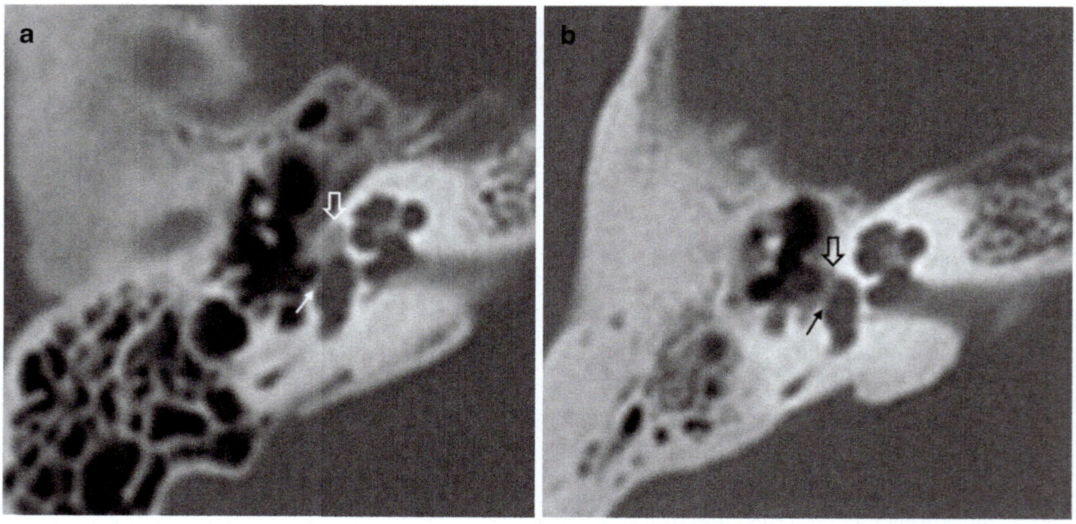

Fig. 8.4 Axial CT images of right ears with otosclerosis: (**a**) typical otosclerotic hypodense focus at the fissula ante-fenestram (empty arrow), dense footplate moderately thickened, (**b**) obliterative thickening of the footplate (arrow), with only small otosclerosis focus at the fissula ante-fenestram (empty arrow)

3. Retrofenestral otosclerosis: CT scan can show retro-fenestral disease invasion which is relevant to the prognosis (Fig. 8.6).
4. Associated abnormalities: like narrow oval window niche (Fig. 8.7), an overhanging facial nerve, or persistent stapedial artery could be found and are of high diagnostic interest for the surgical strategy [7].

Cone Beam-CT is positive to detect active otosclerotic focus that is characteristically hypodense to the surrounding hyperdense otic capsule bone; however, its sensitivity is low for the sclerotic phase of the disease process (hyperdense foci) and for pericochlear foci. When available, cone-beam is highly valuable for follow-up and postoperative prosthesis conditions [22, 23].

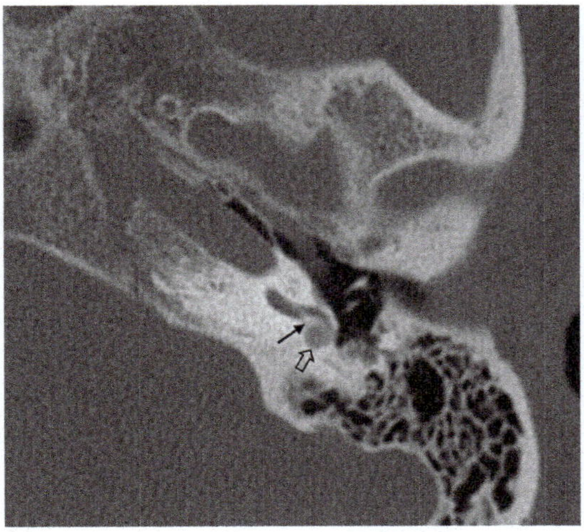

Fig. 8.5 Axial CT image of a left ear, showing otosclerosis of the round window (empty arrow) occupying the entire round window recess and adjacent calcification of the very proximal part of the retrofenestral scala tympani (arrow)

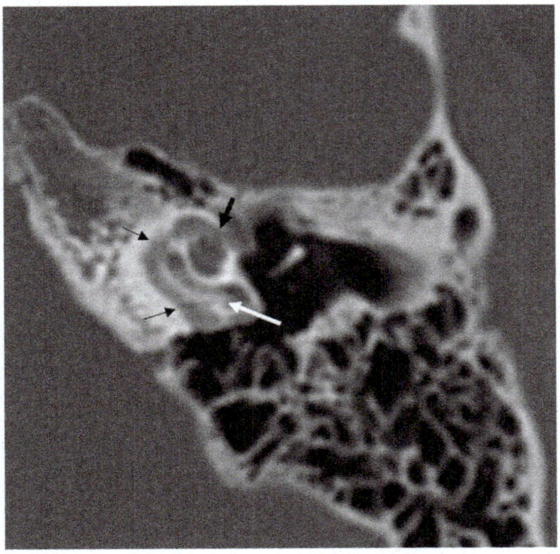

Fig. 8.6 Axial CT image with a complete pericochlear otosclerotic rim (black arrows), coming into close contact with the cochlear endosteum (thick black arrow). In addition, intracochlear calcifications concerning the scala tympani of the basal turn (white arrow)

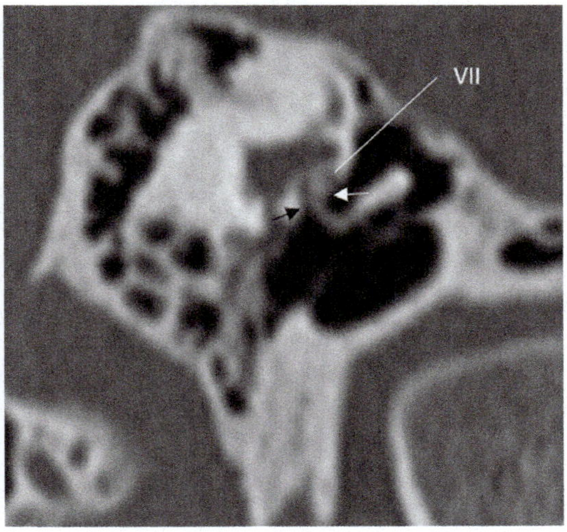

Fig. 8.7 Coronal CT image showing a reduced height of the oval window niche due to a large bony apposition in the superior part of the niche (white arrow), inferior border of the oval niche (black arrow), VII facial nerve

8.9 Stapes Surgery

8.9.1 Indications

1. CHL with at least 25 dB and negative Rinne at 512 Hz is the minimum requirement to propose surgery.
2. Speech discrimination more than 60% in order to obtain a favorable hearing outcome.

8.9.2 Contraindications

1. Stapes surgery of the only hearing ear.
2. Chronic otitis media or externa.
3. Labyrinthine hydrops.
4. Unfavorable systemic disease.
5. Patients above 70 years old as they have more chance of worsening of speech discrimination and perilymphatic fistula complication.
6. Pregnancy.

Informed Consent is mandatory and must be clear.

8.9.3 Surgical Steps (Video 8.1)

1. Elevation of the tympanomeatal flap after assessment of the Malleus head mobility.
2. Curetting the scutum for appropriate exposure of the facial nerve, round window, and pyramidal process.
3. Assessment of the mobility of the ossicles.
4. Separation of the incudostapedial joint.
5. Stapedial tendon sectioning.

6. Removal of the posterior crura by microdrill, micro scissor, or laser.
7. Down fracturing the remaining stapes suprastructure.
8. Measuring the distance between footplate and incus.
9. Fenestration by perforator, microdrill, or laser. The best location is the posterior half of the footplate.
10. Insertion and crimping of the piston. The prosthesis should extend at least 0.25 mm into the vestibule. It is usually 4.25–4.5 mm in length.

8.9.3.1 Stapedectomy vs. Stapedotomy

See Table 8.1 for a comparison between stapedectomy and stapedotomy [24–30].

8.9.3.2 Laser in Stapes Surgery

Using laser in stapes surgery may cause less postoperative SNHL incidence and give better control of hemostasis. However, there is no difference in the result regarding postoperative vertigo and air-bone gap closure [31].

Advantages of stapes laser surgery:

1. Good hemostasis.
2. Increased precision.
3. Less risk of the floating footplate.
4. Decreased risk of perilymph leakage.

Table 8.1 Comparison between stapedectomy and stapedotomy [24–30]

	Stapedotomy	Stapedectomy
Outcome of hearing	Good hearing over all frequencies and better postoperative discrimination score, and better gain in high frequencies	Good hearing in speech frequencies with poor gain at high frequencies hearing (4–8 kHz)
Outcome of tinnitus	High rate of tinnitus suppression	High rate of tinnitus suppression
Postoperative vertigo	Low	High
Floating of footplate	Low	High
Perilymphatic fistula	Rare	4%
Migration of prosthesis	Lower risk	Higher risk
CHL recurrence	4%	12%

See Table 8.2 and Fig. 8.8 for comparison between Argon/KTP laser and CO_2 laser.

Microdrill can be used to perform the fenestration of the footplate during stapes surgery. It

Table 8.2 Comparison between Argon/KTP laser and CO_2 laser

Laser	Advantages	Disadvantages
Argon/ KTP	• Short wavelength (514 nm for Argon, 532 nm for KTP) • Visible light • Good hemostasis • Well absorbed by hemoglobin • Delivered by a fiberoptic handpiece	• Not well absorbed by bone • Higher penetration of radiation • Potential damage to the inner ear structures
CO_2	• Long wavelength (10,000 nm) • Strong bone absorption • Less penetration to surrounding structures • Less risk of inner ear trauma • Available with a fiberoptic micro handpiece	• Invisible, requiring aiming beam (Neon/ helium) • Absorbed by collagen and perilymph. Risk of heating of the perilymph

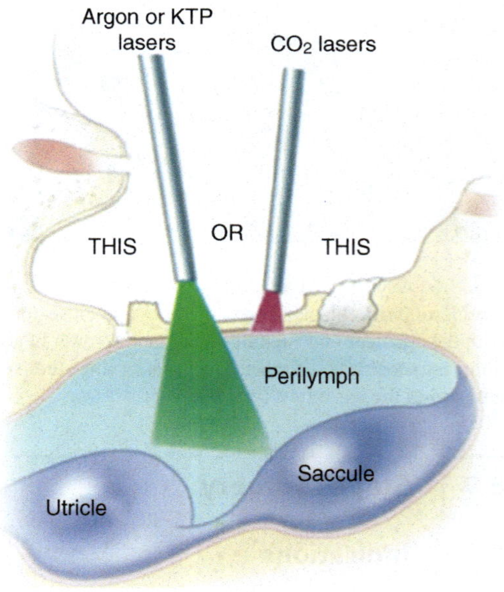

Fig. 8.8 Argon or KTP laser can penetrate till the utricle and saccule. The CO_2 laser is absorbed by perilymph causing heating side effects [7]

gives a hole with regular margins similar to a piston shaft, without causing acoustic trauma to the ear [32]. It is appreciated in obliterative otosclerosis.

8.9.3.3 Prosthesis Selection

- Material: Titanium and Teflon are the most commonly used material for the piston.
- Length: should be 0.5 mm longer than the distance between the footplate and medial edge of the incus. Another 0.25 mm should be added if the piston required bending during insertion.
- Diameter: the larger the diameter, the better the hearing will be, but it can cause more damage to the inner ear. The best diameter is 0.6 mm, with 0.4 mm reserved for narrow OW [33].
- Adequate crimping of the prosthesis to the long process of the incus is essential for energy transmission. It can be crimped by heat, by forceps, or it comes as clipping piston [34].
- Oval window sealing with fat or vein for patient at risk for barotrauma (divers and pilots).

8.9.3.4 Intraoperative Challenges in Stapes Surgery [7]

1. Malleus ankylosis: it may be congenital or acquired. Palpation of malleus should be done before addressing the stapes. Unrecognized malleus fixation can be the cause of failure of air-bone gap closure postoperatively.
2. High jugular bulb: jugular bulb can be laterally located even near the annulus rendering it vulnerable to injury during the elevation of the tympanomeatal flap (Fig. 8.9).
3. Overhanging facial nerve (Fig. 8.10) covering a large part of the footplate, then the surgery should not be done. The laser should be avoided in these cases (see Video 8.2).
4. Obliterative otosclerosis: in which a thick otosclerotic deposit invades and covers the footplate. A large stapedotomy is the procedure of choice in these cases (Fig. 8.11) [35].
5. Incidental disarticulation of the incus: In this case, the incus should be relocated into its anatomical place. However, if the incus can not be relocated, then malleus attachment for the prosthesis is the best solution.
6. Narrow oval window niche (Video 8.3).
7. Round window otosclerosis: A preoperative CT scan is required for diagnosis purposes (see Fig. 8.5).
8. Perilymph oozer and gusher: oozer is usually due to a large vestibular aqueduct and treated by perichondrium or vein seal. Gusher is rare and usually due to a defect of cribrosa of internal auditory meatus. A preoperative CT scan can suspect a Gusher, but not in all cases (Fig. 8.12).

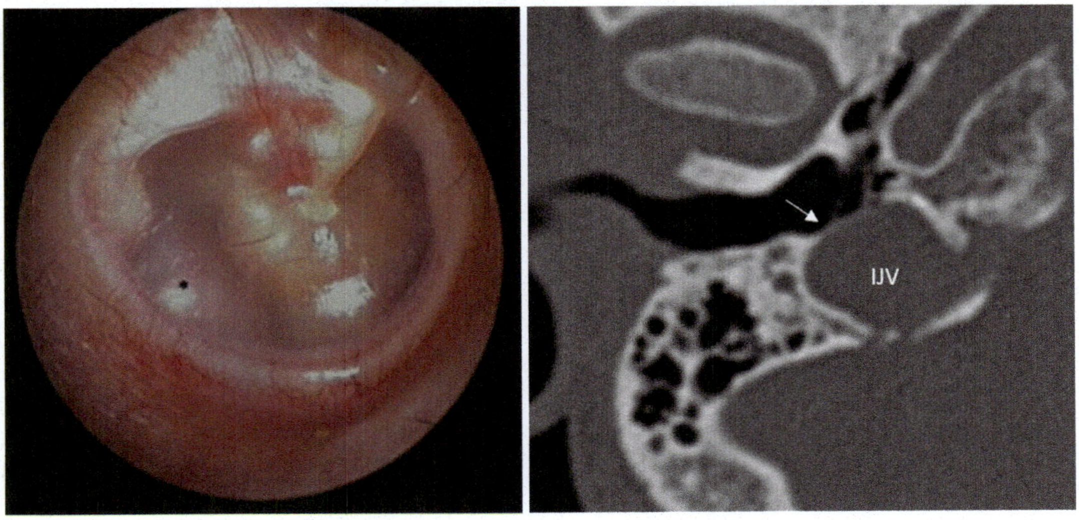

Fig. 8.9 Large jugular bulb (IVJ) coming in close contact with the tympanic membrane (arrow)

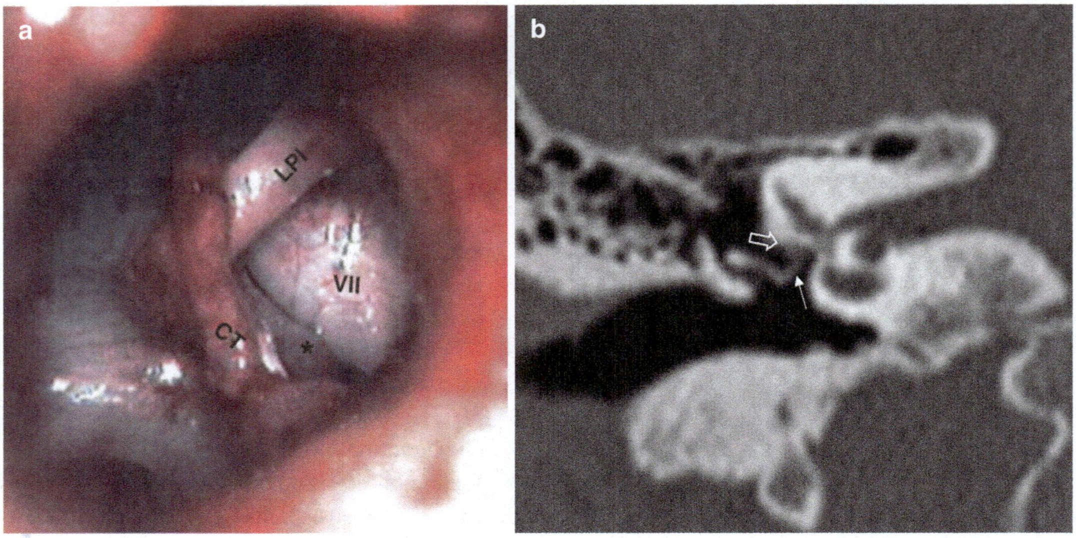

Fig. 8.10 A Left ear stapes surgery challenged by the overhanging facial nerve (VII) that is lying on the crura of the stapes (asterisk in **a**) and narrowing the oval window niche significantly. (**b**) Coronal CT showing a procident facial nerve (empty arrow) in front of the oval window, in proximity to the stapes suprastructure (arrow)

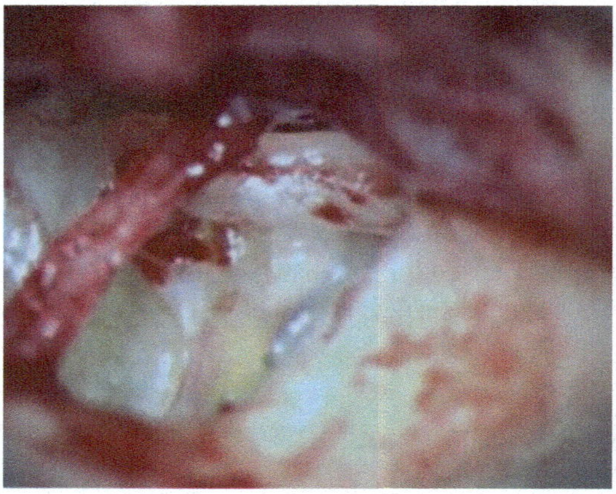

Fig. 8.11 Left middle ear with obliterative otosclerosis

9. Persistent stapedial artery (Fig. 8.13): a rare incident, CT finding of the absence of foramen spinosum should alert the surgeon of this pathology. The procedure should be aborted.

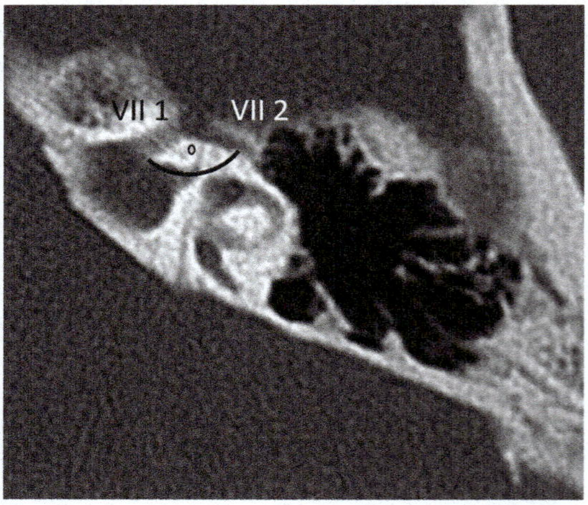

Fig. 8.12 Axial CT of a left ear, showing enlargement of the angle between the first and second portion of the facial nerve, highly suspicious of Gusher syndrome

8.9.4 Outcome of Stapes Surgery

1. Closure of air-bone gap to less than 10 dB in 95% of the cases [36].
2. Improvement in tinnitus in 89% of cases [37].

8.9.5 Complications of Stapes Surgery

1. Taste disturbance: due to chorda tympani injury. Usually, the symptoms are transient, and recovery can happen within 3–6 months [38]. Relevant information for contralateral Stapes surgery.

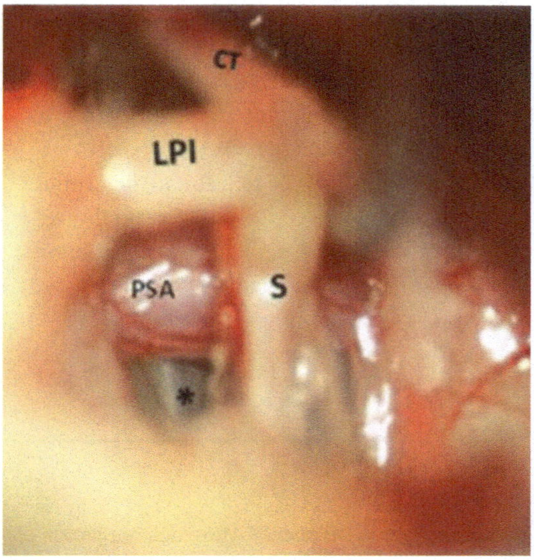

Fig. 8.13 Right ear otosclerosis with the persistent stapedial artery (PSA). The posterior half of the footplate is visible (asterisk) and could be exceptionally accessible for fenestration

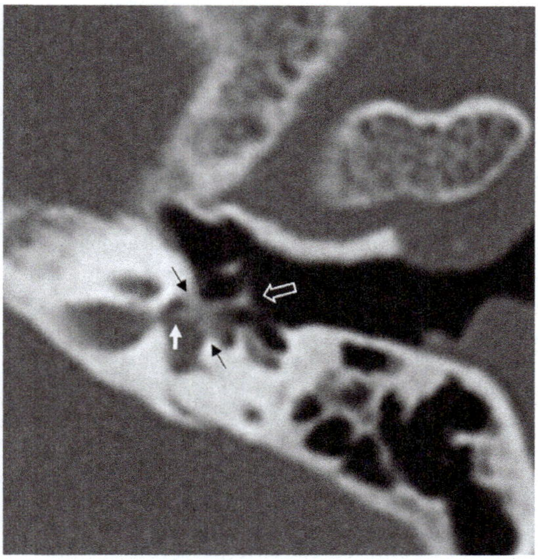

Fig. 8.14 Reformatted CT-Image along the prosthesis axis: stapes prosthesis laterally in contact with the long process of incus and the tympanic membrane (empty arrow), medially the long piston of the stapes prosthesis penetrates deep into the vestibule (white arrow). Thickened footplate between the black arrows

2. Dizziness or vertigo: it can be due to labyrinthitis, which is self-limited and resolves within 3–6 days [39]. Other factors can cause dizziness like the heating effect of laser, long prosthesis, and depressed footplate fragment [40]. Long-lasting dizziness requires exploration to rule out a perilymph fistula.
3. Sensorineural hearing loss: less than 1% in experienced hands [41]. It can be caused by perilymph fistula, granuloma formation, or very long prosthesis that penetrates deep into the vestibule (Fig. 8.14).
4. Perilymph fistula: primary perilymph fistula occurs just after the fenestration and persists long after, while secondary perilymph fistula appears after a period of time of successful sealing. The latter is usually due to the dislocation of the prosthesis. Perilymph fistula indicates explorative tympanotomy.
5. Reparative granuloma: it is a reactive granulation tissue that occurs after the surgery. It can invade the vestibule leading to hearing loss, tinnitus, and dizziness that appear after 7–12 days after the surgery. Most of the cases end in a profound permanent sensorineural hearing loss (Fig. 8.15).

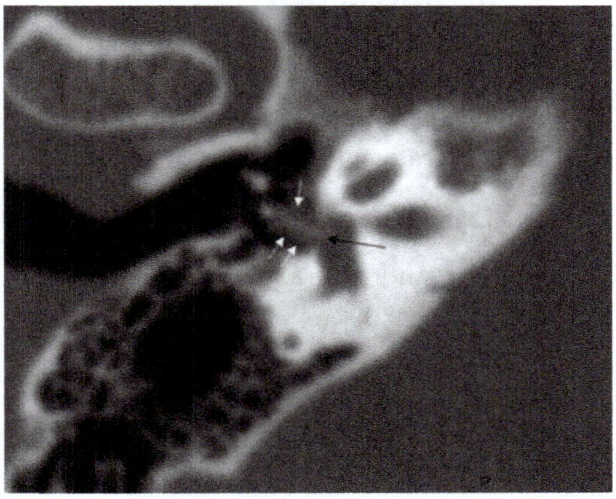

Fig. 8.15 Reformatted CT along the prosthesis axis: hazy condensations around the piston (white arrows) due to the proliferative inflammatory tissue of the granuloma. Intravestibular tip of the prosthesis: black arrow

6. Facial palsy: an immediate post stapedectomy facial palsy is usually due to excessive local anesthesia infiltration. Delayed palsy is usually due to reactivation of the VZ virus or Bell's palsy.
7. Otitis media: Rare, but can cause sensorineural hearing loss. The patient should be admit-

ted to the hospital to receive antibiotics and steroid. Ear packs, if still in the canal, should be removed.

8.9.5.1 Failure in Stapes Surgery

Causes of persistent conductive hearing loss	Causes of recurrent conductive hearing loss
1. Malleus ankylosis 2. Round window otosclerosis 3. Third window 4. Short prosthesis or small diameter prosthesis 5. Prosthesis abutting fenestration margin	1. Resorptive osteitis of the incus 2. Displacement of the prosthesis 3. New bone formation in the oval window 4. Obliteration of the round window by otosclerosis

The most common cause to perform revision stapes surgery is prosthesis displacement followed by incus erosion.

8.10 Conservative Treatment of Hearing Loss in Otosclerosis

1. Hearing aid.
2. BAHA or middle ear implant.
3. Medical treatment: Given in cases of *active* otosclerosis. Signs and symptoms like the presence of Schwartz sign and onset or worsening of tinnitus, vertigo, or hearing loss can indicate active disease. The options for medical therapy include:
   (a) Sodium Fluoride: change the active lesion to an inactive lesion.
   (b) Bisphosphonates: it induces apoptosis in osteoclasts, reducing toxic enzymes' production secondary to abnormal bone metabolism.

Take-Home Messages

- Otosclerosis typically presents with slowly progressive unilateral or bilateral deafness, tinnitus, and vertigo may also occur.
- The hearing loss encountered in these patients can be conductive, sensorineural, or mixed.
- In patients with typical clinical features and uncomplicated conductive hearing loss, audiometry tests are mandatory to establish the diagnosis.
- Imaging study is helpful to determine the disease stages and differential diagnosis, assess associated anatomic abnormalities, and evaluate postoperative prosthesis status.

References

1. Schuknecht HF, Barber W. Histologic variants in otosclerosis. Laryngoscope. 1985;95:1307–17.
2. Altmann F, Glasgold A, Macduff JP. The incidence of otosclerosis as related to race and sex. Ann Otol Rhinol Laryngol. 1967;76:377–92.
3. Cawthorne T. Otosclerosis. J Laryngol Otol. 1955;9:437–56.
4. Precechtel A. Determination of the effect of pregnancy on the activation of otosclerosis. Acta Otolaryngol. 1967;63:121–7.
5. Zehnder AF, Kristiansen AG, Adams JC, Kujawa SG, Merchant SN, McKenna MJ. Osteoprotegrin knockout mouse demonstrate abnormal remodeling of the otic capsule and progressive hearing loss. Laryngoscope. 2006;116:201.
6. Sørensen MS, Jørgensen MB, Bretlau P. Drift barriers in the postcartilaginous development of the mammalian otic capsule. Eur Arch Otorhinolaryngol. 1992;249:56–61.
7. Mansour S, Nicolas K, Ahmad HH. Round window otosclerosis: radiologic classification and clinical correlations. Otol Neurotol. 2011;32:384–92.
8. Moumoulidis I, Axon P, Baguley D, Reid E. A review on the genetics of otosclerosis. Clin Otolaryngol. 2007;32(4):239–47. Review.
9. Niedermeyer HP, Gantumur T, Neubert WJ, Arnold W. Measles virus and otosclerosis. Adv Otorhinolaryngol. 2007;65:86–92.
10. Yoo TJ. Etiopathogenesis of otosclerosis: a hypothesis. Ann Otol Rhinol Laryngol. 1984;93:28–33.
11. Cureoglu S, Schachern PA, Ferlito A, Rinaldo A, Tsuprun V, Paparella MM. Otosclerosis: etiopathogenesis and histopathology. Am J Otolaryngol. 2006;27(5):334–40.
12. Valvassori GE. Imaging of otosclerosis. Otolaryngol Clin N Am. 1993;26:359–71.
13. Hueb MM, Goycoolea MV, Paparella MM, Oliveira JA. Otosclerosis: the University of Minnesota temporal bone collection. Otolaryngol Head Neck Surg. 1991;105:396–405.
14. Schuknecht HF, Kirchner JC. Cochlear otosclerosis: fact or fantasy? Laryngoscope. 1974;84:766–82.

15. van Loon MC, Merkus P, Smit CF, Smits C, Witte BI, Hensen EF. Stapedotomy in cochlear implant candidates with far advanced otosclerosis: a systematic review of the literature and meta-analysis. Otol Neurotol. 2014;35(10):1707–14.
16. Gristwood RE, Venables WN. Otosclerosis and chronic tinnitus. Ann Otol Rhinol Laryngol. 2003;112:398–403.
17. Sando I, Hemenway WG, Miller DR, Black FO. Vestibular pathology in otosclerosis temporal bone histopathological report. Laryngoscope. 1974;84:593–605.
18. Paparella MM, Chasin WD. Otosclerosis and vertigo. J Laryngol Otol. 1966;80:511–9.
19. Hannley MT. Audiologic characteristics of the patient with otosclerosis. Otolaryngol Clin N Am. 1993;26(3):373–87.
20. Bel J, Causse J, Michaux P, Cézard R, Canut Y, Tapon J. Mechanical explanation of the on-off effect (diphasic impedance change) in otospongiosis. Audiology. 1976;15(2):128–40.
21. Lagleyre S, Sorrentino T, Calmels MN, Shin YJ, Escudé B, Deguine O, Fraysse B. Reliability of high-resolution CT scan in diagnosis of otosclerosis. Otol Neurotol. 2009;30(8):1152–9.
22. Révész P, Liktor B, Liktor B, Sziklai I, Gerlinger I, Karosi T. Comparative analysis of preoperative diagnostic values of HRCT and CBCT in patients with histologically diagnosed otosclerotic stapes footplates. Eur Arch Otorhinolaryngol. 2016;273(1):63–72.
23. Ariadna M, Cozma S, Murariu O, Radulescu L, Haba MSC, Vreme RM, Haba D, Iasi/ RO. ECR 2017 diagnostic value of CBCT in otosclerosis. Poster No 2283; 2017.
24. Fisch U. Stapedotomy versus stapedectomy. Otol Neurotol. 2009;30(8):1166–7.
25. Cremers CW, Beusen JM, Huygen PL. Hearing gain after stapedotomy, partial platinectomy, or total stapedectomy for otosclerosis. Ann Otol Rhinol Laryngol. 1991;100:959–61.
26. Spandow O, Soderberg O, Bohlin L. Long-term results in otosclerotic patients operated by stapedectomy and stapedotomy. Scand Audiol. 2000;29:186–90.
27. Persson P, Harder H, Magnuson B. Hearing results in otosclerosis surgery after partial stapedectomy, total stapedectomy and stapedotomy. Acta Otolaryngol. 1997;117:94–9.
28. Fisch U. Stapedectomy versus stapedectomy. Am J Otol. 1982;4:112–7.
29. Esquivel CR, Mamikoglu B, Wiet RJ. Long-term results of small fenestra stapedectomy compared with large fenestra technique. Laryngoscope. 2002;112:1338–41.
30. House HP, Hansen MR, Al Dakhail AAA, House JW. Stapedectomy versus stapedotomy: comparison of results with long-term follow-up. Laryngoscope. 2002;112:2046–50.
31. Wegner I, Kamalski DM, Tange RA, Vincent R, Stegeman I, van der Heijden GJ, Grolman W. Laser versus conventional fenestration in stapedotomy for otosclerosis: a systematic review. Laryngoscope. 2014;124(7):1687–93.
32. Yavuz H, Caylakli F, Ozer F, Ozluoglu LN. Reliability of microdrill stapedotomy: comparison with pick stapedotomy. Otol Neurotol. 2007;28(8):998–1001.
33. Rosowski JJ, Merchant SN. Mechanical and acoustic analysis of middle ear reconstruction. Am J Otol. 1995;16:486–97.
34. Huber AM, Ma F, Felix H, Linder T. Stapes prosthesis attachment: the effect of crimping on sound transfer in otosclerosis surgery. Laryngoscope. 2003;113:853–8.
35. Gierek T, Witkowska M, Zbrowska-Bielska D, Klimczak-Gołab L. Analysis of results of stapedotomy in patients with obliterative otosclerosis. Otolaryngol Pol. 2006;60(3):377–83.
36. Vincent R, Sperling NM, Oates J, Jindal M. Surgical findings and long-term hearing results in 3050 Stapedotomies for primary otosclerosis: a prospective study with the otology-neurotology database. Otol Neurotol. 2006;27:S25–47.
37. Gersdorff M, Nouwen J, Gilain C, Decat M, Betsch C. Tinnitus and otsclerosis. Eur Arch Otorhinolaryngol. 2000;257:314–6.
38. Berling Holm K, Knutsson J, Strömbäck K, Danckwardt Lillieström N, Papatziamos G, Rosenblad A, Von Unge M. Taste disturbance after stapes surgery: an evaluation of frequency, severity, duration, and quality-of-life. Acta Otolaryngol. 2017;137(1):39–43.
39. Birch L, Elbrond O. Stapedectomy and vertigo. Clin Otolaryngol. 1985;10:217–23.
40. Mansour S, Magnan J, Haidar H, et al. Comprehensive and clinical anatomy of the middle ear. Berlin: Springer; 2013. p. 49–81.
41. Glasscock ME III, Storper IS, Haynes DS, Bohrer PS. Twenty-five years of experience with stapedectomy. Laryngoscope. 1995;105:899–904.

Congenital Hearing Loss

9

Abdulsalam Al-Qahtani, Zaid Altamimi,
and Reni K. Chandran

9.1 Introduction

Hearing loss present at birth (congenital hearing loss) is categorized according to the underlying pathology to hereditary (syndromic or non-syndromic), non-hereditary, and idiopathic. Three types of hearing loss can be induced depending on the site of the lesion: conductive, sensorineural, or a combination of both (mixed) [1].

9.2 Neonatal Hearing Screening

Newborn hearing screening programs show that the incidence of congenital hearing loss is 2–4 children per 1000 births, and it is considered as the most frequently occurring birth defect in the US [2, 3]. Mutations in GJB2 account for 50% of people with severe-to-profound congenital autosomal-recessive non-syndromic hearing loss [4].

Neonatal hearing screening programs are available for the early detection of this condition. More than 50% of cases of permanent hearing impairment in childhood can be detected shortly after birth [5]. Using the 1-3-6 model intends to screen all newborns within the first month of birth for early diagnosis and subsequent early management with a better developmental outcome [6]. View the algorithm below to check the steps of the screening. However, passing the neonatal screening does not rule out hearing impairment in childhood. Progressive or late-onset hearing loss can be undetected by neonatal screening programs [6].

A. Al-Qahtani (✉)
Hamad Medical Corporation, Doha, Qatar

Otology Clinical Fellow, Hamad Medical Corporation, Doha, Qatar
e-mail: aalqahtani@hamad.qa

Z. Altamimi
Otology Clinical Fellow, Hamad Medical Corporation, Doha, Qatar
e-mail: Zaltamimi@hamad.qa

R. K. Chandran
Audiology, Hamad Medical Corporation, Doha, Qatar
e-mail: RChandran1@hamad.qa

A. Al-Qahtani et al. (eds.), *Textbook of Clinical Otolaryngology*,
https://doi.org/10.1007/978-3-030-54088-3_9

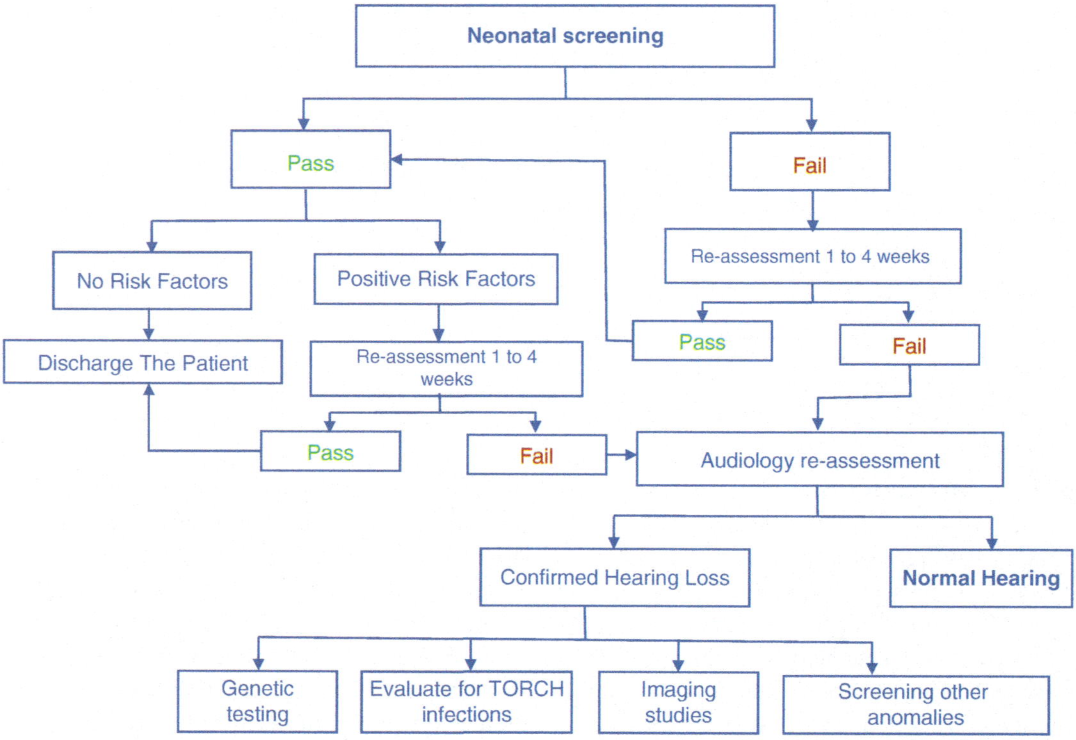

9.3 Evaluation of a Child with Congenital Hearing Loss

The general approach to evaluating the child with suspected congenital hearing loss includes the following:

- **History**: pregnancy history, perinatal and postnatal period, NICU admission, postnatal infection, ototoxic medications, co-existing medical conditions, family history of hearing loss in first- and second-degree relatives, consanguinity, and ethnic origin.
- **Physical examination**: a full head and neck examination should be performed to including any dysmorphic features, the shape, and position of the external ears, neck examination for cysts, sinuses, and scars (branchio-oto-renal syndrome), swelling of the thyroid gland (may indicate Pendred syndrome), and unusual pigmentation of the hair, skin, or eyes (which may indicate an auditory pigmentary disorder).
- **Investigation**: the following should be considered: genetic testing, CT/MRI imaging, thyroid function tests, cardiology evaluation (Echo and ECG, for possible association with Jervell and Lange-Nielsen syndrome or congenital heart conditions), or ophthalmology assessment (electroretinogram if suspected Usher syndrome).

Risk factors for permanent congenital, delayed, or progressive hearing loss in childhood are described in Box 9.1 [5].

Box 9.1 Risk Factors for Permanent Congenital, Delayed or Progressive Hearing Loss in Childhood

- Hearing, speech, language, or developmental delay
- Family history of hearing loss
- Neonatal intensive care unit stay >5 days **or** receiving any of the following treatments: extra corporal membrane oxygenation, assisted ventilation, ototoxic drugs (e.g., gentamycin and tobramycin), loop diuretics, or exchange transfusion for hyperbilirubinemia
- In utero infections (toxoplasmosis, rubella, cytomegalovirus, herpes simplex, or syphilis)
- Craniofacial anomalies, including ear tags, ear pits, and anomalies that involve the outer ear, external auditory canal, and temporal bone
- Physical findings associated with a syndrome known to cause permanent hearing loss (e.g.,, white forelock)
- Syndromes associated with congenital hearing loss or progressive or late-onset hearing loss
- Neurodegenerative disorders or sensorimotor neuropathies
- Confirmed bacterial or viral meningitis
- Head trauma, especially of the basal skull, or temporal bone fractures that require hospitalization
- Chemotherapy

9.4 Categories of Congenital Hearing Loss

1. **Idiopathic (25%).**
2. **Hereditary (50%):**
   - **Non-syndromic (70%)**: more common, the prefix "DFN" to designate non-syndromic DeaFNess, DFN followed by an A implies dominant inheritance, whereas B implies recessive inheritance and X implies X-linked inheritance. Autosomal recessive (AR) in (75–80%), GJ2B mutation (autosomal recessive) coding for the protein gap junction beta 2 (also called connexin 26) results in impaired Potassium (K^+) exchange. Autosomal dominant (AD) in (20–25%), X-linked in (2–4%), and mitochondrial in <1% [5].
   - **Syndromic (30%)**: Divided into AR, AD, and X-linked. The most common syndromic form of hereditary SNHL is Usher syndrome [7], and other AR syndromes include Pendred syndrome and Jervell and Lange–Nielsen Syndrome. The most common AD syndrome is Waardenburg [7], and others include Treacher–Collins Syndrome (Fig. 9.1), Branchio-oto-renal Syndrome (mainly mixed hearing loss), Neurofibromatosis Type 2, and Stickler Syndrome. X-linked includes Alport's syndrome. Box 9.2 describes the features of the most common congenital hereditary hearing loss syndromes.
3. **Non-hereditary (25%)**
   - **Malformations**: arrest in normal development may result in hearing impairment depending on the timing and nature of the developmental insult. About 65% of such abnormalities are bilateral, and 35% are unilateral. Malformations include *Membranous* (Alexander's Aplasia, Scheibe Deformity, and Siebenmann–Bing Dysplasia) and *Osseous and Membranous* (Cochlear Hypoplasia, Mondini, Common Cavity, Cochlear Aplasia, Michel Aplasia, and Small Internal Auditory Canal). Mondini malformation is the most common type of cochlear malformation [1].
     - **Alexander aplasia** is one of the membranous malformations, where cochlear duct differentiation at the level of the basal coil is limited with resultant effects on the organ of Corti and the ganglion cells. Hearing assessment shows high-frequency sensorineural hearing loss with adequate residual hearing in the low frequencies, and amplification devices can be used.
     - **Scheibe aplasia (cochleosaccular dysplasia or Pars Inferior dysplasia)** is one of the membranous malformations, and it is a relatively common cochlear malformation. Scala media is compromised due to the failure of the organ of Corti development affecting the tectorial and the Reissner's membranes. It is

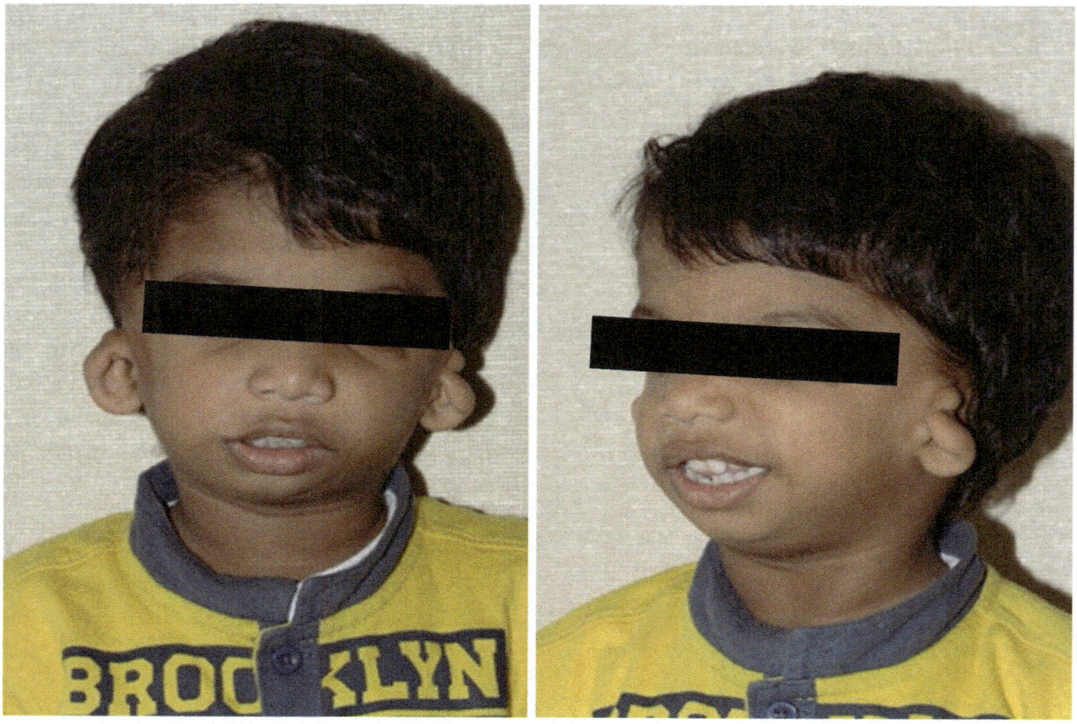

Fig. 9.1 Treacher–Collins syndrome

reported in Jervell and Lange Nielsen, Usher, and Waardenburg syndromes as well as in congenital rubella infants. Amplification devices with rehabilitative intervention are beneficial in many of these children.

- **Michel aplasia** is one of the osseous and membranous malformations, where there is complete agenesis of the petrous portion of the temporal bone resulting in absence of normal inner structures and therefore complete deafness. The developmental arrest occurs early prior to the end of the third gestational week.
- **Mondini deformity** is one of the osseous and membranous malformations, and it is the most common type of cochlear malformation [1]. The developmental arrest occurs at the sixth week of gestation. It presents with an incomplete partition of the cochlea where it contains only about 1.5 turns with only the basal coil and absence of the apical modiolus and interscalar septum. Mondini deformity is associated with enlarged vestibular aqueduct and dilated vestibule. It is seen in Pendred, Waardenburg, Treacher–Collins, and CHARGE syndromes, and it is also seen in congenital cytomegalovirus (CMV) infection.
- **Enlarged Vestibular Aqueduct Syndrome** is defined as a vestibular aqueduct measuring more than 1.5 mm on CT scan. It is thought to be one of the most common congenital causes of sensorineural hearing loss. It presents with early onset bilateral progressive sensorineural hearing loss. It is associated with Pendred syndrome, vestibular anomalies, Mondini malformation, and other cochlear anomalies. Mainstay of treatment is conservative management, including avoidance of head trauma and contact sports.

- **TORCH Infections**: It includes Toxoplasmosis, Other (syphilis, varicella-zoster, parvovirus B19), Rubella, Cytomegalovirus (CMV), and Herpes.
  - Cytomegalovirus: the most common cause of congenital viral deafness [8].
  - Mumps: the most common infectious cause of acquired sensorineural hearing loss.
- **Other perinatal factors**: prematurity, low birth weight, teratogenic drugs, maternal diabetes, hyperbilirubinemia, and neonatal sepsis.

Box 9.2 Overview of Congenital Hearing Loss Syndromes

Syndrome	Features	Comments
Autosomal recessive		
Usher syndrome	Sensorineural hearing loss, retinitis pigmentosa, and vestibular symptoms **Type 1**, profound hearing loss, vestibular symptoms, and retinitis pigmentosa beginning in first decade **Type 2**, stable mild to severe hearing loss and retinitis pigmentosa in first to second decade **Type 3**, progressive hearing loss, variable vestibular symptoms, and variable onset of retinitis pigmentosa	Commonest cause of deafness with blindness, early diagnosis of retinitis pigmentosa possible with electroretinography, and cochlear implants effective
Pendred's syndrome	Sensorineural hearing loss (severe to profound), goiter, and abnormality of the bony labyrinth (Mondini dysplasia or enlarged vestibular aqueduct)	Iodine transport defect diagnosed by perchlorate discharge test in those homozygous for Pendred's syndrome (SLC26A4) and euthyroid goiter
Jervell and Lange-Nielsen syndrome	Profound sensorineural hearing loss with prolongation of QT interval, syncopal episodes, and risk of sudden death	Should have a thorough cardiac evaluation, carriers also at risk for sudden death, and treatment effective
Autosomal dominant		
Waardenburg syndrome	Most common type of AD; hair (white forelock 1), eyes (heterochromia iridis) **Type 1**, white forelock and dystopia canthorum **Type 2**, dystopia absent **Type 3**, upper limb defects **Type 4**, increased incidence of Hirschsprung's disease	Hearing loss caused by defective migration of pigment cells to stria vascularis
Treacher–Collins syndrome	Conductive hearing loss, underdevelopment of facial bones (malar and zygomatic hypoplasia) with malformed ossicles, microtia, cleft palate; micrognathia, downward slanting eyes, coloboma of the eyelid	
Branchio-oto-renal (BOR) syndrome	Hearing loss; preauricular pits; malformed pinnae; Branchial cysts or fistulae; renal anomalies (structural malformations to agenesis)	
X-linked		
Alport's syndrome	Hematuria with progressive renal failure, progressive late-onset high-frequency sensorineural hearing loss; anterior lenticonus and macular flecks	Results from mutations in 1 of 3 collagen genes expressed in glomerular basement membrane

Take-Home Messages

- The most common prenatal cause of hearing loss is intrauterine infection (CMV).
- Mutations in GJB2 account for 50% of severe-to-profound autosomal-recessive non-syndromic deafness.
- The goal of newborn testing is to screen by 1 month of age, diagnose hearing loss by 3 months of age, and initiate intervention by 6 months of age.
- Screening based on risk factors only detects 50% of infants with substantial congenital hearing loss.

References

1. Shibata SB, Eliot Shearer A, Richard JH. Genetic sensorineural hearing loss, Chap. 148. In: Cummings otolaryngology: head & neck surgery. 6th ed. Philadelphia: Elsevier; 2015. p. 2285–300.
2. Parving A. The need for universal neonatal hearing screening–some aspects of epidemiology and identification. Acta Paediatr. 1999;88(432):69–72.
3. White KR. The current status of EHDI programs in the United States. Ment Retard Dev Disabil Res Rev. 2003;9(2):79–88.
4. Smith RJ, Robin NH. Genetic testing for deafness–GJB2 and SLC26A4 as causes of deafness. J Commun Disord. 2002;35(4):367–77.
5. Chi DH, Sabo DL. Pediatric audiology and implantable hearing device, Chap. 100. In: Bailey's head and neck surgery: otolaryngology. 5th ed. Philadelphia: Lippincott Williams & Wilkins; 2014. p. 1507–22.
6. Yoshinaga-Itano C, Sedey AL, Coulter DK, Mehl AL. Language of early- and later-identified children with hearing loss. Pediatrics. 1998;102:1161–71.
7. Smith RJH, Shearer AE, Hildebrand MS, et al. Deafness and hereditary hearing loss overview. 1999 Feb 14 [Updated 2014 Jan 9]. In: Pagon RA, Adam MP, Ardinger HH, et al., editors. GeneReviews® [Internet]. Seattle, WA: University of Washington, Seattle; 1993–2017.
8. Fowler KB, Boppana SB. Congenital cytomegalovirus (CMV) infection and hearing deficit. J Clin Virol. 2006;35:226.

Sensorineural Hearing Loss (SNHL) 10

Aisha Larem, Zaid Altamimi, and Adham Aljariri

10.1 Introduction

Hearing loss can be defined as an impairment in the ability to perceive sound stimulus. It includes three types: Conductive, Sensorineural, and Mixed hearing loss. Sensorineural hearing loss (SNHL) occurs due to defect in the sensory apparatus of the cochlea (sensory), or the peripheral pathways of conduction of nerve impulses (XIII CN) to the brain or in the central auditory pathway or cortex (neural).

Knowledge of growth, development, and functional anatomy of the inner ear is important to be able to identify the pathology and diagnose it. Membranous labyrinth develops from otic placode from the third week of the gestational age (GA) and then it becomes otocysts subdivided into vestibular and cochlear compartments. Cochlea reaches the shape of adult form at 10 weeks and adult size at 20 weeks GA. Cochlea is composed of a 35 mm coiled bony tube with 2.5 turns, and it is divided into scala vestibuli, scala tympani, and scala media. Scala vestibuli and scala tympani contain perilymph, scala media is located between scala vestibuli and tympani, and it contains the endolymph. Scala media is bounded by Reissner's membrane, basilar membrane, osseous spiral lamina, and stria vascularis in the lateral wall, and it contains the organ of Corti. Organ of Corti is the receptor organ for hearing, composed of outer and inner hair cells, supporting cells, and the tectorial membrane. Inner and outer hair cells are differing in morphology and innervation. Inner hair cells' neural innervation is by type I neurons which are predominantly afferent neurons, where 15–20 of these neurons innervate each inner hair cell. Outer hair cells' neural synapses are by type II neurons which are predominantly efferent, where each type II neuron branches to innervate around ten outer hair cells. Sound transduction is defined as converting sound vibrations (mechanical energy) into neural impulse (electrical energy) by the movement of the basilar membrane with the hair cells against the tectorial membrane, stimulating generation of nerve ending impulses in spiral ganglion. The spiral ganglion sends axons into the cochlear nerve. The cochlear nerve transmits auditory information up a series of nuclei to the auditory cortex where perception occurs. These nuclei include: (1) cochlear nucleus, (2) superior olivary nuclei, (3) lateral lemniscus, (4) inferior colliculus, and (5) medial geniculate nuclei.

Sensorineural hearing loss (SNHL) is featured with the following

A. Larem (✉) · Z. Altamimi · A. Aljariri
Hamad Medical Corporation, Doha, Qatar
e-mail: alarem@hamad.qa; ZAITamimi@hamad.qa; AAljariri@hamad.qa

A. Al-Qahtani et al. (eds.), *Textbook of Clinical Otolaryngology*,
https://doi.org/10.1007/978-3-030-54088-3_10

- Normal examination of the external ear canal and tympanic membrane.
- Weber and Rinne's tests show a positive Rinne's test (air conduction (AC) > bone conduction (BC)). Weber's lateralized to the better ear.
- Pure-tone audiometry (PTA) normal air-bone gap with decreased bone conduction.

Identifying the severity of the hearing loss is essential to determine the appropriate intervention. Hearing losses between 26 and 40 dB HL are considered mild, 41 and 55 dB HL moderate, 56 and 70 dB HL moderately severe, 71 and 90 dB HL severe, and >91 dB HL profound [1].

10.2 Etiology of Sensorineural Hearing Loss

Etiologies of SNHL can be divided as a congenital (hereditary, non-hereditary, and idiopathic) or acquired. Figure 10.1 summarizes the most common causes.

10.2.1 Congenital

Congenital etiologies are divided into hereditary, non-hereditary, and idiopathic.

- Hereditary (50%)
  - **Non-syndromic (70%)**: more common, autosomal recessive (AR) in (75–80%), autosomal dominant (AD) in (20–25%), X-linked in (2–4%), and Mitochondrial in <1%. GJ2B mutation (autosomal recessive) coding for the protein gap junction beta 2 (also called connexin 26); results in impaired Potassium (K^+) exchange.
  - **Syndromic (30%)**: Divided to AR, AD, and X-linked. Most common include Usher and Pendred syndromes (both autosomal recessive). Most common AD syndrome is Waardenburg syndrome. X-linked includes Alport syndrome.
    Syndromes' features include [2]
    Waardenburg's syndrome → White forelock, heterochromia of iris.
    Usher syndrome → Retinitis pigmentosa.

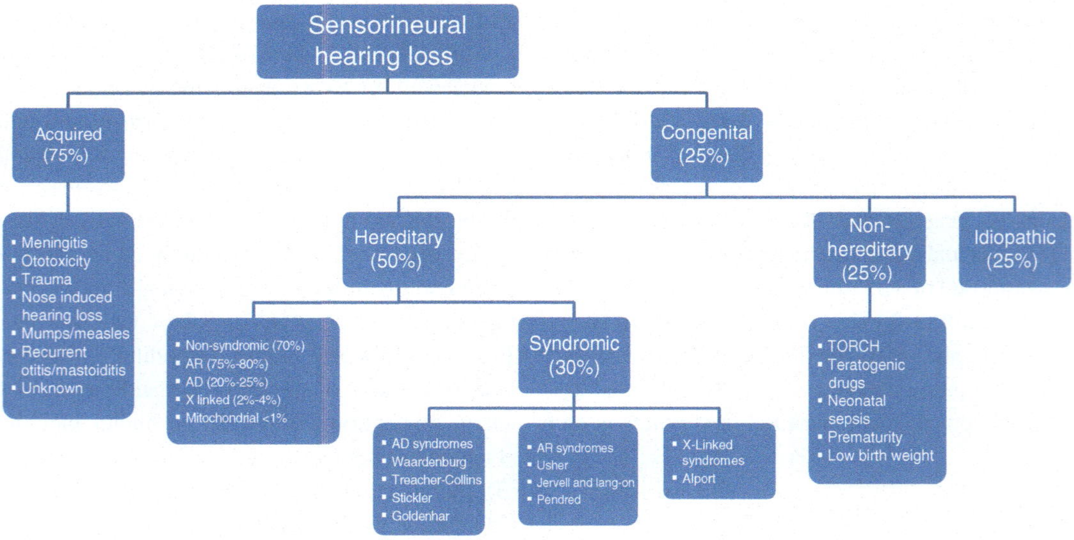

Fig. 10.1 Etiologies of sensorineural hearing loss

Alport's syndrome → Nephritis.
Pendred syndrome → Thyroid goiter.
Jervell and Lange-Nielsen syndrome → Prolonged Q-T intervals and enlarged T waves.

- Non-hereditary (25%)
  - **Malformations** can be **membranous** (Alexander's Aplasia, Scheibe Deformity, Siebenmann–Bing Dysplasia) or **Osseous and Membranous** (Cochlear Hypoplasia, Mondini, Common Cavity, Cochlear Aplasia, Michel Aplasia, Small Internal Auditory Canal). Mondini malformation is the most common type of cochlear malformation.
  - **TORCH Infections**: It includes Toxoplasmosis, Other (syphilis, varicella-zoster, parvovirus B19), Rubella, Cytomegalovirus (CMV), and Herpes.
    - Cytomegalovirus is the most common cause of congenital viral deafness [3].
    - Mumps is the most common infectious cause of acquired sensorineural hearing loss.
  - Other perinatal factors include prematurity, low birth weight, teratogenic drugs, maternal diabetes, hyperbilirubinemia, and neonatal sepsis.
- Idiopathic (25%)

10.2.2 Acquired

The most common causes of acquired sensorineural hearing loss are the following:

1. **Presbycusis.**
2. **Noise-induced hearing loss**.
3. **Post-meningitis.**
4. **Cerebrovascular accident.**
5. **Ototoxic medication exposure.**
6. **Autoimmune inner ear disease** (Cogan's syndrome, relapsing polychondritis, Wegener's granulomatosis, systemic lupus erythematosus, Sjogren's syndrome, and rheumatoid arthritis).
7. **Sudden sensorineural hearing loss**.
8. **Vestibular schwannoma or meningioma**.
9. **Erosive inner ear disease** (cholesteatoma or chronic otitis media).
10. **Trauma to inner ear**.
11. **Endolymphatic hydrops.**

10.2.2.1 Presbycusis

It is an age-related sensorineural hearing impairment. It results from a combination of environmental and genetic factors. Males are affected more often than females. Its features include slow and insidious onset, lack of clarity than a loss of volume, and tinnitus as often the presenting symptoms [4].

- Four types of presbycusis have been identified [5].
  1. **Sensory presbycusis**, characterized by symmetric high frequency hearing loss with a decrease of speech discrimination. The loss affects both hair cells and supporting cells in the basal turn of the cochlea. Figure 10.2 demonstrates pure-tone audiometry with features of Presbycusis in both ears.
  2. **Neural presbycusis**, characterized by a significant loss of speech discrimination. Loss of whole cochlear neurons.
  3. **Strial presbycusis**, characterized by flat pure-tone audiogram with excellent speech discrimination. Associated with atrophy of the stria vascularis in the middle and apical turn of the cochlea.
  4. **Conductive presbycusis (cochlear conductive)**, changes affect the basilar membrane.

Management

Hearing aids or cochlear implants are an excellent option for those who have severe to profound hearing loss with discrimination scores below 40% in both ears [4].

10.2.2.2 Ototoxicity

Ototoxicity can be induced by any route of drug administration (topical, drops, sprays, inhalation, or systemic). Symptoms of ototoxicity include hearing loss (primarily high frequency), tinnitus,

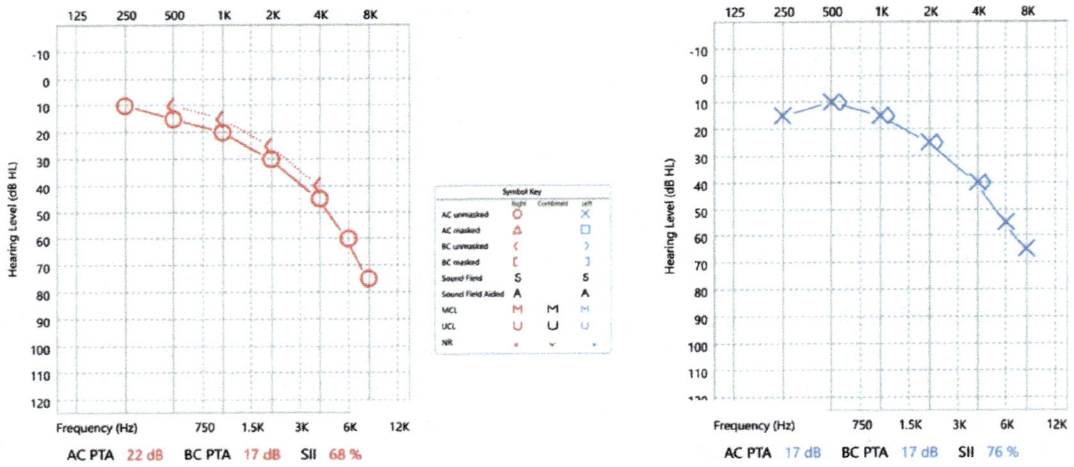

Fig. 10.2 Pure-tone audiometry showing features of Presbycusis in both ears

and balance impairment. The most commonly used drugs causing ototoxicity are the aminoglycosides and platinum-containing chemotherapy agents [4]. Hearing loss may be unilateral or asymmetric and can progress during or after cessation of therapy. Ototoxic drugs inducing low-frequency hearing loss include arsenic and erythromycin. Ototoxic drugs' effects can be permanent (aminoglycoside, cisplatin, carboplatin, or vancomycin) or temporary (salicylates, erythromycin, or quinine). The most common ototoxic drugs are described as follow:

- **Aminoglycosides**

  It can be mainly vestibulotoxic (Streptomycin or Gentamycin) damaging type 1 hair cells of crista ampullaris [6], or mainly cochleotoxic (Neomycin, Kanamycin, or Amikacin) damaging outer hair cells, or vestibulo-cochleo toxic (Tobramycin). The toxicity starts at the basal coil of cochlea (high frequency) and progressing up to the apex. Mitochondrial 12S rRNA gene mutation increases susceptibility to aminoglycosides ototoxicity [7]. Ototoxicity may continue even after the stopping of aminoglycoside [4]. Risk factors include dose, duration, liver and kidney disease, bacteremia, concomitant use of other agents, and genetic predisposition.
- **Anti-neoplastic (chemotherapy)**

  It includes cisplatin and carboplatin. It is highly ototoxic. Cisplatin affects mainly outer hair cells, while carboplatin affects mainly inner hair cells [7]. The main cochlear damage occurs in the basic turn within the outer hair cells. Figures 10.3 and 10.4 show pure-tone audiometry showing and otoacoustic emission findings of bilateral platinum chemotherapy ototoxicity.
- **Loop Diuretics**

  It includes frusemide, ethacrynic acid, and bumetanide. It causes reversible or permanent bilateral hearing loss. Mechanism of toxicity occur by affecting stria vascularis which lead to reductions of endocochlear potential [4].
- **Salicylates (Aspirin)**

  It presents tinnitus more than a loss of hearing. It causes reversible hearing loss.
- **Others**

  It includes industrial chemicals, Vancomycin, Macrolides, and Quinine.

Ototoxicity can be limited and prevented by antioxidants such as *N*-acetyl-cysteine and sodium thiosulfate [8]. It is treated by the cessation of treatment and substitution by a different agent if possible, and hearing rehabilitation can be achieved with applying hearing aid.

10.2.2.3 Noise-Induced Hearing Loss

It can be temporary or permanent hearing loss. Temporary threshold shift (TTS) presents with a brief period of hearing loss after noise exposure, and it is reversible. Permanent threshold shift

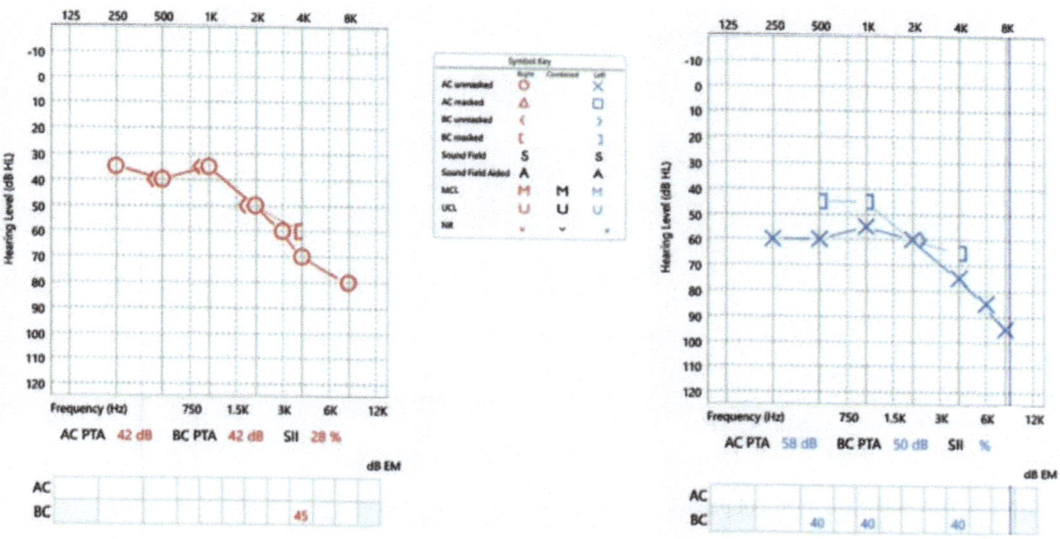

Fig. 10.3 Pure-tone audiometry showing finding of bilateral platinum chemotherapy ototoxicity

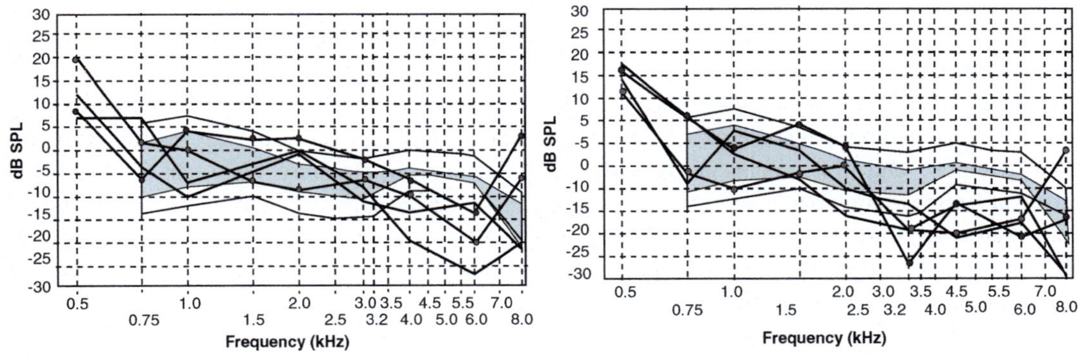

Fig. 10.4 Otoacoustic emission in left and right ears with platinum ototoxicity

(PTS) hearing loss does not return to the previous hearing level [4]. The natural resonance of external auditory canal is from 3 to 5 kHz which may be the reason for a "noise notch" at 4 kHz. Figure 10.5 demonstrates a pure-tone audiometry of patient with noise-induced hearing loss. Acoustic trauma can occur from exposure to intense trauma and lead to immediate hearing loss. The hypothesis of metabolic changes leads to TTS, while the hypothesis of structural changes leads to PTS [9].

Management

Workplace restriction and prevention is better than cure, and measures must be taken for work environments that expose patients to sounds louder than 85 dB for an 8-h period, with each 5-dB increase that must cut exposure into half. Hearing rehabilitation can be achieved by applying hearing aid.

10.2.2.4 Sudden Sensorineural Hearing Loss

It is defined as a unilateral hearing loss of at least 30 dB in at least three contiguous frequencies occurring within 3 days. It can be bilateral in 2%. It is of unknown etiology, possible underlying viral or vascular (ischemic) etiology [10]. Pure-tone audiometry and MRI should be considered to rule out vestibular schwannoma or other intracranial causes such as multiple sclerosis and small vessel ischemic changes. The prevalence of

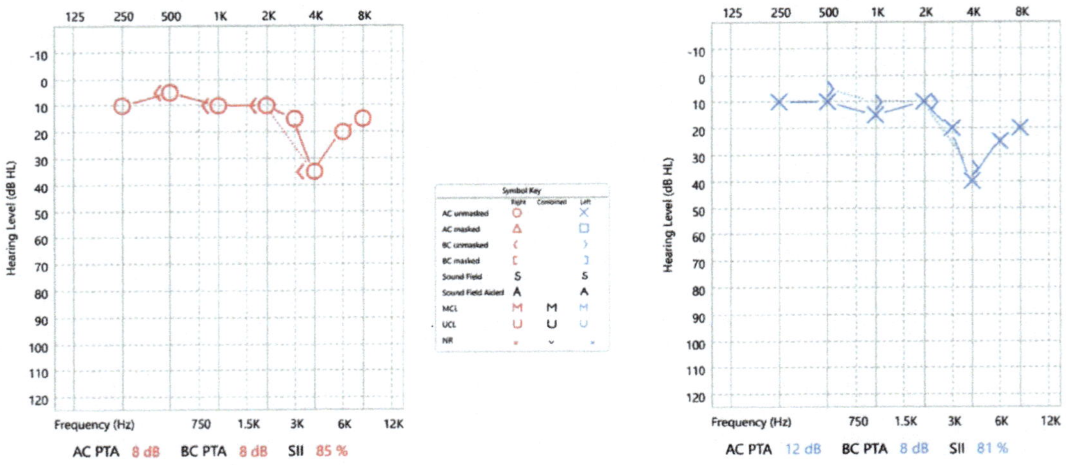

Fig. 10.5 Pure-tone audiometry of patient with noise induced hearing loss

acoustic neuroma among patients with sudden SNHL is less clear, although estimates range from 0.8% [11].

Management

Most recent clinical practice guidelines recommend oral or intratympanic steroids as the first-line treatment, and oral prednisone typically is given at 1 mg/kg/day (up to 60 mg) for 7–14 days and then taper dose over the similar period of time. Intratympanic steroid injection can be used as an initial or salvage treatment [12].

As an adjunct to oral steroids, hyperbaric oxygen and antivirals may be offered. Prognosis is worse with a greater degree of hearing loss, vertigo, advanced age, poorly controlled diabetes, hypertension, and hyperlipidemia [10].

10.2.2.5 Auditory Neuropathy/Dys-Synchrony

It is defined as an abnormal/absent neural transmission in the auditory but evidence of normal outer hair cells function (cochlear microphonic and otoacoustic emissions normal), thought to be caused by abnormal central auditory temporal processing in response to a stimulus. Typically seen in young children, it is mostly related to a genetic cause and has a frequent association with other developmental delays. It may have relatively good pure-tone thresholds but poor speech understanding and auditory development. It exhibits variable response to amplification and/or cochlear implants [13].

10.2.2.6 Autoimmune Inner Ear Disease (AIED)

It is characterized by a subacute progressive fluctuating bilateral sensorineural hearing loss that responds to steroids. One ear is frequently involved initially and worsens before the development of hearing loss in the contralateral side. Patients often describe aural fullness as well as tinnitus [4].

The diagnostic criteria include bilateral sensorineural hearing loss >30 dB at any frequency and progression in at least one ear on two serial audiograms <3 months apart [14]. The hallmark of the disease is the responsiveness of the hearing loss to steroids or cytotoxic drugs [4].

Cogan syndrome is a rare disease of young adults, characterized by triad of autoimmune keratitis, vertigo, and SNHL [4]. Around 15% of cases are associated with other systemic autoimmune diseases including multiple sclerosis, rheumatoid arthritis, and inflammatory bowel disease.

Investigations that help to diagnose AIED include an audiogram and MRI of the internal auditory canal if asymmetric hearing is present. Lab work including anti-HSP-70 (= 68-kDa antigen) can be considered, but it has limited sensitivity and specificity. If other autoimmune diseases are suspected with presence of findings such as arthritis, ocular disease, skin lesions, and kidney disease, a further rheumatological investigation might be required.

Management

It includes a trial of prednisone 60 mg daily for 4–6 weeks, with a close audiological follow-up by repeating PTA frequently. If the patient responds to steroid, then continue until a plateau is reached in the hearing gain, and then a maintenance dose for steroid should be continued for at least 6 months. Regarding non-steroid responders, taper immediately. Methotrexate is used for patients who cannot tolerate steroids or in cases where weaning steroids cause a decline in hearing [15]. Cyclophosphamide and etanercept are considered as a second line. In case profound bilateral SNHL is developed, cochlear implantation is an excellent modality for the restoration of auditory function for this type of pathology.

10.3 Hearing Aids and Auditory Rehabilitation

Hearing aids provide a major role in auditory rehabilitation, where it amplifies the sound to make speech more audible without being uncomfortable. It is mainly indicated for patients with sensorineural hearing loss (SNHL), and it also has a role in the management of conductive hearing loss (CHL), particularly for patients who are not amenable to surgical intervention. Multiple options are available depending on the patient factors, type of hearing loss, unilateral or bilateral, cosmetic appearance, batteries type, and electronic issues. Hearing aids can be either conventional or implantable.

Hearing aid is composed of a microphone, amplifier, receiver, battery, and volume control (see Fig. 10.6).

Hearing aids can be conventional or implantable. The conventional type is more affordable and less invasive but has limitations when it is compared with implantable hearing devices which include insufficient amplification, acoustic feedback, non-linear sound distortion, occlusion effects, poor auditory transduction, and cosmoses. The implantable hearing aids include osseointegrated bone-conducting hearing prostheses and middle ear implants.

1. **Conventional Hearing Aid**:

   It can be categorized to analogue, analogue/digital hybrid, and digital hearing aids. Analogue hearing aid is less common as it has less flexibility than the digital one. The analogue/digital hybrid hearing aids are characterized by digital memory and the ability to control the analogue circuit digitally which makes it more flexible in adjusting gain and acoustic output. The digital hearing aids are computer-controlled devices, via Digital signal processing (DSP) chip, and they have the highest flexibility with improved speech rec-

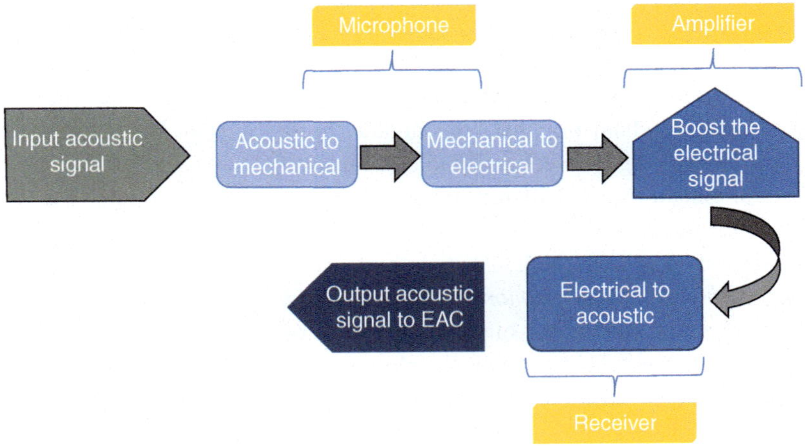

Fig. 10.6 Hearing aid components and function. *EAC* external auditory canal

Table 10.1 Advantages and disadvantages of hearing aids by type

Type of hearing aid	Advantages	Disadvantages
Body Hearing Aids	Low feedback with high level output, easy to manage.	Noticeable, poor sound localization, clothes, and body may rub against the microphone.
Behind the Ear (BTE)	It can be used for severe and profound hearing loss, large case fits larger batteries allows for more amplification and battery life.	Cosmesis, inadequate induces feedback, cannot be used with auricular anomalies.
In the Ear (ITE)	For moderate-to-severe hearing loss, better cosmetically appealing, superior ability to amplify on high-frequency sounds.	Limited gain, feedback problems.
In the Canal (ITC)	More cosmetically appealing and allows for normal acoustics provided by the pinna, superior ability to amplify on high-frequency sounds, helps localization of sound	Gain sufficient for no more than moderate hearing loss, requires dexterity to insert, small size limits output/response controls, venting options limited.
Completely in the Canal (CIC)	Most cosmetically appealing, maximizes pinna and concha effects greater high-frequency gain.	Requires certain fitting criteria, only for moderate hearing loss, small size limits output/response controls, venting options limited, venting options very limited

ognition, sound quality, and comfort via different mechanism, that is, digital noise reduction, digital feedback, and control spectral enhancement. Different types of conventional hearing aid are available which are described in Table 10.1.

Bineural Versus mononeural hearing aid: the general rule is that binaural amplification is the arrangement of choice, unless significant contraindication is present. The main advantages of binaural amplification include better sound localization, speech discrimination, intelligibility in noise, and release from masking, and it also eliminates head shadow effects which reduce high-frequency cues [16]. In addition, patients with binaural hearing loss can have temporary and perhaps a permanent decrease in the auditory function in the unaided ear which can be minimized by fitting a bilateral hearing aid.

Contralateral routing of signal (CROS): it is used in case of single-sided deafness with normal hearing in the other ear. Microphone is fitted on the impaired side and transmitted to a good ear. Bilateral CROS hearing aids also amplify sound to the better hearing ear.

2. **Implantable Hearing Aid**:

   Numerous implantable devices are options for hearing rehabilitation in patients with conductive hearing loss who cannot use a conventional hearing aid.

   (a) *Bone-anchored hearing aids (BAHA)*: They are indicated in cases of chronic otitis media patients with chronically discharging ears, or the presence of a large mastoid bowl or meatoplasty, and they are also indicated in case of congenital anomalies (external ear deformity, aural atresia, and canal stenosis) as well as for single-sided deafness [17].

   Contraindications: Age < 5 years, emotional instability, drug abuse, development delay, average bone conduction threshold (500, 1000, and 3000 Hz) of the indicated ear worse than 45 dB HL, and if maximum speech discrimination of the indicated ear below 60% [17].

   (b) *Middle-ear Implants (MEIs)*: There are two basic types of transducers used in middle ear implantable hearing aids: piezoelectric and electromagnetic. They are used in cases of bilateral moderate-to-severe sensorineural. Its advantages include the elimination of feedback and occlusion effects [18].

Take-Home Messages

- Most common prenatal cause of hearing loss is intrauterine infection (CMV).
- Common causes of perinatal hearing loss are hypoxia, hyperbilirubinemia, infection, and medication toxicity.
- The most common postnatal cause of hearing loss is meningitis.
- Fluctuating hearing loss is seen in perilymphatic fistula, Meniere disease, syphilis, autoimmune induced, sarcoidosis, multiple sclerosis, and migraine-associated hearing loss.

3. **Cochlear implant.**

Acknowledgment Authors of the chapter would like to appreciate the help of Dr. Rani Salim Hammoud, an ENT resident in Hamad medical corporation, for his help and effort in editing the chapter.

References

1. Baiduc RR, Poling GL, Hong O, Dhar S. Clinical measures of auditory function: the cochlea and beyond. Dis Mon. 2013;59(4):147–56. https://doi.org/10.1016/j.disamonth.2013.01.005.
2. Toriello HV, Reardon W, Gorlin RJ. Hereditary hearing loss and its syndromes. 2nd ed. Oxford, UK: Oxford University Press; 2004.
3. Fowler KB, Boppana SB. Congenital cytomegalovirus (CMV) infection and hearing deficit. J Clin Virol. 2006;35:226.
4. Flint PW, Haughey BH, Lund V, et al. Sensorineural hearing loss in adults, Chap 150. In: Cummings otolaryngology: head & neck surgery. 6th ed. Philadelphia: Elsevier; 2015. p. 2319–35.
5. Schuknecht HF. Pathology of the ear. 2nd ed. Philadelphia: Lea & Febiger; 1993.
6. Rybak LP, Ramkumar V. Ototoxicity. Kidney Int. 2007;72:931.
7. Schacht J, Talaska AE, Rybak LP. Cisplatin and aminoglycoside antibiotics: hearing loss and its prevention. Anat Rec (Hoboken). 2012;295(11):1837–50. https://doi.org/10.1002/ar.22578.
8. Sheth S, Mukherjea D, Rybak LP, Ramkumar V. Mechanisms of cisplatin-induced ototoxicity and otoprotection. Front Cell Neurosci. 2017;11:338. https://doi.org/10.3389/fncel.2017.00338.
9. Lim DJ. Effects of noise and ototoxic drugs at the cellular level in the cochlea: a review. Am J Otolaryngol. 1986;7(2):73–99.
10. Kuhn M, Heman-Ackah SE, Shaikh JA, Roehm PC. Sudden sensorineural hearing loss: a review of diagnosis, treatment, and prognosis. Trends Amplif. 2011;15(3):91–105. https://doi.org/10.1177/1084713811408349.
11. Shaia FT, Sheehy JL. Sudden sensori-neural hearing impairment: a report of 1,220 cases. Laryngoscope. 1976;86:389.
12. Chandrasekhar SS, Tsai Do BS, Schwartz SR, Bontempo LJ, Faucett EA, Finestone SA, Hollingsworth DB, Kelley DM, Kmucha ST, Moonis G, Poling GL, Roberts JK, Stachler RJ, Zeitler DM, Corrigan MD, Nnacheta LC, Satterfield L. Clinical practice guideline: sudden hearing loss (update). Otolaryngol Head Neck Surg. 2019;161(1_Suppl):S1–S45.
13. Rance G. Auditory neuropathy/dys-synchrony and its perceptual consequences. Trends Amplif. 2005;9(1):1–43. Review.
14. Mijovic T, Zeitouni A, Colmegna I. Autoimmune sensorineural hearing loss: the otology–rheumatology interface. Rheumatology. 2013;52(5):780–89.
15. Sismanis A, Thompson T, Willis HE. Methotrexate therapy for autoimmune hearing loss: a preliminary report. Laryngoscope. 1994;104:932.
16. Morera C, Manrique M, Ramos A, Garcia-Ibanez L, Cavalle L, Huarte A, Castillo C, Estrada E. Advantages of binaural hearing provided through bimodal stimulation via a cochlear implant and a conventional hearing aid: a 6-month comparative study. Acta Otolaryngol. 2005;125(6):596–606.
17. Kraus EM, Shohet JA, Catalano PJ. Envoy esteem totally implantable hearing system: phase 2 trial, 1-year hearing results. Otolaryngol HNS. 2011;145:100–9.
18. Kozlowski K, Friedland DR. Implantable hearing devices. Curr Surg Rep. 2014;2:59.

Tinnitus and Hyperacusis

11

Aisha Larem, Ma'in Ali Al Shawabkeh,
and Walid Omer

11.1 Introduction

Tinnitus is defined as a perception of sound with no external stimulus [1]. It is considered chronic if it lasts more than 3 months. Tinnitus is divided into two entities: **Subjective tinnitus** in which only the patient can hear it, and **Objective tinnitus,** where others can detect it by either a stethoscope or ear canal microphone [2, 3]. Objective tinnitus can be pulsatile or non-pulsatile. Hyperacusis is considered a central phenomenon that is defined as an unusual tolerance to ordinary environmental sounds. Most of the cases of hyperacusis have unknown pathology. Hyperacusis and tinnitus can coexist with each other.

11.2 Tinnitus

11.2.1 Subjective Non-pulsatile Tinnitus

- Half of the patients have tinnitus in both ears. In those who have it unilateral, it is more common on the left side [3].
- The prevalence increases with age [4].
- Risk factors: age, male sex, lower education and annual income level, more than 15 h per week of noise exposure at work, poor health condition, obesity, hypertension, diabetes, cardiovascular diseases, head trauma, smoking, and alcohol [1, 5].
- Possible etiologies:
  - Certain otologic diseases can present with tinnitus (called syndromic tinnitus). For example, Otosclerosis, Meniere's disease, and vestibular schwannoma [3].
  - Certain medications can cause tinnitus like salicylates, aminoglycosides, quinine, and platinum-based antineoplastic medication [3].
  - Tinnitus is associated with depression and anxiety [6].
  - Look at Table 11.1 for some medical conditions that can lead to tinnitus [7].
- Pathophysiology:
  - Any pathology that can damage the auditory system can lead to tinnitus like:
    - Damage to outer hair cells [8].
    - Disturbance of intracellular calcium level (can be caused by specific medication and noise) [8].
    - Damage to the inner ear can cause the downregulation of the inhibitory pathway leading to spontaneous firing of nerves [9].
- Subtypes:
- Look at Table 11.2 [2].

A. Larem (✉) · M. A. Al Shawabkeh · W. Omer
Hamad Medical Corporation, Doha, Qatar
e-mail: alarem@hamad.qa; MAIGhshoum@hamad.qa; Womer@hamad.qa

A. Al-Qahtani et al. (eds.), *Textbook of Clinical Otolaryngology*,
https://doi.org/10.1007/978-3-030-54088-3_11

Table 11.1 Some medical conditions that can lead to tinnitus

– Sensorineural hearing loss: Sudden sensorineural hearing loss, Meniere's disease, vestibular schwannoma, noise-induced hearing loss, and presbycusis.
– Conductive hearing loss: otitis media, ossicular dislocation, and otosclerosis.
– Endocrine: pregnancy and thyroid disease.
– Metabolic: Vitamin deficiencies and hyperlipidemia.
– Medications: salicylates, aminoglycosides, quinine, platinum-based antineoplastic medication, and antihypertensive medication.
– Head trauma.
– Neurological diseases like meningitis, multiple sclerosis, and stroke.
– Temporomandibular joint (TMJ) syndrome.
– Depression and anxiety.

Table 11.2 Subjective tinnitus subtypes

Hearing loss subtype
Somatic tinnitus subtype
Typewriter tinnitus
Musical tinnitus
Intrusive
Associated with affective disorder

11.2.1.1 Hearing Loss Subtype

- Mainly includes noise-induced hearing loss (NIHL) and presbycusis.
- NIHL:
  - The prevalence of tinnitus in NIHL is 50–70%.
  - Intense sound exposure causes a reduction in blood flow to the cochlea leading to reactive oxygen and nitrogen molecules, which have a damaging effect on the cells.
  - Certain medicines like Vitamin E, salicylates, and *N*-acetylcysteine have antioxidant effects and can give some neuroprotection [2].
- Presbycusis:
  - The prevalence of tinnitus in NIHL is 70%.
  - In those patients, hearing loss is not only attributed to the age, but in fact, it is a combination of the cumulative effect of noise-induced injury to the cochlea, metabolic injury, and vascular injury. Taking in consideration other comorbidities that become more prevalent by aging like diabetes, which can affect the cochlear function [2].

11.2.1.2 Somatic Tinnitus Subtype

- It means the tinnitus in which somatic stimulation can modulate the loudness and pitch of the tinnitus [10].
- Examples:
  - The tinnitus that occurs after the removal of vestibular schwannoma. In some of those patients, tinnitus can be modulated by exaggerating eye movement, leg movement, or cutaneous stimulation of the hand [2].
  - Another example is tinnitus that can occur with the temporomandibular joint disorder. Jaw movement and pressure over the joint can modulate the tinnitus in some of these patients [2].
- Somatic tinnitus can be responsive to acupuncture treatment or electrical stimulation of the ear and scalp [2].

11.2.1.3 Typewriter Tinnitus

- It is chronic intermittent and has staccato quality [2].
- It is believed that it is caused by vascular compression of the ipsilateral auditory nerve [11].
- It can be misdiagnosed by objective tinnitus caused by muscular origin [2].
- It can be responsive to Carbamazepine therapy [11].
- Other types of subjective tinnitus include musical tinnitus, intrusive, and associated with affective disorder [2].
- Evaluation:
  - Identify the features of the tinnitus from history like:
    The laterality.
    Continuous or intermittent.
    Pulsatile or not, the tone.
    Is it hissing, humming, sizzling, buzzing, or roaring.

The effect of the surrounding stimuli on the tinnitus; it is exacerbating or inhibiting the tinnitus.

The effect of the tinnitus on the patient like anxiety, depression, or sleep deprivation.

- Different standardized questionnaires can detect tinnitus severity and the disability that can occur on the individual [3].
- Audio tympanogram [3].
- Other tests like:

  Measurement of loudness and pitch of the tinnitus: it is often not accurate [12].

  Minimal masking level: the intensity of sound needed to mask the tinnitus [13].

  Residual inhibition: the length of time where the tinnitus is absent or decreased after being exposed to one minute of masking [14].
- MRI: especially for unilateral tinnitus [3].

• Management:

• Different devices, medications, and psychotherapy techniques were used to treat tinnitus; some of these methods are:
  - Counseling and reassurance which are considered the key step in management [15].
  - Hearing aid: hearing amplification can decrease tinnitus. Patients with associated hearing loss can benefit from hearing aid in treating this condition [16].
  - Sound therapy: by utilizing specific devices, sound can be used for tinnitus masking or distraction [17].
  - Combination treatment modalities (called tinnitus retraining therapy (TRT)), in which combination of counseling and sound therapy is used [18].
  - Cognitive behavioral therapy (CBT) [19].
  - Some other techniques were used to treat tinnitus like relaxation technique, acupuncture, and some herbal medicines [3].
  - Electromagnetic stimulation [20].
  - Certain medications were used like Tricyclic antidepressants, selective serotonin reuptake inhibitors (SSRI), and benzodiazepine. Local anesthesia like lidocaine can suppress tinnitus, but the effect is short term [3].
  - Intratympanic injection of steroid or local anesthesia [21, 22].
  - Dietary supplements, like vitamins and minerals, were used to treat tinnitus. Vitamin B was found to offer ear protection against noise trauma [3].
  - Lasers [3].
  - Surgery: stapedectomy was found to treat tinnitus caused by otosclerosis [23]. Also, cochlear implantation was found to improve tinnitus in those patients with profound hearing loss [24].

11.2.2 Objective Tinnitus

• It can be pulsatile or non-pulsatile. Look at Table 11.3 [2].

11.2.3 Non-pulsatile Objective Tinnitus

• Caused by otoacoustic emission or patulous Eustachian tube.

• Patulous Eustachian tube:

Table 11.3 Objective tinnitus

Pulsatile		
Synchronous	Non-synchronous	Non-pulsatile
– Arteriovenous malformation or fistula – Persistent stapedial artery – Primary vascular abnormality – Carotid artery stenosis – Atherosclerosis of external carotid subclavian artery – Paraganglioma – Hyperdynamic circulation like pregnancy and hyperthyroidism – Pseudotumor cerebri – Jugular bulb anomaly – Venous hum	– Palatal myoclonus – Tensor tympani/ Stapedial myoclonus	– Otoacoustic emission – Patulous Eustachian tube

- Tuba aperta is another name [3].
- There are two types:
  Patulous ET: in which the ET remains anatomically open [3].
  Semi-patulous ET: in which the ET may open at exercise due to low resistance to airflow [3].
- Symptoms: autophony, hearing loss, a sensation of pressure in the ear, and tinnitus synchronized to breathing [7].
- Causes: weight loss (causing loss of Ostmann's fat pad), radiation, injury to cranial nerve V, or iatrogenic injury to tensor veli palatini muscle during surgery to cleft palate [7].
- Diagnosis: through history and physical examination. Movement of the tympanic membrane with respiration is diagnostic, but it is not always seen. Tympanogram with reflux delay can help in diagnosis but needs an intact TM. Tympanometry can be utilized for diagnosis, and it helps in differentiating between patulous ET and obstructive ET [3].
- Treatment: conservative (it is often self-limited in children). Medical treatment like nasal estrogen drops or oral administration of iodide to induce swelling to the opening of ET [3, 25]. Surgical treatment, for example, grommets insertion was seen to help in alleviating the symptoms [26], and another example is augmentation tympanoplasty with cartilage or tuboplasty [3].

11.2.4 Pulsatile Tinnitus

- It can be divided into synchronous and non-synchronous [3].

11.2.4.1 Synchronous Pulsatile Tinnitus

- It means it synchronizes with the patient's heartbeats.
- Etiology [2].
  - *Arterial causes:*
    Arteriovenous malformation or fistula.
    Persistent stapedial artery.
    Primary vascular abnormality.
    Carotid artery stenosis.
    Atherosclerosis of external carotid subclavian artery.
    Paraganglioma.
    Hyperdynamic circulation like pregnancy and hyperthyroidism.
  - *Venous causes:*
    Pseudotumor cerebri.
    Jugular bulb anomaly.
    Venous hum.
- Investigation:
  - If retrotympanic mass is found during otoscopy, then order CT temporal bone [27].
  - If atherosclerosis of the carotid is suspected, then ask for duplex carotid US [3].
  - If idiopathic intracranial hypertension is suspected, then referral to ophthalmology should be done along with LP for the measurement of CSF pressure [3].
- Treatment:
  - If no pathology is found, then reassurance is recommended.
  - If pathology is found, treat the underlying condition [3].

11.2.4.2 Non-synchronous Pulsatile Tinnitus

- It is not synchronized with the patient's heartbeat.
- Causes:
  - Palatal myoclonus: it is caused by myoclonus of the palate leading to rapid clicking tinnitus [28].
  - Tensor tympani/Stapedial myoclonus: leading to low-frequency tinnitus exaugurated by external sound [29].
- It is essential to differentiate between middle ear myoclonus and palatal muscle myoclonus, with the latter presenting with involuntary movement of the soft palate and suprahyoid muscles. Palatal myoclonus is often associated with CNS lesions so that brain MRI should be done [30].
- Treatment: first conservative and supportive therapy should be tried like relaxation therapy, biofeedback, and tinnitus masking. Certain medications can be used like carba-

mazepine and benzodiazepine. If these trials failed, then surgical therapy can be offered, which includes the division of both tensor tympani and stapedial muscles [3] (Figs. 11.1 and 11.2).

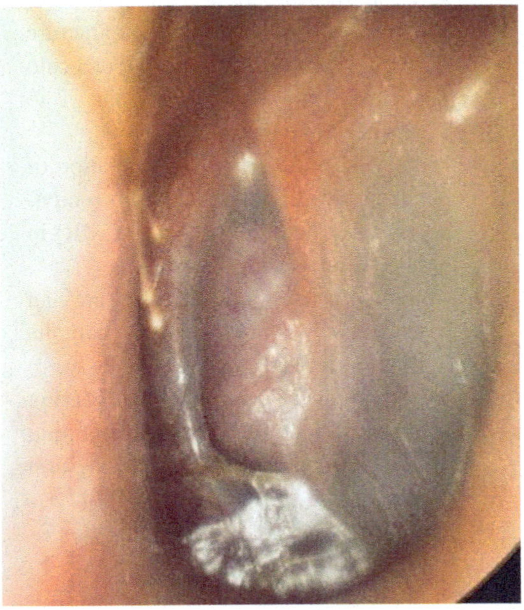

Fig. 11.1 Otoscopic view of aberrant carotid artery

11.3 Hyperacusis

- Defined as unusual tolerance to ordinary environmental sounds [7].
- It is considered a central phenomenon and should be distinguished from recruitment, which is a peripheral phenomenon. Recruitment is not considered part of hyperacusis as the patients will experience rapid growth of loudness upon increasing the tone level [2].
- Prevalence: 8–15% [3].
- Both hyperacusis and tinnitus often occur together [3].
- Most of the cases of hyperacusis have no known pathology. There are some medical conditions that can lead to hyperacusis: look at Table 11.4 [7].
- Pathophysiology is thought to be by GABA central pathways as patients with Benzodiazepine withdrawal experience this phenomenon [31].
- In hyperacusis, patients experience physical discomfort upon exposure to moderate or weak sound stimuli, which generally will not cause any discomfort in a normal person.

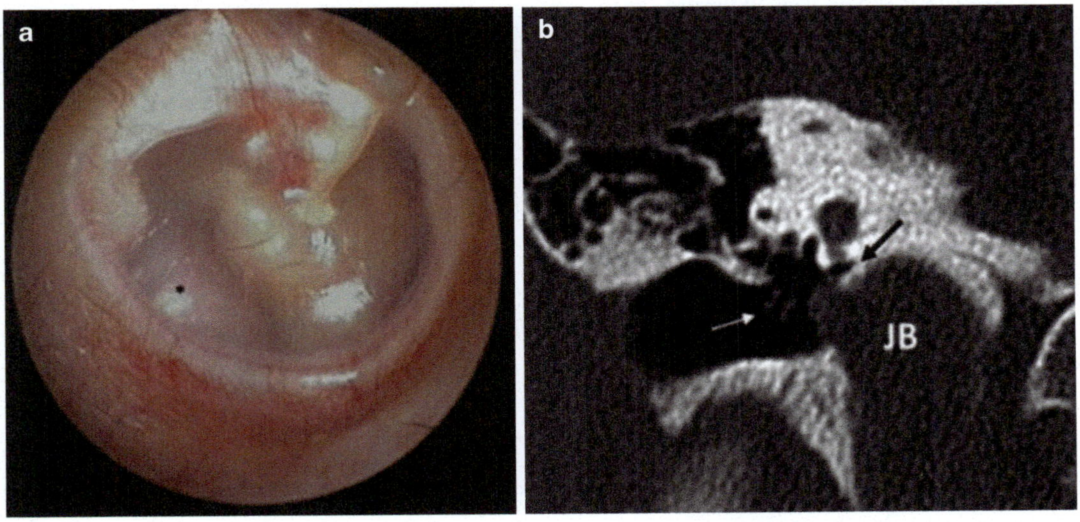

Fig. 11.2 (**a**) Right ear otoscopic image of the typical bluish appearance of the prominent high jugular bulb (asterisk) visible through the tympanic membrane (**b**) coronal CT-reconstruction of a right ear, showing a prominent jugular bulb (JB), protruding in into the hypotympanic cavity up to the level of the round window recess (black arrow). Tympanic aerator (white arrow) inserted through a thin tympanic membrane

Table 11.4 Medical conditions that can lead to hyperacusis

Tinnitus
Bell's palsy
Ramsay hunt syndrome
Lyme disease
Stapedectomy
Perilymphatic fistula
Translabyrinthine excision of a vestibular schwannoma
Head injury
Migraine
Depression
Addison disease
Williams syndrome

- Hyperacusis can have a negative psychological impact on patients. It can lead to misophonia (which means the patient will dislike sounds) or phonophobia (in which patients will have fear from exposure to sounds). In severe cases, patients can become housebound [7].
- Investigation: hyperacusis questionnaires can be utilized. Measurement of loudness discomfort level can be used, but some claim that it is not reliable [3].
- Treatment: Gradual desensitization can be used to treat this condition. Tinnitus retraining therapy (TRT) and cognitive behavioral therapy (CBT) can also be used [32, 33]. It is important to note that in those patients, they may use earplugs as a defense from their increased perception of loudness. However, these earplugs can aggravate the hyperacusis by increasing the central nervous system gain [34].

Take-Home Messages

- Tinnitus is divided into subjective and objective.
- Subjective has different subtypes. Examples are hearing loss subtype, somatic tinnitus, typewriter tinnitus, musical tinnitus, intrusive, and associated with affective disorder.
- Hearing loss subtype includes noise-induced hearing loss and presbycusis. The somatic subtype is modulated through physical stimulation like eye movements, leg movement, and pressure on the temporomandibular joint. Usually, they respond to acupuncture therapy. Typewriter tinnitus has staccato quality and can respond to Carbamazepine therapy.
- History is vital during the evaluation of patients with tinnitus. An audio tympanogram can be ordered. Ask for MRI in cases of unilateral tinnitus.
- Counseling and reassurance are an essential step while managing patients with tinnitus. Different methods were used to treat the condition like hearing aid, sound therapy, tinnitus retraining therapy, and cognitive behavioral therapy.
- Objective tinnitus can be pulsatile or non-pulsatile.
- Non-pulsatile tinnitus includes oto-acoustic emission and Patulous Eustachian tube.
- Patulous Eustachian tube can be caused by weight loss, radiotherapy, and injury to CN V and tensor veli palatini muscle. It presents with autophony, hearing loss, a sensation of pressure in the ear, and tinnitus that is synchronized to breathing.
- Objective non-pulsatile tinnitus can be synchronous or non-synchronous to the patient's heartbeat.
- Synchronous pulsatile objective tinnitus has different etiologies and is usually caused by vascular pathology.
- Non-synchronous pulsatile objective tinnitus is caused by either palatal myoclonus or tensor tympani/stapedial muscle myoclonus. Palatal myoclonus is often associated with CNS lesions so that brain MRI should be done.

- Hyperacusis is a different pathology in which the patient has unusual tolerance to ordinary environmental sounds. It is believed that a central phenomenon causes it.
- Hyperacusis usually coincides with tinnitus. It usually results in a negative psychological effect on the patients. Tinnitus retraining therapy (TRT) and cognitive behavioral therapy (CBT) can be used in treating this condition.

Acknowledgment Authors of the chapter would like to appreciate the help of Dr. Adham Aljariri, an ENT resident in Hamad medical corporation, for his help and effort in editing the chapter.

References

1. McFadden D. Tinnitus: facts, theories, and treatments. Washington, DC: National Academy Press; 1982.
2. Flint P, Haughey B, Lund V, Niparko J, Robbins K, Regan Thomas J, Lesperance M. Cummings otolaryngology. 6th ed. Philadelphia: Elsevier; 2014.
3. Watkinson JC, Clarke RW. Scott-Brown's otorhinolaryngology and head and neck surgery. 8th ed. Boca Raton, FL: CRC Press; 2018.
4. Hoffman HJ, Reed GW. Epidemiology of tinnitus. In: Snow JB, editor. Tinnitus: theory and management. Hamilton: BC Decker; 2004. p. 16–41.
5. Davis A, El Rafaie A. Epidemiology of tinnitus. In: Tyler RS, editor. Tinnitus hand-book. San Diego: Singular; 2000. p. 1–23.
6. Zoger S, Svedlund J, Holgers KM. Relationship between tinnitus severity and psychiatric disorders. Psychosomatics. 2006;47:282–8.
7. Snow JB, Ashley Wackym P. Ballenger's otorhinolaryngology and head and neck surgery. 17th ed. Connecticut: People's Medical Publishing House; 2008.
8. Jastreboff PJ. Phantom auditory perception (tinnitus): mechanisms of generation and perception. Neurosci Res. 1990;8:221–54.
9. Noreña AJ, Eggermont JJ. Changes in spontaneous neural activity immediately after an acoustic trauma: implications for neural correlates of tinnitus. Hear Res. 2003;183:137–53.
10. Ward J, Vella C, Hoare DJ, Hall DA. Subtyping somatic tinnitus: a cross-sectional UK cohort study of demographic, clinical and audiological characteristics. PLoS One. 2015;10(5):e0126254. https://doi.org/10.1371/journal.pone.0126254.
11. Sunwoo W, Jeon YJ, Bae YJ, Jang JH, Koo JW, Song JJ. Typewriter tinnitus revisited: the typical symptoms and the initial response to carbamazepine are the most reliable diagnostic clues. Sci Rep. 2017;7(1):10615. https://doi.org/10.1038/s41598-017-10798-w.
12. Hoare DJ, Edmondson-Jones M, Gander PE, Hall DA. Agreement and reliability of tinnitus loudness matching and pitch likeness rating. PLoS One. 2014;9:e114553.
13. Zagólski O, Stręk P. Tinnitus pitch and minimum masking levels in differentetiologies. Int J Audiol. 2014;53(7):482–9. https://doi.org/10.3109/14992027.2014.893377. Epub 2014 Mar 31.
14. Deklerck AN, Degeest S, Dhooge IJM, Keppler H. Test-retest reproducibility of response duration in tinnitus patients with positive residual inhibition. J Speech Lang Hear Res. 2019;62(9):3531–44. https://doi.org/10.1044/2019_JSLHR-H-18-0514. Epub 2019 Aug 21.
15. Henry JA, Loovis C, Montero M, et al. Randomized clinical trial: group counseling based on tinnitus retraining therapy. J Rehabil Res Dev. 2007;44(1):21–32.
16. Searchfield GD, Kaur M, Martin WH. Hearing aids as an adjunct to counseling: tinnitus patients who choose amplification do better than those that don't. Int J Audiol. 2010;49:574–9.
17. Vernon JA, Meikle MB. Masking devices and alprazolam treatment for tinnitus. Otolaryngol Clin N Am. 2003;36:307–20.
18. Henry JA, Schechter MA, Zaugg TL, et al. Outcomes of clinical trial: tinnitus masking versus tinnitus retraining therapy. J Am Acad Audiol. 2006;17:104–32.
19. Grewal R, Spielmann PM, Jones SE, Hussain SS. Clinical efficacy of tinnitus retraining therapy and cognitive behavioural therapy in the treatment of subjective tinnitus: a systematic review. J Laryngol Otol. 2014;128:1028–33.
20. Dauman R. Electrical stimulation for tinnitus suppression. In: Tyler RS, editor. Tinnitus handbook. San Diego: Singular; 2000. p. 77–98.
21. Cessarani A, Capobianco S, Soi D, et al. Intratympanic dexamethasone treatment for control of subjective idiopathic tinnitus: our clinical experience. Int Tinnitus J. 2002;8:111–4.
22. Sakata H, Kojima Y, Koyama S, et al. Treatment of cochlear tinnitus with trans-tympanic infusion of 4% lidocaine into the tympanic cavity. Int Tinnitus J. 2001;7:46–50.
23. Gersdorff M, Nouwen J, Gilain C, et al. Tinnitus and otosclerosis. Eur Arch Otorhinolaryngol. 2000;257:314–6.
24. Quaranta N, Wagstaff S, Baguley DM. Tinnitus and cochlear implantation. Int J Audiol. 2004;43:245–51.
25. Ikeda R, Oshima T, Oshima H, et al. Management of patulous Eustachian tube with habitual sniffing. Otol Neurotol. 2011;32:790–3.
26. Chen DA, Luxford WM. Myringotomy and tube for relief of patulous Eustachian tube symptoms. Am J Otol. 1990;11:272–3.

27. Weissman JL, Hirsch BE. Imaging of tinnitus: a review. Radiology. 2000;216:342–9.
28. Anis MM, Pollak N. Treatment of palatal myoclonus with botulinum toxin injection. Case Rep Otolaryngol. 2013;2013:231505. https://doi.org/10.1155/2013/231505.
29. Bhimrao SK, Masterson L, Baguley D. Systematic review of management strategies for middle ear myoclonus. Otolaryngol Head Neck Surg. 2012;146:698–706.
30. Oliveira CA, Negreiros J, Cavalcante IC, et al. Palatal and middle-ear myoclonus: a cause for objective tinnitus. Int Tinnitus J. 2003;9:37–41.
31. Richardson M, Flint P, Haughey B, Lund V, Niparko J, Robbins K, Regan Thomas J, Lesperance M. Cummings otolaryngology, head and neck surgery. 5th ed. Philadelphia: Elsevier; 2010.
32. Hazell JWP, Sheldrake JB, Graham RL. Decreased sound tolerance: predisposing factors, triggers and outcomes after TRT. In: Patuzzi R, editor. Proceedings of the Seventh International Tinnitus Seminar. Fremantle: University of Western Australia; 2002. p. 255–61.
33. Jüris L, Andersson G, Larsen HC, Ekselius L. Cognitive behaviour therapy for hyperacusis: a randomized controlled trial. Behav Res Ther. 2014;54:30–7.
34. Formby C, Sherlock LP, Gold SL. Adaptive plasticity of loudness induced by chronic attenuation and enhancement of the acoustic background. J Acoust Soc Am. 2003;114:55–8.

Physiology and Diagnostic Tests of the Vestibular System

12

Walid Omer and Khaled Abdulhadi

12.1 Introduction

- The vestibular system can be regarded as the sixth sense [1].
- Its main functions are to stabilize gaze, posture, and gait during movement (balance in locomotion).
- Usually, the vestibular system input is not consciously perceived, except in abnormal conditions.
- Any disturbance in vestibular input can lead to vertigo (illusion of movement at rest), imbalance (mainly on uneven surfaces and dark areas), and difficulty in reading signs while moving (oscillopsia) [2].

12.2 Anatomy of the Vestibular System

The vestibular system consists of two main organs in the inner ear (Fig. 12.1):

- Otolithic (Otoconial) organs (two on each side):
  - Saccule and utricle.
  - Responds to linear acceleration and gravity (tilt).
  - Saccule (oriented vertically) is more sensitive to vertical acceleration, while the utricle (oriented horizontally) is more sensitive to horizontal acceleration.
  - The sensory neuroepithelium in the otolithic organs is called the macula.
  - The macula consists of hair cells and supporting cells.
  - The hair cells have apical hair bundles that project into a gelatinous material (otolithic membrane) covered by millions of calcium carbonate crystals (Otoconia) [3].
  - Bending of hair bundle happens after head tilt (by the otoconia as a result of gravity) [3, 4].

    Depolarization: Once the bundle is bent in the direction of a hair cell's axis of polarity.

    Hyperpolarization: when tilting the head to the opposite direction, the same cell hyperpolarizes and inhibits the afferent fiber.
- Semicircular canals (three on each side) figure.
  - Horizontal (Lateral), Anterior (superior), and Posterior.
  - Responds to rotational acceleration.
  - Senses head rotation in three-dimensional space.

W. Omer (✉) · K. Abdulhadi
Hamad Medical Corporation, Doha, Qatar
e-mail: Womer@hamad.qa; Khadi@hamad.qa

A. Al-Qahtani et al. (eds.), *Textbook of Clinical Otolaryngology*,
https://doi.org/10.1007/978-3-030-54088-3_12

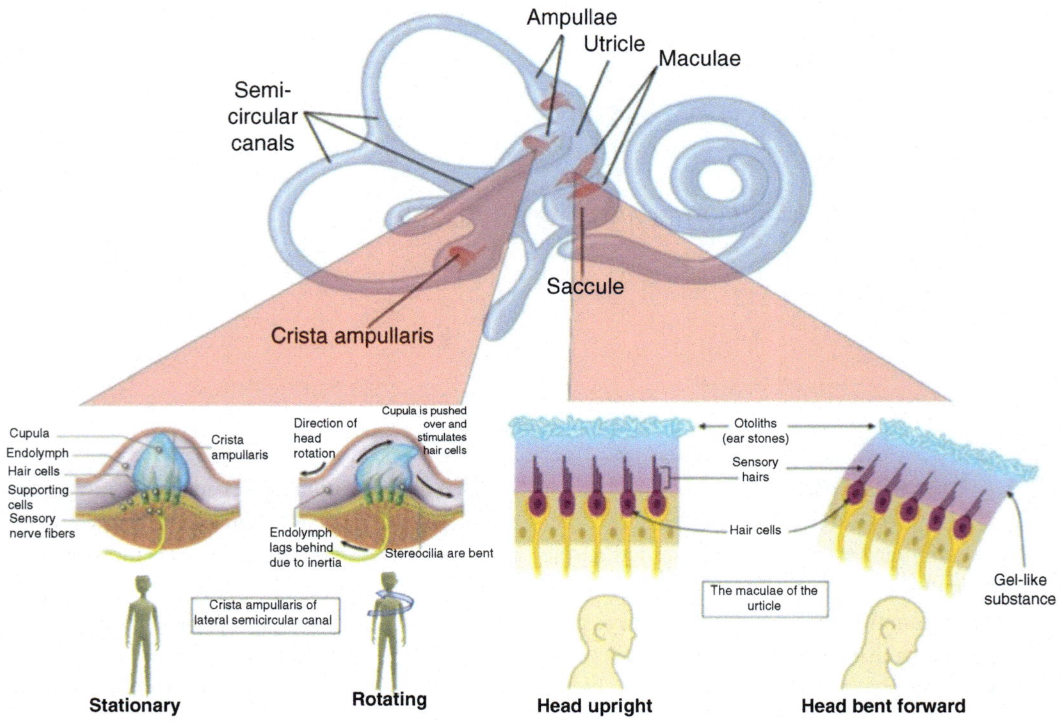

Fig. 12.1 Figure illustrating the anatomy and physiology of the vestibular system

- When the head rotates to one side, endolymph moves, relative to the skull, to the opposite side.
- Deflection of the cupula by endolymph, which in turn bends the hair cells (Stereocilia) in the crista ampullaris (sensory organ of rotation).
- Depending on the direction of endolymphatic fluid and the semicircular canal stimulated, activation or inhibition of nerve firing happens:
  Ampullopetal: toward ampulla (excitatory to the horizontal canal and inhibitory to superior and posterior canal).
  Ampullofugal: away from the ampulla (excitatory to the superior and posterior canal and inhibitory to horizontal canal).
- Planes of the semicircular canals (functional pairs):
  Horizontal: left and right horizontal SCCs.
  RALP: right anterior and left posterior.
  LARP: left anterior and right posterior.

12.3 Vestibular Reflexes

- Sensory input from the eyes (visual), proprioception (somatosensory), and the ears (vestibular) is integrated in the Brainstem (Vestibular Nuclei), which in turn sends afferents compromising the main vestibular reflexes:
  - Vestibulo-ocular reflex: stabilizes gaze during active head rotation (fixation of the retina on the target by acting on the extraocular muscles), when the head moves to one direction, the eyes move to the opposite direction equally (i.e. head movement to the right of 20° leads to eyes move to the left of 20°).
  - Vestibulospinal reflex: Stabilizes posture (acting on the antigravitational muscles).
  - Vestibulocollic reflex: stabilizes the head on the trunk (acting on the neck musculature).

12.4 Nystagmus: Involuntary Repetitive Rhythmic Eye Movement

Alexander law: It is described in individuals with Nystagmus and refers to increase in the amplitude of nystagmus when the eyes move to the direction of the fast phase (the direction of nystagmus is typically named toward the fast phase, and in cases of acute vestibular loss, the fast phase is usually toward the healthy ear) and become slower when looking at the direction of the slow phase.

Ewald's three laws:

- "A stimulation of the semicircular canal causes a movement of the eyes in the plane of the stimulated canal".
- "In the horizontal semicircular canals, an ampullopetal endolymph movement cases a greater stimulation than an ampullofugal one".
- "In the vertical semicircular canals, the reverse is true" [5].

12.5 Vestibular Diagnostic Studies

History taking (the most fundamental part), physical examination, and vestibular function tests are key elements in reaching the correct diagnosis and designing the best management plan.

Vestibular function tests confirm the diagnosis that is suspected by history taking and bedside examination. It is also done to identify three main components in the management of dizzy patient:

1. Identifying the site of the lesion (Central vs. Peripheral)
2. Extent of the lesion (Unilateral vs. Bilateral)
3. The degree of compensation (hence asses the need for vestibular rehabilitation)

12.5.1 Videonystagmography (VNG)/ Electronystagmography (ENG)

- It consists of oculomotor testing (smooth pursuit, saccade, optokinetic, and gaze stabilization testing), positional and positioning testing, and caloric test.
- Videonystagmography refers to recording of the eye movement using infrared cameras, which detect actual eye movements. While ENG (old systems) recodes corneo-retinal potentials.
- It answers two main questions:
  - Is it peripheral or central
  - Localizes the ear

12.5.2 Oculomotor Testing

- Gaze testing: Holding the gaze at the primary gaze and then eyes movement to 30° up, down, right, and left. It tests eye stabilization on the target and is regarded as abnormal in case the eyes move away or off the target. It can be a sign of central dysfunction, and also in acute vestibular dysfunction, gaze stability can be abnormal.
- Smooth Pursuit: It is a system that is activated to fix moving targets on the fovea (it prevents retinal slippage of the images). It is tested by asking the subject to follow a moving target (which is moving smoothly in a sinusoidal pattern on the screen). The smooth pursuit is usually active at targets which are moving at low velocity (less than 60° per second). Abnormal smooth pursuit is indicative of central pathologies.
- Saccade testing: The target here rapidly shifts (jumps) from one place to another on the screen, and the subject moves his eyes so that the target is kept on the fovea. It is testing by rapidly moving target 20° right, left, and center. Abnormal saccade test (dysmetria, slow saccadic velocity, and deconjugate saccades) is indicative of a central pathology.
- Optokinetic test: it is activated to fix images on the retina (not only the fovea) when looking at a moving field (not a specific target like in smooth pursuit or saccade). The subject is tested, while more than 80% of the field of vision is filled with a moving series of objects (example colored strips). Both central and peripheral pathologies can lead to abnormal Optokinetic test.
- Spontaneous nystagmus.

12.5.3 Positional and Positioning (Dix–Hallpike) Testing

- Positional: relates to maintaining the head at the provoking position and is done in the absence of visual fixation where eye movement is recorded at three positions: Supine, head right, or head left.
- Positioning tests: relates to the action of moving the head, and the classical positioning test is Dix–Hallpike, which is Diagnostic of Posterior canal-BPPV. It is done by recording of the eye movement and the resulting nystagmus after positioning the patient.

12.5.4 Caloric Test

- Caloric response was first described by Robert Barany in 1906. For his finding, Barany received a Nobel Prize in 1914.
- It is part of ENG/VNG test battery.
- It tests the function of the lateral semicircular canal only.
- It tests each labyrinth separately (independent of the other canal), which makes it ideal for determining the side of the weakness.
- It is done using warm and cold stimuli with water or air. The degree and symmetry (between both ears) of responsiveness to these stimuli are recorded.
- Method—Patient lying supine and the head is elevated 30° (bringing the horizontal semicircular canal to the vertical plane). Irrigation with warm and cold water or air is done, and the resulting response (Nystagmus) is recorded. Water irrigation (for 30 s) is done at a temperature of 44 °C for warm and 30 °C for cold. Air (for 60 s) is done at a temperature of 49–50 °C for warm and 24 °C for cold (waiting time between each irrigation is 2–3 min).
- Water irrigation gives a more robust response compared to air. Ice water caloric irrigation (ice calorics) is indicated in cases of absent response or when poor irrigation is suspected.
- The mnemonic COWS: cold opposite, warm same describes the resulting direction of the fast phase of nystagmus.
- Outcome Measure in Caloric test.
  - Canal paresis (reduced vestibular response): it compares the response from one side to the other using "Jongkee's formula" RVR = (RC + RW − LC − LW)/TR. Differences 25–27% or more usually considered significant.
  - Unilateral canal paresis is usually a sign of peripheral vestibular pathology, that is, vestibular neuritis. Less commonly is canal paresis with central vestibular pathologies, for example, lesions of the vestibular nerve root-like multiple sclerosis and lateral brainstem infarction.
  - Directional preponderance (DP): Preference of the response (beating of the nystagmus) toward one direction. Generally, 35% or more is usually considered abnormal. The direction preponderance has limited diagnostic value. Both central and peripheral dysfunctions can lead to DP. In peripheral lesions, DP is usually away from the side of the lesion.

12.5.5 Kinetic Rotatory Chair

- It is another part of the vestibular test battery which evaluates vestibulo-ocular reflex (VOR) function.
- Its main indications include:
  - Bilateral vestibular hypofunction (BVH; it is the goal standard for testing BVH).
  - The extent of vestibular compensation.
  - Testing in children.
- Method: Patient seated on the chair and strapped for safety with eye movements recorded during rotation. Rotations are horizontally (to right and left).
- Two main subtypes of kinetic rotatory chair are as follows:
  - Step velocity: the chair accelerates to prespecified velocity (80–240°/s) and keeps rotating at this speed and then suddenly stops (eye recording is done per-rotation and post-rotation).
  - Sinusoidal harmonic acceleration.

- Three main parameters are measured:
  - Gain: Ratio of eye velocity to the head velocity; ideally, it is equal to 1, but in reality, chair testing is normally lower since other factors (e.g., equipment) can lead to this reduction.
  - Phase or time constant.

    Time constant is measured with step velocity and is defined as the time needed for the peak SCEV to reduce to 37% from peak velocity, and normal value is 10–25 s. The phase is measured with the SHA, and it compares SCEV with the maximum chair velocity.
  - Asymmetry: compares SCEV in the right to the left side; normally, there is no asymmetry (both rotations are equal).
- Acute vestibular hypofunction (e.g. vestibular neuritis) leads to reduced gain at all frequencies.
- Bilateral vestibular hypofunction (typically chronic) leads to low normal gain at high frequency and low gain at low frequencies.
- Vestibular compensation is suggested by the absence of asymmetry.

12.5.6 Vestibular Evoked Myogenic potential

- It is an electrophysiological (EMG, electromyography) test of the otolith function.
- cVEMP (cervical) is a test of saccular and inferior vestibular nerve function, while oVEMP (ocular) tests the utricle and superior vestibular nerve.
- cVEMP:
  - cVEMP: VEMP measures VCR (vestibulocollic reflex), which is a reflex that acts on neck muscles to stabilize the head based on inputs from the vestibular system.
  - It is the only vestibular function test that specifically tests the saccule and inferior branch of the vestibular nerve.
  - The test is similar to ABR where electrodes are placed over the ipsilateral SCM; however, the response is larger (200 μV compared to 1 μV for ABR).
  - Pathway: Acoustic Stimuli (95–100 dBnHL) → saccule → inferior vestibular nerve → vestibular nucleus (brainstem) → vestibulospinal tract → sternocleidomastoid muscle.
  - It is generally indicated in cases of Meniere's disease, superior canal dehiscence, vestibular neuritis, and to evaluate saccular and inferior vestibular nerve function.
  - In cases of third window effect (superior semicircular canal dehiscence syndrome and perilymphatic fistula), abnormally low thresholds are detected.
- oVEMP:
  - It is the only vestibular function test that specifically tests utricle and superior vestibular nerve.
  - It is a test of VOR pathway. Both air and bone conduction stimuli can be used (in air, contralateral response is tested, and in bone, conduction bilateral response is tested).
  - Pathway: Acoustic stimuli → utricle → superior vestibular nerve → inferior oblique.

12.5.7 Video Head Impulse Test (vHIT)

- It is the only vestibular test that can test all the semicircular canals (superior, lateral, and posterior).
- It is comprised of rapid head movement (impulses) to the right and left of small amplitude 10–20° with a velocity of 100°/s or more while fixing the eyes at certain point, usually on the wall 1–2 m in front of the patient. Eye movements are recorded with camera goggles.
- A peripheral disorder will result in a corrective saccade. A right-sided lesion will result in a corrective saccade to the left when the head is turned to the right.
- The main advantage of the video head impulse test over the clinical/bedside head impulse is that it can detect overt (corrective saccade that happens after the head movement stops) and

covert saccade (which happens during head movement). In contrast to the bedside test, it only detects the overt saccade.
- A normal test helps to differentiate vestibular neuritis from ischemic brainstem/cerebellar stroke in cases of acute vestibular syndrome.

12.5.8 Computerized Dynamic Posturography

- It is a test of postural stability at different conditions to give a functional assessment of visual, proprioceptive, and vestibular systems.
- Sensory organization test (the main test): it evaluates body sway under the following conditions:
  - Eyes opened: fixed surface and visual surrounding
  - Eyes closed: fixed surface
  - Eyes opened: fixed surface, sway referenced visual surrounding
  - Eyes opened: swayed referenced surface, fixed visual surrounding
  - Eyes closed: swayed referenced surface
  - Eyes opened: swayed referenced surface and visual surrounding
- Uses include vestibular testing to detect functional vestibular impairment, evaluate improvement in function pre- and post-vestibular rehabilitation, and medico-legally to assess malingerers.

Take-Home Messages
- Understanding the physiology of the vestibular system is important in understanding vestibular testing.
- Vestibular test complements history and physical examination, and it does not replace them.
- The vestibular tests help to identify the site and extent of the lesion in addition to assessing the degree of central compensation.

References

1. Goldberg JM, Wilson VJ, Angelaki DE, Cullen KE, Fukushima K. The vestibular system: a sixth sense. Oxford: Oxford University Press; 2012.
2. Grill E, Heuberger M, Strobl R, Saglam M, Holle R, Linkohr B, Ladwig KH, Peters A, Schneider E, Jahn K, Lehnen N. Prevalence, determinants, and consequences of vestibular hypofunction. Results from the KORA-FF4 survey. Front Neurol. 2018;9:1076.
3. Kandel ER, Schwartz JH, Jessell TM, Siegelbaum SA, Hudspeth AJ, editors, Mack S, art editor. Principles of neural science. 5th ed. New York: McGraw-Hill; 2013.
4. Iurato S. Organ of Corti. In: Submicroscopic structure of the inner ear. Oxford: Pergamon; 1967. p. 80–106.
5. Ewald JR. dizziness-and-balance.com/history/ewald.html.

13 Dizziness and Vestibular Disorders

Hassan Haidar and Rawan H. A. Azzam

Key Points

- Vertigo is a common presentation in general practice.
- A careful history is required to elicit features of central or peripheral causes of vertigo.
- Serious causes including stroke need to be considered.
- Physical examination involves a neurological, cardiovascular, eye, and ear examination.
- Treatment is specific to the cause of vertigo.

13.1 Introduction

Dizziness is a common symptom in ENT practice as well as primary care.

The prevalence of vertigo as a function of age lies around 17% and rises up to 39% in those over 80 years of age [1]. Most of the causes are benign, and there are few serious causes that must be considered in diagnosis. Unfortunately, there is no simple and reliable method to identify those patients with serious underlying causes, further increasing the need for a systematic approach to evaluation.

H. Haidar (✉)
Hamad Medical Corporation, Doha, Qatar

ENT Department, Hamad Medical Corporation, Doha, Qatar

R. H. A. Azzam
ENT Department, Hamad Medical Corporation, Doha, Qatar

13.2 Evaluation of a Dizzy Patient

The history and physical examination are the critical elements in determining the underlying cause of the dizziness (Table 13.1).

In the evaluation of a patient who experiences dizziness, our initial efforts must be directed at determining the exact nature of the patient's symptoms because the pathophysiology determines the patient's sensations.

13.2.1 History

The main goal of the history is to determine exactly what the patient means by the term "dizziness". There are generally three things that patients mean by "dizziness", and each requires a distinct process of evaluation:

1. **Vertigo** is defined as the sensation of spinning. Questions such as "does it feel like you're on an amusement ride" and "are you sick to your stomach with the dizziness" suggest that they have vertigo.

A. Al-Qahtani et al. (eds.), *Textbook of Clinical Otolaryngology*,
https://doi.org/10.1007/978-3-030-54088-3_13

Table 13.1 Characteristics of major causes of dizziness

Disorder	Duration	Triggers	Diagnosis
BPPV	Seconds	Turning in bed	Dix–Hallpike
Vestibular Neuritis	3–5 days	Spontaneous, after flu	Unidirectional nystagmus, Positive head thrust test
Meniere's disease	Hours	Salt intake, sleep deprivation, stress	Low-frequency hearing loss, Fluctuating
Migraine-associated dizziness	Minutes to days	Migraine triggers (menses, seasonal changes, sleep deprivation, specific food, stress)	Positive family history, association with migraine headache and symptoms
Stroke	Days to weeks	Spontaneous in patients with cardiovascular risk factors	Associated neurological deficits
Orthostatic hypotension	Seconds	Standing from sitting position	Postural drop in blood pressure
Anxiety Disorder	Minutes to days	Complex visual surround, crowds, stress	Anxiety symptoms
Cerebellar ataxia	Chronic	Alcohol, genetic	Ataxia

2. **Pre-syncope** is a feeling of faintness or lightheadedness. Questions such as "do you feel like you might pass out" or "does it feel similar to when you stand up too fast" are questions which suggest that the patient is describing pre-syncope.
3. **Disequilibrium** is the feeling of being unsteady on one's feet. Typically, this improves quite a bit when there are other sensory cues (such as the ability to touch things) and is much worse when the patient's vision is blocked, or when the surface on which they are walking is very uneven. Questions such as "does it only happen when you're on your feet" and "does it get much better if you touch things" are very useful. Additionally, disequilibrium is probable if the patient notes that the sensation is substantially worse in the dark or when they are in the shower.

Other important points to look after during history taking are:

- The timing of the dizziness whether it appears constantly or in attacks.
- Any associated symptoms (such as hearing change, nausea, etc.).
- The duration of the attacks.
- Provocative causes (such as movement, loud noise, or pressure changes).

The most essential question is whether any neurologic symptoms are present. As there are several potentially dangerous causes of dizziness, one must always maintain a high degree of suspicion (cerebellar hemorrhage or ischemia, brainstem hemorrhage or ischemia, vertebral artery dissection).

One should ask about any weakness or change in sensation of the limbs or face, slurred speech, vision changes, memory loss, or ataxia. These symptoms are indicative of a central insult.

Although rare, compromise of the posterior cerebral circulation may manifest with neck pain (from trauma or vertebral artery dissection) and associated dizziness and requires prompt neurosurgical consultation.

13.2.2 Examination

The examination should focus on the cardiovascular system (cardiac rhythm and orthostatic blood pressure measurements) on the neurologic system (oculomotor function and balance) and the ear examination (vestibular system and hearing).

- **Spontaneous nystagmus**

  Spontaneous nystagmus indicates an imbalance within the vestibular system (central or peripheral). A unidirectional horizontal spontaneous nystagmus is characteristic of an acute peripheral vestibular insult. Spontaneous vertical, pure torsional nystagmus indicates a central lesion.

- **Gaze-evoked nystagmus**

  Unilateral vestibular lesion can result in gaze-evoked nystagmus that only occurs in one direction.

  Central lesions typically lead to gaze-evoked nystagmus that is “multidirectional”.

- **Head Thrust Test**

  The head thrust test is used to assess the vestibulo-ocular reflex (VOR).

  In patients with normal vestibular function, the VOR results in movement of the eyes in the direction opposite to the head movement.

  In peripheral vestibular insult, impairment of the VOR is identified where the eyes move off the target and a voluntary saccade (so-called refixation saccade or catch-up saccades) is observed bringing the patient’s eyes back to the target after the head thrust test.

- **Positional testing**

  Positional testing can trigger peripheral or central nystagmus.

  The Dix–Hallpike test is used to diagnose the posterior semicircular canal in benign paroxysmal positional vertigo (BPPV). The head is turned 45° to the side in the sitting patient, and then he/she is moved to the head-hanging position. If the patient has debris moving in the posterior canal, this will lead to a burst of upbeat-torsional nystagmus lasting about 15 s. Pure vertical nystagmus, particularly persistent downbeat nystagmus, suggests a central lesion, usually involving the midline cerebellum.

- **Gait and balance testing**

  The patient is observed while walking normally, while walking in tandem, and in the Romberg position with eyes opened and closed. Impaired gait and balance can accompany dizziness of any cause.

  Severe gait impairment suggests a neurologic disorder.

  Patients with peripheral vestibular lesions are off-balance but usually can walk with assistance and their imbalance gets exacerbated once they close their eyes.

13.3 Vertigo

Vertigo, the illusion of movement, is due to imbalances of signals to the central vestibular apparatus. This can either be due to peripheral or central causes. Signs and symptoms can usually distinguish peripheral from central causes of vertigo (Table 13.2).

Table 13.2 Common signs and symptoms differentiating central vertigo from peripheral vertigo

	Central vertigo	Peripheral vertigo
Onset	Gradual, slow	Sudden
Intensity	Mild	Severe
Duration	Weeks to months	Intermittent episodes: <1 min for BPPV Continuous lasting for hours or days for vestibular neuritis
Fatigability	Does not fatigue	Fatigues, adaptation
Associated symptoms	Weakness, numbness, falls more likely	Nausea, hearing loss, sweating
Eye closure	Symptoms better with eyes closed	Symptoms worse with eye closed
Nystagmus	Vertical, bilateral	Horizontal
Latency of nystagmus	Short (<5 sec)	Longer (>20 sec)
Ocular fixation	No effect or enhances nystagmus	Suppresses nystagmus (may not suppress during acute phase)
Effect of head position	Little change, associated with more than one position	Worsened by position, often single critical position

13.3.1 Peripheral Vertigo

It relates to damage of the inner ear receptors or to the vestibulocochlear nerve. There may be auditory symptoms. There should be no other signs of damage to the nervous system. The patient is likely to experience nausea or "motion sickness".

The nystagmus is unidirectional either horizontal or rotary.

Head thrust can provide important information. Usually, individuals are able to maintain good focus if the inner ears are intact since the head thrust activates the VOR. Inability to maintain fixation when doing this indicates damage to the inner ear.

13.3.2 Central Vertigo

Central causes include damage to the central nervous system mainly the brain stem. Central vertigo is typically milder than peripheral. The amount of nystagmus is usually greater than the patient's symptoms. Additionally, the nystagmus may be in multiple directions or possibly in a vertical direction. There are often other abnormalities of the central nervous system found by examination.

13.4 Vestibular Disorders

13.4.1 Vestibular Neuritis

Vestibular neuritis is an inner ear disease characterized by a sudden drop in ipsilateral vestibular function and acute onset of severe vertigo without any neurologic deficits.

Epidemiology: Vestibular neuritis accounts for 5–10% of all cases presenting with vertigo, with an annual incidence of approximating 3.5 cases per 100,000 persons. Common age is between 30 and 50 years [2, 3].

Physiopathology: Herpes viral infectious process affecting "Scarpa's" ganglion or the vestibular nerve might be responsible.

The superior vestibular nerve, which supplies the utricle, superior, and horizontal semicircular canals, is more likely to be involved in cases of vestibular neuritis because of the increased length, reduced diameter, and increased bony trabeculae of the bony canal housing it as compared with the inferior vestibular nerve [4–7].

Benign paroxysmal positional vertigo (BPPV) is more common in patients who have suffered from vestibular neuritis because the utricular otoconia might be loosened with the initial neuritis and float into the posterior canal innervated by the superior vestibular nerve which stays functional in the majority of vestibular neuritis patients as evidenced by normal VEMP studies (saccular nerve is branch of superior vestibular nerve).

Clinical manifestations: It is characterized by the acute onset of vertigo with associated nausea, vomiting, and generalized imbalance. The acute phase is often severe and can last from a few hours to several days, while a more subtle sense of imbalance and unsteadiness may linger for weeks. Auditory symptoms are absent.

Patients with accompanying hearing loss are believed to have a slightly different pathophysiological entity termed acute labyrinthitis.

Physical examination: Patients with vestibular neuritis may sway toward the side of the involved ear while standing, but an inability to stand without assistance is indicative of a central lesion.

It is characterised by Spontaneous horizonto-rotatory nystagmus that beats to the contra-lateral side and improves with fixation.

Head thrust testing toward the affected ear will often demonstrate catch-up saccades indicating a peripheral vestibular insult.

Diagnosis: History and physical examination alone are usually adequate for diagnosis and no need for imaging.

Management of the acute phase of vestibular neuritis is primarily medical, while long-term treatment is designed to improve vestibular compensation.

The early administration of steroids may improve the rate and extent of recovery of vestibular function.

Early exercise is encouraged, and patients are instructed on various vestibular exercises designed to enhance ocular stability and improve the tolerance of various head and body movements.

The degree of compensation is somewhat variable and likely depends on a number of factors, including patient age, underlying functional status, and degree of initial vestibular injury. While many patients may be able to compensate with the help of home vestibular exercise programs, others may require formal vestibular rehabilitation.

13.4.2 Meniere's Disease

Meniere's disease (MD) is a clinical syndrome characterized by episodic spontaneous vertigo, fluctuating hearing loss, aural pressure, and tinnitus.

13.4.2.1 Epidemiology

The incidence of MD varies between 4.3 and 15.3 per 100,000 [8, 9].

Affected individuals are usually between the fourth and sixth decades of life, with a female/male ratio of 1.3:1. Bilateral MD at presentation was seen in 11%, with another 14% of unilateral MD becoming bilateral MD.

13.4.2.2 Physiopathology

Endolymphatic hydrops (ELH) is felt to be the underlying histopathologic correlate in MD.

Histopathological studies in human temporal bones have found ELH in most patients with MD [10, 11] .

3 T MRI (3 Tesla MRI) with gadolinium chelate showed ELH in 93% of ears with symptoms attributable to MD [12].

Electrophysiologic studies showing increased SP/AP ratios suggest the presence of ELH [13].

The cause of ELH is multifactorial. Several intrinsic (genetic, anatomic, autoimmune, or vascular) or extrinsic (allergic, viral, or trauma) factors can cause disturbance in the mechanisms involved in the regulation of endolymphatic fluid homeostasis.

13.4.2.3 Diagnosis

History, physical examination, and audiometry alone are enough to establish the diagnosis of MD:

- Two or more spontaneous episodes of vertigo each lasting 20 min to 12 h.
- Low- to medium-frequency sensorineural hearing loss in one ear, defining the affected ear on at least one occasion before, during, or after one of the episodes of vertigo.
- Fluctuating aural symptoms (hearing, tinnitus, or fullness) in the affected ear.
- Not better accounted for by another vestibular diagnosis.

13.4.2.4 Electrophysiologic Studies

Several diagnostic tests have been proposed to study the presence of ELH and complement the clinical diagnosis of MD. Two electrophysiologic tests merit discussion: electrocochleography (ECoG) and VEMPs.

- *Electrocochleography*

  It is an evoked potential in response to a click or tone burst stimuli recorded by an intratympanic or extra tympanic electrode. The SP and AP of the eighth nerve are recorded.

  An increased SP/AP ratio (greater than 0.4) and/or a widened AP width (greater than 3 ms) are considered to be significant for ELH. The sensitivity is 70–90%.
- *The cervical VEMP (cVEMP)*

  The cVEMP is a recording of the vestibulocollic reflex generated in the saccule, carried via the inferior vestibular nerve. It consists of an inhibitory potential of the ipsilateral sternocleidomastoid muscle (SCM) muscle evoked by a brief and loud (>85 dB) monaural click or tone burst stimuli.

  Patients with MD were shown to have increased cVEMP thresholds or absent reflex compared with controls.
- *Caloric Testing and Head-thrust Testing*

  Significant caloric weakness is present in 42–73% of patients with MD.

  Caloric testing is useful in: (1) assessment of contralateral function before an ablative procedure, (2) assessment of residual function after an ablative procedure, and (3) assessment of ipsilateral function; if residual function is good, we favor a non-destructive procedure.

13.4.2.5 Management

The initial management of MD includes a low-salt diet and avoidance of caffeine derivatives and alcohol.

- *Diuretics and low-sodium diet* are effective in controlling the symptoms of MD in most of patients.
- *Intratympanic dexamethasone* can control vertigo in more than 90% of patients. Although more than half of the patients responded to one or two injections, some patients may require more than four injections.
- *Intratympanic gentamicin* is a destructive treatment that results in chemical labyrinthectomy. Gentamicin is a selective vestibulotoxic aminoglycoside antibiotic that causes apoptotic cell death of the vestibular dark cells, resulting in partial or complete ablation of peripheral vestibular function. Hearing deterioration occurs in 10–35% of patients and depends on host genetic susceptibility to aminoglycosides affect. When hearing is poor, it is a reasonable option that offers effective vertigo control with minimal morbidity; however, in patients with serviceable hearing, many physicians feel reluctant to use it.
- *Endolymphatic sac surgery:* The efficacy of sac surgery has been, and continues to be, debated. There is no evidence of its superiority to natural history of the disease.
- *Vestibular nerve sectioning*: Selective sectioning of the vestibular nerve performed via retrosigmoid approach offers more than 95% control of vertigo. It is an excellent option in patient with refractory vertigo and serviceable hearing.
- *Labyrinthectomy*: When conservative procedures fail to control vertigo, the treating otologist needs to consider neural or labyrinthine destructive procedures to ablate all residual vestibular function in the hope of controlling the ongoing vestibulopathy.

13.4.3 Benign Paroxysmal Positional Vertigo

Benign paroxysmal positional vertigo (BPPV) is the most common peripheral vestibular end-organ disease and is typified by a sudden, transient vertigo which is accompanied by characteristic nystagmus.

13.4.3.1 Epidemiology

BPPV is the most common vestibular disorders with an estimated lifetime prevalence of 2.4% in the general adult population. More than 30% of patients attending a dizzy clinic are diagnosed with BPPV.

Although this disorder affects people across their lifespan, it tends to affect individuals aged 50–70 years.

13.4.3.2 Pathophysiology of BPPV

The otoconia from the utricle dislodge and settle within one of the three semicircular canals, changing the fluid-filled canal dynamics from detecting rotation of the canals to detecting gravitation forces on the head.

The debris may be found within the long arm of the canal (canalithiasis) or in the short arm of the canal or attached to the cupula (cupulolithiasis).

The reasons for detachment are many but include increasing age, trauma, and infection.

95% of BPPV cases involve the PSC, and 5% involve the lateral semicircular canal (LSC).

13.4.3.3 Diagnosis and Treatment of PSC-BPPV

The diagnosis of BPPV is based on history and findings on positional testing. Patients who complain of vertigo with rolling in bed or getting out of bed are most likely to have BPPV.

- Dix–Hallpike diagnostic maneuver is the diagnostic maneuver. During this maneuver, the patient's head is turned 45° to one side while he is seated. The patient is then moved quickly to a supine position with the neck slightly extended and the head remaining turned. The diagnostic criteria for posterior canal BPPV are vertigo associated with the characteristic nystagmus—ipsidirectional torsional and up beating nystagmus is seen when the undermost ear is affected. With a latency of 30–45 s before onset and a duration of less than 60 s. The nystagmus is noted to reverse direction when the patient is brought back up to a sitting position. The nystagmus diminishes with repeated positional testing in the same sitting.
- Epley therapeutic maneuver is canalith repositioning maneuver described by Epley and consists of a series of four head positions designed to use the effects of gravity to treat canalithiasis. With each head position, the debris settles to the lowest portion of the canal, moving the debris away from the ampulla, into the common crus, and then into the utricle.

  Repeating the maneuver 2–3 times is significantly more effective than performing it once.

  There is no need for postintervention postural and activity restrictions.

  It is effective in more than 90% of cases.
- The Semont therapeutic maneuver is another PSC canalith repositioning maneuver whereby the patient is rapidly moved from lying on one side to lying on the other. The Semont maneuver is less effective and not currently favored because the high velocity which is anxiety provoking. Practically, it is often tried when Epley maneuver fails.

13.4.3.4 Diagnosis and Treatment of LSC-BPPV

LSC-BPPV can be diagnosed with supine positional testing (head centered supine, right ear down, and then left ear down). This maneuvre provokes a bidirectional/bipositional horizontal nystagmus. The identification of the involved ear in LSC-BPPV can be especially difficult because the canals are coplanar, and nystagmus is seen in both positions regardless of the involved ear.

Two distinct subtypes of LSC-BPPV exist based on nystagmus direction during supine positional testing:

- Geotropic LSC-BPPV

  It is caused by canaliths moving within the long arm of the LSC.

  During supine positional testing, nystagmus is horizontal and beats toward the ground and is worse with the affected ear down. The nystagmus has a short latency and prolonged duration with poor fatigability.

  Treatment of geotropic LSC-BPV consists of 360° log roll maneuvers toward the unaffected ear at 90° increments every 30–60 s, beginning with the patient in the supine position and laterally rotated toward the affected ear. Repositioning treatments can alleviate symptoms in 75–100% of patients
- Apogeotropic LSC-BPPV

  It is very rare and is caused by otoconial debris that adheres to the cupula of the lateral canal (cupulolithiasis) or otoconia trapped in the proximal segment of the lateral canal.

  During supine positional testing, the nystagmus beating is away from the undermost ear. Nystagmus is usually worse with the affected ear uppermost.

  Treatment of apogeotropic LSC-BPPV consists of the Lempert 360° roll maneuver toward the unaffected ear. The efficacy of canalith repositioning for apogeotropic LSC-BPPV is less than 50%.

13.4.3.5 Surgical Treatment of BPPV

If repositioning therapy is not successful, surgery is an option for PSC-BPPV. Plugging of the involved semicircular canal has been used in cases of resistant PSC-BPPV.

However, this treatment has been more difficult for LSC-BPPV because of the difficulty in locating the correct side.

13.4.4 Migraine-Associated Vertigo

Migraine-associated vertigo (MAV) is defined as vertigo or dizziness caused by migraine.

13.4.4.1 Prevalence

Ten percent of the population has migraine headaches [14],and 1/3 of them experience dizziness [15]. It affects women approximately three times more frequently than men. MAV is 10 times more common than Meniere's disease.

13.4.4.2 Clinical Manifestations

- The most common symptoms of MAV are rotational vertigo, intolerance of head motion or visual motion, sensation of motion sickness, floating, rocking, tilting, walking on an uneven surface, and lightheadedness.
- The onset of symptoms could be gradual or abrupt and usually, but necessarily, associated with migraine symptoms like headache, photophobia, phonophobia, nausea, and/or aura.
- MAV is usually triggered by migraine triggers: menses, sleep deprivation, fasting, dehydration, change of season, caffeine (or change in the pattern of caffeine intake), chocolate, alcohol, aged cheeses, nitrites…
- The duration of symptoms is usually few hours but may range from minutes to days.

13.4.4.3 Diagnosis

It is based on the identification of the following three clinical criteria:

1. Episodic vestibular symptoms of at least moderate severity.
2. History of migraine, or migrainous symptoms during some attacks of vertigo, or migraine triggers of vertigo in more than 50% of attacks.
3. Other causes are ruled out by appropriate investigations. The most useful tests include audiometry (to exclude Meniere's disease or labyrinthitis) and videonystagmography (to exclude peripheral vestibular hypofunction). In cases where doubt remains, brain imaging is warranted.

13.4.4.4 Treatment

MAV is managed similarly to migraine:

- *Trigger avoidance.*
- *Pharmaceutical Prophylactic* is favored when attacks are frequent or severe. Three groups of medications can be employed: anticonvulsants, antihypertensives, and antidepressants. In our practice, treatment most commonly starts with the antidepressant, venlafaxine, followed by the anticonvulsant, topiramate, and then b-blockers (e.g. propranolol).

Benign paroxysmal vertigo of childhood (BPVC) is a vertiginous disorder of childhood attributable to migraine and has a prevalence of 3%. It typically occurs in children 3–8 years old. Attacks are sudden in onset and are typically brief, lasting only a few seconds to minutes. The affected child may remain still, refusing to move, or may grab onto something for support, and nystagmus is often noted during the attack. There is often associated anxiety, pallor, nausea, sweating, and occasionally vomiting. At the completion of the attack, the child usually resumes normal activity. Physical examination and all imaging studies typically are normal. After a few years, the episodes of BPVC cease. Children affected with BPVC may develop classic migraines later in life [16–18].

13.4.5 Superior Canal Dehiscence Syndrome

Typical symptoms include hyperacusis for bone-conducted sounds with autophony, and vertigo induced by loud sounds (Tullio phenomenon) or increased pressure in the middle ear (Hennebert sign) or intracranial space (e.g. during strenuous activities) (see Chap. 13).

13.4.6 Perilymph Fistula

Perilymphatic fistula results from a small leak between the inner ear and the air-filled middle ear. The sudden change in inner ear pressure due to leakage of this fluid may trigger episodes of vertigo as well as producing some chronic damage to hair cells. Changing pressure in the external ear (such as with insufflation through an otoscope) may also precipitate attacks in both of these conditions. This has been termed "Hennebert's sign". Although this has also been suggested as a "fistula test", this is not specific for perilymph fistula. Precipitation of attacks by changes in pressure (airplanes, driving in mountains, and Valsalva) is more characteristic of perilymph fistula (see Chap. 14).

13.5 Central Causes of Vertigo

The central causes of vertigo include cerebrovascular disease (including transient ischemic attacks), multiple sclerosis, Chiari malformation, and any other conditions directly damaging the caudal brain stem or the vestibulocerebellum.

13.5.1 Chiari Malformation

Chiari malformation is defined by protrusion of the lower portion of the cerebellum through the foramen magnum. This compresses the caudal brain stem and vestibular areas and can cause dizziness and imbalance. It is often associated with an occipital headache and downbeat nystagmus, which strongly suggest an abnormality at the craniocervical junction. Coughing, sneezing, straining, or neck extension can all make these symptoms worse.

13.5.2 Vertebrobasilar Insufficiency

Dizziness and imbalance are common problems in elderly patients.

Although BPPV accounts for majority of cases of vertigo in this population, the presentation of an elderly patient with vertigo, including position-dependent vertigo, must address the possibility of vertebrobasilar ischemia.

Vertigo can be the presentation of vertebrobasilar ischemia, and in fact, vertigo is the most common initial isolated symptom and sign of ischemia in the posterior circulation.

Typical vertebrobasilar patients are older and have multiple vascular risk factors.

Vertebrobasilar insufficiency typically causes multiple cranial nerve symptoms (e.g. visual abnormalities, diplopia or oscillopsia, dizziness, or dysphagia) and may culminate in frank syncope.

Typically, vertigo in vertebrobasilar TIAs is abrupt in onset and usually lasts several minutes. When the vertigo is accompanied by other symptoms of brainstem ischemia (e.g. visual symptoms, drop attacks, extremity numbness, or dysarthria), one would assume that vertigo derives from vertebrobasilar ischemia.

13.5.3 Vertebral Artery Dissection

Vertebral artery dissection is a rare but serious condition that can result from neck trauma. This may occlude branches that go to the vestibular area of the brain stem or cerebellum and cause vertigo. Any new onset of vertigo after neck trauma should evoke the diagnosis of vertebral arerty dissection.

13.6 Disequilibrium

This is a common type of dizziness in the elderly. This is due to disturbance of sensory or motor control systems that are necessary to maintain the upright posture.

- **Sensory disequilibrium:** The vast majority of cases of disequilibrium are due to sensory difficulties. This typically occurs with gradual decrease in sensory acuity in several systems. Usually, there is diminished sensitivity to joint position in the feet, along with some decreased sensitivity of the inner ear balance organ. The symptoms typically are exacerbated in situations where the vision is obstructed.

This kind of deficit usually shows dramatic improvement when the patient touches or holds onto a stationary object (replacing the loss of sensitivity in feet with the sensitivity of the hands). These patients improve with a cane or other gait-assistive device.

- **Motor disequilibrium**: Patients with Parkinson's disease or cerebellar disease often have disequilibrium due to motor difficulties. This limits their ability to respond to the changing conditions of ambulation. Slowed responses in Parkinson's disease or incoordination and cerebellar disease may make the patient entirely unable to walk safely. The patient perceives this as disequilibrium.

Take-Home Messages

- Assessment of a dizzy patient starts by obtaining a proper history and examination in order to reach a diagnosis and offer the best management.
- Vertigo is due to imbalances of signals to the central vestibular apparatus. It can either be due to peripheral or central causes. Signs and symptoms can usually distinguish peripheral from central causes of vertigo.
- Peripheral vertigo is due to damage of the inner ear receptors or to the vestibulocochlear nerve.
- Central vertigo is due to damage to the central nervous system mainly the brain stem. It is typically milder than peripheral vertigo.
- Vestibular disorders include vestibular neuritis, Meniere's disease, benign paroxysmal positional vertigo, and migraine-associated vertigo.
- Vestibular neuritis is an inner ear disease characterized by a sudden drop in ipsilateral vestibular function and acute onset of severe vertigo without any neurologic deficits.
- Meniere's disease (MD) is characterized by episodic spontaneous vertigo, fluctuating hearing loss, aural pressure, and tinnitus.
- Benign paroxysmal positional vertigo (BPPV) is the most common peripheral vestibular end-organ disease and characterized by a sudden, transient vertigo accompanied by a characteristic nystagmus. 95% of BPPV cases involve the PSC, and 5% involve the LSC.
- Migraine-associated vertigo is diagnosed based on excluding other causes, history of migraine, and presence of vestibular symptoms.

References

1. Davis A, Moorjani P. The epidemiology of hearing and balance disorders. In: Luxon LM, Furman JM, Martini A, Stephens D, editors. Textbook of audiological medicine. London: Dunitz M; 2003. p. 89–99.
2. Neuhauser H. Epidemiology of vertigo. Curr Opin Neurol. 2007;20:40–6.
3. Sekitani T, Imate Y, Noguchi T, et al. Vestibular neuronitis: epidemiological survey by questionnaire in Japan. Acta Otolaryngol Suppl. 1993;503:9–12.
4. Theil D, Arbusow V, Deurfuss T, et al. Prevalence of HSV-1 LAT in human trigeminal, geniculate, and vestibular ganglia and its implication for cranial nerve syndromes. Brain Pathol. 2001;11(4):408–13.
5. Baloh RW, Ishiyama A, Wackym P, et al. Vestibular neuritis: clinical–pathological correlation. Otolaryngol Head Neck Surg. 1996;114:586–92.
6. Schuknecht HF, Kitamura K. Vestibular neuronitis. Ann Otol Rhinol Laryngol. 1981;78:1–19.
7. Nadol JB. Vestibular neuritis. Otolaryngol Head Neck Surg. 1995;112:162–72.
8. Arenberg IK, Balkany TJ, Goldman G, et al. The incidence and prevalence of Meniere's disease–a statistical analysis of limits. Otolaryngol Clin N Am. 1980;13:597.
9. Stahle J, Stahle C, Arenberg IK. Incidence of Meniere's disease. Arch Otolaryngol. 1978;104:99.
10. Rauch SD, Merchant SN, Thedinger BA. Menière's syndrome and endolymphatic hydrops: double-blind temporal bone study. Ann Otol Rhinol Laryngol. 1989;98:873–83.
11. Merchant SN, Adams JC, Nadol JB. Pathophysiology of Menière' syndrome are symptoms caused by endolymphatic hydrops? Otol Neurotol. 2005;26: 74–81.

12. Pyykkö I, Nakashima T, Yoshida T, Zou J, Naganawa S. Meniere's disease: a reappraisal supported by a variable latency of symptoms and the MRI visualisation of endolymphatic hydrops. BMJ Open. 2013;3(2):e001555.
13. Lamounier P, Gobbo DA, de Souza TSA, de Oliveira CACP, Bahmad F. Electrocochleography for Ménière's disease: is it reliable? Braz J Otorhinolaryngol. 2014;80:527–32.
14. Stewart W, Shechter A, Rasmussen B. Migraine prevalence. A review of population based studies. Neurology. 1994;44(Suppl 4):S17–23.
15. Selby G, Lance JW. Observations on 500 cases of migraine and allied vascular headache. J Neurol Neurosurg Psychiatry. 1960;23:23–32.
16. Niemensivu R, Pyykko I, Erna K. Vertigo and imbalance in children. Arch Otolaryngol Head Neck Surg. 2005;131:996–1000.
17. Lempert T, Neuhauser H. Migrainous vertigo. Neurol Clin. 2005;23:715–30.
18. Ralli G, Atturo F, deFilippis C. Idiopathic benign paroxysmal vertigo in children, a migraine precursor. Int J Pediatr Otorhinolaryngol. 2009;73:S16–8.

Perilymphatic Fistula

14

Aisha Larem, Ma'in Ali Al Shawabkeh, and Adham Aljariri

14.1 Introduction

Perilymphatic fistula is an abnormal connection between the labyrinth and structures surrounding it [1]. It is a condition that can present with a variety of non-specific symptoms; it is considered a diagnostic challenge. A proper history and physical examination is a key element during workup of those patients. Treatment options vary depending on the severity and response to medical therapy and conservative measures.

14.2 Clinical Manifestations

It has a wide range of symptoms:

1. Hearing loss [2]
    (a) It is the most common symptom.
    (b) It can show high frequency, low frequency, or even a flat sensorineural hearing loss.
    (c) It tends to fluctuate.
    (d) It can sometimes present with conductive hearing loss.
2. Vertigo [2]
    (a) It is the most common reason for seeking medical advice.
    (b) It can resemble Benign paroxysmal positional vertigo (BPPV) or Meniere's disease.
    (c) It can mimic disequilibrium in certain occasions. For example, patients may present with disequilibrium upon exposure to loud voices (Tullio's phenomenon) or by increasing Cerebrospinal fluid (CSF) pressure (during lifting or blowing of the nose).
3. Tinnitus [3]
    (a) Other symptoms of perilymphatic fistula usually accompany tinnitus.

14.3 Workup

- Diagnosis of the perilymphatic fistula is usually tricky, but it is mainly based on history, physical examination findings, and exclusion of other diagnoses.
- Some tests that can be used are as follows:
    - Audiometry: it can show high frequency, low frequency, or flat sensorineural hearing loss. A low-frequency conductive hearing

A. Larem (✉)
Hamad Medical Corporation, Doha, Qatar

Otology Clinical Fellow, Hamad Medical Corporation, Doha, Qatar
e-mail: alarem@hamad.qa

M. A. Al Shawabkeh
Otology Clinical Fellow, Hamad Medical Corporation, Doha, Qatar
e-mail: MAIGhshoum@hamad.qa

A. Aljariri
Hamad Medical Corporation, Doha, Qatar
e-mail: AAljariri@hamad.qa

A. Al-Qahtani et al. (eds.), *Textbook of Clinical Otolaryngology*,
https://doi.org/10.1007/978-3-030-54088-3_14

loss can be seen in superior semicircular canal dehiscence. It is recommended to do the test in lateral decubitus while the affected ear is up [4, 5].
- Fistula test: the presence of nystagmus upon applying pressure on the external auditory canal is considered a positive fistula test. Hennebert sign is the presence of a positive fistula test without any middle ear pathology [5].
- Measuring of postural sway upon applying pressure on the external auditory canal [5].
- Electronystagmography/videonystagmography: It can show unilateral weakness. It can also be used to increase the sensitivity of a fistula test [6].
- Some other methods were utilized to help in diagnosis, like measuring Beta 2 transferrin and using fluorescein to detect perilymphatic fistula. However, their utilization has been questioned and still in doubt [7, 8].
- Exploration: it is considered unreliable for spontaneous perilymphatic fistula. However, its reliability is increased in the presence of a temporal bone fracture or stapedectomy surgery in a patient's history [3].

14.4 Management

- Conservative: Bed rest, head elevation, and avoid straining [3].
- Surgical management in case of failure to respond to conservative therapy. It consists of patching the otic capsule. Some surgeons patch the oval and round window regardless of the intraoperative findings as the detection rate of the perilymphatic fistula is quite low. Fat, perichondrium, fascia, and temporalis muscle can be used for patching [3, 9].

14.5 Etiologic Causes

Look at Table 14.1.

Table 14.1 Location and the probable etiologic causes of perilymphatic fistula

Otic capsule	Oval window	Round window
• Cholesteatoma • Temporal bone fracture • Superior semicircular canal dehiscence	• Barotrauma • Head trauma • Stapedectomy • Acoustic trauma	• Barotrauma • Mondini dysplasia

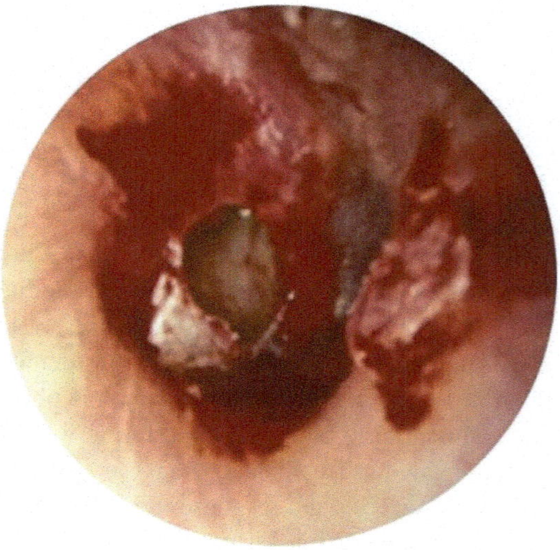

Fig. 14.1 Traumatic rupture of the tympanic membrane caused by barotrauma

14.5.1 Barotrauma (Fig. 14.1)

- Pressure changes can cause damage to the inner ear by three mechanisms:
  - Alternobaric trauma: it occurs in cases of increased pressure or asymmetrical pressure of the middle ear. It usually occurs more during the ascent of the divers or ascent of the planes. Conditions that affect the functions of the eustachian tube (URTI, sinusitis) can increase individual's susceptibility to these kinds of trauma [10].
  - Atmospheric barotrauma: it occurs in cases of the increase of the air pressure, which can cause middle ear and inner ear damage. It usually gives long-lasting symptoms as compared to the alternobaric trauma [10].

- Inner ear decompression sickness: it occurs due to the formation of bubbles in the labyrinth or its blood supply. It happens in deep water divers who use mixed gases like oxyhelium [3].

14.5.2 Acoustic Trauma

- Explosive blast produces sound more than 200 dB, which can cause tympanic membrane (TM) perforation and disruption of the ossicles. Inner ear injury can happen, especially if conductive mechanisms are not disrupted [1].

14.5.3 Trauma

- It can happen in cases of head trauma or penetrating injury with or without temporal bone fracture. However, it is rare to have a perilymphatic fistula after trauma in normal temporal bone anatomy. Look at Fig. 14.2 [10, 11].

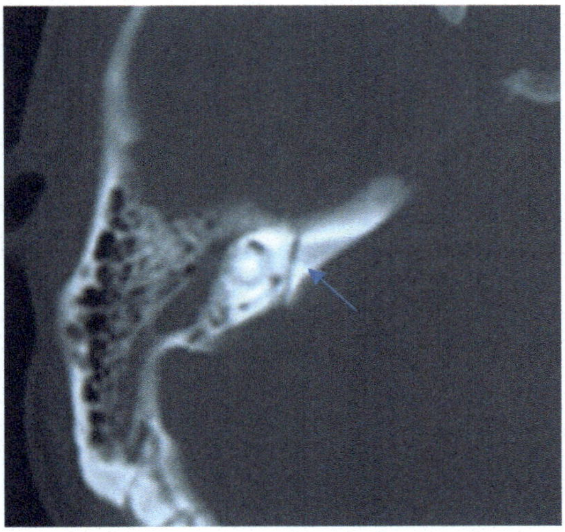

Fig. 14.2 Axial CT scan of left temporal transverse fracture (arrow) (Image Reprinted with permission from Elsevier: Elsevier books, Skull base imaging, Bert De Foer, Abdellatif Bali, Anja Bernaerts, Joost van Dinther, Erwin Offeciers, Jan W. Casselman, Jan 1, 2018)

14.5.4 Stapedectomy

- Perilymphatic fistula can happen after stapedectomy. It can be a primary or secondary one.
  - Primary: if it presents at the end of the procedure.
  - Secondary: if it manifests months or years after the procedure.
- It is more common in stapedectomy than stapedotomy.
- It is more common in revision surgeries.
- The use of gelatin sponge to seal the stapedectomy presents the highest risk of developing the fistula [10].

14.5.5 Superior Semicircular Canal Dehiscence

- Prevalence: It can be seen in 4–8% in high-resolution CT [2].
- Pathogenesis: It is often multifactorial (congenital and acquired factors) [10].
- Symptoms: Patients can have only vestibular symptoms, only auditory symptoms, or a combination of both [10, 12]. They often present with hearing loss, autophony (they can hear their voice), pulsatile tinnitus, and hearing the movement of their eyes (due to increased bone conduction). They can present with the Tullio phenomenon (vertigo and imbalance after exposure to loud voices). They might complain of vertigo and imbalance after conditions that increase Cerebrospinal fluid (CSF) pressure. Pure tone audiometry shows conductive hearing loss (CHL) with a larger air-bone (AB) gap at low frequencies [10].
- Diagnosis: High-resolution CT scan. Dehiscence can be seen in coronal view, Stenvers view (in the plane of orthogonal), or Poschl view (in the place of the SSC) [13]. CT usually overestimates the size of the dehiscence. To improve the specificity, then 0.5 mm CT scan should be reformatted to the Poschl plane [14] Fig. 14.3.

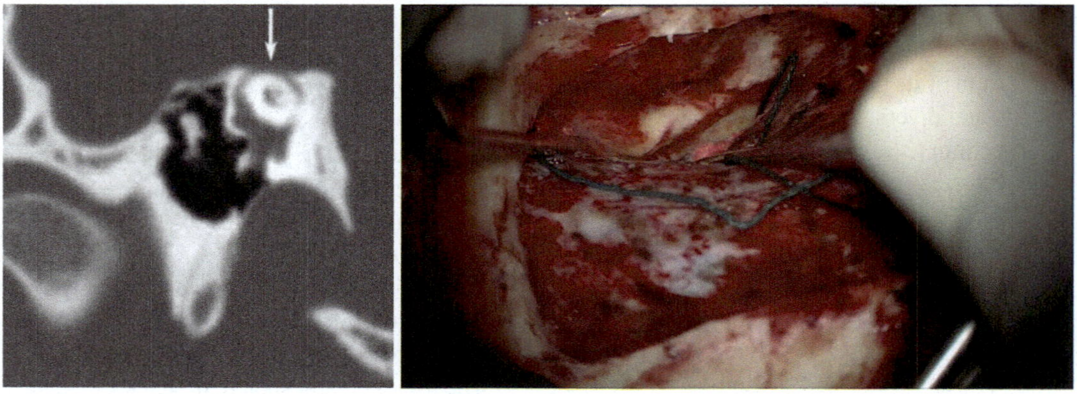

Fig. 14.3 Coronal CT scan of left IAM demonstrating left superior semicircular canal dehiscence, and next image shows SCC intraoperatively

- VEMP: it has high sensitivity and specificity (around 90%). Patients with SSC dehiscence will have a lower threshold in the affected ear for both air and bone conduction [1].
- Treatment: if patients have mild symptoms, then conservative measures should be taken. Insertion of ventilation tubes can relieve pressure symptoms. If symptoms are severe, then surgical correction should be considered [10].
- Surgical Approaches [10].
  - Middle cranial fossa craniotomy: gives a good exposure. Disadvantages are risks of craniotomy, more extended hospital stay, and temporal bone retraction.
  - Endoscopic middle cranial fossa: it has less hospital stay but still has risks of craniotomy.
  - Transmastoid: avoid craniotomy risks but do not have direct exposure to the SSC.

14.5.6 Mondini Malformation [2] (Fig. 14.4)

- It is the most common malformation of the cochlea.
- The cochlea has only 1.5 turns.
- The modiolus is hypoplastic and lacking the interscalar septum.
- Patients usually have variable auditory functions depending on the organ of Corti formation and the number of neurons.
- Now it is subtyped into three types: *Type 1*, entire modiolus and interscalar septa are lacking (it has a cystic appearance), *Type 2*, normal base turn with a cystic apex (Mondini type), and *Type 3*, where the modiolus is deficient (it has partial septation on the interscalar at the periphery of the cochlea).

14.5.7 Congenital Perilymphatic Fistula

- It is an abnormal communication between the inner ear and the middle ear. It is associated with micro-fissures around the round window or oval windows and dysplasia of labyrinthine or internal auditory meatus. It is usually suspected if a child presents with progressive or fluctuating sensorineural hearing loss (SNHL) [10, 15].

14.5.8 Perilymphatic Fistula in Children

- It can be seen in temporal bone anomalies and children who have severe or profound sensorineural hearing loss (SNHL). It can present with recurrent meningitis or Cerebrospinal fluid (CSF) behind the TM [10].

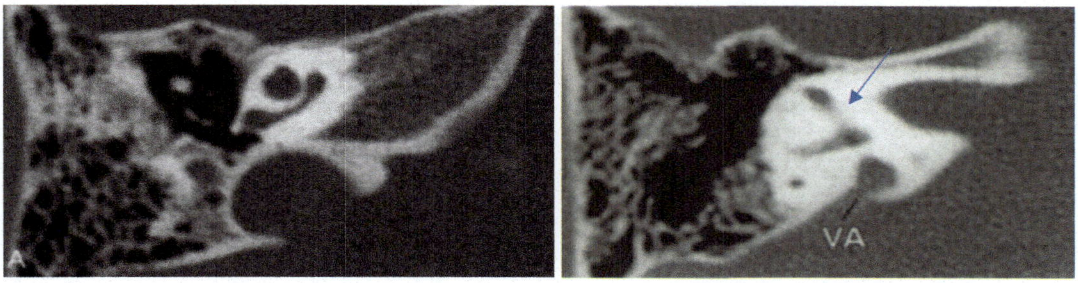

Fig. 14.4 Axial HRCT of the right temporal bone showing type II incomplete partition of the cochlea (Mondini malformation) with failure of segmentation of the middle and apical turns (arrow) associated with enlarged vestibular aqueduct (VA)

Take-Home Messages

- Perilymphatic fistula is a diagnostic challenge.
- Different images and diagnostic modalities should be used judiciously not to overwhelm the patient with unnecessary tests.
- Consider conservative management first.

References

1. Flint P, Haughey B, Lund V, Niparko J, Robbins K, Regan Thomas J, Lesperance M. Cummings otolaryngology. 6th ed. Philadelphia: Elsevier; 2014.
2. Watkinson JC, Clarke RW. Scott-Brown's otorhinolaryngology and head and neck surgery. 8th ed. Boca Raton, FL: CRC Press; 2018.
3. Snow JB, Ashley Wackym P. Ballenger's otorhinolaryngology and head and neck surgery. 17th ed. Connecticut: People's Medical Publishing House; 2008.
4. Kita AE, Kim I, Ishiyama G, Ishiyama A. Perilymphatic fistula after penetrating ear trauma. Clin Pract Cases Emerg Med. 2019;3(2):115–8. https://doi.org/10.5811/cpcem.2019.1.37404.
5. Hazell JW, Fraser JG, Robinson PJ. Positional audiometry in the diagnosis of perilymphatic fistula. Am J Otol. 1992;13(3):263–9.
6. Hornibrook J. A balance test for chronic perilymph fistula. Int J Otolaryngol. 2012;2012:163691. https://doi.org/10.1155/2012/163691.
7. Daspit CP, Churchill D, Linthicum FH Jr. Diagnosis of perilymph fistula using ENG and impedance. Laryngoscope. 1980;90(2):217–23.
8. Delaroche O, Bordure P, Lippert E, Sagniez M. Perilymph detection by beta2-transferrin immunoblotting assay. Application to the diagnosis of perilymphatic fistulae. Clin Chim Acta. 1996;245(1):93–104.
9. Gehrking E, Wisst F, Remmert S, Sommer K. Intraoperative assessment of perilymphatic fistulas with intrathecal administration of fluorescein. Laryngoscope. 2002;112(9):1614–8.
10. Hughes GB, Sismanis A, House JW. Is there consensus in perilymph fistula management? Otolaryngol Head Neck Surg. 1990;102:111–7.
11. Mikulec AA, McKenna MJ, Ramsey MJ, et al. Superior semicircular canal dehiscence presenting as conductive hearing loss without vertigo. Otol Neurotol. 2004;25:121–9.
12. Sequeira SM, Whiting BR, Shimony JS, et al. Accuracy of computed tomography detection of superior canal dehiscence. Otol Neurotol. 2011;32:1500–5.
13. Belden CJ, Weg N, Minor LB, Zinreich SJ. CT evaluation of bone dehiscence of the superior semicircular canal as a cause of sound- and/or pressure-induced vertigo. Radiology. 2003;226:337–43.
14. Zuniga MG, Janky KL, Nguyen KD, et al. Ocular versus cervical VEMPs in the diagnosis of superior semicircular canal dehiscence syndrome. Otol Neurotol. 2013;34:121–6.
15. Weber PC, Bluestone CD, Perez B. Outcome of hearing and vertigo after surgery for congenital perilymphatic fistula in children. Am J Otolaryngol. 2003;24:138–42.

Temporal Bone Trauma

15

Hassanin Abdulkarim, Abdulsalam Al-Qahtani,
and Ahmed Elsotouhy

Key Points
In this chapter, we will learn:

- Three main conditions involved in temporal bone trauma.
- Types of temporal bone fractures and their clinical presentation, investigations, and management plans.
- Middle ear trauma and its clinical presentation, investigations, and management plans.
- Barotrauma causes, clinical presentation, investigations, and management plans.

15.1 Temporal Bone Fractures

15.1.1 Introduction

- Temporal bone is the strongest bone of the body and at the same time one of the most complex bone as it contains many important structures, including the vestibulocochlear apparatus, carotid artery, jugular vein, and the facial nerve. Also, it is surrounded by the brain and other cranial nerves.
- Temporal bone as part of skull base has many foramina and openings causing weakness points which are involved by head trauma leading the fracture to follow these weak points.
- Temporal bone may involve none or all of these structures, and also can involve other structures like cranial nerve (6th, 9th, 10th, and 11th).
- The head is the most commonly injured part of the body (75% of all motor vehicle accidents).
- Approximately 30% of head traumas have skull fracture, and the ear is the most frequently sensory organ damaged.
- Temporal bone injury happens in up to 22% of all skull fractures and is caused mainly by motor vehicle accidents (around 30%).
- Temporal bone fracture is a common manifestation of head trauma, and 90% of temporal bone fractures are associated with intracranial injuries and 9% with cervical spine injury.
- Bilateral temporal bone fractures are present in 8–29% of all fractures.
- These can be due to blunt or penetrating trauma, and stab and gunshot wounds are the most common penetrating wounds. Gunshot wounds medial to the geniculate ganglion are usually fatal because it is associated with big vessels bleeding.

H. Abdulkarim (✉) · A. Al-Qahtani · A. Elsotouhy
Hamad Medical Corporation, Doha, Qatar
e-mail: habdulkarim@hamad.qa; aaa2009@qatar-med.cornell.edu; aelsetouhy@hamad.qa

A. Al-Qahtani et al. (eds.), *Textbook of Clinical Otolaryngology*,
https://doi.org/10.1007/978-3-030-54088-3_15

15.1.2 Types

- Ulrich was the first to classify temporal bone fractures into longitudinal and transverse fractures in 1926 [1].
- Ghorayeb and Yeakley studied 150 temporal bone fractures and found the majority is actually oblique or mixed [2].
- Other classification is otic capsule involvement or sparing.
- Ishman and Friedland classified them into petrous and non-petrous involvement, where the petrous-involved fractures have greater correlation with sensorineural hearing loss (SNHL) presence [3].
- All these classifications are arbitrary but useful to predict the type of injury expected. Although temporal bone fractures are irregular and non-uniform in their pathway.
- Despite the recent classifications, Ulrich's is the most commonly used due to its simplicity.

15.1.2.1 Longitudinal Fractures

Longitudinal fractures involve 80% of all temporal bone fractures. They are usually caused by a lateral force over the mastoid or temporal squama (temporal or parietal blows). The fracture line parallels the long axis of the petrous pyramid. It starts in the pars squamosa (mastoid or external auditory canal), extends through the posterosuperior bony external canal, continues across the roof of the middle ear space anterior to the labyrinth, and ends anteromedially in the middle cranial fossa in close proximity to the foramen lacerum and ovale (Table 15.1).

15.1.2.2 Transverse Fractures

Transverse fractures involve 20% of all temporal bone fractures. They are usually caused by a frontal, parietal, and less likely occipital blow. The fracture line runs at a right angle to the long axis of the petrous pyramid and starts in the middle cranial fossa (close to the foramen lacerum and spinosum). It then crosses the petrous pyramid transversely and ends at the foramen magnum. It may also extend through the internal auditory canal and injure the nerves directly (Table 15.1).

Table 15.1 Comparison of longitudinal and transverse temporal bone fractures with their main corresponding features

Feature	Longitudinal fractures	Transverse fractures
Incidence	80%	20%
Mechanism	Temporal or parietal trauma	Frontal or occipital trauma
CSF otorrhea	Common	Occasional
Tympanic membrane perforation	Common	Rare
Facial nerve damage	20% (temporary and delayed)	50% (severe, permanent, and immediate)
Hearing loss	Common (CHL)	Common (SNHL)
Hemotympanum	Common	Possible
Nystagmus and vertigo	Common (mild and temporary)	Common (severe and prolonged)
Otorrhagia	Common	Rare

15.1.2.3 Oblique or Mixed Fractures

They are a mixture of both longitudinal and transverse.

15.1.3 Clinical Presentation

15.1.3.1 Bleeding

Into the ear canal from skin and tympanic membrane laceration, hemotympanum (Fig. 15.1), external auditory canal fractures.

15.1.3.2 Hearing Loss

Conductive hearing loss (*CHL*) due to ossicular chain disruption [4, 5]:

- Incudostapedial joint separation (82%)
- Incus dislocation (57%)
- Fracture of the stapes crura (30%)
- Fixation of the ossicles in the attic (25%)
- Incudomalleolar joint separation (<3%)

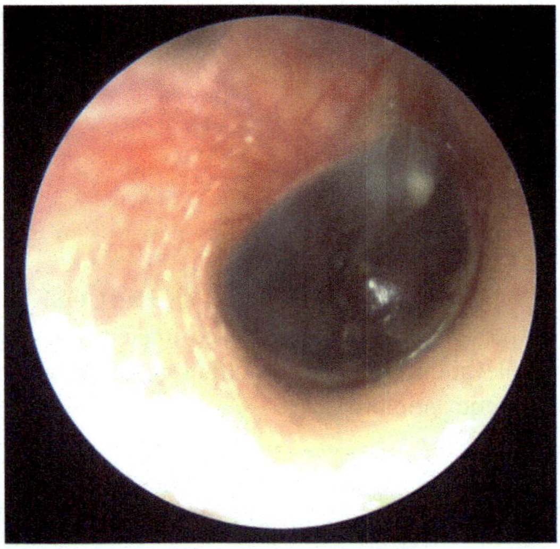

Fig. 15.1 Right ear hemotympanum

Also, it could be due to effusion of the middle ear by blood or cerebrospinal fluid (CSF), ear canal filled by debris, blood, or discharge.

Sensorineural hearing loss (*SNHL*) may occur as a result of concussive damage to the inner ear, and cochlear and vestibular structures are usually destroyed, producing a profound sensorineural hearing loss and tinnitus.

Rarely, a mixed hearing loss may occur.

15.1.3.3 Facial Nerve Paralysis

Twenty percent of longitudinal fractures and 50% of transverse fractures injure the facial nerve and cause paralysis. The injury site is usually the horizontal segment of the nerve distal to the geniculate ganglion in longitudinal fractures. The injury site is from the internal auditory canal to the horizontal segment distal to the geniculate ganglion in transverse fractures.

15.1.3.4 Vertigo and Nystagmus

Vertigo occurs but is not related to the severity of the fracture.

The intensity of the vertigo will decrease after 7–10 days and then continues to decrease steadily over the following 1–2 months, leaving an unsteady feeling that lasts approximately 3–6 months.

15.1.3.5 CSF Otorhinorrhea

It is common but usually temporary.

15.1.4 Physical Examination

- Ear examination: auricle, ear canal, and tympanic membrane complete examination including Rinne and Weber's tests.
- Look for battle sign and Racoon eyes for other skull base fractures.
- Nystagmus and fistula test.
- Dix–Hallpike test.
- Facial nerve examination and other cranial nerves.

15.1.5 Investigations

- Hearing tests: pure tone audiometry and even auditory brainstem response.
- Fluid collection from the ear or nose and testing for Beta2 transferrin.
- CT scan: High-resolution Ct scan (HRCT) is the imaging of choice in temporal bone fractures, best to identify temporal bone fractures type, direction, presence (pneumolabyrinth) or absence of otic capsule involvement, complications like hemotympanum, tympanic membrane perforation, ossicular injury, perilymphatic fistula, CSF leak, cochlea-vestibular injury, facial nerve injury, and vascular injury (Figs. 15.2, 15.3, 15.4, and 15.5).
- Angiography can be requested if major vascular injury is suspected.
- Magnetic resonance imaging (MRI) cannot identify temporal bone fracture. MRI has both poor sensitivity and specificity in this respect. It is best used to identify and assess the intracranial contents and/or a nerve palsy, bleeding inside the otic capsule, vestibular apparatus, vestibular nucleus, and brainstem. It also can identify nerve compression and herniation of intracranial contents into the mastoid cavity.

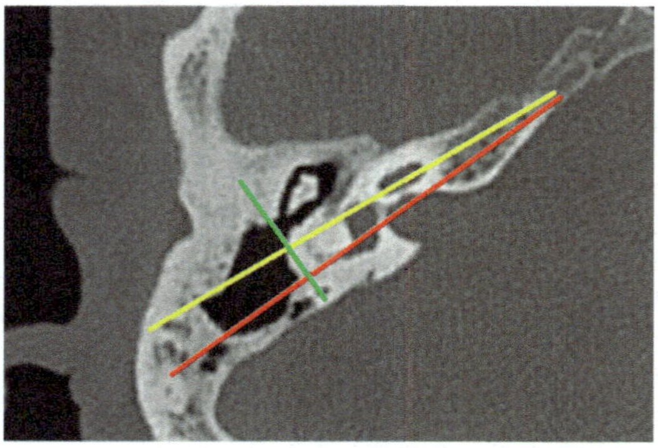

Fig. 15.2 Axial CT of temporal bone showing the axis of temporal bone (yellow line) the line of longitudinal fractures (red line) and transverse fractures line (green line)

- Nerve conduction study for facial nerve like electromyography (EMG) or electroneurography (ENoG).

15.1.6 Treatment

15.1.6.1 Medical

- Most middle ear effusion (Fig. 15.6), CSF, or perilymphatic fistula can be treated by head elevation, avoidance of straining and prophylactic antibiotics.

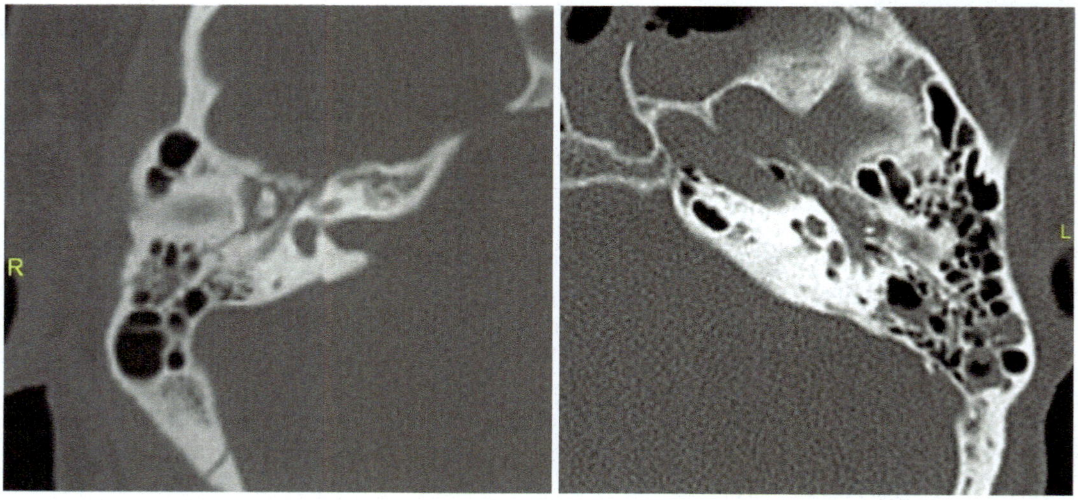

Fig. 15.3 Axial CT sections of the temporal bones in two different patients (Right and Left) showing longitudinal fractures associated with hemotympanum and hemomastoid

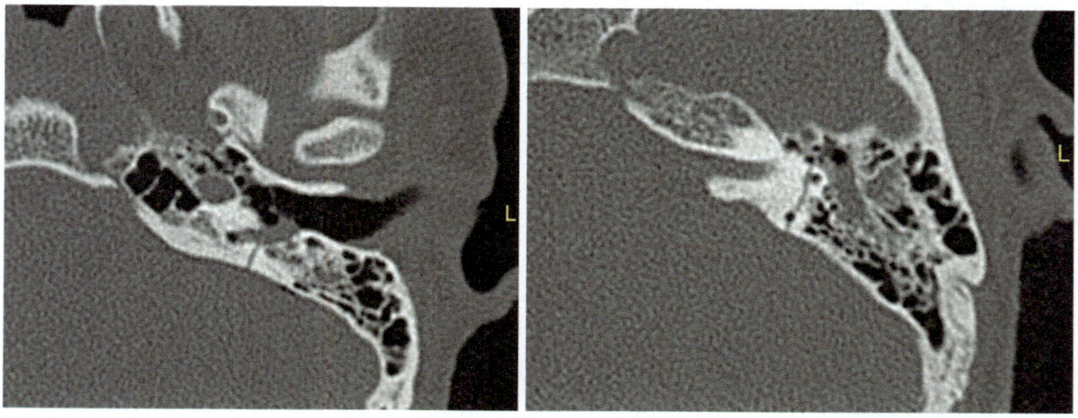

Fig. 15.4 Transverse fractures are seen involving the left temporal bone and passing through the superior semicircular canal

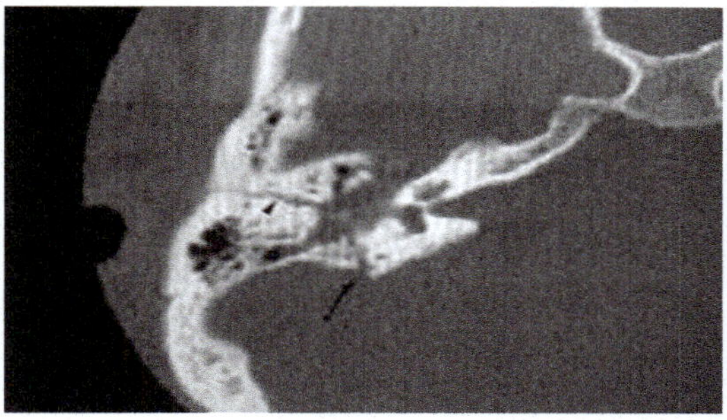

Fig. 15.5 Axial non-contrast CT with bone windows demonstrates a complex fracture with a transverse (arrow) and oblique (arrowhead) component

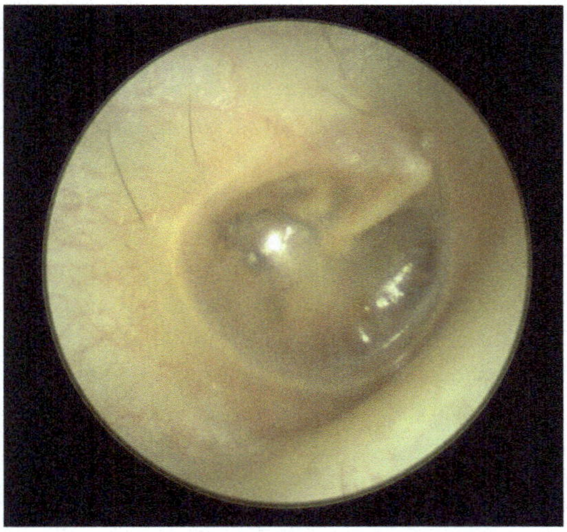

Fig. 15.6 Right middle ear effusion

- Small tympanic membrane perforation (Fig. 15.7) can heal spontaneously within 4 weeks by water avoidance and antibiotics ear drops if contamination of middle ear happened.
- Corticosteroid therapy for facial nerve weakness or sensorineural hearing loss might be necessary.
- Epley for posttraumatic benign paroxysmal positional vertigo and vestibular rehabilitation.
- Antibiotics for meningitis and CSF leak (controversial).

15.1.6.2 Surgical

- Myringoplasty with or without ossiculoplasty for non-healing perforations of the ear drum or to repair ossicular chain disruption.

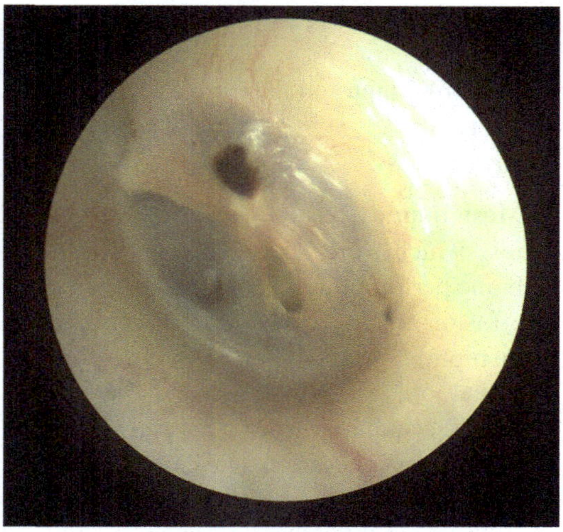

Fig. 15.7 Left traumatic tympanic membrane perforation

- Middle ear exploration for repair of perilymphatic fistula from round or oval window.
- Facial nerve decompression for complete immediate facial nerve paralysis or >90% degeneration by ENoG.
- Cochlear Implant, but before considering it, labyrinthitis ossificans must be considered when bilateral severe sensorineural hearing loss is present.

15.2 Middle Ear Trauma

15.2.1 Introduction

- Middle ear trauma or injury to inner ear compartment or both happens in up to 33% with severe head trauma and over 50% of temporal bone fractures [6, 7].
- Injury can be shown as hemotympanum, decreased hearing, CSF otorrhea, perilymph fistula, and otic capsule injury.
- Inner ear injury is more frequently seen with temporal bone fractures with facial paralysis and CSF otorrhea.
- Middle ear trauma can also happen after blunt trauma to the ear canal (punched ear, slap, direct fall to the ear, road traffic accidents, and sport injury) or by penetrating injury by Q-tip and gun shot or even by welding spark.

15.2.2 Clinical Presentation

Otalgia from injury to the ear canal, middle ear, or inner ear.

Hearing loss:

- Most injuries result in conductive hearing loss which can be mild in tympanic membrane perforation or hemotympanum or CSF effusion or can be severe in ossicular chain disruption (most commonly at the incudostapedial joint).
- Sensorineural hearing loss happens as a result of cochlear concussion, otic capsule fractures, or by impingement of cochlear nerve in the auditory canal fracture.

Vertigo: due to concussion or perilymph fistula.

Otorrhea: which can be clear fluid (CSF or perilymph), bloody, or purulent (from infection by contamination).

Tinnitus: due to inner ear involvement.

Rhinorrhea: clear or bloody by escape of ear fluids to the nose through Eustachian tube or by an independent direct fracture of the anterior skull base. Usually aggravated by Valsalva manoeuver or bending the head down.

Facial paralysis: unlikely to happen in isolated middle ear injury, usually as part of temporal bone trauma.

15.2.3 Physical Examination

- Ear examination: auricle, ear canal, and tympanic membrane complete examination including Rinne and Weber's tests.
- Look for battle sign and Racoon eyes for other skull base fractures.
- Nystagmus and fistula test.
- Facial nerve examination and other cranial nerves.

15.2.4 Investigations

- Hearing tests: pure tone audiometry and even auditory brainstem response.
- Fluid collection from the ear or nose and testing for Beta2 transferrin.
- CT scan: for skull fractures and ossicular chain disruption (preferably by temporal bone CT with thin cuts). Angiography can be requested if major vascular injury is suspected.
- MRI: only for facial nerve injury (preoperatively), otherwise wouldn't add anything to CT.
- Nerve conduction study for facial nerve like EMG or ENoG.

15.2.5 Treatment

15.2.5.1 Medical

- Most middle ear effusion (Fig. 15.6), CSF, or perilymphatic fistula can be treated by head elevation avoidance of straining and prophylactic antibiotics.
- Small tympanic membrane perforation can heal spontaneously within 4 weeks by water avoidance and antibiotics ear drops if contamination of middle ear happened.
- Corticosteroid therapy for facial nerve weakness or sensorineural hearing loss might be necessary.

15.2.5.2 Surgical

- Tympanoplasty with or without ossiculoplasty for non-healing perforations (Fig. 15.7) of the ear drum or to repair ossicular chain disruption.
- Middle ear exploration for repair of perilymphatic fistula from round or oval window.
- Facial nerve decompression for complete facial nerve paralysis or >90% degeneration by ENoG.

15.3 Barotrauma

15.3.1 Introduction

- The middle ear is an air-filled space. The middle ear pressure is preserved from the atmospheric pressure by the function of Eustachian tube and the tympanic membrane.
- The Eustachian tube acts as a valve to eliminate the extra pressure of the middle ear to the

nasopharynx passively with the help of absorption of gases through middle ear mucosa and also allows air to pass through the nasopharynx to equalize the pressure of the middle ear actively by the contraction of the soft palate muscle.

- Any severe changes to the middle ear pressure without these protective mechanisms will cause damage to the middle ear structures in a condition called barotrauma.
- The Eustachian tube consists of two parts bony [posterolateral] and cartilaginous [inferomedial] parts lined by respiratory mucosa.
- Eustachian tube opens temporarily during swallowing and yawning allowing air to pass from the nasopharynx to the ear by the contraction of tensor veli palatini muscle. And this muscle also helps to isolate the nasopharynx during the swallowing to prevent oropharynx content to go to the nasopharynx and the ear, thus preventing spread of infection to the middle ear, and also helps to keep the Eustachian tube closed all the time to prevent the eardrum from moving with respiration like what happens in the condition called patulous Eustachian tube.
- Eustachian tube dysfunction happens mainly due to mucosal edema causing dysfunction like in infection by an upper respiratory tract infection, allergy, or acid reflux, or by mechanical obstruction in conditions like adenoid enlargement in children and nasopharyngeal tumor in the adults.

15.3.2 Etiology

There are many causes of barotrauma

(a) Flying

The most common is flying. The atmospheric pressure decreases as the airplane is ascending and increases during descend. Middle ear pressure has to be equalized during these events to compensate that change. As long as these changes are gradual, normal equalization happens by swallowing, Valsalva, or middle ear gas absorption.

If for any reasons the change in altitude is fast, the pressure equalization mechanism fails to equalize and barotrauma happens. Injury happens by stretching, bruising, or even bleeding from the tympanic membrane and middle ear mucosa.

In more severe conditions, ear drum perforation, ossicles fractures or dislocation, and injury to inner ear by round and oval window membrane rupture with perilymph fistula occur [8, 9].

(b) Diving, the other common condition is Diving; the mechanism is similar to flying but usually the pressure change is more severe [10].

(c) Blast injury

Blast injury has become more frequently seen after the increased number of wars and terrorist attacks. After a blast explosion, a pressure wave travels to a certain distance causing movement of the structures in its way. This pressure changing causes the barotrauma.

Because of the high energy of the blast, most of the presentation is severe (i.e. tympanic membrane perforation, ossicles fractures or dislocation, or inner ear fistula) [11].

(d) Decompression chamber: it occurs due to difference in volume and circulation of both cochlea and vestibule (vestibule has 30% more volume and 25% less circulation than the cochlea) which reduces any compensation to pressure changes and causes barotrauma, and most of the symptoms are sensorineural hearing loss (SNHL) and vertigo [12].

(e) Sky diving: although a fast descent happens and the middle ear pressure should change, but symptoms doesn't seem to occur frequently [13].

15.3.3 Clinical Presentation

1. *Ear block* or pressure feeling in the ear (most common).
2. *Hearing loss*

   (a) Conductive hearing loss: in case of serous effusion (Fig. 15.6) or bleeding in the middle ear (Fig. 15.7), ear drum perforation, and ossicles injury.
   (b) SNHL: inner ear trauma or perilymphatic fistula.
3. *Vertigo*
4. *Otalgia*
5. *Tinnitus*: most commonly pulsating but can be constant, frequently temporary but sometimes can be persistent.

15.3.4 Diagnosis

- Diagnosis is made by good history (any scenario of sudden pressure change) and confirmed by physical examination.
- Hearing test (Rinne and Weber's) or pure tone audiometry to differentiate between CHL and SNHL is recommended.
- Radiological investigations are usually not needed.

15.3.5 Treatment

- Most of simple conditions of barotrauma just need conservative treatment (observation and symptomatic treatment), and even edema, bleeding or effusion, tympanic membrane perforation, and minor fistula heal spontaneously.

15.3.5.1 Medical

- Analgesic for pain management.
- Decongestant to open Eustachian tube although no good evidence to fasten the recovery.
- Antibiotics: only when ear drum perforation and contamination of middle ear.
- Steroid: no evidence of benefit except with SNHL or facial nerve injury.

15.3.5.2 Surgical Treatment

- Myringoplasty for tympanic membrane perforation.
- Ossiculoplasty for ossicular chain fracture or dislocation.
- Middle ear exploration and patching of fistula from the round or oval window, although hearing restoration results are not promising despite early intervention.
- Myringotomy with or without ventilation tube: useful for both prevention and treatment of barotrauma as it helps draining the fluids and correcting the hearing; tubes are beneficial for hyperbaric treatment patients and contraindicated for divers as it will open the middle ear to water.

15.3.6 Prevention

Avoidance is the best choice of treatment for barotrauma and can be achieved by

- Canceling or postponing flying or diving in cases of cold or allergies when ear equalization maneuvers fail.
- Swallowing or Valsalva maneuver during the flight or dive.
- Chewing gum or sucking hard candies for adults, and sucking infant bottle is helpful to equalize the pressure during the flight.
- Decongesting 30 min before the takeoff or diving to reduce edema around the Eustachian tube.
- Surfactant inhalation prior to diving is under research.
- Special ear plugs designed to reduce pressure changes.
- Balloon dilatation of Eustachian tube (controversial with lack of evidence).
- Myringotomy with ventilation tube.

Take-Home Messages

- Temporal bone fracture is part of other skull fractures during head trauma, and because of its important contents and surrounding structures, it might cause serious life-threatening injuries.
- Many classifications have been defined, but Ulrich's classification is the most easy and convenient to use.
- Although classified into longitudinal and transverse, the majority in real life is a mixed type.
- Most fractures are diagnosed by CT scan.
- Barotrauma is a common condition usually caused by flying, scuba diving, and blast injury.
- Most of barotrauma are self-limited and can be treated symptomatically.
- Prevention is the most important part of the treatment of barotrauma.

References

1. Ulrich K. Verletzungen des Gehorlorgans bel Schadelbasisfrakturen (Ein Histologisch und Klinissche Studie). Acta Otolaryngol Suppl. 1926;6:1–150.
2. Ghorayeb BY, Yeakley JW. Temporal bone fractures: longitudinal or oblique? The case for oblique temporal bone fractures. Laryngoscope. 1992;102(2):129–34.
3. Ishman SL, Friedland DR. Temporal bone fractures: traditional classification and clinical relevance. Laryngoscope. 2004;114(10):1734–41.
4. Diaz R, Brodie HA. Middle ear and temporal bone trauma. In: Cummings CW, Haughey BH, Thomas JR, Harker LA, Flint PW, editors. Otolaryngology-head and neck surgery, vol. 4. 4th ed. Philadelphia: Elsevier Mosby; 2005. p. 2057–2079/139.
5. Hough JV, Stuart WD. Middle ear injuries in skull trauma. Laryngoscope. 1968;78(6):899–937.
6. Ort S, Beus K, Isaacson J. Pediatric temporal bone fractures in a rural population. Otolaryngol Head Neck Surg. 2004;131:433.
7. Zimmerman WD, Ganzel TM, Windmill IM, et al. Peripheral hearing loss following head trauma in children. Laryngoscope. 1993;103:87.
8. Brown TP. Middle ear symptoms while flying. Ways to prevent a severe outcome. Postgrad Med. 1994;96:135.
9. Rosenkvist L, Klokker M, Katholm M. Upper respiratory infections and barotraumas in commercial pilots: a retrospective survey. Aviat Space Environ Med. 2008;79:960.
10. Moon RE. Treatment of diving emergencies. Crit Care Clin. 1999;15:429.
11. Breeze J, Cooper H, Pearson CR, et al. Ear injuries sustained by British service personnel subjected to blast trauma. J Laryngol Otol. 2011;125:13.
12. Bessereau J, Tabah A, Genotelle N, et al. Middle-ear barotrauma after hyper-baric oxygen therapy. Undersea Hyperb Med. 2010;37:203.
13. Gutovitz S, Weber K, Kaciuban S, et al. Middle ear pressure and symptoms after skydiving. Aviat Space Environ Med. 2008;79:533.

Cerebellopontine Angle Pathologies

16

Jacques Magnan, Hassan Haidar, and Zaid Altamimi

16.1 Introduction

Cerebellopontine angle (CPA) pathologies spectrum includes cranial nerves (5th–12th) pathologic lesions, dura lesions, and vasculature pathologies (malformations, and vascular loop conflict). In this chapter, the pathologies divided in two main categories, the CPA tumors and the neurovascular conflicts. The clinical presentation of the CPA tumors is variable depending on the size, site, and the displacement of the neurovascular structure. It can be asymptomatic, or more often symptomatic. It may present with otological signs (vertigo, tinnitus, or unilateral hearing loss) or specific disorders of cranial nerves. CPA tumors are usually benign and vestibular schwannomas are the most common. Functional pathologies associated with neurovascular conflicts of CPA include trigeminal neuralgia (TN), hemifacial spasm (HFS), and glossopharyngeal neuralgia (GN).

J. Magnan
Head & Neck Surgery Department, Hospital NORD and University Aix-Marseille, Marseille, France

H. Haidar (✉)
Hamad Medical Corporation, Doha, Qatar

Otolaryngology Department, Hamad Medical Corporation, Doha, Qatar

Z. Altamimi
Otolaryngology Department, Hamad Medical Corporation, Doha, Qatar
e-mail: Zaltamimi@hamad.qa

16.2 Anatomy of the Cerebellopontine Angle

The cerebellopontine angle (CPA) is a wedged angular space between the pons anterior-medially and the cerebellum posterior-medially and closed anterior-laterally by the posterior surface of the temporal bone. The roof is the tentorium, the floor is the occipital bone surrounding the foramen magnum. The CPA is filled by cerebrospinal fluid (CSF) and crossed by the cranial nerves (V to XII) and many vascular structures (Figs. 16.1 and 16.2).

16.2.1 Vascular Structures of CPA

The three major arteries of the cerebellum: the SCA, AICA, and PICA originate from the vertebrobasilar tree and pass through the CPA between the cranial nerves towards the cerebellum; from up to down.

1. **Superior cerebellar artery (SCA)** arises near the termination of the basilar artery. It passes lateralward, immediately below the oculomotor nerve, which separates it from the posterior cerebral artery, winds around the cerebral peduncle, close to the trochlear nerve, to arrive at the upper surface of the cerebellum (Fig. 16.2).

A. Al-Qahtani et al. (eds.), *Textbook of Clinical Otolaryngology*,
https://doi.org/10.1007/978-3-030-54088-3_16

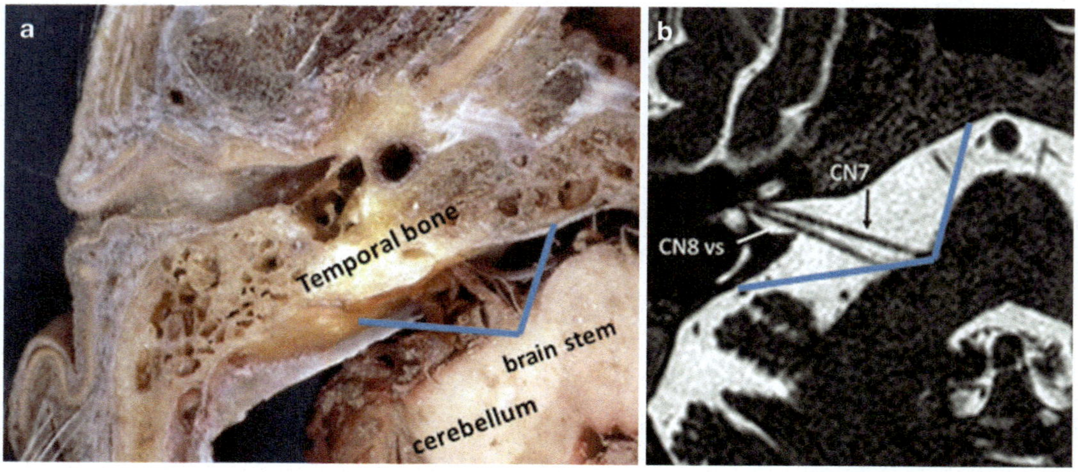

Fig. 16.1 (**a**) Gross anatomy, cross-sectional view of the right cerebellopontine angle of Mingazini demonstrating the wedge-shaped space of the CPA within the posterior fossa between the posterior surface of the temporal bone, brain stem, and cerebellum (blue triangle). (**b**) T2 CISS MRI at the same level showing the CPA full of CSF and crossed by the cochleovestibular nerve (CN8) and facial nerve (CN 8) at this level of cut to enter the internal auditory canal of the temporal bone. *VS* vestibular segment of the cochleovestibular nerve

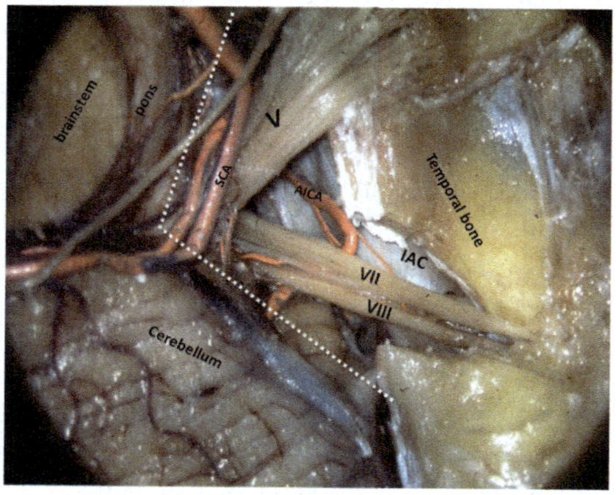

Fig. 16.2 Superior view of the right CPA (between white lines), the space between the pons anterior-medially and the cerebellum posterior-medially and closed anterior-laterally by the posterior surface of the temporal bone. The CPA is crossed by the cranial nerves (V to XII) and many vascular structures. V: trigeminal nerve; VII: facial nerve; VIII: vestibule-cochlear nerve; AICA: antero-inferior cerebellar artery; SCA: superior cerebellar artery; IAC: internal auditory canal

2. **The anterior inferior cerebellar artery (AICA)** arises from the basilar artery; as it moves posteriorly within the CPA it takes a long loop laterally to the porus acusticus (medial opening of the internal auditory canal) before turning back towards the cerebellum. In 20% of cases, the AICA actually passes inside of the internal auditory canal. The AICA either above or below the CN VII and VIII and in 25% of individuals, it passes between them (Fig. 16.2).
3. **The posterior inferior cerebellar artery (PICA)** is the largest branch of the vertebral artery. It is one of the three main arteries that supply blood to the cerebellum. It winds backward around the brain stem, passing between the origins of the lower cranial nerves, to the cerebellum.

Two important venous structures cross the CPA:

1. **The petrosal vein (of Dandy)** is a bulky vein that brings returning venous blood from the cerebellum and lateral brain stem to the superior. It is generally encountered in the area of the trigeminal nerve posterior to it. The petrosal vein often carries enough venous blood that its obstruction can lead to venous infarction and cerebellar edema, and it should be preserved if at all possible.
2. **The vein of Labbé** carries returning venous blood from the inferior and lateral surface of the temporal lobe to the superior petrosal sinus, tentorial venous lakes, or the transverse sinus. Sudden occlusion of the vein of Labbé carries a high risk of venous infarction of the temporal lobe and rapid cerebral edema.

16.2.2 Cranial Nerves in the CPA (Fig. 16.3)

1. **Trigeminal Nerve**: The point where the roots of the trigeminal nerve emerge in the brainstem is called "REZ" (Root Entry Zone), an anatomical landmark of great functional hierarchy. The cisternal (Vc) or pre-ganglionar segment occupies the upper floor sector of the cerebellopontine angle, above the acoustic-vestibulo-facial bundle, heading upwards and laterally, from the posterior fossa to the apex of the petrous portion of the temporal bone, where it finds Meckel's space region. During this course, surrounded by cerebrospinal fluid, it presents close relations, with the accessory superior petrous vein and superior cerebellar artery.

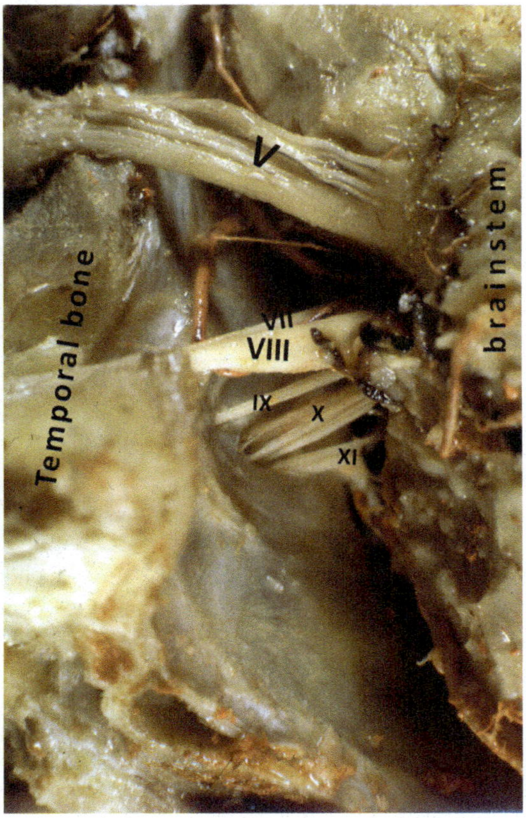

Fig. 16.3 Posterior view of left CPA anatomy after removal of the cerebellum showing cranial nerves (CN) V–XII and its anatomical relations. V: trigeminal nerve; VII: facial nerve; VIII: cochleovestibular nerve; IX: glossopharyngeal nerve; X: vagus nerve; XI: accessory nerve

2. **The facial nerve** arises from the brainstem lateral of the pontomedullary sulcus 2–3 mm anterior to the root entry zone of the vestibulocochlear nerve. The foramen of Luschka (i.e., the opening of the lateral recess of the fourth ventricle) is located just inferior and posterior to the root exit zones of the efferent motor facial nerve and the root entry zone of the afferent sensorial vestibulocochlear nerve. As the facial nerve leaves the brain stem, the fibers are sheathed in oligodendroglia derived from the central nervous system. Within a few millimeters of leaving the brain stem, however, the nerve loses its oligodendroglial ensheathment and becomes ensheathed instead by Schwann cells (transitional zone or Obersteiner–Redlich zone). Throughout the remainder of its peripheral course, it remains within its Schwann cell investment. It passes directly across the cerebellopontine angle for about 15 mm, accompanied by the vestibulocochlear nerve. It consistently enters the internal auditory canal by crossing the anterior superior margin of the porus acusticus.
3. **The vestibulocochlear nerve** arises from the brainstem slightly posterior to the facial nerve. It remains sheathed in oligodendroglia for approximately 15 mm (almost to the point at which it passes into the internal auditory canal). It has the longest oligodendroglial investment of any peripheral nerve. The junction between oligodendroglia and Schwann cells (i.e., the Obersteiner–Redlich zone) occurs just medial to the porus acusticus. Because vestibular schwannomas arise from Schwann cells, they arise most commonly within the most lateral portions of the cerebellopontine angle or the internal auditory canal. The nervus intermedius (nerve of Wrisberg) leaves the brain stem between facial and vestibulocochlear nerves. At some point within the cerebellopontine angle, the nervus intermedius crosses over to become associated with the facial nerve. It may do so as several separate rootlets. The point where the nervus intermedius crosses to become associated with the facial nerve shows considerable variation, but in 22% of individu-

als, it is adherent to the vestibulocochlear nerve for 14 mm or more. As the vestibulocochlear and facial nerve reaches the porus acusticus (medial opening of the internal auditory canal), they pass together with the nervus intermedius and sometimes a loop of AICA.

4. **Lower cranial nerves** include the glossopharyngeal (IX), vagus (X), spinal accessory nerves (XI). Inferior and a bit anterior to the foramen of Luschka is the olive, and just posterior to the olive lie the rootlets of origin for cranial nerves IX, X, and XI. They cross inferiorly in a fan-shaped pattern the CPA towards the jugular foramen.
5. **The hypoglossal nerve** exits the brain stem through a series of small rootlets anterior to the olive.

16.2.3 Internal Auditory Canal

The internal auditory canal is approximately 8.5 mm in length (range 5.5–10.5 mm), lined with dura, and filled with spinal fluid surrounding the acousticofacial nerve bundle. Its medial end is oval in shape and is referred to as the porus acusticus. Its lateral end is a complicated structure referred to as the fundus or lamina cribrosa. The fundus is divided into a superior and inferior half by the transverse crest.

The upper half is further subdivided into an anterior and posterior segment by a vertical crest (Bill's Bar). The vertical crest separates the macula cribrosa superior, which allows passage of the superior vestibular nerve posteriorly, from the meatal foramen, which allows the entry of the facial nerve anteriorly into the fallopian canal.

The inferior half of the fundus is a single oval-shaped space, the anterior portion of which is occupied by a rounded depression (tractus spiralis foraminosus) filled with small openings to accommodate the terminal branches of the cochlear nerve. The posterior portion is filled with a macula crista inferior through which pass the terminal ends of the inferior vestibular nerve.

16.2.4 Surgical Endoscopical Anatomy of the CPA (Fig. 16.4)

The surgical CPA can then be divided into three zones comprising each one a nerve, vessels and its distinct pathologies:

1. **Inferior zone**: inferior external occupied by the lower cranial nerves and the PICA born from the ipsilateral vertebral artery.
2. **Middle zone**: more medial than the inferior zone, consists of the acousticofacial bundle which crosses this space in a straight line. It is the zone of the AICA which may form several loops there and engage itself towards the porus and sometimes deep in the meatus.
3. **Superior zone**: is located more medially at the anterior tip of the CPA, well inside of the middle zone. It contains the trigeminal nerve. The other occupying permanent structure of this space is the vein of Dandy, a very bulky vein joining the higher petrous sinus. The artery of this territory is the SCA.

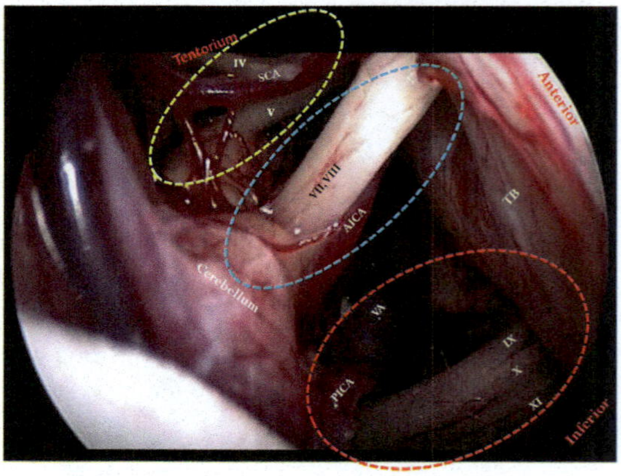

Fig. 16.4 Panoramic view of left cerebellopontine angle in surgical position showing the three zones; inferior zone in red containing the lower cranial nerves (IX, X, XI) and postero-inferior cerebellar artery (PICA) and vertebral artery (VA), middle zone in blue containing the acoustic-facial bundle (VII, VIII) and antero-inferior cerebellar artery (AICA), superior zone in yellow containing trigeminal nerve, Dandy vein, and superior cerebellar artery (SCA). TB: posterior surface of temporal bone; IV: fourth cranial nerve

16.3 Cerebellopontine Angle (CPA) Tumors

Lesions of the cerebellopontine angle (CPA) comprise 10% of all intracranial tumors.

The differential diagnosis of cerebellopontine angle (CPA) includes vestibular schwannoma (85%), meningioma (3–15%), epidermoid cyst (2–6%), facial and lower cranial nerve schwannomas (2–3%), arachnoid cyst (1%), and other rare tumors (include lipomas, dermoid tumors, paraganglioma, chordoma, trigeminal schwannoma, malignancies, and metastatic lesions (primaries from glial tumors, breast, lung, prostate)).

16.3.1 Vestibular Schwannoma (VS)

It is a benign tumor of the Schwann cell that most commonly arises from the Schwann cells of the inferior vestibular nerve (Fig. 16.5). It is misnomer as acoustic neuroma since it is not a neuroma and typically does not originate from the cochlear nerve. They comprise about 6% of all intracranial tumors, about 30% of posterior fossa tumors, and about 85% (most common) of tumors in the region of the cerebellopontine angle. The incidence is increasing, 20 new cases per million population, per year. There are no causative risk factors or exposures. Bilateral vestibular schwannomas are associated with autosomal dominant neurofibromatosis type 2 (NF2). The histology of vestibular schwannoma composed of Antoni A tissue (uniform compact spindle cells with parallel palisading nuclei and verocay bodies), and Antoni B tissue (less cellular, fatty, and less uniform). Vestibular schwannomas stain positive with S-100 and vimentin. It is a benign condition with a very rare malignant degeneration (<1%).

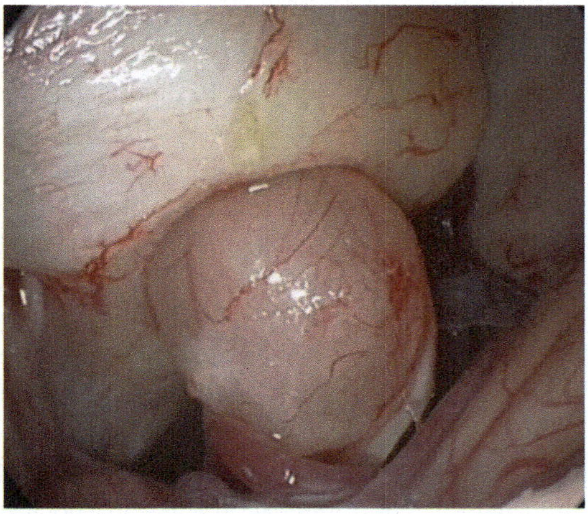

Fig. 16.5 Left CPA with medium-size vestibular schwannoma

16.3.1.1 Clinical Presentation

1. Most of the asymptomatic patients are diagnosed incidentally on imaging studies performed for separate indications. The symptom of vestibular schwannomas depends upon the size and location of the tumor. Although most vestibular schwannomas grow slowly, the growth rate of schwannoma is variable and difficult to predict. Tumor size either remains static, increases or rarely regresses. Usually, it is a slow increment, 1–2 mm/year. Three separate growth patterns can be distinguished within acoustic tumors, as follows:
   (a) No growth or very slow growth.
   (b) Slow growth (i.e., ≥2 mm/year on imaging studies).
   (c) Fast growth (i.e., ≥1.0 cm/year on imaging studies).

   Tumors that arise within the internal auditory canal may produce earlier symptoms in the form of hearing loss or vestibular disturbance by compressing the adjacent nerves and vascular structure. While if it grows medially in the CPA, the tumors can continue to grow until they reach 2–3 cm in size before any symptoms appear.
2. Most vestibular schwannoma (VS) cases prove at the otological stage with unilateral auditory or vestibular dysfunction. The most common presenting symptom is a unilateral, progressive, high frequency sensorineural hearing loss that develops in approximately 95%. From 5% to 25% of patients with VS present with sudden sensorineural hearing loss. The hearing loss occurs through direct

injury to the cochlear nerve or interruption of the cochlear blood supply. For this reason, any patient with unilateral sensorineural hearing loss needs further investigation to rule out VS. There is a poor correlation between the tumor size and the hearing status as patients with large tumors may have normal hearing and patients with small tumors may be severe hearing loss in the affected ear.

The second most common symptom is unilateral tinnitus (75%) of patients with VS. The presence of unilateral tinnitus alone is enough reason to evaluate the patient for VS tumor. Vertigo and disequilibrium are uncommon presenting symptoms among patients with VS. Vertigo attacks are correlated with smaller tumors, whereas chronic disequilibrium is correlated with larger tumors.

Other reported symptoms include decreased sensation of the ear canal and concha bowl (Hitselberger sign) and it is due to injury of the sensory fibers of the facial nerve.

3. Expansion of the tumor within the CPA may lead to the neurological stage which is becoming less and common. Increased intracranial pressures, brainstem compression, and cranial nerve dysfunction induce headache, facial weakness, unilateral facial numbness, visual loss, dysphagia, hoarseness, and hydrocephalus. Facial weakness is sufficiently uncommon (<1%) that facial weakness associated with a small- or medium-size tumor should raise suspicion that it is not a vestibular schwannoma.
4. Bilateral vestibular schwannomas strongly suggest the presence of neurofibromatosis type 2 (NF-2), an autosomal dominant neurocutaneous disorder associated with a mutation on the long arm of chromosome 22 that code for the protein merlin. It is characterized by the development of multiple schwannomas, meningiomas, and ependymomas. The occurrence of bilateral vestibular schwannomas is almost considered the pathognomonic of this disorder. Such patients typically with family history present clinically in the second and third decades of life, much earlier than those with the sporadic intracranial schwannoma.

Neurofibromatosis Type 2

- Autosomal dominant
- Mutation in NF2 gene (22q12.2) which codes for the protein neurofibromin 2 (or merlin): regulation of contact-dependent inhibition of cellular proliferation
- Diagnosis requires one of the following:
  - Bilateral VS, or
  - Unilateral VS with a family history of NF2, or
  - Multiple brain tumors with a family history of NF2

16.3.1.2 Diagnosis

Different evaluation tools can be used to diagnose VS including audiologic and electrophysiologic evaluations, vestibular tests, but the key assessment is the imaging study.

Pure-tone audiometry and word discrimination evaluation in VS patients typically present with asymmetric sensorineural hearing loss with disproportionately poorer than expected word discrimination test. Rollover phenomenon is seen in VS cases as increased sound intensity results in decreased word discrimination ability.

Electrophysiologic testing by auditory brainstem response (ABR) represents the most sensitive and specific audiologic test with sensitivity reach up to 85–90% in medium and large tumors, but it is not as sensitive as MRI as it may miss tumors <1 cm in size. ABR findings suggestive of retro-cochlear lesion are prolonged interaural wave V latency, interaural wave I–III, and interaural I–V latencies.

Vestibular assessment is mainly done by caloric test and vestibular evoked myogenic potential (VEMP), which can help to determine the nerve of origin (superior vs. inferior vestibular nerve) of VS that may add prognostic information. The prognosis for hearing preservation with surgical resection is more difficult with a tumor in inferior vestibular nerve due to proximity to the cochlear nerve and possible shared blood supply. The caloric test in VS identifies a unilateral vestibular weakness in the tumor side, which indicates that the tumor has affected or originates from the superior vestibular nerve. Myogenic potential (VEMP) testing that shows an absent or reduced VEMP response with normal caloric testing indicates VS originating from the inferior vestibular nerve.

Magnetic resonance imaging (MRI) is the gold standard in the evaluation of patients with unilateral auditory and vestibular dysfunction. It appears in MRI with contrast as isointense T1 with contrast shows intense enhancement that can appear as "ice cream cone" or "mushroom" shape (Figs. 16.6, 16.7, and 16.8). MRI imaging can detect down to a 1–2 mm sized tumor with contrast administration. CT with contrast indicated if MRI is unavailable or contraindicated, may miss tumors <1 cm. Table 16.1 shows the differential diagnosis of CPA tumors along with their MRI findings.

16.3.1.3 Management

Vestibular schwannoma management goal is to preserve life with avoidance of any serious neurologic sequelae as facial paralysis, optimally achieved with complete tumor removal and preserving the facial and hearing functions. VS management includes one of the following three primary treatment options: (1) surgical excision of the tumor, (2) arresting tumor growth using stereotactic radiation therapy, or (3) careful serial observation.

The selection of treatment options depends on multiple factors including mainly the tumor size and the age, but also medical status of the patient, tumor progression, hearing status, and patient preference (see Fig. 16.9).

Observation

Although VS most often is a slow growing tumor the growth rate of schwannoma is variable and difficult to predict. A tumor is considered to be growing when its size is superior to 2 mm per year. Simple observation without any therapeutic intervention has been used in the following groups of patients:

- Elderly patients (>65 years).
- Patients with small tumors (<1.5 cm), especially if their hearing is good.
- Patients with medical conditions that significantly increase the risk of the operation.
- Patients with a tumor on the side of an only hearing ear.

The observation should be followed with serial MRIs every 6 months for the first year, and yearly thereafter if no growth is detected then resume on observation. Individuals who are being observed ultimately require therapeutic intervention in between 15% and 40%. In young patients, the growing tumor potential is higher. It is the reason why they are better served by tumor removal as the hearing-preservation approach may be lost. The management and observation strategy of vestibular schwannomas is summarized in Fig. 16.9.

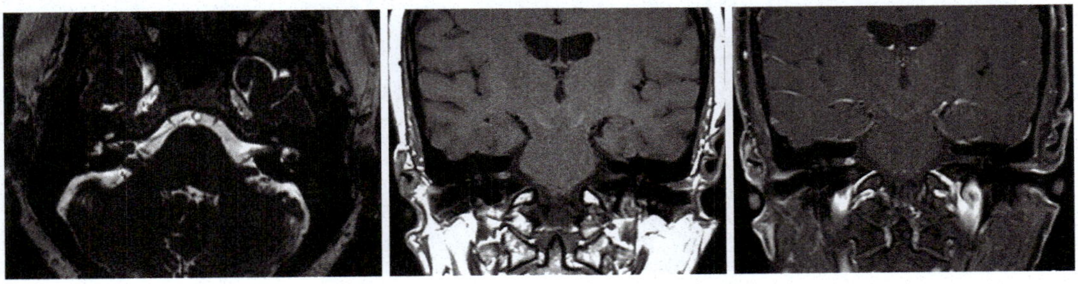

Fig. 16.6 Axial T2 CISS and coronal T1 WI MRI before and after IV contrast administration showing a small right intracanalicular soft tissue signal intensity lesion that shows homogenous post-contrast enhancement representing right-sided intracanalicular vestibular schwannoma

Stereotactic Radiation Therapy

It aims to prevent tumor growth and does not eliminate it. Stereotactic radiotherapy is indicated for tumors less than 2.5 cm (including CAI), elderly, and poor surgical candidates with asymptomatic growing tumors. It is contraindicated for cystic tumors, big tumor, or small no growing tumor.

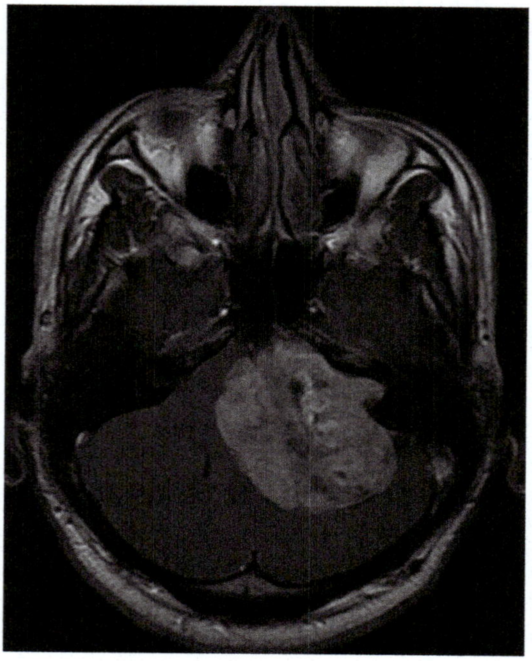

Fig. 16.7 Axial post-contrast T1 WI MRI showing large left cerebellopontine mass lesion extending to the middle line and distorting the brainstem and widening the left internal auditory canal with rather homogenous enhancement representing large left vestibular schwannoma

Current modalities for radiation for vestibular schwannoma include (1) single fraction Gamma-knife given using rigid frame fixed to patient's head, (2) hypofractionated linear accelerator photon radiation therapy (cyber-knife) with image-guided system, and (3) proton beam.

Advantages of radiation therapy include the benefit of no hospitalization and the rapid return to normal activity, lower immediate posttreatment morbidity, and mortality, i.e., lower risk of facial nerve injury and stroke. Overall long-term outcomes are similar to surgery.

Disadvantages of radiation therapy include delayed sensorineural hearing loss due to blood vessel fibrosis and treatment failure with a high risk of facial paralysis after required salvage surgery and a rare risk of malignant degeneration (<0.1%).

Surgery

Surgical removal remains the treatment of choice for tumor eradication. Surgery considered a better choice for younger healthy patients and larger tumors (the distance between the porus acusticus and the middle line is 2.5–3 cm). The goal of surgical intervention is to have a complete resection of the tumor while preserving facial nerve and auditory function. Tumor size and location play a major role in determining the complications rate; larger tumors have more risk for facial nerve dysfunction and hearing loss.

Different surgical approaches were described for resection of vestibular schwannoma (Fig. 16.10). The surgical approach is selected based on tumor size, location, and auditory function

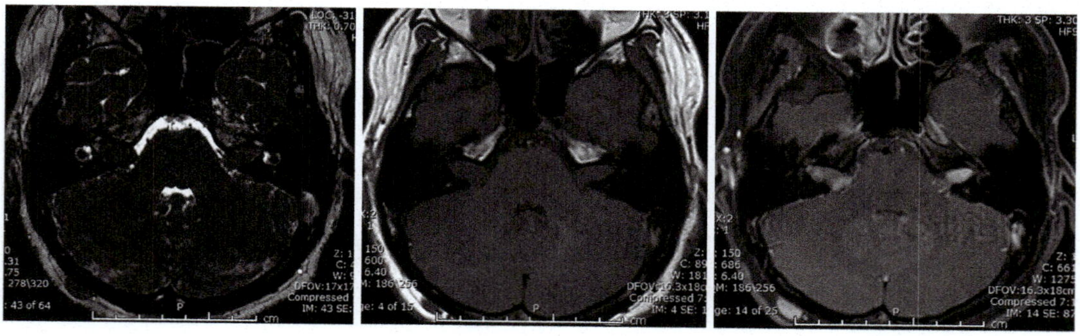

Fig. 16.8 Axial T2 CISS, axial T1 WI MR before and after IV contrast administration showing bilateral intracanalicular soft tissue lesions extending into the CP angle cisterns and showing homogenous enhancement pattern representing bilateral vestibular schwannomas in a known patient with NF type 2

Table 16.1 Differential diagnosis of cerebellopontine angle lesions with their CT and MRI findings

Tumor	CT	MRI T1	MRI T2	MRI T1 with contrast	Notes
Schwannoma (vestibular 85%, facial 1%)	Isodense, heterogeneous enhancement	Isointense	Iso/ hyperintense	Strong enhancement, with cystic areas	Usually centered into IAC
Meningioma (3–15%)	Hypodense, homogeneous Enhancement, calcifications	Isointense	Isointense	Strong enhancement	Dural tail, often eccentric to IAC
Paraganglioma	Erosion of caroticojugular spine	Isointense	Isointense	Strong enhancement	Salt and pepper appearance
Epidermoid (2–6%)	Hypointense	Hypointense	Hyperintense	Non-enhancing	Restricted diffusion on DWI, cause bone erosion
Cholesterol granuloma	Isodense, with smooth expansion of bone	Hyperintense	Hyperintense	Non-enhancing	
Mucocele	Hypodense	Hypointense	Hyperintense	Rim-enhancing	
Lipoma	Hyperdense	Hyperintense	Hypointense	Non-enhancing	Suppresses with fat saturation
Arachnoid cyst	Hypodense	Hypointense	Hyperintense	Non-enhancing	Dark on T2 FLAIR

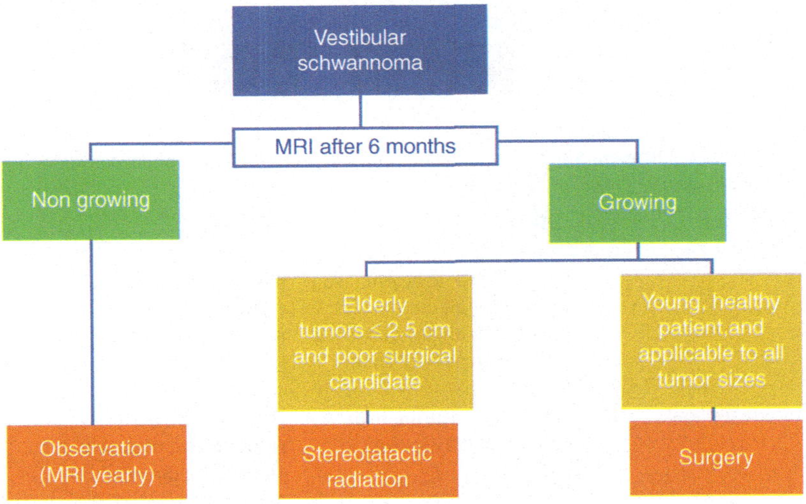

Fig. 16.9 Management strategy of vestibular schwannoma

in the operated side (Fig. 16.11). Each approach is discussed and compared in detail in Table 16.2. The combined approach typically involves an enlarged retrosigmoid (suboccipital) and translabyrinthine approaches. This combined appraoch is used in resection of CPA tumors that are greater than 4–3 cm which needs wide exposure.

Different considerations go into deciding which approach should be used, which summarized in the following:

1. *Preoperative auditory function*: Translabyrinthine approach is preferred if no serviceable hearing. For patients that have a serviceable hearing (discrimination score >50%), the common approaches include the retrosigmoid alone or combined with retrolabyrinthine approach and the middle cranial fossa approach. Normal preoperative ABR and abnormal caloric test findings favor hearing conservation.

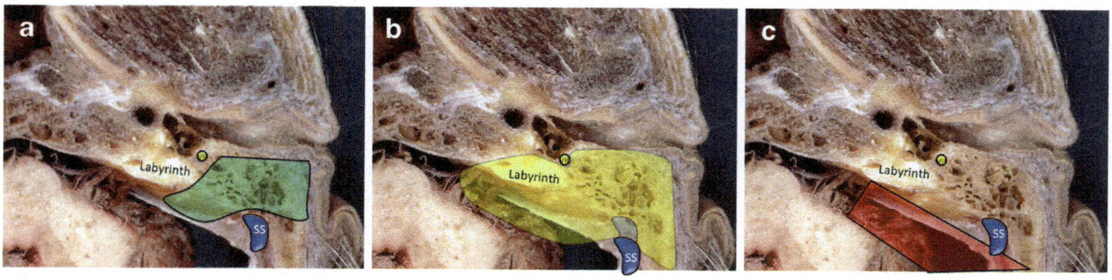

Fig. 16.10 (**a**) Retrolabyrinthine approach; (**b**) Translabyrinthine approach, notice that the sigmoid sinus posterior retraction provides wider view of the CPA; (**c**) retrosigmoid approach

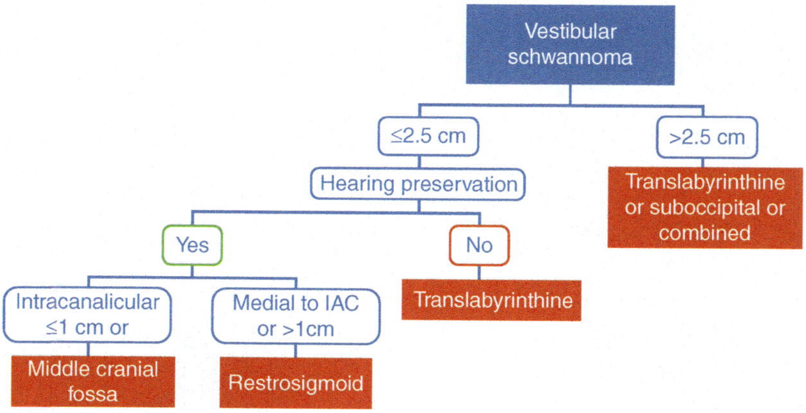

Fig. 16.11 The surgical approach in vestibular schwannoma is selected based on tumor size, location, and auditory function in the operated side

Table 16.2 Different surgical approaches for reresection of vestibular schwannoma: indications, advantages, and disadvantages

Approach	Indications	Advantages	Disadvantages
Translabyrinthine	Approach of choice for non-serviceable hearing; can be used for all tumor sizes; preferred with any vestibular schwannomas over 2 cm	Excellent exposure with most direct access to CPA; consistent facial nerve identification distally with lowest risk of injury; no cerebellar retraction	Sacrifices hearing; needs abdominal fat to close; contraindicated in acute or chronic otitis media
Retrosigmoid	Serviceable hearing with tumor medially located to IAC	Potential for hearing preservation; remove tumors of all sizes; direct and quicker exposure of the brainstem	Limited access to lateral IAC; recurrence of tumor; headache; intradural drilling of IAC; and need for endoscope
Suboccipital (with large craniotomy and sitting position)	Serviceable hearing with tumor medially located to IAC/large tumors	Large exposure; no need suction	Cerebellar retraction; higher incidence of headache; potential of air embolism
Middle cranial fossa	Serviceable hearing with small intracanalicular (intra-IAC)	Potential for hearing preservation possible; exposure of entire IAC; no intradural drilling; low postoperative headache rates	Higher risk of facial nerve injury; Requires retraction of temporal lobe (small risk of aphasia or seizure); poor exposure to posterior fossa
Retrolabyrinthine	Serviceable hearing	Combined with retrosigmoid offers the best conditions for preservation of hearing and facial nerve function; less cerebellar retraction	Limited exposure to the CPA; needs abdominal fat to close

2. *Tumor size*: Hearing conservation surgery is more achievable with smaller tumors (<1.5 cm) and the use of cochlear monitoring.
3. *Tumor location*: The tumor lies within the lateral portions of the internal auditory canal cannot be reached by the retrosigmoid approach without endoscope-assisted procedure.
4. *Relevant anatomical variations*: Translabyrinthine approach is much more difficult with high-riding jugular bulb, anteriorly placed sigmoid sinus, and contracted sclerotic mastoid.
5. *Surgeon preference.*

Both ablative and hearing-preservation surgical approaches have complications, including the following:

1. *Abdominal subcutaneous hematoma*: from the site of fat harvest, with a rate of 3.2%.
2. *Hemorrhage* into the posterior fossa in the immediate postoperative period can produce brainstem compression and death. The mortality rate for surgical excision of vestibular schwannoma has declined to less than 1%.
3. *Cerebellar injuries* (rare).
4. *Facial nerve*: surgical approaches must offer preservation of facial nerve function (House Brackmann grade I or II) in over 95% of patients with tumors less than 1.5 cm; however, this rate decreases as tumor size increases. Consequently, partial resection with complementary radiotherapy on the residual piece is questionable in large tumors to preserve the facial function. Incidence of delayed facial palsy varies from 10% to 30%, the vast majority have complete recoveries.
5. *Lower cranial nerve injury* is rare but can be a risk in large tumor.
6. *Cerebrospinal fluid leak*: the incidence has been reported from 1% to 10% of cases.
7. *Aseptic meningitis and meningitis: the reported rate is between 1% and 8% of cases.*
8. *Postoperative headache*: It is more common with suboccipital approach, found in more than 30% of patients and very rare in minimally retrosigmoid approach.
9. *The ventriculoperitoneal shunt*: It is becoming rare. The resection of the tumor restores the CSF system. But it can be required facing a resistant postoperative CSF leak.

<u>NF-2 management</u> is more complex and required a multidisciplinary center since the patient is young with great risk of deafness along with the loss of other special senses and locomotion. Radiotherapy requires higher doses to avoid growing which is harmful for hearing preservation or rehabilitation. Generally, remove the larger tumor with less hearing first. If able to preserve the cochlear nerve at the time of surgery, consider a cochlear implant. Consider the placement of auditory brainstem implant at the time of initial surgery if the cochlear nerve sacrificed. Observe the only hearing ear with serial MRI or CT if the patient is bearing auditory implant.

In conclusion, It is important to discuss with the patient and the family the outcome and the prognosis of the surgical removal of the tumor, hence the patient would have a realistic expectation. The key point is not the hearing (except in cases of only one hearing side) but the facial nerve functioning. Hearing-preservation rates and long-term facial nerve outcome are largely tied to the size of the tumor. Regarding tinnitus, in 25–60% of patients, it is improved or abolished; on the other hand, it can get worse in only 6–20%. Recurrence of the tumor is variable but is generally reported at less than 1%, except in cases of voluntary partial removal. Even in such cases the tumor is still growing in 10–25%. MRI Surveillance for postoperative tumor recurrence should persist every year for 5 years then at 10 years postoperatively.

16.3.2 Other Cerebellopontine Angle Tumors

16.3.2.1 Meningiomas

Meningioma represents the second most common CPA tumor (3–15%). It arises from cap (endothelial) cells from the arachnoid layer (arachnoid villi) of the meninges. Histopathology examination usually shows calcified psammoma

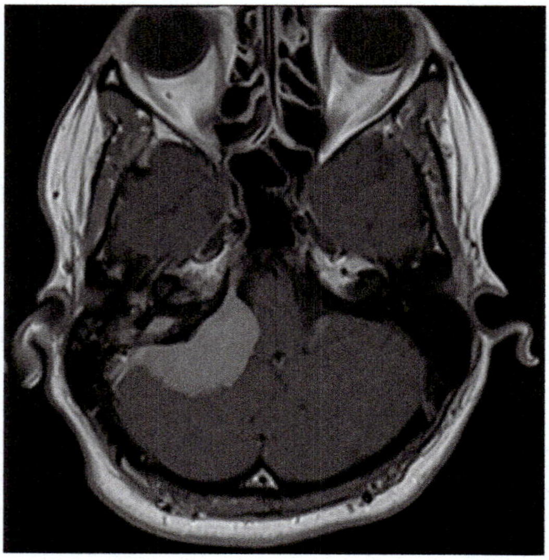

Fig. 16.12 Axial view T1 WI MR after IV contrast administration showing right CPA lesion with a dural tail (sessile and broad-based) and showing homogenous enhancement pattern representing right CPA meningioma

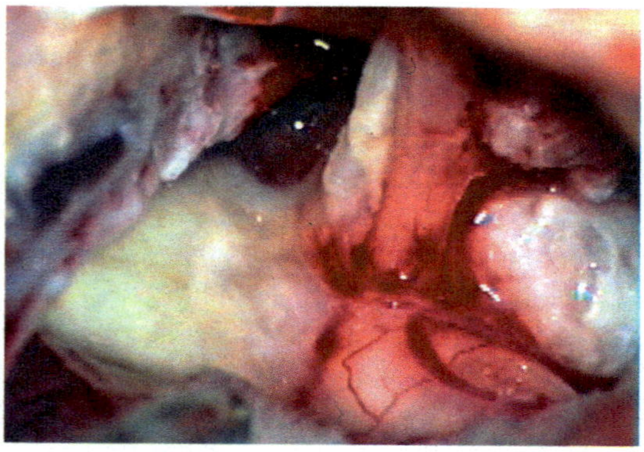

Fig. 16.13 Intraoperative image of epidermoid cyst during translabyrinthine approach showing cholesteatoma surrounding the acoustic-facial bundle

bodies. It is more common among middle-aged women. Meningiomas associated with hereditary tumor syndromes such as NF2, where patients develop multiple meningiomas. Around 2–5% has a malignant nature.

Presentation depends upon their size and location; it is similar to vestibular schwannoma, generally larger than VS before causing hearing loss or vestibular symptoms.

Imaging can often distinguish meningioma from VS; meningiomas are homogeneous, denser, contain calcifications and hyperostosis, and have dural tail appearance (sessile and broad-based) (see Fig. 16.12).

Management options are the same as vestibular schwannoma and include surgical excision, stereotactic radiation therapy, and external beam radiation. Microsurgical resection is considered the gold standard of treatment.

16.3.2.2 Epidermoid Cysts

Epidermoid cysts are congenital intradural lesions developed from sequestered ectodermal epithelial cell rests; it is also called congenital cholesteatoma of the CPA. It represents approximately 5% of all masses in the CPA region (third most common).

Symptoms are similar to other tumors of the CPA; however, they may cause earlier hemifacial spasm and progressive facial paralysis compared with the other CPA lesions.

The diagnosis is mainly intraoperative (see Fig. 16.13). MRI imaging features include dark on T1, extremely bright T2 signal, non-enhancing on contrast, and restricted diffusion on diffusion weighted image (DWI) (see Fig. 16.6). The primary and only treatment of these lesions is surgical excision (see Fig. 16.14).

16.3.2.3 Facial and Lower Cranial Nerve Schwannomas

Schwannomas can develop on the 5th through the 12th cranial nerves; however, they are far less common than VS. They account for 2–3% of tumors within the CPA.

Facial nerve schwannoma usually involves geniculate ganglion, and facial nerve function generally not impaired until the tumor is quite large. MRI is the method of choice to diagnose facial nerve schwannoma, characterized by enhancing dumbbell-shaped expansion of the intratemporal facial nerve and/or enhanced enlargement of the geniculate ganglion region (see Fig. 16.15).

Management Plan

Preoperative facial nerve function is the most important factor determining the treatment approach (**see algorithm** Fig. 16.16):

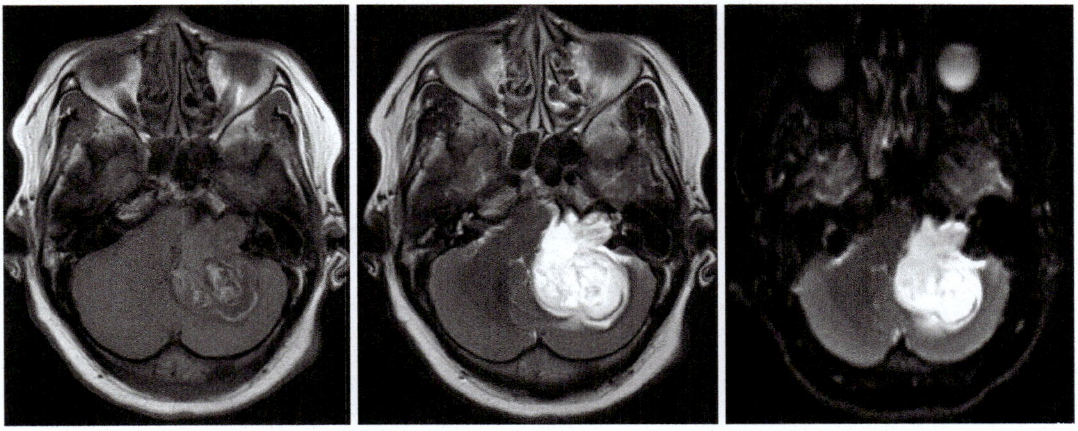

Fig. 16.14 Axial view MRI T1, T2, DWI respectively, showing extensive left epidermoid cyst involving all CPA

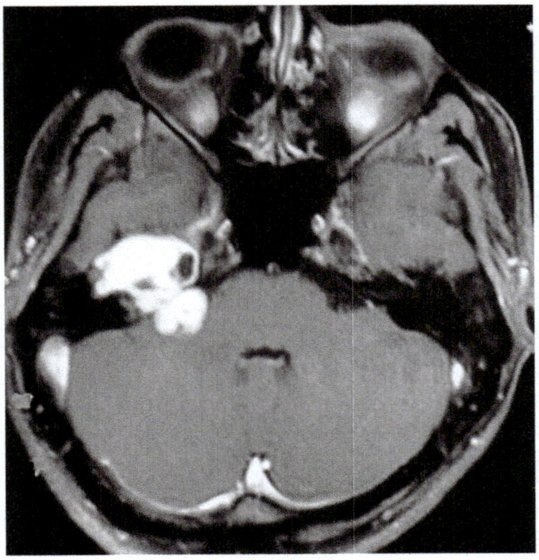

Fig. 16.15 Post-contrast T1 MRI showing right-sided enhancing lesion with cystic change suggestive of facial nerve schwannoma involving the cerebellopontine angle, meatus, labyrinthine segment, and geniculate ganglion

- Normal nerve function or weakness HB III or less → Clinical and radiological follow-up
- Growing facial nerve tumors → decompression of the facial nerve in the temporal bone to delay facial palsy and/or radiotherapy to reduce growing potential and prevent facial palsy
- Facial palsy HB grade IV or more → Surgical excision + reconstruction
- Symptomatic facial nerve tumors → surgical excision

16.3.2.4 Arachnoid Cysts (1%)

Arachnoid cysts are congenital malformation of the arachnoid that results in a thin-walled sac filled with CSF, and these lesions comprise less than 1% of CPA tumors. It is typically asymptomatic but can cause compression symptoms. The relationships between the image of the cyst and the symptoms are often questionable.

The diagnosis is based on MRI, characterized by non-enhancing lesion that is hypointense on T1 and hyperintense on T2.

Management generally is through observation or minimally invasive surgery for symptomatic lesions via incision and drainage using a retrosigmoid approach.

16.3.2.5 Others

Other rare tumors include lipomas, paraganglioma, chordoma, malignancies, and metastatic lesions with primaries from glial tumors, breast, lung, and prostate.

16.4 Neurovascular Conflicts of CPA

The complex and changing vascular system of the CPA can come in contact with cranial nerves passing in the CPA and cause vascular compression and irritation of the nerve (neurovascular conflict). Usually, it is caused by an abnormal course of a vascular loop, vertebrobasilar doli-

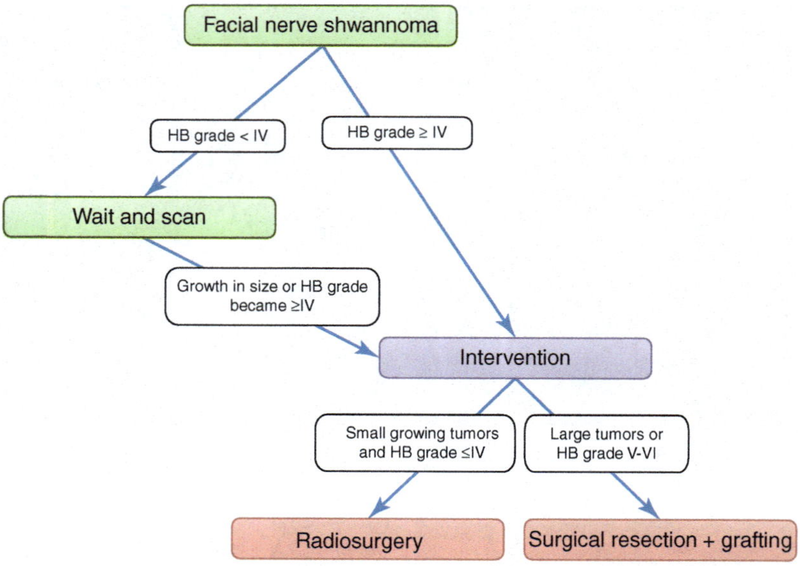

Fig. 16.16 Algorithm showing management plan for facial nerve schwannoma

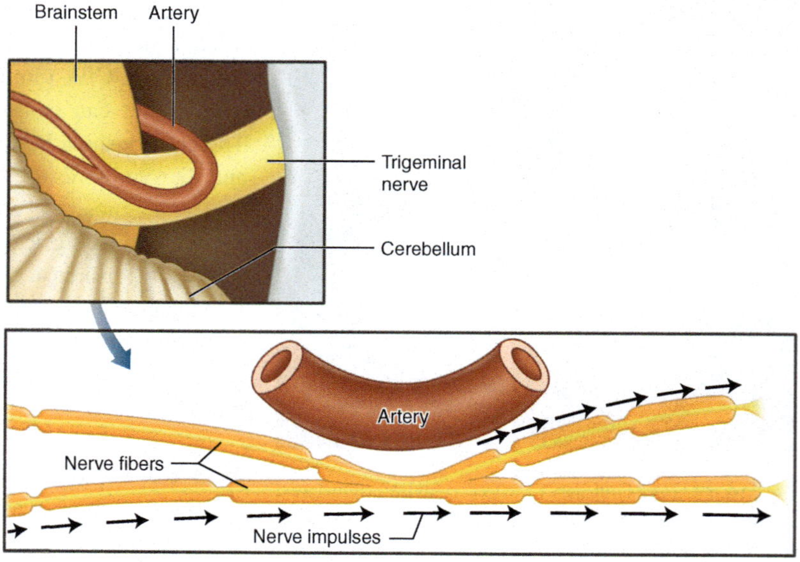

Fig. 16.17 Vascular compression of the respective nerves at the exit zone from the brainstem causes demyelination of the root entry/exit zone of the nerve with resultant lateral transmission of an impulse from one axon to another resulting in exaggerated hyperactivity of the nerve (ephaptic transmission)

choectasia (elongation and dilatation of vertebral and basilar artery), or rarely aneurysmal dilations of an artery.

16.4.1 Pathogenesis

Vascular compression of the respective nerves at the REZ (root exit zone or root entry zone) from the brainstem is the principal factor involved in the genesis of cranial nerve hyperactivity through demyelination with the neural short circuit (ephaptic transmission) and nuclear hyperactivity (see Fig. 16.17).

16.4.2 Hemifacial Spasm (HFS)

HFS refers to a condition where patients develop unilateral facial movement disorder characterized by non-voluntary, unilateral, and intermittent twitching of muscles innervated by the facial nerve mainly involving the orbicularis oculi muscle (90%). More than 95% of the cases are caused

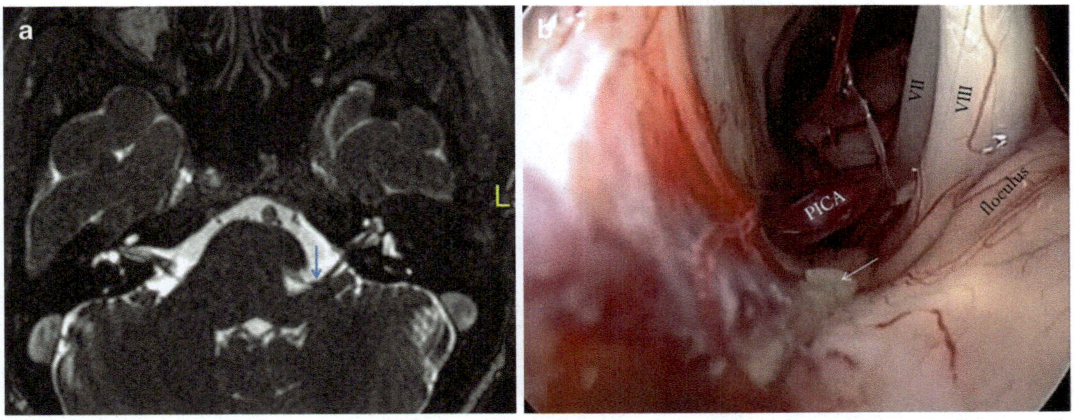

Fig. 16.18 A case of left-sided hemifacial spasm. (**a**) T2-MRI showing the vascular compression of the facial nerve at its exit from brain stem (blue arrow). (**b**) Operative view showing the postero-inferior cerebellar artery (PICA) is high and in contact with the facial nerve (VII). The white arrow corresponds to Foramen of Luschka which is located posterior and inferior to the facial nerve exit. VIII: vestibulocochlear nerve

by neurovascular compression. The most common offending vessel in the hemifacial spasm (HFS) is the PICA accounting for more than 50% of the cases, while the other eliciting vessels may include vertebral artery, AICA, isolated or associated and rarely veins.

The diagnosis is based on MRI assessment in T2 axial and coronal with thin slices 0.4 mm MRI. In this sequence, the CSF is white and both nerves and vessels can be clearly identified by contrast. Angio MRI is not useful, showing only vessels without the location of the cranial nerves (see Fig. 16.18).

Medical management is the only palliative with transitory effect and includes medications, such as carbamazepine, and botulinum toxin injections. Surgical decompression is the unique curative treatment, highly successful where the offending vessel is gently displaced and separated from the involved cranial nerve by the Teflon pad.

16.4.3 Trigeminal Neuralgia (TN)

Trigeminal neuralgia also termed *tic douloureux*, is recognized by brief paroxysmal, strong, and sharp pain strictly limited to one side of the face and localized in the distribution of the trigeminal nerve. The attack is precipitated by stimuli to the distribution of the trigeminal nerve, such as the wind blowing, eating, washing, shaving, cold, warmth, and draught which defines the trigger zone. Its incidence is around 5 per 100,000 individuals. There is a relatively higher incidence of suicide in TN due to the severe nature of the pain.

A positive response to neuropathic pain medications, such as carbamazepine or gabapentin, often supports the diagnosis of typical trigeminal neuralgia and potentially predicts a good outcome for microvascular decompression (MVD) surgery.

MRI is the key for the diagnosis and require precise and thin slices in the trigeminal area using axial, coronal, and sagittal incidences along the nerve in T2 but also in TI gadolinium to visualize venous structures; the most frequent vessel which offends the trigeminal nerve is the superior cerebellar artery (Fig. 16.19), then AICA, dolicho basilar or vertebral artery. Veins are associated in 25% of compression or irritation of the trigeminal nerve, it usually occurs near the root entry zone which can be located on all the course of the nerve from the Meckel cave entrance to the pons.

All patients presenting with trigeminal neuralgia should have an MRI scan as part of their evaluation to exclude intracranial tumoral pathology (meningioma).

The medication of choice is carbamazepine in trigeminal neuralgia, it is effective in reducing the symptoms in 70% of patients, and other medications used include gabapentin, valproate, and baclofen. In the case of failed medical management, surgical procedures to cure the patient

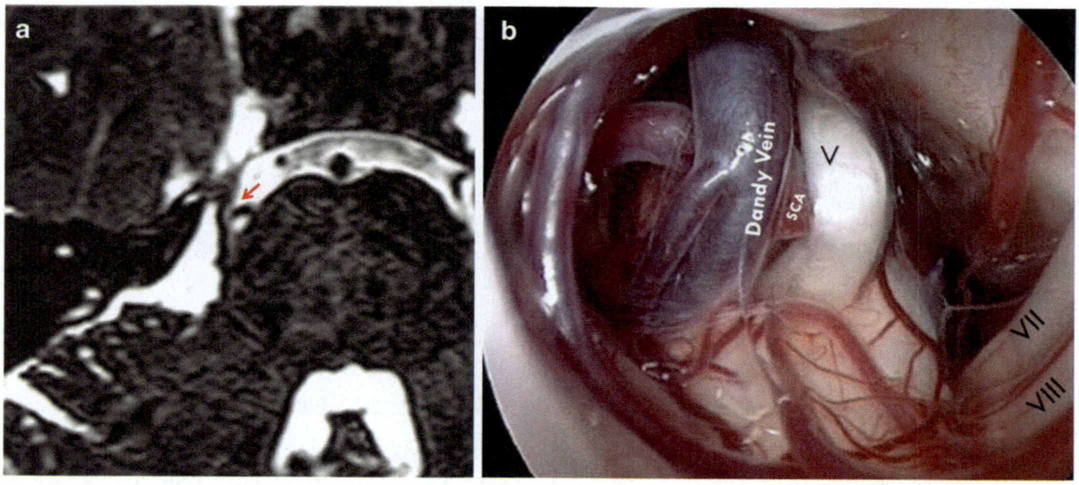

Fig. 16.19 A case of right-sided trigeminal neuralgia. (**a**) T2-MRI showing the vascular compression of the trigeminal nerve in its cisternal segment (red arrow). (**b**) Operative view showing the superior cerebellar artery (SCA) pushing down the trigeminal nerve (V) and causing significant compression. VII: facial nerve, VIII: vestibulocochlear nerve

is indicated. The endoscope-assisted microvascular decompression (MVD) treats the cause of the disorder. All other procedures are previous treatment proposed when trigeminal neuralgia was considered as idiopathic, it incluided radiofrequency thermocoagulation, balloon compression, stereotactic radiation, and percutaneous rhizotomies. Although percutaneous procedures offer a less invasive route to the Gasserian ganglion for partial rhizotomy, MVD offers the only opportunity to identify an offending vessel through a nondestructive procedure with a more lasting result.

16.4.4 Vascular Compression of the Vestibulocochlear Nerve

Vascular compression of the vestibulocochlear nerve (CN VIII) can induce nerve symptoms such as vertigo and unilateral tinnitus (pulsatile is only 20%). The relationship between the vascular compression and the symptoms is a "thorny issue" because of the lack of specificity of clinical signs and the frequency of AICA loop in contact with the auditory nerve. MRI must be done with thin slices 0.4 mm to show the distortion of the vestibulocochlear nerve. ABR abnormality must confirm the involvement of the auditory nerve (I–III inter-peak prolonged latency of more than 0.2 ms compared to the opposite). The most frequent offending vessel is the anterior inferior cerebellar artery (AICA). This syndrome is controversial, and some physicians argue its existence. Nevertheless, reports of efficacious microvascular decompression of the vestibulocochlear nerve suggest that surgical treatment of vascular loop syndrome may be useful for some patients.

16.4.5 Glossopharyngeal Neuralgia (GN)

GN is rare and characterized by paroxysms of repetitive stabbing pain localized unilaterally in the base of the tongue, soft palate, and throat in the lateral and posterior parts of the pharynx and radiating to the ipsilateral ear. Neuralgia can be triggered by swallowing, yawning, coughing, or chewing, and usually lasts for a few seconds.

Take-Home Messages

- Vestibular schwannomas account for approximately 85% of tumors found within the CPA.
- Bilateral vestibular schwannomas are associated with autosomal dominant neurofibromatosis type 2 (NF2).
- Vestibular schwannomas stain positive with S-100 and vimentin. It is a benign condition with a very rare malignant degeneration (<1%).
- The most common presenting symptoms of vestibular schwannoma is a unilateral, progressive, high frequency sensorineural hearing loss.
- Magnetic resonance imaging (MRI) is the gold standard in the evaluation of patients with unilateral auditory and vestibular dysfunction.
- Imaging can often distinguish meningioma from VS; meningiomas are homogeneous, denser, contain calcifications and hyperostosis, and have dural tail.
- The major etiology of cerebellopontine neurovascular conflict is the pulsatile compression of a vascular structure on the origin of the nerve.

Further Reading

Brackmann DE, Cullen RD, Fisher LM. Facial nerve function after translabyrinthine vestibular schwannoma surgery. Otolaryngol Head Neck Surg. 2007;136(5):773–7.

Brunori A, Scarano P, Chiappetta F. Non-acoustic neuroma tumor (NANT) of the cerebello-pontine angle: a 15-year experience. J Neurosurg Sci. 1997;41:159–68.

Magnan J. Endoscope-assisted microsurgery of trigeminal, facial and auditory nerves in Surgery of lateral skull base: a 50-year endeavour. Acta Otorhinolaryngol Ital. 2019;39(Suppl 1):117–21.

Magnan J, Parikh B, Miyazaki H. Functional surgery of cerebellopontine angle by minimally invasive retrosigmoid approach. New Delhi: Jayppee Brothers Medical Publishers; 2013.

Matthies C, Samii M. Management of 1000 vestibular schwannomas (acoustic neuromas): clinical presentation. Neurosurgery. 1997;40(1):1–9.

Sanna M. Atlas of microsurgery of the lateral skull base. New York: Thieme; 2008.

Sanna M, Taibah A, Russo A, Falcioni M, Agarwal M. Perioperative complications in acoustic neuroma (vestibular schwannoma) surgery. Otol Neurotol. 2004;25(3):379–86.

Zanoletti E, Mazzoni A, Martini A, et al. Surgery of the lateral skull base: a 50-year endeavour. Acta Otorhinolaryngol Ital. 2019;39(Suppl 1):S1–S146.

Lateral Skull Base Pathologies

17

Zaid Altamimi, Hassan Haidar,
and Abhishek Menon

17.1 Introduction

The temporal bone, petrous apex, and jugular foramen are complex anatomic regions of the lateral skull base with distinct pathologies. The diversity and complexity of pathologies arising in the skull base need a multidisciplinary skull base team approach to facilitate management and to avoid significant morbidity and mortality. In this chapter, we discuss the anatomy, common pathologies, diagnostics, and management of jugular foramen, petrous apex, and other temporal bone lesions. The most common lesion seen involving the jugular fossa is a glomus jugulare paraganglioma followed by schwannomas and meningiomas [1]. Cholesterol granuloma is the most common pathologic lesion found in the petrous apex.

Thorough knowledge of the jugular foramen, petrous apex, and temporal bone anatomy is essential for the diagnosis and proper management of their pathologies.

Jugular foramen is one of the most important foramina of the lateral skull base. It contains the lower cranial nerves and major vascular structures. Tumors that develop within it, or extend into it, provide significant diagnostic and surgical challenges. The jugular foramen is separated by the jugular spine and a fibrous band into two fibro-osseous compartments (Fig. 17.1).

1. *Pars vascularis*: posterolateral vascular compartment, which is larger and receives the internal jugular vein, vagus nerve (CN X) with Arnold's branch, the spinal nerve (CN XI), and posterior meningeal artery. The cranial nerves are medial to the internal jugular.
2. *Pars nervosa*: anteromedial nervous compartment, which is smaller and receives the glossopharyngeal nerve (CN IX), the Jacobson's branch, and the inferior petrosal sinus.
   (a) Posterior to the jugular fossa lies the small canal of Arnold's nerve.
   (b) Medial to the jugular fossa, there is the groove of the inferior petrosal sinus and the opening of the cochlear aqueduct.

The petrous apex is a pyramid-shaped structure formed by the medial portion on the temporal bone. It is obliquely positioned within the skull base, with its apex pointing anteromedially and its base located posterolaterally. It is bounded by inner ear structures laterally, the petro-occipital fissure medially, the petrosphenoidal fissure and the internal carotid artery (ICA) anteriorly, and the posterior cranial fossa posteriorly. The middle cranial

Z. Altamimi · H. Haidar (✉) · A. Menon
Hamad Medical Corporation, Doha, Qatar
e-mail: Zaltamimi@hamad.qa

A. Al-Qahtani et al. (eds.), *Textbook of Clinical Otolaryngology*,
https://doi.org/10.1007/978-3-030-54088-3_17

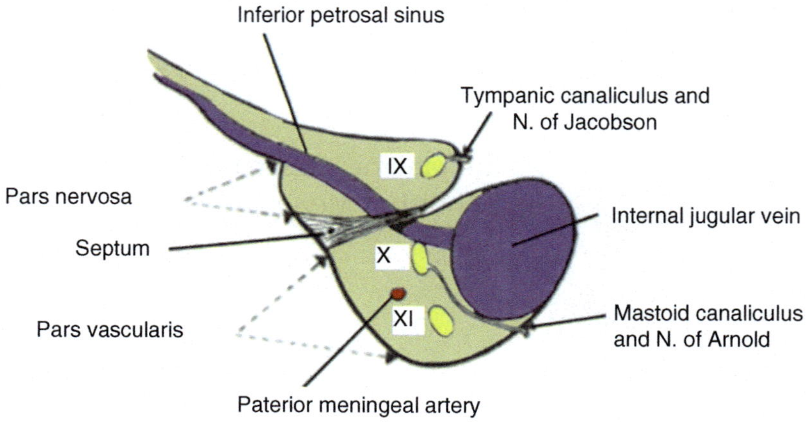

Fig. 17.1 Jugular foramen compartments anatomy and its contents

fossa, Meckel's cave, and ICA form the superior surface. The inferior surface is formed by the jugular bulb and the inferior petrosal sinus. The anterior portion of the petrous apex is filled with marrow in approx. 60% of temporal bones, pneumatized in 33% and sclerotic in 7%.

17.2 Jugular Foramen Tumors

The most common lesion seen involving the jugular fossa is a glomus paragangliomas, other lesions include meningiomas, schwannoma of lower cranial nerves, metastatic tumors, chordoma, and chondrosarcomas. Most of the jugular fossa tumors are slow growing. The clinical manifestations are arising by the compressing effect on the nerves that lie within the fossa and the tumor extension. The signs and symptoms are usually unilateral and can be related to the affected cranial nerves.

17.2.1 Paraganglioma

Paragangliomas, also called glomus tumors, are rare benign, slow-growing tumors, although they are locally destructive, that arise from parasympathetic ganglia chief cells which are arranged in well-defined nests "zellballen." Embryologically it is derived from the neural crest.

They occur more frequently on the left side, females are more frequently affected than males (3:1), and two-third of the patients are in their fourth to fifth decade at the time of presentation. Bilateral in 10% of patients, and multicentric in 5–15%. It has the ability to secrete catecholamines in 1–3%. Malignancy defined by the presence of metastasis occurs in 3–5% of the cases [2]. In 10% it is a familial form of an autosomal dominant disorder, multicentricity may occur in as many as 78% [3]. The hereditary susceptibility is carried on chromosomes 11 and 1 by the PGL loci that are responsible for the SDH gene (succinate dehydrogenase), where the SDH subunit D gene (SDHD) is a critical component of a cellular oxygen-sensing system in the mitochondrial matrix, and its mutation leads to chronic hypoxia stimulation cell proliferation [4]. Glomus tumors considered the most common benign tumor of the temporal bone and middle ear of adults.

They occur in a variety of places in the head and neck. Most common types include:

1. *Carotid body*: the most common type of paragangliomas (65%).
2. *Glomus tympanicum*: usually originate on the promontory of the cochlea. It arises from the tympanic branch of CN IX (Jacobson nerve).
3. *Glomus jugulare*: the most common type of jugular foramen paragangliomas. The incidence, in general, is 0.1 per 100,000. It arises from the adventitia of the jugular bulb, and glomus jugulare tumors are frequently supplied by the ascending pharyngeal artery.
4. *Glomus vagale*: it arises from paraganglia around the vagus nerve at the base of skull.

17.2.1.1 Clinical Presentation

They are usually large at the time of presentation. The symptoms vary and depend on the involvement and extent of the tumor which can affect the lower cranial nerves including VII through XII. Pulsatile tinnitus is the most common presenting symptom [5]. Other symptoms are summarized in Fig. 17.2. Secretory glomus tumors cause flushing, diarrhea, palpitations, hypertension, and headache. If suspect secreting tumor, do 24-h urine catecholamines (vanillylmandelic acid, metanephrine) or plasma-free metanephrines (most sensitive, but high false positives); and order abdominal CT for positive lab tests to rule out pheochromocytoma.

In at least 10% of those with jugular paragangliomas can have multiple ipsilateral cranial nerves involvement. Table 17.1 shows different types of the associated cranial nerve syndromes.

The special signs which might be found with glomus tumors include:

- **Brown's sign**: reddish-blue hue of glomus tympanicum behind intact eardrum, blanches on pneumatic otoscopy. Presents in 10–30%.
- **Aquino sign**: the pulsatile nature of the tumor can be diminished with ipsilateral carotid artery compression.
- **Objective tinnitus** may be apparent if auscultation over the mastoid or infra-auricular area reveals an audible bruit.
- **Rising sun sign**: reddish middle ear mass.

17.2.1.2 Diagnostic Tests

Imaging scans provide essential information to diagnose paragangliomas of all types. Magnetic resonance imaging (MRI) is the best diagnostic test for paragangliomas with the characteristic appearance of "*salt and pepper*"; pepper refers to the signal voids of huge feeding arteries, and salt represents subacute hemorrhage within the tumor [6]. The MRI provides information about tumor size, local extent, regional anatomy, and intracranial extension that are essential in planning surgery.

High-resolution computed tomography (HRCT) of the temporal bone can be used as an initial image. It appears as follows:

- **Glomus tympanicum**: temporal bone CT shows an enhancing mass in middle ear/mastoid/hypotympanum (see Fig. 17.3).
- **Glomus jugulare**: temporal bone CT shows "*Phelp sign*" as a destruction of the carotico-jugular spine that separates the jugular bulb from the petrous carotid artery. The tumor can have irregularly eroded margins with a "*moth-eaten*" appearance. Figure 17.4 shows the MRI and CT appearance of glomus jugulare.

Angiography is not routinely ordered for diagnosis, but it demonstrates the vascularity of paragangliomas and may be used for preoperative embolization. These tumors are highly vascular for which biopsy is contraindicated in most circumstances.

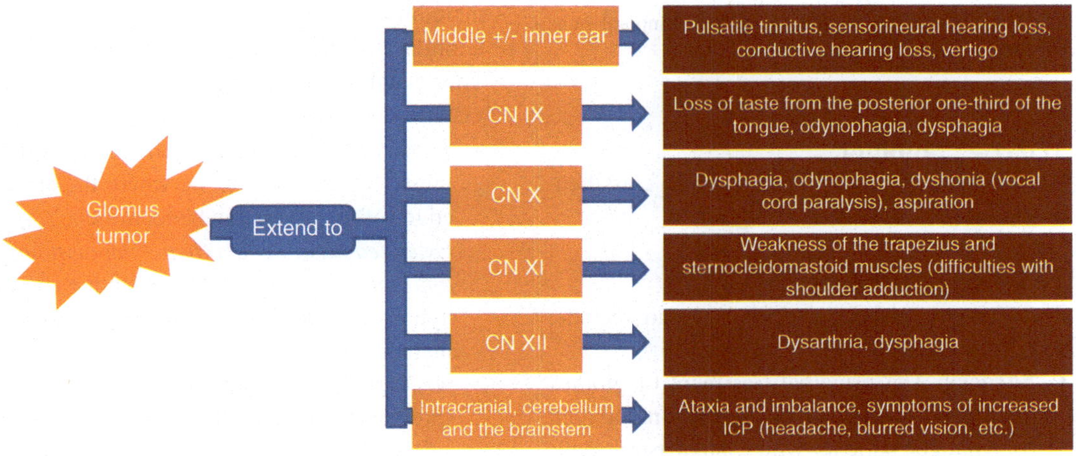

Fig. 17.2 Symptoms of glomus tumor depending on its extension. *CN* cranial nerve, *ICP* intracranial nerve

Table 17.1 Cranial nerves syndromes associated with glomus tumors

Syndrome	Involved cranial nerves (CN)	Clinical manifestations
Vernet syndrome	CN IX–XI	Ipsilateral palsy lead to: dysphonia/hoarseness; soft palate dropping, deviation of the uvula towards the normal side; dysphagia; loss of sensory function from the posterior 1/3 of the tongue; decrease in the parotid gland secretion; loss of gag reflex; sternocleidomastoid and trapezius muscles paresis
Collet–Sicard syndrome	CN IX–XII	Same as Vernet syndrome with addition of CN XII palsy which lead to: dysarthria; unilateral tongue weakness, atrophy and fasciculations
Villaret syndrome	CN IX–XII and sympathetic chain	Ipsilateral paralysis of the last four cranial nerves (IX, X, XI, XII) and Horner syndrome (enophthalmos, ptosis, and miosis)

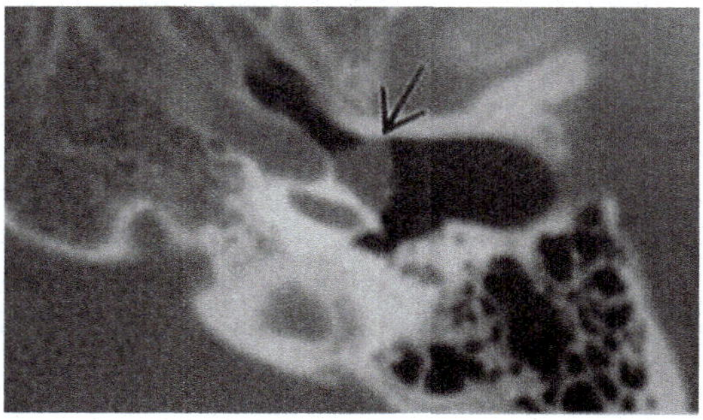

Fig. 17.3 Axial CT section of the left temporal bone showing small glomus tympanicum

17.2.1.3 Staging

Glomus tumors are classified by Fisch classifications, which is described in Fig. 17.5.

17.2.1.4 Treatment

The treatment modalities of glomus tumor include:

- **Surgery**: The principal treatment of glomus tumors is typically surgical excision. Favored for younger patients with cranial nerve deficits. It can be achieved by different approaches, as discussed below.
- **Radiotherapy** (stereotactic or external beam radiotherapy): as a primary or adjuvant therapy with subtotal resection. It can arrest tumor growth rate by causing obliterative endarteritis in the vessels [7].
- **Observation**: may observe if not growing, older patients, and poor surgical candidates. Alpha- and beta-blockers drugs used for secreting tumors as an adjunctive treatment.

Surgery

Complete excision is the favorable outcome after the surgical intervention, but a trend to do a subtotal resection in extensive tumors to spare functioning cranial nerves with possible adjuvant radiation therapy if subsequent tumor progression.

A variety of surgical approaches have been described for the management of glomus tumor that depends mainly on the localization, size, and extension of the tumor. Preoperative preparation and different approaches include the following [1]:

- All approaches need neck dissection for proximal carotid artery and internal jugular vein control.
- Preoperative embolization 1 or 2 days before surgery to decrease intraoperative blood loss, shorten the duration of the procedure, and reduce postoperative morbidity; embolize external carotid artery branches commonly including ascending pharyngeal artery.
- Glomus tympanicum approaches → Transcanal or hypotympanotomy approach via an extended facial recess approach.
  - *Transcanal*: mainly for small localized glomus tympanicum tumors, where the entire edges of the tumor can be identified.
  - *Extended facial recess (hypotympanotomy) approach*: For larger glomus tumors with hypotympanum and mastoid extension. It includes a complete mastoidectomy via a postauricular incision, then facial recess (posterior tympanotomy) opened with a sacrifice of the chorda tympani nerve to

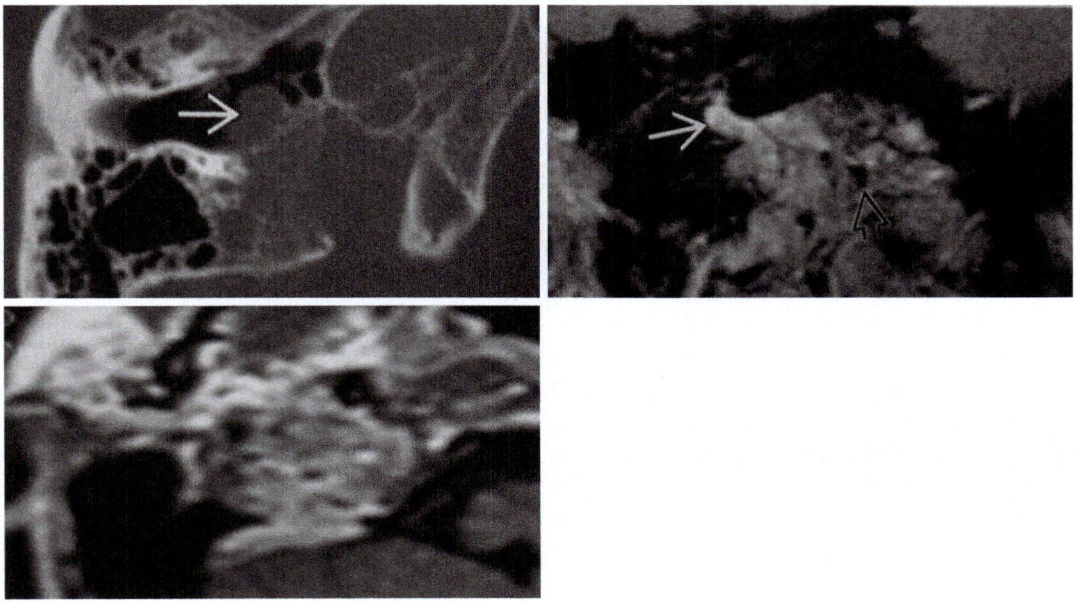

Fig. 17.4 Axial CT, coronal T2WI, and contrast-enhanced axial T1 MRI showing permeative bony destructing lesion centered into the right jugular fossa with erosion of the jugular spine and wall of the petrous carotid canal and extension into the hypotympanic space while showing characteristic salt and pepper pattern in MR images

Fig. 17.5 Fisch staging system (includes both glomus tympanicum and jugulare)

Fisch staging system (Includes both glomus tympanicum and jugulare)

- **Type A involves promontory only.**
- **Type B involves hypotympanum but no erosion over jugular bulb.**
- **Type C erodes bone over jugular bulb:**
  - **C1 erodes carotid foramen.**
  - **C2 involves vertical carotid canal.**
  - **C3 extension to horizontal carotid.**
  - **C4 extension to cavernous sinus.**
- **Type D intracranial extension:**
  - **De extradural, Di intradural**
  - **D1 <2 cm intracranial.**
  - **D2 >2 cm intracranial.**
  - **D3 unresectable.**

allow full exposure to the posterior mesotympanum and hypotympanum with skeletonization of the sigmoid sinus and exposure of the jugular bulb through the retrofacial air cells.

- Glomus jugulare approaches → transmastoid-transcervical exposure ± Fisch type A infratemporal fossa approach with anterior rerouting of the facial nerve to further increase exposure (can cause some degree of permanent facial weakness).
  - *Infratemporal fossa Type (ITF) A Approach*: The development of this approach, as pioneered by Fisch, has

allowed the excision of lateral skull base lesions which were previously deemed unresectable. This approach is used for the removal of tumors where the jugular foramen involves the vertical segment of the petrous internal carotid artery, primarily class C and D glomus temporal tumors. The key point of this approach is the anterior transposition of the facial nerve, which provides optimal control of the infralabyrinthine and jugular foramen regions, as well as the vertical portion of the internal carotid artery (see Fig. 17.6).

- For intracranial extension, a combined otologic and neurosurgical approach is recommended.

17.2.2 Other Jugular Foramen Tumors

- Schwannoma of lower cranial nerves.
- Meningiomas (see Fig. 17.7).
- Metastatic tumors.
- Chordoma.
- Chondrosarcomas.

17.3 Petrous Apex Lesions

The most common lesion seen involving the petrous apex is a cholesterol granuloma [8], and other findings and lesions include asymmetric marrow, effusion, epidermoid cyst, petrous apicitis, metastatic tumors, chordoma, and chondrosarcomas. Petrous apex presents symptoms including hearing loss, facial paresis and paralysis, dizziness, otorrhea, trigeminal paresthesia, and diplopia.

17.3.1 Cholesterol Granuloma

The most common cystic lesion of the petrous apex. Defined as a slowly expansive pathogenesis from obstruction of air cell drainage →

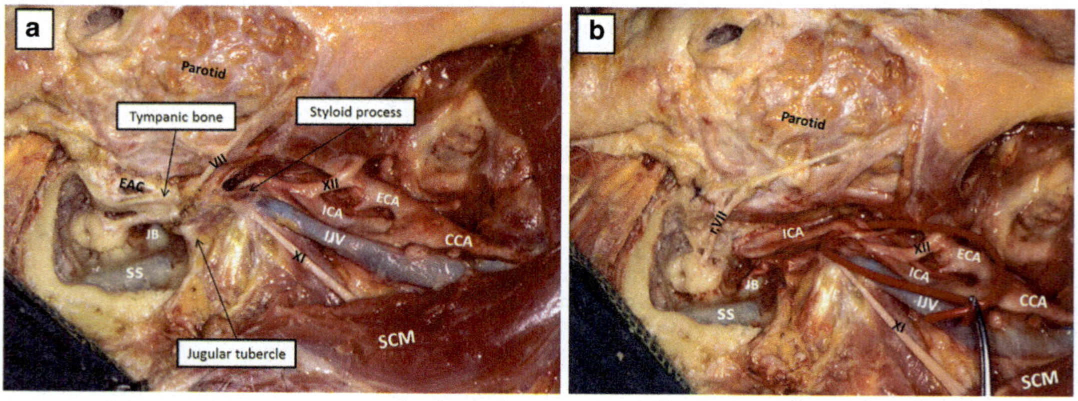

Fig. 17.6 Left side ITF type A. (**a**) A standard, curvilinear postauricular incision extended into the upper neck. The anterior flap is elevated superficial to periosteum over the mastoid and deep to platysma in the neck. The external auditory canal (EAC) is transected at the bony cartilaginous junction, and the flap continued forward over the parotid for 2–3 cm. The facial nerve (VII) is dissected from the parotid. The upper neck is next dissected and great vessels (*IJV* internal jugular vein, *CCA* common carotid artery, *ECA* external carotid artery, *ICA* internal carotid artery) and cranial nerves exposed in the neck. The vagus and accessory nerves (XI) are identified as they exit the jugular foramen and the hypoglossal (XII) is noted as it crosses the carotid bifurcation. The sternocleidomastoid muscle (SCM) is dissected from the lateral and medial mastoid tip and mobilized with the postauricular flap. A well-beveled canal wall down mastoidectomy is next performed and the sigmoid sinus (SS) and jugular bulb (JB) are completely skeletonized. The entire tympanic and mastoid course of the facial nerve is identified and decompressed to 270° of its circumference, from the geniculate ganglion to the stylomastoid foramen. (**b**) The bony EAC and the tympanic bone are removed, the facial nerve is anteriorly transposed, and the styloid process removed to allow complete exposure of internal carotid artery (ICA)

hemorrhage → RBC breakdown → foreign body reaction to cholesterol crystals [9]. Other features include the following:

- Clinical findings: Usually asymptomatic, it may expand to compress CNs and brainstem.
- MRI findings show nonenhancing lesion with T1 and T2 hyperintensity from both high fluid and fat content (see Fig. 17.8).

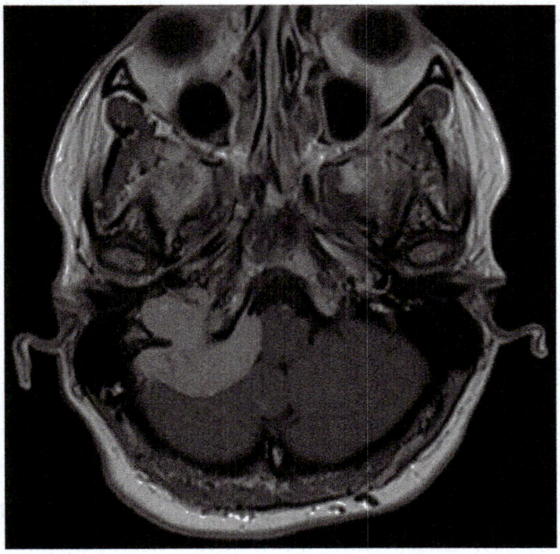

Fig. 17.7 MRI T1 with contrast shows dumbbell shape meningioma of the right jugular foramen

- Management:
  - Observe if not causing symptoms.
  - Surgical decompression for cranial neuropathies, brainstem compression
    - Transnasal approaches provide the widest access for lesions with extension medial to the carotid.
    - Lateral approaches: Infracochlear and infralabyrinthine afford only narrow access but provides a route for aeration and drainage through connection with middle ear/mastoid.

17.3.2 Asymmetric Marrow

It is a variant of normal anatomy; it is found in around 5–10% of individuals as an asymptomatic imaging finding. It appears on MRI as nonenhancing T1 hyperintense asymmetry. CT scan demonstrates normal, noneroded bone. No follow-up or treatment is required.

17.3.3 Effusion/Trapped Fluid

It occurs in a pneumatized petrous apex that trapped effusion. It is seen on imaging studies and in most cases is asymptomatic.

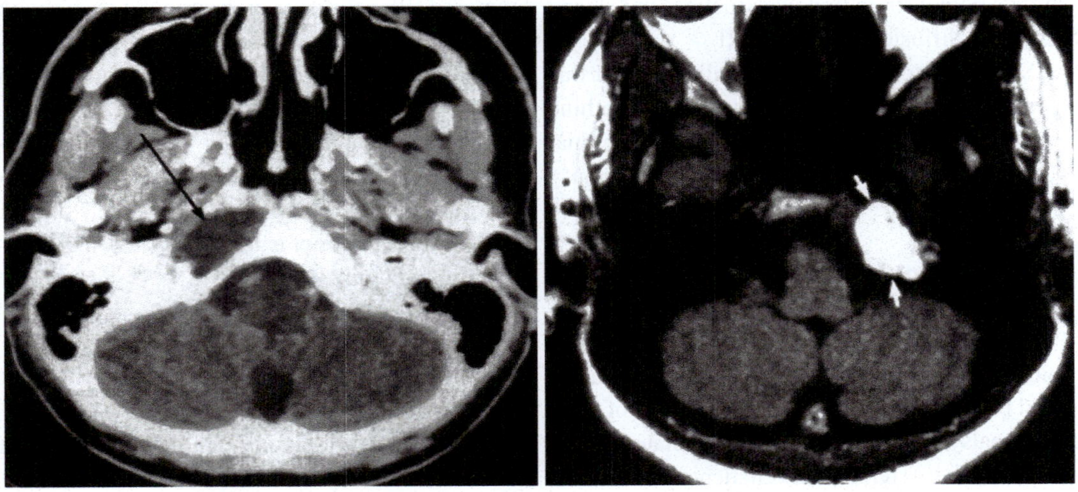

Fig. 17.8 Axial CT and T1 MRI in two different patients showing expansile lesion in the right and left petrous apices respectively displaying CT hypodensity and high T1-WI signal intensity due to fatty contents representing cholesterol granuloma

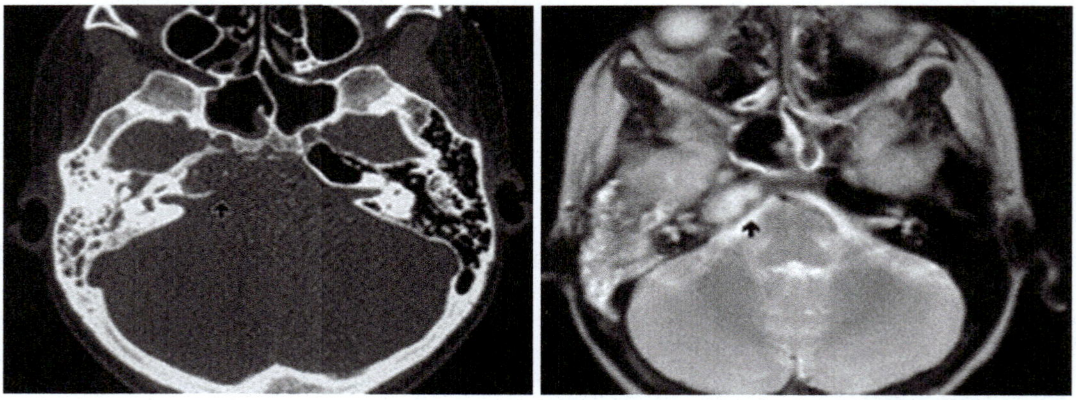

Fig. 17.9 Axial HRCT and T2WI MR showing evidence of right-sided otomastoiditis with opacification of pneumatized right petrous apex and erosion of its posteromedial wall denoting petrous apicitis

CT shows petrous apex air cell opacification with present septations; MRI demonstrates a T1 hypointense, T2 hyperintense area with no enhancement.

Most cases are asymptomatic with no required intervention. For symptomatic patients, prolonged antibiotics with a corticosteroid can be used, and rarely surgical drainage is required.

17.3.4 Cholesteatoma/Epidermoid Cyst

Epithelial cyst within the petrous apex. Imaging studies demonstrate bone destruction on CT and restricted diffusion on DWI MRI.

Surgical excision is quite challenging in this area, if patient has a dead ear. A translabyrinthine or transcochlear approach will give optimal access for the eradication of the cholesteatoma.

17.3.5 Petrous Apicitis

Petrous apicitis is a rare complication of otomastoiditis especially in individuals with a pneumatized petrous apex. There is a classic triad of sixth nerve palsy, deep facial pain, and ipsilateral otorrhea, which is referred to as Gradenigo syndrome, although it may not be present in every patient [8].

CT scan demonstrates air cell coalescence; T1 intermediate signal may have an enhancing ring with abscess; otherwise does not enhance; T2 high signal (see Fig. 17.9).

Treatment is achieved by antibiotics if no improvement surgical drainage should occur by mastoidectomy and drainage.

17.3.6 Chordoma

It is a malignancy of the primitive notochord that usually arises from the midline with extension from clivus to petrous apex. It has a locally aggressive behavior. Skull base chordomas account for only 0.1–0.2% of all intracranial tumors [10]. CT shows a destructive lesion with calcification foci and enhances on T1 with contrast, which may be difficult to differentiate from chondrosarcoma.

The optimal treatment involves radical surgery plus adjuvant radiotherapy. Chordoma carries a poor prognosis with a high rate of recurrence, even after extensive surgery and adjuvant radiotherapy [10].

17.3.7 Chondrosarcoma

It is a rare cartilaginous tumor. It arises from skull base synchondroses, most commonly from the petroclival region [10]. It presents as a destructive lesion that invades bone and extends into soft tissues and can manifest with headache and diplopia. The lesion is located in the central or paramedian skull base. The diagnosis of chondrosarcoma is radiological; CT shows irregular bone destruction, may have "popcorn" calcifications, and enhances on T1 with contrast.

Treatment is surgical resection; both radiation therapy and chemotherapy are of no benefit as primary therapy, but radiotherapy (proton beam) may be of benefit in cases of subtotal resection and recurrent tumor [11].

17.3.8 Metastasis

The petrous apex is the most common site of metastatic spread within the temporal bone [8]. Breast cancer is the most common primary metastatic cancer, followed by lung, prostate, kidney, and melanoma primary cancers.

17.4 Diffuse Temporal Bone/Other Skull Base Lesions

17.4.1 Fibrous Dysplasia

It is a focal condition where medullary bone is replaced by fibro-osseous tissue. Usually monostotic (localized to one site), progressive external auditory canal occlusion with conductive hearing loss rarely causes sensorineural hearing loss. Diagnosis is usually made by CT scan, which shows "ground glass" expansive mass; treatment is mainly observation, may consider canaloplasty for conductive hearing loss or cholesteatoma formation behind canal stenosis, and radiotherapy should be avoided.

17.4.2 Eosinophilic Granuloma

It is the most common form of Langerhans cell histiocytosis, known as the localized form, it carries the best prognosis [12]. It typically affects mastoid, the external auditory canal (EAC), and petrous apex, and may involve entire temporal bone; it affects older children and young adults. It presents as painful postauricular swelling, or with granulation and otorrhea of EAC. CT scan shows areas of bony destruction, and MRI T1 with contrast shows enhancement. Treatment is conservative, surgical excision, or low-dose radiotherapy for inaccessible or recurrent lesions.

17.4.3 Rhabdomyosarcoma

It is the most common temporal bone malignancy of children. It affects the middle ear and mastoid. It is divided into four histologic types: embryonal, botryoid, alveolar, and pleomorphic. The embryonal type is the most common. It presents with chronic otalgia and otorrhea that fails to respond to appropriate medical therapy. Treatment includes limited surgical intervention, external beam radiotherapy, and chemotherapy.

17.4.4 Endolymphatic Sac Tumor

It is a rare malignancy of the inner ear, originating from the endolymphatic sac on the posteromedial wall of the temporal bone. It is slow growing, but locally destructive tumor with a low risk of distant metastases.

It is histologically shown as papillary adenomas. It has an association with Von-Hippel–Lindau (VHL) syndrome (seen in 10–30% of VHL patients); therefore, these patients require screening [10].

The diagnosis is mainly by imaging; CT scan shows a soft tissue mass on the posterior petrous face with a destruction of adjacent regions of the temporal bone with a characterizing expansile appearance. MRI shows retrolabyrinthine lesion with hyperintense T1, heterogeneous T2 signal, and T1 with contrast reveals heterogeneous enhancement (see Fig. 17.10).

The treatment is best achieved with early and complete tumor resection. Different lateral skull base approaches can be used according to tumor localization, tumor size, and invasion. It is a highly vascularized tumor with a higher risk of bleeding. Radiotherapy can be utilized depending on the disease stage [10].

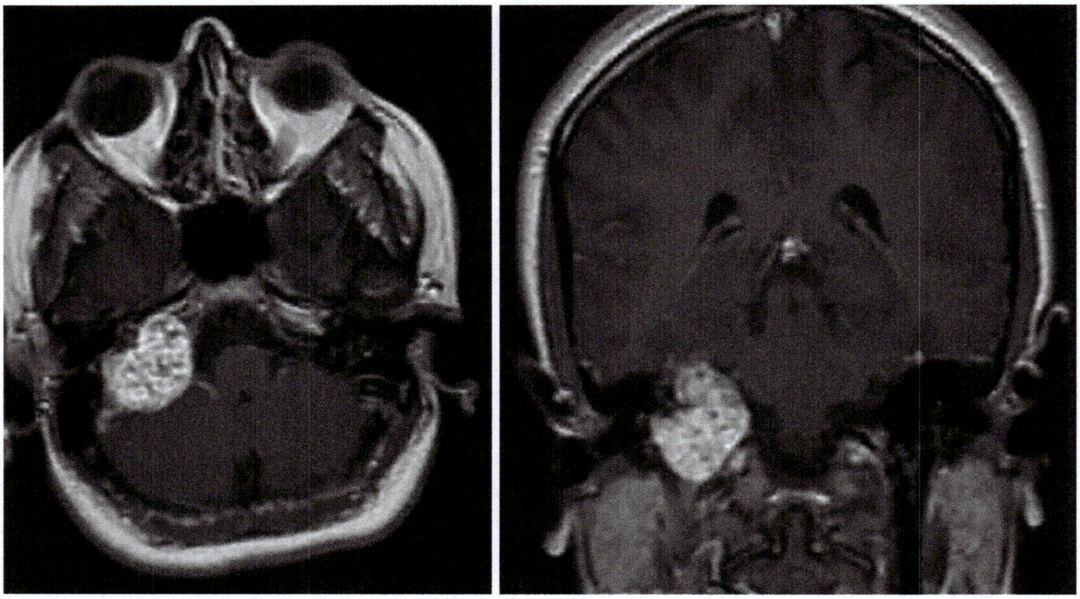

Fig. 17.10 Axial and coronal MRI T1 with contrast reveals heterogeneous enhancement of right ear endolymphatic sac tumor

17.4.5 Osteopetrosis

It is a rare disorder of bone remodeling with a symmetrical increase in bone density because of defective function of the osteoclasts. It presents in two types, an autosomal dominant (AD) type and an autosomal recessive (AR) type. The AD, also known as Albers-Schonberg disease, is the more common type, affecting the head and mandible including the temporal bone and ossicles but it spars the otic capsule. It presents with cranial neuropathies due to compression at neural foramina. The AR, also known as malignant infantile osteopetrosis, is more severe with higher morbidity and mortality.

The treatment focuses on symptomatic management, and decompression interventions of the facial nerve and the cochlear nerve may be of benefit. Bone marrow transplantation also has been described for malignant osteopetrosis.

Take-Home Messages

- Glomus tumors considered the most common benign tumor of the temporal bone and middle ear of adults. Glomus jugulare is the most common type involving the jugular fossa.
- Glomus tumors can present with different types of associated cranial nerve syndromes, including Vernet syndrome, Collet–Sicard syndrome, and Villaret syndrome.
- Jugular foramen lesions surgical excision is quite challenging and might require advance approaches such as transmastoid-transcervical, and infratemporal fossa approach.
- Cholesterol granuloma is the most common pathologic lesion found in the petrous apex.

- Petrous apicitis can present with classic triad of sixth nerve palsy, deep facial pain, and ipsilateral otorrhea, which is referred to as Gradenigo syndrome.
- The petrous apex is the most common site of metastatic spread within the temporal bone, and most commonly metastasize from breast cancer.
- Fibrous dysplasia is characterized by "ground glass" on CT scan. Radiotherapy should be avoided as it carries a risk of malignant transformation.

References

1. Ramina R, Maniglia JJ, Fernandes YB, Paschoal JR, Pfeilsticker LN, Neto MC, Borges G. Jugular foramen tumors: diagnosis and treatment. Neurosurg Focus. 2004;17(2):E5.
2. Borba LA, Araújo JC, de Oliveira JG, Filho MG, Moro MS, Tirapelli LF, Colli BO. Surgical management of glomus jugulare tumors: a proposal for approach selection based on tumor relationships with the facial nerve. J Neurosurg. 2010;112(1):88–98.
3. Fish JH, Klein-Weigel P, Biebl M, et al. Systematic screening and treatment evaluation of hereditary neck paragangliomas. Head Neck. 2007;29(9):864–73.
4. Drovdlic CM, Myers EN, Peters JA, et al. Proportion of heritable paraganglioma cases and assodated clinical characteristics. Laryngoscope. 2001;111:1822–7.
5. Fayad JN, Keles B, Brackmann DE. Jugular foramen tumors: clinical characteristics and treatment outcomes. Otol Neurotol. 2010;31:299–305.
6. Weissman JL, Hirsch BE. Imaging of tinnitus: a review. Radiology. 2000;216:342–9.
7. Willen SN, Einstein DB, Maciunas RJ, et al. Treatment of glomus jugulare tumors in patients with advanced age: planned limited surgical resection followed by staged gamma knife radiosurgery: a preliminary report. Otol Neurotol. 2005;26:1229–34.
8. Isaacson B, Kutz JW, Roland PS. Lesions of the petrous apex: diagnosis and management. Otolaryngol Clin N Am. 2007;40(3):479–519.
9. Jadder RK, Cho M. A new theory to explain the genesis of petrous apex cholesterol granuloma. Otol Neurotol. 2003;24:96–106.
10. Zanoletti E, Mazzoni A, Martini A, et al. Surgery of the lateral skull base: a 50-year endeavour. Acta Otorhinolaryngol Ital. 2019;39(Suppl 1):S1–S146. https://doi.org/10.14639/0392-100X-suppl.1-39-2019.
11. Lustig LR, Sciubba J, Holliday MJ. Chondrosarcoma of the skull base and temporal bone. J Laryngol Otol. 2007;121:725–35.
12. Bayazit Y, Sirikci A, Bayaram M, Kanlikama M, Demir A, Bakir K. Eosinophilic granuloma of the temporal bone. Auris Nasus Larynx. 2001;28(1):99–102.

The Facial Nerve

18

Hassan Haidar and Suzan Mohamed

18.1 Introduction

The facial nerve can be affected anywhere along its course. A comprehensive assessment considering all differential diagnoses is critical to optimal management, as prompt and appropriate therapy leads to better outcomes. The chapter will cover the anatomy, pathology, investigation, and intervention. Information is organized to cover the most common pathology followed by least common and then rare conditions.

18.2 Facial Nerve Anatomy

The facial nerve runs from the brain stem to facial muscles, and it has seven segments: intracranial → meatal segment → meatal foramen → labyrinthine segment→ tympanic segment → mastoid segment → extratemporal segment [1].

In the parotid, the facial nerve divides into five branches (extratemporal branches): temporal, zygomatic, buccal, marginal mandibular, and cervical.

The Narrowest segment of nerve (0.68 mm) occurs at meatal foramen [2] and is the presumed site of nerve injury in Bell's palsy and therefore is site of facial nerve decompression.

Dehiscence is the most common variation of facial nerve, and the most frequent dehiscent areas are: tympanic segment > geniculate (middle fossa) > mastoid (adjacent to retrofacial cells).

In the brainstem, three nuclei give rise to the facial nerve:

1. Facial motor (voluntary facial movement),
2. Superior salivatory (parasympathetic efferents for tearing and salivation),
3. Nucleus of the solitary tract (sensory afferents for taste).

The facial nerve trunk consists of approximately 10,000 nerve fibers, approximately 7000 of which are myelinated motor fibers. The remaining 3000 fibers are somatosensory and secretomotor, and are known as the Nervus Intermedius.

The facial nerve sheath consists of several layers. The endoneurium, closely adherent to the layer of Schwann cells of the axons, surrounds each nerve fiber. The perineurium, which is the intermediate layer surrounding groups of fascicles, provides tensile strength to the nerve and is believed to represent the primary barrier to the spread of infection. The outermost layer of the nerve is the epineurium. This outer layer contains the vasa nervorum, which provides the blood supply to the nerve.

H. Haidar (✉)
Hamad Medical Corporation, Doha, Qatar

S. Mohamed
Otolaryngology Department, Hamad General Corporation, Doha, Qatar
e-mail: SMohamed50@hamad.qa

A. Al-Qahtani et al. (eds.), *Textbook of Clinical Otolaryngology*,
https://doi.org/10.1007/978-3-030-54088-3_18

18.3 House–Brackmann Scale

The House–Brackmann Facial Nerve Grading System is widely used to characterize the degree of facial paralysis. In this scale, grade I is assigned to normal function, and grade VI represents complete paralysis. Intermediate grades vary according to function at rest and with effort (Fig. 18.1).

18.4 Facial Nerve Injury and Regeneration

18.4.1 Facial Nerve Injury Classification (Fig. 18.2)

1. **Neuropraxia**
   (a) Axon and supporting tissues remain intact
   (b) No Wallerian degeneration
   (c) Complete recovery
2. **Axonotmesis**
   (a) Loss of continuity of the axon
   (b) Wallerian degeneration occurs
   (c) Complete recovery, no synkinesis
3. **Neurotmesis**
   (a) Injury involves endoneurium
   (b) Wallerian degeneration occurs
   (c) Increasing risk of synkinesis and incomplete recovery with increasing Sunderland class

In facial palsy, there can be a combination of injuries occurring at the same time. Electrodiagnostic testing is useful to demonstrate the most prevalent degree of injury.

Electrodiagnostic testing can determine percentage of fibers stimulable (neuropraxia) versus non-stimulable (axonotmesis and neurotmesis).

Unfortunately, no current testing can distinguish between axonotmesis from neurotmesis. More rapid degeneration indicates more severe injury and most likely neurotmesis.

Wallerian degeneration is a process that occurs before nerve regeneration and can be described as a cleaning or clearing process that essentially prepares the distal stump for reinnervation. Schwann cells proliferate and form endoneurial tubes with the remaining connective tissues that guide regeneration of the axon to its final destination.

Electrical stimulation can promote nerve regeneration [3].

When nerve fibers are damaged, they may aberrantly regenerate. During regeneration, excessive collateral branching of the axons occurs, not only at the site of the lesion but also along the entire course of the nerve. These extra-axons may result in synkinesis. **An example of abnormal neural regrowth** is "crocodile tears," or increased lacrimation associated with eating. It occurs when efferent fibers normally targeted to travel with the chorda tympani nerve to the submandibular and sublingual glands are misdirected through the greater superficial petrosal nerve to the lacrimal gland. This results in parasympathetic innervations of the lacrimal gland as well as the normal target, the salivary glands. As a result,

House–Brackmann Classification

° I: Normal function
° II: Slight weakness but symmetric at rest, good forehead motion
° III: Obvious weakness but symmetric at rest, impaired forehead motion, able to close eye, may have synkinesis or contracture
° IV: Symmetric at rest, incomplete eye closure, no forehead motion
° V: Asymmetry at rest, barely perceptible movement
° VI: Asymmetry at rest, no movement

Fig. 18.1 House–Brackmann classification of facial palsy

Sunderland Classification of Facial Nerve Injuries

° Class I: Neuropraxia; compression of axon, no axonal disruption
° Class II: Axonotmesis; disruption of axon; endoneurium, perineurium, and epineurium still intact
° Class III: Neurotmesis; disruption of endoneurium surrounding axon; perineurium and endoneurium still intact, risk for synkinesis
° Class IV: Neurotmesis; disruption of perineurium and endoneurium, epineurium still intact

Fig. 18.2 Sunderland classification of facial nerve injuries when eating, instead of getting the normal salivary response to increase the salivation, the neuronal signal causes tearing of the lacrimal gland.

These abnormal movements can be more distressing than the facial palsy itself. Botulinum toxin injection and facial reanimation are among the proposed methods of treatment.

18.5 Facial Nerve Function Tests

It is used to assess integrity of nerve in cases of complete facial paralysis (for paresis not used because nerve is intact).

18.5.1 Electroneuronography (ENoG: Evoked EMG)

It records facial muscle compound action potentials (CAP) in response to transcutaneous electrical stimulation (stimulating electrode placed at the region of stylomastoid foramen).

It provides an objective measure of action potential amplitudes from normal and paralyzed sides.

It should NOT be done until 2–3 days after injury (wait for Wallerian degeneration to occur).

It predicts prognosis and determines the criteria for surgical intervention in traumatic/Bell's palsy (>90% denervation). In Bell's palsy: middle fossa decompression is suggested if >90% degeneration compared to normal side within 2 weeks.

18.5.2 Electromyography (EMG)

It determines the level of spontaneous muscle activity, and it is useful in predicting prognosis for acute or long-standing paralysis.

Fibrillation → Seen in denervated muscle ~2 weeks after injury.

Silence → Muscle atrophy (long-standing denervation).

- Polyphasic potentials → seen with muscle reinnervation ~6 weeks after injury
- Normal voluntary action potentials indicate at least partial nerve continuity.

18.5.3 Nerve Excitability Test (NET)

It compares the lowest current stimulation threshold required to cause minimal muscle contraction on each side of the face (difference >3.5 mA considered significant); it requires subjective observation by tester.

18.5.4 Maximum Stimulation Test (MST)

It compares muscle movement on each side of face in response to suprathreshold current stimulation, stimulation probe placed in the region of nerve branch to be tested; it requires subjective grading by tester.

18.6 Unilateral Facial Nerve Weakness (Fig. 18.3)

18.6.1 Congenital Facial Palsy

Congenital causes include obstetric, developmental facial paralysis, Möbius syndrome, and idiopathic mandibular division palsy.

- ***Obstetric injury***, often with forceps delivery, is the commonest cause of congenital cause; most recover within a month.
- ***Idiopathic marginal mandibular nerve palsy*** (congenital unilateral lower lip palsy/CULLP) causes unilateral weakness of depressor anguli oris and is associated with other major congenital anomalies in 10% of children, most commonly the cardiovascular system. It affects about one in 160 live births.
- ***Möbius syndrome*** is a rare condition of unknown origin. Children usually present at an early age with facial and ocular symptoms which include incomplete eye closure, mask-like face, inability to follow gaze, drooling, and difficulty sucking. The facial nerve is always involved, the abducens nerve is involved in 75–100% of cases, and the hypoglossal nerve is commonly implicated. Other cranial nerves may be involved. The condition is often bilateral.

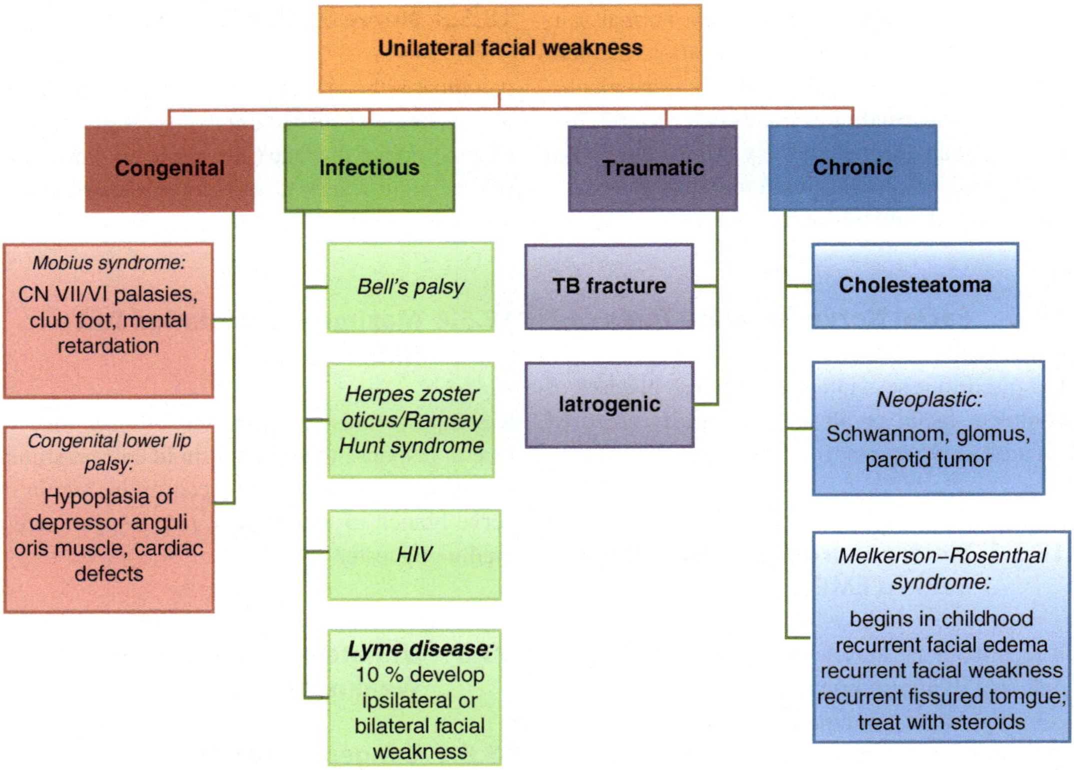

Fig. 18.3 Causes of unilateral facial palsy

Limb abnormalities may be present in up to 25% of cases.

- ***Goldenhar's syndrome*** comprises hemifacial microsomia, epibulbar dermoid cysts, and vertebral anomalies, and may have facial nerve weakness.

18.6.2 Bell's Palsy

It is the most common cause of unilateral facial weakness/paralysis, and idiopathic but viral etiology is suspected.

Risk factors: Diabetes, pregnancy, and prior history (10% recur).

18.6.2.1 Clinical

- Acute unilateral weakness or paralysis develops within 48 h.
- May have viral prodrome, hyperacusis, decreased tearing, numbness/pain of ear/face/neck, and taste changes
- **ENoG** can be considered for patients with ***complete*** paralysis, and it is used to determine candidacy for surgical intervention.

18.6.2.2 Treatment

- ***High-dose steroids*** (prednisone 1 mg/kg) increase the rate of recovery.
- No evidence of improvement with addition of antivirals to steroids [4]
- Eye care if difficulty with eye closure to prevent exposure keratitis (saline drops, lacrilube ointment, and eye bubble)
- ***Surgery***: Middle fossa decompression for patients under 65 with >90% neuronal degeneration within 2 weeks of onset

18.6.2.3 Prognosis

More than 90% of patients will completely recover [5].

It shows poor prognosis with advanced age and complete paralysis.

18.6.3 Traumatic Facial Palsy

Trauma is the second commonest cause and may be due to temporal bone fracture, penetrating wounds, or obstetric injury.

18.6.3.1 Blunt Trauma

- Longitudinal versus transverse (see chapter TB fracture)
- Facial paralysis is more likely with transverse fractures
- Most commonly injured at perigeniculate region
- Management analogous to Bell's palsy
  - Medical: High-dose steroids (prednisone 1 mg/kg)
  - Surgical: Consider decompression for patients with immediate complete paralysis and >90% neuronal degeneration on ENoG within 2 weeks of onset. If no hearing, perform translabyrinthine exploration; if hearing is still present, combined middle fossa/transmastoid exploration is performed.

18.6.3.2 Penetrating Trauma

- Gunshots, knives, ...
- High risk of nerve transection
- Nerve injury to facial nerve branches medial to a line drawn vertically through the lateral canthus of the eye may retain facial movement because of the degree of arborization
- Injury to the frontal and marginal mandibular nerves manifesting with weakness should always be repaired as the likelihood of spontaneous recovery is poor. Nerve repair should ideally be done within 72 h to permit identification of the distal ends of the severed nerves by electrical stimulation; beyond 72 h neurotransmitter stores may become depleted.

> **Surgical Pearl**
> At birth, the facial nerve exits in the stylomastoid foramen on the lateral aspect of the skull, just inferior to the tympanic membrane and external ear canal. This makes the facial nerve vulnerable to traumatic injury during difficult delivery.

18.6.4 Herpes Zoster Oticus/Ramsay Hunt Syndrome

Herpes zoster oticus: Reactivation of herpes zoster virus (normally dormant in geniculate ganglion) with cutaneous lesions in distribution of nervus intermedius (CN VII).

Since the vestibulocochlear nerve is in proximity to the geniculate ganglion, it may also be affected, and patients may also suffer from tinnitus, hearing loss, and vertigo. Involvement of the trigeminal nerve can cause numbness of the face.

Ramsay Hunt syndrome: Herpes zoster oticus + facial paralysis, 18% of adult facial palsies.

18.6.4.1 Clinical

- Shingles in external auditory canal, pinna, anterior 2/3 s of tongue, and soft palate;
- Facial paresis/paralysis with Ramsey Hunt syndrome,
- May have associated hearing loss (50% of patients, due to involvement of CN VIII), also tinnitus and vertigo/disequilibrium

18.6.4.2 Diagnosis

- Audiogram may show sensorineural hearing loss;
- MRI to evaluate the course of facial nerve

18.6.4.3 Treatment

- Treatment with prednisone and acyclovir 800 mg five times a day started within the first 3 days of facial paralysis may increase the probability of complete recovery [6]
- Consider anticonvulsants (carbamazepine, gabapentin, lyrica) for postherpetic neuralgia

Prognosis: Increased risk of residual facial weakness compared to Bell's palsy.

18.6.5 Acute Otitis Media and Mastoiditis

It is typically seen in children who appear toxic with otoscopic findings of middle ear empyema.

The palsy is often progressive in over a 2–3-day interval.

It can be adequately treated with wide myringotomy and systemic antibiotics.

18.6.6 Chronic Otitis Media

Facial nerve dysfunction associated with chronic suppurative otitis media (mucosal inflammation or cholesteatoma) reflects a toxic neuritis, external compression, or intraneural compression from edema or abscess.

18.6.6.1 Treatment

Treatment includes mastoidectomy as soon as possible with surgical removal of irreversible disease in the middle ear and mastoid, as well as decompression of the involved segment.

18.6.7 Malignant Otitis Externa

It affects elderly patients with uncontrolled diabetes mellitus or in others who are immunocompromised and typically present with symptoms of otorrhea and progressive disabling otalgia lasting few weeks.

The pathognomonic signs are otoscopic evidence of ear canal inflammation or granulation tissue at the bony–cartilaginous junction.

Facial palsy reflects advanced skull base extension of the osteomyelitis.

18.6.7.1 Diagnosis

- MRI is very helpful for establishing extent of disease and monitoring response to therapy.

18.6.7.2 Treatment

- Systemic antipseudomonal antibiotics
- Operative debridement of the tympanic bone, the mastoid, and the skull base is indicated only when medical treatment fails

18.6.8 Facial Nerve Neoplasms

Facial nerve tumors are rare lesions.

Less than 5% of facial palsy is caused by a neoplasm [7].

Despite the rarity of facial nerve tumors, the presence of a progressive, persistent, or recurrent facial nerve function deficit should always arouse suspicion of a facial nerve lesion and warrants MRI with gadolinium. Other clues for facial nerve tumors are hemifacial spasm antecedent to the palsy, associated dysfunction of regional cranial nerves, prolonged otalgia or facial pain, mass in the middle ear, external ear canal, digastric region, or parotid gland.

Schwannomas are the most commonly identified histopathologically, followed by hemangiomas and meningiomas.

Facial nerve schwannomas can arise from any segment of the facial nerve and are usually located in a multisegment manner, intratemporally and particularly in the geniculate ganglion (Fig. 18.4).

The number of cases with isolated intraparotid locations is limited [8].

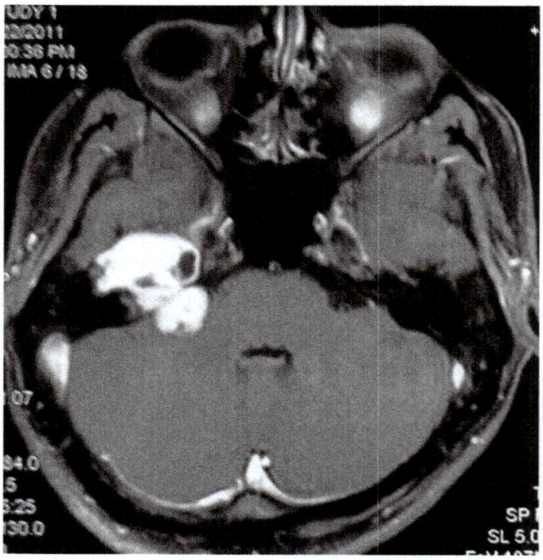

Fig. 18.4 Postcontrast T1 MRI showing right sided enhancing lesion with cystic change suggestive of facial nerve schwannoma involving the cerebellopontine angle, meatus, labyrinthine segment, and geniculate ganglion

Facial Nerve Schwannomas

- Most common primary neoplasm of facial nerve.
- Slowly growing tumors, average 1 m per year.
- Multisegmental involvement with geniculate ganglion most commonly affected [9].
- Iso to hypointense on T1, iso to hyperintense on T2 with homogenous enhancement.
- Cystic change in 20% of cases (Fig. 18.4) [9].
- CT may show bone remodeling and scalloping if intratemporal in location.
- Management: Observation, Radiosurgey, rarely excision (**see algorithm** Fig. 18.5).

Facial Nerve Hemangioma

- Venous vascular malformation of the facial nerve.
- Predilection for the geniculate ganglion.
- Facial palsy out of proportion to the size of the lesion.
- Heterogeneously hyperintense T2 mass with punctuate foci of hypointensity which enhances.
- CT scan: honey comb appearance.

18.6.8.1 Management Plan

Preoperative facial nerve function is the most important factor determining the treatment approach (**see algorithm** Fig. 18.5):

- Normal nerve function or weakness HB III or less → Clinical and radiological follow-up.
- Growing facial nerve tumors → Radiosurgery.
- Facial palsy HB grade IV or more → Surgical excision+ reconstruction.
- Symptomatic facial nerve tumors → surgical excision.

18.6.8.2 Surgery

In most cases, excision of the involved facial nerve segment is required for total tumor resection. In such cases, reconstruction with a nerve graft is required. Postoperative facial nerve function is usually not better than HB Grade 3 [10].

The most important factor determining postoperative facial nerve function is the grade and duration of facial nerve paralysis before surgery [11]. Long-standing complete facial palsy implies very bad prognosis for postoperative facial nerve function.

18.6.9 Iatrogenic Facial Paralysis

The facial nerve can be injured by direct mechanical disruption from a rotating burr, transection with a sharp instrument, accidental evulsion (eg,

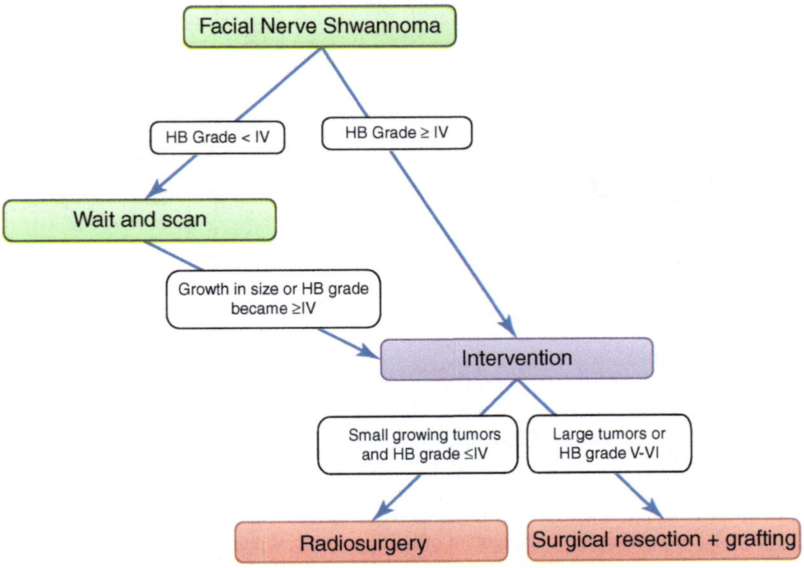

Fig. 18.5 Algorithm showing management plan for facial nerve schwannoma

from traction), or a crushing injury. A rotating surgical burr can produce thermal injury without directly contacting the facial nerve. Thermal injury is more likely when diamond burrs are used than when cutting burrs are employed.

18.6.9.1 Parotid Surgery

- Most common surgery with iatrogenic FN injury.
- The likelihood of facial weakness correlates with tumor location deep to the plane of the facial nerve, previous parotid surgery, and previous sialadenitis.
- All parotid surgery is best undertaken with facial nerve monitoring, and at the end of the procedure, the main trunk should be stimulated to confirm continuity.
- If there is no response, the nerve and its branches should be closely inspected for areas of discontinuity and repaired immediately.

18.6.9.2 Ear Surgery

- The incidence of FN palsy is less than 1%.
- Most commonly during mastoidectomy followed by cochlear implantation.
- Very rare in tympanoplasty or stapedectomy
- Mechanism—direct mechanical injury or heat generated from drilling
- Most common area of injury: second genu, followed by mastoid segment
- Management: (Fig. 18.6)
  - Recognized at surgery:
    Complete or more than 50% transaction → Primary repair
    Less than 50% disruption: decompression (1 cm from each side of injury)
    No return of function should be anticipated before 4 months
  - Recognized immediate postoperatively:
    Remove the mastoid dressing and ear pack and wait for few hours for LA-induced weakness to wear off
    Paralysis persists and surgeon unsure about integrity of facial nerve → Re-explore as soon as possible
    Sure about integrity of facial nerve → High-dose steroids ×10 days

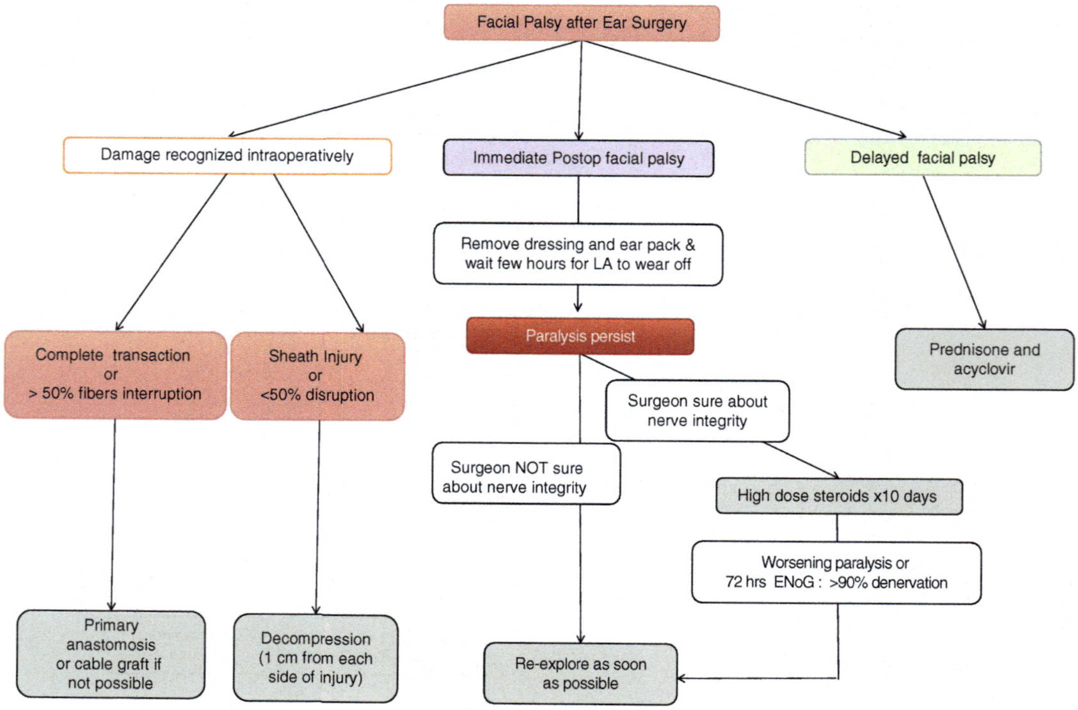

Fig. 18.6 Algorithm for management of iatrogenic facial palsy after ear surgery

72 h—ENoG to assess degree of degeneration: >90% degeneration → re-explore
<90% degeneration—monitor
If worsening paralysis occurs, re-explore
- Delayed palsy
Incidence of 1%
Reactivation of HSV or VZV is postulated as the underlying mechanism
Combined use of prednisone and acyclovir should be considered
Overall prognosis appears to be good

Intraoperative Facial Nerve Monitoring
- Intraoperative monitoring uses facial electromyography, with or without a stimulating probe.
- Muscle relexants must be avoided to permit muscle stimulation and neural monitoring, and this fact must be communicated to the anesthesiologist.
- Intraoperative monitoring is not a substitute for anatomic knowledge and good surgical technique. Facial nerve monitoring is cost effective and beneficial for neurotologic, mastoid, amd parotid surgery, and its use can reduce the risk of iatrogenic facial nerve injury.
- Intraoperative monitoring is not a substitute for anatomic knowledge and good surgical technique. Improper set up, equipment failure, or misuse may lead to worse outcomes than if facial monitoring was not used.

18.7 Bilateral Facial Nerve Paralysis (Fig. 18.7)

18.7.1 Melkersson–Rosenthal Syndrome

Melkersson–Rosenthal syndrome is a rare disease of childhood and early adolescence characterized by recurrent facial paralysis, swelling of the face and lips (usually the upper lip), and fissured tongue.

Melkersson–Rosenthal syndrome is idiopathic disease, but there may be a genetic predisposition. Crohn's disease or sarcoidosis can have similar manifestations.

Diagnosis is mainly based on clinical features. Biopsy of the lip is useful in diagnosis as well as in differentiating between the different types of the disease.

Treatment is symptomatic and may include NSAIDs and corticosteroids to reduce swelling.

18.8 Facial Nerve Reanimation Strategies

The aims of facial nerve reanimation strategies are to protect the eye, restore facial symmetry, facilitate a spontaneous, dynamic smile, and improve speech. Operative procedures may be static or dynamic (Fig. 18.8). The patinet should wait at least 12 months for the first sign of facial movment after any kind of facila nerve surgery. At the end of this period, failure to have any sign of facial movment imposes the need for another facial reanimation strategy (dynamic or static).

18.8.1 Static Procedures

Static procedures do not reproduce the dynamic movement of the face, although it may be ameliorated. Static procedures may be very beneficial to provide corneal protection, improve the nasal airway, prevent drooling, and improve facial asymmetry at rest. They are potentially indicated in the elderly, the unfit, those unwilling or unfit to undergo prolonged surgery, and those with established paralysis without viable facial musculature. Static procedures to correct functional disabilities include temporary or permanent tarsorrhaphy; insertion of gold weights, brow lift or suspension; forehead skin excision; unilateral facelift type procedures; and static slings.

18.8.2 Dynamic Procedures

Dynamic procedures attempt to improve facial symmetry at rest and to provide synchronous facial movement, preferably in a spontaneous manner.

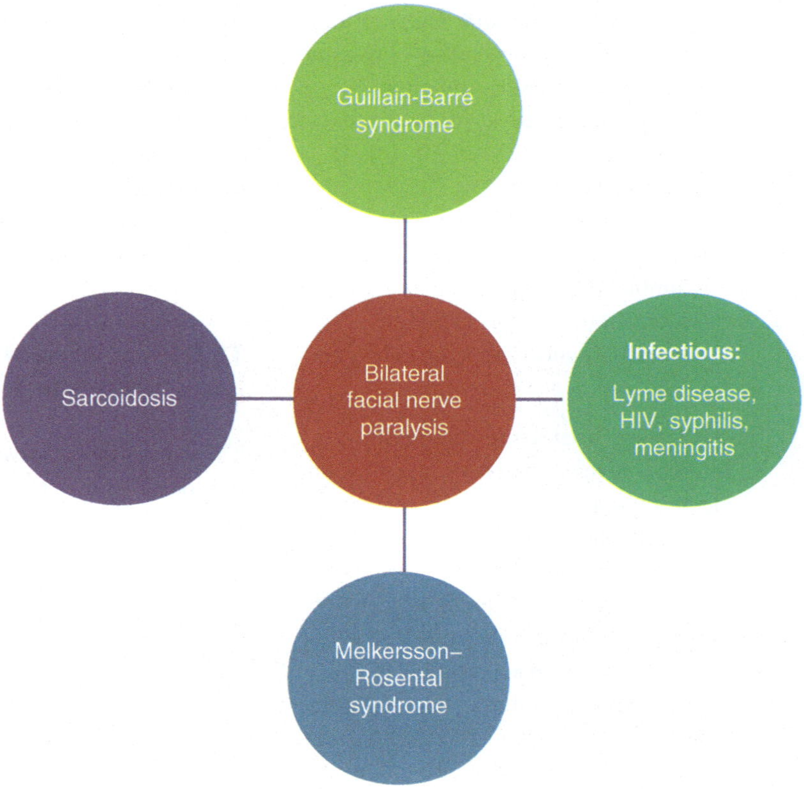

Fig. 18.7 Most common causes of bilateral facial paralysis

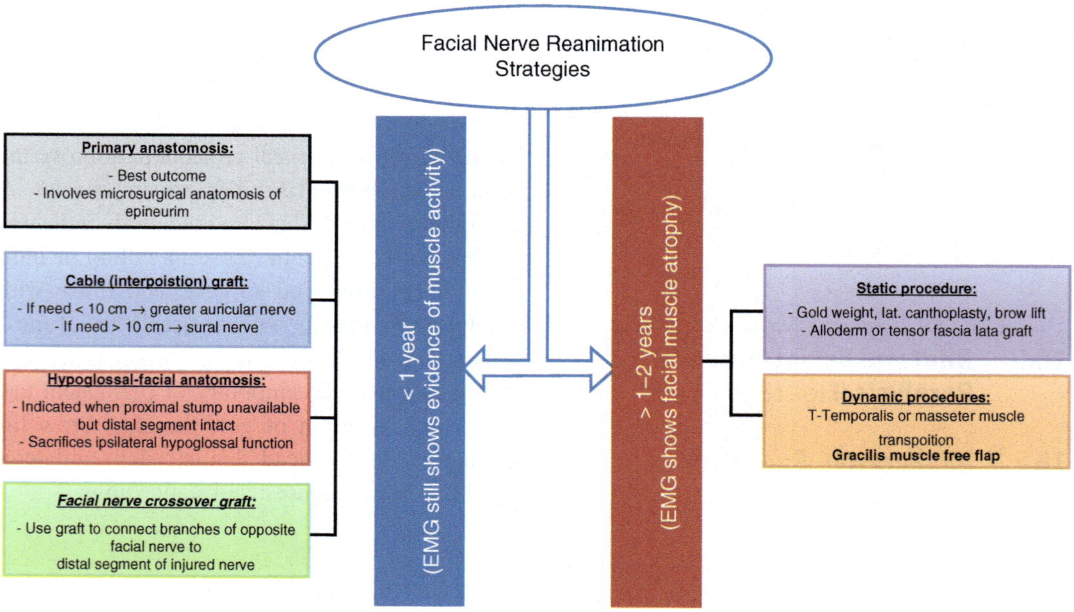

Fig. 18.8 Facial nerve reanimation strategies

18.9 Hemifacial Spasm

Hemifacial spasm is a movement disorder of muscles innervated by the facial nerve, which is almost always unilateral. The cause in most cases is a compression of the facial nerve in the cerebellopontine angle by an artery, most commonly by PICA (postero-inferior cerebellar artery) (Fig. 18.9). The root exit zone of the facial nerve (REZ) corresponds to a junctional area between central and peripheral myelin.At this level, the facial nerve is sensitive to compression from a vascular loop; vascular compression at the REZ of the facial nerve is the most acceptable underlying physiopathology of a hemifacial spasm.

18.9.1 Diagnosis

By the clinical features.

Magnetic resonance imaging using CISS sequence is helpful to identify the offending artery and to rule out other intracranial cause (Fig. 18.10).

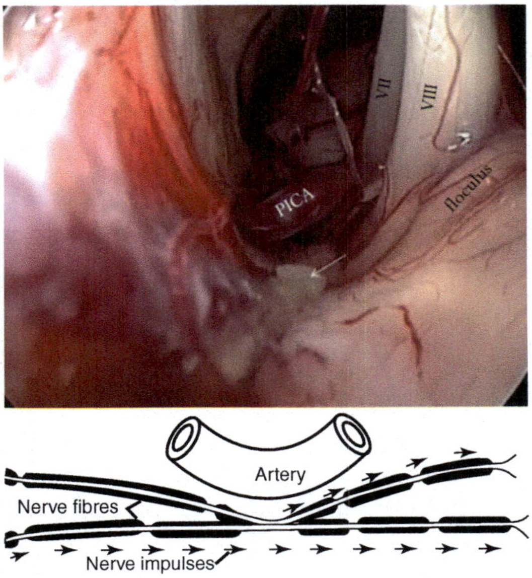

Fig. 18.9 Left CPA endoscopy showing compression of the facial nerve(VII) by PICA (postero-inferior cerebellar nerve)

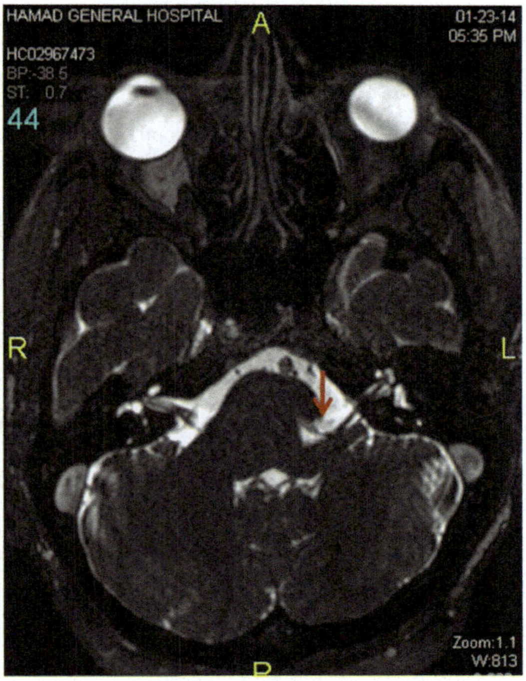

Fig. 18.10 CISS T2 sequence MRI showing vascular loop (red arrow) in contact with facial nerve exit zone

18.9.2 Treatment

Local injection of botulinum toxin masks the symptoms for few months.

Microvascular decompression surgery via retrosigmoid approach with interposition of an insulating material (Teflon pad) between the nerve and the offending artery. The cure rate is above 95% with very low morbidity.

Take Home Massages

- Facial nerve is one of the complex cranial nerve due to his complex function and anatomical course.
- Facial nerve palsy can be unilateral or bilateral; cases can vary from idiopathic, infectious, neoplastic, or iatrogenic.
- Prognosis of facial nerve recovery depends on primary pathology, type of injury, and duration of palsy.
- Facial nerve function test can give an idea about the type of injury and help to plan the appropriate nerve reanimation strategy.

References

1. May M, Schaitkin BM, editors. The facial nerve. 2nd ed. New York: Thieme; 2000.
2. Fisch U, Esslen E. Total intratemporal exposure of the facial nerve. Pathologic findings in Bell's palsy. Arch Otolaryngol. 1972;95(4):335–41.
3. Willand MP, Nguyen MA, Borschel GH, Gordon T. Electrical stimulation to promote peripheral nerve regeneration. Neurorehabil Neural Repair. 2016;30(5):490–6.
4. Sullivan FM, Swan IR, Donnan PT, et al. Early treatment with prednisolone or acyclovir in Bell's palsy. N Engl J Med. 2007;357(16):1598–607. https://doi.org/10.1056/NEJMoa072006.
5. Peitersen E. The natural history of Bell's palsy. Am J Otol. 1982;4(2):107–11.
6. Murakami S, Hato N, Horiuchi J, Honda N, Gyo K, Yanagihara N. Treatment of Ramsay Hunt syndrome with acyclovir-prednisone: significance of early diagnosis and treatment. Ann Neurol. 1997;41(3):353–7.
7. Jackson CG, Glasscock ME, Hughes F, et al. Facial paralysis of neoplastic origin, diagnosis and management. Laryngoscope. 1980;90:1581–95.
8. Caughey RJ, May M, Schaitkin BM. Intraparotid facial nerve schwannoma: diagnosis and management. Otolaryngol Head Neck Surg. 2004;130:586–92.
9. Thompson AL, et al. Magnetic resonance imaging of facial nerve schwannoma. Laryngoscope. 2009;119(12):2428–36.
10. Falcioni M, Russo A, Taibah A, Sanna M. Facial nerve tumors. Otol Neurotol. 2003;24:942–7.
11. Chao WC, Liu TC, Ng SH, Wu CM. Facial nerve schwannoma. Otolaryngol Head Neck Surg. 2009;141:146–7.

19 External Ear Malignancies

Aisha Larem, Ma'in Ali Al Shawabkeh,
and Zeynel A. Dogan

19.1 Introduction

Generally speaking, malignant neoplasms of the auricle are common, and that can be attributed to sun exposure, especially in men. It constitutes 5% of all other cutaneous malignancies. Fair skin, chronic immunosuppressive therapies, radiotherapy, and certain skin conditions are examples of risk factors that can increase the individual susceptibility to this type of malignancies. Cutaneous malignancies are considered the most common malignant tumor of the ear canal. Primary malignancies of the external auditory canal (EAC) are rare; they are usually an extension of the cutaneous malignancies of the sun-exposed area of the auricle.

A. Larem (✉)
Hamad Medical Corporation, Doha, Qatar

HMC, Doha, Qatar
e-mail: alarem@hamad.qa

M. A. Al Shawabkeh
HMC, Doha, Qatar
e-mail: MAIGhshoum@hamad.qa

Z. A. Dogan
ENT(ORL-HNS), Head and Neck Department,
St. Anna Hospital—University of Dusseldorf,
Dusseldorf, Germany

19.2 Malignancy of Auricle

19.2.1 Actinic Keratosis

- Solar keratosis and senile keratosis are other terms for this condition.
- It is premalignant [1].
- It is caused by sun exposure.
- Risk factors: Fair skin, chronic immunosuppressive therapies, and increasing age [1].
- Appearance: erythematous raised patch that has flat top with sandpaper [2].
- It has 5% of malignant transformation into squamous cell carcinoma (SCC) [2].
- Treatment: curettage, cryotherapy, topical tretinoin, 5-fluorouracil, laser, dermabrasion, or excision [2].

19.2.2 Lentigo Maligna

- Hutchinson's freckle is another term for this condition.
- It is a melanoma in situ [2].
- Appearance: macular spot, which is brown to black with irregular boundaries that enlarge overtime slowly [3].
- It has 5% of malignant transformation into an invasive melanoma [2].
- It has high recurrence rates [2].
- Treatment: Surgical excision. Moh's technique can be utilized in anatomically essential regions [2].

A. Al-Qahtani et al. (eds.), *Textbook of Clinical Otolaryngology*,
https://doi.org/10.1007/978-3-030-54088-3_19

19.2.3 Keratoacanthoma

- Appearance: a volcano-like bump that is affecting an area of the pinna and grows rapidly, reaching maximum size in 1–2 months [2].
- Risk factors: sun exposure, male, and fair skin [4].
- Common in male, middle-age to elderly patients [4].
- Treatment: excision [4].

19.2.4 Basal Cell Carcinoma (BCC)

- The least aggressive skin cancer, with a low incidence of metastasis (below 0.1%)
- The most common skin cancer in the head and neck area [5]
- Risk factors: Sun exposure, radiotherapy, immunosuppression therapy, and specific conditions like:
  - Xeroderma Pigmentosum, which is an autosomal-recessive genetic disease. The patient has a defect in the DNA repair mechanism after UV damage; he will have multiple BCC. In addition, they will have corneal opacification and neurological deficits [2, 6].
  - Nevoid basal cell carcinoma syndrome: It is an autosomal-dominant disorder. Patients will have multiple BCC along with odontogenic keratocyte formation, intracranial calcification, palmar pitting, and ribs abnormalities [2, 7].
- Appearance: a pearly skin lesion with rolled borders and telangiectasias [8].
- Histology: It has different subtypes like superficial, nodular, pigmented, infiltrative, morpheaform (sclerosis), and basal squamous. Morpheaform (sclerosis) and basal squamous have a more aggressive clinical course than the others. Basal squamous has the worst clinical picture [8].
- Treatment: Surgical excision with 4–5 mm margins. Radiotherapy can also be used. Moh's micrographic mapping can be utilized [5].
- BCC and SCC have the same staging.
- Look at Fig. 19.1:

19.2.5 Squamous Cell Carcinoma

- It is considered the most common malignancies for auricle [2].
- It has a capacity for metastasis and local destruction.
- The high metastasis and recurrence rates can be related to its close relation to structures underneath it, which will make the resection more difficult. Some believe that this is due to its close approximation to the external auditory canal [2].
- Risk factors: sun exposure, fair skin, radiation exposure, immunosuppression therapy, preexisting lesions, scars, and burns [9].
- Appearance: An indurated erythematous patch, its border cannot be distinguished. It has an area of an ulceration that can bleed easily (see Fig. 19.2) [9].

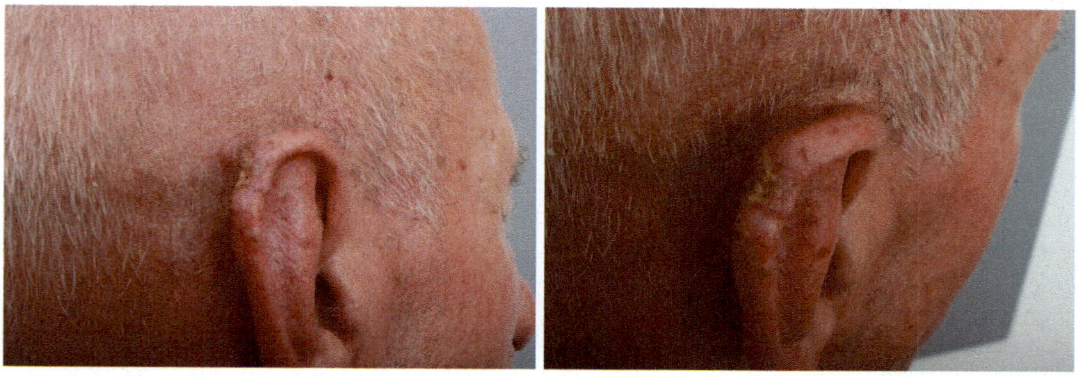

Fig. 19.1 Patient with BCC of upper part of helix of the right ear

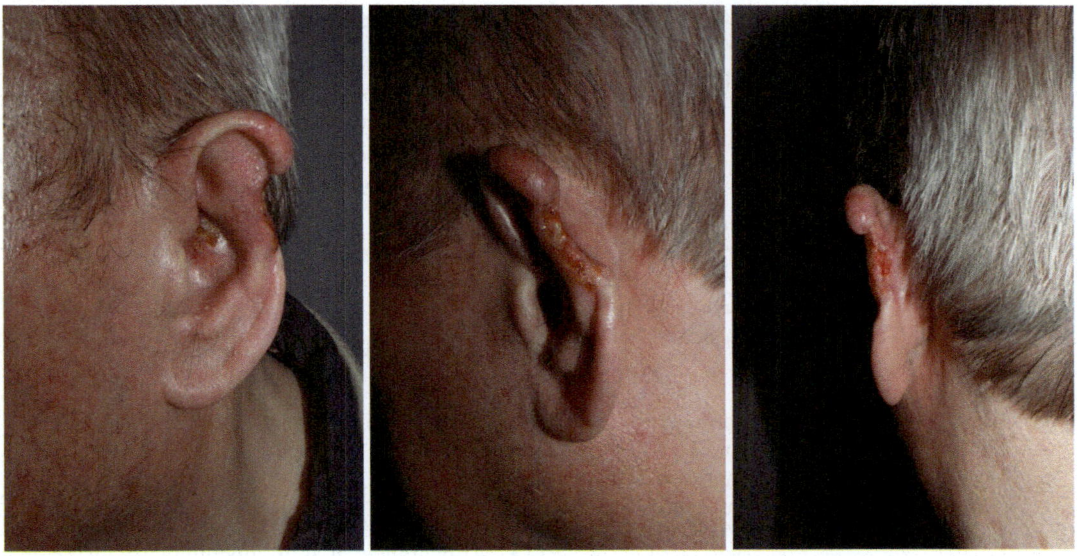

Fig. 19.2 Patients with SCC of the left auricle, note the ulcerative lesion

- Most common location: Helix then posterior pinna, antihelix, and triangular fossa [2].
- Can spread through the lymphatic system. For lesion in the auricle, it can spread to pre-auricular within parotid and postauricular LN. Level II–V lymph nodes can be involved as well [2].
- Staging system: see Table 19.1.
- Treatment: Excision with 6 mm margins circumferentially, which might require auriculectomy. Radiotherapy might be indicated postoperatively. Close follow-up of the patient is required to monitor the resected area and to detect any new lesion in sun-exposed areas. See Figs. 19.3 and 19.4 [2, 10].

Table 19.2 shows a comparison between BCC and SCC.

19.2.6 Melanoma

- It arises from the melanocytes.
- It can arise from the sun-exposed area, lentigo maligna lesion, or even from a nevus.
- Twenty to 30% of melanoma are located in the head and neck region, and 10–15% are in the auricle [2].
- It occurs mainly in the elderly, especially on the left side of the face due to sun exposure during driving [2, 5].
- The most common location in auricle is the helix followed by the lobule [11].
- Histology: It has four subtypes: superficial spreading, nodular, lentigo maligna, and acral lentiginous. Superficial spreading is the most common type [5].
- It has 12–36% chance of lymph node spread. The lymphatic drainage is determined by sentinel lymph node sample [2].
- Treatment: some believe a total auriculectomy with parotidectomy and neck dissection is required for all auricular lesions [12].
- Excisional margins:

In situ	5 mm
Depth less than 1 cm	1 cm
Depth between 1 and 2 cm	Between 1 and 2 cm
Depth more than 2 cm	2 cm

- In general, auricle has a worse prognosis than other parts of the body [11].
- Staging: there are three staging systems available, TNM from AJCC, Clark, and Breslow.

Table 19.1 Tumor-Node-Metastasis (TNM) staging adapted from AJCC Cancer Staging Manual 8th Edition

Tx	Primary tumor cannot be identified
Tis	Carcinoma in situ
T1	Tumor smaller than 2 cm in greatest dimension
T2	Tumor 2 cm or larger, but smaller than 4 cm in greatest dimension
T3	Tumor 4 cm or larger in maximum dimension or minor bone erosion or perineural invasion or deep invasion*
T4a	Tumor with gross cortical bone/marrow invasion
T4b	Tumor with skull base invasion and/or skull base foramen involvement
Clinical N (cN)	
Nx	Regional lymph nodes cannot be assessed
N0	No regional lymph node metastasis
N1	Metastasis in a single ipsilateral lymph node, 3 cm or smaller in greatest dimension and ENE(−)
N2a	Metastasis in a single ipsilateral node larger than 3 cm but not larger than 6 cm in greatest dimension and ENE(−)
N2b	Metastasis in multiple ipsilateral nodes, none larger than 6 cm in greatest dimension and ENE(−)
N2c	Metastasis in bilateral or contralateral lymph nodes, none larger than 6 cm in greatest dimension and ENE(−)
N3a	Metastasis in a lymph node larger than 6 cm in greatest dimension and ENE(−)
N3b	Metastasis in any node(s) and ENE(+)
Pathological N (pN)	
Nx	Regional lymph nodes cannot be assessed
N0	No regional lymph node metastasis
N1	Metastasis in a single ipsilateral lymph node, 3 cm or smaller in greatest dimension and ENE(−)
N2a	Metastasis in single ipsilateral or contralateral node 3 cm or smaller in greatest dimension and ENE(+)
N2b	Metastasis in multiple ipsilateral nodes, none larger than 6 cm in greatest dimension and ENE(−)
N2c	Metastasis in bilateral or contralateral lymph nodes, none larger than 6 cm in greatest dimension and ENE(−)
N3a	Metastasis in a lymph node larger than 6 cm in greatest dimension and ENE(−)
N3b	Metastasis in a single ipsilateral node larger than 3 cm in greatest dimension and ENE(+);*or* multiple ipsilateral. Contralateral, or bilateral nodes, any with ENE(+)
M	
M0	No distant metastasis
M1	Distant metastasis

19.2.7 Rhabdomyosarcoma

- It is considered a disease of pediatrics [13].
- Auricular rhabdomyosarcoma is extremely rare. Temporal bone involvement represents less than 7% of all rhabdomyosarcoma cases [13, 14].
- Appearance: like a polypoid lesion [14]

19.2.8 Merkel Cell Carcinoma

- Considered neuroendocrine cells [15].
- It is a rare tumor [15].
- Risk factors: elderly, fair skin, sun exposure, and immunocompromised [15].
- Appearance: it is a subcutaneous lesion that has reddish-blue or pink color [15].
- Histology: small round cells, stain positive for neurons specific enolase, cytokeratin (CK), and chromogranin, which can help of other cutaneous malignancies [15].
- It has a high rate of metastasis [16].
- Had 30–50% local recurrence rate, and 50–80% lymph node spread [2].
- Male and young age patients have a worse prognosis [2].
- It has 55% 3-year survival rate [2].
- Treatment: complete surgical excision with a wide surgical margin (2 cm margin for those more than 2 size) and elective neck dissection. Postoperative radiotherapy is indicated for aggressive malignancy [15].
- It is considered radiosensitive and chemosensitive [15].

19.3 Malignancy of EAC

19.3.1 Spread

The bony ear canal limits tumor growth. However, it can still spread through the following:

1. Fissures of the Santorini: an embryologic remnant that leaves small anterior

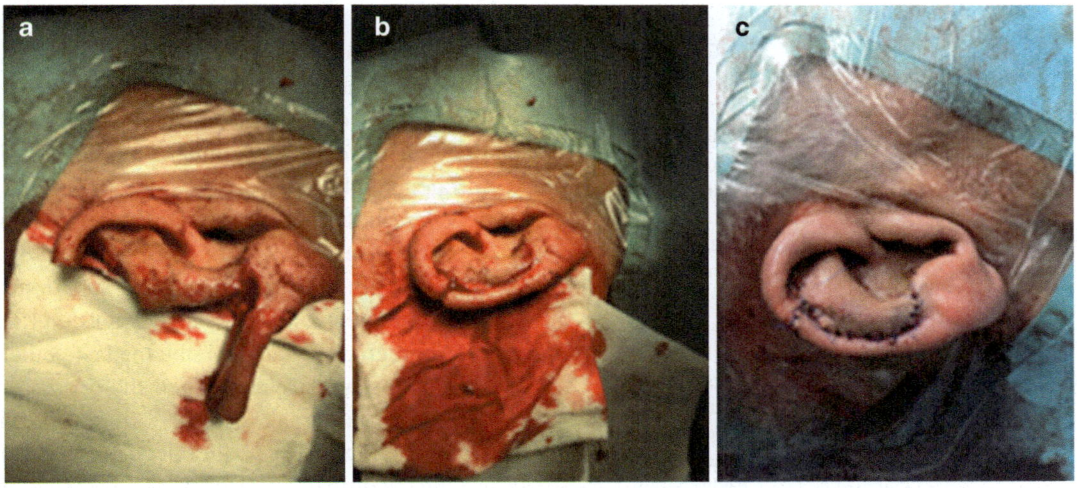

Fig. 19.3 Steps of the resection of auricular SCC with reconstruction: (**a**) Resection of the SCC with wide margin. (**b**) Utilizing the surrounding tissue as a flap for closure. (**c**) The shape of the auricle at the end of the procedure

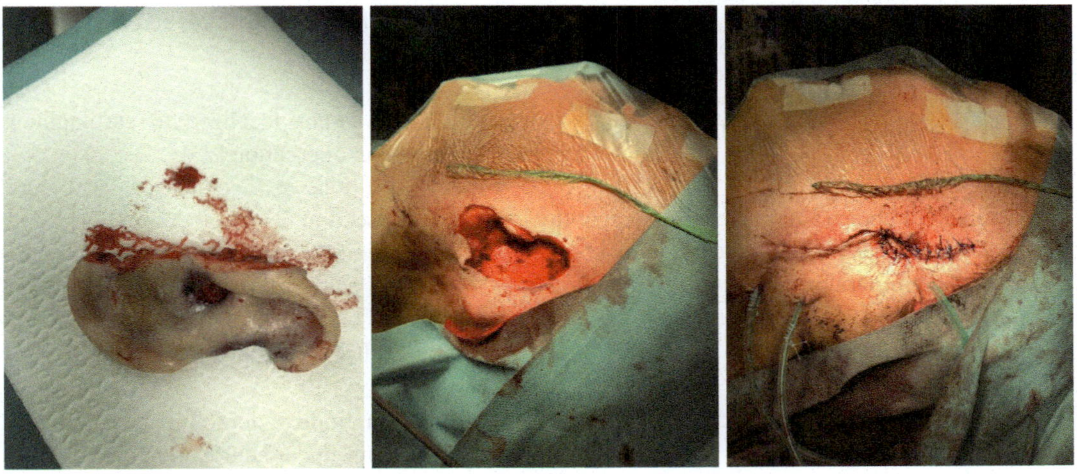

Fig. 19.4 Complete left auricular excision for a patient with SCC of left auricle

dehiscence in the cartilaginous part of the ear canal, which connects to parotid inferiorly [17].
2. Bony and cartilaginous junction part of the ear canal.
3. Huschke's foramen (Foramen tympanicum): a defect found in the tympanic ring in the inferior anterior margin and opens into the temporomandibular joint (TMJ). It is found in 5% [17].

19.3.2 Basal Cell Carcinoma

- It is the second most common primary malignant tumor of the EAC. SCC is considered the most common [18].
- BCC in this location tends to have an aggressive course and has high recurrence rates with high mortality rates [19].
- Treatment: Even with aggressive treatment, it is common to have a local recurrence.

Table 19.2 Comparison between BCC and SCC

	BCC	SCC
Aggressiveness	Low incidence of metastasis	It has a capacity for metastasis and local destruction
Appearance	A pearly skin lesion with rolled borders and telangiectasias	Indurated erythematous patch, and its border cannot be distinguished. It has an area of ulceration that can bleed easily
Treatment	Surgical excision with 2–4 mm margins. Radiotherapy can also be used. Moh's micrographic mapping can be utilized	Excision with 1 cm margins circumferentially, which might require auriculectomy. Radiotherapy might be indicated postoperatively. Close follow-up of the patient is required to monitor the resected area and to detect any new lesion in sun-exposed areas

Treatment of choice is complete excision with negative margins, and that necessitates subtotal or total temporal bone resection depending on the extension of the disease [19].

19.3.3 Squamous Cell Carcinoma

- It is an aggressive disease [20].
- It constitutes 80% of the malignant tumor of EAC. However, it occurs less common than those in the auricle [2].
- Signs and symptoms:
  - Ear pain: which can resemble otitis externa or media; so, the persistence of pain despite treatment should raise the suspicion of such a condition [21, 22].
  - Bloody otorrhea [20].
  - Hearing loss [20]
  - Other symptoms or signs are cervical lymphadenopathy and cranial nerve involvement. Facial paralysis and vertigo occur in cases at an advanced stage [2, 22].
- Imaging:
- Assess the following: the EAC, middle ear, mastoid, facial nerve, sigmoid sinus, jugular bulb, carotid canal, tegmen, middle and posterior cranial fossa, TM joint, and parotid and infratemporal fossa [5].
  - CT scan: to look for erosion and extension of the disease [5].
  - MRI with contrast to look for soft tissue involvement and intracranial extension [5].
  - Angiography can be obtained if other imaging modalities showed the possibilities of internal carotid artery (ICA) involvement. The balloon occlusion test can be utilized to check the patency of ICA in the contralateral side [5].
- Investigation: Biopsy of the lesion: obtain a deep biopsy [5].
- Staging: There are several staging systems available
- Treatment:
  - T1 and tumor localized to cartilaginous part: sleeve resection [23].
  - T1 with bone involvement or T2: Lateral bone resection (± radiotherapy) [23]
  - T3: lateral temporal bone resection plus subtotal petrosectomy followed by radiotherapy, or subtotal temporal bone resection plus postoperative radiotherapy [5, 24].
  - T4 with limited dural involvement "less than 1 cm" and no intraparenchymal extension: subtotal or lateral temporal bone resection with postoperative radiotherapy [5, 24].
- See Table 19.3 for the type of temporal bone resection.
- Neck management:
- If the node is positive, then a modified radical neck dissection is performed.
- If the node is negative, then selective neck dissection for level II, III, Va, and parotidectomy (either superficial if facial nerve function is not affected or total if facial nerve function is affected) [5, 24]
- The patient is considered inoperable in case of:

Table 19.3 Types of temporal bone resection [25]

Sleeve resection	Removal of the cartilaginous part of the ear canal along with the skin over the bony part
Lateral bone resection	Removal of the cartilaginous and bony EAC with the TM, malleus, and incus
Subtotal temporal bone resection	Same as lateral bone resection with the contents of the middle ear, mastoid, otic capsule, and middle ear medial wall
Total bone resection	Same as subtotal bone resection with petrous apex and neurovascular bundle

- ICA encasement.
- Extension to petrous apex
- Dural involvement of more than 1 cm intraparenchymal extension [24].

19.3.4 Rhabdomyosarcoma

- A rare malignant tumor [2].
- EAC rhabdomyosarcoma is usually an extension from the middle ear [2].
- Appearance: polyps causing destruction of the bone and neurological deficit like facial nerve palsy [2].

19.3.5 Melanoma

- It usually arises as a primary tumor [26].
- EAC melanoma is considered a high-risk lesion as the tumor will be hidden in the ear canal, so it will grow to a significant thickness [26].
- Treatment: Complete surgical excision with negative margin (total or subtotal temporal bone resection), neck dissection, and postoperative radiotherapy [26].

19.3.6 Langerhans Cell Histiocytosis

- Symptoms: mass in the ear canal, ear pain, ear discharge, bloody ear discharge, and hearing loss [2].
- This usually involves the medial bony part of the EAC [2].
- CT will show EAC soft tissue along with bony erosion [2].

19.3.7 Malignant Ceruminous Tumors

19.3.7.1 Ceruminous Adenoid Cystic Carcinoma

- Constitutes around 2.4% of all primary malignant tumor of EAC [27].
- They arise from the ceruminous gland [27].
- Symptoms: ear pain and mass in the ear canal [27].
- They have an indolent course and tend to have a perineural invasion, which is considered a hallmark feature of this tumor [28].
- Treatment: complete surgical excision with negative margin along with parotidectomy (to remove the tumor cells that spread through the fissures) and neck dissection with postoperative radiotherapy [2].

19.3.7.2 Ceruminous Adenocarcinoma

- Less frequent than adenoid cystic carcinoma with EAC [2].
- They are classified as low and high grade.
- Symptoms are similar to ceruminous adenoid cystic [2].
- Treatment: complete surgical excision with negative margin with postoperative radiotherapy [2].

19.3.7.3 Ceruminous Mucoepidermoid Carcinoma

- Rare tumor, appears less frequent than the previous two [2].
- Symptoms: ear pain and mass in the lateral part of the ear canal, ear discharge, bloody ear discharge, hearing loss, and facial nerve paralysis [2].
- Treatment: complete surgical excision [2].

Take Home Massages

Auricular Malignancies

- Actinic keratosis is a premalignant condition that can be treated by curettage, cryotherapy, or some local applicants.
- Keratoacanthoma is considered a low-grade skin tumor.
- BCC is the least aggressive skin cancer and the most common skin cancer in the head and neck. Histologically, it has different subtypes like superficial, nodular, pigmented, infiltrative, morpheaform (sclerosis), and basal squamous (last two have an aggressive clinical course). It is treated by surgical excision with 2–4 mm margins.
- SCC is the most common malignancy of the auricle. It is treated by excision with 1 cm margins circumferentially.
- Melanoma can arise de novo or from pre-existing lentigo maligna lesion. It has four subtypes: superficial spreading (most common), nodular, lentigo maligna, and acral lentiginous. TNM, Breslow, and Clerk are some staging systems in use. It is treated by surgical excision with surgical margin depending on the thickness of the tumor.
- Merkel cell carcinoma is considered a neuroendocrine cell tumor that can affect the auricle. It has a high rate of metastasis. Thirty to 50% local recurrence rate and 50% to 80% lymph node spread rate. It is treated by complete surgical excision with a wide surgical margin (up to 3 cm) and elective neck dissection. Postoperative radiotherapy is indicated for aggressive types.

EAC Malignancy

- BCC of the EAC tends to have an aggressive course and has high recurrence rates.
- SCC constitutes 80% of the malignant tumor of EAC. There are different staging systems like Manolidis Staging System, Stell–McCormick Staging System, and Arriaga (University of Pittsburgh) Revised by Moody. It is treated by temporal bone resection like (sleeve, lateral, subtotal, and total). However, in cases like ICA encasement, an extension to petrous apex, dural involvement more than 1 cm, and intraparenchymal extension, the tumor will be considered inoperable.
- Rhabdomyosarcoma, melanoma, and langerhans cell histiocytosis are other tumors that can affect EAC.
- Malignant ceruminous tumors can affect the ear canal. Ceruminous adenoid cystic carcinoma, ceruminous adenocarcinoma, and ceruminous mucoepidermoid carcinoma are examples of those tumors.

Acknowledgment Authors of the chapter would like to appreciate the help of Dr. Adham Aljariri, an ENT resident in Hamad medical corporation, for his help and effort in editing the chapter.

References

1. Goldenberg G, Perl M. Actinic keratosis: update on field therapy. J Clin Aesthet Dermatol. 2014;7(10):28–31.
2. Quinton G. Fundamental otology: pediatric and adult practice reference. 1st ed. New Delhi: Jaypee Brothers Medical Publishers; 2012.
3. Kasprzak JM, Xu YG. Diagnosis and management of lentigo maligna: a review. Drugs Context. 2015;4:212281 . Published 2015 May 29. https://doi.org/10.7573/dic.212281.
4. Zito PM, Scharf R. Keratoacanthoma. [Updated 21 Feb 2019]. In: StatPearls [Internet]. Treasure Island, FL: StatPearls Publishing; 2019. https://www.ncbi.nlm.nih.gov/books/NBK499931.
5. Watkinson JC, Clarke RW. Scott-Brown's otorhinolaryngology and head and neck surgery. 8th ed. Boca Raton, FL: CRC Press; 2018.
6. Black JO. Xeroderma pigmentosum. Head Neck Pathol. 2016;10(2):139–44. https://doi.org/10.1007/s12105-016-0707-8. Epub 2016 Mar 14. Review. PubMed PMID: 26975629; PubMed Central PMCID: PMC4838978.

7. Martinez MF, Romano MV, Martinez AP, González A, Muchnik C, Stengel FM, Mazzuoccolo LD, Azurmendi PJ. Nevoid basal cell carcinoma syndrome: PTCH1 mutation profile and expression of genes involved in the hedgehog pathway in Argentinian patients. Cells. 2019;8(2):pii: E144. https://doi.org/10.3390/cells8020144. PubMed PMID: 30754660; PubMed Central PMCID: PMC6406887.
8. Flint P, Haughey B, Lund V, Niparko J, Robbins K, Regan Thomas J, Lesperance M, editors. Cummings otolaryngology. 6th ed. Philadelphia: Elsevier; 2014.
9. Parekh V, Seykora JT. Cutaneous squamous cell carcinoma. Clin Lab Med. 2017;37(3):503–25. https://doi.org/10.1016/j.cll.2017.06.003. Review. PubMed PMID: 28802498.
10. Motley R, Preston P, Lawrence C. Multi-professional guidelines for the management of the patient with primary cutaneous squamous cell carcinoma. London: British Association of Dermatologists. http://www.bad.org.uk/library- media/documents/SCC_2009.pdf.
11. Narayan D, Ariyan S. Surgical considerations in the management of malignant melanoma of the ear. Plast Reconstr Surg. 2001;107(1):20–4. PubMed PMID: 11176596.
12. Pack GT, Conley J, Oropeza R. Melanoma of the external ear. Arch Otolaryngol Head Neck Surg. 1970;92(2):106–13.
13. Crozier E, Rihani J, Koral K, Cope-Yokoyama S, Rakheja D, Ulualp SO. Embryonalrhabdomyosarcoma of the auricle in a child. Pediatr Int. 2012;54(6):945–7. https://doi.org/10.1111/j.1442-200X.2012.03621.x. PubMed PMID: 23279030.
14. Raney RB, Lawrence W, Maurer HM, et al. Rhabdomyosarcoma of the ear in childhood. A report from the Intergroup Rhabdomyosarcoma Study-I. Cancer. 1983;51(12):2356–61.
15. Brady M, Spiker AM. Cancer, Merkel cell of the skin. [Updated 19 Mar 2019]. In: StatPearls [Internet]. Treasure Island, FL: StatPearls Publishing; 2019.
16. Wang TS, Byrne PJ, Jacobs LK, Taube JM. Merkel cell carcinoma: update and review. Semin Cutan Med Surg. 2011;30(1):48–56. https://doi.org/10.1016/j.sder.2011.02.001.
17. Lovin B, Gidley P. Squamous cell carcinoma of the temporal bone: a current review. Laryngoscope Investig Otolaryngol. 2019;4(2):684–92. https://doi.org/10.1002/lio2.330.
18. Breen JT, Roberts DB, Gidley PW. Basal cell carcinoma of the temporal bone and external auditory canal. Laryngoscope. 2018;128(6):1425–30. https://doi.org/10.1002/lary.26785. Epub 2017 Aug 29. PubMed PMID: 28850700.
19. Vandeweyer E, Thill MP, Deraemaecker R. Basal cell carcinoma of the external auditory canal. Acta Chir Belg. 2002;102(2):137–40. PubMed PMID: 12051089.
20. Lobo D, Llorente JL, Suárez C. Squamous cell carcinoma of the external auditory canal. Skull Base. 2008;18(3):167–72. https://doi.org/10.1055/s-2007-994290.
21. Zainuddin N, Abdullah O. Squamous cell carcinoma of the external auditory canal in a patient with non-resolving ear discharge. Malays Fam Physician. 2015;10(2):52–4. Published 2015 Aug 31.
22. Yin M, Ishikawa K, Honda K, Arakawa T, Harabuchi Y, Nagabashi T, Fukuda S, Taira A, Himi T, Nakamura N, Tanaka K, Ichinohe M, Shinkawa H, Nakada Y, Sato H, Shiga K, Kobayashi T, Watanabe T, Aoyagi M, Ogawa H, Omori K. Analysis of 95 cases of squamous cell carcinoma of the external and middle ear. Auris Nasus Larynx. 2006;33(3):251–7. Epub 2006 Jan 20. PubMed PMID: 16431060.
23. Shinomiya H, Uehara N, Teshima M, Kakigi A, Otsuki N, Nibu KI. Clinical management for T1 and T2 external auditory canal cancer. Auris Nasus Larynx. 2019;46(5):785–9. https://doi.org/10.1016/j.anl.2019.02.004. Epub 2019 Feb 21. PubMed PMID: 30799138.
24. Visnyei K, Gill R, Azizi E, Culliney B. Squamous cell carcinoma of the external auditory canal: a case report and review of the literature. Oncol Lett. 2013;5(5):1587–90. https://doi.org/10.3892/ol.2013.1241.
25. Allanson BM, Low TH, Clark JR, Gupta R. Squamous cell carcinoma of the external auditory canal and temporal bone: an update. Head Neck Pathol. 2018;12(3):407–18. https://doi.org/10.1007/s12105-018-0908-4.
26. Gowthami C, Kumar P, Ravikumar A, Joseph LD, Rajendiran S. Malignant melanoma of the external auditory canal. J Clin Diagn Res. 2014;8(8):FD04–FD6. https://doi.org/10.7860/JCDR/2014/8841.4719.
27. Ebelhar AE, West DS, Aouad RK. Ceruminous adenoid cystic carcinoma of external auditory canal. J Int Adv Otol. 2017;13(2):292–4. https://doi.org/10.5152/iao.2017.3929. PubMed PMID: 28816699.
28. Prasad V, Shenoy VS, Rao RA, Kamath PM, Shihab H. Adenoid cystic carcinoma—a rare differential diagnosis for a mass in the external auditory canal. J Clin Diagn Res. 2015;9(1):MD01–MD2. https://doi.org/10.7860/JCDR/2015/10374.5369.

Cochlear Implant and Other Implantable Hearing Devices

20

Hassanin Abdulkarim, Abdulsalam Al-Qahtani, and Ali Al-Saadi

Key Points

In this chapter, we will learn:

- What is a cochlear implant device?
- Pathophysiology and causes of sensorineural hearing loss
- Indications and cocntraindications for cochlear implant surgery
- Investigations needed for diagnosis
- Surgery of cochlear implant and its complications
- Short description about other implantable hearing devices (middle ear and bone anchored)

20.1 Introduction

- Cochlear implants are surgically implanted prosthetic devices that use electrical stimulation to the cochlear nerve to provide hearing. It collects sound through the external device microphone and then changes to electrical impulse to the internal device's electrodes (Fig. 20.1a, b).
- Simulating the physiology of the ear, the sound collected from the external device microphone is processed and changed to electrical current passing to the inner device's corresponding electrodes tonotopically.
- Cochlear implantation has become a routine procedure worldwide for the management of severe-to-profound sensorineural hearing loss. It is a phenomenal example of success that was made possible through collaboration among engineers, surgeons, scientists, and the medical community.
- As of 2012, more than 300,000 implants have been performed worldwide, and this number is in constant rise every year.
- Patient candidacy is through an evaluation of a big team made of ENT surgeons, audiologists, psychologists, speech and language therapists, and social workers.

20.2 History of the Procedure

- In 1957, Djourno and Eyries observed that activation of the auditory nerve with an electrified device gives auditory stimulation in a patient.
- 1963, Doyle and Doyle's early experiments in scala tympani implantation [1].
- In 1972, the first House/3M single-channel implant was done [2].

H. Abdulkarim · A. Al-Qahtani (✉) · A. Al-Saadi
Hamad Medical Corporation, Doha, Qatar
e-mail: habdulkarim@hamad.qa; aaa2009@qatar-med.cornell.edu; aalsaadi1@hamad.qa

A. Al-Qahtani et al. (eds.), *Textbook of Clinical Otolaryngology*,
https://doi.org/10.1007/978-3-030-54088-3_20

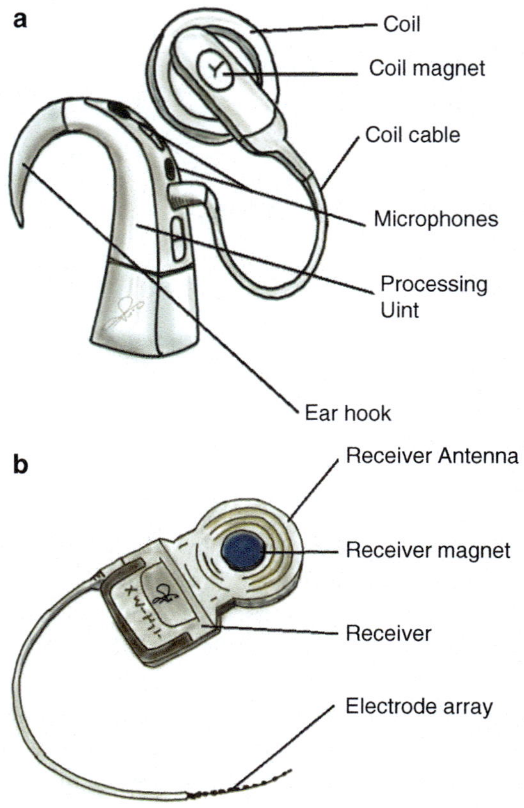

Fig. 20.1 Cochlear implant device components. (**a**) Components of external device. (**b**) Component of internal device

- In 1984, multichannel devices were introduced.
- In 2008, image-guided minimally invasive cochlear implantation was developed and is still under research.

20.3 Etiology

Common etiologies that result in congenital and delayed-onset hearing loss needing cochlear implant:

- Pediatric
  - Idiopathic
  - Genetic hearing loss (dominant or recessive)
  - Acquired usual infectious: bacterial and postviral meningitis
- Adult patients
  - Progressive hearing loss that began in childhood
  - Viral-induced sudden hearing loss
  - Ototoxicity
  - Otosclerosis (cochlear)
  - Ménière disease
  - Trauma
  - Autoimmune conditions
  - Presbycusis
  - Bacterial infections

20.4 Pathophysiology

- Severe-to-profound deafness patients had a direct or indirect injury to the organ of Corti, causing hair cell degeneration or dysfunction.
- Success of cochlear implantation depends on stimulation of surviving spiral ganglion neurons.
- The number of surviving neuron populations needed for successful implantation remains unknown till now. However, studies do report better postimplantation performance with higher residual spiral ganglion cells [3].
- Also, delayed loss of residual hearing in implantation done is connected with intracochlear fibrosis; thus, interventions aimed at reduction of cochlear trauma and inflammation, that is, perioperative steroids and hearing preservation approaches, are routinely used successfully [3].

20.5 Diagnosis and Selection

In adults, most of the patients reaching for cochlear implantation are already following with an ENT surgeon or audiologist regarding his sensorineural hearing loss with hearing aid use, so the final decision to proceed for cochlear implant is an eventual expected step of the management.

For children, most of the developed countries have a neonatal screening program right after birth to early pick deafness in neonates.

From these programs, diagnosis of SNHL (sensorineural hearing loss) is made, investigations and radiological imaging are requested, and hearing aid fitting is also done.

Failure of benefits from hearing augmentation is later on referred for cochlear implant programs.

Candidates will be further referred to psychologists and social workers to assess readiness and address expectations of the patient or the parents for the procedure.

20.6 Indications

Any patient with moderate-to-profound sensorineural hearing loss or a patient who still struggles to hear and understand despite appropriately fit hearing aids is a candidate for cochlear implant.

Although cochlear implants are mainly used for those with bilateral hearing loss, they may also be used in patients with severe unilateral sensorineural hearing loss, with or without tinnitus.

Candidates do not need to be totally deaf. Indeed, most patients have some hearing, and the sentence recognition scores can be up to 60% in best-aided conditions.

The clinical scenarios indicating cochlear implant are as follows:

- Congenital hearing loss and prelingual deafness
- Acquired hearing loss and postlingual deafness
- Severe hearing loss that can be aided and that deteriorates to profound loss in childhood, adolescence, or adulthood (perilingual) and coexists with various degrees of language development.

Generally, the candidacy for implantation is considered separately for adults and children as outlined in the 1995 National Institutes of Health (NIH) consensus statement on cochlear implantation [4, 5].

Prelingually deafened adults, although potentially suitable for cochlear implantation, must be counseled in regard to realistic expectations, as language and open-set speech discrimination outcomes are less predictable.

Children are considered suitable for cochlear implantation at age of 1 year, and because of meningitis-related deafness with progressive cochlear ossification, occasional earlier implantation is necessary [6].

Differences between cochlear implants in children and adults include:

- The best candidates for cochlear implants are postlingual (had speech and language skills before losing their hearing), and most adult candidates for a cochlear implant fall into this category.
- Adults typically perceive more of a mechanical sound after implantation; the sound typically becomes more natural after 4–8 weeks.
- Adults with bilateral hearing loss benefit from bilateral implants, which improve speech perception, allow better hearing in conditions with significant background noise, enhance sound localization, and allow the patient to hear sound coming from either side without having to turn one's head [7–10].

20.7 Contraindication

- Contraindications to cochlear implantation may include deafness due to lesions of the eighth cranial nerve or brain stem (those patients may benefit from brain stem implant although controversial).
- In addition, chronic infections of the middle ear and mastoid cavity or tympanic membrane perforation can be contraindications (relative).
- Cochlear aplasia as demonstrated on CT scans remains an absolute contraindication.
- Certain medical conditions such as specific hematologic, pulmonary, and cardiac conditions also may be contraindications.
- The lack of realistic expectations regarding the benefits of cochlear implantation and/or a lack of strong desire to develop enhanced oral communication skills poses a strong contraindication for implant surgery.

20.8 Evaluation

20.8.1 History

Obtain a detailed otological history including family history of hearing loss, patient's developmental history, and immunizations.

20.8.2 Physical Examination

Conduct a comprehensive physical including general ENT with focus on otologic exam. Pay specific attention for any infectious, chronic ear component that will influence the decision and sequences of procedures to make the ear safe before implantation.

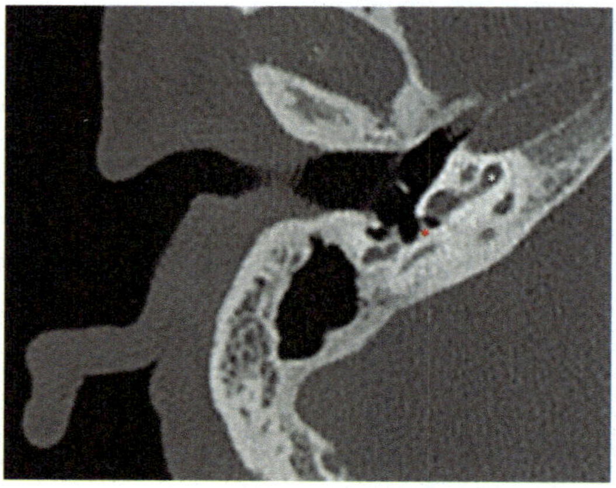

Fig. 20.2 Axial cut of temporal bone CT scan showing basal turn of the cochlea (white asterisk) and a bony ridge obscuring the round window niche (red asterisk)

20.9 Investigations

20.9.1 Laboratory Studies

1. CBC (complete blood count) count
2. Electrolytes
3. Clotting time studies
4. Immunologic workup for patient has rapidly progressive hearing loss or other signs or symptoms of autoimmune hearing loss like a Western blot analysis for antibodies to the heat shock protein. Thyroid and renal function for Pendred and Alport syndrome
5. Genetic testing such as the test for connexin 26 mutations

20.10 Imaging Studies

1. High-resolution CT scanning of the temporal (imaging of choice)

   This study helps determine the absence of malformations that contraindicate implantation (e.g., cochlear aplasia, absence of the auditory nerve). Additional relative contraindications, such as chronic otitis media, are revealed with high-resolution CT (Figs. 20.2, 20.3, 20.4, and 20.5).

   CT scanning also reveals abnormalities that alter the standard insertion procedure of the electrode array. These abnormalities include Mondini dysplasia, common cavity, and cochlear ossification. Suspect cochlear ossification in patients with a history of meningitis (Figs. 20.2, 20.3, 20.4, and 20.5).
2. High-resolution T2-weighted fast spin echo MRI is complementing and even replacing CT scanning because of its increased ability to reveal cochlear ossification with identification of nerves inside internal auditory canal (Fig. 20.6a, b).
3. Plain film radiography of the cochlea in the anteroposterior plane (transorbital) is useful to confirm correct placement of the electrode array is used to provide evidence and confirmation of correct initial placement in the event that delayed implant malfunction arises and electrode migration is suspected (Fig. 20.7).
4. Intraoperative fluoroscopy to confirm electrode placement and also guides the right trajectory of placement in cases of malformed cochlear anatomy.

20.11 Treatment

20.11.1 Medical Therapy

Steroid therapy preoperatively and can be extended till activation of the implant postoperatively for prevention of delayed loss of residual hearing and intracochlear fibrosis postop.

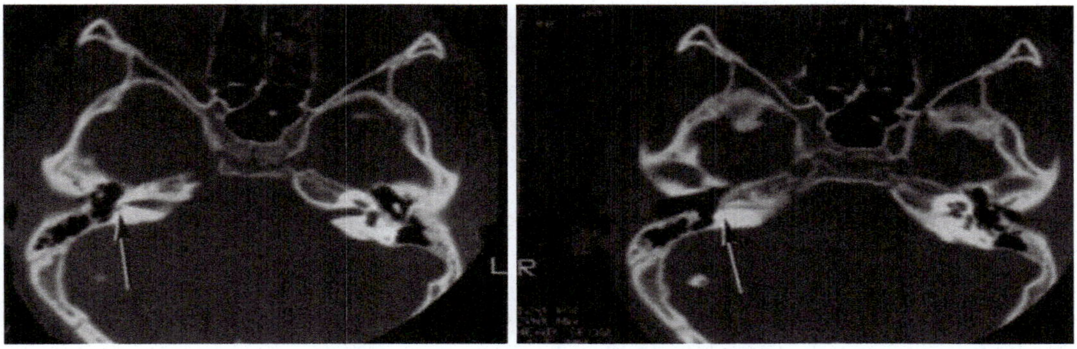

Fig. 20.3 Total absence of the right inner ear structures is noted with a flattening of the medial wall of the right inner cavity in a patient with Michel anomaly

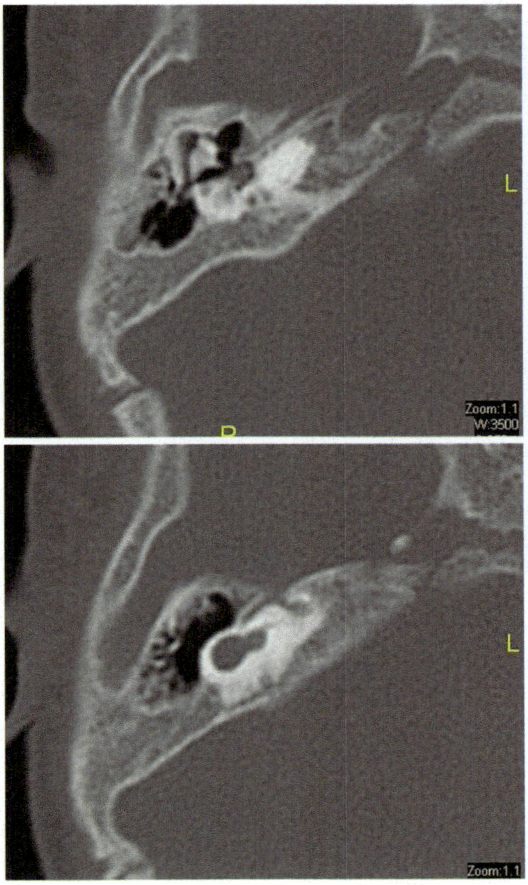

Fig. 20.4 Axial HRCT of the right temporal bone showing marked hypoplasia of the right cochlea associated with small malformed vestibule and semicircular canals

Prophylactic antibiotics intra- and postoperative.

Immunization against *Streptococcus pneumoniae* and *Haemophilus influenzae* if not taken in the immunization schedule.

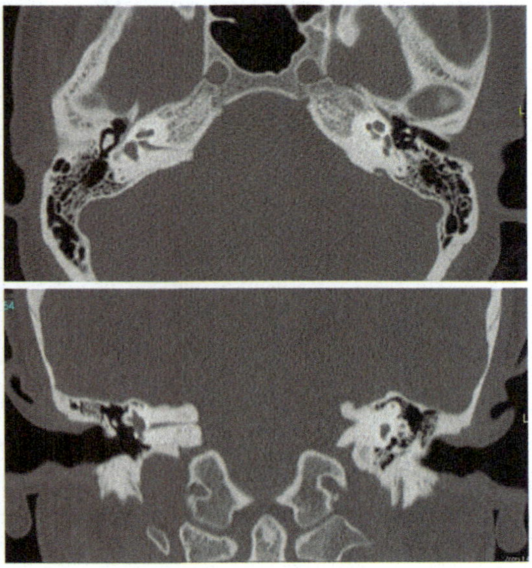

Fig. 20.5 Axial and coronal HRCT of the temporal bones showing tight stenosis of the right internal auditory canal with normal appearing osseous labyrinth

20.11.2 Surgical Therapy

Cochlear implant surgery is the treatment of choice for patient with moderate-to-profound sensorineural hearing loss without benefit from hearing aids.

Unilateral versus bilateral implant has always been a debate regarding the benefits versus cost.

Bilateral implants showed benefits in the aspects of improved speech perception, allowed better hearing in conditions with significant background noise, and enhanced sound localization [11, 12].

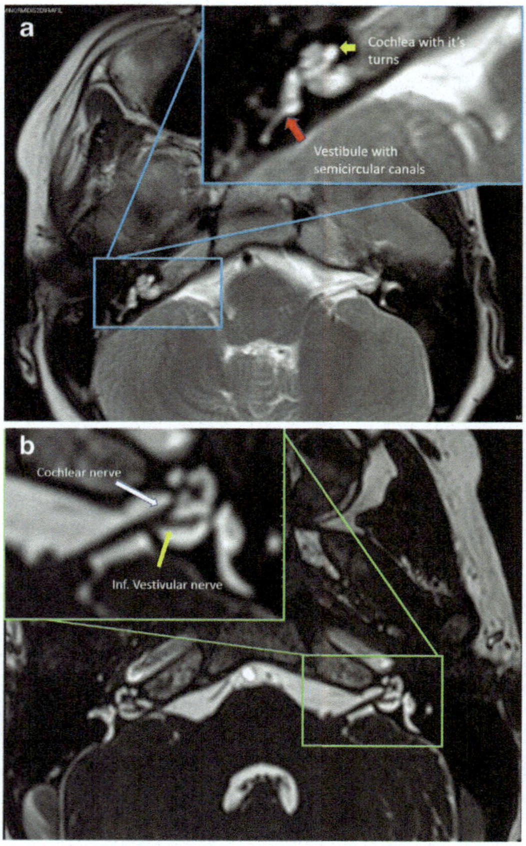

Fig. 20.6 T2 axial cut of temporal bone MRI showing internal auditory canal and inner ear structures

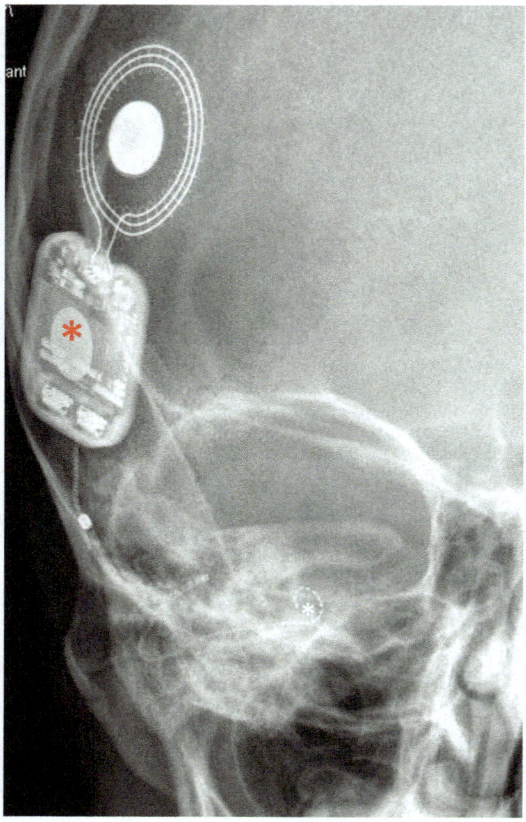

Fig. 20.7 Transorbital x-ray postoperatively showing inner device (red asterisk) and the electrodes array turn inside the cochlea (white asterisk)

20.12 Procedure

20.12.1 Step 1: Flap Marking and Incision Design

Facial nerve monitoring is recommended.

Hair shaving is optional according to the surgeon's preference.

Using the dummies (or mock ups) and specific implant templates, marking of the location of the external and internal devices is made.

Incision is in or at a parallel line to the postauricular crease according to the surgeon preference up to 2 cm posterior to the crease.

Elevation of anterior and posterior flaps.

Periosteum elevation anteriorly and posteriorly.

20.12.2 Step 2: Mastoidectomy and Posterior Tympanotomy

A cortical mastoidectomy is done till reaching the mastoid antrum by identifying the short process of incus and lateral semicircular canal.

Thinning of posterior canal wall is done.

Thinning of facial nerve surrounding bone is done with generous irrigation till hue of the facial nerve is seen.

Posterior tympanotomy is done to enter the facial recess enough to visualize the round window (Fig. 20.8a).

20.12.3 Step 3: Cochlear Implant Receiver Well Drill Out with Tie-Down Holes

Using internal device's templates, the receiver well is drilled usually superior and posterior to the mastoidectomy area.

Holes are drilled around the well to be used for fixation after device placement.

20.12.4 Step 4: Cochleostomy

Size of cochleostomy is variable according to cochlear implant manufacturer recommendations.

Location is over the basilar turn of the cochlea anteroinferior to the round window.

Some surgeons including author prefer to do cochleostomy through round window (Fig. 20.8b).

20.12.5 Step 5: Implant Tie Down and Electrode Insertion

The electrode is inserted through the cochleostomy to the maximum length possible.

Once inserted, the device is fixed to the well by sutures or tie.

Cochleostomy is sealed by subcutaneous tissue (Fig. 20.8c).

20.12.6 Step 6: Telemetry, Closure, and Radiograph

Telemetry, impedance, and NRT (neural response telemetry) testing are done.

Closure of the layers and wound is done.

Mastoid pressure bandage is applied for 24–72 h.

20.12.7 Postoperative Details

Observe for nystagmus and facial weakness.

Radiological testing as preferred (Fig. 20.7).

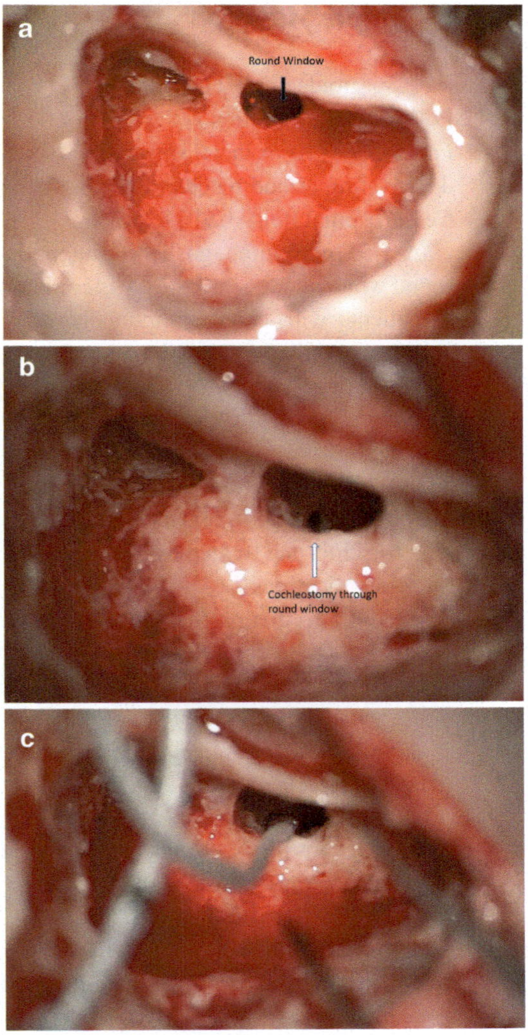

Fig. 20.8 Surgical steps of cochlear implant surgery. (**a**) Cortical mastoidectomy and posterior tympanotomy. Showing the short process of incus (white asterisk) and chorda tympani (red asterisk) and the shadow of round window niche (black arrow). (**b**) Cochleostomy made through the round window (white arrow). (**c**) Insertion of electrodes array through the cochleostomy

20.12.8 Follow-Up

Visit within 5–7 days to check for hematoma and wound, to be repeated at the 2 weeks postoperative.

Arrange a visit within 3–5 weeks postoperatively with the audiologist for device stimulation.

20.13 Complications

- Same as mastoidectomy [13, 14]
  1. Postoperative infection
  2. Facial paralysis or facial spasm (treated by deactivating offending electrode)
  3. Cerebrospinal fluid (CSF) leakage

     A CSF/perilymph gusher through the round window or cochleostomy is common in patients with cochlear anomalies (like enlarged vestibular aqueduct syndrome, common cavity, and wide internal auditory canal syndrome). Leak is best managed by packing the round window with fascia or muscle after implant insertion.
  4. Meningitis. Usually prevented by preoperative vaccine, and treated by antibiotics.
  5. Flap complications
     (a) Seroma formation best avoided by use of a mastoid compressive dressing for at least 2 days. If developed, it can be evacuated using large bore needle aspiration with mastoid pressure dressing applied for another 2–3 days.
     (b) Implant migration: good fixation of the device to the well and sealing the cochleostomy area with tissue or muscle.
     (c) Necrosis of the flap: sometimes closure under tension will affect the blood supply of the skin and subcutaneous tissue causing necrosis.

         Can be prevented by good supra- and subperiosteal flaps and closed in different directions.
  6. Device failure: perform telemetry and consider communication with the implant manufacturer before explanation and reimplantation.

20.14 Outcome and Prognosis

- The overall prognosis for hearing improvement and improved quality of life in the properly selected patient is excellent.

20.15 Future and Controversies

- The future of cochlear implantation is exciting and is now upon us.
- Bilateral cochlear implantation has demonstrated significant benefits for patients in a number of areas, which include hearing in noise, speech perception outcomes, and sound directionality.
- In the future, patients can expect faster and better coding strategies, which result in better speech perception.
- Improvement in chip design and battery design will likely pave the way for totally implantable cochlear implants as microphones become integrated to middle- or external-ear structures.
- Nanotechnology is rapidly providing hope for smaller, more robust, electrode array designs with a virtually endless number of electrode contact sites.
- Image-guided minimally invasive cochlear implantation

20.16 Conclusion

- Team-based approach for selection of cochlear implant candidates.
- Cochlear implants are surgically implanted devices to convert sound to electrical impulse through the cochlear nerve.
- Thorough evaluation makes better hearing results.
- Bilateral cochlear implantation showed better hearing results and sound localization.

20.17 Implantable Hearing Aids

The majority of cases of SNHL require only acoustic amplification to address communication skills. This is generally accomplished with conventional air conduction hearing aids. Despite improvements in conventional hearing aid technology, only 15% of the 20 million hearing-impaired people in the United States who could benefit from amplification utilize these devices [15].

The development of semi-implantable and totally implantable hearing aids has in part been an attempt to compensate for limitations of conventional hearing aids.

Implantable hearing aids comprise two types: middle ear aids and bone-anchored devices.

20.17.1 Middle Ear Implantable Hearing Aids

Given the costs and risks of surgical placement, an implantable hearing aid (IHA) should ideally provide significant benefits over conventional hearing aids, including

1. Better appearance
2. Improved fidelity
3. Broader frequency response
4. Less distortion
5. Reduction or elimination of feedback
6. Better speech understanding

The devices should not

1. Interfere with residual hearing
2. Limit patient activities
3. Predispose patients to infection

Several IHA designs are currently under investigation and development, with at least few already receiving approval by the FDA for clinical use.

However, despite many potential advantages over conventional aids, IHAs have met with limited success to date.

Conventional hearing aids work by amplifying airborne sound prior to its reaching the middle ear. Microphone converts an incoming acoustic signal into an electrical signal that is amplified, filtered, processed to adjust dynamic range, and then transduced by a speaker back into airborne sound waves that then drive the middle ear and inner ear in the normal physiologic manner. Though usually adequate, this approach has many limitations.

First, nonlinearities in the transduction process cause distortion and limit the useful dynamic range of the aid.

Second, because the impedance mismatch between the air-filled external auditory canal and fluid-filled cochlea is only partly compensated by the middle ear mechanism, much of the amplified airborne sound is reflected back from the tympanic membrane. This limits the acoustic power and perceptual loudness a hearing aid can generate, and increases problems with hearing aid “squeal” due to feedback of sounds reaching the hearing aid’s microphone.

The potential for feedback limits the useful amplification of a conventional hearing aid and mandates a tight hearing aid mold fit in the ear canal or placement of the microphone outside the canal, resulting in discomfort, otitis externa, autophony, ear fullness (the occlusion effect), and visibility of the hearing aid. All of these factors conspire to reduce patient acceptance of conventional aids.

In contrast to conventional air-conducting hearing aids, middle ear IHAs are designed to directly drive the ossicular chain, reducing impedance mismatch, feedback, autophony, and distortion of the amplified signal while offering increased functional gain. Some IHA designs require no ear canal components, averting the risk of otitis externa and reducing autophony and ear fullness.

There is also a cosmetic advantage to not having a visible apparatus within the ear, though most IHAs do require an external processor that is visible behind the ear.

Middle ear IHAs may be completely or partially implantable.

Partially implantable devices consist of an external microphone and speech processor, which is connected to an inductive transmitter with an external coil that transmits electrical energy transcutaneously to the internal device. Batteries to power the system are contained within the external device.

The internal device consists of a receiving coil, processing electronics, and mechanical driver (Fig. 20.9).

A fully implantable system houses all of these components within the implanted portion of the device and is periodically recharged via a transcutaneous inductive link (Fig. 20.10).

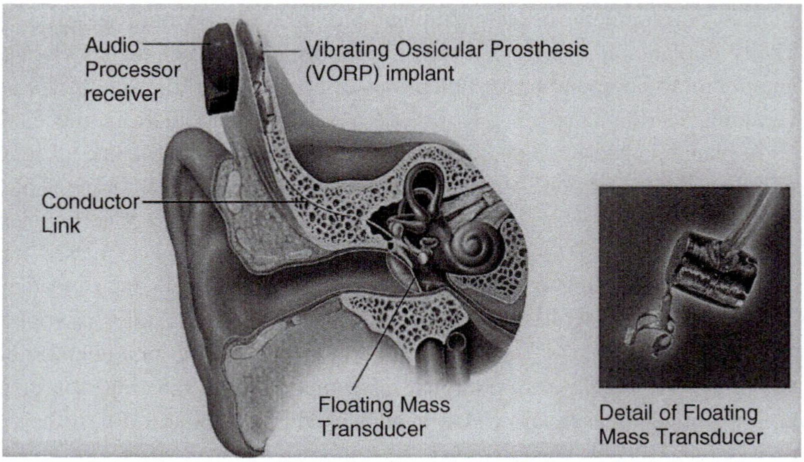

Fig. 20.9 Partially implantable IHA components (Vibrant Med-El (formerly Vibrant Soundbridge))

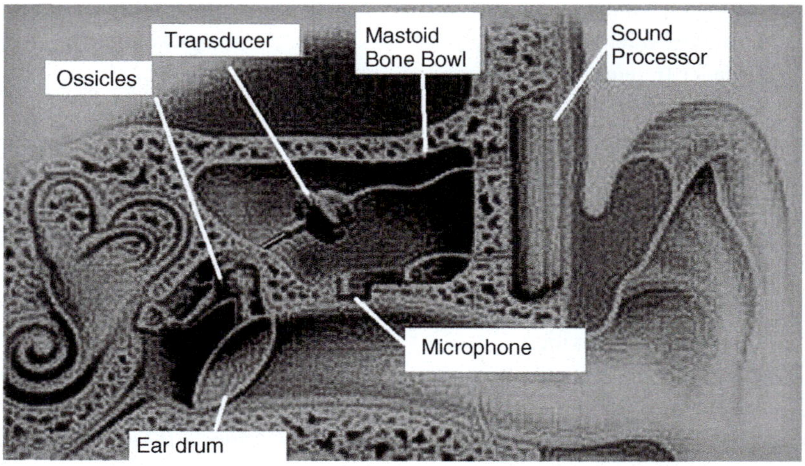

Fig. 20.10 Fully implantable IHA components (the Totally Implantable Communication Assistance aid, or TICA®)

Most IHAs employ either piezoelectric or electromagnetic actuators for converting electrical signals to mechanical movement of the ossicular chain.

20.17.2 Bone-Anchored Hearing Devices

Conductive and mixed hearing losses are highly prevalent disorders that often may be addressed with standard tympanoplasty and/or ossiculoplasty techniques or rehabilitated with traditional hearing aids.

However, there remains a large subset of these patients who are unsuitable surgical candidates for correction of their deficit or who are unable to tolerate a traditional hearing aid.

This group includes patients with

1. Chronically draining ears.
2. Discomfort from the sound levels required from a traditional hearing aid.
3. Patients unable to tolerate a hearing aid because of a large mastoid bowl or meatoplasty following chronic ear surgery.
4. Patients with otosclerosis, tympanosclerosis, or canal atresia and who have a contraindication to surgical repair may defy traditional approaches.
5. Patients who have undergone external auditory canal closure following extensive skull

base surgery also are not amenable to traditional hearing aids.
6. Single-sided deafness also are candidates.

Application of osteointegration technology to bone-anchored hearing aids represents a refinement of conventional bone-conducting hearing aids.

The utility of conventional bone-conducting devices is now considered limited.

The bone conductor must be applied with steady pressure to the mastoid cortex (usually via a headband or eyeglasses). Patients often experience pain, headache, and skin irritation at the contact site. Furrowing of the skull due to pressure is not unusual in children who use bone conductors. Further, sound fidelity is limited by soft tissue attenuation, variable placement of the vibrator, and flaccidity of the securing device (e.g., eyeglass frames).

The success of this technology relies on two basic principles: the creation of a permanent percutaneous connection and the placement of an osseointegrated titanium abutment upon which a transducer is coupled.

Titanium is the most notable among several materials that have found clinical application in anchoring dental prostheses. This is because of its ability to create a corrosion-resistant oxide layer on the surface of the implant that confers osseointegration potential. Because the implant may be worn for several decades or longer, the toxicity and carcinogenicity of the oxide coating take on particular importance.

To date, pure titanium appears free of the adverse sequelae seen with other metals and thus continues to represent an ideal implant material [16–18].

Currently, the only commercially available osseointegrated hearing aid is the Bone-Anchored Hearing Aid (the BAHA™, manufactured by Cochlear Corporation, formerly by Entific and Nobel Biocare).

The BAHA™ consists of a pure titanium implant and a sound processor. The processor couples directly to the titanium implant via a skin penetrating abutment, utilizing a force-fit, plastic coupling) (Fig. 20.11).

In addition to implantation for purely conductive or mixed hearing losses, emerging data indicate the value of BAHA amplification for patients

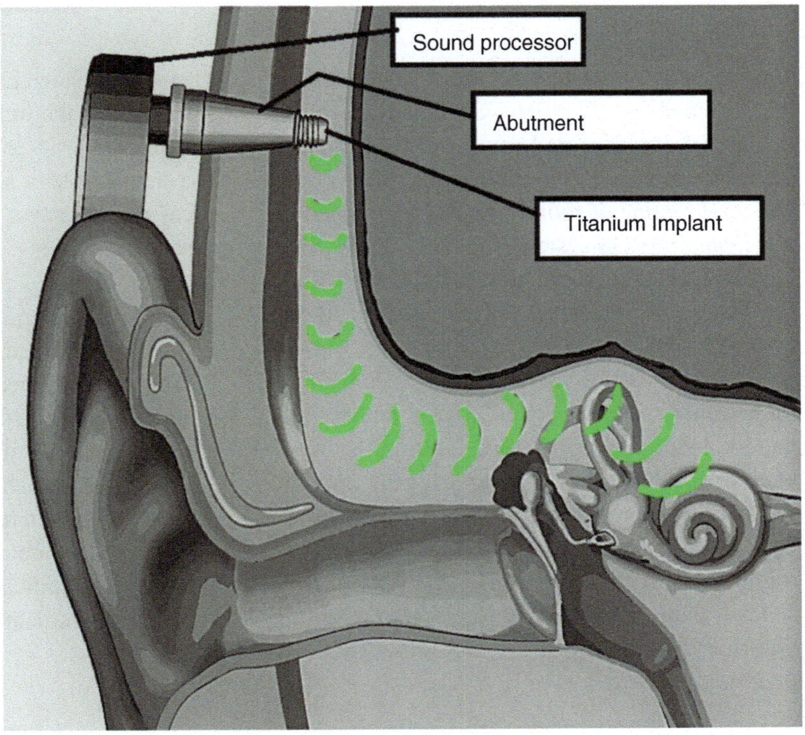

Fig. 20.11 BAHA components

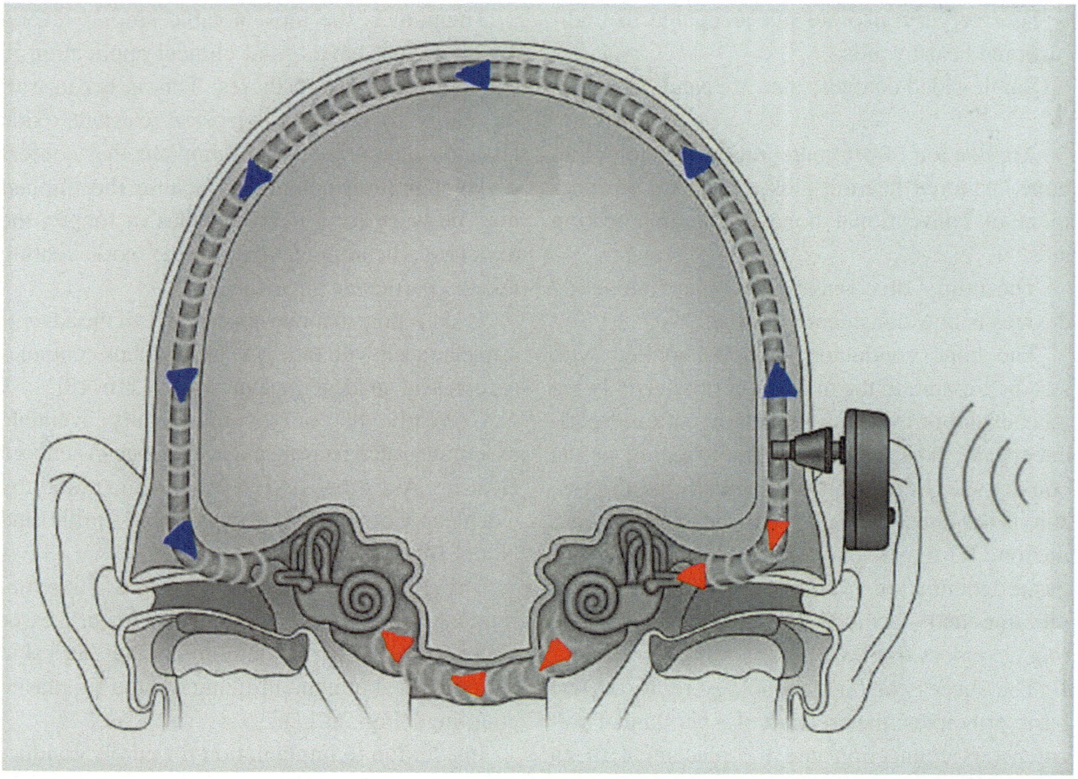

Fig. 20.12 BAHA sound waves pathways to both ipsilateral and contralateral ears

with unilateral profound SNHL. The BAHA on the deafened ear effectively expanded the sound field for the patient and improved the patient's speech understanding in noise, much like a contralateral routing of sound (CROS) hearing aid or transcranial CROS system (Fig. 20.12) [19, 20].

However, in contrast to CROS, BAHA does not require the placement of an earmold in the better hearing ear.

BAHA hearing results show subjective improvement in both sound quality and speech understanding in noise [21]. The main drawback of BAHA is the possibility for the implant to dislodge from the skull after apparent successful, complete osseointegration, unrelated to trauma or other obvious cause. Tjellstrom (personal communication, September 2005) reported the rate was 6.0% in adults and 5.7% in children.

He recommended placing a new implant 7 mm above or below the first site as a short outpatient procedure under a local anesthesia, removing only a small circle of skin and leaving the former surgical site otherwise intact.

Take Home Messages

- Cochlear implant surgery is the main surgical treatment for severe SNHL after the failure of hearing aid.
- Surgery itself is the main step of the treatment, but results depend mainly on the postoperative rehabilitation program.
- Future technological advances will make a significant development in the cochlear implant's devices, surgery, and results.

Question
Which is the absolute contraindication for cochlear implant surgery?
(a) Mondini displasia
(b) Cochlear ossification
(c) Cochlear aplasia
(d) Otosclerosis

Answer
(c)

References

1. Doyle J, Doyle D. Electrical stimulation of the nerve deafness. Bull Los Angel Neurol Soc. 1963;28:148–50.
2. House WF, Urban J. Long term results of electrode implantation and electronic stimulation of the cochlea in man. Ann Otol Rhinol Laryngol. 1973;82(4):504–17. [Medline].
3. Quesnel AM, Nakajima HH, Rosowski JJ, Hansen MR, Gantz BJ, Nadol JB Jr. Delayed loss of hearing after hearing preservation cochlear implantation: human temporal bone pathology and implications for etiology. Hear Res. 2016;333:225–34. [Medline].
4. National Institutes of Health. NIH consensus statement. Cochlear Implants Adults Child. 1995;13(2):1–30.
5. Evaluation of Revised Indications (ERID) for cochlear implant candidacy for the adult CMS population. ClinicalTrials.gov. https://clinicaltrials.gov/ct2/show/NCT02075229. Accessed 13 Oct 2017.
6. Gantz BJ, McCabe BF, Tyler RS. Use of multichannel cochlear implants in obstructed and obliterated cochleas. Otolaryngol Head Neck Surg. 1988;98(1):72–81. [Medline].
7. Green JD Jr, Marion MS, Hinojosa R. Labyrinthitis ossificans: histopathologic consideration for cochlear implantation. Otolaryngol Head Neck Surg. 1991;104(3):320–6. [Medline].
8. Seyyedi M, Viana LM, Nadol JB Jr. Within-subject comparison of word recognition and spiral ganglion cell count in bilateral cochlear implant recipients. Otol Neurotol. 2014;35(8):1446–50. [Medline].
9. Basura GJ, Eapen R, Buchman CA. Bilateral cochlear implantation: current concepts, indications, and results. Laryngoscope. 2009;119:2395.
10. Bichey BG, Miyamoto RT. Outcomes in bilateral cochlear implantation. Otolaryngol Head Neck Surg. 2008;138:655.
11. Smulders YE, van Zon A, Stegeman I, et al. Comparison of bilateral and unilateral cochlear implantation in adults: a randomized clinical trial. JAMA Otolaryngol Head Neck Surg. 2016; 142:249.
12. National Institute on Deafness and Other Communication Disorders. National Institute of Health. National strategic research plan, vol. 5. US Department of Health and Human Services; 1996.
13. Tambyraja RR, Gutman MA, Megerian CA. Cochlear implant complications: utility of federal database in systematic analysis. Arch Otolaryngol Head Neck Surg. 2005;131(3):245–50. [Medline].
14. Rubinstein JT, Gantz BJ, Parkinson WS. Management of cochlear implant infections. Am J Otol. 1999;20(1):46–9. [Medline].
15. Esselman GH, Coticchia JM, Wippold FJ 2nd, Fredrickson JM, Vannier MW, Neely JG. Computer-stimulated test fitting of an implantable hearing aid using three-dimensional CT scans of the temporal bone: preliminary study. Am J Otol. 1994;15:702–9.
16. Johansson CB. On tissue reactions to metal implants. Ph.D. Thesis, Biomaterials/Handicap Research. Goteborg: University of Goteborg; 1991.
17. Eriksson E, Branemark P. Osseointegration from the perspective of the plastic surgeon. Plast Reconstr Surg. 1994;93:626–37.
18. von Ludinghausen M, Meister P, Probst J. Metallosis after osteosynthesis. Pathol Eur. 1970;5:307–14.
19. Vaneecloo FM, Ruzza I, Hanson JN, et al. The monaural pseudo-stereophonic hearing aid (BAHA) in unilateral total deafness: a study of 29 patients. Rev Laryngol Otol Rhinol (Bord). 2001;122:343–50.
20. Niparko JK, Cox KM, Lustig LR. Comparison of the bone anchored hearing aid implantable hearing device with contralateral routing of offside signal amplification in the rehabilitation of unilateral deafness. Otol Neurotol. 2003;24:73–8.
21. Wazen JJ, Spitzer JB, Ghossaini SN, et al. Transcranial contralateral cochlear stimulation in unilateral deafness. Otolaryngol Head Neck Surg. 2003;129: 248–54.

Part III

Rhinology/Allergy

21 Radiology of Paranasal Sinuses

Umais Momin, Ahmed Shaikh, Mashael Alhail,
Hamad Al Saey, Sara Ashkanani,
and Shanmugam Ganesan

21.1 Introduction

Imaging of paranasal sinuses forms an important component of examination and preoperative planning for any surgical intervention. Evaluation of the paranasal sinuses involves assessment of two components: the sinus contents, including the mucosa, and the bony walls including vessels. Normal sinus mucosa is very thin and is not seen on CT or MRI, and CT or MRI readily reveals the presence of a normally aerated sinus, mucosal thickening (chronic sinusitis, retention cysts, or polyps), or an air-fluid level.

CT scan is the modality of choice for assessment of normal anatomy and pathology of sinuses and is routinely performed prior to any sinus surgeries. With the advent of multidetector computed tomography (MDCT), imaging of paranasal sinuses prior to functional endoscopic sinus surgery (FESS) has become mandatory. Multiplanar imaging, particularly coronal reformations, offers precise information regarding the anatomy of the sinuses and its variations, which is an essential requisite before surgery.

The success of functional endoscopic surgery depends on adequate knowledge of the complicated anatomy of the paranasal sinuses. Certain anatomic variations are thought to be predisposing factors for the development of sinus diseases, and thus, it becomes necessary for the surgeon to be aware of these variations, especially if the patient is a candidate for functional endoscopic sinus surgery (FESS).

U. Momin
Department of Clinical Imaging, Hamad Medical Corporation, Doha, Qatar
e-mail: Umomin@hamad.qa

A. Shaikh (✉) · M. Alhail · H. Al Saey · S. Ashkanani
Otolaryngology-Head and Neck Surgery Division, Department of Surgery, Hamad Medical Corporation, Doha, Qatar

Department of Otolaryngology-Head and Neck Surgery Division, Weill Cornell Medicine-Qatar, Doha, Qatar
e-mail: malhail@hamad.qa; Halsaey@hamad.qa; sashkanani@hamad.qa

S. Ganesan
Otolaryngology-Head and Neck Surgery Division, Department of Surgery, Hamad Medical Corporation, Doha, Qatar
e-mail: sganesan@hamad.qa

21.2 Technique of CT Scan for FESS

At our institution, we performed the scan with multidetector computed tomography (MDCT) with the patient in supine position with 1 mm thick overlapping axial slices.

Axial images of the sinuses are acquired with 0.5 mm collimation, and from this raw data, sagittal and coronal reformations are obtained using both soft tissue and bone window algorithms.

A. Al-Qahtani et al. (eds.), *Textbook of Clinical Otolaryngology*,
https://doi.org/10.1007/978-3-030-54088-3_21

21.2.1 Anatomy and Its Variation

The lateral nasal wall contains three bulbous projections, namely the superior, middle, and inferior turbinates (conchae), which divide the nasal cavity into superior, middle, and inferior meatuses.

The superior meatus drains the posterior ethmoid air cells.

The middle meatus drains the frontal sinus via the nasofrontal recess, the maxillary sinus via the maxillary ostium (Hiatus semilunaris), and the anterior ethmoid air cells via the ethmoid cell ostia.

The nasolacrimal duct drains into the inferior meatus.

Sphenoethmoidal recess is a small area above superior concha and receives the opening of sphenoid air sinus.

CT scan is the gold-standard investigation in all sinus diseases [1, 2].

21.3 Ostiomeatal Unit

The osteomeatal unit (OMU) (Fig. 21.1) includes the

1. Maxillary sinus ostium
2. Ethmoid infundibulum
3. Anterior ethmoid air cells, and
4. Frontal recess

The UP prevents the direct contact of the inspired air with the maxillary sinus, acting like a shield, and plays a role in mucociliary activity. The UP is a thin, semi-circular bony process of variable length and covered with the mucosa.

21.3.1 Ethmoidal Cells [3–5]

Ethmoidal cells according to pneumatization are classified as

1. Agger nasi
2. Onodi cells
3. Hilar cells
4. Bulla ethmoidalis

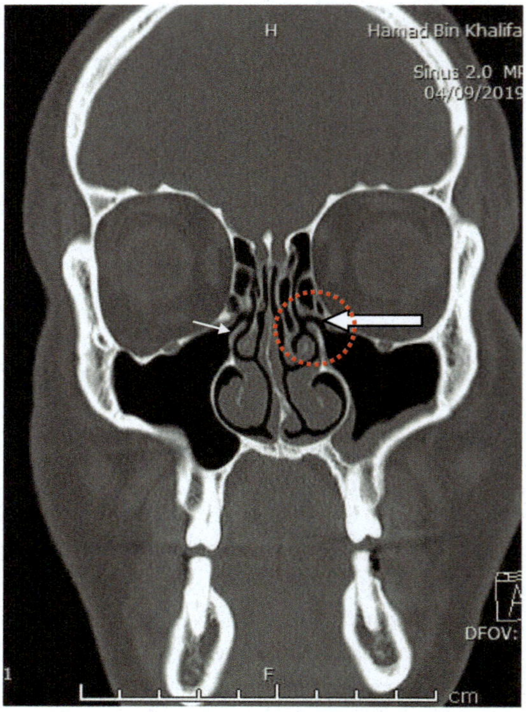

Fig. 21.1 Uncinate Process, UP (arrow), Maxillary infundibulum (block arrow), and OMU (dotted circle)

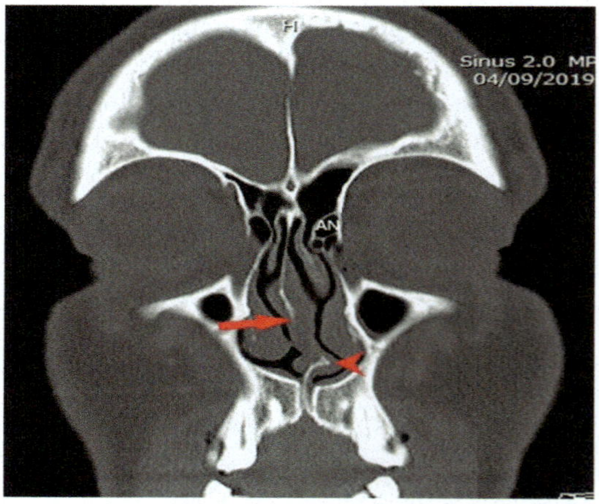

Fig. 21.2 AN (agger nasi) cell, deviated nasal septum (red arrow), and septal spur (red arrow head)

21.3.2 Agger Nasi Cells Fig. 21.2

This cell is present in nearly all patients and is an ethmoturbinal remnant. It is the most anterior ethmoidal air cell and extends anteriorly into the lacrimal bone [6, 7]. A good view of frontal recess [8, 9] is obtained when the agger nasi cells are opened. Thus, its size may directly influence the patency of the frontal recess and the anterior middle meatus. It forms the anterior and inferior wall of the frontal recess, and the surgical access to recess is via the agger nasi.

21.3.3 Onodi Cells Fig. 21.3

These are posterior ethmoidal cells extending into the sphenoid bone, either adjacent to or impinging upon the optic nerve [10]. When these Onodi cells abut or surround the optic nerve, the nerve is at risk when surgical excision of these cells is performed. It is also a potential cause of incomplete sphenoidectomy.

21.3.4 Haller Cells Fig. 21.4

These are also called infraorbital ethmoid cells and are pneumatized ethmoid air cells. These cells contribute to the narrowing of the infundibulum and may compromise the ostium of the maxillary sinus, thus contributing to recurrent maxillary sinusitis [11–13].

These cells may contribute to narrowing of the infundibulum (Fig. 21.5).

Ethmoid bulla (Fig. 21.6) is the largest anterior ethmoid air cells.

It is the roof of the hiatus semilunaris and posterior ethmoid infundibulum.

The relationship of ethmoid bulla with lamina papyracea in lateral, and the relationship of frontal cranial fossa in superior with base should be clarified in preoperative CT.

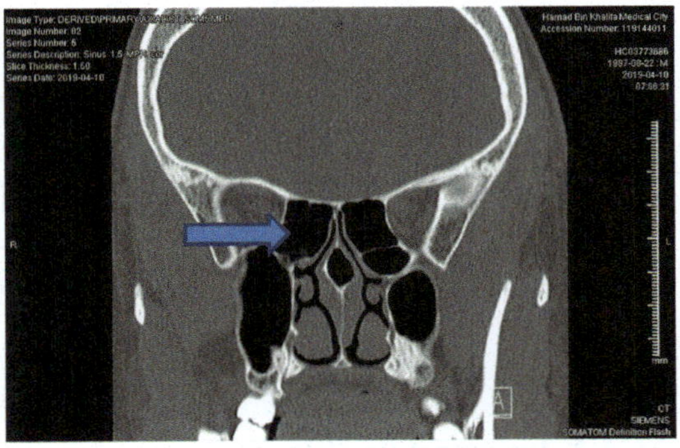

Fig. 21.3 Onodi cell (blue arrow)

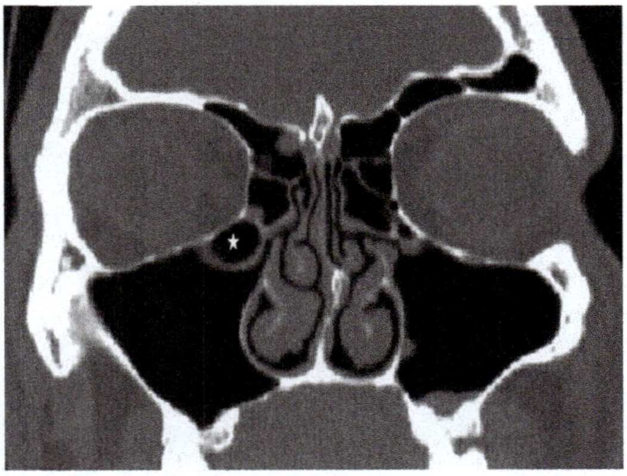

Fig. 21.4 CT shows right Haller cell (star)

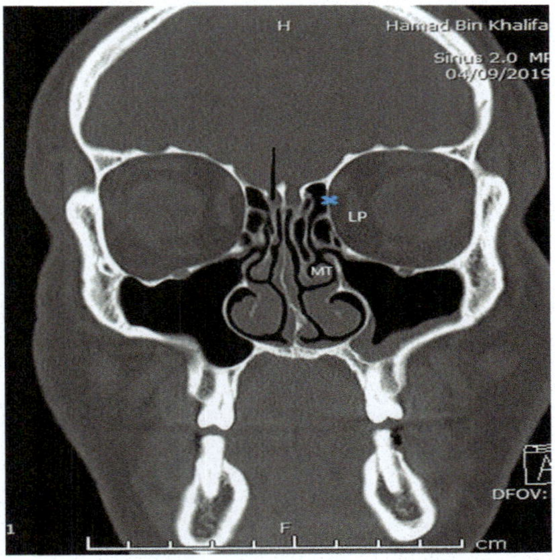

Fig. 21.5 MT (Middle turbinate), LP (lamina papyracea), olfactory cleft (black arrow), and Concha Bullosa (white arrow)

The sphenoethmoidal recess, also called the posterior ostiomeatal unit, drains the posterior sinuses (posterior ethmoidal and sphenoid) (Fig. 21.7).

Concha Bullosa [14] (Fig. 21.5): Pneumatization of middle turbinate by the extension of ethmoid sinus cell.

Paradoxical turbinates (Fig. 21.8) occur as the convexity of the middle turbinate is directed toward the medial wall of the maxillary sinus.

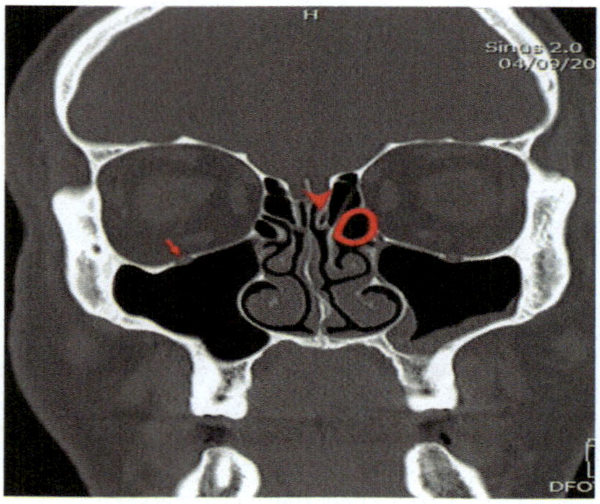

Fig. 21.6 Ethmoid bulla, EB (red circle), superior turbinate (arrow head), and inferior orbital nerve (red arrow)

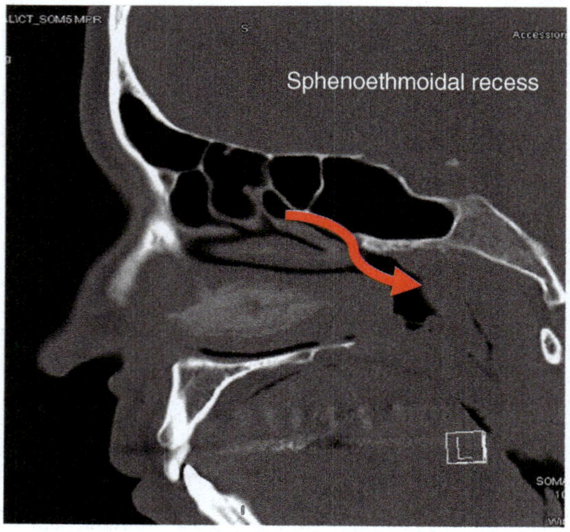

Fig. 21.7 Red arrow sphenoethmoidal recess

21.4 The Frontalethmoidal (Kuhn) Cells [15]

There are various accessory air cells in the frontoethmoidal region that may or may not be present. It is important to work out the drainage pathway of the frontal sinus around these cells.

Frontalethmoidal air cells, also known as Kuhn air cells, are categorized into four types depending on their number and degree of extension into the frontal sinus.

Type 1 (most common): Single cell superior to the ANC that does not extend into the frontal sinus (i.e., remains below the "beak").

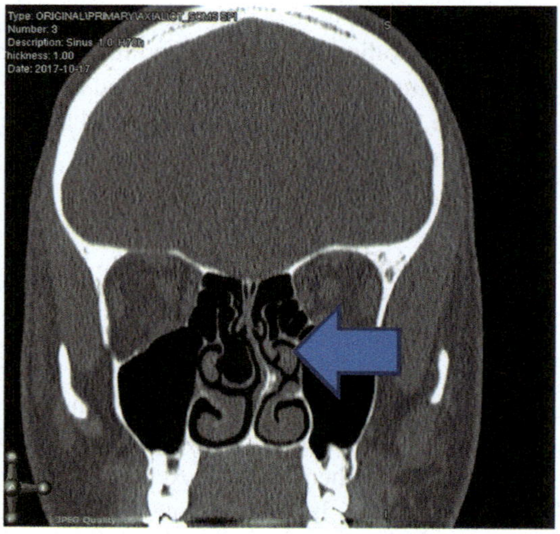

Fig. 21.8 Paradoxical middle turbinate (arrow)

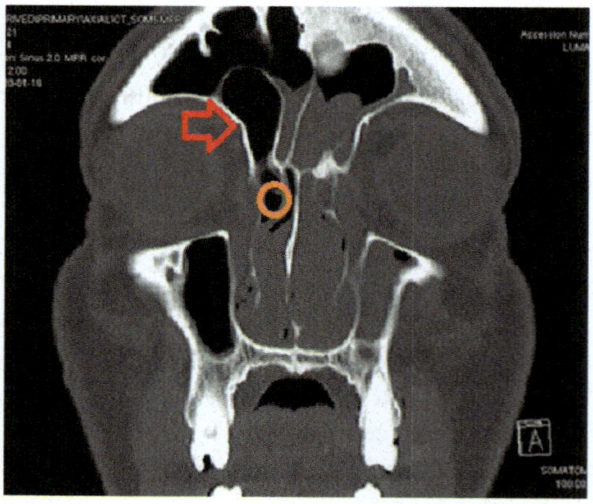

Fig. 21.9 Type 3 frontal cell (red arrow) and Agger nasi (yellow)

Type 2: Two or more cells superior to the ANC that may or may not extend into the frontal sinus.

Type 3: Single frontal cell superior to the ANC that extends into the frontal sinus (Fig. 21.9).

Type 4: Completely contained in the frontal sinus.

Radiological characteristics of some diseases are as follows.

21.4.1 Inverted Papilloma

- Inverted papilloma are benign tumors of unknown etiology characterized by strong potential for local destruction, high rate of recurrence, and malignant potential.

- They display characteristic radiological findings [16].

CT characteristics include (Fig. 21.10)

- Heterogeneous enhancement
- Sclerosis and erosion of the bones

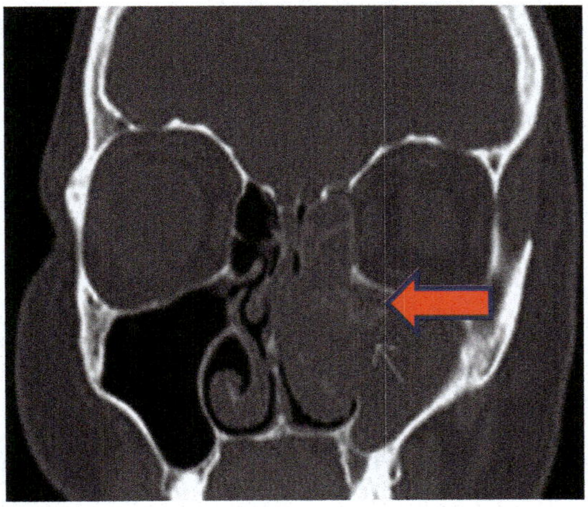

Fig. 21.10 Osteogenesis marked with arrow

- Periosteal thickening
- Osteoblastic rimming and immature bone formation which helps in prediction of site of attachment

21.4.2 Osteitis Sign (Fig. 21.11)

- Presence of thickening of sinus wall compared to the contra lateral site
- Osteogenesis and thickening of the bone or sclerosis

MRI pattern includes (Fig. 21.12)

- Convoluted cerebriform pattern on MRI
- T1 and T2
- **T1**: isointense to muscle
- **T2** generally hyperintense to muscle alternating hypointense lines
- **T1 C+ (Gd)** heterogeneous enhancement alternating hypointense lines

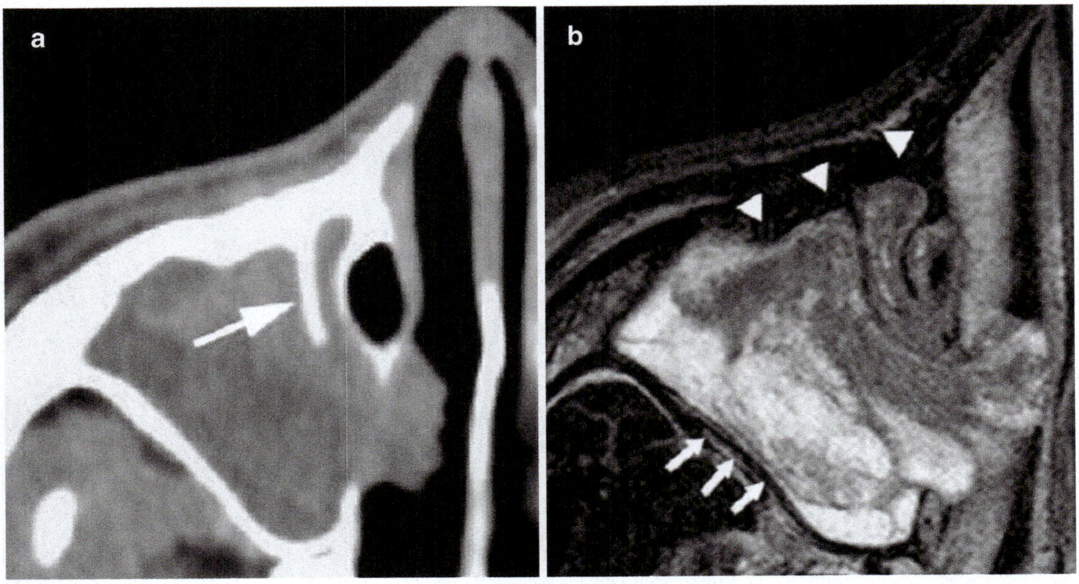

Fig. 21.11 Osteitis sign (white arrow). (**a**) CT sinus. (**b**) MRI sinuses

21.5 Allergic Fungal Sinusitis (Fig. 21.13) [20–24]

Allergic fungal sinusitis (AFS) represents distinct forms of chronic rhinosinusitis with nasal polyposis characterized by high recurrence.

Imaging characteristic of AFS includes:

Double-density shadow on CT sinus, and the high-density shadow is produced by high-density minerals, that is, manganese, aluminum, and calcium concentrated by fungal concretions.

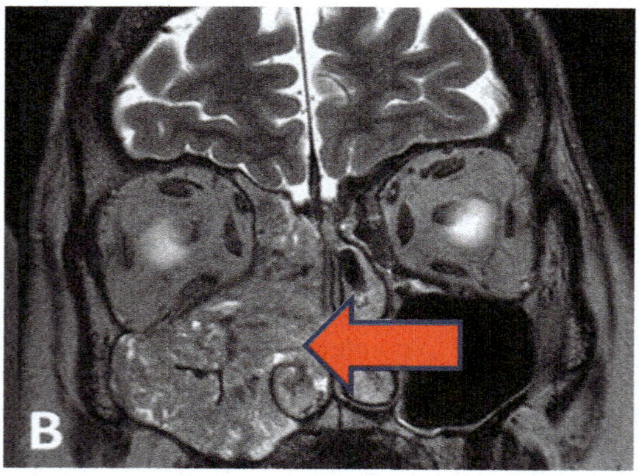

Fig. 21.12 MRI T2-weighted image showing cribriform pattern [17]

Expansile destruction of the paranasal sinuses.

MRI characteristic of allergic fungal sinusitis (Fig. 21.14):

Hypointensity on T1WI and T2WI is the most common finding.

T1: hypointense inflamed mucosal thickness. It can have multiple T1 appearances.

T2: usually a hyperintense peripheral inflamed mucosal thickness.

Low T2 signal or signal void is due to high concentration of metals such as iron, magnesium, and calcium concentrated by fungi and high protein and low water content in allergic mucin.

T1 C+ (Gd):

- An inflamed mucosal lining has contrast enhancement
- No enhancement in the canter

21.5.1 Neoplasms (Fig. 21.15a, b) [23, 24]

Various nasal neoplasms include lymphoma, squamous cell carcinoma, and esthesioneuroblastoma (Fig. 21.16).

They all show extensive bony destruction with enhancement on contrast.

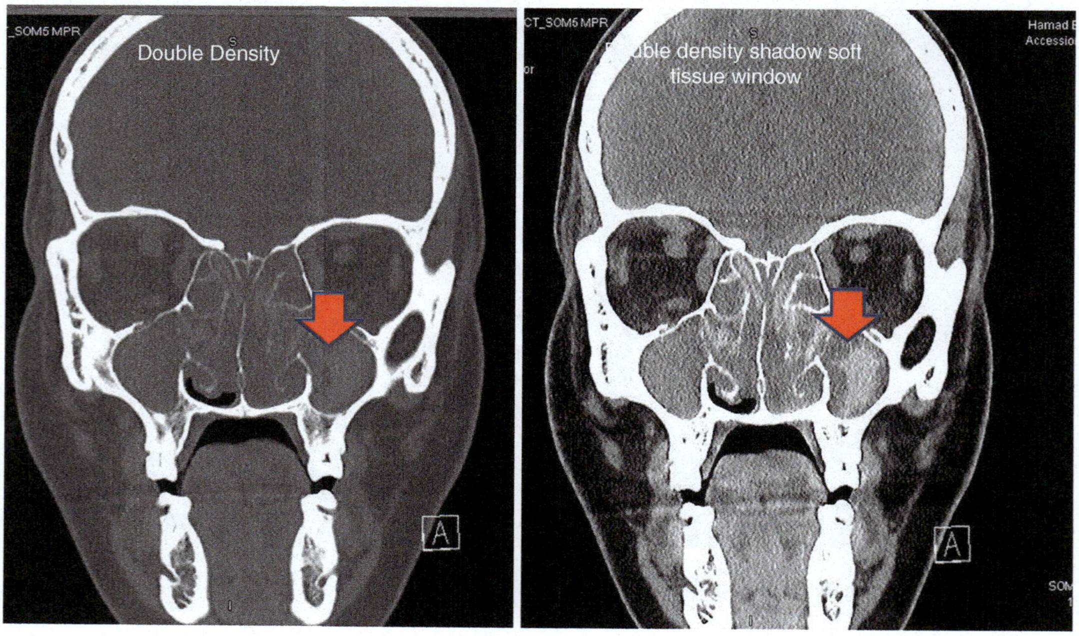

Fig. 21.13 Coronal CT scan showing double density (red arrow) allergic fungal sinusitis [17–19]

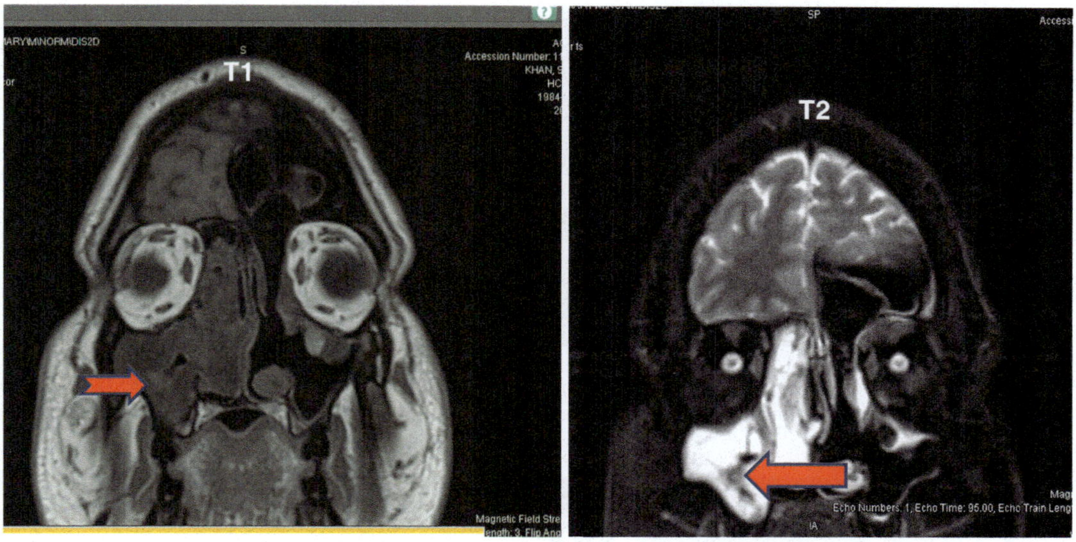

Fig. 21.14 T1 and T2 images of MRI AFS flow void seen in the maxillary sinus (arrow) T2-weighted images with hyperintense inflamed sinus mucosa

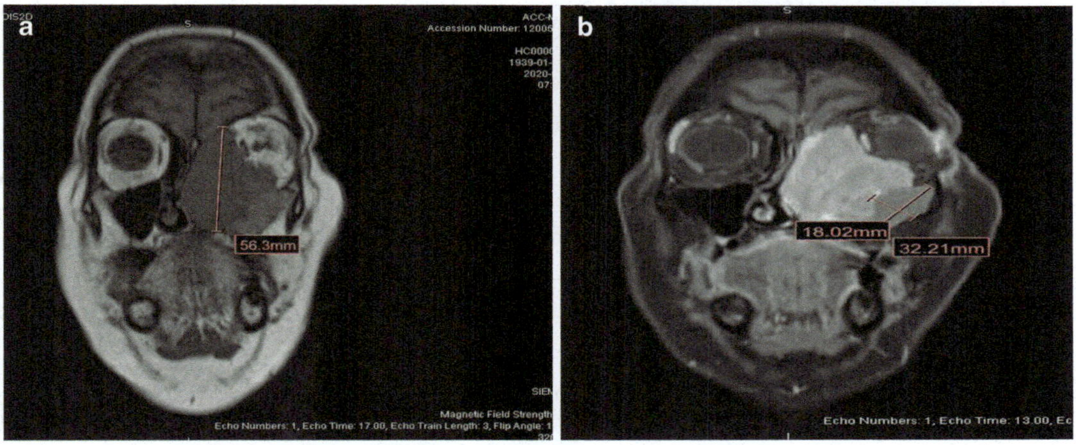

Fig. 21.15 (**a**) Precontrast MRI T1 image showing mass lesion with extensive destruction. (**b**) Postcontrast enhancing lesion MRI T1 image with excessive destruction

21.6 Vessels in Paranasal Sinuses

Major vessels seen on the plane CT scan are anterior ethoidal artery, posterior ethmoidal artery, sphenopalatine artery, and carotid artery.

21.7 Anterior Ethmoidal Artery (Fig. 21.17)

Anterior ethmoidal artery (AEA) is a branch of ophthalmic artery given in the orbit. It exists between the superior oblique and medial rectus.

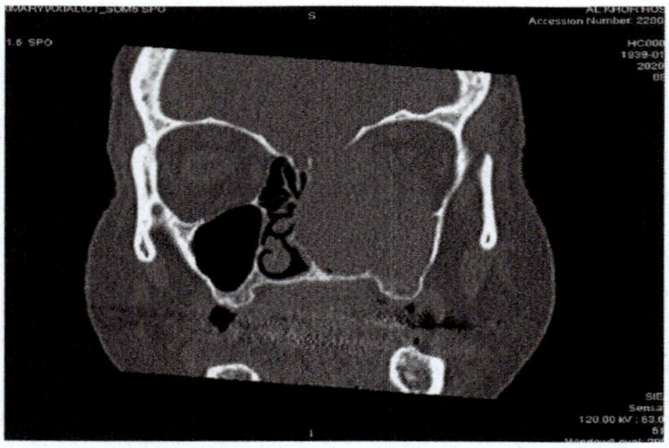

Fig. 21.16 Heterogeneous mass with destruction of skull base and lamina papyracea (Lymphoma)

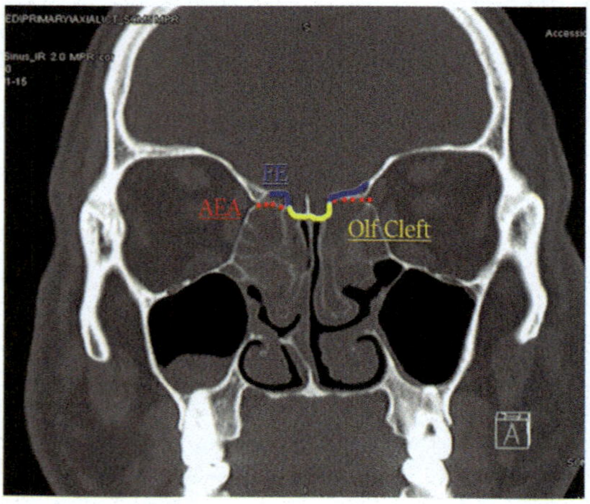

Fig. 21.17 Anterior ethmoidal artery (AEA, red mark) with olfactory cleft (yellow) and fovea ethmoidalis (blue)

In its intranasal route, the anterior ethmoid artery lies inside a bony canal called anterior ethmoidal canal that leaves the orbit through the anterior ethmoidal foramen.

Anterior ethmoidal artery is seen at the anterior ethmoidal roof as marked in the image.

21.8 Posterior Ethmoidal Artery (Fig. 21.18)

The posterior ethmoidal artery (PEA) is a branch of ophthalmic artery passes through the posterior ethmoidal canal and enters the dura at the posterior margin of the cribriform plate and supplies the dura of the medial third of the floor of the anterior cranial fossa. PEA is seen at the roof of posterior ethmoidal cells and most of the time is covered with bone.

21.9 Sphenopalatine Artery (Fig. 21.19)

Sphenopalatine artery (SPA) is a terminal branch of the internal maxillary artery originating from the external carotid artery system. The SPA is the major blood vessel to the nasal cavity mucosa: supplying the superior, middle, and inferior turbinate; lateral nasal wall; and nasal septum. The

Fig. 21.18 Image showing PEA at the skull base (red dots)

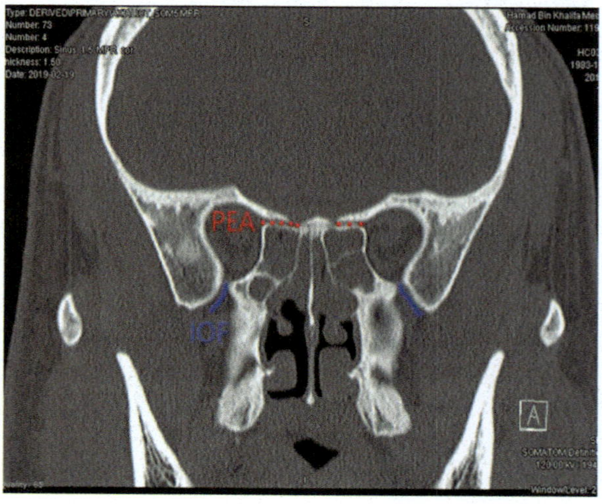

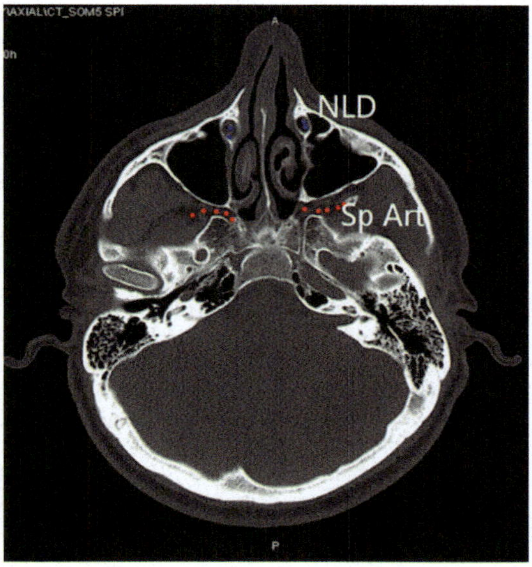

Fig. 21.19 Sphenopalatine artery exiting from the sphenopalatine foramen (red). *NLD* nasolacrimal duct

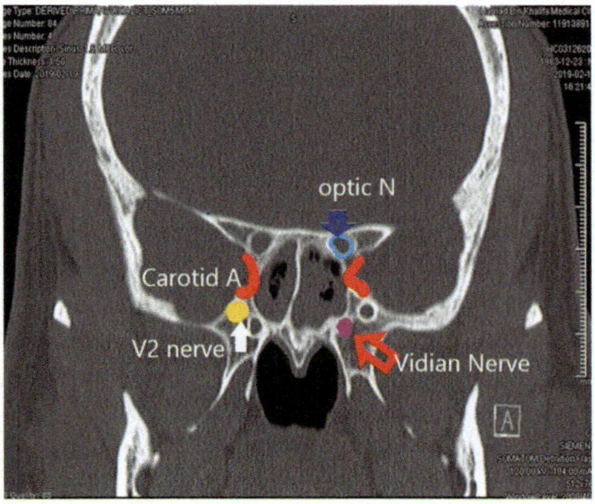

Fig. 21.20 Optic nerve (blue arrow), carotid artery (red), Vidian nerve (red arrow), and V2 (white arrow)

sphenopalatine artery travels within the pterygopalatine fossa and enters the nasal cavity through the sphenopalatine foramen within the superior meatus between the middle turbinate and the posterior end of the superior turbinate on the lateral nasal wall.

Lateral sphenoid wall shows following important structures (Fig. 21.20):

1. Optic nerve
2. Carotid artery
3. Vidian nerve
4. V2 Division of trigeminal nerve in foramen rotundum marked

Take Home Messages
- It is important to study the CT sinuses prior to any surgical intervention for anatomical variations.
- Allergic fungal sinusitis has characteristic appearance on CT scan and MRI scan.
- CT sinus in chronic rhinosinusitis forms one of the criteria for diagnosis.
- Anatomical variations of vessels in the nasal cavity are common, and dehiscence of vessels should be studied before FESS.
- The aim of this chapter is to highlight the clinically relevant sinonasal anatomy and variants.

References

1. Loevner LA, Sonners AI. Imaging of neoplasms of the paranasal sinuses. Magn Reson Imaging Clin N Am. 2002;10:467–93.
2. Earwaker J. Anatomic variants in sinonasal CT. Radiographics. 1993;13:381–415.
3. Joe JK, Ho SY, Yanagisawa E. Documentation of variations in sinonasal anatomy by intraoperative nasal endoscopy. Laryngoscope. 2000;110:229–35.
4. Ly N, McCaig LF. National hospital ambulatory medical care survey: 2000 outpatient department summary. Adv Data 2002:1–27; 2000 Imaging of the paranasal sinuses 33.
5. Lanza DC, Kennedy DW. Adult rhinosinusitis defined. Otolaryngol Head Neck Surg. 1997;117:S1–7.
6. Daniels DL, Mafee MF, Smith MM, et al. The frontal sinus drainage pathway and related structures. AJNR Am J Neuroradiol. 2003;24:1618–27.
7. Beale TJ, Madani G, Morley SJ. Imaging of the paranasal sinuses and nasal cavity: normal anatomy and clinically relevant anatomical variants. Semin Ultrasound CT MR. 2009;30:2–16.
8. Lee WT, Kuhn FA, Citardi MJ. 3D computed tomographic analysis of frontal recess anatomy in patients without frontal sinusitis. Otolaryngol Head Neck Surg. 2004;131:164–73.
9. Kantarci M, Karasen RM, Alper F, et al. Remarkable anatomic variations in paranasal sinus region and their clinical importance. Eur J Radiol. 2004;50:296–302.

10. Yousem DM, Grossman RI. Neuroradiology. 3rd ed. Philadelphia: Mosby; 2010.
11. Kennedy DW, Zinreich SJ, Rosenbaum AE, et al. Functional endoscopic sinus surgery. Theory and diagnostic evaluation. Arch Otolaryngol. 1985;111:576–82.
12. Bolger WE, Butzin CA, Parsons DS. Paranasal sinus bony anatomic variations and mucosal abnormalities: CT analysis for endoscopic sinus surgery. Laryngoscope. 1991;101:56–64.
13. Sarna A, Hayman LA, Laine FJ, et al. Coronal imaging of the osteomeatal unit: anatomy of 24 variants. J Comput Assist Tomogr. 2002;26:153–7.
14. Zinreich SJ, Mattox DE, Kennedy DW, et al. Concha bullosa: CT evaluation. J Comput Assist Tomogr. 1988;12:778–84.
15. Jeon TY, Kim HJ, Chung SK, et al. Sinonasal inverted papilloma: value of convoluted cerebriform pattern on MR imaging. AJNR Am J Neuroradiol. 2008;29:1556–60.
16. Crist W, Gehan EA, Ragab AH, et al. The third intergroup rhabdomyosarcoma study. J Clin Oncol. 1995;13:610–30.
17. Veress B, Malik OA, el-Tayeb AA, et al. Further observations on the primary paranasal aspergillus granuloma in the Sudan: a morphological study of 46 cases. Am J Trop Med Hyg. 1973;22:765–72.
18. Zinreich SJ, Kennedy DW, Malat J, et al. Fungal sinusitis: diagnosis with CT and MR imaging. Radiology. 1988;169:439–44.
19. Allphin AL, Strauss M, Abdul-Karim FW. Allergic fungal sinusitis: problems in diagnosis and treatment. Laryngoscope. 1991;101:815–20.
20. Chakrabarti A, Denning DW, Ferguson BJ, et al. Fungal rhinosinusitis: a categorization and definitional schema addressing current controversies. Laryngoscope. 2009;119:1809–18.
21. Aribandi M, McCoy VA, Bazan C 3rd. Imaging features of invasive and noninvasive fungal sinusitis: a review. Radiographics. 2007;27:1283–96.
22. de Shazo RD, Chapin K, Swain RE. Fungal sinusitis. N Engl J Med. 1997;337:254–9.
23. Siddiqui AA, Shah AA, Bashir SH. Craniocerebral aspergillosis of sinonasalorigin in immunocompetent patients: clinical spectrum and outcome in 25 cases. Neurosurgery. 2004;55:602–11; discussion: 611–613.
24. de Shazo RD, O'Brien M, Chapin K, et al. A new classification and diagnostic criteria for invasive fungal sinusitis. Arch Otolaryngol Head Neck Surg. 1997;123:1181–8.

Allergic and Non-allergic Rhinitis

22

Mona Al-Ahmad, Mohammed Hassab,
and Ali Al Ansari

22.1 Allergic Rhinitis

Mona Al-Ahmad

Key Points

- After reviewing this chapter, students should be able to:
- Identify the different variants of allergic rhinitis
- Understand the proposed pathogenesis of allergic rhinitis
- Mention the diagnostic tools used for allergic rhinitis
- Describe the different therapeutic options used in managing allergic rhinitis

22.1.1 Introduction

Prevalence of allergic rhinitis (AR) has been generally reported in a range from 10 to 30% with an approximate 7–10% belonging to non-allergic rhinitis (NAR) [1–4]. Among patients presenting with symptoms of allergic rhinitis, a prevalence for local allergic rhinitis (LAR) can be expected in 7–30% of patients [5–8]. There are a number of physiological, functional, and immunological relationships between the upper (nose, nasal cavity, paranasal sinuses, pharynx, and larynx) and lower (trachea, bronchial tubes, bronchioles, and lungs) respiratory tracts. Therefore, AR is frequently associated with asthma, which is found in 15–38% of patients with AR [9]. Furthermore, AR is considered as a risk factor for the development of asthma [9].

22.1.2 Definition

AR is an inflammatory, IgE-mediated disease characterized by rhinorrhea, sneezing, nasal congestion, and/or nasal itching. The condition is frequently accompanied by conjunctivitis; allergic rhinoconjunctivitis, and symptoms reverse spontaneously or after treatment. Other associated symptoms include itching of the palate, postnasal drip, and cough [10].

Clinical history is an important part of assessment of AR patients and should include family,

M. Al-Ahmad
Microbiology Department, Faculty of Medicine, Kuwait University, Kuwait City, Kuwait

M. Hassab (✉)
Department of Otorhinolaryngology, Faculty of Medicine, University of Alexandria, Alexandria, Egypt

A. Al Ansari
ORL-HNS (ENT), Hamad Medical Corporation, Doha, Qatar

A. Al-Qahtani et al. (eds.), *Textbook of Clinical Otolaryngology*,
https://doi.org/10.1007/978-3-030-54088-3_22

environmental, and occupational information and questions regarding loss of smell (hyposmia or anosmia), snoring, sleep problems, postnasal drip or chronic cough, sedation, asthma, and conjunctivitis. A record of frequency, severity, duration, persistence or intermittence and seasonality of symptoms should be included as well. Color and lateralization of rhinorrhea, timing and lateralization of nasal obstruction, intake of other drugs, and concomitant symptoms must be explored. Assessment of quality of life should be evaluated including potential indoor/outdoor allergic triggers as well as effect of previous therapy [11].

Clinical history alone is not a good predictor to determine the clinical relevance of a certain allergen, being patients' own assessment of AR or clinical history alone inferior to the combination of skin prick test (SPT) and clinical history [12]. Standard questions to match the clinical symptoms with a specific allergen have a high specificity (>80%) but a decreased sensitivity (11–56%) when SPT is the only diagnostic method used [13].

AR is classified by many ways depending on clinical symptoms. It can be classified according to:

1. Temporal pattern of exposure to a triggering allergen as seasonal (e.g., pollens), perennial/year round (e.g., dust mites). Recently, the terms of intermittent (symptoms <4 days/week or for <4 consecutive weeks) and persistent (symptoms >4 days/week or for >4 consecutive weeks) AR are used instead [10].
2. Episodic (environmental from exposures not normally encountered in the patient's environment, e.g., visiting a home with pets).
3. Frequency of symptoms.
4. Severity of symptoms: mild (no disturbance of sleep; no impairment of daily activities, leisure, or sport; no impairment of school or work; symptoms present but are not troublesome), moderate or severe (disturbance of sleep; impairment of daily activities, leisure, or sport; impairment of school or work; troublesome symptoms) [10].

22.1.3 Pathophysiology

Numerous inflammatory cells infiltrate the nasal mucosa lining of AR patients once they are exposed to an allergen (most commonly airborne are house dust mite, cockroaches, animal dander, molds, and pollens). These cells include mast cells, CD4-positive T cells, B cells, macrophages, and eosinophils. Helper (Th2) CD4 cells release cytokines (mostly IL-4, IL-5, IL-13) that promote immunoglobulin (IgE) production by plasma cells. Cross-linking of IgE molecules on mast cells and basophils, on second allergen exposure, results in clinical symptoms of AR: itching, rhinorrhea, and mucous secretion.

Patients who have a symptomatic sensitization to aeroallergens seem to present with immediate allergic reactions that are not followed by the typical late-phase response. It has been observed that low levels of IL-5 confirmed by mRNA testing but not of IL-4 or IFN-γ on allergen stimulated peripheral blood mononuclear cells from SPT positive asymptomatic patients and a reduced IL-5 inhibition driven by Treg cells was described in symptomatic SPT positive patients but not in asymptomatic or non-atopic patients [14–17]. This laboratory findings correlate with the in vivo findings of a decreased intradermal delayed response to skin test, decreased eosinophils in nasal mucosa, and decreased blood eosinophil-to-lymphocyte ratio in asymptomatic SPT positive patients [18–20].

A higher number of asymptomatic patients is found in polysensitized patients [21]. Neither the extent of SPT patterns nor levels of specific IgE (sIgE) can make an efficient differentiation between symptomatic and asymptomatic patients [22–24]. Symptomatic AR patients have much higher levels of sIgE and skin reactivity, compared to asymptomatic ones, but these values do not lead to a significant difference [25, 26]. A family history of atopy has been related with a 15–30% increased possibility of presenting respiratory symptoms among patients presenting with positive SPT [21, 25, 27].

22.1.4 Diagnosis

The basic diagnosis of AR consists of a detailed medical history followed by confirmation of sensitization with in vivo SPT and/or in vitro sIgE test. If properly performed, they yield confirmatory evidence for the diagnosis of specific allergy in patients with AR. Nasal examination including endoscopic examination is essential to confirm the diagnosis of allergic rhinitis and rule out other pathologies. Anterior rhinoscopy often shows hypertrophied turbinates with pale or bluish mucosa. Allergic shiners (blue-gray discoloration below the eyelids) and a transverse nasal crease are typical in AR patients. As AR is a risk factor for the development of asthma, the clinical examination of patients should include screening for asthma [10, 11].

SPT is an essential test to confirm sensitization in IgE-mediated allergic disease like AR. A recent meta-analysis showed that this technique is reasonably accurate in identifying patients with suspected AR symptoms (sensitivity range of 68–100% and specificity range of 70–91%) [28]. There are some reported factors that may affect the accuracy of SPT like type of testing device, skill of the tester, skin reactivity, stability of test reagents and its potency [25, 28].

In vitro tests, on the other hand, assess antigen-specific IgE by testing the patient's serum. It is also a safer option if the patient is unable to do SPT, like in the case of treatment with antihistamine medication. However, these tests are expensive compared with skin testing.

A problem can be encountered, as not only non-allergic rhinitis patients can present with positive sensitization to allergens that mismatch with the clinical symptoms and sensitization, but also patients with local allergic rhinitis (LAR) can present with clinical symptoms and negative SPT [11, 29, 30].

The prevalence of asymptomatic sensitization in general population ranges from 1 to 5% for a single allergen and up to 8–30% when a panel of aeroallergens is used, with a range of 10–50% of individuals presenting with positive SPT being asymptomatic [24]. Asymptomatic sensitization is also denoted as latent and it is a risk factor for a later development of symptoms including asthma, with studies showing that 20–60% of these patients become symptomatic during a follow-up period of 2–24 years [24, 25].

In a national USA survey, including individuals between 6 and 59 years and testing with 10 allergens, up to 71.3% of patients with positive SPT were positive to more than one allergen [31].

Among possible causes of false-positive SPT are staff-related causes as violent technique, puncture vs. prick technique and pressure over the lancet among others, lancet characteristics, toxic reactions to the extract (allergen, impurities, additives) or concomitant physical urticarial [24, 32, 33]. The role of cross-reactivity with allergens that are clinically irrelevant (i.e., profilin) must also be considered [24, 34].

The rate of allergen sensitization increases with age in pediatric population reaching a peak before the age of 20–34 years, and this is opposite to the burden of rhinitis symptoms in sensitized patients that decrease with age [35–37].

22.1.5 Diagnostic Scenarios When Standard Testing Is Not Enough

1. **False-positive results in patients with only non-allergic rhinitis with or without asthma**:

   If discordance between SPT or sIgE and clinical history is found, further testing including the time-consuming and specialized staff required nasal provocation test (NPT) may be indicated. Over the last decade, an increasing number of studies on local allergic rhinitis has proven the need to reconsider patients classified as non-allergic rhinitis by means of NPT [29, 38–40].
2. **Polysensitized patients with a mix of real allergy and only sensitization**:

   As discussed above, both SPT and sIgE determination alone is only able to detect allergen sensitization. A recent meta-analysis using NPT as gold standard has shown an estimate sensitivity and specificity for skin prick testing of 85% and 77%, respectively [28]. Although trained and specialized staff are required for the time-consuming NPT, it is the option of choice in allergic rhinitis to confirm clinical relevance to a certain allergen [29, 41, 42]. A recent EAACI position paper has extensively discussed the present recommended methodology for NPT performance [41]. Polysensitized patients who have a positive SPT results might be the result of a subclinical cross-sensitization. This issue has been shown by means of NPT to multiple allergens (Cupressus Vs cypress pollen), when only the monosensitized patients presented NPT as opposed to the 64 polysensitized [38]. Relevant clinical history is important in patients sensitized to panallergens such as profilin or polcalcin, as they can have no real clinical relevance on the patient symptoms [43].

3. **Patients with local allergic rhinitis diagnosed as non-allergic**:

   Despite the time-consuming and specialized staff required, NPT needs to be implemented especially in patients where clinical symptoms and SPT or sIgE mismatch and this has been proved both for indoor and outdoor allergens: There is a large number of publications proving the underdiagnosed prevalence of LAR for indoor allergens as HDM and also for molds or cats that are considered as outdoor sensitization [5, 39, 40, 44–46]. Moreover, there is evidence as well for pollen-induced allergic patients [5, 38, 47, 48]. In a recent review on AR or NAR patients subjected to diagnostic local nasal provocation from 1946 to 2015, it was concluded that positive NPT was shown in 26.5% of patients previously considered non-allergic, and that AR defined by SPT or sIgE may lead to 13.7% of patients without accurate sensitization to allergens or non-allergic etiologies [49]. A pediatric study showed that LAR was present in 29.2% (7/24) of the patients presenting with negative SPT or sIgE, leading to the conclusion that LAR is substantially present in chronic, difficult-to-treat rhinitis patients presenting with negative SPT or sIgE [5].

22.1.6 Clinical Approach to Improve Diagnosis

22.1.6.1 Component-Resolved Diagnosis

The implementation of novel molecular diagnostic testing may improve the sensitivity and specificity of sIgE testing for AR and LAR patients, with in vitro results being progressively closer to the results of nasal and bronchial testing but still not being able to replace them as confirmatory test [26, 50]. Given the difficulties, and the time consumption in performing NPT, component-resolved diagnosis is gaining field on this topic [51]. This improvement may be important due to the increased regulatory demands in many countries, like the EU [52].

Component-resolved diagnosis (CRD) will continue gaining role on a proper decision regarding the need and composition of allergen immunotherapy (AIT) for the future, especially at the time that component-based AIT becomes a routine practice. This topic has been recently reviewed and there are World Allergy Organization (WAO) and European Allergy, Asthma and Clinical Immunology (EAACI) consensus document and guidelines [53–55]. It has been proved useful not only in identification of clinically relevant allergens but more important to determine the presence of panallergens such as profilin or polcalcins that can be a confounding factor for proper AIT leading therefore to significant changes in the decision to implement AIT [56, 57].

Recently, a sort of “atopic molecular march” has been described with an evolution from monomolecular to polymolecular sensitization determined as molecular spreading, and it has been described for children presenting with starting molecules Phl p1 or Der p1/p2/p23 [58, 59]. Furthermore, it has been hypothesized that early allergen immunoprophylaxis targeting these initiator molecules might prevent AR and asthma on preclinical stages [53].

22.1.6.2 Basophil Activation Test

Basophil activation test (BAT) measures basophil response to allergen cross-linking IgE on basophil granulocytes. In addition to clinical history, SPT, and specific IgE determination, BAT can be a part of the diagnostic evaluation of patients with IgE-mediated allergic response like AR [60]. Furthermore, BAT has proven useful in LAR, as well, as more sensitive and less time consuming alternative to detection of nasal specific IgE for HDM, being able to diagnose at least 50% of LAR to HDM with one study was a determinant factor to differentiate symptomatic and asymptomatic patients sensitized to HDM [22, 61].

22.1.7 Treatment

Treatment of allergic rhinitis should be tailored to each patient's condition taking into considerations several factors including age of the patient, nature and severity of symptoms, presence of comorbidities, and quality of life. Guideline-directed treatment plan (such as ARIA recommendations) proved to be effective [10]. Therapeutic measures for managing AR include education and environment control, pharmacotherapy, and immunotherapy:

Education and Environmental Control: It is essential to explain to the patient the nature of his disease, underlying etiology, and the need for extended medical care. Suggestions to avoid and minimize exposure to allergens and irritant factors such as tobacco smoke are discussed with the patients. Measure such as bedding and pillow covers, high efficiency vacuuming of carpets may be useful for house dust mite control. The potential role of pets should be highlighted [10, 11].

Pharmacotherapy: The most effective treatment of allergic rhinitis includes the use of modern generation **intranasal corticosteroid (INC) sprays** with minimum bioavailability and/or non-sedating **oral second generation H1 antihistamines**. While INC sprays are efficacious for all allergic rhinitis symptoms, oral H1 antihistamines relieve mostly rhinorrhea, sneezing, and itching but not nasal blockage. Intranasal corticosteroid (INC) sprays have a slow onset of action and it may take few days for their therapeutic effect to be felt by the patient. Hence, they may be initially prescribed in combination with oral antihistamine. Long-term use of INC sprays may be associated with minor side effects such as nasal dryness and bleeding and can be minimized by educating the patient the proper technique of application. **Oral decongestants** such as pseudoephedrine combined with an antihistamine and/or INC sprays are used in patients with nasal congestion. However, they can cause significant side effects such as irritability, tremors, insomnia, palpitations, and hypertension. They should be avoided in patients with heart disease, hypertension, glaucoma, urinary retention problems, and thyrotoxicosis. **Antileukotrienes** such as montelukast may be used in patients with asthma associated with allergic rhinitis. Short burst of **oral corticosteroids** may be used in patients with severe allergic flare-up. **Intranasal H1 antihistamines** such as azelastine are effective for controlling nasal symptoms. They need to be applied twice daily and their main side effect is inducing a bitter taste. **Nasal anticholinergics** such as ipratropium bromide 0.03% are effective in controlling rhinorrhea, but do not relief other nasal symptoms. They block muscarinic receptors, leading to a decrease in the parasympathetic function. They are usually used in combination with INC sprays or with an antihistamine. Minor side effects include headache, epistaxis, and nasal dryness. They should be used with caution in patients with narrow-angle glaucoma and in prostatic hypertrophy. **Intranasal sodium cromoglycate** is a mast cell stabilizer and was shown to be effective in the prevention and treatment of allergic rhinitis but is less effective than INC sprays and oral antihistamines. They require application four times daily and ocular formulas are helpful in treating allergic conjunctivitis [10, 11].

Two to four weeks after use of the initial therapy, patients should be reevaluated for the efficacy of this treatment in controlling their symptoms and for the presence of side effects. Based upon this evaluation, maintenance treatment is designed. During follow-up visits, and based upon the patients' response, treatment may be either maintained or stepped down. Modification of the maintenance treatment will also be required during allergic flare ups or respiratory tract infections [10, 11].

Immunotherapy: AIT is a highly effective treatment modality for patients with AR. Unlike other pharmacological treatments, AIT is considered an immune modulating therapy with long-lasting efficacy in the management of AR [62]. It has a well-established efficacy for inhalant allergen sensitization, including patients presenting with LAR [29].

AIT prescription should be based on the clinically relevant allergens and not merely on potentially irrelevant SPT or sIgE sensitization [63]. In polysensitized patients, single-allergen products are recommended when an allergen is clearly responsible for the main symptoms load. The use of AIT for 2 products as single-AIT formulations in parallel is the preferred form of administration when 2 allergens are responsible for the main impact [51, 64]. The fine-tuning of the clinically relevant allergens in polysensitized patients can therefore increase the implementation of these recommendations.

Take Home Messages

- Allergic rhinitis is a common disease with a prevalence as high as 30%.
- It is the commonest chronic rhinitis encountered and has a significant impact on the patients' health, quality of life, and work performance.
- The diagnosis of AR is attained mainly through a detailed medical history. In vivo SPT and/or in vitro sIgE test confirm the diagnosis.
- Therapeutic measures for managing AR include education and environment control, pharmacotherapy, and immunotherapy:
- Treatment should be tailored to each patient's condition taking into considerations age of the patient, nature and severity of symptoms, presence of comorbidities, and quality of life. Guideline-directed treatment plan (such as ARIA recommendations) proved to be effective.

22.2 Non-allergic Rhinitis

Mohammed Hassab and Ali Al Ansari

Key Points

- After reviewing this chapter, students should be able to:
- Identify the different variants of non-allergic rhinitis
- Understand the proposed pathogenesis of the different variants of non-allergic rhinitis
- Describe the therapeutic options used in managing the different variants of non-allergic rhinitis

Non-allergic rhinitis includes a heterogeneous group of patients with rhinitis resulting from different pathophysiologic mechanisms other than allergy or infection.

Prevalence: Although the prevalence of allergic rhinitis is well investigated, the prevalence of non-allergic rhinitis is less known. Non-allergic rhinitis tends to occur more in adults, with the typical age of presentation between 30 and 60 years. It is suggested that it is responsible for 50% of cases of chronic rhinitis. A Danish study found that 25% of rhinitis was non-allergic. The disease was found to be more prevalent in women. In the United States, non-allergic rhinitis is estimated to affect around 19 million people [65–68].

The variants of non-allergic rhinitis include:

22.2.1 Idiopathic (Vasomotor) Rhinitis

This is the most frequent form of non-allergic rhinitis encountered. All chronic rhinitis patients without an obvious underlying etiology are grouped together under this variant. Accordingly, this variant is a diagnosis of exclusion. To make this diagnosis, all other causes of non-allergic rhinitis have to be excluded. The patients suffer from perennial nasal congestion, rhinorrhea, and/

or sneezing with no identifiable etiology. It is non-IgE-mediated, non-infectious, and not associated with nasal eosinophilia. The exact pathophysiology of this variant remains to be poorly understood. It is thought to be due to autonomic imbalance with parasympathetic hyperactivity and sympathetic hypoactivity. Parasympathetic hyperactivity results in an increase of acetylcholine and vasoactive intestinal peptide (VIP). Sympathetic hypoactivity results in a decrease of norepinephrine and neuropeptide Y. This imbalance results in excessive nasal secretions and nasal congestion. Other hypotheses suggest hyperactivity of C-fiber, or the release of excessive amounts of neuropeptides (substance P and neurokinins) that promote nasal congestion and nasal secretion production. Topical steroids are initially given for a period of 6 weeks. Ipratropium bromide 0.03% is effective against anterior rhinorrhea, but does not affect other nasal symptoms. This molecule blocks muscarinic receptors, leading to a decrease in the parasympathetic function. Minor side effects include headache, epistaxis, and nasal dryness.

If symptoms persist, intranasal capsaicin has been shown to be an effective treatment (Fig. 22.1) [69–72].

22.2.2 Drug-Induced Rhinitis

1. **Rhinitis Medicamentosa**: This is not an infrequently encountered condition where an individual overuses local vasoconstrictor drops or sprays (oxymetazoline, xylometazoline, naphazoline, etc.) to maintain his nasal airway patent. Initially, the instillation of the vasoconstrictor drops/spray, which is alpha adrenergic agonist, shrinks and decongests the nasal mucosa by constricting the blood vessels. However, rebound congestion occurs after a few hours resulting in nasal blockage and driving the patient to further instill more drops or spray. Over time, increasing amounts of the local medication will be needed to decongest the nasal mucosa and relieve the blockage and the patient becomes addicted to its use. As a result of this, the nasal mucosal blood vessels lose the alpha adrenergic tone and the normal nasal cycle is suppressed. The cilia are decreased in number and squamous metaplasia occurs.

   Diagnosis: The patient gives a typical history of nasal blockage and congestion that is only relieved by the instillation of vasoconstrictor drops/sprays. This problem may have been running for weeks, months, and even years. On examination, the nasal mucosa is usually dry, reddish, and thinned out. Occasionally, an underlying primary cause of nasal obstruction, such as a significantly deviated nasal septum, is detected.

   Treatment: It is critical to explain to the patient the cause of the problem and importance of getting off the use of these local vasoconstrictor agents. Short burst of systemic steroids, topical intranasal steroids, and systemic decongestant drugs may be prescribed

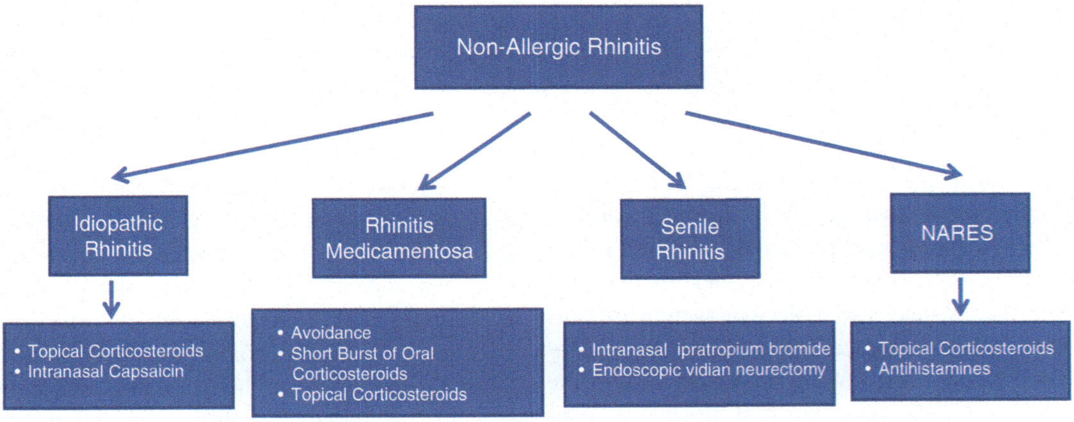

Fig. 22.1 Main therapeutic measures in different forms of non-allergic rhinitis

to help to wean the patient off the local vasoconstrictors. In the subset of patients with an obvious cause of nasal blockage, such as a significantly deviated nasal septum, a septoplasty may be considered but only several weeks after the patient has stopped using the local vasoconstrictors. Similarly, radiofrequency reduction of the inferior turbinate or an inferior turbinoplasty procedure may be considered in select cases (Fig. 22.1) [66, 67, 73].
2. **Cocaine Abuse**
3. **Aspirin and NSAIDs Intolerance**: This may result in an intense eosinophilic rhinitis with the patient suffering from profuse watery rhinorrhea. In the variant of Aspirin Exacerbated Respiratory Disease (AERD), the patient has eosinophilic rhinosinusitis with nasal polyposis, asthma, and aspirin intolerance. The patient's symptoms and asthma are worsened by aspirin and/or NSAIDs intake. The disease results from a defect in the arachidonic acid metabolism with inhibition of the cyclooxygenase pathway and preferential increase in the lipoxygenase pathway with excessive leukotriene production. Avoidance of these drugs is important in this group of patients [65–67].
4. **Others**: Antihypertension medications such as ACE inhibitors, beta blockers, methyldopa, reserpine, guanethidine, phentolamine, chlorpromazine, oral contraceptives, and neostigmine (used in treatment of myasthenia gravis) can produce nasal obstruction [66, 67].

22.2.3 Occupational

This arises in response to airborne particles in the work environment. Occupational rhinitis can result from allergic or irritant responses, which elicit eosinophilic or neutrophilic inflammation. Numerous chemical agents have been identified. These include high molecular weight irritants such as grain dust, flour, fish and seafood proteins, latex, and low molecular weight irritants such as isocyanates, aldehydes, ninhydrin, chlorine, wood dust, and many others. Complete avoidance is the most essential measure in managing this variant of rhinitis [74].

22.2.4 Hormonal

- **Rhinitis of Pregnancy**: During pregnancy, the elevated levels of estrogen may induce an inflammatory process in the nasal mucosa causing bothersome nasal obstruction. Saline irrigations may help in alleviating this condition, which resolves spontaneously after delivery [75].
- **Honeymoon rhinitis, epistaxis of vicarious menstruation**, and rhinitis associated with the use of contraceptive pills all are associated with hormonal pathophysiology [75].
- **Hypothyroidism and acromegaly may be associated with inflammatory changes in the nasal mucosa** [66, 67].

22.2.5 Non-allergic Rhinitis with Eosinophilia Syndrome (NARES)

This was first described by Jacobs et al. in 1981. In this rhinitis variant, patients present with perennial symptoms of paroxysmal sneezing, profuse watery rhinorrhea, and itching in the nasopharynx. Their nasal smears show profound eosinophilia while their allergy testing (skin prick test, total and specific IgE) is negative. These patients respond well to topical corticosteroids [76–78].

22.2.6 Senile Rhinitis

Typically, this occurs in the elderly where the patient suffers primarily from persistent watery rhinorrhea with clear watery drops trickling down from the nose. Intranasal ipratropium bromide given up to six times daily is reported to control the condition. Its parasympatholytic effect decreases submucosal gland secretion. Ipratropium bromide should be used with caution in patients with narrow-angle glaucoma, prostatic hypertrophy, or bladder neck obstruction. Injection of botulinum toxin type A (BTA) into the nasal cavities is another suggested treatment modality. Endoscopic vidian neurectomy has been reintroduced and seems to have excellent results, although the treatment is not without potential serious side effects (Fig. 22.1) [79–81].

22.2.7 Gustatory Rhinitis

This is a condition characterized by sudden onset of excessive bilateral watery rhinorrhea occurring immediately after the ingestion of foods (often, hot and spicy). This is usually not associated with sneezing or itching or any other symptoms. Intranasal ipratropium bromide is usually an effective treatment [82].

22.2.8 Atrophic Rhinitis

This could be either primary or secondary. In **primary atrophic rhinitis**, there is atrophy of the nasal mucosa and underlying bone, with the nasal cavity becoming wide and containing foul-smelling crusts. Typically, the condition occurs in young females. Interestingly, the patients complain of nasal obstruction, cacosmia, and possibly mild epistaxis with separation of the crusts. It has been suggested to result from Klebsiella ozaenae infection, although its role as a primary pathogen is not confirmed. **Secondary atrophic rhinitis** can result from nasal granulomas, radiation, and trauma including surgical resection [66, 67].

Take Home Messages

- Non-allergic rhinitis includes a heterogeneous group of patients.
- It roughly constitutes 50% of patients with chronic rhinitis.
- It includes drug-induced rhinitis, hormonal rhinitis, senile rhinitis, occupational rhinitis, gustatory rhinitis, NARES, atrophic rhinitis, and idiopathic rhinitis.
- Treatment plan of non-allergic rhinitis varies from one variant to another.

References

1. Bauchau V, Durham SR. Prevalence and rate of diagnosis of allergic rhinitis in Europe. Eur Respir J. 2004;24(5):758–64.
2. Nathan RA, Meltzer EO, Derebery J, Campbell UB, Stang PE, Corrao MA, et al. The prevalence of nasal symptoms attributed to allergies in the United States: findings from the burden of rhinitis in an America survey. Allergy Asthma Proc. 2008;29(6):600–8.
3. Zhang Y, Zhang L. Prevalence of allergic rhinitis in China. Allergy Asthma Immunol Res. 2014;6(2):105–13.
4. Hellings PW, Klimek L, Cingi C, Agache I, Akdis C, Bachert C, et al. Non-allergic rhinitis: position paper of the European Academy of Allergy and Clinical Immunology. Allergy. 2017;72(11):1657–65.
5. Tsilochristou O, Kyriakakou M, Manolaraki I, Lakoumentas J, Tiligada E, Maragkoudakis P, et al. Detection of local allergic rhinitis in children with chronic, difficult-to-treat, non-allergic rhinitis using multiple nasal provocation tests. Pediatr Allergy Immunol. 2019;30(3):296–304.
6. Bozek A, Scierski W, Ignasiak B, Jarzab J, Misiolek M. The prevalence and characteristics of local allergic rhinitis in Poland. Rhinology. 2019;57(3):213–8.
7. Cheng KJ, Xu YY, Liu HY, Wang SQ. Serum eosinophil cationic protein level in Chinese subjects with nonallergic and local allergic rhinitis and its relation to the severity of disease. Am J Rhinol Allergy. 2013;27(1):8–12.
8. Rondon C, Campo P, Galindo L, Blanca-Lopez N, Cassinello MS, Rodriguez-Bada JL, et al. Prevalence and clinical relevance of local allergic rhinitis. Allergy. 2012;67(10):1282–8.
9. Leynaert B, Bousquet J, Neukirch C, Liard R, Neukirch F. Perennial rhinitis: an independent risk factor for asthma in nonatopic subjects: results from the European Community Respiratory Health Survey. J Allergy Clin Immunol. 1999;104(2 Pt 1):301–4.
10. Brozek JL, Bousquet J, Baena-Cagnani CE, Bonini S, Canonica GW, Casale TB, et al. Allergic rhinitis and its impact on asthma (ARIA) guidelines: 2010 revision. J Allergy Clin Immunol. 2010;126(3):466–76.
11. Scadding GK, Kariyawasam HH, Scadding G, Mirakian R, Buckley RJ, Dixon T, et al. BSACI guideline for the diagnosis and management of allergic and non-allergic rhinitis (Revised Edition 2017; First edition 2007). Clin Exp Allergy. 2017;47(7):856–89.
12. Smith HE, Hogger C, Lallemant C, Crook D, Frew AJ. Is structured allergy history sufficient when assessing patients with asthma and rhinitis in general practice? J Allergy Clin Immunol. 2009;123(3):646–50.
13. Murray AB, Milner RA. The accuracy of features in the clinical history for predicting atopic sensitization to airborne allergens in children. J Allergy Clin Immunol. 1995;96(5 Pt 1):588–96.

14. Nakai Y, Ohashi Y, Kakinoki Y, Tanaka A, Washio Y, Nasako Y, et al. Allergen-induced mRNA expression of IL-5, but not of IL-4 and IFN-gamma, in peripheral blood mononuclear cells is a key feature of clinical manifestation of seasonal allergic rhinitis. Arch Otolaryngol Head Neck Surg. 2000;126(8):992–6.
15. Ohashi Y, Nakai Y, Tanaka A, Kakinoki Y, Masamoto T, Kato A, et al. Allergen-induced synthesis of interleukin-5, but not of IgE, is a key mechanism linked to symptomatic episodes of seasonal allergic rhinitis in sensitized individuals. Scand J Immunol. 1998;47(6):596–602.
16. Assing K, Nielsen CH, Poulsen LK. Immunological characteristics of subjects with asymptomatic skin sensitization to birch and grass pollen. Clin Exp Allergy. 2006;36(3):283–92.
17. Ling EM, Smith T, Nguyen XD, Pridgeon C, Dallman M, Arbery J, et al. Relation of CD4+CD25+ regulatory T-cell suppression of allergen-driven T-cell activation to atopic status and expression of allergic disease. Lancet. 2004;363(9409):608–15.
18. Bodtger U, Poulsen LK, Malling HJ. Asymptomatic skin sensitization to birch predicts later development of birch pollen allergy in adults: a 3-year follow-up study. J Allergy Clin Immunol. 2003;111(1):149–54.
19. Braunstahl GJ, Fokkens WJ, Overbeek SE, KleinJan A, Hoogsteden HC, Prins JB. Mucosal and systemic inflammatory changes in allergic rhinitis and asthma: a comparison between upper and lower airways. Clin Exp Allergy. 2003;33(5):579–87.
20. Yenigun A, Sezen S, Calim OF, Ozturan O. Evaluation of the eosinophil-to-lymphocyte ratio in pediatric patients with allergic rhinitis. Am J Rhinol Allergy. 2016;30(2):e21–5.
21. Fuiano N, Fusilli S, Passalacqua G, Incorvaia C. Allergen-specific immunoglobulin E in the skin and nasal mucosa of symptomatic and asymptomatic children sensitized to aeroallergens. J Investig Allergol Clin Immunol. 2010;20(5):425–30.
22. Zidarn M, Robic M, Krivec A, Silar M, Resch-Marat Y, Vrtala S, et al. Clinical and immunological differences between asymptomatic HDM-sensitized and HDM-allergic rhinitis patients. Clin Exp Allergy. 2019;49(6):808–18.
23. Bokanovic D, Aberer W, Hemmer W, Heinemann A, Komericki P, Scheffel J, et al. Determination of sIgE to rPhl p 1 is sufficient to diagnose grass pollen allergy. Allergy. 2013;68(11):1403–9.
24. Bodtger U. Prognostic value of asymptomatic skin sensitization to aeroallergens. Curr Opin Allergy Clin Immunol. 2004;4(1):5–10.
25. Bousquet J, Anto JM, Bachert C, Bousquet PJ, Colombo P, Crameri R, et al. Factors responsible for differences between asymptomatic subjects and patients presenting an IgE sensitization to allergens. A GA2LEN project. Allergy. 2006;61(6):671–80.
26. Gellrich D, Hogerle C, Becker S, Groger M. Is quantitative sIgE serology suitable for distinguishing between silent sensitization and allergic rhinitis to dermatophagoides pteronyssinus? J Investig Allergol Clin Immunol. 2019;29(2):124–31.
27. Lau S, Nickel R, Niggemann B, Gruber C, Sommerfeld C, Illi S, et al. The development of childhood asthma: lessons from the German Multicentre Allergy Study (MAS). Paediatr Respir Rev. 2002;3(3):265–72.
28. Nevis IF, Binkley K, Kabali C. Diagnostic accuracy of skin-prick testing for allergic rhinitis: a systematic review and meta-analysis. Allergy Asthma Clin Immunol. 2016;12:20.
29. Campo P, Eguiluz-Gracia I, Bogas G, Salas M, Plaza Seron C, Perez N, et al. Local allergic rhinitis: implications for management. Clin Exp Allergy. 2019;49(1):6–16.
30. Lockey RF. "ARIA": global guidelines and new forms of allergen immunotherapy. J Allergy Clin Immunol. 2001;108(4):497–9.
31. Nelson HS. Allergen immunotherapy (AIT) for the multiple-pollen sensitive patient. Expert Rev Clin Pharmacol. 2016;9(11):1443–51.
32. Andersen HH, Lundgaard AC, Petersen AS, Hauberg LE, Sharma N, Hansen SD, et al. The Lancet weight determines wheal diameter in response to skin prick testing with histamine. PLoS One. 2016;11(5):e0156211.
33. Werther RL, Choo S, Lee KJ, Poole D, Allen KJ, Tang ML. Variability in skin prick test results performed by multiple operators depends on the device used. World Allergy Organ J. 2012;5(12):200–4.
34. van Ree R, Aalberse RC. Specific IgE without clinical allergy. J Allergy Clin Immunol. 1999;103(6):1000–1.
35. Govaere E, Van Gysel D, Massa G, Verhamme KM, Doli E, De Baets F. The influence of age and gender on sensitization to aero-allergens. Pediatr Allergy Immunol. 2007;18(8):671–8.
36. Suh MJ, Park JA, Chang SW, Kim JH, Lee KH, Hong SC, et al. Chronological changes in rhinitis symptoms present in school-aged children with allergic sensitization. PLoS One. 2019;14(1):e0210840.
37. Kerkhof M, Droste JH, de Monchy JG, Schouten JP, Rijcken B. Distribution of total serum IgE and specific IgE to common aeroallergens by sex and age, and their relationship to each other in a random sample of the Dutch general population aged 20-70 years. Dutch ECRHS Group, European Community Respiratory Health Study. Allergy. 1996;51(11):770–6.
38. Sin AZ, Ersoy R, Gulbahar O, Ardeniz O, Gokmen NM, Kokuludag A. Prevalence of cypress pollen sensitization and its clinical importance in Izmir, Turkey, with cypress allergy assessed by nasal provocation. J Investig Allergol Clin Immunol. 2008;18(1):46–51.
39. Demirturk M, Gelincik A, Ulusan M, Ertek B, Buyukozturk S, Colakoglu B. The importance of mold sensitivity in nonallergic rhinitis patients. Int Forum Allergy Rhinol. 2016;6(7):716–21.
40. Shin YS, Jung CG, Park HS. Prevalence and clinical characteristics of local allergic rhinitis to house dust mites. Curr Opin Allergy Clin Immunol. 2018;18(1):10–5.

41. Auge J, Vent J, Agache I, Airaksinen L, Campo Mozo P, Chaker A, et al. EAACI position paper on the standardization of nasal allergen challenges. Allergy. 2018;73(8):1597–608.
42. Gosepath J, Amedee RG, Mann WJ. Nasal provocation testing as an international standard for evaluation of allergic and nonallergic rhinitis. Laryngoscope. 2005;115(3):512–6.
43. San Nicolo M, Braun T, Eder K, Berghaus A, Groger M. Clinical relevance of IgE to profilin and/or polcalcin in pollen-sensitized patients. Int Arch Allergy Immunol. 2016;169(2):101–7.
44. Ha EK, Na MS, Lee S, Baek H, Lee SJ, Sheen YH, et al. Prevalence and clinical characteristics of local allergic rhinitis in children sensitized to house dust mites. Int Arch Allergy Immunol. 2017;174(3–4):183–9.
45. Al Ahmad M, Arifhodzic N, Nurkic J, Jusufovic E, Hanoun AL, Rodriguez T. Role of nasal challenge and local eosinophilia in indirect exposure to cat in allergic rhinitis patients. Eur Ann Allergy Clin Immunol. 2018;50(3):125–31.
46. Al-Ahmad M, Jusufovic E, Arifhodzic N, Nurkic J, Hanoun AL. Sensitization to cat: when is nasal challenge needed? Int Arch Allergy Immunol. 2019;179(2):108–13.
47. Blanca-Lopez N, Campo P, Salas M, Garcia Rodriguez C, Palomares F, Blanca M, et al. Seasonal local allergic rhinitis in areas with high concentrations of grass pollen. J Investig Allergol Clin Immunol. 2016;26(2):83–91.
48. Krajewska-Wojtys A, Jarzab J, Gawlik R, Bozek A. Local allergic rhinitis to pollens is underdiagnosed in young patients. Am J Rhinol Allergy. 2016;30(6):198–201.
49. Hamizan AW, Rimmer J, Alvarado R, Sewell WA, Kalish L, Sacks R, et al. Positive allergen reaction in allergic and nonallergic rhinitis: a systematic review. Int Forum Allergy Rhinol. 2017;7(9):868–77.
50. Comite P, Minale P, Ferrero F, Mussap M, Ciprandi G. Der p 1 IgE measurement for distinguishing between sensitization and allergy. Immunol Lett. 2015;166(2):145–6.
51. Demoly P, Passalacqua G, Pfaar O, Sastre J, Wahn U. Management of the polyallergic patient with allergy immunotherapy: a practice-based approach. Allergy Asthma Clin Immunol. 2016;12:2.
52. Klimek L, Hammerbacher AS, Hellings PW, Fokkens WJ, Hoffmann HJ, Muraro A, et al. The influence of European legislation on the use of diagnostic test allergens for nasal allergen provocation in routine care of patients with allergic rhinitis. Rhinology. 2015;53(3):260–9.
53. Matricardi PM, Dramburg S, Potapova E, Skevaki C, Renz H. Molecular diagnosis for allergen immunotherapy. J Allergy Clin Immunol. 2019;143(3):831–43.
54. Canonica GW, Ansotegui IJ, Pawankar R, Schmid-Grendelmeier P, van Hage M, Baena-Cagnani CE, et al. A WAO-ARIA-GA(2)LEN consensus document on molecular-based allergy diagnostics. World Allergy Organ J. 2013;6(1):17.
55. Matricardi PM, Kleine-Tebbe J, Hoffmann HJ, Valenta R, Hilger C, Hofmaier S, et al. EAACI molecular allergology user's guide. Pediatr Allergy Immunol. 2016;27(Suppl 23):1–250.
56. Stringari G, Tripodi S, Caffarelli C, Dondi A, Asero R, Di Rienzo Businco A, et al. The effect of component-resolved diagnosis on specific immunotherapy prescription in children with hay fever. J Allergy Clin Immunol. 2014;134(1):75–81.
57. Moreno C, Justicia JL, Quiralte J, Moreno-Ancillo A, Iglesias-Cadarso A, Torrecillas M, et al. Olive, grass or both? Molecular diagnosis for the allergen immunotherapy selection in polysensitized pollinic patients. Allergy. 2014;69(10):1357–63.
58. Hatzler L, Panetta V, Lau S, Wagner P, Bergmann RL, Illi S, et al. Molecular spreading and predictive value of preclinical IgE response to Phleum pratense in children with hay fever. J Allergy Clin Immunol. 2012;130(4):894–901.
59. Posa D, Perna S, Resch Y, Lupinek C, Panetta V, Hofmaier S, et al. Evolution and predictive value of IgE responses toward a comprehensive panel of house dust mite allergens during the first 2 decades of life. J Allergy Clin Immunol. 2017;139(2):541–9.
60. Knol EF. Requirements for effective IgE cross-linking on mast cells and basophils. Mol Nutr Food Res. 2006;50(7):620–4.
61. Gomez E, Campo P, Rondon C, Barrionuevo E, Blanca-Lopez N, Torres MJ, et al. Role of the basophil activation test in the diagnosis of local allergic rhinitis. J Allergy Clin Immunol. 2013;132(4):975–6.e1–5.
62. WHO position paper. Allergen immunotherapy: therapeutic vaccines for allergic diseases. Arerugi. 1998;47(7):698–704.
63. Bousquet J, Pfaar O, Togias A, Schunemann HJ, Ansotegui I, Papadopoulos NG, et al. ARIA Care pathways for allergen immunotherapy. Allergy. 2019;74(11):2087–102.
64. Calderon MA, Cox L, Casale TB, Moingeon P, Demoly P. Multiple-allergen and single-allergen immunotherapy strategies in polysensitized patients: looking at the published evidence. J Allergy Clin Immunol. 2012;129(4):929–34.
65. Bachert C, van Cauwenberge P, Olbrecht J, van Schoor J. Prevalence, classification and perception of allergic and non-allergic rhinitis in Belgium. Allergy. 2006;61(6):693–8.
66. Corriveau MN, Claus B. Allergic and nonallergic rhinitis. In: Kennedy DW, Hwang PH, editors. Rhinology: diseases of nose, sinuses, and skull base. New York: Thieme Medical Publishers, Inc.; 2012. p. 82–91.
67. Fokkens W, Saleh H, Georgalas C. Nonallergic rhinitis: definition, classification, and management. In: Georgalas C, Fokkens W, editors. Rhinology and skull base surgery. New York: Thieme Medical Publishers, Inc.; 2013. p. 229–45.

68. Fokkens WJ. Thoughts on the pathophysiology of non-allergic rhinitis. Curr Allergy Asthma Rep. 2002;2(3):203–9.
69. Van Rijswijk JB, Blom HM, Fokkens WJ. Idiopathic rhinitis, the ongoing quest. Allergy. 2005;60(12):1471–81.
70. Blom HM, Godthelp T, Fokkens WJ, KleinJan A, Mulder PG, Rijntjes E. The effect of nasal steroid aqueous spray on nasal complaint scores and cellular infiltrates in the nasal mucosa of patients with non-allergic, noninfectious perennial rhinitis. J Allergy Clin Immunol. 1997;100(6 Pt 1):739–47.
71. Dolovich J, Kennedy L, Vickerson F, Kazim F. Control of the hypersecretion of vasomotor rhinitis by topical ipratropium bromide. J Allergy Clin Immunol. 1987;80(3 Pt 1):274–8.
72. Van Rijswijk JB, Boeke EL, Keizer JM, Mulder PG, Blom HM, Fokkens WJ. Intranasal capsaicin reduces nasal hyperreactivity in idiopathic rhinitis: a double-blind randomized application regimen study. Allergy. 2003;58(8):754–61.
73. Graf P. Rhinitis medicamentosa: a review of causes and treatment. Treat Respir Med. 2005;4(1):21–9.
74. Slavin RG. Occupational rhinitis. Ann Allergy Asthma Immunol. 1999;83(6 Pt 2):597–601.
75. Ellegård EK, Karlsson NG, Ellegård LH. Rhinitis in the menstrual cycle, pregnancy, and some endocrine disorders. Clin Allergy Immunol. 2007;19:305–21.
76. Jacobs RL, Freedman PM, Boswell RN. Non-allergic rhinitis with eosinophilia (NARES syndrome): clinical and immunologic presentation. J Allergy Clin Immunol. 1981;67(4):253–62.
77. Rondon C, Fernandez J, Canto G, Blanca M. Local allergic rhinitis: concept, clinical manifestations, and diagnostic approach. J Investig Allergol Clin Immunol. 2010;20(5):364–71.
78. Moneret-Vautrin DA, Hsieh V, Wayoff M, Guyot JL, Mouton C, Maria Y. Nonallergic rhinitis with eosinophilia syndrome a precursor of the triad: nasal polyposis, intrinsic asthma, and intolerance to aspirin. Ann Allergy. 1990;64(6):513–8.
79. Malmberg H, Grahne B, Holopainen E, Binder E. Ipratropium (Atrovent) in the treatment of vasomotor rhinitis of elderly patients. Clin Otolaryngol Allied Sci. 1983;8(4):273–6.
80. Sapci T, Yazici S, Evcimik MF, et al. Investigation of the effects of intranasal botulinum toxin type A and ipratropium bromidenasal spray on nasal hypersecretion in idiopathic rhinitis without eosinophilia. Rhinology. 2008;46(1):45–51.
81. Robinson SR, Wormald PJ. Endoscopic vidian neurectomy. Am J Rhinol. 2006;20(2):197–202.
82. Georgalas C, Jovancevic L. Gustory rhinitis. Curr Opin Otolaryngol Head Neck Surg. 2012;20(1):9–14.

23 Acute Sinusitis and Its Complications

Matthew Kim, Aaron Pearlman, Ashutosh Kacker, and Michael G. Stewart

Key Points

- AVRS accounts for most cases of ARS.
- AVRS and AR can predispose for development of ABRS.
- Diagnosis of ARS (including AVRS and ABRS) is primarily clinical.
- Initial management of ARS consists of supportive therapy.
- Antibiotics should be considered after 7 days of symptoms or double-worsening.
- Further evaluation, including imaging, should be considered in patients with treatment failure or suspected complications.
- Management of orbital complications usually entails parenteral antibiotics and multidisciplinary evaluation, with surgery typically reserved for Chandler grades III-V.
- Management of intracranial complications entails parenteral antibiotics, surgery, and multidisciplinary evaluation.
- Episodes of RARS are managed similarly to ABRS, with surgery reserved for patients with frequent infections.
- Immunologic testing and imaging (to evaluate for anatomic factors and rule out CRS) may be helpful in RARS.

23.1 Introduction

Rhinosinusitis is one of the most commonly diagnosed and treated disease entities within otorhinolaryngology. Contemporary understanding of rhinosinusitis as more than simply an anatomic or infectious pathologic process has led to a more sophisticated nosology in the realm of rhinosinusitis, including distinctions based on chronicity and etiology, with even more specific classifications based on pathophysiologic mechanisms now coming to fruition. While this paradigm shift is best evidenced by current concepts surrounding the diagnosis and management of chronic rhinosinusitis, there has been a similar evolution in philosophy with regard to diagnosis of acute rhinosinusitis and the role and timing of antibiotic therapy. This chapter reviews the evaluation and treatment of acute viral rhinosinusitis, acute bacterial rhinosinusitis, and recurrent acute rhinosinusitis. Orbital and intracranial complicates of acute bacterial rhinosinusitis and their management are also reviewed.

M. Kim · A. Pearlman · A. Kacker · M. G. Stewart (✉)
Department of Otolaryngology—Head and Neck Surgery, Weill Cornell Medical College and NewYork-Presbyterian Hospital, New York, NY, USA
e-mail: mk3183@cumc.columbia.edu; anp2022@med.cornell.edu; ask9001@med.cornell.edu; mgs2002@med.cornell.edu

A. Al-Qahtani et al. (eds.), *Textbook of Clinical Otolaryngology*,
https://doi.org/10.1007/978-3-030-54088-3_23

23.1.1 Classification

- Acute rhinosinusitis (ARS) refers to inflammation of the nasal cavity and paranasal sinuses lasting up to 4 weeks. The term "rhinosinusitis" is preferred over sinusitis because there is almost always a component of rhinitis with sinusitis
  - 4–12 weeks: subacute rhinosinusitis
  - >12 weeks: chronic rhinosinusitis (CRS)
- Acute bacterial rhinosinusitis (ABRS) refers to secondary bacterial infection of the paranasal sinuses
- Acute invasive fungal sinusitis refers to a life-threatening, fulminant fungal infection seen in immunocompromised individuals (see chapter on fungal sinusitis)

23.1.2 Epidemiology

- One of the most common health complaints prompting medical evaluation and antibiotic prescription
  - Global prevalence 6–15%
- Associated with significant healthcare expenditures and decreased productivity
- Majority of cases occur in association with viral upper respiratory tract infection
  - Allergic rhinitis is also common predisposing factor.
- Other risk factors include:
  - Age (<15 or >45 years)
  - Smoking history
  - Anatomic variants (deviated nasal septum, concha bullosa, nasal polyposis)
  - Nasal foreign bodies (including nasal cannula, nasogastric tube)

23.1.3 Pathophysiology

- Most frequently caused by viral infection
  - Symptom onset within 24 h of infection
  - Most common pathogens: rhinovirus > influenza > parainfluenza > adenovirus

Table 23.1 Causes of ARS (descending frequency)

Acute rhinosinusitis
Viral
Rhinovirus
Influenza
Parainfluenza
Adenovirus
Bacterial
Streptococcus pneumoniae
Haemophilus influenzae
Moraxella catarrhalis
Staphylococcus aureus
Fungal
Aspergillus spp.
Zygomycetes (*Rhizopus*, *Rhizomucor*, *Mucor*, *Absidia*)

- Progression to ABRS in 0.5–2%
  - Mucosal edema → ↓mucociliary clearance → mucus stasis → bacterial superinfection
  - Most common pathogens: *Streptococcus pneumoniae* > *Haemophilus influenzae* > *Moraxella catarrhalis* > *Staphylococcus aureus* (Table 23.1)

23.1.4 Clinical Presentation

- Acute viral rhinosinusitis (AVRS) and ABRS present with similar symptoms
- Nasal symptoms
  - Congestion/obstruction
  - Purulent rhinorrhea/postnasal drip
  - Facial pain/pressure
  - Decreased olfaction
- Extranasal symptoms
  - Fever
  - Fatigue
  - Cough
  - Ear pressure/fullness
  - Throat pain
  - Dental pain
  - Halitosis
  - Headache
- Features suggestive of ABRS
  - Lack of improvement after 7–10 days
  - "Double sickening or worsening" (worsening after a period of improvement)

23.1.5 Diagnostic Evaluation

- Exam findings
  - Facial exam: edema/erythema, tenderness
  - Anterior rhinoscopy: mucosal edema, turbinate hypertrophy, copious clear or purulent rhinorrhea
  - Oral exam: postnasal drainage, pharyngeal erythema
- Nasal endoscopy helpful in certain cases
  - Severe symptoms
  - Unilateral disease
  - Failure to respond to treatment
  - Suspected mass
  - Recent surgery
  - Immunocompromised patient
  - Suspected complicated infection
- Diagnosis based primarily on history and exam
  - Routine imaging NOT indicated
  - Imaging indicated under special circumstances
    - Suspected orbital or intracranial complication
    - Suspected recurrent acute rhinosinusitis
  - Comparison of imaging modalities
    - Ultrasonography: not recommended
    - Plain film radiography (X-ray): historically used, not recommended
    - Computed tomography (CT): excellent bony resolution, radiation exposure
    - Magnetic resonance imaging (MRI): excellent soft tissue resolution, no radiation exposure, sensitive for intracranial and orbital infection
- Cultures
  - Not required for diagnosis, but can have treatment implications
  - Middle meatal cultures correlate well with maxillary sinus aspiration
  - Nasal or nasopharyngeal swab cultures not clinically useful

23.1.6 Treatment

- Symptomatic relief
  - Indicated for both AVRS and ABRS
  - Systemic agents: analgesics/antipyretics, decongestants, mucolytics
  - Topical agents (sprays): steroids, saline, decongestants (limit use to 3–5 days)
- Antimicrobial therapy for ABRS
  - Watchful waiting appropriate up to 7 days after diagnosis
  - Antibiotics typically started for clinical worsening or persistent symptoms after 7 days
  - First-line antibiotic choice is amoxicillin or amoxicillin/clavulanate
    - Alternatives in Penicillin-allergic patients: third-generation cephalosporin ± clindamycin, doxycycline, fluoroquinolone
      - Macrolides and trimethoprim-sulfamethoxazole no longer recommended for initial therapy due to increasing prevalence of resistance
  - Duration of treatment 5–10 days
  - Risk of antibiotic therapy
    - Allergic reactions
    - GI upset
    - Development of bacterial resistance
- Treatment failure: worsening or failure to improve after 7 days of initial treatment
  - Consider alternate diagnoses
    - Facial pain and headache syndromes
    - Rhinitis
    - Nasal airway obstruction
  - Evaluate for possible complications of ABRS (see below)
  - Middle meatal cultures
  - Change antibiotic
    - High-dose amoxicillin/clavulanate
    - Respiratory fluoroquinolone
  - Failure of multiple antibiotic courses
    - Imaging to evaluate for anatomic abnormality or complicated ABRS
    - Middle meatal culture
  - Relapse after treatment
    - Mild → longer course of same antibiotic
    - Moderate to severe → consider change in antibiotic and/or imaging
- Oral steroids not recommended for routine use
  - Not helpful as monotherapy

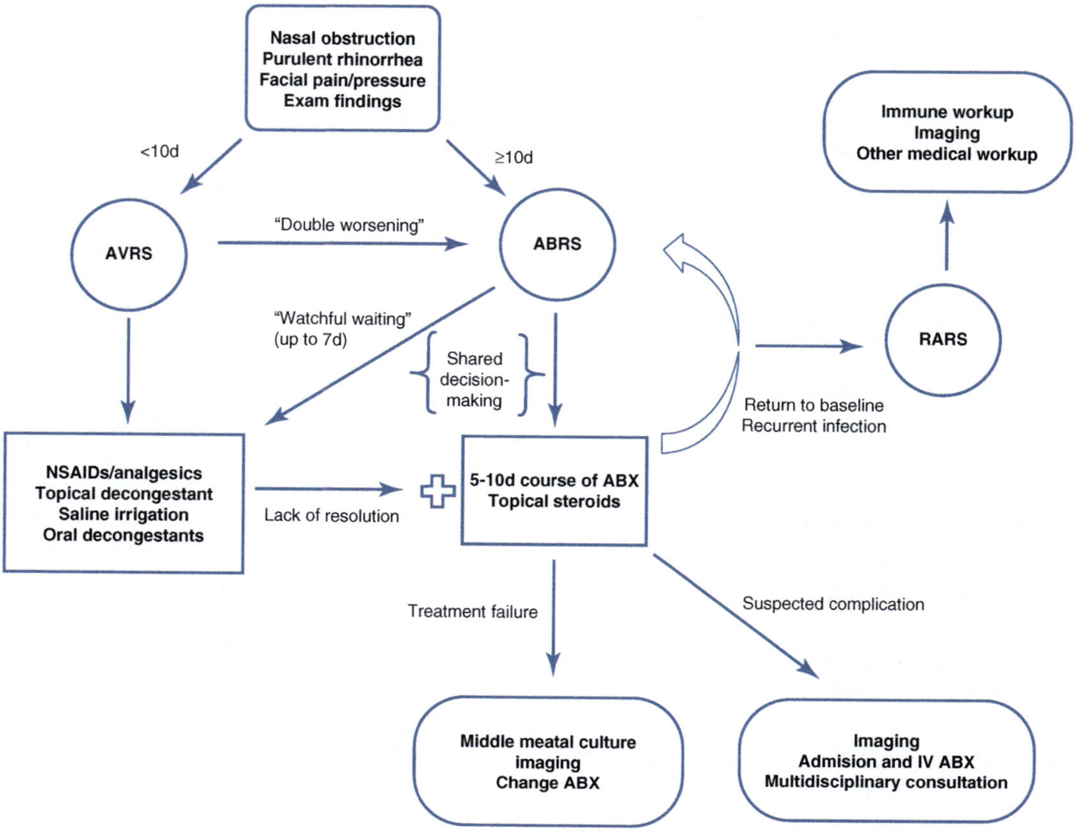

Fig. 23.1 ARS treatment algorithm

- May shorten time to symptom resolution when used in conjunction with antibiotics
  - Risk of adverse effects
- Oral antihistamines not recommended for ABRS
  - May be helpful in allergic patients for AVRS
  - Can lead to nasal dryness
  - Can cause drowsiness and xerostomia (Fig. 23.1)

23.1.7 Complications

- Suspect in patients with atypical signs and symptoms:
  - Persistent high fever
  - Periorbital edema/erythema, proptosis, diplopia/extraocular motility impairment, vision changes
  - Cranial nerve palsy
  - Headache, meningeal signs
  - Altered mental signs
- Predisposing factors
  - Winter months (increased incidence of AVRS)
  - Age
    - Infant: highest risk of meningitis
    - 3–6 years: highest rate of hospitalization for complication of ABRS
    - 10–29 years: highest risk of intracranial complication
      - Teenage males likely to have simultaneous orbital and intracranial complications
- Orbital complications
  - Most common complication of acute rhinosinusitis
    - Due to two-way communication between ethmoid and ophthalmic venous plexuses

        - Valveless ophthalmic veins communicate anteriorly with facial veins and posteriorly with cavernous sinus

      Periorbita is the only soft tissue barrier between orbit and sinonasal cavity

        - Fuses anteriorly with tarsal plates to form orbital septum

      Usually polymicrobial

        - Viridans streptococci and staphylococci are most common organisms

  - Chandler classification system of orbital complications

      I: Preseptal orbital cellulitis

        - Periorbital edema/erythema
        - No chemosis or ocular symptoms
        - Can occur in absence of sinusitis
          - Infection of eyelid and orbital adnexa
          - Trauma
          - Foreign body

      II: Postseptal orbital cellulitis

        - Proptosis, chemosis, ophthalmoplegia
        - Can have decreased visual acuity later in disease course

      III: Orbital subperiosteal abscess

        - Symptoms similar to group II
        - Usually normal vision unless abscess very large

      IV: Orbital abscess

        - Symptoms similar to group III
        - Usually complete ophthalmoplegia and decrease in vision

      V: Cavernous sinus thrombosis

        - Symptoms similar to group IV
        - Additional involvement of V1 and V2
        - Bilateral eye symptoms
        - Can have associated meningismus, frank meningitis, or sepsis

  - Orbital apex syndrome

      Presents similar to cavernous sinus thrombosis with frank optic nerve involvement

      Trigeminal involvement would be limited to V1 branches

  - Superior orbital fissure (Rochon–Duvigneaud) syndrome

      Similar to orbital apex syndrome but spares optic nerve

  - Evaluation

      Comprehensive ophthalmologic exam

      Imaging

        - CT is the gold standard
          - IV contrast useful if concern for abscess or cavernous sinus thrombosis
        - MRI is better for cavernous sinus thrombosis

  - Management

      Medical therapy—oral agents—is usually sufficient (Chandler I–II)

      Intravenous antibiotics (Chandler II–V)

        - High-dose penicillin/beta-lactamase inhibitor (e.g., ampicillin/sulbactam) or third-generation cephalosporin
        - Adjunct medications: systemic/topical steroids and decongestants, saline irrigations, mucolytics

      Surgery (Chandler IV–V)

        - Subperiosteal abscess (III): size >2 cm and age >9 years more likely to require surgical intervention
        - Lack of improvement over 48–72 h on medical therapy alone also indication for surgery
        - Lateral and superior abscesses likely require external orbitotomy

      Anticoagulation for cavernous sinus thrombosis is controversial

        - Thought to stop progression of thrombosis, decrease clot propagation, and allow better antibiotic penetration
        - Risk includes systemic or intracranial hemorrhage and septic embolization

- Frontal bone osteomyelitis with subperiosteal abscess ("Pott's puffy tumor")
  - Suppurative infection of diploic veins
  - Causes bone demineralization and necrosis
  - Requires medical and surgical therapy

      Prolonged IV antibiotics for osteomyelitis

- Intracranial complications
  - More common in males and children >7 years
  - CRS thought to increase risk due to chronic mucosal/bony changes that decrease mucociliary clearance and hinder antibiotic penetration
    - Initial symptoms may not be characteristic of ARS
      - Persistent headache and fever are typical presenting complaints
  - Mechanism: septic thrombophlebitis or direct bony extension (neurovascular foramina, congenital dehiscence, traumatic fracture)
  - Microbiology
    - Meningitis mostly due to *Streptococcus pneumoniae*
    - Abscess often polymicrobial, including anaerobes
  - May be asymptomatic until late in course due to involvement of non-eloquent frontal lobe
    - Seizures, focal neurologic deficits are late findings and portend poor prognosis
    - Can present synchronously and in conjunction with orbital complications
  - MRI with contrast is radiographic study of choice
    - CT often also obtained for bony anatomy and surgical planning
  - Epidural abscess
    - Most common intracranial complication
    - Generally associated with frontal sinusitis
      - Headache, fever, orbital pain, frontal pain
    - Favorable prognosis
  - Subdural abscess
    - Also usually a sequela of frontal sinusitis
    - Usually unilateral
    - Tendency to spread over cerebral cortex and into interhemispheric region
    - Higher morbidity and mortality
      - Can have rapid progression
      - Headaches, fever, letharg → coma
      - Meningismus and focal neurologic deficits
  - Intracerebral abscess
    - Less common
    - Typically involves frontal and parietal lobes
      - Frontal sinusitis > sphenoid/ethmoid sinusitis
    - Fever, headache, lethargy, vomiting
      - Seizures, focal deficits are late findings
      - Can also have mood swings and behavioral changes
    - Lumbar puncture contraindicated before imaging obtained
      - Risk of brain herniation
  - Venous sinus thrombosis
    - Sagittal sinus thrombosis can occur secondary to frontal sinusitis
    - Meningeal signs and significant neurologic complications
    - Often in conjunction with other intracranial complications
  - Meningitis
    - Typically secondary to ethmoiditis or sphenoiditis
    - Headache, neck stiffness, fever
    - Can present with sepsis or cranial neuropathy
    - Often in conjunction with other intracranial complications
  - Management
    - Broad-spectrum intravenous antibiotics with good intracranial penetration
      - Often 4–8 week course of antibiotics
    - Systemic steroids and anticonvulsants
    - Neurosurgical drainage usually indicated
    - Sinus surgery to address culprit sinuses
      - Frontal sinus trephination can be useful adjunct to endoscopic techniques
    - Repeat imaging critical to monitor treatment response and prior to discharge to ensure continued resolution without treatment escalation

23.1.8 Recurrent Acute Rhinosinusitis

- Predisposing factors
  - Viral ARS
  - Allergic rhinitis
  - Immunodeficiency
  - Anatomy (e.g., deviated nasal septum, concha bullosa)
- Confirming true ABRS episodes is important
  - Endoscopy reveals purulence during acute episode
  - Imaging between episodes can confirm complete resolution and reveal anatomic anomalies
- Management
  - Immunologic testing
    Immunoglobulin deficiencies
    - Combined variable immunodeficiency (CVID)
    - IgA deficiency
    - Specific antibody deficiency
  - Role of antibiotics and topical steroids limited to use during ARS episodes
  - Surgery may be beneficial in select patients
    Appropriateness criteria
    - ≥4 episodes per year
    - ARS confirmed by endoscopy or imaging
    - Shared decision-making
    - Failed trial of nasal steroid or loss of productivity

    Extent of surgery unclear
    - Addressing anatomic variants predisposing to recurrent infection can be helpful
  - Balloon sinuplasty may also be beneficial
    Less evidence than for ESS, for this indication

Take Home Messages
- ARS can be characterized by causative pathogen (virus, bacteria, fungus).
- Diagnosis is chiefly clinical.
- Treatment depends on etiology and symptom duration.
- Complications of ABRS warrant special attention.

Further Reading

Clayman GL, Adams GL, Paugh DR, Koopmann CF Jr. Intracranial complications of paranasal sinusitis: a combined institutional review. Laryngoscope. 1991;101(3):234–9.

Fokkens WJ, Lund VJ, Hopkins C, et al. European position paper on rhinosinusitis and nasal polyps 2020. Rhinology. 2020;58(Suppl S29):1–464.

Orlandi RR, Kingdom TT, Hwang PH, et al. International Consensus Statement on Allergy and Rhinology: Rhinosinusitis. Int Forum Allergy Rhinol. 2016;6(Suppl 1):S22–209.

Peña MT, Preciado D, Orestes M, Choi S. Orbital complications of acute sinusitis: changes in the post-pneumococcal vaccine era. JAMA Otolaryngol Head Neck Surg. 2013;139(3):223–7.

Rosenfeld RM, Andes D, Bhattacharyya N, Cheung D, Eisenberg S, Ganiats TG, Gelzer A, Hamilos D, Haydon RC III, Hudgins PA, Jones S, Krouse HJ, Lee LH, Mahoney MC, Marple BF, Mitchell CJ, Nathan R, Shiffman RN, Smith TL, Witsell DL. Clinical practice guideline: adult sinusitis. Otolaryngol Head Neck Surg. 2007;137(3 Suppl):S1–31.

Rosenfeld RM, Piccirillo JF, Chandrasekhar SS, et al. Clinical practice guideline (update): adult sinusitis. Otolaryngol Head Neck Surg. 2015;152(2 Suppl):S1–S39.

Fungal Sinusitis

24

Daniel B. Spielman, Zhong Zheng, Abtin Tabaee, and Michael G. Stewart

Key Points

- Fungal rhinosinusitis represents a group of distinct clinical entities linked by the presence of pathogenic fungi within the paranasal sinuses that are implicated in the pathophysiology. Given the unique features of each disorder, it is more appropriate to think of the different forms of fungal rhinosinusitis as separate diseases.
- The following represent the different forms of fungal rhinosinusitis: fungus ball (mycetoma), allergic fungal rhinosinusitis, acute invasive fungal sinusitis, chronic invasive fungal sinusitis, and granulomatous invasive fungal sinusitis.
- Can be categorized based on different variables:
  - Chronicity: Acute (acute invasive fungal sinusitis) vs chronic (chronic invasive fungal, granulomatous, fungus ball, allergic fungal sinusitis)
  - Role of fungi: Infection (acute and chronic invasive fungal sinusitis) vs inflammatory trigger (allergic fungal sinusitis, granulomatous, fungus ball)
  - Host status: Immunocompetent (allergic fungal sinusitis, fungus ball, granulomatous) vs immunosuppressed (acute and chronic invasive fungal sinusitis)
  - Presence of tissue invasion: Invasive (acute and chronic invasive fungal sinusitis) vs noninvasive (allergic fungal sinusitis, granulomatous, fungus ball)
- Evaluation includes clinical assessment, imaging, tissue culture and histopathology.
- Multimodality treatment is indicated and differs for the different types of fungal rhinosinusitis.

24.1 Introduction

Fungal pathogens have the potential to cause a wide spectrum of sinonasal disease, affecting both immunocompetent and immunosuppressed patients. Fungal rhinosinusitis represents a group of distinct disease entities ranging from benign noninvasive mycetoma formation to acutely ful-

D. B. Spielman · Z. Zheng · A. Tabaee
M. G. Stewart (✉)
Department of Otolaryngology—Head and Neck Surgery, Weill Cornell Medical Center and New York-Presbyterian Hospital, New York, NY, USA
e-mail: dbs9010@nyp.org; atabaee@med.cornell.edu; mgs2002@med.cornell.edu

A. Al-Qahtani et al. (eds.), *Textbook of Clinical Otolaryngology*,
https://doi.org/10.1007/978-3-030-54088-3_24

minant tissue invasion. While certain species of fungi may be more aggressive, the clinical phenotype that develops is the result of a complex interplay between the host immune system and the characteristics of the pathogen. Proper diagnosis is essential and is based on multimodality evaluation. A high suspicion is essential to detect acute invasive fungal sinusitis in immunosuppressed patients as the risk of lethal disease may be mitigated by early medical and surgical therapy. This chapter reviews each form of fungal rhinosinusitis including clinical presentation, diagnostic testing, and treatment modalities.

24.2 Fungus Ball (Mycetoma)

Demographics/Epidemiology

- Mass of fungal hyphae and associated inflammatory changes within the lumen of the involved paranasal sinus. Absence of tissue invasion.
- Occurs in immunocompetent individuals. No relation to atopic disease.
- Most commonly in the maxillary sinus followed by the sphenoid sinus.

Disease Pathophysiology

- Overgrowth of fungal debris, ostial obstruction secondary to inflammatory changes, and bony changes of the involved sinus can occur over long periods of time. Secondary bacterial infection may occur.
- *Aspergillus fumigatus* and dematiaceous species are the most common fungi present.

Clinical Presentation, Symptoms, Disease Course

- Symptoms may be limited or absent. Inflammatory changes of the involved sinus occur slowly and may be subclinical.
- Initial detection may be based on an incidental finding on imaging.
- Endoscopic examination of the middle meatus and sphenoethmoid recess may be normal. Mild nonspecific inflammatory changes may be noted.

Diagnostic Testing

- Imaging studies in combination with intraoperative findings and tissue pathology are diagnostic.
- Computed tomography (see Fig. 24.1):
  - Complete or near complete opacification of a single sinus without inflammatory changes in the other sinuses.
  - Heterogenous opacification on imaging with hypoattenuation of the surrounding mucosa and hyperattenuation of the fungal ball.
  - Focal areas of calcification and hyperdensity are common secondary to the presence of heavy metals including iron, magnesium, and manganese.
  - Thickening and sclerosis of the surrounding bony walls may occur. Focal areas of thinning and erosion may also occur.
- Magnetic resonance imaging:
  - Hypointense inflammatory changes on T1 and T2 due to absence of free water.

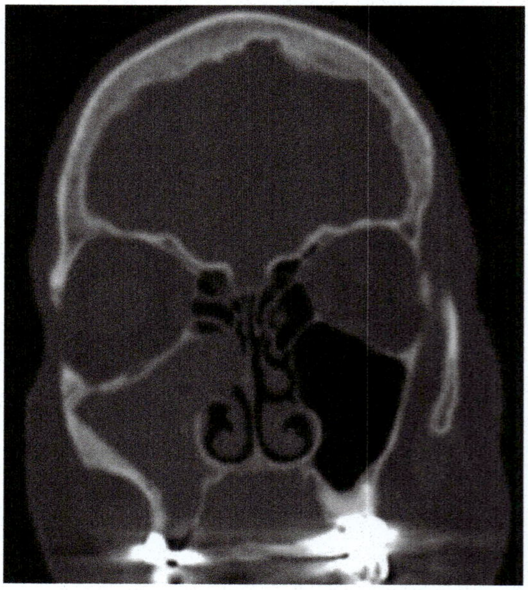

Fig. 24.1 Fungus ball. CT scan is notable for unifocal, complete opacification of the right maxillary sinus by polypoid soft tissue with focal areas of hyperdensity. Osteitic changes of the maxillary sinus walls, and widening/expansion of the natural maxillary ostial region are also noted

Presence of paramagnetic metals may be seen on MRI.

Treatment Principles

- Treatment is based on endoscopic antrostomy of the involved sinus and clearance of the fungal debris within the sinus cavity. Creation of a wide antrostomy and aggressive irrigation of the cavity at the time of surgery can facilitate healing. Tissue biopsy and culture should be performed to confirm diagnosis.
- Antibiotic therapy may be indicated if there is secondary bacterial infection.
- Antifungal therapy is not indicated.

24.3 Allergic Fungal Sinusitis (AFS)

Demographics/Epidemiology

- First described by B Safirstein in 1976, followed by a case series by AA Katzenstein in 1983
- Most commonly affects younger, immunocompetent, atopic patients
- Male predominance (1.5–2.6:1) [1]
- More common in temperate, warm, and high humidity environments (e.g., Mississippi river basin and southern United States)
- Subtype of chronic rhinosinusitis, representing 5–10% of cases, depending on the region

Disease Pathophysiology

- Multifactorial with an interplay of host and environmental factors
- Inflammatory mediated, in contrast to infectious variants of fungal sinusitis
- Similar to allergic bronchopulmonary aspergillosis (ABPA) in the lower airway
- Eosinophilic Th-2 inflammatory pathway activation, similar to other subtypes of CRSwNP
- Immune barrier hypothesis
  - Chronic fungal colonization and proliferation, impaired nasal epithelial barrier function, activation of type 2 inflammation, development of nasal polyposis
- Associated with immunocompetent state, atopy, comorbid allergic rhinitis, eosinophilia, and asthma
- Common fungal species
  - Dematiaceous family—*Bipolaris, Alternaria, Curvularia, Exserohilum, Fusarium*
  - *Aspergillus* spp.

Clinical Presentation, Symptoms, Disease Course

- Indolent course with progressive nasal obstruction, rhinorrhea, postnasal drainage, facial pressure, hyposmia/anosmia
- Commonly asymmetric presentation, but may be bilateral
- Significant nasal polyposis
- Pain is not common
- Characterized by progressive bony demineralization, expansion, remodeling, and erosion
- Facial dysmorphia if significant bony remodeling
- Orbital complications
  - Proptosis, diplopia, or acute visual loss if orbital extension and optic nerve compression
- Intracranial complications (which are rare)
  - Meningitis, epidural, or subdural abscesses

Diagnostic Testing

- Endoscopy
  - Polypoid changes of nasal mucosa, mucoid discharge, mucosal crusting, and eosinophilic mucin may be seen
- CT sinus without contrast (see Fig. 24.2):
  - Opacification of involved sinuses, commonly asymmetric
  - Characteristic heterogeneous signal intensity within sinus cavity with central areas of hyperattenuation
  - Accumulation of ferromagnetic debris (iron, magnesium, manganese, etc.) within allergic fungal mucin
- MRI (see Fig. 24.3):
  - Better soft tissue resolution

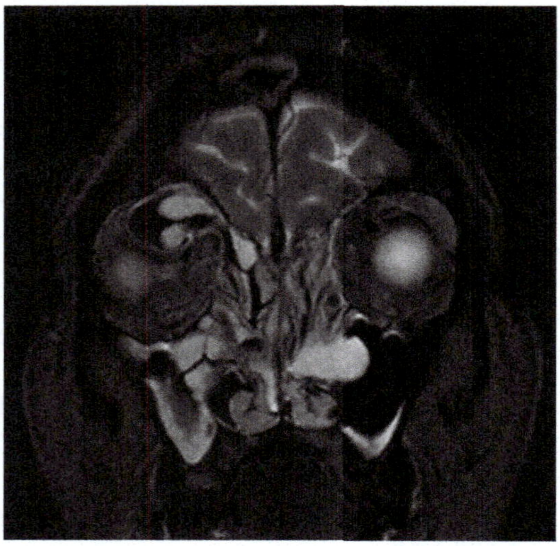

Fig. 24.3 Allergic fungal sinusitis. Coronal T2 fat suppressed MRI scan demonstrates diffuse inflammatory changes with mixed signal characteristics including areas of relative hypointensity. Right frontal-orbital dehiscence with inferior displacement of the orbital contents by a heterogenous inflammatory collection is noted

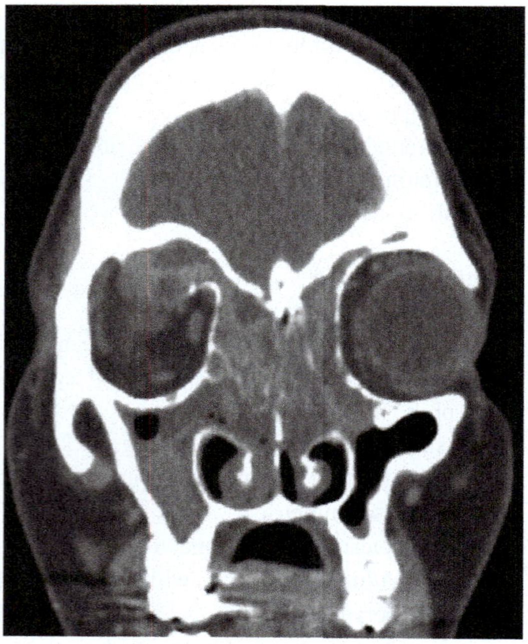

Fig. 24.2 Allergic fungal sinusitis. CT is notable for extensive paranasal sinus opacification, right frontal-orbital dehiscence, and a possible orbital collection. Heterogenous density of the inflammatory tissue in the paranasal sinuses is noted

  - Useful to assess areas of concern for orbital or intracranial extension
  - Low water content of allergic mucin, combined with high water content of edematous sinonasal mucosa readily appreciated on T2 weighted images
- Elevated level of total serum IgE (>1000 IU/ml) [2]
- Hypersensitivity on skin testing or radioallergosorbent test (RAST) to fungal antigens
- Definitive diagnosis requires pathologic specimen obtained at time of surgery
- Bent and Kuhn criteria
  - Major criteria
    - Nasal polyposis
    - Type I hypersensitivity to fungal antigen on skin testing or RAST
    - Characteristic CT findings
    - Eosinophilic mucin
    - Noninvasive fungal elements in sinus content
  - Minor criteria
    - Bone erosion
    - Unilateral disease
    - Charcot–Leyden crystals
    - Peripheral eosinophilia
    - Positive fungal culture
- Histology
  - Eosinophilic mucin
    - Thick tenacious and viscous consistency
    - Light tan to brown or green in color
- Noninvasive fungal hyphae within sheets of eosinophils or Charcot–Leyden crystals (derived from eosinophils breakdown products) [3]
- Fungal stains can help identify fungal elements
- Fungal culture
  - Not a major diagnostic criterion
  - May be isolated in other subtypes of rhinosinusitis
  - Low sensitivity for fungal growth

Treatment Principles

- Endoscopic sinus surgery
  - An important component of multidisciplinary management

- Allows for pathology and culture necessary for diagnosis
- Creation of large antrostomies to allow complete clearing of polypoid inflammatory tissue, fungal debris, and eosinophilic mucin
- Allows postoperative surveillance, debridement, and access to topical therapy
- Commonly have expanded sinuses and bony thinning due to chronic remodeling. Need for careful surgical technique near the orbit and skull base to avoid injury

- Postoperative medical therapy
  - Topical corticosteroid irrigation
    Intranasal sprays vs. large volume saline irrigations with dissolved steroids
    Extrapolated from CRSwNP data
    Improve mucosal edema and patient-reported outcomes [4]
  - Systemic corticosteroid
    Short burst courses in the perioperative period can prevent exacerbation and early recurrence, and are generally well tolerated [5, 6]
    Risks of therapy include weight gain, hyperglycemia, mood disturbances, insomnia, gastric ulceration, and rarely adrenal insufficiency or avascular necrosis of the hip
  - Immunotherapy [4, 7]
    Systemic desensitization (e.g., allergy shots) to fungal antigens is an option in recalcitrant cases
    May decrease rate of recurrence and reduce steroid requirement
    May start 6 weeks postoperatively after sufficient mucosal healing
  - Systemic antifungal
    Lack of evidence for routine use
    Reserved for patients refractory to topical and systemic corticosteroid, or as steroid-sparing alternative to wean off long-term steroid dependence [4]
    Potential for hepatotoxicity with oral antifungal therapy
  - Topical antifungal
    Recent, controlled studies have demonstrated lack of efficacy. Not recommended for routine use in AFS [3, 6]
  - Monoclonal antibodies
    Data extrapolated from CRSwNP literature
    Gan et al. [8]– improvement in SNOT-22 and endoscopy scores and reduction in steroid and antifungal therapy requirements in AFS patients treated with omalizumab (monoclonal antibody to IgE). Monoclonal antibodies to IL3, 4, and 5 may have potential roles in AFS management
    May be a consideration in patients with AFS and lower airway disease refractory to surgery and topical steroid therapy

24.4 Acute Invasive Fungal Sinusitis (AIFS)

Epidemiology

- AIFS is a rapidly progressive fungal infection of the sinonasal mucosa, deep tissues and with the potential to spread into the structures surrounding the paranasal sinuses.
- Occurs primarily in immunosuppressed patients including poorly controlled diabetes mellitus (especially with ketoacidosis), hematologic malignancies, stem cell and solid organ transplant patients. An absolute neutrophil count <1000/μL is a risk factor.

Pathophysiology

- Two groups of fungi—belonging to the genus Aspergillus or the order Mucorales (*Rhizopus* spp., *Rhizomucor* spp., *Absidia* spp., and *Mucor* spp.)
- Invasion of fungi into vessel walls causes endothelial damage and thrombosis. Angioinvasion and tissue necrosis are the hallmarks of histologic diagnosis

Clinical Presentation

- Symptoms—Symptoms are nonspecific and may mimic acute rhinosinusitis. Atypical symptoms may include facial paresthesias, facial hypesthesia, facial edema, and vision changes. Facial hypesthesia most commonly

occurs from infraorbital nerve (V2) involvement.
- The presence of sinusitis type symptoms in an immunocompromised host should raise the concern for AIFS especially if the symptoms are asymmetric, atypical, or fulminant.
- Onset is acute and disease progression can be rapid.
- The underlying immunosuppression often means a reduced inflammatory response, and patients may be surprisingly asymptomatic.

Diagnostic Testing

- Nasal endoscopy—Mucosal edema, pallor, ulceration, or necrosis often involve the middle turbinate and septum but can be isolated anywhere within the sinonasal cavity. Areas of involvement are often insensate. In one study, nearly 30% of patients with AIFS had normal findings on nasal endoscopy [9].
- Imaging—Both CT scan and MRI have utility in diagnosis. Imaging should be performed in all patients with high clinical suspicion, even if nasal endoscopy is negative. Conflicting data exist about which modality is more sensitive and specific [10, 11].
- Contrast CT—hypoattenuating lesion with lack of contrast uptake by devascularized and necrotic tissue. Bony dehiscence including peri-orbital, nasolacrimal duct and skull base regions is best assessed on CT. Soft tissue changes of the orbit and pterygopalatine fossa are concerning for spread outside of the paranasal sinuses.
- MRI—greater soft tissue definition to determine the extent of surrounding involvement in the pterygopalatine fossa, orbit, intracranial cavity, and retroantral fat.
- Histopathology—essential to obtain definitive diagnosis.
  - Evaluate platelets and coagulopathy status before performing a bedside biopsy.
  - Patients with suspicious findings on imaging, but no lesions on nasal endoscopy, should be taken to the operating room for sinusotomy and biopsy.
  - Permanent pathology section is the gold standard for diagnosis, but processing time is lengthy.
  - Sensitivity of frozen section is 84% while the negative predictive value is 0.72 [12]. Taking multiple biopsies increases the likelihood of obtaining a correct diagnosis.
  - The characteristic histopathologic findings include fungal elements invading the mucosa, submucosa, vessel walls with thrombosis, and tissue necrosis. Fungal stains including methenamine silver are necessary. Mucor hyphae are broad, irregular, non-septated with 90° branching. *Aspergillus* hyphae have 45° branching patterns with septations.
- Cultures—sensitivity is 55% and should not be used for diagnostic purposes because the time required for processing unnecessarily delays treatment. Tissue cultures should be obtained in the operating room to guide antifungal therapy.
- Laboratory markers
  - Elevated CRP is a predictor of worse prognosis [13].
  - Positive serum galactomannan test suggests the presence of invasive aspergillosis, although sensitivity is limited and it will not detect species of the Mucorales order.
- Diagnostic criteria
  - Symptoms <4 weeks
  - Sinonasal mucosal thickening or supportive findings on imaging and/ or nasal endoscopy
  - Tissue pathology consistent with invasive fungal sinusitis
- The foundation of treatment is multimodality therapy aimed at reversing the underlying immunosuppressed state, surgical debridement of necrotic, nonviable tissue and systemic antifungal therapy.
- Medical Therapy—Treatment should begin with intravenous antifungal medication but can be transitioned to oral after disease control.
  - Empiric treatment of mucormycosis or AIFS of unknown pathogen: amphotericin B (coverage of both mucormycosis and aspergillus).

  - First-line treatment of confirmed invasive aspergillus: voriconazole.
  - Alternative, salvage antifungal agents: itraconazole, posaconazole, micafungin, or caspofungin.
  - Reversal of immunosuppression is essential for treatment success. Infusion of granulocyte colony stimulating factor is recommended in neutropenic patients.
  - Blood glucose levels must be corrected in diabetics.
  - Nasal saline irrigations postoperatively; consider the addition of topical amphotericin B although efficacy is unclear.
- Surgical Therapy
  - Urgent surgery is indicated in all patients able to tolerate surgical intervention. The objective is to resect all gross disease using intraoperative frozen section to confirm negative margins. Disease restricted to the sinonasal cavity can typically be addressed endoscopically. Advanced disease may require open approaches. Serial debridements with short interval periods of time for surveillance and managing disease progression. Orbital exenteration may be indicated in 21% of cases [14].
  - Patient counseling regarding the life-threatening nature of the infection, implications of serial surgical debridements, and realistic goals associated with extended surgery (e.g., orbital exenteration) are important considerations.

Prognosis
- The ability to achieve reversal of the underlying immunosuppression combined with surgery and antifungal therapy is the best overall predictor of survival [15].
- Time to treatment predicts mortality. This supports the need for active vigilance in the assessment of immunosuppressed patients with sinusitis.
- Mortality is approximately 50%.

24.5 Chronic Invasive Fungal Sinusitis (CIFS)

Epidemiology
- CIFS affects immunosuppressed individuals although cases in immunocompetent patients have been reported. In contrast to AIFS, these patients do not generally have neutropenia or uncontrolled diabetes.
- Common Risk Factors—diabetes, chronic renal disease, chronic liver disease, and long-term corticosteroid use.

Pathophysiology
- Most frequently caused by Aspergillus molds, especially *Aspergillus fumigatus*, but cases of Candida and Mucor species have been reported. These same fungal species commonly exist and can be cultured in noninvasive forms of inflammatory CRS.
- The true pathophysiology or impetus for invasive disease is unknown, but is likely related to the interaction between the host immune system and the pathogen.
- The presence of mixed disease in some cases suggests the potential that an infection may evolve from one disease state to another in response to host factors.

Clinical Presentation
- Indolent course often developing over several months. Patients present with both nasal and extranasal symptoms, including facial pain/edema and orbital symptoms. Some present with orbital apex syndrome.

Diagnostic Testing
- Nasal Endoscopy—There is no singular pathognomonic finding. Purulence, mucosal edema, pallor, ulceration, and necrosis may be present. Disease may be restricted to a particular sinus, making nasal endoscopy unremarkable.
- Imaging—unilateral mucosal thickening often presenting as a mass lesion with surrounding

bony destruction that can be indistinguishable from a malignancy.
- Noncontrast CT scan—lesion is hyperattenuated with surrounding bony destruction.
- MRI—lesion is hypoattenuated on T1 and T2-weighted sequences. Involvement of surrounding soft tissue structures, such as the preantral or orbital fat, suggests invasive disease.
- Biopsy—The gold standard for diagnosis is histopathologic analysis, therefore biopsy is essential.
  - Histopathology reveals fungal hyphae in the setting of non-granulomatous chronic inflammation with mixed cellularity.
  - PCR can corroborate a diagnosis and identify a pathogen.
- Cultures—culture data may contribute to selecting appropriate medical therapy, but does not serve a role in diagnostic purposes.
  - Cultures are positive in approximately 50% of cases.
- Diagnostic criteria
  - Symptoms >12 weeks
  - Sinonasal mucosal thickening or lesion on imaging or endoscopy
  - Hyphal forms on histopathologic exam with invasion of the mucosa or bone in the setting of non-granulomatous inflammation. Necrosis may be present but is not requisite.

Treatment Principles
- Medical Management—Treatment is individualized with extensive variability in the literature. Most advocate the use of systemic antifungal medications, although one study by Li et al. demonstrates successful cure in some patients with surgical therapy alone [16].
  - Antifungal medication: Voriconazole is the first-line agent for aspergillus, but if the species cannot be cultured or the patient's clinical status worsens, other agents should be considered, including amphotericin B, posaconazole, itraconazole, micafungin, and caspofungin.
  - Topical nasal saline irrigation should be performed postoperatively. Topical amphotericin B may be added to nasal irrigations although there is limited supportive literature.
  - Duration of therapy is variable without clear guidelines, typically 3–4 months. Endoscopic and imaging surveillance should be performed before discontinuing treatment.
- Surgical Management—endoscopic sinus surgery is indicated in all cases for both diagnostic and therapeutic benefit. The treatment paradigm mirrors that of AIFS, with a goal of resecting all gross and microscopic disease followed by prolonged systemic antifungal therapy.

Prognosis
- In contrast to AIFS, the prognosis of CIFS is excellent. Published cure rates range from 89–100% with rare reports of mortality.

24.6 Granulomatous Invasive Fungal Sinusitis (GIFS)

Epidemiology
- The least prevalent subtype of fungal sinusitis. True incidence is unknown.
- Most commonly occurs in the Middle East, Northern Africa, and India. It is likely underdiagnosed in these regions, comprising 30% of cases of fungal sinusitis in some areas. Very uncommonly reported in North America.
- Affects immunocompetent individuals; M > F, more common in ages 20–35 years old. There is no known risk factor.

Pathophysiology
- Infection is caused by fungal invasion into surrounding tissues evoking a granulomatous response with associated necrosis.
- *Aspergillus flavus* is isolated almost exclusively. *Aspergillus fumigatus* has been reported.

Clinical Presentation
- Indolent course developing over several months with a similar presentation to CIFS. Most commonly patients exhibit orbital manifestations, including diplopia and propto-

sis. Cavernous sinus syndrome has also been reported.

Diagnostic Evaluation

- Nasal endoscopy—GIFS is not easily differentiated from AIFS or CIFS on nasal endoscopy. Endoscopic findings can range from a normal nasal cavity to mucosal edema, pallor, ulceration, or necrosis.
- Imaging—CT and MRI provide valuable information about the extent of bony erosion and soft tissue involvement respectively. The imaging findings are the same as those for CGIS.
- Biopsy—essential for definitive diagnosis.
  - Histopathologic findings—chronic granulomatous inflammation with invasive fungal hyphae in the mucosa and within the cytoplasm of multinucleated giant cells.
- Cultures—Intraoperative cultures should be taken to help guide medical therapy, in the event of resistance or poor clinical response. Culture data does not reveal an isolate in many cases and therefore has no role in diagnosis.
- Diagnostic Criteria
  - Symptoms >12 weeks
  - Sinonasal mucosal thickening or lesion on imaging or endoscopy
  - Hyphal forms on histopathologic exam with invasion of the mucosa or bone in the setting of granulomatous inflammation.

Treatment Principles

- Medical Management
  - Nasal saline irrigation; consider addition of topical amphotericin B
  - Systemic antifungal therapy—voriconazole is the first-line therapy. Alternative options for patients with worsening clinical status include amphotericin B, posaconazole, itraconazole, and micafungin.
  - Duration of therapy—continuation of systemic antifungals is recommended for a minimum of 3 months although there is no standard treatment protocol. Close surveillance should be performed, especially before discontinuing therapy.
- Surgical Management—endoscopic sinus surgery is indicated to achieve source control. Open procedures are not necessary unless there is involvement of the orbit, palate, or intracranial cavity.

Prognosis

- Outcome data is extremely limited and exists only in the form of case reports.

Take Home Messages

- The diagnosis of allergic fungal rhinosinusitis is described by the Bent and Kuhn criteria. Nasal endoscopy may reveal nasal polyposis, mucosal edema, and allergic mucin. Imaging demonstrates heterogeneous sinus opacification potentially with surrounding bony demineralization and asymmetry.
- Maintaining a high index of suspicion for acute invasive fungal sinusitis in evaluating immunosuppressed patients is essential. Symptoms of invasive disease may be mild or indistinguishable from chronic rhinosinusitis.
- In patients with invasive fungal sinusitis, nasal endoscopy may be normal early in the disease course. Abnormal findings include mucosal pallor, edema, and/or necrosis. CT or MRI, and tissue biopsy should be obtained for further evaluation.
- Histopathology is the gold standard in diagnosis of invasive fungal sinusitis. If inaccessible at bedside, sinusotomy and biopsy in the operating room should be considered.
- Surgical therapy is indicated in treatment of all forms of fungal sinus disease. Steroids play an important role in the management of allergic fungal sinusitis, while systemic antifungals are essential in the treatment of invasive disease.

References

1. Tyler MA, Luong AU. Current understanding of allergic fungal rhinosinusitis. World J Otorhinolaryngol. 2018;4:179–85.
2. Luong AU, Marple BF. Allergic fungal sinusitis. Curr Allergy Asthma Rep. 2004;4:465–70.
3. Ryan MW, Clark CM. Allergic fungal rhinosinusitis and the Unified Airway: the role of antifungal therapy in AFRS. Curr Allergy Asthma Rep. 2015;15:75.
4. Gan EC, Thamboo A, Rudmik L, et al. Medical management of allergic fungal rhinosinusitis following endoscopic sinus surgery: an evidence-based review with recommendations. Int Forum Allergy Rhinol. 2014;4:702–15.
5. Plonk DP, Luong A. Current understanding of allergic fungal rhinosinusitis and treatment implications. Curr Opin Otolaryngol Head Neck Surg. 2014;22:221–6.
6. Hoyt AEW, Borish L, Gurrola J, et al. Allergic fungal rhinosinusitis. J Allergy Clin Immunol Pract. 2016;4:599–604.
7. Patadia MO, Welch KC. Role of immunotherapy in allergic fungal rhinosinusitis. Curr Opin Otolaryngol Head Neck Surg. 2015;23:21–8.
8. Gan EC, Habib AR, Rajwani A, et al. Omalizumab therapy for refractory allergic fungal rhinosinusitis patients with moderate or severe asthma. Am J Otolaryngol. 2015;36:672–7.
9. Payne SJ, Mitzner R, Kunchala S, Roland L, McGinn JD. Acute invasive fungal rhinosinusitis: a 15-year experience with 41 patients. Otolaryngol Head Neck Surg. 2016;154:759–64.
10. Middlebrooks EH, Frost CJ, de Jesus RO, Massini TC, Schmalfuss IM, Mancuso AA. Acute invasive fungal rhinosinusitis: a comprehensive update of CT findings and design of an effective diagnostic imaging model. AJNR Am J Neuroradiol. 2015;36:1529–35.
11. Groppo ER, El-Sayed IH, Aiken AH, Glastonbury CM. Computed tomography and magnetic resonance imaging characteristics of acute invasive fungal sinusitis. Arch Otolaryngol Head Neck Surg. 2011;137:1005–10.
12. Ghadiali MT, Deckard NA, Farooq U, Astor F, Robinson P, Casiano RR. Frozen-section biopsy analysis for acute invasive fungal rhinosinusitis. Otolaryngol Head Neck Surg. 2007;136:714–9.
13. Cho HJ, Jang MS, Hong SD, Chung SK, Kim HY, Dhong HJ. Prognostic factors for survival in patients with acute invasive fungal rhinosinusitis. Am J Rhinol Allergy. 2015;29:48–53.
14. Turner H, Soudry E, Nayak JV, Hwang PH. Survival outcomes in acute invasive fungal sinusitis: a systematic review and quantitative synthesis of published evidence. Laryngoscope. 2013;123:1112–8.
15. Roxbury CR, Smith DF, Higgins TS, et al. Complete surgical resection and short-term survival in acute invasive fungal rhinosinusitis. Am J Rhinol Allergy. 2017;31:109–16.
16. Li Y, Li Y, Li P, Zhang G. Diagnosis and endoscopic surgery of chronic invasive fungal rhinosinusitis. Am J Rhinol Allergy. 2009;23(6):622–5. https://doi.org/10.2500/ajra.2009.23.3361.

Chronic Rhinosinusitis in Adults

25

Shanmugam Ganesan, Ahmed Shaikh, Hamad Al Saey, Mansour Al Sulaiti, Emaad Alduhirat, and Nafil Arimbrathodi

25.1 Introduction

Chronic rhinosinusitis (CRS) has been a major cause of morbidity in the community, with a significant financial burden on the health care system worldwide. CRS is a prevalent disease with varied presentations. For the last two decades, we have seen the development of many guidelines, definitions and management protocols. The most widely accepted definitions and the management guidelines were first published in European Position Paper on Rhinosinusitis and Nasal polyps (EPOS) in 2005 and subsequently in 2007 and 2012. Most recently, in February 2020, EPOS 2020 was published with the updated and latest evidence-based guidelines for the management of CRS.

CRS affects approximately 5–12% of the general population according to recent data, and the prevalence of doctor-diagnosed CRS is 2–4% [1]. Etiology and management differ between adult and pediatric CRS patients, and this chapter primarily focuses on adult CRS.

25.2 Definition

Distinguishing between rhinitis and sinusitis is challenging, both physiologically and pathophysiologically, and hence the term rhinosinusitis is accepted globally [1].

Chronic rhinosinusitis (with or without nasal polyps) in adults is defined [1–4] as:

- Inflammation of the nose and the paranasal sinuses characterized by two or more symptoms, one of which should be either
  - nasal blockage/obstruction/congestion or nasal discharge (anterior/posterior nasal drip):
  - ± facial pain/pressure
  - ± reduction or loss of smell

and either

- endoscopic signs of:
  - nasal polyps, and/or.
  - mucopurulent discharge primarily from the middle meatus

S. Ganesan (✉) · A. Shaikh · H. Al Saey · M. Al Sulaiti
Otolaryngology-Head and Neck Surgery Division, Department of Surgery, Hamad Medical Corporation, Doha, Qatar

Department of Otolaryngology-Head and Neck Surgery, Weill Cornell Medicine-Qatar, Doha, Qatar
e-mail: sganesan@hamad.qa; Halsaey@hamad.qa; Malsulaiti1@hamad.qa

E. Alduhirat · N. Arimbrathodi
Otolaryngology-Head and Neck Surgery Division, Department of Surgery, Hamad Medical Corporation, Doha, Qatar
e-mail: EAlDuhirat@hamad.qa; NArimbrathodi@hamad.qa

A. Al-Qahtani et al. (eds.), *Textbook of Clinical Otolaryngology*,
https://doi.org/10.1007/978-3-030-54088-3_25

  - and/or
  - edema/mucosal obstruction primarily in the middle meatus
  - and/or
- CT changes:
  - mucosal changes within the ostiomeatal complex and/ or sinuses

25.3 Duration of Disease

25.3.1 Acute

- <12 weeks
- with complete resolution of symptoms

25.3.2 Chronic

- ≥12 weeks
- without complete resolution of symptoms

25.4 Classification

CRS has been classified [1, 2, 4–6] into

- Chronic rhinosinusitis with nasal polyps (CRSwNP): bilateral, endoscopically visualized polyps in the middle meatus.
- Chronic rhinosinusitis without nasal polyps (CRSsNP): no visible polyps in the middle meatus, if necessary following decongestant [2].

Based on recent EPOS 2020, the following new classification has been introduced as follows:

Primary (Table 25.1) and secondary (Table 25.2), each divided into localized and diffuse based on anatomical distribution. In the primary CRS, either type 2 or non-type 2 based on endotype dominance [1].

The severity of the disease can be divided into MILD and MODERATE/SEVERE based on visual scale (VAS) score (0–10 cm) [7, 8]:

- MILD = VAS 0–3
- MODERATE = VAS >3–7
- SEVERE = VAS >7–10

To evaluate the total severity, the patient is asked to indicate on a VAS question:

How troublesome are your symptoms of rhinosinusitis?

A VAS > 5 affects the patient QOL • only validated in adults with CRS [2, 3, 7–9].

Table 25.1 Primary CRS classification

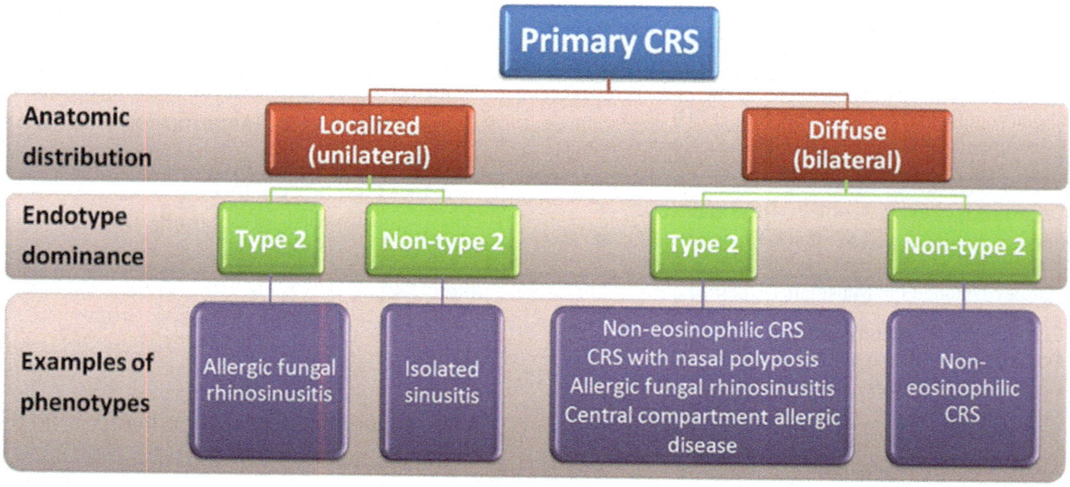

Courtesy: W.J. Fokkens, V.J. Lund, C. Hopkins, P.W. Hellings et al European Position Paper on Rhinosinusitis and Nasal Polyps 2020 [1]. *CRS* chronic rhinosinusitis

Table 25.2 Classification of secondary CRS

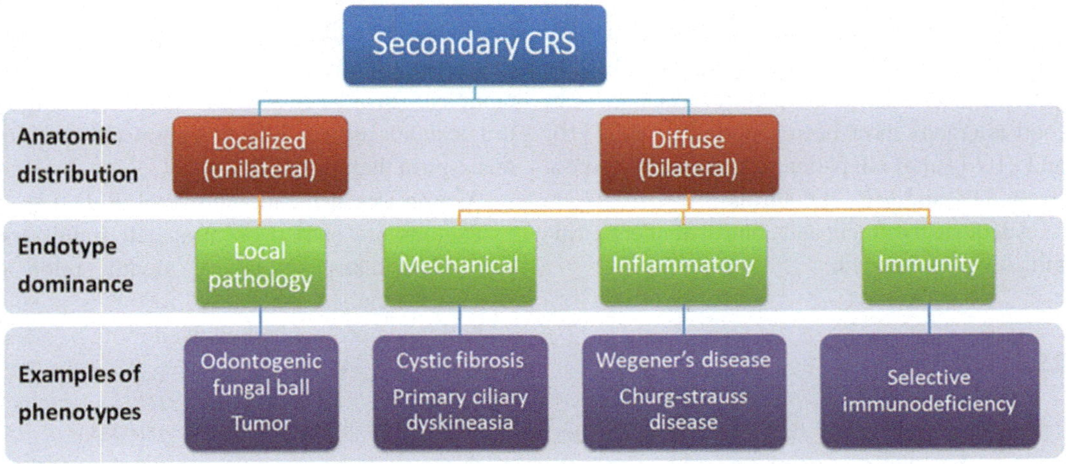

Courtesy: *W.J. Fokkens, V.J. Lund, C. Hopkins, P.W. Hellings* et al *European Position Paper on Rhinosinusitis and Nasal Polyps 2020* [1]. *CRS* chronic rhinosinusitis

25.5 Pathophysiology

The emerging view was that CRS is considered as a syndrome with a multifactorial etiology resulting from a dysfunctional interaction between the host immune system and the various environmental factors [1, 2].

25.6 Diseases Associated with Chronic Rhinosinusitis

25.6.1 Ciliary Impairment

Ciliary function plays an essential role in the clearance of the sinuses and the prevention of chronic inflammation. Secondary ciliary dyskinesia is common in patients with CRS, and most of the time, it is reversible. CRS is a well-known problem in patients with Kartagener's syndrome and primary ciliary dyskinesia (PCD). PCD has a strong association with CRSwNP in 15–30% of patients [1]. Patients with cystic fibrosis (CF), the resultant inability of the cilia to transport the viscous mucus causes ciliary malfunction and consequently CRS and it is irreversible. 40% of patients with CF present with nasal polyps [1, 2, 10]. The treatment is currently symptomatic.

25.6.2 Allergy

At the sinus ostia site, swelling of nasal mucosa in allergic rhinitis has been postulated to hinder airflow and block the sinus ostia, resulting in mucus accumulation and infection. A significant overlap of symptoms between AR and CRS has been seen. A number of studies report allergy markers are more prevalent in CRS populations. Benninger et al. reported 54% of CRS patients had positive skin prick results. CRS patients undergoing sinus surgery had a prevalence of positive skin prick tests ranges from 50% to 84%, of which the majority (60%) have multiple positive allergens [1, 2, 4].

Between 0.5% and 4.5% of subjects with allergic rhinitis have NP [11, 12], which compares with the normal population. Kern found, in 25.6% of patients with allergy compared to 3.9% in a control population, the presence of NP [8,

13]. The prevalence of allergy in patients with NP has been reported from 10% [14], to 54% [15] and 64% [15]. Despite some reports that have implicated atopy as being more prevalent in patients with NP, positive intradermal tests to food allergens have been reported in 70% [16] and 81% [16] of NP patients compared to respectively 34% and 11% of controls.

Adequate treatment and control of allergic rhinitis is recommended.

25.6.3 Asthma

There is a correlation between CRSwNP and asthma, but their interrelationship is poorly understood [1, 12, 16]. The prevalence of asthma is around 25% in patients with CRS compared to 5% in the general population. Studies of radiological abnormalities of the sinuses in asthma patients showed a high prevalence of abnormal sinus mucosa and a stronger association with asthma in patients with CRS and allergic rhinitis asthma is reported by 26% of patients with CRSwNP, compared to 6% of controls [12]. 7% of asthmatic patients have NP [16], with a prevalence of 13% in non-atopic asthma and 5% in atopic asthma women who have nasal polyps are 1.6 times more likely to be asthmatic and 2.7 times to have allergic rhinitis.

25.6.4 Aspirin Sensitivity

In patients with aspirin sensitivity, 36–96% have CRSwNP. HLA A1/B8 has been reported as having a higher incidence in patients with asthma and aspirin sensitivity.

Aspirin-exacerbated respiratory disease (AERD) is a clinical condition which results in adverse upper and lower respiratory symptoms, particularly rhinitis, bronchospasm, and/or laryngospasm, following exposure to cyclooxygenase-1 (COX-1) inhibiting drugs, namely aspirin or nonsteroidal anti-inflammatory drugs (NSAIDs). The aspirin challenge test is the gold standard for the diagnosis of AERD. Aspirin desensitization and continuous aspirin therapy have been highly efficacious in those patients with poor control of their disease. After the diagnosis of AERD is made, disease management is based upon either complete avoidance of all COX-1-inhibiting drugs and/or aspirin desensitization and continuous aspirin therapy [1, 2, 13].

Aspirin Desensitization protocol: Ref. [13].

Patients are started of mast cell stabilizers, e.g., Montelukast sodium, 2 months prior to desensitization.

Following protocol is followed:

Dose	Day 1 (mg)	Day 2 (mg)
08:00 am	40	160
11:00 am	60	160–325
02:00 pm	100	325

The patients are given 325 mg BID as a maintenance dosage.

Aspirin desensitization followed by daily aspirin therapy has been established as an effective treatment for patients with chronic rhinosinusitis with polyposis with AERD, and it is a class A recommendation.

25.6.5 Immunocompromised State

Immunological testing should be an integral part of the diagnostic pathway of patients with CRS. Higher incidences of CRS have been reported in immunocompromised patients. More than half of HIV patients have CRS as reported by Porter et al. [14].

25.6.6 Immune Deficiencies

Immunodeficiencies are more common with CRS; the most common immunodeficiency found is Common Variable Immunodeficiency (10%) and selective IgA deficiency (6%). Meta-analysis with CRS patients from 13 studies found that 23% of patients with difficult-to-treat CRS cases and 13% of individuals with recurrent CRS had immunoglobulin deficiencies. The prevalence of immune deficiencies could be up to 50% in “difficult-to-treat cases” of CRS according to a recent study [15, 16].

25.6.7 Gastroesophageal Reflux Disease

Gastro-esophageal reflux disease (GERD) is a common gastrointestinal disorder that affects approximately 10% of populations and is hypothesized as a possible factor for CRS. A meta-analysis study in 2016 gathered 32 publications that assessed the prevalence or incidence of CRS in a GERD population. They concluded that CRS subjects had a greater prevalence of intranasal *Helicobacter pylori* and acid reflux than subjects without CRS [17].

Grade of Recommendation for Proton pump inhibitor: D (level of evidence III).

25.6.8 Allergic Fungal Rhinosinusitis (Figs. 25.1 and 25.2)

Allergic fungal rhinosinusitis (AFRS) is characterized by the presence of eosinophilic mucin, noninvasive fungal hyphae, and a type 1 hypersensitivity to fungi. It represents 5–10% of CRS cases [1].

Bent-Kuhn [18] five *major criteria* includes:

- Nasal polyposis
- Eosinophilic mucin without fungal invasion into sinus tissue
- Fungi on staining
- Type 1 hypersensitivity to fungi
- Characteristic radiological findings

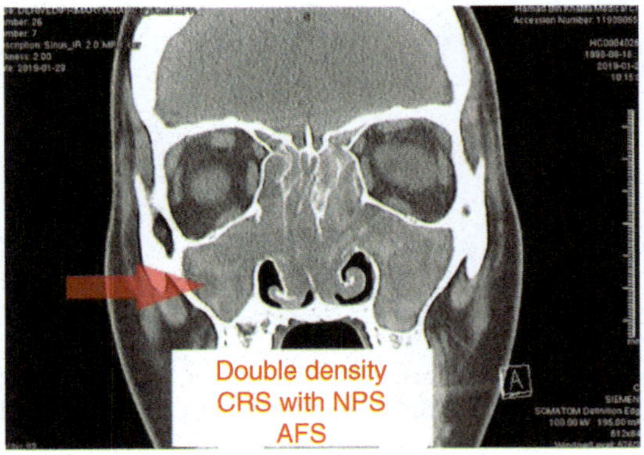

Fig. 25.1 CT coronal view demonstrating chronic rhinosinusitis with nasal polyposis (Bilateral/diffuse) allergic fungal sinusitis (AFS)

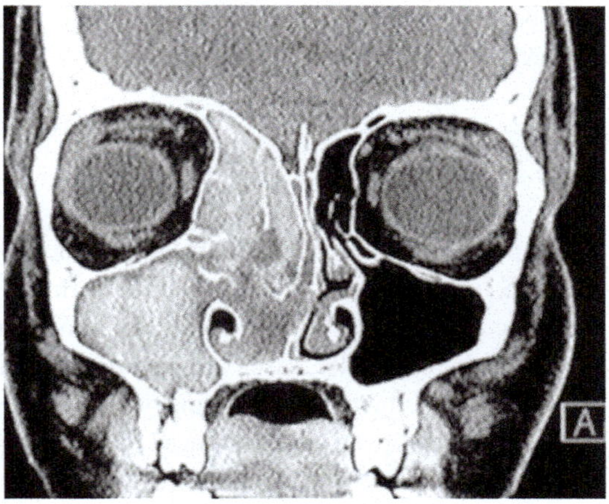

Fig. 25.2 Unilateral allergic fungal sinusitis

Minor criteria includes:

- Bone erosion
- Charcot–Leyden crystals
- Positive fungal culture
- Eosinophilia
- Absence of immunodeficiency status or diabetes

Generally agreed management plan for AFRS:

- Surgery
- Medical treatment alone is not adequate
- Oral steroids
- Nebulized topical steroids
- Allergen-specific Immunotherapy in selected cases
- An oral antifungal may reduce recurrence but do not improve symptoms [1]

Surgeons should have a low threshold in suspecting AFRS in CRS cases, and the patients must be counseled for high recurrence rate, multiple surgeries, and long-term follow-up.

25.6.9 Pregnancy and Endocrine State

Nasal congestion occurs in roughly one-fifth of women during pregnancy [19]. Several theories were proposed. In addition to direct hormonal effects on the nasal mucosa by estrogen, progesterone and placental growth hormone, indirect hormonal effects, such as vascular changes, may also be involved. This leads to nasal congestion and eventual nasal mucosal edema.

25.6.10 Biofilms

Many pathogenic bacteria colonize the surface of the NPS forming biofilms. They are not a primary etiologic agent in NP but add more inflammation significantly. Clinically, cases of biofilm-resistant NP are correlated with severe forms of the disease and worse postoperative outcomes. Methicillin-resistant *Staphylococcus aureus* (MRSA) appears to pose a significant risk to the disease. The importance of minimizing future resistance patterns due to increasing prevalence of *S. aureus* and antimicrobial resistance in chronic sinonasal disease highlights the importance of using culture directed antimicrobial therapy [20–22].

25.6.11 Environmental Factors

Smoking, along with laryngopharyngeal reflux and secondary smoke appears to be the significantly independently associated with CR. *H. pylori* DNA has been detected in between 11% [23] to 33% of sinus samples from patients with CRSsNP but not from controls.

25.6.12 Nasal Anatomic Variants

Anatomic variants have been suggested as risk factors for CRS, systematic review analyzing the role of septal deviations in CRS demonstrated a significant association of septal deviation and rhinosinusitis [24].

25.6.13 Diagnosis

25.6.13.1 Anterior Rhinoscopy

Anterior rhinoscopy alone is of limited value but remains the first step in examining a patient with these diseases.

25.6.13.2 Nasal Endoscopy

This may be performed without and with decongestion [5, 23, 24]. Nasal endoscopy affords significantly better illumination and visualization compared to anterior rhinoscopy for the examination of the middle and superior meati as well as the nasopharynx and mucociliary drainage pathways and sinus ostia.

25.6.14 Imaging [25] (Fig. 25.3)

Due to the optimal display of air-bone and soft tissue, CT scanning is the method of choice for paranasal sinuses. It should not be considered, however, as the primary step in the diagnosis of the condition, except where some unilateral signs and symptoms corroborate history and endoscopic examination after the failure of medical therapy.

MRI has no radiation risk and improved soft tissue definition over CT scan with the ability to differentiate between soft tissue masses and secretions that are retained/obstructed. MRI thus assists CT in the diagnosis of neoplastic processes.

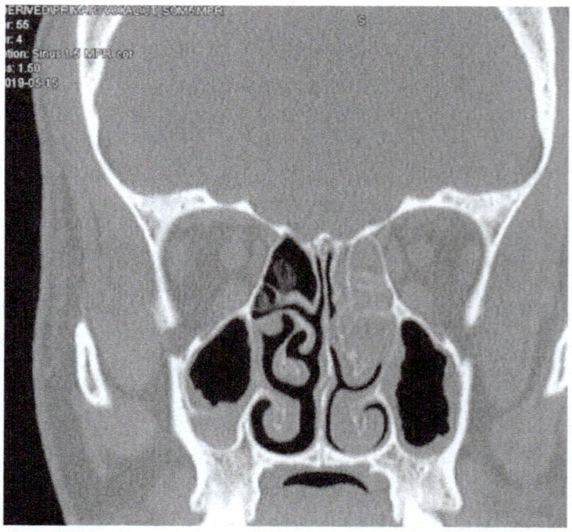

Fig. 25.3 Chronic rhinosinusitis without nasal polyposis, CORONAL CT Sinus with opacification of ethmoid sinuses

25.6.15 Grading of Nasal Polyp [1, 2, 4]

- 0—Absence of polyps;
- 1—polyps in middle meatus only;
- 2—polyps beyond middle meatus but not blocking the nose completely;
- 3—polyps completely obstructing the nose.

A wide range of other diagnostic tests are available to assist with the differential diagnosis and to define predisposing etiological factors, but many are only available in research departments.

25.6.16 Nasomucociliary Clearance [26, 27]

The use of saccharin, dye, or radioactive particles to measure mucociliary transit time has been available for almost 30 years. It enables one to recognize early changes in sinosinus homeostasis. Although a crude measure, it has the advantage of considering the entire mucociliary system and is useful if normal (<35 min). However, it does not distinguish between the primary or secondary causes of ciliary dysfunction if it is prolonged. Nasomucociliar clearance was also tested using a mixture of vegetable charcoal powder and 3% saccharin to show a delay in CRS patients compared to normal.

25.6.17 Rhinomanometry (Active Anterior and Posterior)

Measuring nasal airway resistance by measuring nasal flow at constant pressure is again of limited use in chronic rhinosinusitis and nasal polyposis, but can be useful in verifying that increased nasal congestion results from decreased inflammation in the middle tissue, rather than mechanical obstruction [4, 5, 7, 23].

25.6.18 **Treatment** (Figs. 25.4 and 25.5)

25.6.19 Intranasal Corticosteroids

Topical and systemic glucocorticoids may affect eosinophilic function by either directly decreasing eosinophilic viability and activation [24, 27, 28] or indirectly decreasing the secretion of chemotactic cytokines by nasal mucosa and polyp epithelial cells.

Meta-analyses have shown results significantly favorable to the topical steroid group.

Drug-related events include epistaxis, dry nose, nasal burning, and nasal irritation.

Cochrane review [29] done to assess the effects of intranasal corticosteroids in people with chronic rhinosinusitis has the following results.

It included 2738 pts and 18 RCT.

1. Improvement for nasal blockage > rhinorrhea > anosmia > facial pain.
2. There was an increased risk of epistaxis with intranasal corticosteroids (risk ratio (RR) 2.74, 95% CI 1.88 to 4.00; 2508 participants; 13 studies; high-quality evidence.

- None of the studies treated or followed up patients long enough to provide meaningful data on the risk of osteoporosis or stunted growth (children).

Different type of sprays does not have any difference in outcome (Fluticasone v/s mometasone).

Systemic Steroids:

Cochrane review related to the use of systemic steroids for a short period has the following outcomes:

- Eight RCTs (474 randomized participants)
- Disease-specific health-related quality of life: improved quality of life after treatment (2–3 weeks) in the group receiving oral

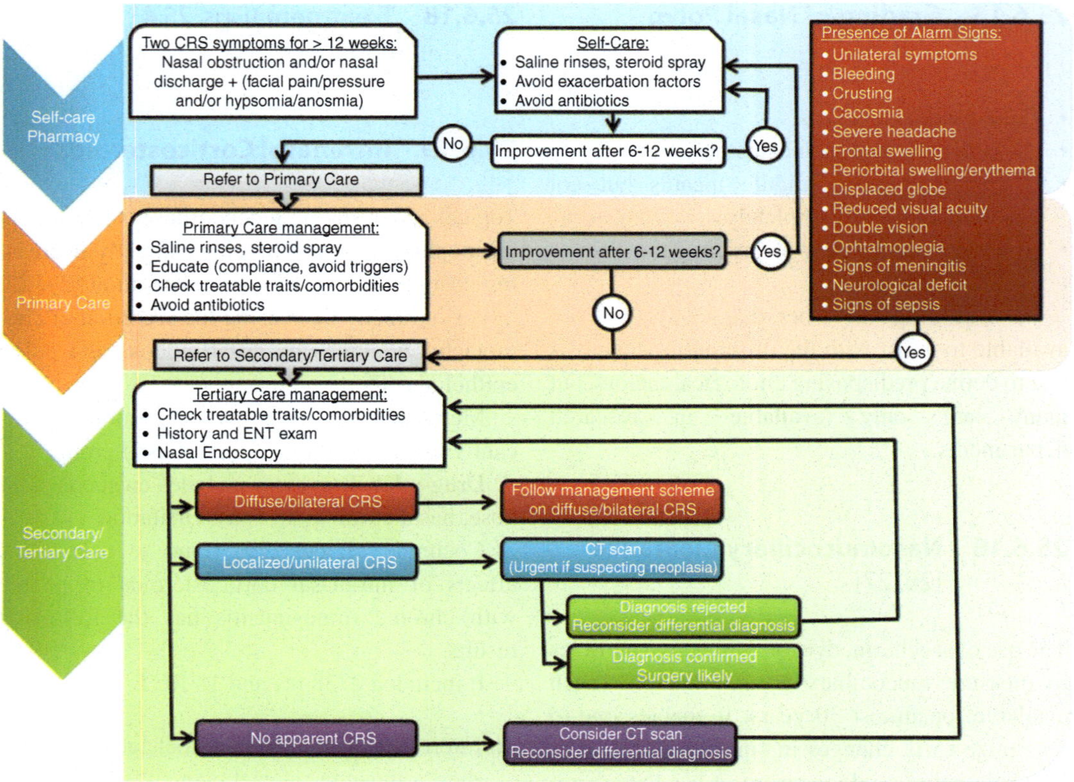

Fig. 25.4 Care Pathway for chronic sinusitis (CRS)

steroids compared with the group who received placebo (standardized mean difference)

- *Disease severity*: nasal blockage, nasal discharge, facial pressure, hyposmia; all improved
- *Adverse events*: gastrointestinal disturbances (risk ratio (RR) 3.45, 95% CI and insomnia (RR 3.63, 95% CI
- There was no significant impact of oral steroids on mood disturbances at the dosage used in the included
- At 3–6 months after the end of the oral steroid treatment period, there is little or no improvement in health-related quality of life or symptom severity for patients taking an initial course of oral steroids compared with placebo or no treatment.

Hence the steroids were recommended for short periods in acute exacerbations.

25.6.20 Long-Term Antibiotics

Patient with normal IgE levels macrolides have demonstrated some improvement with RCTs when used for >12 weeks. Level of evidence for macrolides in all patients with CRSsNP isIb, and strength of recommendation C, because the two double-blind placebo-controlled studies are contradictory; indication exists for better efficacy in CRSsNP patients with normal IgE with the level of evidence 1a. No RCTs exist for other antibiotics.

Cochrane review [30] on the use of systemic antibiotics

25.6.21 Antibiotics Versus Placebo

- Three studies compared antibiotic treatment with placebo (176 participants).
- At the end of treatment, the SNOT-20 score was lower in the group receiving 3 months of treatment with macrolide antibiotics than the placebo group.

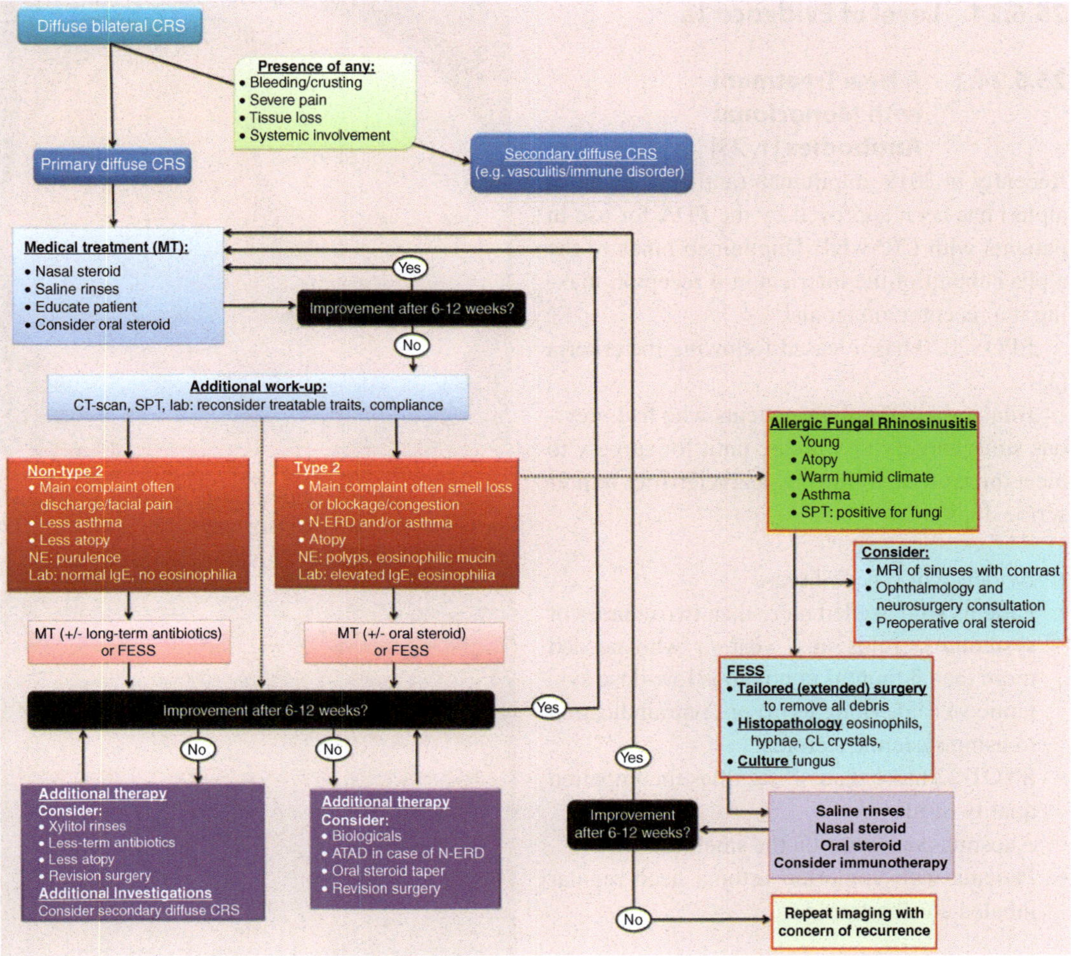

Fig. 25.5 Management pathway for CRS

25.6.22 Topical Antibiotics in CRS [30, 31]

There is a low level of evidence for the efficacy of topical antibacterial therapy in seven uncontrolled trials. However, three placebo-controlled trials failed to show any additive effect of topical antibiotics as compared to saline alone. Topical antibacterial therapy cannot be recommended in the treatment of CRS.

25.6.23 Level of Evidence Ib

25.6.23.1 Nasal Irrigation with Saline [32]

Isotonic or hypertonic saline solutions delivered by bottle, spray, pump, or nebulizer are frequently used in the treatment of sinus disease, mainly as a supplement to other therapies. Nasal saline irrigations were judged beneficial in the treatment of the symptoms of chronic rhinosinusitis when used as the sole modality of treatment in a Cochrane report.

All outcome parameters were significantly better in the nasal douches group than in the nasal spray group.

Recent EPOS2020 guideline advised using nasal saline irrigation with isotonic saline or Ringer's lactate with or without the addition of xylitol, sodium hypochlorite, and/or xyloglucan. It advised against the use of baby shampoo and hypertonic saline solution due to side effects [1].

25.6.24 Level of Evidence 1a

25.6.24.1 A New Treatment with Monoclonal Antibodies [1, 23]

Recently in 2019, dupilumab (anti-IL-4 receptor alpha) has been approved by the FDA for use in patients with CRSwNP. Dupilumab binds to the alpha subunit of the interleukin-4 receptor, making it a receptor antagonist.

EPOS2020 has released following the criteria [1].

Bilateral nasal polyps patients who had previous sinus surgery or who are unfit for surgery to meet three of the following characteristics to prescribe dupilumab.

- Evidence of type 2 disease
- Patients who needed more than two courses of systemic steroids in 1 year or who needed more than 3 months continuous low-dose systemic steroids (long term) or contraindication to using systemic steroids
- SNOT-22 more than 40 signifies the impaired quality of life
- Anosmia confirmed on the smell test
- Patients with comorbid asthma need regular inhaled corticosteroids

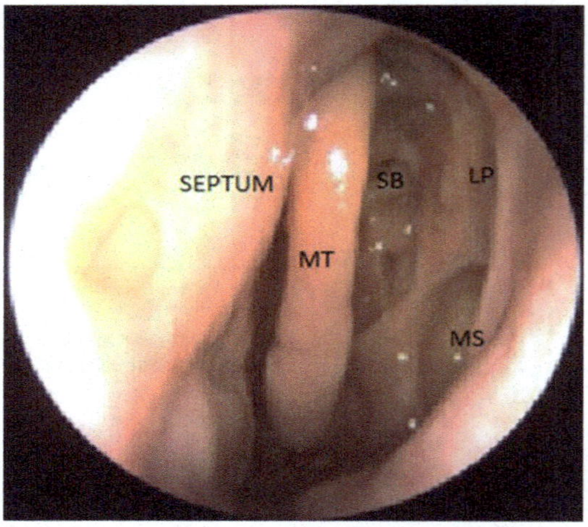

Fig. 25.6 Healed Sinonasal cavity post FESS (*MT* middle turbinate, *MS* maxillary sinus, *SB* skull base, *LP* Lamina Papyracea)

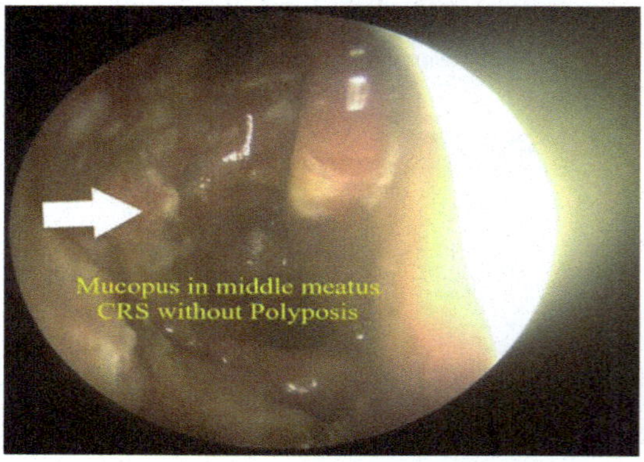

Fig. 25.7 CRSsNP: pus and inflammation in middle meatus

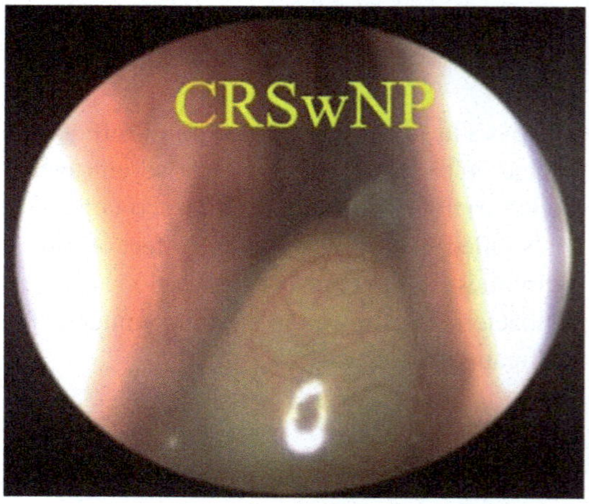

Fig. 25.8 CRSwNP: nasal polyp seen in middle meatus (grade II)

25.6.25 Functional Endoscopic Sinus Surgery [33] (Figs. 25.6, 25.7, and 25.8)

FESS has become an established surgical strategy, comprising several specific techniques, in the treatment of patients with CRS refractory to medical treatment. Despite its wide use, there is still a paucity of evidence regarding the effectiveness of FESS when compared to medical treatment and more conventional sinus surgery techniques.

Large prospective studies and case series have shown that endoscopic sinus surgery is effective and safe for the management of patients of CRS without NP who have failed medical treatment there is a significant amount of well-designed level II-level III evidence collected from tens of thousands of patients, that endoscopic sinus surgery is safe and is associated with improvements in symptoms scores (especially nasal obstruction and discharge), disease-specific and generic QOL as well as objective measures.

Although not fully evidence-based, the extent of surgery is frequently tailored to the extent of disease, which may appear as a reasonable approach. In primary paranasal sinus surgery, surgical conservatism is recommended. The decision to preserve or resect the anterior lower half of the middle turbinate can be left to the discretion of the surgeon based on its disease status. There is not enough data to support the use of balloon catheters as an alternative to standard endoscopic sinus surgery techniques.

(Please refer to Chap. 26: Steps of FESS and complications.)

25.6.26 Resistant/ Refractory CRS [34]

This is a small subset of CRS patients who fail multiple FESS procedures; FESS is successful, with reported success rates of 90% for primary FESS. However, success in revision cases falls to 69.8%. Recent research suggests the etiopathogenesis of this small but significant number of patients of rCRS (Refractory CRS) [35–37].

Inflammatory load theory: This theory suggests that grade of inflammation positively correlates with disease severity, and it has been postulated that grade of eosinophilia correlates with inflammation and higher CT scan scores.

It was found that a higher grade of mucosal eosinophilia consistently predicted a worse prognosis with more probable recurrence of the disease. The factors that contribute to the overall inflammatory load are:

1. Biofilms
2. Eosionophilic mucous
3. Inflammatory polyps
4. Fungal antigens and *Staphylococcus aureus*
5. Osteitic bone

The inflammatory load is the most important predictor of long-term outcome. Patients with a high inflammatory load have a higher probability of being refractory to standard FESS. Although the definitive management of these rCRS patients remains uncertain in the literature, many reports point out a role for more radical or extended surgeries in this group.

The summary of treatment with level of evidence and grade of recommendation is provided as follows (Table 25.3).

Table 25.3 Level of evidence [1, 2, 4]

Treatment	Level of evidence	Recommendation
Topical steroids	Ia	A
Oral steroids in CRS with nasal polyps	Ia	A
Oral antibiotics short term	Ib	A
Oral antibiotics long term	Ib	A (if IgE normal)
Topical saline irrigation	Ia	A
Grade of recommendation		**Interventions**
A	1A	Systemic review of randomized controlled trials
	1B	Individual randomized control trial
B	2A	Systemic review of cohort studies
	2B	Individual cohort studies
B	3A	Systemic review of case control studies
	3B	Individual case control study
C	4	Case series
D	5	Expert opinion without explicit critical appraisal or base on physiology or bench research

Reference: Oxford Centre for Evidence-Based Medicine—Levels of Evidence (March 2009)

Take Home Messages

- Chronic rhinosinusitis (CRS) comprises a group of disorders that arise from complex inflammatory processes with varied presentations.
- Environmental and exogenous factors play major role in etiology.
- Tremendous burden on healthcare system with significant negative impact on patients physical, psychological, and social functioning.
- The chapter is intended for all clinicians who are likely to diagnose and manage adult patients with CRS and applies to all settings.
- Aim to improve diagnostic accuracy, reduce inappropriate use of radiological investigations and antibiotics use.
- There are many guidelines for management of CRS and the recommendation by EPOS2020 paper is the latest and has been widely used.
- EPOS2020 steering group has introduced a new classification for CRS: Primary and Secondary CRS with localized and diffuse subgroups, based on anatomical distribution and endotype dominance.
- No standardized therapy for CRS and it should be treated with appropriate medical therapy. Surgery is considered for patients who have failed medical treatment.
- Substantial level 1a evidence suggests that topical corticosteroids improve outcomes in patients with CRS, including subgroups with and without nasal polyps.
- Topical saline nasal irrigation with isotonic saline is highly recommended—Level 1a evidence.
- Dupilumab, (anti IL-4Receptor alpha) monoclonal antibody has been introduced in 2019 to treat patients with CRS with polyps who meet the criteria.
- Endoscopic sinus surgery aims to eradicate the inflammatory tissues and osteitis, improve adequate drainage and ventilation, restore mucociliary function, increase the access for topical, and to improve the quality of life.
- Approximately 15–20% of patients require revision sinus surgery.

References

1. Fokkens WJ, Lund VJ, Hopkins C, Hellings PW, Kern R, Reitsma S, Toppila-Salmi S, Bernal-Sprekelsen M, Mullol J, et al. European position paper on rhinosinusitis and nasal polyps 2020. Rhinology. 2020;58(Suppl S29):1–464. https://doi.org/10.4193/Rhin20.600.
2. Fokkens WJ, Lund VJ, Mullol J, Bachert C, Alobid I, Baroody F, Cohen N, Cervin A, Douglas R, Gevaert P, Wormald PJ, et al. European position paper on rhinosinusitis and nasal polyps 2012. Rhinol Suppl. 2012;23(3):1–298.
3. Fokkens W, Lund VJ, Mullol J. European position paper on rhinosinusitis and nasal polyps 2007. Rhinol Suppl. 2007;20:1–136.
4. Meltzer EO, Hamilos DL. Rhinosinusitis diagnosis and management for the clinician: a synopsis of recent consensus guidelines. Mayo Clin Proc. 2011;86(5):427–43.
5. Meltzer EO, Hamilos DL, Hadley JA, Lanza DC, Marple BF, Nicklas RA, et al. Rhinosinusitis: establishing definitions for clinical research and patient care. J Allergy Clin Immunol. 2004;114(6 Suppl):155–212.
6. Fokkens W, Lund V, Bachert C, Clement P, Helllings P, Holmstrom M, et al. EAACI position paper on rhinosinusitis and nasal polyps executive summary. Allergy. 2005;60(5):583–601.
7. Lim M, Lew-Gor S, Darby Y, Brookes N, Scadding G, Lund VJ. The relationship between subjective assessment instruments in chronic rhinosinusitis. Rhinology. 2007;45:144–7.
8. Remenschneider AK, D'Amico L, Gray ST, Holbrook EH, Gliklich RE, Metson R. The EQ-5D: a new tool for studying clinical outcomes in chronic rhinosinusitis. Laryngoscope. 2015;125:7–15.
9. van Oene CM, van Reij EJ, Sprangers MA, Fokkens WJ. Quality-assessment of disease specific quality of life questionnaires for rhinitis and rhinosinusitis: a systematic review. Allergy. 2007;62:1359–71.
10. Desrosiers M, Evans GA, Keith PK, Wright ED, Kaplan A, Bouchard J, et al. Canadian clinical practice guidelines for acute and chronic rhinosinusitis. J Otolaryngol Head Neck Surg. 2011;40(Suppl 2):S99–S193.

11. Hamilos DL, Leung DY, Wood R, Cunningham L, Bean DK, Yasruel Z, et al. Evidence for distinct cytokine expressionin allergic versus nonallergic chronic sinusitis. J Allergy Clin Immunol. 1995;96(4):537–44.
12. Slavin RG. Sinusitis in adults and its relation to allergic rhinitis, asthma, and nasal polyps. J Allergy Clin Immunol. 1988;82(5 Pt 2):950–6.
13. Simon RA, Dazy KM, Waldram JD. Update on aspirin desensitization for chronic rhinosinusitis with polyps in aspirin-exacerbated respiratory disease (AERD). Curr Allergy Asthma Rep. 2015;15(3):508. https://doi.org/10.1007/s11882-014-0508-7.Review.
14. Porter JP, Patel AA, Dewey CM, Stewart MG. Prevalence of sinonasal symptoms in patients with HIV infection. Am J Rhinol. 1999;13(3):203–8.
15. Schwitzguébel AJ-P, Jandus P, Lacroix J-SS, et al. Immunoglobulin deficiency in patients with chronic rhinosinusitis: systematic review of the literature and meta-analysis. J Allergy Clin Immunol. 2015;136:1523–31.
16. Mazza JM, Lin SY. Primary immunodeficiency and recalcitrant chronic sinusitis: a systematic review. Int Forum Allergy Rhinol. 2016;6:1029–33.
17. Leason SR, Barham HP, Oakley G, et al. Association of gastro-oesophageal reflux and chronic rhinosinusitis: systematic review and meta-analysis. Rhinology. 2017;55:3–16.
18. Bent JP 3rd, Kuhn FA. Diagnosis of allergic fungal sinusitis. Otolaryngol Head Neck Surg. 1994;111(5):580–8.
19. Brozek JL, Akl EA, Alonso-Coello P, Lang D, Jaeschke R, Williams JW, et al. Grading quality of evidence and strength of recommendations in clinical practice guidelines. Part 1 of 3. An overview of the GRADE approach and grading quality of evidence about interventions. Allergy. 2009;64(5):669–77.
20. Cohen M, Kofonow J, Nayak JV, Palme JN, Chiu AG, Leid JG, et al. Biofilms in chronic rhinosinusitis: a review. Am J Rhinol Allergy. 2009;23(3):255–60.
21. Rachelefsky GS, Goldberg M, Katz RM, Boris G, Gyepes MT, Shapiro MJ, et al. Sinus disease in children with respiratory allergy. J Allergy Clin Immunol. 1978;61(5):310–4.
22. Grove R. Chronic hyperplastic sinusitis in allergic patients: a bacteriologic study of 200 operative cases. J Allergy Clin Immunol. 1990;11:271–6.
23. Orlandi RR, Smith TL, Marple BF, Harvey RJ, Hwang PH, Kern RC, Kingdom TT, Luong A, Rudmik L, Senior BA, Toskala E, Kennedy DW. Update on evidence-based reviews with recommendations in adult chronic rhinosinusitis. Int Forum Allergy Rhinol. 2014;4(Suppl 1):S1–S15. https://doi.org/10.1002/alr.21344. Review.
24. Rosenfeld RM, Piccirillo JF, Chandrasekhar SS, Brook I, Ashok Kumar K, Kramper M, Orlandi RR, Palmer JN, Patel ZM, Peters A, Walsh SA, Corrigan MD. Clinical practice guideline (update): adult sinusitis. Otolaryngol Head Neck Surg. 2015;152(2 Suppl):S1–S39. https://doi.org/10.1177/0194599815572097.
25. Emanuel IA, Shah SB. Chronic sinusitis, computed tomography relationships. Otolaryngol Head Neck Surg. 2000;123(6):687–91.
26. Hamilos DL, Leung DY, Wood R, Meyers A, Stephens JK, Barkans J, et al. Chronic hyperplastic sinusitis: association of tissue eosinophilia with mRNA expression of granulocyte-macrophage colony stimulating factor and interleukin-3. J Allergy Clin Immunol. 1993;92(1 Pt 1):39–48.
27. Desrosiers M, Evans GA, Keith PK, et al. Canadian clinical practice guidelines for acute and chronic rhinosinusitis. Allergy Asthma Clin Immunol. 2011;7(1):2. https://doi.org/10.1186/1710-1492-7.
28. Scadding GK, Durham SR, Mirakian R, Jones NS, Drake-Lee AB, Ryan D, Dixon TA, Huber PA, Nasser SM, British Society for Allergy and Clinical Immunology. BSACI guidelines for the management of rhinosinusitis and nasal polyposis. Clin Exp Allergy. 2008 Feb;38(2):260–75. https://doi.org/10.1111/j.1365-2222.2007.02889.x.
29. Chong LY, Head K, Hopkins C, Philpott C, Schilder AGM, Burton MJ. Intranasal steroids versus placebo or no intervention for chronic rhinosinusitis. Cochrane Database Syst Rev. 2016;(4):CD011996.
30. Head K, Chong LY, Piromchai P, Hopkins C, Philpott C, Schilder AGM, Burton MJ. Systemic and topical antibiotics for chronic rhinosinusitis. Cochrane Database Syst Rev. 2016;(4):CD011994. https://doi.org/10.1002/14651858.CD011994.pub2.
31. Sedaghat AR, Hoehle LP, Gray ST. Chronic rhinosinusitis control from the patient and physician perspectives. Laryngoscope Investig Otolaryngol. 2018;3(6):419–33. https://doi.org/10.1002/lio2.208.
32. Chong LY, Head K, Hopkins C, Philpott C, Glew S, Scadding G, Burton MJ, Schilder AGM. Saline irrigation for chronic rhinosinusitis. Cochrane Database Syst Rev. 2016;(4):CD011995.
33. Khalil H, Nunez DA. Functional endoscopic sinus surgery for chronic rhinosinusitis. Cochrane Database Syst Rev. 2006;(3):CD004458. https://doi.org/10.1002/14651858.CD004458.pub2.
34. Wang DY, Wardani RS, Singh K, Thanaviratananich S, Vicente G, Xu G, et al. A survey on the management of acute rhinosinusitis among Asian physicians. Rhinology. 2011;49(3):264–71.
35. Collins MM, Loughran S, Davidson P, Wilson JA. Nasal polyposis: prevalence of positive food and inhalant skin tests. Otolaryngol Head Neck Surg. 2006;135(5):680–3.
36. Pang YT, Eskici O, Wilson JA. Nasal polyposis: role of subclinical delayed food hypersensitivity. Otolaryngol Head Neck Surg. 2000;122(2):298–301.
37. Szucs E, Ravandi S, Goossens A, Beel M, Clement PAR. Eosinophilia in the ethmoid mucosa and its relationship to the severity of inflammation n chronic rhinosinusitis. Am J Rhinol. 2002;16:131–4.

Functional Endoscopic Sinus Surgery

26

Emad Al Duhirat, Hamad Al Saey, Mansour Al Sulaiti, Shanmugam Ganesan, and Ahmed Shaikh

26.1 Introduction

Indications for ESS:

- Chronic rhinosinusitis (CRS) with or without nasal polyposis not responding to medical therapy
- Allergic fungal sinusitis
- Orbital decompression
- Endoscopic Dacryocystorhinostomy (DCR)
- Sinus mucoceles
- Cerebrospinal fluid leak and skull base reconstruction
- Control of epistaxis
- Choanal atresia/stenosis
- Neoplastic diseases
- Part of skull base surgery

Majority of rhinologists agree that ESS for chronic rhinosinusitis should be a "disease-directed" and mucosal-sparing operation, giving the sinuses the chance to normally restore the mucosa and the drainage pathways [1–3].

It is important to review the CT scan before the surgery thoroughly to assess the important structures and landmarks to plan a safe surgery; in order not to forget any important detail, the following mnemonic can be followed:

CLOSE

- C: *C*ribriform plate
- L: *L*amina papyracea
- O: *O*nodi cell
- S: *S*phenoid sinus
- E: Anterior *E*thmoid artery

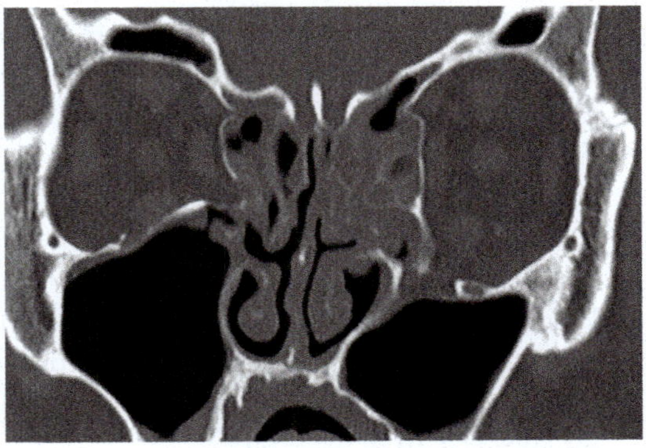

Orbital fat herniation

E. Al Duhirat (✉)
Otolaryngology-Head and Neck Surgery Division, Department of Surgery, Hamad Medical Corporation, Doha, Qatar
e-mail: EAlDuhirat@hamad.qa

H. Al Saey · M. Al Sulaiti · S. Ganesan
Otolaryngology-Head and Neck Surgery Division, Department of Surgery, Hamad Medical Corporation, Doha, Qatar

Department of Otolaryngology-Head and Neck Surgery Division, Weill Cornell Medicine-Qatar, Doha, Qatar
e-mail: Halsaey@hamad.qa; Malsulaiti1@hamad.qa; sganesan@hamad.qa

A. Shaikh
Hamad Medical Corporation, Doha, Qatar
e-mail: Ashaikh4@hamad.qa

A. Al-Qahtani et al. (eds.), *Textbook of Clinical Otolaryngology*,
https://doi.org/10.1007/978-3-030-54088-3_26

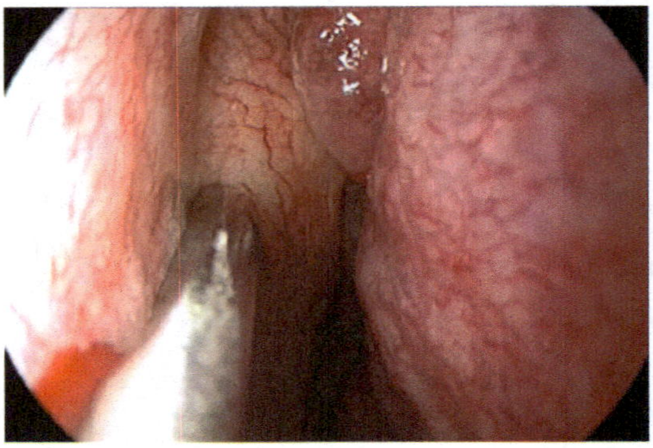

Palpating the uncinate

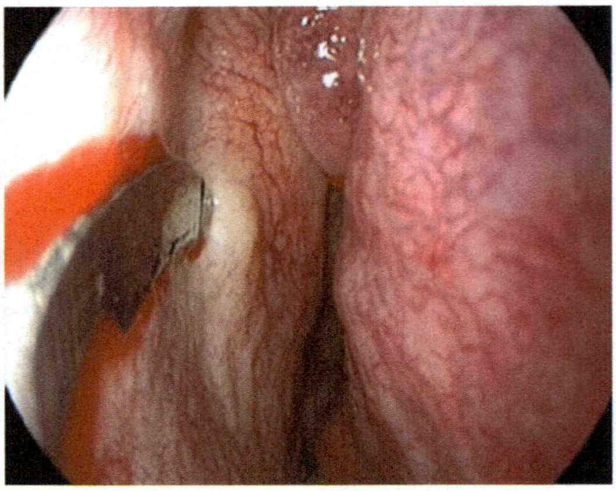

Anterior-to-posterior uncinectomy using sickle knife

26.2 Uncinectomy

The uncinate is a sickle-shaped bone divided into three parts: the middle portion of the uncinate process attaches to the lacrimal bone and lamina papyracea, and the horizontal portion attaches to the ethmoidal process of the inferior turbinate and palatine bone. The superior portion of the uncinate extends to a varying degree into the frontal recess and may insert into the lamina papyracea, skull base, middle turbinate, or combination of these [4–7].

It projects posteriorly forming a gutter (the infundibulum), and it has a free edge that creates a space between this free edge and the bulla ethmoidalis (hiatus semilunaris) [7].

26.2.1 The Anterior Posterior Approach

- Incise the uncinate process at the level of its middle and inferior third using a sickle knife or a Freer's elevator.
- Extend the incision inferiorly and posteriorly along its horizontal aspect.
- Remove the uncinate with a straight biting Blakesley forceps [8].
- Enlarge the incision superiorly (if indicated) to open the infundibulum toward the frontal outflow tract after making sure that there is a safe distance from the orbit.
- Remaining superior and inferior attachments of the uncinate can be cut with a through-cutting forceps.
- Identify the natural ostium of the maxillary sinus, the recessus terminalis, if any, and the frontal recess.
- This anteroposterior approach has a higher risk of orbital penetration. Exposed orbital fat should be left alone and should not be manipulated [9–12].

26.2.2 The Posterior Anterior Approach

- Identify the uncinate process, hiatus semilunaris, and infundibulum using an angled probe.
- Gently fracture the uncinate process with the angled probe.
- Pass the pediatric backbiter into the middle meatus which is easier to be introduced about the midway up the middle portion of the uncinate before it is slid down the free edge until it comes to rest on the transition of the middle and horizontal parts of the uncinate.
- Rotate the backbiter so that the biting blade is opened upward, in the vertical plane of the meatus.
- Then rotate it horizontally to engage the posterior free edge of the uncinate process.
- The uncinate is cut using sequential bites of the backbiter.
- The upper uncinate process (most superior extension) can be dislocated with a ball probe

and gently dissected with a biting forceps if exposure of the frontal recess is indicated.

- In order to expose the natural ostium of the maxillary sinus and avoid its blockage, the tail of the uncinate needs to be removed either using a backbiter, side biter, or microdebrider, with paying attention not to injure the inferior turbinate.

This approach is safer as one moves away from the orbit when dissecting, and thus the risk of inadvertently entering the orbit is reduced [13–17].

26.3 Complications of Uncinectomy

The two areas at risk during uncinectomy are the orbit and the nasolacrimal duct.

- Gently use the backbiter anteriorly while going toward the lacrimal sac/duct (the bony resistance will increase here): medialize the uncinate before biting.
- An uncinate process that is atelectatic and pressed against the lamina has a higher risk of injury to the orbit especially when using the anterior-to-posterior approach [18–20].

26.4 Middle Meatal Antrostomy

- When the uncinate process is intact, the height of the lower one-third of the middle turbinate approximates the location of the natural ostium.
- Once the most anterior-inferior aspect of the uncinate has been removed, the natural ostium of the maxillary sinus can be seen.
- The ostium lies at the junction of the anterior and inferior walls of the ethmoidal bulla.
- A curved suction, with its tip directed infero-laterally away from the lamina papyracea, can be passed through the natural ostium into the maxillary sinus.
- The superior border of the natural ostium demarcates the junction of the medial orbital floor with the lamina papyracea.

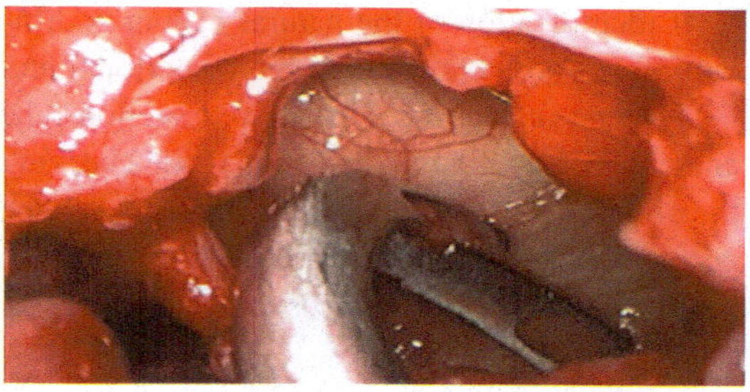

Widening the maxillary antrum anteriorly using backbiter

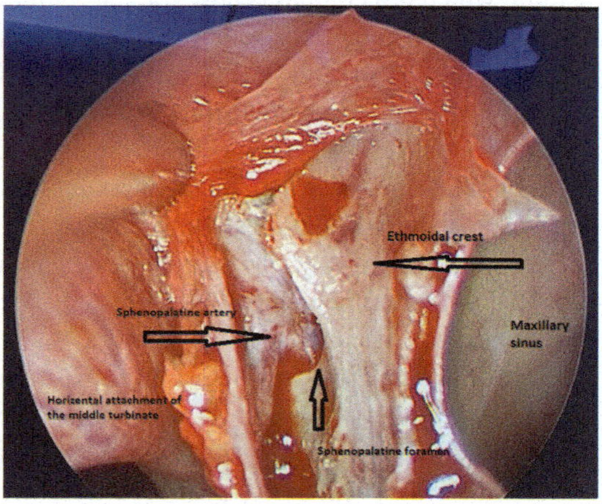

Relation of the posterior wall of the maxillary sinus to sphenopalatine artery

An accessory ostium is located within the posterior fontanelle of the maxillary sinus behind the natural ostium. Cadaveric studies have shown that 10% of the general population have an accessory ostium [21].

- There is no absolute need to enlarge the maxillary ostium for just inflammatory diseases.
- In advanced disease (such as allergic fungal rhinosinusitis and nasal polyps) and revision surgery, a wide antrostomy may be justified [22–24].

This can be achieved by widening the ostium toward the posterior fontanelle. Widening the ostium will uncover the medial orbital floor, which corresponds to the superior horizontal bony ridge of the antrostomy. Keeping the dissection below the level of the medial orbital floor helps in guiding the surgeon to a safe direction below the level of the skull base [25–27].

If identification of the natural ostium is difficult or not possible, palpate the posterior fontanelle area with the tip of a curved suction tube and enter smoothly into the sinus while checking the orbit during that. Entering the sinus should be performed pointing toward the floor of the sinus cavity while leaning on posterior third of the inferior turbinate.

Inability of the surgeon to locate the proper natural maxillary sinus ostium at surgery may result in the creation of a posterior fontanelle ostium, which is a common cause for ESS failure [28–30], because of the circular flow of mucus from the natural ostium of the maxillary sinus into the posterior fontanelle ostium [16, 17].

Identifying the posterior wall of the maxillary sinus should be done by the surgeon as it is an important landmark demarcating approximately the anterior wall of the sphenoid sinus which is almost 7 cm from the columella, adjacent to the nasal septum posteriorly.

Does enlarging the maxillary sinus ostium affect the long-term results. The role of nitric oxide (NO) in the sinuses is the main reason for this controversy [31]. NO is produced by nitric oxide synthase (NOS) in the mucosa of the sinuses [32, 33]. NO is believed to enhance the mucosa defense by stimulating the ciliary motility and by inhibiting infection by bacteria, viruses, and fungi [34]. Kennedy et al. [11] described the natural size of the maxillary ostium to be 5 mm by 5 mm; enlarging the ostium may in some patients cause dilution of the concentration of the sinus NO to allow colonization of the sinus by bacteria [35].

26.5 Mega-Antrostomy

In this surgery, the posterior part of the antrostomy is lowered to the floor of the nose with preserving the nasolacrimal duct.

In patients who have persistent chronic maxillary sinus infections and in cystic fibrosis patients (abnormal ciliary movement), the antrostomy can be lowered to the floor of the nose thereby to facilitate gravity-dependent drainage and better sinus irrigation.

26.6 Anterior Ethmoid

The anterior ethmoids are the cells that lie anterior to the basal lamella, consist of the ethmoid bulla, agger nasi cell, and the cells that lie against the medial orbital wall anterior to the basal lamellae.

The ethmoid bulla, visible directly behind the free edge of the middle and horizontal portions of uncinate process, the bulla ethmoidalis, like all sinuses, drains via a natural ostium. This is usually found on its posteromedial aspect in the retro-bulla recess, surrounded by the following:

- The lamina papyracea laterally.
- Posteriorly the vertical aspect of the basal lamella of the middle turbinate and the retro-bulbar recess.
- Anteriorly the ethmoid infundibulum and the vertical aspect of the uncinate process.

Steps of opening the ethmoid bulla:

- Enter the ethmoidal bulla, at a safe distance from the orbit, medially and inferiorly.
- Use a J-curette or a straight-forward suction device to do so.
- Inferior and medial walls are resected, while the posterior wall is attempted to keep intact.
- Follow the anterior wall of the ethmoid bulla, and identify the frontal recess, the roof of the

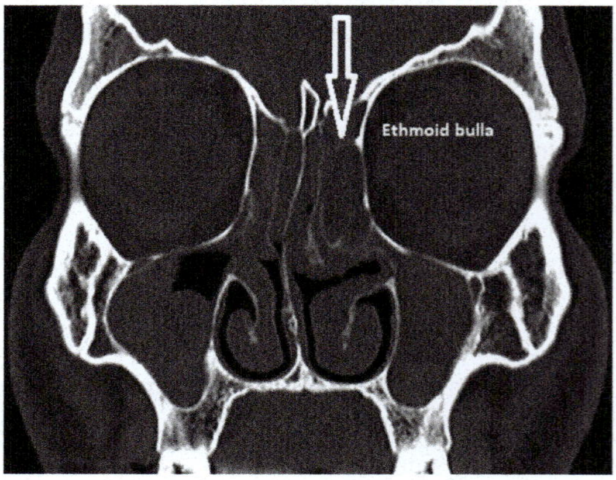

CT scan coronal section showing opacified left ethmoid bulla

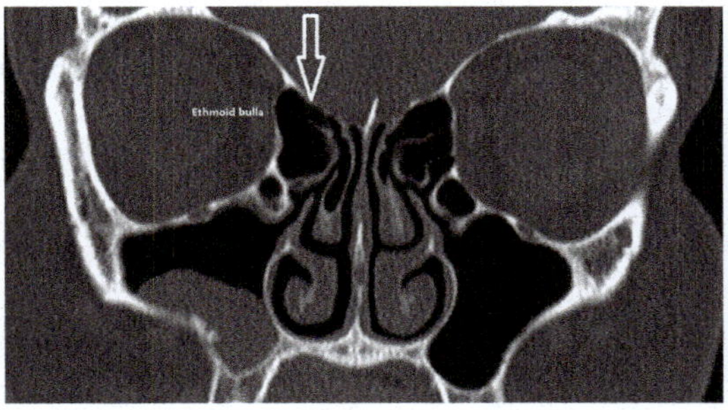

CT scan coronal section showing the right ethmoid bulla

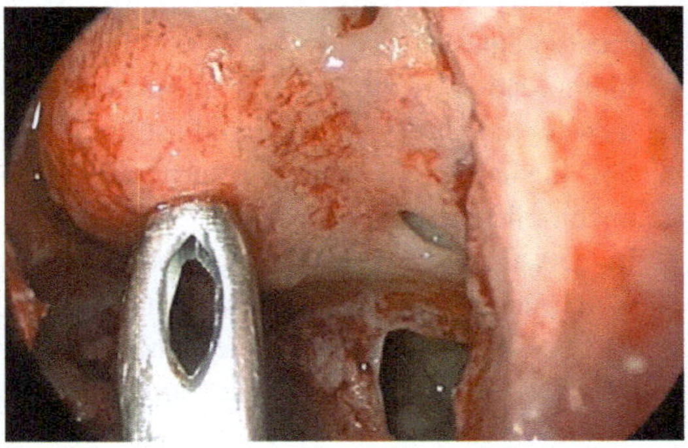

Anatomical identification of the left ethmoid bulla

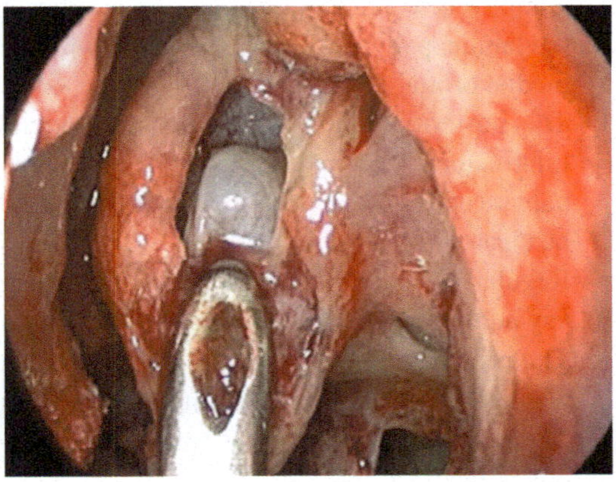

Dissection the left ethmoid bulla

ethmoid, and the anterior ethmoid artery (located at the most superior attachment of the anterior wall of the bulla at the roof or right behind).

- Identify the lamina papyracea. The floor of the orbit and the maxillary strut are helpful landmarks to identify the papyracea.

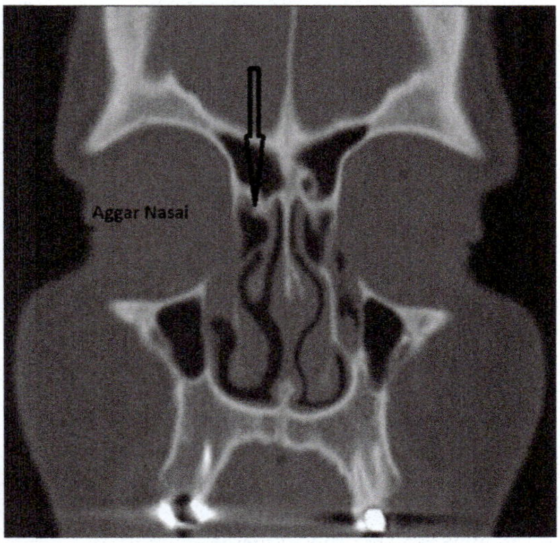

CT scan coronal section showing the right agger nasi

- The retrobulbar recess lies behind the bulla, and the skull base forms its superior limit.
- If a posterior ethmoidectomy is to be performed in addition to opening the bulla, none of its anterior wall is retained. Removing the bulla entirly gives improved access to the posterior ethmoid complex but also allows the lamina papyracea to be identified.
- The superior wall of the ethmoid bulla can extend up to the skull base or may be separated from it by one or more suprabullar cells [36].

The agger nasi cell is the most anterior ethmoid cell and is present in 98.5% of patients [37]. It is usually seen on the CT scan anterior to the middle turbinate [37, 38].

The major part of the agger nasi cell is placed anterior to the uncinate, and the posterior half of the agger nasi cell is closely related to the upper extension of the uncinate process [39].

Mostly the uncinate/medial wall of agger nasi cell attached to the lamina papyracea. The anterior wall of the agger nasi is formed by the insertion of the middle turbinate into the medial orbital wall anteriorly (the "axilla" of the middle turbinate). The agger nasi is positioned between the nasal bones, the lacrimal bones, and the ascending process of the maxilla.

Safe exenteration of agger nasi cells may be accomplished with angled forceps parallel to the lamina papyracea which allows exposure of the frontal outflow tract. If the microdebrider is used, then the opening is pointed perpendicular or away from the lamina papyracea until the latter is clearly identified.

26.7 Posterior Ethmoid

The posterior ethmoid cells are bounded

- Anteriorly by the basal lamella of the middle turbinate.
- Posteriorly by the anterior wall of the sphenoid sinus.
- Medially by the superior turbinate.
- Laterally by the orbital apex.
- Superiorly by the skull base.

Enter the superior meatus through the ground lamella in a region. To do this, mark the transition from the posterior horizontal ground lamella to the vertical ground lamella at the point where it turns vertically, next to the middle turbinate or through the basal lamella at the middle third (below imaginary horizontal line drawn at the level of the posterior medial orbital floor to the nasal septum), then the microdebrider or straight Blakesley is pushed through the ground lamella.

Widen this point until the superior meatus and anterior edge of the superior turbinate are identified with certainty.

The low, medial entry through the basal lamella minimizes the potential risk of damage to the skull base which may occur if entry is made higher on its vertical portion or above the level of the posterior medial orbital floor [25, 40].

Once the posterior ethmoids are entered through the ground lamella, the superior meatus and superior turbinate are identified and the recess that one can see from the nasal cavity between the superior and middle turbinates as seen from the septal side. This space is the common outflow tract for the posterior ethmoid cells.

The safe way to perform complete ethmoidectomy is

- Early identification of the lamina papyracea.
- Remove the inferior anterior and posterior ethmoid cells until the sphenoid face is reached.
- Identify the skull base at the posterior ethmoid or sphenoid sinus roof.
- Dissect along the skull base from a posterior to anterior direction.
- It is safer to make the superior ethmoid dissection after sphenoidotomy. This allows safer identification of the posterior ethmoid roof and the posteromedial orbital wall, by following the sphenoid roof (planum) and the lateral sphenoid wall; this is done retrogradely (posteroanterior).
- Identification of the superior turbinate makes it easier to identify the sphenoid ostium which lies medial to the superior turbinate in an uncomplicated case [41–44].
- In revision and severe polyposis cases in which the superior turbinates can't be identified or the anatomy is distorted, the posterior medial orbital floor provides an important landmark to help the surgeon in finding the level of initial entry into the sphenoid sinus ostium area, next to the posterior nasal septum. An inferior ethmoidectomy should be completed to identify the inferior portion of the lamina papyracea and its junction with the medial orbital floor [23–25].
- The posterior ethmoid air cells that extend inferolaterally along the slope of the lamina papyracea into the retromaxillary area should be cleared [45].
- Regularly palpate the eye prior to removing any additional ethmoidal cells.
- The posterior ethmoidal artery and nerve can be identified in the sphenoethmoidal recess, in front and above the anterior wall of the sphenoid sinus.

Be aware that the skull base slants downwards as the posterior ethmoid is approached.

- Identify the presence of an Onodi cell preoperatively as well as intraoperatively to avoid injury to the orbital apex.
- Dissect from "known to unknown" during ethmoidectomy and check around (especially) behind the bony partitions before removing them.

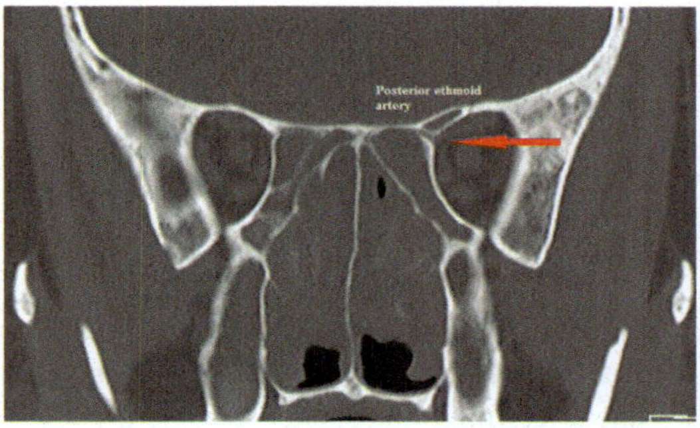

CT scan coronal section showing the posterior ethmoid artery

- The roof of the maxillary sinus is an important landmark so keep it in mind when dissecting through the ethmoid cavity.
- Learn to "zoom out." To avoid getting lost in the ethmoid cavity, intermittently bring the endoscope out of the ethmoid cavity anterior to the middle turbinate to get an overall picture of where dissection is occurring and to reorient yourself during ethmoidectomy to the proper direction.
- Avoid mucosal stripping.

26.8 Sphenoethmoidal Cell (Onodi Cell)

The posterior most ethmoidal air cell extends posteriorly to lie superolateral to the sphenoid sinus and thus in close proximity to the optic nerve and internal carotid artery [46].

The incidence of Onodi cell can be as high as 42% [47].

On the coronal cut of a CT scan identify the solid bony rim of the posterior choanae, the cell sitting directly above this is the sphenoid sinus. Any horizontal bony septation above this cell would be suspicious that there may be Onodi cell present.

26.9 The Anterior Ethmoid Artery

Runs from lateral to medial across the fovea ethmoidalis at a 45° angle. Mostly it is found behind the upward continuation of the bulla ethmoidalis. When a suprabullar recess is present, the anterior

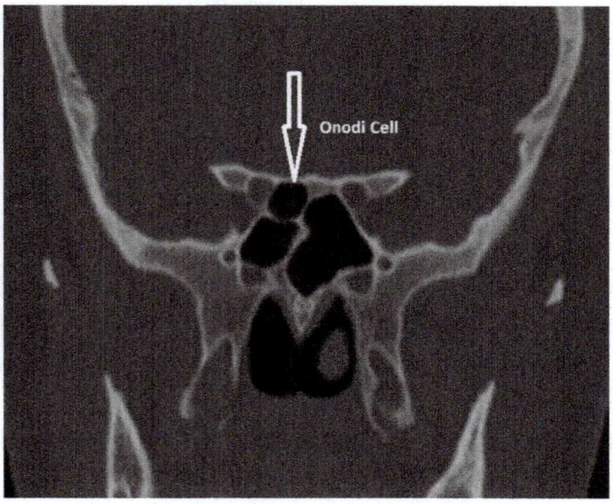

CT scan coronal section showing Onodi cell

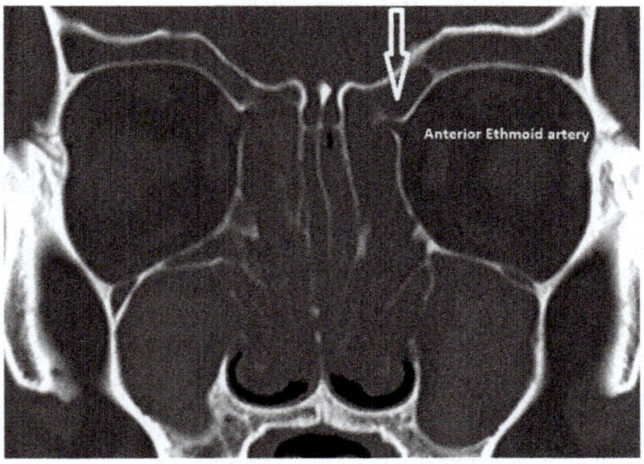

CT scan coronal section showing the anterior ethmoid artery

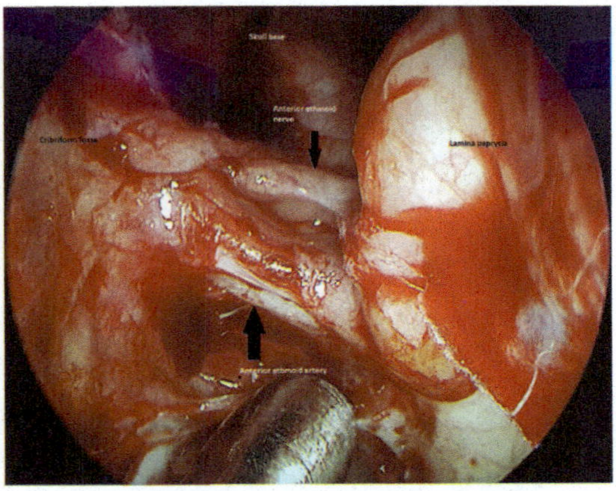

Anatomical dissection of the anterior ethmoid artery and nerve

ethmoidal artery will be in the frontal recess. The anterior ethmoidal artery may lie hanging in a mesentery from the skull base in 14–43% of patients. Reviewing the CT preoperatively is an important step to locate the anterior ethmoid artery and avoid its injury [48].

26.10 The Middle Turbinate

The middle turbinate should be preserved. And not to be destabilized during surgery. The most common cause for destabilization of the middle turbinate is fracturing its anterior vertical insertion from the skull base or cutting the horizontal portion of the basal lamellae.

Excessive manipulation may fracture the turbinate's insertion to the skull base and makes it floppy, which might lead to lateralization of the middle turbinate and obstruction of the middle meatus and frontal recess postoperatively.

Resection of the inferior portion of the basal lamellae may injure a branch of the sphenopalatine artery. Bleeding in this area can be controlled using bipolar/monopolar diathermy.

26.11 Concha Bullosa (Middle Turbinate Pneumatization)

Identified in 35% (range 14–53%) of patients.

Resection the lateral lamella of the middle turbinate (concha bullosa) improves access to the middle meatus and to clear the disease inside the concha bullosa if found.

- A scalpel or sickle knife is used to incise the anterior face of the concha bullosa vertically.
- Endoscopic scissor is used to complete the incision inferiorly to the lateral insertion of the turbinate on the lateral nasal wall, care must be taken as a branch of the sphenopalatine artery might be encountered here.
- To complete the superior incision posteriorly as high as possible, keeping in mind down slope of the skull base and the turbinate.

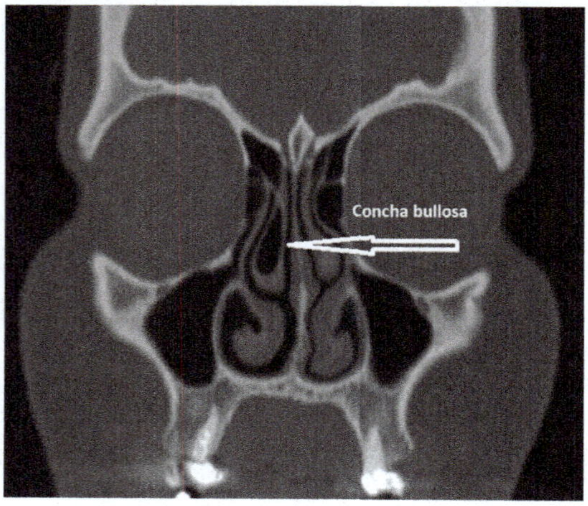

CT scan coronal section showing right concha bullosa

26.12 Sphenoidectomy

Sphenoid sinuses are paired and most posteriorly located, endoscopic approaches are least morbid and most preferred approaches. The sphenoid sinus is also the gateway to many extended endonasal procedures, including approaches to pituitary lesions, other sellar and parasellar lesions, and petroclival lesions amenable to an endonasal approach.

The two main endoscopic pathways to the sphenoid sinus are the transseptal and transethmoid approaches. Both require identification of the natural sphenoid ostium.

26.12.1 Anatomical Landmarks

Superior Turbinate: the most consistent landmark for identification of natural osteum of sphenoid sinus. The ST is identified after lateralization of middle turbinate. The sphenoid osteum is seen 5–10 mm above and medial to the attachment of ST.

Planum Sphenoidale: The sphenoid ostium is on average 11 mm inferior to the skull base and is approximately halfway between the floor of the sphenoid sinus and planum sphenoidale.

Choana: The sphenoid ostium is typically found 2 cm superior to the arch of the choana.

Onodi Cells: pneumatized posterior most ethmoidal cell which is always lateral and superior to the sphenoid sinus.

Posterior septal branch of the sphenopalatine artery [49]: This artery serves as the vascular pedicle for nasoseptal reconstructive flaps. The vessel runs 2–6 mm inferior to the sphenoid ostium, within the mucosa superior to the choana.

Bolger's parallelogram [50]: parallelogram which is traditionally used for identification of sphenoid osteum; it is defined by following landmarks.

Surgical steps:

Endoscopic transethmoid approach:

1. Complete ethmoidectomy is done.
2. The basal lamellae of middle turbinate is identified.
3. A window is made through the basal lamella to expose the superior turbinate.
4. The sphenoid osteum is located after lateralizing the superior turbinate.
5. The floor of the orbit when maxillary antrostomy is done can be used as marker as the superior limit when searching for the sphenoid ostium, as the sphenoid ostium lies below the level of the floor of the orbit.
6. The inferior part of ST can be removed for further widening of the sphenoid osteum using true cutting instrument.
7. When enlarging the sphenoid osteum, the nasoseptal branch of sphenopalatine artery may get injured and can cause troublesome hemorrhage.

Endoscopic transnasal approach:

1. Lateralization of the middle turbinate is carefully performed with a Freer elevator placed onto the inferior aspect of the turbinate is done till inferior part of ST is visible.

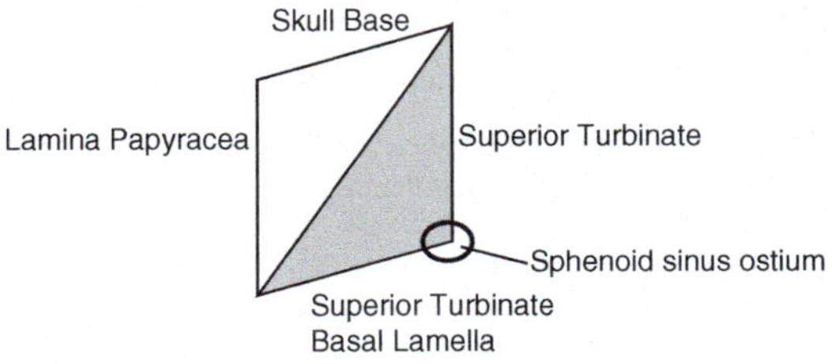

Bolger's parallelogram

2. Lateralization of ST to expose the sphenoid osteum.
3. Sphenoid osteum is widened medially and inferiorly.
4. This approach is used in isolated sphenoid sinus diseases or for transsphenoid approach for sellar or parasellar lesions [44, 49–52].

Frontal sinus:

Excellent understanding of frontal sinus anatomy is imperative to achieve optimal surgical outcomes. There are many endoscopic approaches and surgeries for sinus depending upon the anatomy, relationship of the frontal osteum to the surrounding structures, and extent of frontal sinus disease.

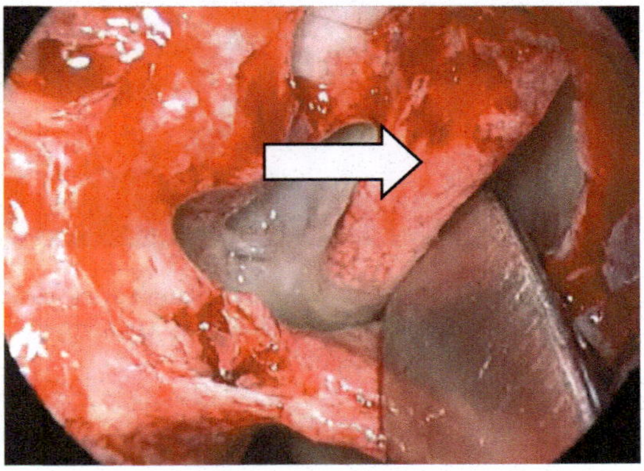

Arrow superior turbinate

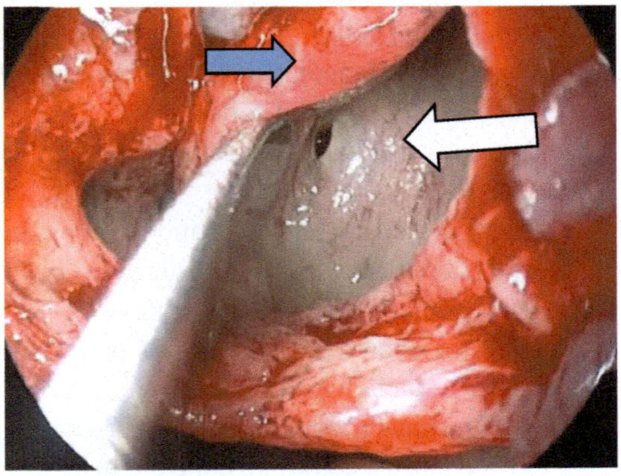

White arrow (natural sphenoid ostium), blue arrow (superior turbinate)

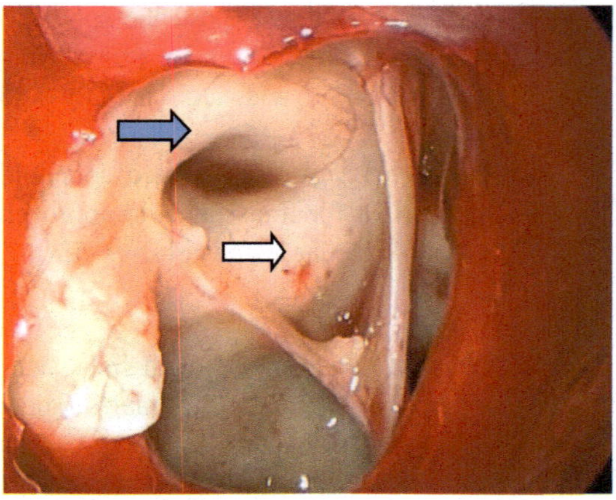

White arrow (carotid artery), blue arrow (optic nerve)

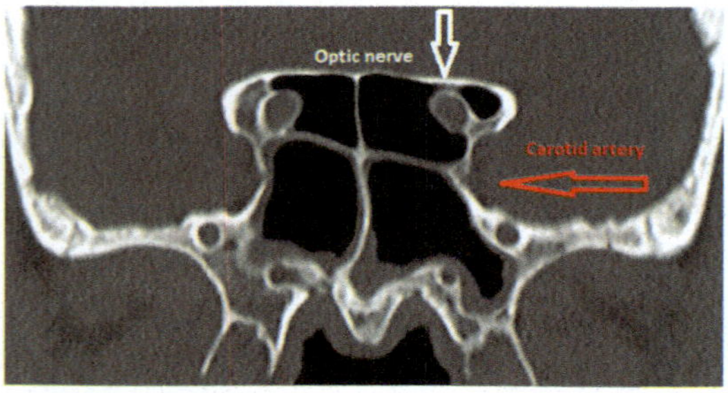

CT scan coronal section showing the relation of the optic nerve (white arrow) and the carotid artery (red arrow) to the lateral wall of the sphenoid sinus

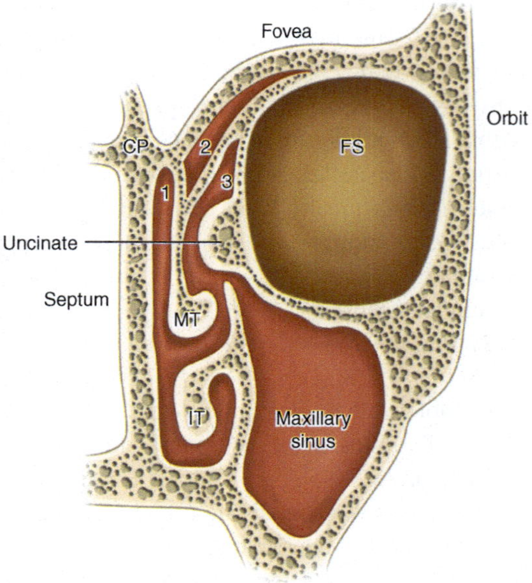

MT : Middle turbmate
IT : Inferior turbmate

Attachments of the uncinate

Frontal sinus anatomy [53]:

1. Following are the relation of frontoethmoidal recess:
   - Anterior: uncinate, agger nasi, and Kuhn-type frontal cells
   - Posterior: ethmoid bulla, suprabullar, and supraorbital ethmoid cells
   - Lateral: uncinate, agger nasi, lamina papyracea
   - Medial: attachment of the middle turbinate and lateral lamellae of the cribriform plate

   The frontal sinus outflow tract is dependent on the anatomic relationships of various structures, including the uncinate process, middle turbinate, agger nasi, and frontoethmoid cells. Most commonly, the uncinate process ascends from its inferior and anterior attachments to the inferior turbinate and lacrimal bone, respectively, to blend in with the medial wall of the agger nasi cell (1 in Figure above) In such cases—85% of the time—the frontal sinus will drain between the uncinate process and the middle turbinate. In the remaining cases (no 2 and 3 in Figure above), the uncinate attaches to the middle turbinate or the skull base, resulting in the frontal sinus draining directly into the infundibulum.
2. The axilla of the middle turbinate as it attaches to the lateral nasal wall marks the anteroinferior limit of the agger nasi region.
3. The slope of the posterior table of the frontal sinus as it joins the ethmoid skull base determines the anterior-to-posterior dimension of the frontal.
4. The anterior ethmoid artery is often at the posterior margin of the frontal recess.
5. Type of Frontal Cells (Kuhn's Classification):

Bent and Kuhn divided the frontal infundibulum cells into four categories, according to their relationship to the agger nasi cell and the orbital roof.

- Type 1 was defined as a single anterior ethmoid cell within the frontal recess above the agger cell.
- Type 2 was defined as a strand of two or more anterior ethmoid cells above the agger nasi cells.

- Type 3 represented a single cell located above the agger nasi and extending superiorly from the recess, through the ostium, up into the frontal sinus with occupation of nearly 50% of the sinus.
- Type 4 described as a single, but isolated cell existing completely within the frontal sinus and has no connection to the frontal recess.

Surgical approach [53–55]:

1. The approach to the frontal sinus starts with uncinectomy.
2. The frontal recess is approached from a posterior-to-anterior and a medial-to-lateral direction.
3. 45°/30° endoscope is used for precise visualization.
4. The anterior ethmoid artery is often identified at the posterior border of the supraorbital ethmoid cell or at the posterior aspect of the frontal recess.
5. The frontal sinus most commonly drains between the middle turbinate and the agger nasi-uncinate complex; the drainage pathway is most frequently medial and posterior to the posterior wall of the agger nasi.
6. After the agger nasi and any Kuhn frontal cells are removed, the opening to the frontal sinus may be enlarged anteriorly and laterally using a Hosemann frontal sinus punch.
7. Endoscopic frontal procedures can be described by the following classification, based on Wolfgang Draf's initial work in 1991 for endonasal frontal recess dissections:
   - Draf I: Removal of the superior uncinate with preservation of the agger nasi.
   - Draf IIa: Removal of all cells within the frontal recess.
   - Draf IIb: Draf IIa dissection plus removal of the ipsilateral floor of the frontal recess, i.e., from septum to lamina papyracea.
   - Draf III: Bilateral Draf IIb dissection plus removal of the intersinus septum and the superior nasal septum to create a single common opening, i.e., from lamina papyracea of one side to other side.

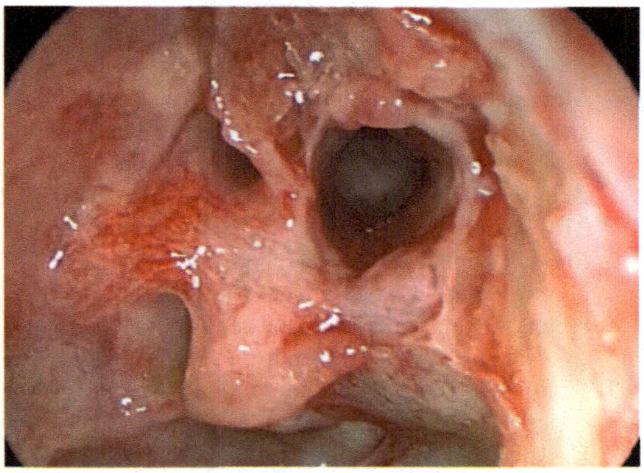

Frontoethmoidal recess

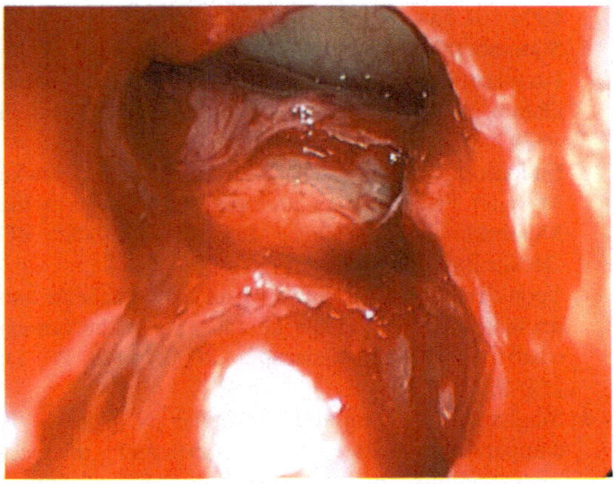

Frontal sinus

Take Home Messages

- Anatomical orientation of the nose and paranasal sinuses is the most important step before performing an endoscopic sinus surgery.
- It is important to review the CT scan before the surgery thoroughly assessing the CLOSE mnemonic.
- Different approaches and extent of surgery should be kept in mind for successful surgical outcome and to be able to manage any anatomical variation during the surgery.

References

1. Messerklinger W. Uber die drainage der menschlichen nasennebenholen unter normalen und pathologischen bendingungen II: die stirnhole und ihr ausfuhrungssystem. MonatsschOhrenheilkd. 1967;101:313–26.
2. Messerklinger W. Endosckopiche diagnose und chirurgie der rezidivierenden sinusitis. In: Krajina Z, editor. Advances in nose and sinus surgery. Zagreb, Yugoslavia: Zagreb University; 1985.
3. Stammberger H. Endoscopic endonasal surgery—concepts in treatment of recurring rhinosinusitis. Part I. Anatomic and pathophysiologic considerations. Otolaryngol Head Neck Surg. 1986;94:143–7.
4. Wake M, Takeno S, Hawke M. The uncinate process: a histological and morphological study. Laryngoscope. 1994;104:364–9.
5. Stammberger H, Kennedy D, Bolger W, et al. Paranasal sinuses: anatomic terminology and nomenclature. Ann Otol Rhinol Laryngol. 1995;104(Suppl 167):7–16.
6. Endoscopic anatomy. In Stammberger H, Hawke M (eds) Functional endoscopic sinus surgery: the Messerklinger technique. Philadelphia, PA: BC Decker Publishers; 1991. pp 61–90.
7. Yoon JH, Kim KS, Jung DH, et al. Fontanelle and uncinated process in the lateral wall of the human nasal cavity. Laryngoscope. 2000;110(2 Pt 1):281–5.
8. Singhania AA, Bansal C, Chauhan N, Soni S. A comparative study of two different uncinectomy techniques: swing-door and classical. Iran J Otorhinolaryngol. 2012;24:63–7.
9. Stammberger H. Functional endoscopic sinus surgery: the Messerklinger technique. Philadelphia, PA: BC Decker; 1991.
10. Fokkens WJ, Lund VJ, Mullol J, et al. EPOS 2012: European position paper on rhinosinusitis and nasal polyps 2012. A summary for otorhinolaryngologists. Rhinology. 2012;50(1):1–12.
11. Kennedy DW, Ramakrishnan VR. Functional endoscopic sinus surgery: concepts, surgical indications, and techniques. In: Hwang PH, Kennedy DW, editors. Rhinology diseases of the nose, sinuses, and skull base. New York: Thieme; 2012. p. 305–35.
12. Otori N, Yanagi K, Moriyama H. Maxillary and ethmoid sinuses in skull base surgery. In: Stamm A, editor. Transnasal endoscopic Skull Base and brain surgery tips and pearls. New York: Thieme; 2011. p. 109–14.
13. Levine HL. Functional endoscopic sinus surgery: evaluation, surgery, and follow-up of 250 patients. Laryngoscope. 1990;100(1):79–84.
14. Casiano R. Basic endoscopic sinonsal dissection. In: Casiano R, editor. Endoscopic sinonasal dissection guide. New York: Thieme; 2012. p. 19–58.
15. Wormald PJ. Surgery of the bulla ethmoidalis, middle turbinate, and posterior ethmoids and sphenoidotomy, including three- dimensional reconstruction of the posterior ethmoids. In: Wormald PJ, editor. Endoscopic sinus surgery anatomy, three-dimensional reconstruction, and surgical technique. 2nd ed. New York: Thieme; 2007. p. 101–14.
16. Simmen D, Jones N, Brine HR. Applied anatomy for endoscopic sinus and skull base surgery. In: Simmen D, Jones N, editors. Manual of endoscopic sinus and skull base surgery. 2nd ed. New York: Thieme; 2014. p. 80–90.
17. Saleh H, Nouraei R. Basic surgical techniques in endoscopic sinus surgery. In: Georgalas C, Fokkens W, editors. Rhinology and skull base surgery from the lab to the operating room: an evidence-based approach. Stuttgart: Georg Thieme Verlag KG; 2013. p. 331–25.
18. Wormald PJ, McDonogh M. The 'swing-door' technique for uncinectomy in endoscopic sinus surgery. J Laryngol Otol. 1998;112(6):547–51.
19. Levine HL. Functional endoscopic sinus surgery: evaluation, surgery, and follow-up of 250 patients. Laryngoscope. 1990;100(1):79–84.
20. Joe JK, Ho SY, Yanagisawa E. Documentation of variations in sinonasal anatomy by intraoperative nasal endoscopy. Laryngoscope. 2000;110(2 Pt 1):229–35.
21. Jog M, McGarry GW. How frequent are accessory sinus ostia. J Laryngol Otol. 2003;117(4):270–2.
22. Lee JM, Chiu AG. Role of maximal endoscopic sinus surgery techniques in chronic rhinosinusitis. Otolaryngol Clin North Am. 2010;43:579–89. ix
23. Schaefer SD. An anatomic approach to endoscopic intranasal ethmoidectomy. Laryngoscope. 1998;108(11 Pt 1):1628–34.
24. May M, Schaitkin B, Kay SL. Revision endoscopic sinus surgery: six friendly surgical landmarks. Laryngoscope. 1994;104(6 Pt 1):766–7.
25. Casiano RR. A stepwise surgical technique using the medial orbital floor as the key landmark in performing endoscopic sinus surgery. Laryngoscope. 2001;111:964–74.
26. Harvey RJ, Shelton W, Timperley D, et al. Using fixed anatomical landmarks in endoscopic skull base surgery. Am J Rhinol Allergy. 2010;24:301–5.
27. Wuttiwongsanon C, Chaowanapanja P, Harvey RJ, et al. The orbital floor is a surgical landmark for the Asian anterior skull base. Am J Rhinol Allergy. 2015;29:e216–9.
28. Owen R, Kuhn F. The maxillary sinus ostium: demystifying the middle meatal antrostomy. Am J Rhinol. 1995;9(6):313–20.
29. Richtsmeier WJ. Top 10 reasons for endoscopic maxillary sinus surgery failure. Laryngoscope. 2001;111(11 Pt 1):1952–6.
30. Parsons DS, Stivers FE, Talbot AR. The missed ostium sequence and the surgical approach to revision functional endoscopic sinus surgery. Otolaryngol Clin North Am. 1996;29(1):169–83.
31. Kirihene RK, Rees G, Wormald PJ. The influence of the size of the maxillary sinus ostium on the

nasal and sinus nitric oxide levels. Am J Rhinol. 2002;16(5):261–4.
32. Moncada S, Palmer RMJ, Higgs EA. Nitric oxide: physiology, pathophysiology, and pharmacology. Pharmacol Rev. 1991;43(2):109–42.
33. Nathan CF, Hibbs JB Jr. Role of nitric oxide synthesis in macrophage antimicrobial activity. Curr Opin Immunol. 1991;3(1):65–70.
34. Schlosser RJ, Spotnitz WD, Peters EJ, Fang K, Gaston B, Gross CW. Elevated nitric oxide metabolite levels in chronic sinusitis. Otolaryngol Head Neck Surg. 2000;123(4):357–62.
35. Sathananthar S, Nagaonkar S, Paleri V, Le T, Robinson S, Wormald PJ. Canine fossa puncture and clearance of the maxillary sinus for the severely diseased maxillary sinus. Laryngoscope. 2005;115(6):1026–9.
36. Cashman EC, Macmahon PJ, Smyth D. Computed tomography scans of paranasal sinuses before functional endoscopic sinus surgery. World J Radiol. 2011;3:199–204.
37. Bolger WE, Butzin CA, Parsons DS. Paranasal sinus bony anatomic variations and mucosal abnormalities: CT analysis for endoscopic sinus surgery. Laryngoscope. 1991;101:56–64.
38. Stammberger HR, et al. Paranasal sinuses: anatomic terminology and nomenclature. Ann Otol Rhinol Laryngol. 1995;104(Suppl 167):7–16.
39. Kim KS, Kim HU, Chung IH, et al. Surgical anatomy of the nasofrontal duct: anatomical and computed tomographic analysis. Laryngoscope. 2001;111:603–8.
40. Edelstein DR, Uberatore L, Dushkin S, Han JC. Applied aoalDmy of the posterior sinuses in relation ID the optic nerve, trigemina nerve and carotid artery. Am J Rhinol. 1995;9:321–33.
41. Gupta T, Aggarwal A, Sahni D. Anatomical landmarks for locating the sphenoid ostium during endoscopic endonasal approach: a cadaveric study. Surg Radiol Anat. 2013;35:137–42.
42. Eweiss AZ, Ibrahim AA, Khalil HS. The safe gate to the posterior paranasal sinuses: reassessing the role of the superior turbinate. Eur Arch Otorhinolaryngol. 2012;269:1451–6.
43. Kim HU, Kim SS, Kang SS, Chung IH, Lee JG, Yoon JH. Surgical anatomy of the natural ostium of the sphenoid sinus. Laryngoscope. 2001;111:1599–602.
44. Orlandi RR, Lanza DC, Bolger WE, Clerico DM, Kennedy DW. The forgotten turbinate: the role of the superior turbinate in endoscopic sinus surgery. Am J Rhinol. 1999;13:251–9.
45. Herzallah IR, Saati FA, Marglani OA, Simsim RF. Retromaxillary pneumatization of posterior ethmoid air cells: novel description and surgical implications. Otolaryngol Head Neck Surg. 2016;155:340–6.
46. Elwany S, Elsaeid I, Tbabet H. Endoscopic anatomy of the spbenoid slnus. J Laryngol Otol. 1999;113:122–6.
47. Kainz J, Stammberger H. Danger areas of the posterior rhlno basls. AD endoscopic and anatomical-surgical study. Acta Otolaryngol. 1992;112:852–61.
48. Floreani SR, Nair SB, Switajewski MC, Wonnald PJ. Endoscopic : anterior ethmoidal artery ligation: a cadaver study. Laryngoscope. 2006;116:1263–7.
49. Halawi AM, Simon PE, Lidder AK, et al. The relationship of the natural sphenoid ostium to the skull base. Laryngoscope. 2015;125(1):75–9.
50. Bolger WE, Keyes AS, Lanza DC. Use of the superior meatus and superior turbinate in the endoscopic approach to the sphenoid sinus. Otolaryngol Head Neck Surg. 1999;120(3):308–13. Review.
51. Miwa T, Furukawa M, Tsukatani T, et al. Impact of olfactory impairment on quality of life and disability. Arch Otolaryngol Head Neck Surg. 2001;127(5):497–503.
52. Pinna Fde R, Ctenas B, Weber R, et al. Olfactory neuroepithelium in the superior and middle turbinates: which is the optimal biopsy site? Int Arch Otorhinolaryngol. 2013;17(2):131–8.
53. Barham HP, et al. Frontal sinus surgery and sinus distribution of nasal irrigation. Int Forum Allergy Rhinol. 2016;6(3):238–42.
54. Timperley DG, et al. Lateral frontal sinus access in endoscopic skull-base surgery. Int Forum Allergy Rhinol. 2011;1(4):290–5.
55. Chin D, et al. The outside-in approach to the modified endoscopic Lothrop procedure. Laryngoscope. 2012;122(8):1661–9.

Complications of Functional Endoscopic Sinus Surgery

27

Shanmugam Ganesan, Emad Al Duhirat, Hamad Al Saey, Mansour Al Sulaiti, Maryam Abdulraheem, Rafia Zahid, and Ahmed Shaikh

27.1 Introduction

Functional endoscopic sinus surgery (FESS) is an effective treatment modality for sinus diseases, especially for patients who fail appropriate medical therapy. The outcomes of FESS have improved over time because of multiple factors like technologic advances, improved surgical training, and a better understanding of the disease's pathophysiology. The outcome and complications of surgery are affected by multiple factors, including patient-related factors, pathology, and surgeon-related factors.

The reported complications of FESS are not uncommon. A literature review reveals a range of significant complications between 0.3% and 22.4% (median 7.0%) [1]. The bloody surgical field decreases the visualization and is associated with higher complication rates. It is always safer to abort the procedure and plan elective second surgery if proper hemostasis cannot be achieved. Using image guidance during the surgery decreases the incidence of complications significantly [2]. The global relative ratio of complications on the right side is reported to be 55–86% and found to be more common than the left side [3, 4].

Proper preoperative preparation, including thorough history taking, physical examination, and detailed interpretation of the CT scans, will alert the surgeon to the presence of any anatomical variations, which might increase the chance of damage to any vital structures including the orbit and skull base.

27.2 Increased Risk of Complications

- Revision surgery
- Anatomic variations
- Advanced sinus disease
- Severe comorbidities
- Increased intraoperative bleeding
- Inexperienced surgeon
- Increased risk on the right side (right handed surgeon)
- Extended endoscopic sino-neurosurgery

S. Ganesan (✉) · H. Al Saey · M. Al Sulaiti
Otolaryngology-Head and Neck Surgery Division, Department of Surgery, Hamad Medical Corporation, Doha, Qatar

Department of Otolaryngology-Head and Neck Surgery Division, Weill Cornell Medicine-Qatar, Doha, Qatar
e-mail: sganesan@hamad.qa; Halsaey@hamad.qa; Malsulaiti1@hamad.qa

E. Al Duhirat · M. Abdulraheem · R. Zahid · A. Shaikh
Otolaryngology-Head and Neck Surgery Division, Department of Surgery, Hamad Medical Corporation, Doha, Qatar
e-mail: EAlDuhirat@hamad.qa; mabdulraheem1@hamad.qa; rzahid1@hamad.qa; ashaikh4@hamad.qa

A. Al-Qahtani et al. (eds.), *Textbook of Clinical Otolaryngology*,
https://doi.org/10.1007/978-3-030-54088-3_27

27.3 Prevention of Complications

- Knowledge, skill, and experience of the surgeon
- Patient checklist prior to surgery, which includes:
  - Sinus-skull base anatomy imaging
  - Maxillary-to-ethmoid sinus ratio
  - Slope of the skull base
  - Cribriform plate/Olfactory cleft
  - Anterior and posterior ethmoidal arteries location
  - Lamina papyracea
  - Optic nerve and carotid artery positions in the sphenoid sinus
  - Presence of Onodi cell
  - Anatomic variations/Asymmetric skull base

Multiple ways were used to categorize the complications of FESS, either to the severity or to location (Table 27.1).

Table 27.1 FESS complications

Localization/ overall type of injury	"Minor complication"	"Major complication"
Orbital complicaton	• Orbital emphysema • Ecchymosis of the eylid	• Orbital hematoma • Reduced visual acuity/blindness • Enophthalmos • Injury of the nasolacrimal duct
Intracranial complication	• Uncomplicated CSF fistula	• CSF leak • (Tension-) pneumocephalus • Encephalocele • Brain abscess • Meningitis • Intracranial (subarachnoid) hemorrhage • Direct injury of brain tissue
Bleeding	• Minor bleeding (stopped with nasal packing, no need for blood transfusion)	• Injury of the ant. ethmoidal artery • Injury of the sphenopalatine artery • Injury of internal carotid artery • Bleeding in need of transfusion

Table 27.1 (continued)

Localization/ overall type of injury	"Minor complication"	"Major complication"
Other	• Synechiae • Slight exacerbation of preexisting bronchial asthma • Hyposmia • Local infection (osteitis) • Postoperative MRSA-Infection • Atrophic rhinitis • Paraffinoma • Myospherulosis • Temporal irritation of the infraorbital nerve • Hypoesthesia of the lip or teeth	• "Toxic shock syndrome" • Anosmia • Severe exacerbation of a preexisting bronchial asthma or bronchospasm • Death

Courtesy of Hosemann et al.: Danger points, complications, and medicolegal aspects in endoscopic sinus surgery [5]

27.4 Intraoperative Complications

27.4.1 Intranasal Complications

Diffuse mucosal bleeding, which affects the operation flow and its safety, occurs mainly in the setting of active inflamed mucosa and nasal polyposis in the absence of proper preoperative and intraoperative preparation. About 5% of the endoscopic sinus surgery is affected by diffuse bleeding, and about 1.4% of the procedures are canceled [6, 7]. The rate of peri- or postoperative bleeding is supposed to be around 2% altogether; transfusion was needed in about 0.2% of cases [8, 9].

- A preoperative systemic steroid (e.g., 30 mg/day prednisone for 5 days) and possibly adding topical cortisone treatment can lead to less bleeding, which reduces the duration of surgery [5].
- Lifting the head and the upper part of the patient's body for about 10–20°.

- Applying local, drug-induced vasoconstriction [10–13].
- Topical vasoconstriction by epinephrine (usually 1:1000) [14]. Optic nerve damage and blindness after the application of pads of adrenaline have been reported [15]. The risk of side effects is 0.05%, and it was concluded that the topical application of epinephrine 1:1000 is safe in adults who have no prior cardiac damage. 0.05% oxymetazoline is used, with subsequent use of 0.1% oxymetazoline for children; in selected cases, epinephrine 1:2000 can be used [16, 17].
- Controlled hypotension by anesthesia.
- 50–60 or 80 mmHg for elderly individuals, and a decrease of the systolic blood pressure less than 100 mmHg [3, 18]. Note, the mean arterial blood pressure must not be decreased to less than 85% of the initial. Also, note that dangerous complications like organ ischemia have been seen in 0.02–0.06% of cases [19, 20, 22].
- Heart rate and blood loss have been shown to have a relationship, and there is a recommendation for a pulse rate of 60 per minute [5].
- The insertion of 3% H_2O_2 using saturated cotton wool strips is recommended to suppress capillary bleeding [23].
- Use of tranexamic acid.
  - Tranexamic acid is applied: perioperative administration (3 × 1 g daily for 5 days, starting 2 h before the operation) is recommended [24].
  - Tranexamic acid (10 mg/kg) is administered intravenously at the beginning of the sinus surgery, leading to a significant improvement of the hemostasis in the surgical area [25].
- Rinsing the surgical field with 40° hot water is also helpful [26].

27.4.2 Arterial Injury

Arterial bleeding sources are the sphenopalatine artery, anterior ethmoid artery, and the posterior ethmoid artery. Knowing their anatomy will help to avoid their injury.

Sphenopalatine artery: In 80%, the sphenopalatine foramen is located in the superior nasal meatus or the transition area between the middle nasal meatus and the superior nasal meatus, directly behind or below the ethmoidal crest of the palatine bone. Several ostia are found in about 13% of cases [27, 28]. In 97% of cases, the SPA is divided into two or more branches. In 64% of cases, 3–10 branches may enter the lateral nasal wall [29, 30]. The nasoseptal branch of the sphenopalatine artery traverses through the lower third of the anterior wall of the sphenoid sinus and the surgeons entering the sphenoid sinus should avoid injury to the vessel. In approximately 3% of pituitary surgery, postoperative bleeding occurs from this vessel [5].

Resection of the middle turbinate near its posterior insertion site along the lateral nasal wall, aggressive enlargement of the maxillary ostium in a posterior direction, and enlargement of the sphenoid ostium in an inferior direction all may cause bleeding from the sphenopalatine artery or one of its branches. Generally bleeding from the sphenopalatine artery is managed by identification of the vessel and its branches and controlled by clipping or electrocautery methods (Fig. 27.1).

The anterior ethmoid artery: Cadaveric studies showed variability of the location of the anterior ethmoid artery. The distance from nostrils to the anterior ethmoid artery at the skull base is approximately 6–7 cm, and the distance to the

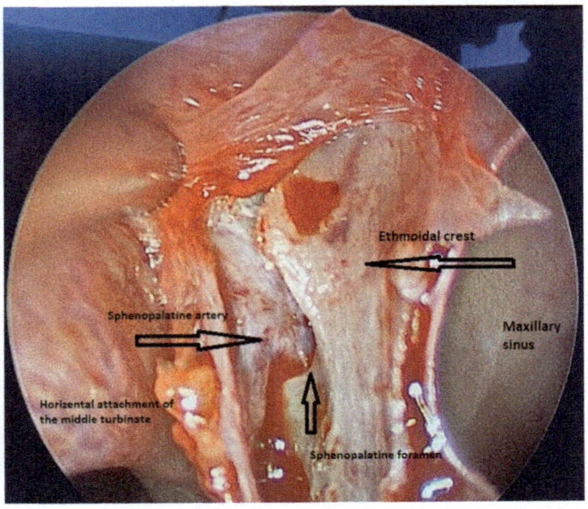

Fig. 27.1 Sphenopalatine artery

posterior ethmoid artery is approximately 7–8 cm [31–33].

The artery could be identified endoscopically within the posterior wall of the most superior suprabullar ethmoidal cell and approximately 11 mm posterior to the common wall between the posterior wall of the frontal infundibulum and this superior-most suprabullar cell [31–35]. According to anatomical studies, arteries are missing in about 5–10% of cases. The anterior ethmoid artery traverses the skull base around 12 mm anterior to the posterior ethmoid artery (Figs. 27.2, 27.3, and 27.4).

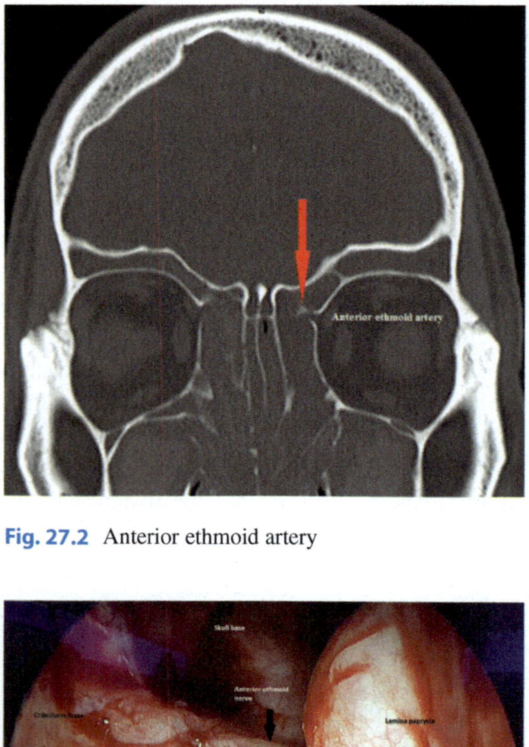

Fig. 27.2 Anterior ethmoid artery

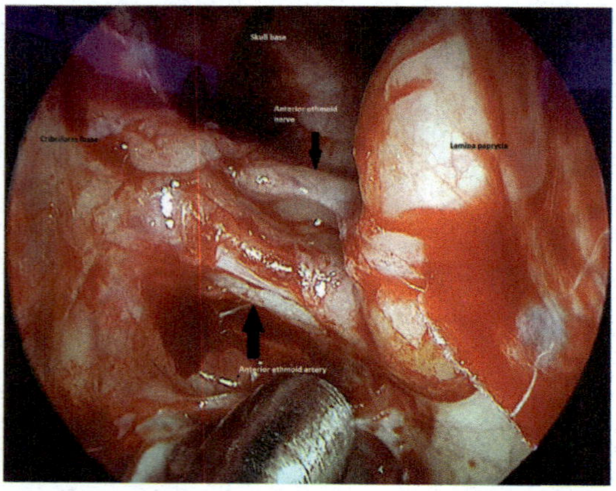

Fig. 27.3 Anatomical dissection of the anterior ethmoid artery

Since the blood flows through the anterior ethmoid artery from a postero-lateral to an antero-medial direction, the angle between the lamina papyracea to the artery is 60° and its disruption must be managed to avoid retraction of the artery into the orbit. Bipolar cautery is preferred to control the bleeding, to avoid transmitting the electrical current to the skull base and orbit. The external approach can also be used for control.

The posterior ethmoid artery: It runs 5 mm anterior to the sphenoethmoid angle, which is formed by the junction of the anterior sphenoid wall and the posterior ethmoid roof. It is smaller than the anterior ethmoidal arteries, runs symmetrical and linear in most cases with bony dehiscences noted in approximately 60% of cases. The distance to the optic nerve is 8–9 mm. According to literature, absence of arteries is noted in 2–34% of cases. The artery is most commonly injured during sphenoid sinus entry or during manipulations of the posterior ethmoid bone [5]. Bipolar cautery is preferred to control the bleeding, to avoid transmitting the electrical current to the skull base and orbit (Fig. 27.5).

27.4.3 Intraorbital Complications

The most common orbital complication of the endoscopic sinus surgery is a trauma of the lamina papyracea [36]. The incidence of a periorbital injury is around 2% [6, 8].

27.4.4 Orbital Emphysema

Postoperative emphysema of the eyelid may occur following nose-blowing, sneezing, or after anesthesia with mask ventilation. In several cases, there have been two likely observations—either a surgical defect or a history of fracture in lamina papyracea.

Mainly, in the upper eyelid, the emphysema develops. Orbital emphysema usually managed conservatively and resorbed within a week. Nose-blowing and sneezing are advised to the patient to be avoided (Fig. 27.6) [38, 39].

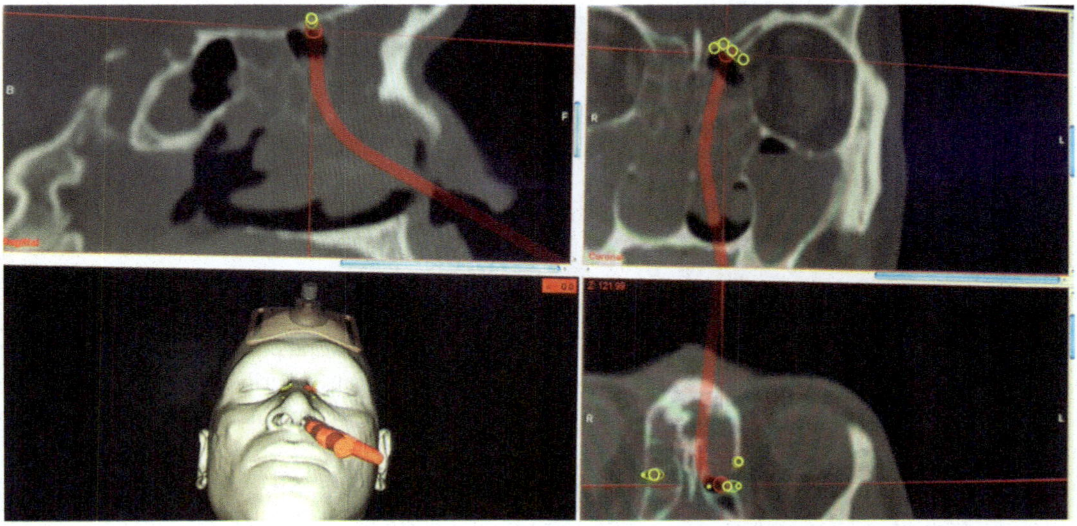

Fig. 27.4 Navigation assisted localization of the anterior ethmoid artery

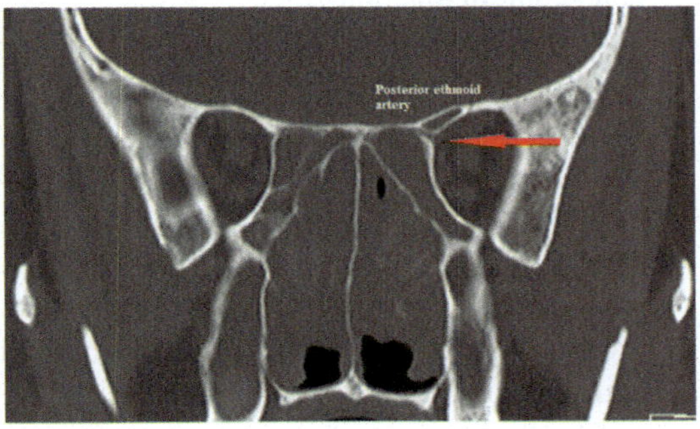

Fig. 27.5 Posterior ethmoid artery

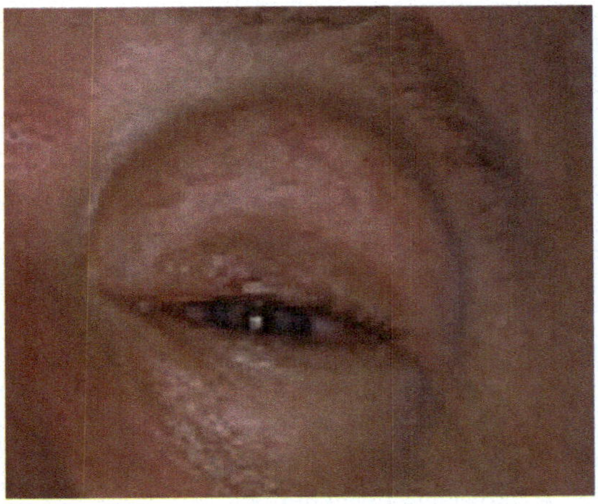

Fig. 27.6 Orbital emphysema due to injury to lamina papyracea. (Courtesy of Kevin C. Welch, MD, James N. Palmer, MD Department of Otorhinolaryngology, Division of Rhinology, University of Pennsylvania [37])

27.4.5 Orbital Fat Exposure

Injury to the lamina papyracea may occur during uncinectomy, or aggressive lateral dissection during ethmoidectomy. The injury most likely occurs due to aggressive debrider powered instrumentation or in the presence of hypoplastic-atelectatic maxillary sinus.

Routine palpation of the globe is vital while operating in this region, watching for any movement by performing intraoperative pressure test described by Draf and Stankiewicz [5]. In case orbital fat is seen, manipulation of the fat within the ethmoid sinus should be avoided to prevent further injury. Uses of suction manipulation and powered instrumentation should be avoided. No repair of this defect is needed. If needed, a silicon sheet can be placed temporarily on the area of the defect. Serial examinations of the eye should be performed during the remainder of surgery to ensure that intraorbital hemorrhage has not developed. Nasal packing should usually be avoided in such cases (Fig. 27.7).

27.4.6 Intraorbital Hematoma

The incidence of orbital hematoma is around 0.1% [40, 41]. The average orbital volume in a confined cavity is 26 cc and an increase in vol-

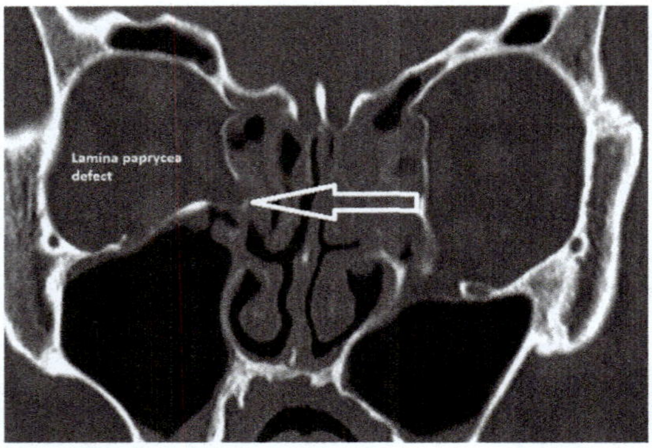

Fig. 27.7 Right orbital content prolapse

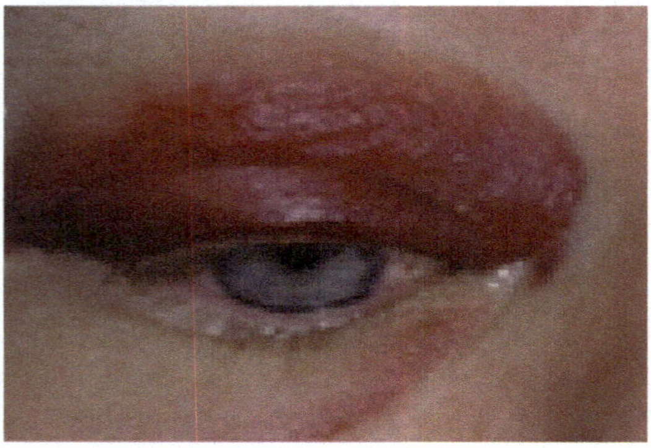

Fig. 27.8 Orbital hematoma as a result of anterior ethmoid artery injury. (Courtesy of Kevin C. Welch, MD, James N. Palmer, MD Department of Otorhinolaryngology, Division of Rhinology, University of Pennsylvania [37])

ume of 4 cc results in 6 mm proptosis. Normal intraocular pressure is 12–22 mmHg.

Intraorbital hemorrhage has 50% the risk of permanent blindness with manifest retrobulbar hematoma with accompanying loss of vision [37, 41, 42]. Bleeding into the orbit occurs from injury to intraorbital vessels or retraction of a bleeding from anterior or posterior ethmoid arteries causing an acute increase in the intraorbital pressure and retinal ischemia. Injury to orbital or ophthalmic veins results in slow process of accumulation of blood. The retina can tolerate up to 90 min of ischemia before irreversible damage happens (Fig. 27.8).

Signs and symptoms of intraorbital hemorrhage include:

- Tense globe
- Increased intraocular pressure
- Progressive proptosis with chemosis
- Conjunctival vessels congestion and subconjunctival hemorrhage
- Pupillary dilation
- Loss of pupillary reflex
- Eye pain
- Limitation of eye mobility
- Visual field loss and loss of vision

The list of managing a slowly expanding intraorbital hematoma and proptosis occurring mainly in the postoperative period, most likely secondary to venous bleeding includes the following:

- Head end of the bed raised
- Cooling compresses applied
- Removal of nasal packing if any
- Gentle eye massage applied provided if there is no contraindication
- Administration of systemic steroids (dexamethasone 0.2 mg/kg IV)
- Mannitol 20% (1–2 g/kg IV over 20–30 min)
- Acetazolamide (10–15 mg/kg IV) can reduce edema and aqueous humor production
- Topical Timolol eye drops 0.5%, 1–2 drops twice daily, can help reduce intraocular pressure through decreasing the production of aqueous humor
- Antibiotics
- Immediate ophthalmic consultation with a serial examination of visual acuity and intraocular pressures is mandatory [37]
- CT scan

A rapidly developing intraorbital hematoma occurring either intraoperatively or in the recovery room, most likely secondary to anterior ethmoidal injury is managed as follows [5].

- Stop the procedure if it happens during surgery
- Elevate the head end of the bed
- Cooling compresses applied with ice
- Normalize the blood pressure
- Remove nasal packing
- Control nasal bleeding if any
- Consult the ophthalmologist
- Ocular massage helps to redistribution of hematoma (controversial)

A lateral canthotomy (reduction of IOP by approximately 14 mmHg) and cantholysis (reduction of IOP by approximately 30 mmHg) must be performed to increase orbital volume and reduce the pressure [37]:

- Intraocular pressure more than 40 mmHg
- Loss of pupillary reflex
- Cherry red macula

Additional following procedures can be performed if needed:

- Medial orbital wall decompression (reduction of IOP by approximately 10 mmHg)
- Orbital floor decompression
- Control of bleeding by endoscopic or external artery ligation (Fig. 27.9)

Flowchart algorithm (Fig. 27.10):

27.4.7 Extraocular Muscle Injury

The medial rectus muscle is the most susceptible muscle to injury during endoscopic sinus surgery, especially in the posterior ethmoid sinus resulting in irreversible diplopia and exotropia. It is likely to occur with an incidence of approximately 1/1000 [35]. Other eye muscles are less often injured; the inferior rectus muscle may be damaged in surgeries involving the maxillary sinus, and the superior oblique (trochlea) muscle may be lacerated in extended endonasal frontal sinus surgery [43].

The use of powered instruments (microdebrider) in sinus surgery has been associated with greater risks of injury to the extraocular muscles [44]. Injuries may range from muscle contusion to complete transection. Strabismus surgery is not always successful in restoring the full range of motion of the globe, but if any surgery to be

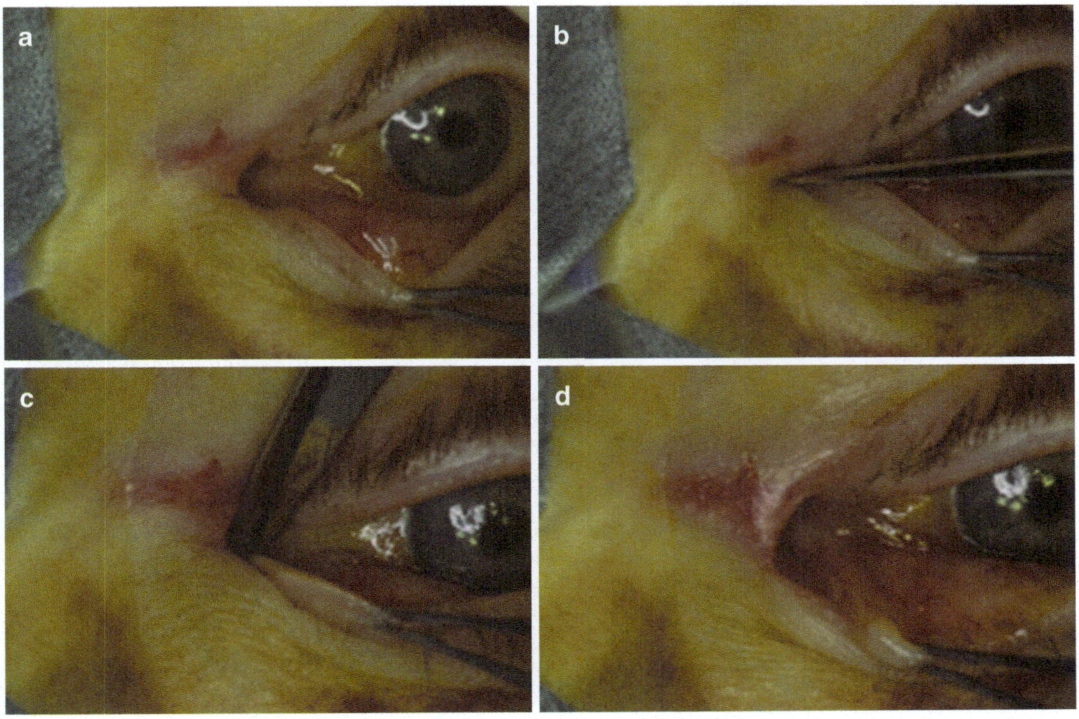

Fig. 27.9 Steps of lateral canthotomy and cantholysis. (**a**) Lateral canthus incision. (**b**) Retraction of the inferior lid shows the extent of incision. (**c**) The inferior crus of the lateral canthal tendon is divided. (**d**) The lower lid is retracted to show the final result. (Courtesy of R. Gausas, MD, Philadelphia, PA [37])

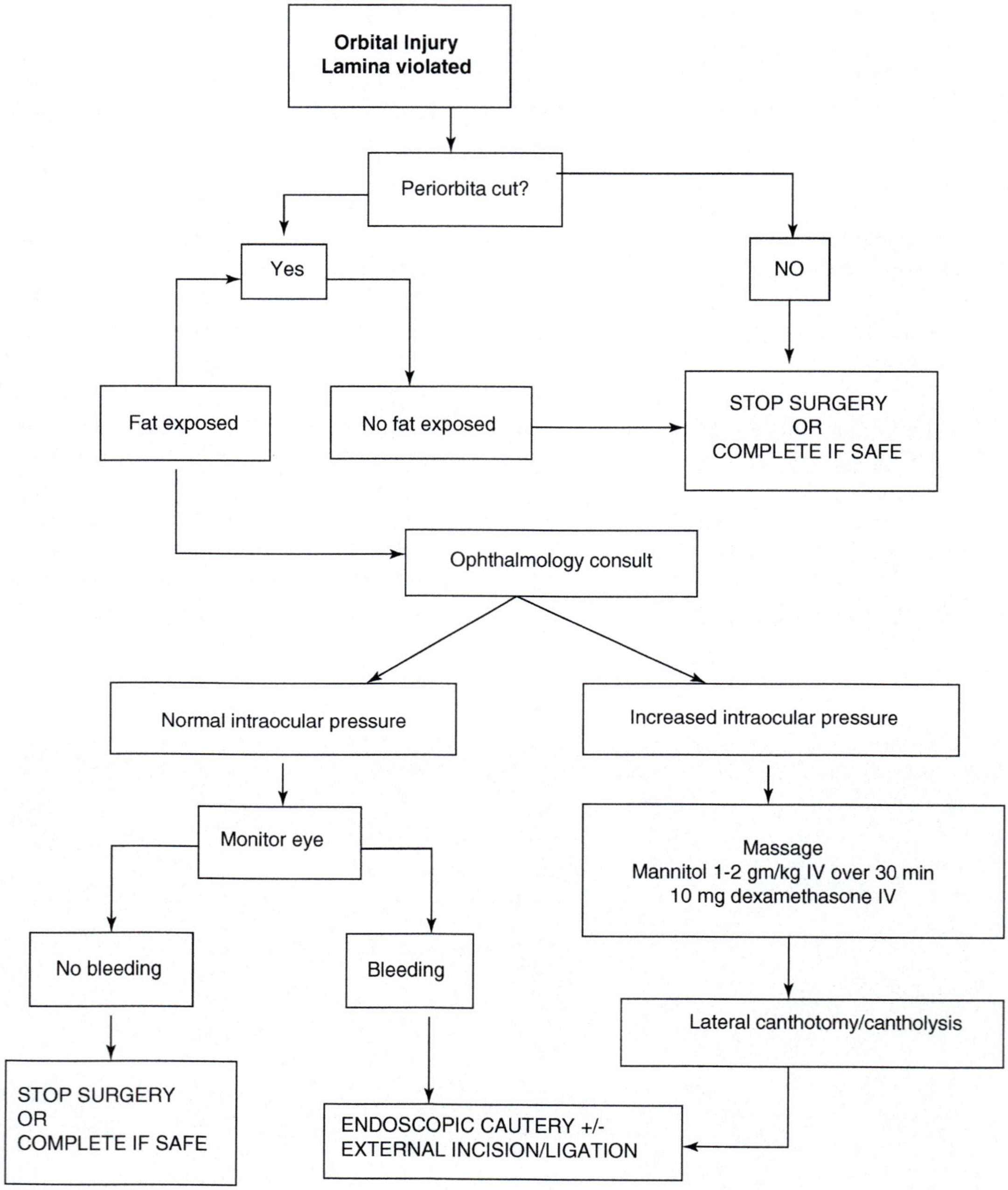

Fig. 27.10 Algorithm for addressing intraoperative orbital bleeding. (Courtesy of Kevin C. Welch, MD, James N. Palmer, MD Department of Otorhinolaryngology, Division of Rhinology, University of Pennsylvania [37])

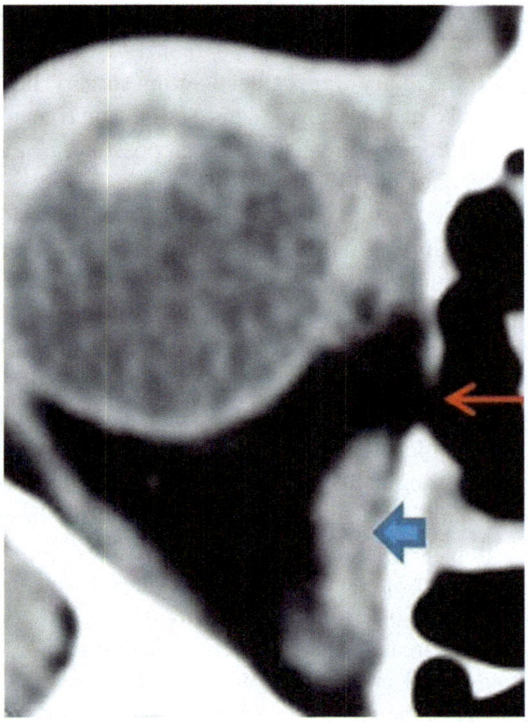

Fig. 27.11 Postoperative CT scan showing the destruction of the lamina papyracea (red arrow) and complete transection of the medial rectus muscle (blue arrow). (Courtesy of Hosemann et al.: Danger points, complications, and medicolegal aspects in endoscopic sinus surgery [5])

done should be performed within 2–3 weeks from injury after the resolution of the edema (Fig. 27.11).

27.4.8 Optic Nerve Injury

The optic nerve typically forms an indentation in the lateral wall of the sphenoid sinus, and approximately 5% of these have dehiscent bone; this can occur unilaterally or bilaterally. Failing to recognize the Onodi cell can place patients at risk for optic nerve injury during a posterior ethmoidectomy. Onodi cells present in 8–14% of the general population and considered to be a posterior ethmoid cell that pneumatizes lateral and superior to the sphenoid sinus [45].

Optic nerve injury can happen at the level of the orbital apex or the superolateral sphenoid sinus, which might cause a partial loss of vision or blindness.

If an injury to the optic nerve is suspected,

- Normalize the blood pressure
- A high-dose systemic corticosteroid (dexamethasone 0.5–1 mg/kg body weight IV) should be given
- Administration of methylprednisolone 4 × 250 mg per day for 3 days (controversial)
- Ophthalmologic consultation to assess the visual acuity
- A postoperative CT scan is necessary to evaluate the location and extent of this injury
- MRI scan helps to evaluate the optic nerve sheath or disruption
- Optic nerve decompression in specific cases may be considered (Fig. 27.12)

27.4.9 Intracranial Complications

All suspected and proven intracranial complications must be managed jointly with the neurosurgery team.

A pneumocephalus is the presence of gas (air) in the cranial cavity. Largely, it is based on the extracranial and intracranial space communication. In subdural, epidural, intraventricular, subarachnoid, or intracerebral spaces, air may be present.

Intracranial pressure increases gradually, causing a tension pneumocephalus to develop.

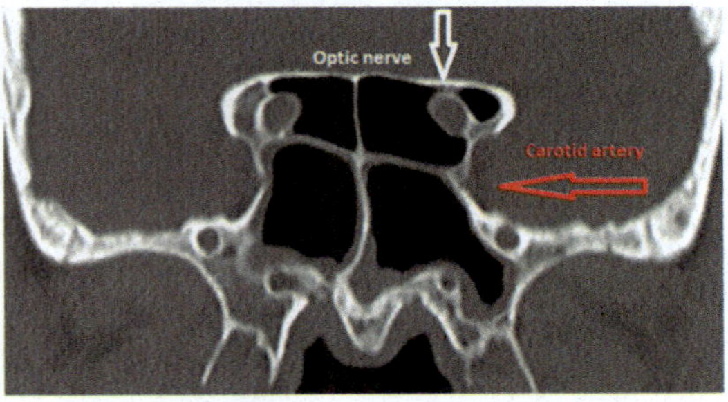

Fig. 27.12 CT scan coronal section showing the optic nerve (dehiscent) within the sphenoid sinus (white arrow), carotid artery bulging inside the sphenoid sinus (red arrow)

Symptoms include:

- An altered state of consciousness.
- Restlessness.
- Headache.
- Nausea and vomiting.
- Eye motility disorders.
- Ataxia.
- Spasms (Fig. 27.13).

27.4.10 Cerebrospinal Fluid Leak

The incidence of iatrogenic endoscopic sinus surgery injury to the skull base and CSF leak is 0.5% [10, 44]. The rate of unexpected dura exposure is 0.2% [5].

Although the injury may occur anywhere along the skull base, the cribriform plate, posterior wall of the frontal sinus, roof of the posterior ethmoid, and roof of the sphenoid sinus are the most common areas. The weakest area of the skull base and most liable to injury is at the junction of the anterior ethmoid artery and the middle turbinate along the anterior ethmoid roof [46]. The weakest area of the skull base at the lateral lamella of the olfactory fossa is 0.05–1 mm thin and is susceptible for injury. The surgeons should be aware of the asymmetric skull base and the incidence is approximately 10% [5].

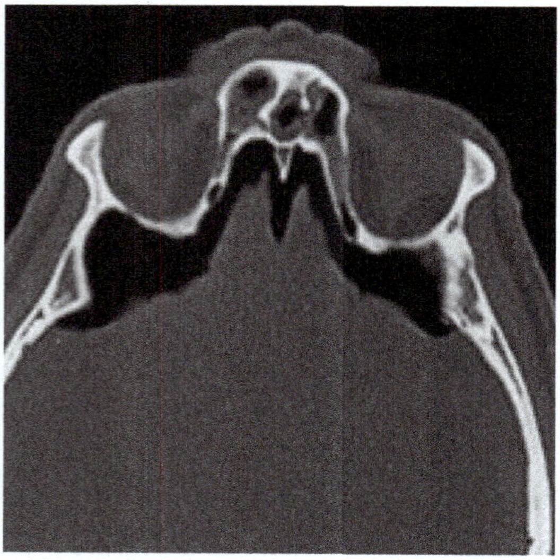

Fig. 27.13 Axial CT scan showing tension pneumocephalus post sinus surgery complicated by skull base perforation (Mount Fuji sign). (Courtesy of Hosemann et al.: Danger points, complications, and medicolegal aspects in endoscopic sinus surgery [5])

If the injury is recognized during surgery, better to be managed in the same setting and if managed properly, greater than 90% possibility of a good outcome [47, 48].

Once the patient is awake, a CT scan should be obtained to assess for pneumocephalus or intracranial injury.

Although many surgeons believe that antibiotics cover should be used either oral or intravenous in case of skull base injury and CSF leak, a meta-analysis by Brodie and colleagues showed no significant differences in the rates of ascending meningitis in patients treated with and without antibiotics in traumatic anterior skull base CSF leaks [49].

Bernal-Sprekelsen and colleagues found an incidence of ascending meningitis in 29% of patients treated conservatively [50]. Furthermore, trans-nasal endoscopic repair of CSF leaks has been reported to be successful in 90% to 97% of patients [47, 51].

Literature evidence showed various successful techniques described either underlay or onlay, depending on the size of the defect for repairing the fistula. In general, autologous grafts are preferred which includes mucosa, fascia, fat, cartilage, bone, or perichondrium with or without pedicled flaps. Defects more than 5 mm in diameter are closely in several layers partly with cartilage or bone. Fibrin glue does not need to be routinely applied in every case [5]. In cases where the site of leak is difficult to localize, 10% intrathecal fluorescein (FDA non-approved product) can be used to identify the leak. Appropriate informed consent must be obtained for using fluorescein. Most surgeons prefer nasal packing for 3–7 days with bed rest, antibiotics as a prophylaxis to prevent ascending infection, sleep with head end elevation (40–70°), to avoid lifting heavy objects and blowing nose for a certain period. In addition, patients are advised to sneeze with an open mouth and laxatives are prescribed for patients with constipation. Lumbar drains are not routinely placed except in cases with increased intracranial pressure, large defect repair and revision cases (Fig. 27.14).

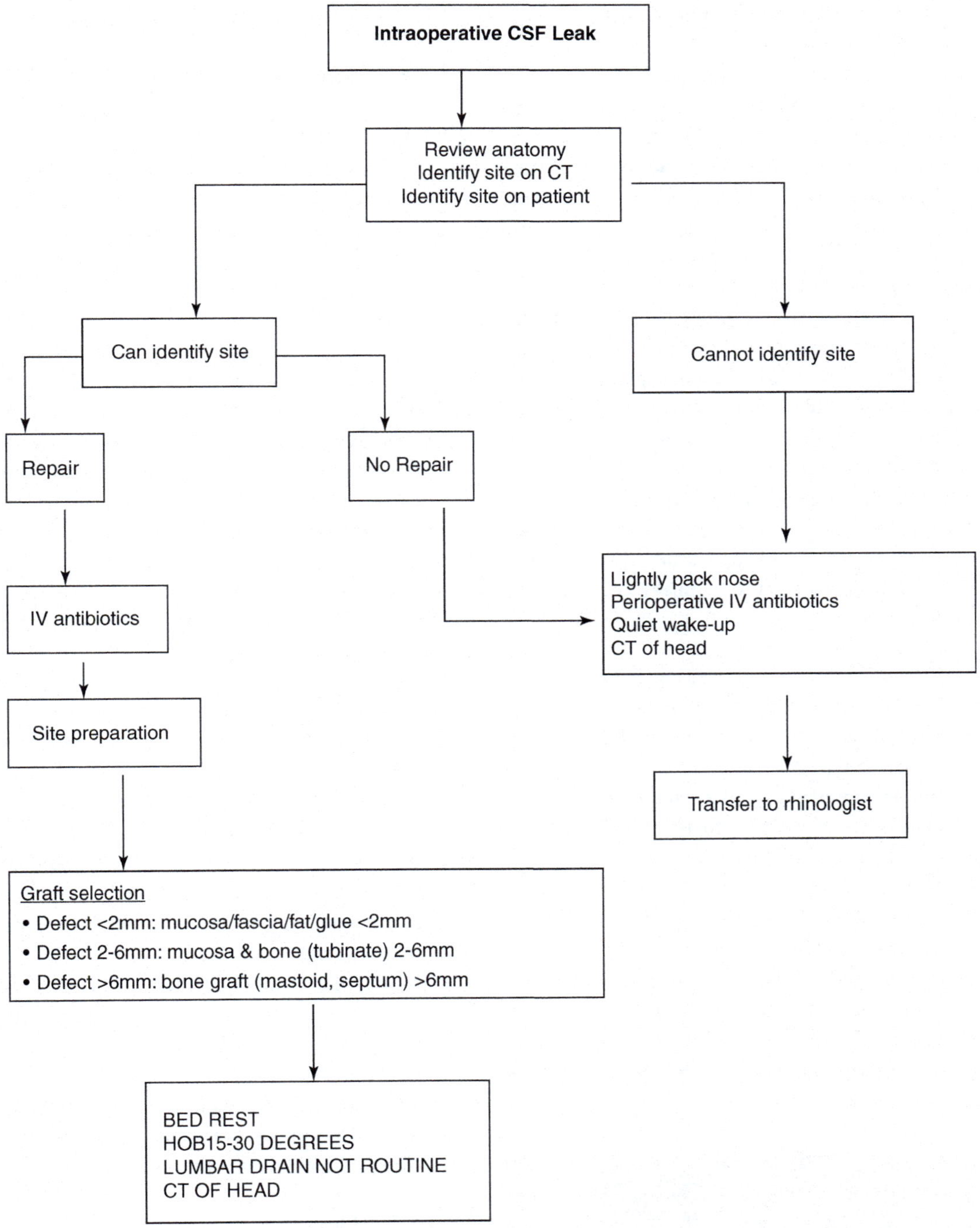

Fig. 27.14 Algorithm for addressing intraoperative CSF leak. (Courtesy of Kevin C. Welch, MD, James N. Palmer, MD Department of Otorhinolaryngology, Division of Rhinology, University of Pennsylvania [37])

27.4.11 Internal Carotid Artery Injury

Exact incidence of carotid artery injuries in paranasal surgery is unknown. Review of literature has shown a rate of 0.3% in surgery of diffuse chronic rhinosinusitis [8]. A rate of 1% for pituitary surgery [52]. For sinoneurosurgical procedures, the rate quoted is approximately 0.3–0.9%. Mortality rate is 17% [5].

The internal carotid artery (ICA) indents the lateral sphenoid sinus wall, with 7% of these being dehiscent. 1% of inter-sphenoid septum will insert on the bony canal of the carotid artery [37].

Injury to the ICA may occur when the sphenoid sinus is entered too far laterally, or the carotid canal is penetrated when surgical dissection is performed along the lateral sphenoid wall, and the carotid canal is penetrated (Fig. 27.15).

Internal carotid artery injury management plan:

- Immediate tight nasal packing and pharyngeal packing to tamponade the bleeding
- Several suctions and multiple IV lines must be established
- Initiate aggressive fluid resuscitation, and emergency blood transfusion should begin to maintain cerebral perfusion
- Maintain normotension
- Compression of same side of ICA with or without cervical incision
- Consult and involve neurosurgery team help
- Definitive treatment is performed by the interventional radiologist, who uses angiography to identify the site and extent of vascular injury (Fig. 27.16)

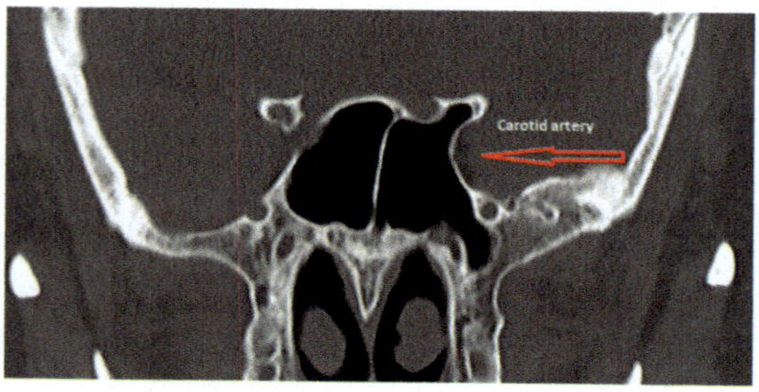

Fig. 27.15 CT scan coronal section showing the carotid artery relation to the lateral wall

27.5 Postoperative Complications

27.5.1 Intranasal Complications

27.5.1.1 Epistaxis

The prevalence of epistaxis following sinus surgery is 2% [8].

It is typically seen either immediately following surgery because of inadequate hemostasis or 5–7 days after surgery when the crusts get dislodged.

In cases where excessive bleeding is absent at the end of surgery, nasal packing should not be placed at the end of surgery [53, 54] as packing materials may cause delayed restoration of normal sinus drainage and increased patient discomfort. Mild cases of postoperative epistaxis can often be managed with topical decongestant sprays.

Epistaxis treatment protocols use a stepwise treatment approach based on the severity and site of bleeding.

- Vital signs monitoring
- Blood tests for Hg level and coagulation profile
- Intravenous access for fluid replacement and blood/blood products transfusion if needed
- Identify the site of bleeding and try to cauterize if bleeding source is identified
- Packing with absorbable or non-absorbable nasal packs may be needed
- Bleeding that is not controlled with conservative measures, examination under anesthesia must be performed and cauterization or ligation of vessels should be performed
- Embolization or external ligation in case of failure of the previous methods must be discussed as the available options

27.5.1.2 Sinusitis

The possibility of sinusitis after sinus surgery is high and reaches up to 16% of patients [29]. Bare mucosal surfaces, intranasal bacterial colonization, and decreased mucociliary clearance of nasal secretions contribute to sinus infection during the healing period.

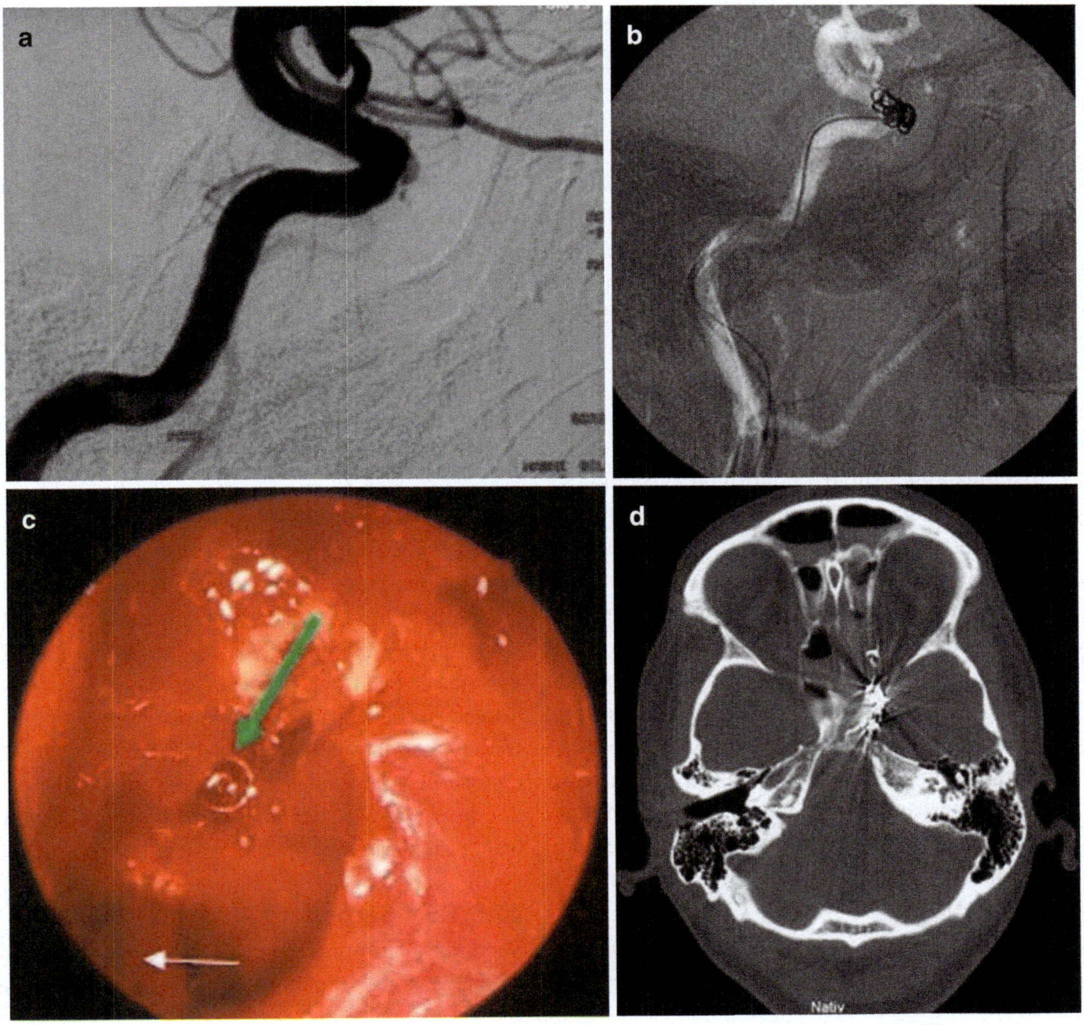

Fig. 27.16 Laceration of the left-sided internal carotid as a complication of sinus surgery. (**a**) Angiogram locating the lesion site (Anterior genu). (**b**) Occlusion of the artery by coils. (**c**) Revision surgery shows the coil. (**d**) Post-treatment CT scan. (Courtesy of Hosemann et al.: Danger points, complications, and medicolegal aspects in endoscopic sinus surgery [5])

27.5.1.3 Synechiae

The most common complication of sinus surgery is synechia formation. Synechiae occur in about 10% of cases, however, in most cases (60–90%) functionally unapparent [7, 8, 55]. One to three percent of incidence of symptomatic synechiae are documented [3, 56].

In a series of patients undergoing revision sinus surgery, adhesions were found to be present in 56% of cases and were felt to be a contributing factor for failure in up to 31% of patients [57].

In case of trauma to the middle turbinate mucosa, an adhesion may form between the middle turbinate and the lateral nasal wall, obstructing sinus drainage pathways. Adhesions may also form between the inferior turbinate and the nasal septum. The generally acknowledged postoperative basic care consists of rinsing with saline and mechanical cleaning, and topical steroids are essential for synechia formation avoidance [58]. Non-absorbable/absorbable nasal packing can help to avoid synechiae. Specific placeholders have been developed with the same intention.

After an ethmoidectomy, in 10–40% of cases, scar-induced lateralization of a detached vertical lamella of the middle turbinate is noted. A lateral synechia may occur in the area of the medial orbital wall in up to 7% of cases [59].

Literature has shown many recommendations to prevent scar-induced lateralization of a "floppy turbinate," also known as a conserved, mobile vertical lamella of the middle nasal turbinate. Such recommendations are shown below:

- Special supporting septum foils (splints) for about 14 days.
- Establishing a small, "controlled synechia" to the nasal septum, possibly using fibrin glue. Olfactory impairment was not observed.
- Suturing of the middle turbinate to the nasal septum. An olfactory impairment was not observed.
- By using a branch, the fixation of the lamella using customary clips introduces an artificial pouch in the mucous membrane of the septum. Using an absorbable clip in the mucous membrane of the septum in which the lamella of the turbinate is pinned can create a similar effect. This clip consists of polylactides.
- Absorbable, cortisone-releasing stents may be inserted into the ethmoid (Fig. 27.17).

Myospherulosis is a foreign body reaction to petrolatum or lanolin found in some antibiotic ointments used to coat packing material placed in the nose, which might result in granulation tissue formation. This complication may be avoided by the use of water-soluble antibiotic gels, instead of petrolatum-containing ointments, in patients undergoing sinonasal surgery [60].

27.5.1.4 Anosmia

Postoperative anosmia in about 0.07–1% of endoscopic sinus surgery [8]. In rhinoneurosurgical surgery, the rate of postoperative anosmia is approximately 2% [61].

27.5.1.5 Hyposmia

Postoperative deficits in smell may occur secondary to scarring of olfactory mucosa, direct mechanical trauma, progressive inflammation of the olfactory cleft mucosa, and modification of the nasal air flow passage. Hosemann et al. quoted in their article that the rate of postoperative hyposmia is about 3% and the rate of smell distortion is around 9% [5]. It is imperative to document any complaints related to smell and taste preoperatively for medicolegal purpose.

27.5.1.6 Secondary Atrophic Rhinitis

Secondary atrophic rhinitis may occur after extensive sinus surgery or revision multiple sinus

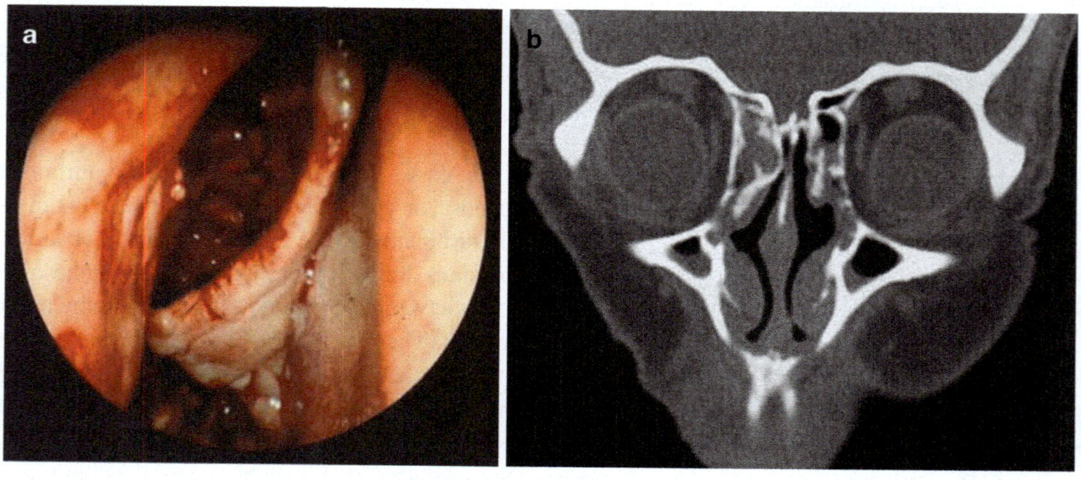

Fig. 27.17 (**a**) Intraoperative floppy turbinate. (**b**) CT scan shows the lateralization of the middle turbinate. (Courtesy of Hosemann et al.: Danger points, complications, and medicolegal aspects in endoscopic sinus surgery [5])

surgeries, due to stripping of larger areas of mucous membranes and resections of both middle and superior turbinates. Patients usually complain of nasal obstruction in the presence of roomy wide nasal cavities and excessive accumulation of crusting noted on endoscopic examination. In general, the rate of postoperative atrophic rhinitis after routine CRS surgery is roughly between 0.08% and 0.4% [5].

27.5.2 Orbital Complications

27.5.2.1 Corneal Abrasion

Keeping the eyes exposed during the endoscopic sinus surgery to serve as a landmark and to check for orbital complications is an essential part of the draping method for sinus surgery; nevertheless, this might expose the eye for trauma or dryness.

Corneal abrasion presents with eye pain and foreign body sensation during the immediate postoperative period. Ophthalmology consultation should be done.

27.5.2.2 Nasolacrimal Duct System Injury

The surgeons should be familiar with the nasolacrimal duct system to avoid complications. The lacrimal sac is approximately 7 mm wide and extends 4–8 mm cranially beyond the axilla of the middle turbinate. The distance between the free edge of the uncinate process and the anterior edge of the lacrimal sac is 5 mm (0–9 mm) and the maxillary sinus optimum is approximately 4 mm (0.5–18 mm) [5].

Epiphora following endoscopic sinus surgery has been reported by experienced surgeons between 0.3% and 1.7% of cases. In 3% of cases, inadvertently injuries of the lacrimal ducts are described [40].

Injury to the nasolacrimal duct can occur while enlarging the maxillary ostium too far anteriorly using microdebrider or back-biting forceps, uncinectomy, and surgery on the anterior frontal recess.

Nasolacrimal duct injury symptoms appear directly after surgery or within 2–3 weeks. Patients present with persistent tearing (epiphora) or lacrimal sac infection (dacryocystitis) [62]. All patients need closure follow-up and ophthalmology consultation if needed. Persistent symptomatic patients need dacryocystorhinostomy.

27.5.3 Intracranial Complications

27.5.3.1 Cerebrospinal Fluid Leak

Persistent, unilateral, and watery rhinorrhea following sinus surgery may alert for CSF leak. A CT scan is needed to evaluate the integrity of the skull base, looking for the presence of a bony defect or pneumocephalus, and a sample of nasal fluid should be collected for beta-2 transferrin assay.

27.5.3.2 Meningitis

Postoperative meningitis is rare, although it represents the most frequent intracranial complication in paranasal sinus surgery. In rhino-neurosurgical procedures, the postoperative rate of meningitis is about 1–3% [63, 64].

When suspecting meningitis, a CT scan has to be ordered immediately, followed by a lumbar puncture. Symptoms or findings are, e.g., fever, laboratory diagnostics indicating major inflammation, headache and neck pain, and impaired consciousness. An active cerebrospinal fluid fistula needs to be detected, and the patient should also be monitored intensively [65].

Rarely (0.9%), a frontal brain abscess was reported after rhino-neurosurgical surgery. Mainly responsible are *Staphylococcus aureus*, gram-negative bacteria, or polymicrobial colonization.

Most studies imply that the prophylactic administration of antibiotics does not reduce the risk of meningitis or brain abscess in skull base surgery [66]. When antibiotics are used in routine cases, the following antibiotics are recommended as monotherapy: ceftazidime, amoxicillin/clavulanic acid, or cefazolin. Vancomycin or clindamycin are recommended if there is intolerance [67, 68].

27.6 Revision Surgery

Despite the progress in the FESS techniques and the technological advances, 10–15% of the patients will undergo revision surgery [21, 69, 70]. Major complications after revision FESS rate was 0.46% and was found to be similar to primary cases [1].

Take Home Messages

- The best management of complications is avoidance, and in order to avoid complications, surgeons should have good anatomical knowledge.
- Study preoperative imaging thoroughly.
- Training in hands-on cadaveric dissection courses.
- It is always safer to abort the procedure and plan elective second surgery if proper hemostasis cannot be achieved.
- Informed consent and documentation for medicolegal purpose.
- Remember learning curve.
- Know your limitations and call for help.
- The percentage of significant complications between 0.3% and 22.4% (median 7.0%).
- The most common complication of sinus surgery is synechiae formation.
- The most common orbital complication of the endoscopic sinus surgery is a trauma of the lamina papyracea.
- Meningitis is the most frequent intracranial complication in paranasal sinus surgery.

References

1. Krings JG, Kallogjeri D, Wineland A, Nepple KG, Piccirillo JF, Getz AE. Complications of primary and revision functional endoscopic sinus surgery for chronic rhinosinusitis. Laryngoscope. 2014;124:838–45.
2. Dalgorf DM, Sacks R, Wormald PJ, et al. Image-guided surgery influences perioperative morbidity from endoscopic sinus surgery: a systematic review and meta-analysis. Otolaryngol Head Neck Surg. 2013;149(1):17–29.
3. Castillo L, Verschuur HP, Poissonnet G, Vaille G, Santini J. Complications of endoscopically guided sinus surgery. Rhinology. 1996;34(4):215–8.
4. Vanden Abeele D, Clemens A, Tassignon MJ, van de Heyning PH. Blindness due to electrocoagulation following functional endoscopic sinus surgery. J Laryngol Otol. 1996;110(3):261–4.
5. Hosemann W, Draf C. Danger points, complications and medico-legal aspects in endoscopic sinus surgery. GMS Curr Top Otorhinolaryngol Head Neck Surg. 2013;12:Doc06. https://doi.org/10.3205/cto000098.
6. Aletsee C, Deglmann M, Dieler R. Chirurgische Eingriffe an den Nasennebenhöhlen bei Sinusitiden und benignen Tumoren. Indikationen, Konzepte und Komplikationen einer Weiterbildungseinrichtung. [Paranasal sinus surgery in chronic sinus disease and benign tumors indications, concepts and complications at a teaching institution]. Laryngorhinootologie. 2003;82(7):508–13.
7. Nguyen QA, Cua DJ, Ng M, Rice DH. Safety of endoscopic sinus surgery in a residency training program. Ear Nose Throat J. 1999;78(12):898–902, 904.
8. Dalziel K, Stein K, Round A, Garside R, Royle P. Endoscopic sinus surgery for the excision of nasal polyps: a systematic review of safety and effectiveness. Am J Rhinol. 2006;20:506–19.
9. Vleming M, Middelweerd RJ, de Vries N. Complications of endoscopic sinus surgery. Arch Otolaryngol Head Neck Surg. 1992;118:617–23.
10. Fokkens W, Lund V, Mullol J, European Position Paper on Rhinosinusitis and Nasal Polyps Group. European position paper on rhinosinusitis and nasal polyps 2007. Rhinol Suppl. 2007;20:1–136.
11. Cinčikas D, Ivaškevičius J, Martinkėnas JL, Balseris S. A role of anesthesiologist in reducing surgical bleeding in endoscopic sinus surgery. Medicina (Kaunas). 2010;46:730–4.
12. Nair S, Collins M, Hung P, Rees G, Close D, Wormald PJ. The effect of beta-blocker premedication on the surgical field during endoscopic sinus surgery. Laryngoscope. 2004;114(6):1042–6.
13. Romlin B, Petruson K, Nilsson K. Moderate superficial hypothermia prolongs bleeding time in humans. Acta Anaesthesiol Scand. 2007;51(2):198–201.
14. Wigand ME. Endoscopic surgery of the paranasal sinuses and anterior skull base. 2nd ed. Stuttgart: Thieme; 2008.
15. Huang TW, Liu CM, Cheng PW, Yang CH. Posterior ischemic optic neuropathy following endoscopic sinus surgery. Otolaryngol Head Neck Surg. 2003;129:448–50.
16. Higgins TS, Hwang PH, Kingdom TT, Orlandi RR, Stammberger H, Han JK. Systematic review of topical vasoconstrictors in endoscopic sinus surgery. Laryngoscope. 2011;121(2):422–32.
17. Anderhuber W, Walch C, Nemeth E, Semmelrock HJ, Berghold A, Ranftl G, Stammberger H. Plasma adren-

aline concentrations during functional endoscopic sinus surgery. Laryngoscope. 1999;109:204–7.
18. Sieskiewicz A, Olszewska E, Rogowski M, Grycz E. Preoperative corticosteroid oral therapy and intraoperative bleeding during functional endoscopic sinus surgery in patients with severe nasal polyposis: a preliminary investigation. Ann Otol Rhinol Laryngol. 2006;115(7):490–4.
19. Blackwell KE, Ross DA, Kapur P, Calcaterra TC. Propofol for maintenance of general anesthesia: a technique to limit blood loss during endoscopic sinus surgery. Am J Otolaryngol. 1993;14(4):262–6.
20. Crawley BK, Barkdull GC, Dent S, Bishop M, Davidson TM. Relative hypotension and image guidance: tools for training in sinus surgery. Arch Otolaryngol Head Neck Surg. 2009;135(10):994–9.
21. Smith LF, Brindley PC. Indications, evaluation, complications, and results of functional endoscopic sinus surgery in 200 patients. Otolaryngol Head Neck Surg. 1993;108:688–96.
22. Sartcaoglu F, Celiker V, Basgul E, Yapakci O, Aypar U. The effect of hypotensive anaesthesia on cognitive functions and recovery at endoscopic sinus surgery. Eur J Anaesthesiol. 2005;22:157–9.
23. Leunig A. Vermeidung von und Umgang mit Blutungen während endoskopischer Nasennebenhöhlenchirurgie. [Avoiding and dealing with bleeding during endoscopic sinus surgery]. Laryngorhinootologie. 2006;85(4):249–52.
24. Yaniv E, Shvero J, Hadar T. Hemostatic effect of tranexamic acid in elective nasal surgery. Am J Rhinol. 2006;20(2):227–9.
25. Alimian M, Mohseni M. The effect of intravenous tranexamic acid on blood loss and surgical field quality during endoscopic sinus surgery: a placebo-controlled clinical trial. J Clin Anesth. 2011;23(8):611–5.
26. Solares CA, Ong YK, Carrau RL, Fernandez-Miranda J, Prevedello DM, Snyderman CH, Kassam AB. Prevention and management of vascular injuries in endoscopic surgery of the sinonasal tract and skull base. Otolaryngol Clin North Am. 2010;43(4):817–25.
27. Midilli R, Orhan M, Saylam CY, Akyildiz S, Gode S, Karci B. Anatomic variations of sphenopalatine artery and minimally invasive surgical cauterization procedure. Am J Rhinol Allergy. 2009;23(6):e38–41.
28. Pádua FG, Voegels RL. Severe posterior epistaxis-endoscopic surgical anatomy. Laryngoscope. 2008;118(1):156–61.
29. Schwartzbauer HR, Shete M, Tami TA. Endoscopic anatomy of the sphenopalatine and posterior nasal arteries: implications for the endoscopic management of epistaxis. Am J Rhinol. 2003;17(1):63–6.
30. Simmen DB, Raghavan U, Briner HR, Manestar M, Groscurth P, Jones N. The anatomy of the sphenopalatine artery for the endoscopic sinus surgeon. Am J Rhinol. 2006;20:502–5.
31. Aziz ZS, Zaya NE, Bass RM. Anatomic measurements of the anterior and posterior ethmoid arteries in cadaveric heads using endoscopic sinus instrumentation. Ear Nose Throat J. 2014;93:E11–5.
32. Zong Y, Li X, Jiang Y, Xu J, Li J. Transnasal approach to the anterior skull base: an endoscopic anatomic study. J Craniofac Surg. 2014;25:1041–3.
33. Moon HJ, Kim HU, Lee JG, Chung IH, Yoon JH. Surgical anatomy of the anterior ethmoidal canal in ethmoid roof. Laryngoscope. 2001;111:900–4.
34. Simmen D, Raghavan U, Briner HR, et al. The surgeon's view of the anterior ethmoid artery. Clin Otolaryngol. 2006;31:187–91.
35. Jang DW, Lachanas VA, White LC, Kountakis SE. Supraorbital ethmoid cell: a consistent landmark for endoscopic identification of the anterior ethmoidal artery. Otolaryngol Head Neck Surg. 2014;151:1073–7.
36. Rombout J, de Vries N. Complications in sinus surgery and new classification proposal. Am J Rhinol. 2001;15(6):363–70.
37. Welch KC, Palmer JN. Intraoperative emergencies during endoscopic sinus surgery: CSF leak and orbital hematoma. Otolaryngol Clin North Am. 2008;41(3):581–96.
38. Han JK, Higgins TS. Management of orbital complications in endoscopic sinus surgery. Curr Opin Otolaryngol Head Neck Surg. 2010;18(1):32–6.
39. Tzifa KT, Skinner DW. Peri-orbital surgical emphysema following functional endoscopic sinus surgery, during extubation. J Laryngol Otol. 2001;115(11):916–7.
40. Bhatti MT, Stankiewicz JA. Ophthalmic complications of endoscopic sinus surgery. Surv Ophthalmol. 2003;48:389–402.
41. Ramakrishnan VR, Palmer JN. Prevention and management of orbital hematoma. Otolaryngol Clin North Am. 2010;43(4):789–800.
42. Stankiewicz JA. Blindness and intranasal endoscopic ethmoidectomy: prevention and management. Otolaryngol Head Neck Surg. 1989;101(3):320–9.
43. Thacker NM, Velez FG, Demer JL, Wang MB, Rosenbaum AL. Extraocular muscle damage associated with endoscopic sinus surgery: an ophthalmology perspective. Am J Rhinol. 2005;19(4):400–5.
44. Bhatti MT, Giannoni CM, Raynor E, Monshizadeh R, Levine LM. Ocular motility complications after endoscopic sinus surgery with powered cutting instruments. Otolaryngol Head Neck Surg. 2001;125(5):501–9.
45. Onodi A. The optic nerve and the accessory sinuses of the nose. New York: William Wood & Co.; 1910.
46. Kainz J, Stammberger H. The roof of the anterior ethmoid: a place of least resistance in the skull base. Am J Rhinol. 1989;3:191–9.
47. Hegazy HM, Carrau RL, Snyderman CH, Kassam A, Zweig J. Trans-nasal endoscopic repair of cerebrospinal UID rhinorrhea: a meta-analysis. Laryngoscope. 2000;110(7):1166–72.
48. Banks CA, Palmer JN, Chiu AG, O'Malley BW Jr, Woodworth BA, Kennedy DW. Endoscopic closure of CSF rhinorrhea: 193 cases over 21 years. Otolaryngol Head Neck Surg. 2009;140(6):826–33.

49. Brodie HA. Prophylactic antibiotics for posttraumatic cerebrospinal fluid fistulae. A meta-analysis. Arch Otolaryngol Head Neck Surg. 1997;123:749–52.
50. Bernal-Sprekelsen M, Bleda-Vazquez C, Carrau RL. Ascending meningitis secondary to traumatic cerebrospinal fluid leaks. Am J Rhinol. 2000;14:257–9.
51. Lanza DC, O'Brien DA, Kennedy DW. Endoscopic repair of cerebrospinal fluid fistulae and encephaloceles. Laryngoscope. 1996;106:1119–25.
52. Gondim JA, Almeida JP, Albuquerque LA, Schops M, Gomes E, Ferraz T, Sobreira W, Kretzmann MT. Endoscopic endonasal approach for pituitary adenoma: surgical complications in 301 patients. Pituitary. 2011;14(2):174–83.
53. Orlandi RR, Lanza DC. Is nasal packing necessary following endo-scopic sinus surgery? Laryngoscope. 2004;114(9):1541–4.
54. Mo JH, Han DH, Shin HW, Cha W, Chang MY, Jin HR. No packing versus packing after endoscopic sinus surgery: pursuit of patients' comfort after surgery. Am J Rhinol. 2008;22(5):525–8.
55. Kinsella JB, Calhoun KH, Bradfield JJ, Hokanson JA, Bailey BJ. Complications of endoscopic sinus surgery in a residency training program. Laryngoscope. 1995;105:1029–32.
56. Re M, Massegur H, Magliulo G, Ferrante L, Sciarretta V, Farneti G, Macrì G, Mallardi V, Pasquini E. Traditional endonasal and microscopic sinus surgery complications versus endoscopic sinus surgery complications: a meta-analysis. Eur Arch Otorhinolaryngol. 2012;269(3):721–9.
57. Ramadan HH. Surgical causes of failure in endoscopic sinus surgery. Laryngoscope. 1999;109(1):27–9.
58. Rudmik L, Soler ZM, Orlandi RR, Stewart MG, Bhattacharyya N, Kennedy DW, Smith TL. Early postoperative care following endoscopic sinus surgery: an evidence-based review with recommendations. Int Forum Allergy Rhinol. 2011;1(6):417–30.
59. Khalil HS, Eweiss AZ, Clifton N. Radiological findings in patients undergoing revision endoscopic sinus surgery: a retrospective case series study. BMC Ear Nose Throat Disord. 2011;11:4.
60. Sindwani R, Cohen JT, Pilch BZ, Metson RB. Myospherulosis following sinus surgery: pathological curiosity or important clinical entity? Laryngoscope. 2003;113(7):1123–7.
61. de Almeida JR, Snyderman CH, Gardner PA, Carrau RL, Vescan AD. Nasal morbidity following endoscopic skull base surgery: a prospective cohort study. Head Neck. 2011;33(4):547–51.
62. Serdahl CL, Berris CE, Chole RA. Nasolacrimal duct obstruction after endoscopic sinus surgery. Arch Ophthalmol. 1990;108(3):391–2.
63. Ransom ER, Chiu AG. Prevention and management of complications in intracranial endoscopic skull base surgery. Otolaryngol Clin North Am. 2010;43(4):875–95.
64. Kraus DH, Gonen M, Mener D, Brown AE, Bilsky MH, Shah JP. A standardized regimen of antibiotics prevents infectious complications in skull base surgery. Laryngoscope. 2005;115(8):1347–57.
65. Singh A, Germanwala AV. Management of postoperative complications of skull base surgery. Op Tech Otolaryngol Head Neck Surg. 2011;22:237–45.
66. Horowitz G, Fliss DM, Margalit N, Wasserzug O, Gil Z. Association between cerebrospinal fluid leak and meningitis after skull base surgery. Otolaryngol Head Neck Surg. 2011;145(4):689–93.
67. Snyderman CH, Carrau RL, Kassam AB, Zanation A, Prevedello D, Gardner P, Mintz A. Endoscopic skull base surgery: principles of endonasal oncological surgery. J Surg Oncol. 2008;97(8):658–64.
68. Brown SM, Anand VK, Tabaee A, Schwartz TH. Role of perioperative antibiotics in endoscopic skull base surgery. Laryngoscope. 2007;117(9):1528–32.
69. Chandra RK, Palmer JN, Tangsujarittham T, Kennedy DW. Factors associated with failure of frontal sinusotomy in the early follow-up period. Otolaryngol Head Neck Surg. 2004;131:514–8.
70. Musy PY, Kountakis SE. Anatomic findings in patients undergoing revision endoscopic sinus surgery. Am J Otolaryngol. 2004;25:418–22.

28 Neoplasms of the Sinonasal Cavity

Andrew Tassler, Charles A. Riley, Chetan Safi, and Michael G. Stewart

Key Points

- Majority of malignant tumors of the sinonasal cavity come from the maxillary sinus (50–70%), followed by nasal cavity (15–30%), ethmoid cavity (10–20%), and rarely the frontal and sphenoid sinuses.
- Nasal endoscopy and cross-sectional imaging to determine vascularity of lesions and invasion of vital structures such as orbit and brain.
- CT is helpful in determining bony erosion while MRI can assess for perineural spread, vascular anatomy, and dural invasion.
- Unilateral paranasal sinus disease and polyposis could be an indication of a neoplastic process.
- Squamous cell carcinoma is the most common paranasal sinus malignancy and accounts for approximately 75% of cases.
- Most sinonasal malignancies will require multimodality therapy.

28.1 Introduction

Though sinonasal neoplasms are not routinely encountered, the differential diagnosis for these lesions can be vast. Most sinonasal masses present with similar symptoms of nasal obstruction, epistaxis, nasal discharge, and/or facial pain. Additionally, due to limited anatomic real estate, both benign and malignant lesions can cause compressive effects leading to orbital and intracranial complications as well as possible regional cervical metastases. Diagnostic workup for each lesion will be slightly varied but ultimately will comprise of some combination of nasal endoscopy, CT, MRI, and/or biopsy via an endoscopic or image guided approach. Furthermore, treatment for these lesions will involve a combination of surgical therapy, chemotherapy, and or radiation therapy.

28.2 Sinonasal Cavity Tumor Epidemiology

1. Uncommon tumors with wide range of histopathology.
   (a) Congenital malformations to benign tumors to high-grade malignancies.
2. Most common malignancy is squamous cell carcinoma (SCCA).
   (a) Scca of sinonasal cavity is a rare malignancy which occurs with the frequency of

A. Tassler · C. A. Riley · C. Safi · M. G. Stewart (✉)
Department of Otolaryngology—Head and Neck Surgery, Weill Cornell Medical College and NewYork-Presbyterian Hospital, New York, NY, USA
e-mail: ant9025@med.cornell.edu; mgs2002@med.cornell.edu

A. Al-Qahtani et al. (eds.), *Textbook of Clinical Otolaryngology*,
https://doi.org/10.1007/978-3-030-54088-3_28

approximately 1:200,000 in the United States.

3. Malignant tumors of the sinonasal cavity represent less than 1% of all cancers, and about 3% of cancers of the upper aerodigestive tract.
4. Majority of malignant tumors of the sinonasal cavity come from the maxillary sinus (50–70%), followed by nasal cavity (15–30%), ethmoid cavity (10–20%), and rarely the frontal and sphenoid sinuses.

28.3 History and Presentation

1. Causative factors
   (a) SCCA
      - Nickel, aflatoxin, mustard gas, hydrocarbons
      - Fibers found in wood and textile industries
   (b) Adenocarcinoma
      - Woodworking, furniture making, leather-related occupational exposure
   (c) Human Papilloma Virus (HPV) may be a co-factor
   (d) Chronic infection/inflammation
   (e) Previous radiation
2. History
   (a) Sinonasal tumors can be a diagnostic challenge because they present with symptoms that mimic common inflammatory sinonasal disease
   (b) Results in delayed diagnosis and higher stages at presentation
   (c) Most common symptoms include nasal obstruction, nasal discharge, facial pain, congestion, epistaxis, smell disturbance, epiphora, hypesthesia, pain, aural fullness, hearing loss, otalgia, and neck swelling
3. Physical exam
   (a) Nasal cavity mass, midface and periorbital edema, proptosis, middle ear effusion, loose dentition, trismus, malocclusion, cranial nerve deficits including CN I, II, III, IV, V1, V2, and VI
4. Nasal endoscopy
   (a) Evaluate extent of tumor
   (b) Determine origin/base
   (c) Determine vascularity of tumor
   (d) Perform valsalva during examination
      - Expansion of tumor suggests intracranial extension
5. Biopsy
   (a) Tumors may be biopsied during nasal endoscopy, unless there is concern for intracranial extension or increased vascularity
   (b) Consider diagnostic imaging such as computed tomography (CT) or magnetic resonance imaging (MRI) prior to biopsy
      - Evaluate for intracranial (i.e., encephalocele) or vascular lesions
   (c) Safest way to perform biopsy is in the operating room (OR)
      - Allows frozen section confirmation of adequate specimen
      - Controlled airway and facilitates control of bleeding
   (d) Nodal disease warrants fine-needle aspiration to assess for regional spread

28.4 Imaging

1. Computed tomography
   (a) Evaluate tumor involvement of paranasal sinuses, bony skull base, and retro-orbital/orbital apex region
   (b) CT defines bony invasion
   (c) CT does not define soft tissue well
   (d) Malignant tumors cause bony destruction; benign tumors cause tissue remodelling and hyperostosis
2. Magnetic resonance imaging
   (a) Clarifies tumor versus inflammatory mucosa/secretions
      - Tumor typically is bright on T1 and enhances with contrast
      - Inflammatory mucosa/secretions are bright on T2
   (b) Assess for perineural spread
   (c) Defines vascular anatomy
   (d) Helpful to determine dural invasion, infratemporal and intracranial extension
   (e) CT and MRI are complimentary, particularly in the workup of sinonasal malignancies

3. Positron Emission Tomography (PET)
   (a) Assesses regional and distant disease for malignant tumors

28.5 Differential Diagnosis of Neoplasms

1. Benign
   (a) Osteoma
      - Most commonly found in frontal > ethmoid > maxillary sinus
      - Benign, slow growing, usually asymptomatic
      - Manage with observation typically, unless it is obstructing sinus outflow tract
      - Multiple osteoma lesions associated with Gardner syndrome
        - Malignant degeneration of intestinal polyp
   (b) Fibrous dysplasia
      - Hamartomatous lesion in which medullary bone is replaced by fibro-osseous tissue
      - Slow growing, painless
      - Destroys bone, with eggshell-thin cortex from destruction of cortical bone
      - Ground-glass expansive mass on CT
      - May obliterate sphenoid or frontal sinuses
      - Treatment of asymptomatic disease involves observation with serial imaging
   (c) Inverting papilloma
      - Arises from proliferation of cells in Schneiderian mucosa
        - Associated with HPV 6, 11 and Epstein–Barr Virus (EBV)
        - Benign pathology but locally aggressive
      - More common in males, in sixth to seventh decades of life
      - Symptoms.
        - Unilateral polyp, unilateral nasal congestion/obstruction, epistaxis, rhinorrhea
      - Histopathology
        - Endophytic growth of epithelium
      - On CT imaging, hyperostotic bone can be identified at site of origin
      - Approximately 10% risk of transformation to SCCA (highest risk in smokers)
      - Krouse Staging System
        - Stage T1—limited to one area of the nasal cavity
        - Stage T2—involvement of the medial wall of the maxillary or ethmoid sinuses and/or osteomeatal unit
        - Stage T3—involvement of the superior, inferior, posterior, anterior, or lateral walls of the maxillary sinus
        - Stage T4—tumors with extra-sinonasal spread or malignancy
   (d) Juvenile Nasopharyngeal Angiofibroma (JNA)
      - Most common vascular mass in nose
      - Benign but aggressive; slow growing, may spread intracranially but does not metastasize
      - May have hormonal component
      - Most common presentation is unilateral epistaxis in teenage male; other symptoms include rhinorrhea, congestion/obstruction, anosmia, headache, facial swelling, and proptosis
      - Endoscopy demonstrates vascular lesion emanating from sphenopalatine area; avoid biopsy
      - Staging System—Radkowski
        - Stage 1A—limited to nose or nasopharynx
        - Stage 1B—extension into at least one paranasal sinus
        - Stage 2A—minimal extension through the sphenopalatine foramen; includes minimal part of medial pterygomaxillary fossa
        - Stage 2B—full occupation of pterygomaxillary fossa with Holman-Miller sign; lateral or anterior displacement of maxillary artery branches; may have superior extension with orbital bone erosion
        - Stage 2C—extension through pterygomaxillary fossa into the cheek,

temporal fossa, or posterior to the pterygoids
    - Stage 3A—skull base erosion with minimal intracranial extension
    - Stage 3B—skull base erosion with minimal intracranial extension, involving cavernous sinus
- University of Pittsburgh Medical Center Staging System for JNA
    - Stage 1—within the nasal cavity, medial pterygoid fossa
    - Stage 2—Within paranasal sinuses, lateral pterygoid fossa; no residual vascularity
    - Stage 3—Skull base erosion, orbit, or infratemporal fossa; no residual vascularity
    - Stage 4—Skull base erosion, orbit, or infratemporal fossa; residual vascularity
    - Stage 5—Intracranial extension, residual vascularity
      M—medial extension
      L—lateral extension
- Expansion of pterygopalatine fossa present on CT/MRI
    - Holman-Miller sign—anterior bowing of posterior wall of maxillary sinus
    - Findings are pathognomonic for JNA
- Very vascular tumor
    - Primary blood supply from internal maxillary artery from external carotid artery
    - Also receives blood supply from internal carotid artery, ethmoid arteries, contralateral arteries
    - Do not biopsy in clinic
- Treatment includes embolization before surgical resection
    - Endoscopic, midface de-gloving, and transfacial approaches can be performed
    - Success with resection is dependent on surgeon preference
    - Recurrence rates with the various approaches are about equal

2. Malignant
    (a) Squamous cell carcinoma
        - Approximately 75% of all paranasal sinus malignancies
        - Smoking exposure is a risk factor
        - Overall low (<10%) risk for occult neck disease
        - AJCC Paranasal sinus cancer staging
            - Maxillary
              Ohngren's line
                - Imaginary angled sagittal plane from medial canthus of eye to the angle of the mandible
                - Infrastructural lesions, anterior/inferior, have better outcomes; more amenable to resection
                - Suprastructural lesions, posterior/superior, present at more advanced stages, more likely to involve skull base and perineural invasion; less amenable to resection

              T1—tumor limited to maxillary sinus mucosa without bone involvement

              T2—tumor causing erosion of bone such as hard palate; extension of tumor into middle meatus

              T3—tumor invades of the following: posterior wall of maxillary sinus, orbital floor, subcutaneous tissues, pterygopalatine fossa, ethmoid sinuses

              T4a—moderately advanced local disease
                - Tumor invades orbit, skin of face, pterygoid plates, infratemporal fossa, cribriform plate, sphenoid sinus, frontal sinus
                - T4b—advanced local disease
                - Tumor invades orbital apex, dura, brain, nasopharynx, clivus
            - Ethmoid sinus T stage

T1—Tumor within one subsite without bony invasion

T2—Tumor invading two adjacent subsites or extending into nasoethmoid complex

T3—Tumor invades orbital floor, medial orbital wall, maxillary sinus, palate, or cribriform plate

T4a—Moderately advanced local disease.

- Tumor invades orbit, skin of face, pterygoid plates, infratemporal fossa, cribriform plate, sphenoid sinus, or frontal sinus

T4b—advanced local disease.

- Tumor invades orbital apex, dura, brain, nasopharynx, clivus

(b) Intestinal-Type Adenocarcinoma (ITAC)
- Risk factors
  - Wood-dust exposure
  - Leather-related occupational exposure
- Presents more commonly in the ethmoid sinuses

(c) Adenoid cystic carcinoma
- Minor salivary gland origin in the paranasal sinuses
  - More common in minor than major salivary glands
  - Insidious growth
- Significant propensity to invade along nerves, resulting in pain and paresthesia
- Distant metastases common but can be delayed
- Good 5-year survival but poor 10-year survival

(d) Esthesioneuroblastoma
- Rare malignancy
- Arises from olfactory epithelium
- Bi-modal frequency
  - Presents in teenagers and elderly
- Kadish System
  - A—tumors limited to the nasal cavity
  - B—extension into paranasal sinuses
  - C—extension beyond paranasal sinuses
  - D—Metastatic disease
- Hyams histopathologic grading system
  - Grading is based on mitosis, necrosis, pleomorphism, and type of tissue architecture
  - Grade 1 and 2—Homer-Wright pseudorosettes
  - Grade 3 and 4—Flexner–Wintersteiner rosettes
- Most common treatment includes surgical resection with postoperative radiation

(e) Lymphoma
- Risks
  - Irradiation, EBV, immunosuppression
- Symptoms
  - Nodal mass, fever, night sweats, nasal obstruction, epistaxis, exophthalmos
- Workup
  - Imaging and biopsy
  - Maintain index of suspicion
- Treatment
  - Non-surgical: chemotherapy, radiation therapy

(f) Malignant mucosal melanoma
- Sinonasal cavity is most common site of mucosal melanoma
- Very aggressive and high grade
  - All lesions are at least T3 and Stage III
- Surgery and radiation are mainstays of treatment
- Poor 2-year survival, around 25%.
- Local recurrence and distant metastasis are common
- Less aggressive or palliative surgical approach can be used given poor prognosis

(g) Nasopharyngeal Carcinoma (NPC)
- Causes of NPC
  - Genetic factors

    Family clusters: 15% of NPC patients have a first-degree family member with NPC

HLA-B, C, and D haplotypes are associated with increased risk
  - Environmental factors
    High-nitrosamine diet of salted fish, eggs, and vegetables
  - Epstein–Barr virus (EBV)
    Elevated IgA Viral capsid antigen (VCA) and IgA Early Antigen (EA)
    EBV DNA is useful screening tool for early asymptomatic NPC
    - Earlier detection and better outcomes
- Demographics
  - 75% male
  - Highest world incidence if in Guangzhou, China
    Southern China, Northern Africa, Southeast Asia at higher risk
  - 99% of patients with NPC have symptoms at diagnosis
- Symptoms
  - Neck mass—level V and level II
  - Otitis media with effusion and/or Eustachian tube dysfunction
  - Unilateral hearing loss
  - Hemoptysis
  - Nasal congestion
  - Cranial nerve palsy
    CN V > VI > XI > X > XII
- World Health Organization Classification of NPC
  - Type I—keratinizing SCC
    5-year survival is 35%
  - Type II—nonkeratinizing carcinoma (EBV+)
  - Type III—undifferentiated carcinoma (EBV+)
    5-year survival is 60%
- Workup
  - MRI to evaluate tumor extent and skull base involvement
  - PET to evaluate distant disease
  - Audiogram
  - EBV serology
    IgA VCA—highly sensitive
    IgA EA—highly specific
- Staging for NPC
  - T1—Confined to nasopharynx or extends to oropharynx or nasal cavity
  - T2—Tumor extends to the parapharyngeal space
  - T3—Tumor involves sinuses and/or skull base
  - T4—Intracranial or infratemporal involvement, or cranial nerve or orbital involvement
  - N0—No nodal disease
  - N1—Unilateral cervical lymph nodes <6 cm, or retropharyngeal nodes <6 cm above the supraclavicular fossa
  - N2—Bilateral cervical LN <6 cm above supraclavicular fossa
  - N3a—Lymph node >6 cm
  - N3b—Supraclavicular lymph node
- Treatment options
  - Stage I-II: Radiation alone
  - Stage III–IV: Chemoradiation
  - Persistent disease: Salvage surgery
  - Recurrent disease: Reirradiation or salvage surgery

28.6 Factors Associated with Survival

1. Histological findings of primary tumor (Table 28.1)
   (a) Worst: melanoma
   (b) Best: minor salivary gland tumors
2. T stage
3. Presence/Extent of intracranial involvement
4. Positive margins
5. Prior radiation
6. Nodal disease
7. Distant disease

28.7 Treatment

1. Benign sinonasal tumors
   (a) Dependent on extent of disease and pathology

Table 28.1 Overall survival based on histopathologic diagnosis

Histopathology	5-Year OS
Squamous cell carcinoma	30–50%
Intestinal-type adenocarcinoma	60–70%
Adenoid cystic carcinoma	≈60%
Esthesioneuroblastoma	78%
Mucosal melanoma	<30%
Undifferentiated carcinoma	75%
Neuroendocrine carcinoma	65%

OS overall survival

(b) Observation, partial resection, complete resection with margins
(c) Radiation for symptomatic tumors when surgery not possible

2. Malignant sinonasal tumors
   (a) Consideration of nearby neurovascular structures
   - Brain, eye, important arteries and veins

   (b) Oncologic outcomes and morbidity improving over last several decades
   (c) Endoscopic approaches
   - Low morbidity
   - Comparable, if not better, outcomes in properly selected patients
   - May be performed for definitive resection of disease, debulking, or palliation
   - Dependent on surgeon technical skill

   (d) Transfacial open approaches
   - Lateral rhinotomy
     – Requires external incision with some resultant morbidity and cosmetic deformity
     – Provides excellent visualization of maxillary, ethmoid, and sphenoid sinuses as well as medial orbit
   - Midface de-gloving
     – Requires transfixion and intercartilaginous incisions bilaterally with gingivobuccal incisions
     – Excellent visualization for inferior nasal cavity and medial maxillary walls
     – Allows bilateral exposure
     – No external incisions
   - Facial translocation
     – Used for wide exposure of middle cranial base, infratemporal fossa, pterygopalatine fossa, and nasopharynx

   (e) Low-grade cancers
   - Single-modality primarily, with surgical resection for early maxillary or nasal cavity tumors versus primary radiation
     – Radiation field and dose are limited by orbital and intracranial complications such as blindness, keratitis, and brain necrosis

   (f) High-grade cancers
   - Multimodal therapy with either primary radiation therapy with surgical salvage or primary surgical excision with postoperative radiation therapy

   (g) Unresectable disease or non-operative patients
   - Primary radiation, chemotherapy, or combination chemoradiation

   (h) Obtaining local control is most important factor that impacts survival
3. Management of neck disease
   (a) N0 neck
   - Elective neck dissection is generally not indicated
   - <10% of exam-negative necks contain occult disease

   (b) N1–N3 Neck
   - Neck dissection indicated

28.8 Complications from Tumor Treatment

1. Hemorrhage
   (a) Venous vs arterial; potentially life-threatening
   (b) Increased risk in vascular tumors; consider pre-operative embolization
2. Intradural vs extradural nerve injury
3. Positive margins
4. Wound infection, sinonasal mucocele, chronic rhinosinusitis
5. Orbital complications

   (a) Optic nerve compression, retrobulbar hematoma, blindness, diplopia, epiphora
6. Intracranial infections
   (a) Meningitis, cerebritis
      - Most significant complication
      - Life-threatening
7. Cerebrospinal fluid leak
   (a) Prevented by achieving watertight closure
   (b) Vascularized intranasal or locoregional flap
   (c) Use of lumbar drain dependent on surgeon- and institution-specific variables
8. Intracranial complications
   (a) Stroke
   (b) Pneumocephalus
      - Occurs from trapped air that enters into nasal cavity from sinonasal tract
      - High risk of brain herniation
      - Treat with emergent aspiration, re-exploration to identify and repair communication between sinonasal cavity and brain
9. Neurologic complications
   (a) Hypesthesia, paresthesia, seizure, anosmia

Take Home Messages

- Malignant tumors of the sinonasal cavity represent less than 1% of all cancers, and about 3% of cancers of the upper aerodigestive tract.
- Sinonasal tumors can be a diagnostic challenge because they present with symptoms that mimic common inflammatory sinonasal disease.
- CT and MRI can complement each other in determining vascular anatomy, bony erosion into the orbit or skull base, as well as meningeal involvement and perineural spread of tumor.
- Surgical resection of sinonasal masses can involve an interdisciplinary team with multiple endoscopic and open approaches available.
- Sinonasal malignancies generally require multimodality therapy for adequate treatment.
- Complications from sinonasal tumor treatment can include epistaxis, optic nerve compression, cerebrospinal fluid leak, stroke, pneumocephalus, hypoesthesia/paresthesias, or tumor recurrence.

Recommended Readings

1. Weymuller EA, Davis GE. Malignancies of the paranasal sinus. In: Flint PW, Haughey BH, Lund V, Niparko JK, Robbins KT, Thomas JR, Lesperance MM, editors. Cummings otolaryngology head and neck surgery. Philadelphia, PA: Elsevier Saunders; 2010. p. 1121–32.
2. Nicolai P, Castelnuovo P. Benign tumors of the sinonasal tract. In: Flint PW, Haughey BH, Lund V, Niparko JK, Robbins KT, Thomas JR, Lesperance MM, editors. Cummings otolaryngology head and neck surgery. Philadelphia, PA: Elsevier Saunders; 2010. p. 717–27.
3. Virk JS, Chan J, Dimitrov L, Williamson A, Sandison A, Weir J, Clarke P. Sinonasal cancer: an overview of the emerging subtypes. J Laryngol Otol. 2020;12:1–6.
4. López F, Lund VJ, Suárez C, Snyderman CH, Saba NF, Robbins KT, Vander Poorten V, Strojan P, Mendenhall WM, Rinaldo A, Ferlito A. The impact of histologic phenotype in the treatment of sinonasal cancer. Adv Ther. 2017;34(10):2181–98.
5. Llorente JL, López F, Suárez C, Hermsen MA. Sinonasal carcinoma: clinical, pathological, genetic and therapeutic advances. Nat Rev Clin Oncol. 2014;11(8):460–72.
6. Turner JH, Reh DD. Incidence and survival in patients with sinonasal cancer: a historical analysis of population-based data. Head Neck. 2012;34(6):877–85, 877.
7. Sanghvi S, Khan MN, Patel NR, Yeldandi S, Baredes S, Eloy JA. Epidemiology of sinonasal squamous cell carcinoma: a comprehensive analysis of 4994 patients. Laryngoscope. 2014;124(1):76–83.
8. Choussy O, Ferron C, Védrine PO, Toussaint B, Liétin B, Marandas P, Babin E, De Raucourt D, Reyt E, Cosmidis A, Makeiff M. Adenocarcinoma of ethmoid: a GETTEC retrospective multicenter study of 418 cases. Laryngoscope. 2008;118(3):437–43.
9. Kang JH, Cho SH, Kim JP, Kang KM, Cho KS, Kim W, Seol YM, Lee S, Park HS, Hur WJ, Choi YJ. Treatment outcomes between concurrent chemo-

radiotherapy and combination of surgery, radiotherapy, and/or chemotherapy in stage III and IV maxillary sinus cancer: multi-institutional retrospective analysis. J Oral Maxillofac Surg. 2012;70(7):1717–23.
10. Robin TP, Jones BL, Gordon OM, Phan A, Abbott D, McDermott JD, Goddard JA, Raben D, Lanning RM, Karam SD. A comprehensive comparative analysis of treatment modalities for sinonasal malignancies. Cancer. 2017;123(16):3040–9.
11. Snyderman CH, Carrau RL, Kassam AB, Zanation A, Prevedello D, Gardner P, Mintz A. Endoscopic skull base surgery: principles of endonasal oncological surgery. J Surg Oncol. 2008;97(8):658–64.
12. Lund VJ, Howard D, Wei W, Spittle M. Olfactory neuroblastoma: past, present, and future? Laryngoscope. 2003;113(3):502–7.
13. Lu VM, Ravindran K, Phan K, Van Gompel JJ, Smith TR, Donaldson AM, Quinones-Hinojosa A, Mekary RA, Chaichana KL. Surgical outcomes of endoscopic versus open resection for primary sinonasal malignancy: a meta-analysis. Am J Rhinol Allergy. 2019;33(5):608–16.
14. Dong D, Wang Y, Li C, Zhang H, Zhao Y, Lai J. Fibro-osseous lesions of paranasal sinus and craniofacial region: a retrospective study of 282 cases. Laryngoscope. 2020;14
15. Lisan Q, Laccourreye O, Bonfils P. Sinonasal inverted papilloma: From diagnosis to treatment. Eur Ann Otorhinolaryngol Head Neck Dis. 2016;133(5):337–41.
16. López F, Triantafyllou A, Snyderman CH, Hunt JL, Suárez C, Lund VJ, Strojan P, Saba NF, Nixon IJ, Devaney KO, Alobid I. Nasal juvenile angiofibroma: current perspectives with emphasis on management. Head Neck. 2017;39(5):1033–45.

Cerebrospinal Fluid Rhinorrhea

29

Hamad Al Saey, Ahmed Shaikh, Sara Ashkanani,
Mansour Al Sulaiti, Emad Al Duhirat,
and Shanmugam Ganesan

29.1 Introduction

Cerebrospinal fluid (CSF) rhinorrhea is result of abnormal communication between subarachnoid space and sinonasal cavities. It results from the breakdown of layers separating the nasal cavity from subarachnoid space. Rhinorrhea is a common rhinology complaint and should be differentiated from CSF leak.

Anatomy: CSF is ultrafiltrate of plasma which contains electrolyte, glucose, and proteins. It is present in the subarachnoid space helps in maintaining the hemostasis of neural tissue and maintains the chemical environment of brain. It is produced by choroid plexus; the further flow is as follows [1].

H. Al Saey (✉) · A. Shaikh · S. Ashkanani
M. Al Sulaiti · E. Al Duhirat · S. Ganesan
Otolaryngology-Head and Neck Surgery Division, Department of Surgery, Hamad Medical Corporation, Doha, Qatar

Department of Otolaryngology-Head and Neck Surgery Division, Weill Cornell Medicine-Qatar, Doha, Qatar
e-mail: Halsaey@hamad.qa; sashkanani@hamad.qa; Malsulaiti1@hamad.qa; EAlDuhirat@hamad.qa; sganesan@hamad.qa

A. Al-Qahtani et al. (eds.), *Textbook of Clinical Otolaryngology*,
https://doi.org/10.1007/978-3-030-54088-3_29

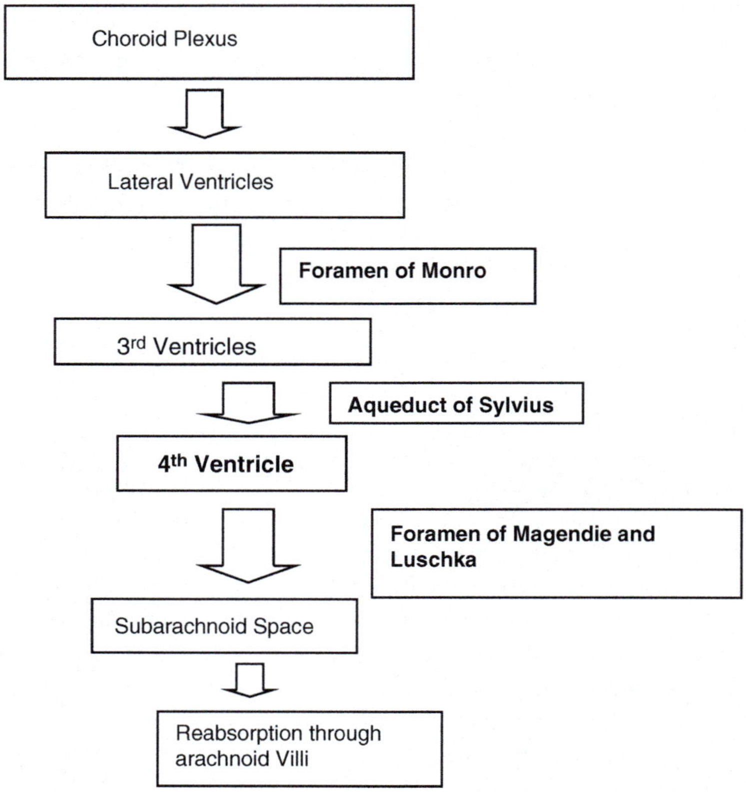

Total Volume of CSF : 140 ml
Production: 0.33ml/ minute
Normal CSF pressure: 5 to 15 cm of H_20
Neurological Symptoms occur when ICP (intracranial pressure) > 15 to 20 cm of H_20

29.2 Aetiology

CSF rhinorrhea has been classified according to the aetiology as follows [2]:

1. Posttraumatic: 80% of CSF leaks are from nonsurgical head trauma, 2% of all head trauma, 30% of all basilar skull base fractures have CSF leak [3].
2. Iatrogenic: 16% of all leaks are from surgical trauma [5].
3. Spontaneous: 14–46% of all cases of CSF rhinorrhea [6, 7].
4. Idiopathic.

29.3 Diagnosis

Patients of CSF rhinorrhea present with unilateral watery discharge (90%) with salt or sweet taste in the throat. Rhinorrhea is positional with increase in leaning forward or standing position sometimes referred to as tea pot sign.

Other symptoms include headache, decrease in vision, and sometimes dizziness and tinnitus.

Confirmation of CSF rhinorrhea can be done by the following test.

- *Ring sign*: CSF combined with the blood leave a ring sign or a halo sign. The nasal secretions mixed with blood when placed on filter paper or bed sheets leave a central clearance of CSF and peripheral blood termed as halo sign. This is immediate indicator of CSF and gives a clue, but reliability of this sign is poor [8].

- *Glucose testing*: Testing clear rhinorrhea for glucose is a quick option for diagnosis; it was traditionally considered that the glucose in the nasal secretions is because of presence of CSF. Recent studies have indicated that glucose is also present in 50% cases of acute viral rhinitis, diabetes mellitus, and endotracheal secretions of ICU patients. It has 80% specificity and low sensitivity [8].
- *Beta-2 transferrin*: Beta-2 transferrin is a glycoprotein that is present in CSF, but is not detected in nasal secretions or surrounding tissue. It is used as a marker for CSF rhinorrhea. It is detected by using immunofixation, sodium dodecyl sulfate polyacrylamide gel electrophoresis, and isoelectric phoresis. It has high sensitivity and high specificity. Beta-2 transferrin is also present in vitreous and perilymph [8, 9].
- *Beta trace proteins*: Similar to beta-2 transferrin, beta trace protein is also present in high concentration in CSF; it is produced by leptomeninges and choroid plexus. The reported sensitivity and specificity of the test is 100%. Bacterial meningitis and renal insufficiency can affect the level of beta trace proteins in CSF.

Once CSF leak has been confirmed, localization of the leak is essential for preoperative planning.

Radiological investigations are used for confirmation and localization of site of leak.

29.3.1 High-Resolution Computed Tomography (HRCT)

HRCT is first choice for localization of site of leak. It is best modality to delineate the osseous anatomy for surgical planning. If patient has multiple osseous defects, then it becomes challenging to determine which defect is definite source of CSF leak. If only one osseous defect is identified and corresponds to clinical symptoms, then no additional further imaging is needed to proceed surgery.

29.3.2 Computed Tomography Cisternography [10]

CTC is performed by instilling intrathecal nonionic myelographic iodinated contrast (fluorescein). Sinuses are scanned both in prone and supine position. There is increase in >50 Hounsfield units around the osseous defect in positive study around site of leak (Fig. 29.1).

When introduced in 1977, CTC was considered the study of choice to evaluate CSF fistulae, but it is now selectively used as a problem-solving tool in specific scenarios, primarily in the setting of multiple osseous defects on CT, to determine the site of leak. CTC has a wide range of reported sensitivities of 33–100% and specificity of approximately 94% [10]. The main limitation of CTC is that patients have to be actively leaking, or able to elicit a leak, at the time of examination. Low rates of sensitivity are predominantly attributed to imaging in the absence of an active leak, with other potential causes being obscuration of small leak in the setting of high-density contrast media adjacent to high-density bone and high viscosity of contrast media prohibiting leakage through a fistulous tract. The disadvantages of CTC include high radiation dose related to multiple scans, inherent risk of a lumbar puncture, and potential adverse outcome from iodinated contrast.

29.3.3 Magnetic Resonance Cisternogram

MRC is a common imaging modality used for CSF leak diagnosis. It is a noninvasive study capable of both leak confirmation and site localization by the inherent bright signal of CSF on

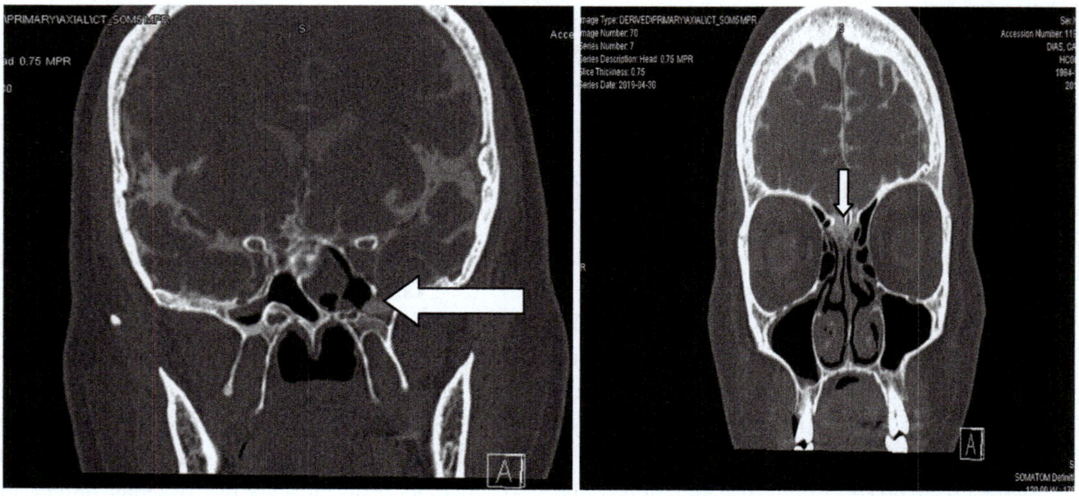

Fig. 29.1 CT cisternography demonstrating the leak from lateral sphenoid recess (Sternberg's canal horizontal arrow) and cribriform plate (vertical arrow)

T2-weighted images passing from intracranial into paranasal sinuses, as well as by the identification of herniated soft tissue in skull base defects [10].

Magnetic resonance (MR) cisternography (MRC) is performed by acquiring heavily T2-weighted (T2w) images to increase conspicuity of the contrast between CSF and the adjacent skull base. The spatial resolution of HRCT is far superior to that of MR imaging, but the advent of thin-slice images that can be reformatted into multiple planes significantly improves MR imaging of the skull base. MRC should continue to be used in conjunction with HRCT because MR imaging cannot provide the exquisite osseous detail of CT [10].

29.3.4 Radionuclide Cisternography

RNC is a nuclear medicine study in which a radioisotope is injected intrathecally via lumbar puncture, and pledgets are placed in the nasal cavities for several hours at a time, then removed and measured for radioactive tracer. This study may be able to better detect a CSF leak that is too slow or intermittent to produce a sufficient sample for beta-2 transferrin testing. It is an invasive study, however, and therefore carries the potential risks inherent to any other lumbar puncture with intrathecal injection. RNC is considered a diagnostic or confirmatory study rather than a localization study. The tracer may exit the skull base at the location of the fistula but contact the pledget at a second separate site. In addition, it cannot guarantee that the CSF is from a rhinologic leak and not an otologic leak that has traveled down the Eustachian tube into the nasopharynx.

The available data indicate that this is a more invasive, more expensive, and less accurate test than beta-2 transferrin or beta trace protein. Based on these facts, RNC should not be routinely employed to confirm the presence of a CSF leak [10].

29.4 Spontaneous CSF Leaks

Spontaneous CSF leaks represent distinct group of pathologies, by definition spontaneous leak is defined as CSF rhinorrhea in absence of any preceding event. Most of these patients show clinical signs and radiographic features of increased intracranial pressure. Accurately diagnosing patients with spontaneous CSF leaks is critical for the successful repair of these patients because multiple studies have identified increased ICP as a negative risk factor for successful repair [6–8, 11]. Although repair of nasal CSF leaks using endoscopic techniques has high success rates, patients with spontaneous CSF leaks have historically had a significantly lower success rate. There is strong correlation between the spontaneous leak and benign intracranial hypertension.

Patients are generally obese middle-aged women who present with spontaneous clear rhinorrhea. The diagnosis is confirmed by beta-2 transferrin.

After diagnosing CSF rhinorrhea by beta-2 transferrin, next is localization of the skull base defect and site of CSF fistula. High-resolution computed tomography (CT) is the initial radiographic test of choice, allowing for evaluation of the bony integrity of the skull base and paranasal sinuses. Patients with spontaneous CSF leaks have characteristic CT findings that support the diagnosis. The bone of the skull base is broadly attenuated and thin. Arachnoid pits secondary to the bony impressions from the arachnoid villi in the skull base are present in 63% of patients with spontaneous CSF leaks. The most common sites of skull base dehiscence are the lateral recess of the sphenoid and the ethmoid roof. Pneumatization of the lateral recess of the sphenoid is reported in 91% of patients with spontaneous CSF leaks, in comparison with 23–43% in normal patients [12]. Dehiscence of the ethmoid roof or cribriform plate is seen in 14% of patients with spontaneous CSF leaks [13]. The presence of multiple skull base defects is common and may be present in 31% of these patients.

Magnetic resonance imaging (MRI) is a useful adjunct in the evaluation of patients with CSF rhinorrhea. Patients with spontaneous CSF leaks have the highest rate of meningoencephalocele formation, ranging from 50 to 100% [1, 9]. MRI is effective in assessing the contents of meningoencephalocele. Another benefit of MRI in the evaluation of patients with spontaneous CSF leaks is the recognition of the empty sella. Empty sella syndrome is a common radiographic finding seen in both spontaneous CSF leaks and IIH [3, 4, 14]. Increased ICP are exerted on sites of inherent structural weakness including the fascia of the sellar diaphragm. The resulting herniation of the meninges and CSF through the sellar diaphragm produces the appearance of an empty sella on MRI. The presence of empty sella syndrome has been associated with both increased ICP and spontaneous CSF leaks [9, 15, 16].

29.5 Traumatic CSF Rhinorrhea

Approximately 80% of CSF leaks result from nonsurgical trauma, 16% from surgical procedures, and the remaining 4% are nontraumatic. Of the traumatic leaks, more than 50% are evident within the first 2 days, 70% within the first week, and almost all present within the first 3 months. Delayed presentation may result from wound contraction or scar formation, necrosis of bony edges or soft tissue, slow resolution of edema, devascularization of tissues, posttreatment tumor retraction, or progressive increases in intracranial pressure (secondary to brain edema or other process). As with most maxillofacial trauma, traumatic CSF leaks occur most commonly in young males and complicate 2% of all head traumas, and 12–30% of all basilar skull fractures. Anterior skull base leaks are more common than middle or posterior leaks, due to the firm adherence of the dura to the anterior basilar skull. The most common sites of CSF rhinorrhea following accidental trauma are the sphenoid sinus (30%), frontal sinus (30%), and ethmoid/cribriform (23%), When looking at surgical trauma, the most common sites of CSF leak following FESS are ethmoid/cribriform (80%), followed the frontal sinus (8%) and sphenoid sinus (4%). After neurosurgical procedures, the most common site of CSF leak is the sphenoid sinus (67%) because of the high number of pituitary tumors that are addressed via transsphenoidal approach [17–19].

29.6 Management of CSF Leaks

29.6.1 Conservative Management

Conservative treatment consists of strict bed rest and elevation of the head at least 30°. In addition, patients should be advised to refrain from coughing, sneezing, nose blowing, and straining or

Valsalva maneuvers. Stool softeners are recommended, as well as antiemetics to avoid emesis or retching, antitussives to avoid coughing, and strict blood pressure management. The goal of these measures is to reduce active flow through the leak, reduce CSF pressure, and allow healing of the defect to seal the leak, avoiding surgical intervention; the overall rate of cessation with conservative treatment was 39.5% when used for 3 days. Resolution with conservative treatment of CSF fistulas involving temporal bone origin was 60%, whereas anterior skull base defects resolved 26.4% of the time with conservative treatment. If conservative management is extended to 7 days, resolution rates improve to 85%.

29.6.2 Prophylactic Antibiotics

Cochrane Database review was performed to address these deficiencies. The analysis included 208 patients from four randomized controlled trials and an additional 2168 patients from 17 nonrandomized controlled trials. The analysis concluded that the evidence does not support the use of prophylactic antibiotics to reduce the risk of meningitis in patients with basilar skull fractures or basilar skull fractures with active CSF leak. Analysis of both randomized and nonrandomized controlled trials failed to show a benefit or adverse effects of prophylactic antibiotic use in patients with active CSF leak; therefore, the current available literature suggests that prophylactic antibiotics do not decrease the risk of meningitis. It should be stated that perioperative antibiotics are indicated for surgical repair of CSF leaks, and in certain circumstances (such as active bacterial rhinosinusitis or grossly contaminated tract leading to the intracranial cavity) antibiotic coverage is reasonable [4, 13, 20].

29.6.3 Cerebrospinal Fluid Diversion

If there is persistence of the leak with conservative treatment, CSF diversion (most commonly with a lumber drain but occasionally serial lumbar punctures) is pursued. Lumbar drains are passive devices yet they require active management. Average drainage rates are around 10 mL per hour. Optimal drainage lowers CSF pressure to decompress the leak; however, if drainage is too high, severe headaches and pneumocephalus may result from drawing of air through the skull base defect into the cranial vault. There is also the added risk of meningitis. The benefits are that the addition of CSF diversion to conservative measures raises success rates to 70–90% with the average duration of drainage being 6.5 days. Another benefit of this treatment is that it can be performed at the bedside, even if patients are not stable enough to go to the operating room. Lumbar drains can also be used as an adjunctive treatment to increase the success rates following a variety of surgical repairs.

29.6.4 Surgical Management

Open intracranial approaches have historically been used for CSF leak repair, but in recent decades these have largely been replaced by endonasal endoscopic approaches, given their high success rate and lower morbidity profile. Commonly utilized endoscopic repair techniques for CSF leak are numerous, including free tissue grafts, vascularized flaps, and tissue sealants, as well as various multilayer combinations of these methods. Studies have shown that vascularized flaps are superior in the setting of large dural defects or high-flow CSF leaks [7, 8]; otherwise, implementation of a specific repair technique is directed more by surgeon preference than by evidence-based guidance.

29.6.5 Transcranial Approach

Although CSF rhinorrhea was initially described in the seventeenth century, it was not until 1926 that Dand [21] reported the first successful repair by using a bifrontal craniotomy for access and a fascia lata graft for repair. After craniotomy the brain is retracted and the site of the defect is identified. Multiple tissues can be used for repair including fascia lata grafts, muscle plugs, and pedicled galeal or pericranial flaps. Tissue sealants, such as fibrin glue, can be used to hold the graft in position; however, this will only last a few weeks, leading the authors to prefer suture closure to the dura distal to the defect, which more securely holds the graft in place. Reported success rates vary; however, recurrence rates as high as 27% have been reported. The clear advantage of this approach is that it provides direct access to the defect and allows for repair of multiple sites; however, with high reported failure rates, the morbidity of a craniotomy, and brain retraction (including potential hematoma, seizures, and anosmia), extracranial techniques are now preferred in most circumstances. At present these techniques are mostly used in patients who require a craniotomy and exposure of the skull base to treat associated intracranial pathology.

29.6.6 Endoscopic Repair

There are a variety of different graft materials available for endoscopic repair of CSF leaks, including fat, bone, allografts, free mucosal grafts, and vascularized grafts, as well as glues or sealants to secure these materials in place. Following an extensive literature search on the topic of endoscopic repair for CSF rhinorrhea, the overall success rate ranges from 70 to 100% on first attempt and 86 to 100% on second for all reported repair materials. Endoscopic techniques have emerged as the preferred approach to the repair of skull base defects since their initial description by Wigand in 1981. This initial report described repair of a defect encountered during sinus surgery. In 1989, the first report of the use of rigid transnasal endoscopy for the endonasal repair of CSF rhinorrhea was described. Following identification and localization of the skull base defect, standard endoscopic techniques are used to expose the defect site. This approach provides excellent exposure of the ethmoid roof, cribriform plate, and the sphenoid sinus. The choice of graft material has been a source of debate for some time; however, based on a recent meta-analysis, it appears that graft material does not affect success rate as long as sound surgical technique is used. Graft choices include temporalis fascia, fascia lata, muscle plugs, mucosal grafts (with or without bone), autogenous fat, free cartilage grafts (from the nasal septum or auricle), and free bone grafts (from the nasal septum, calvarium, or iliac crest). For small defects, free mucosal or free fascial grafts can be placed in an overlay fashion.

Overlay, underlay, combined, and the obliteration techniques can be used for CSF closure. Overlay grafts are placed over the defect and these are outside the bony cranial cavity. The underlay grafts could be of two types (these are inside the bony cranial cavity). The epidural underlay graft is between the bone and the dura matter. The intradural underlay graft is placed in the subdural space. The combined techniques can be used. In a meta-analysis of the literature, both techniques yielded similar results. In the epidural underlay technique, the intact dura is separated from the edge of the skull base defect to expose an adequate buttress for the stabilization of the graft. The free graft should be designed in such a way that it can be pushed few millimeters between the bone and the dura on all the sides of the defect. Bone or cartilage underlay grafts are advocated for large bony defects associated with herniating brain or meninges. The inlay technique is technically more demanding than the overlay technique. Inlay grafting is also suited to repair defects of the posterior wall of the frontal sinus, the cribriform plate, the ethmoid roof, and the sphenoid sinus in some cases. The onlay (overlay) technique is recommended if there is a risk of nerves or vessels injury. It is also indicated when an inlay technique is not technically possible. The graft is placed generally over the dural lesion and over the exposed bony margins, which have been denuded of the mucosa. The graft is supported in place with layers of Gel foam/Gel film or Surgicel; followed by a packing, overlay grafts (79%) are more frequently used as compared to inlay grafts (12%). As an alternative, a vascularized haddad flap (nasoseptal flap) can be used designed over the nasal septal branch of sphenopalatine artery (Fig. 29.2a–c).

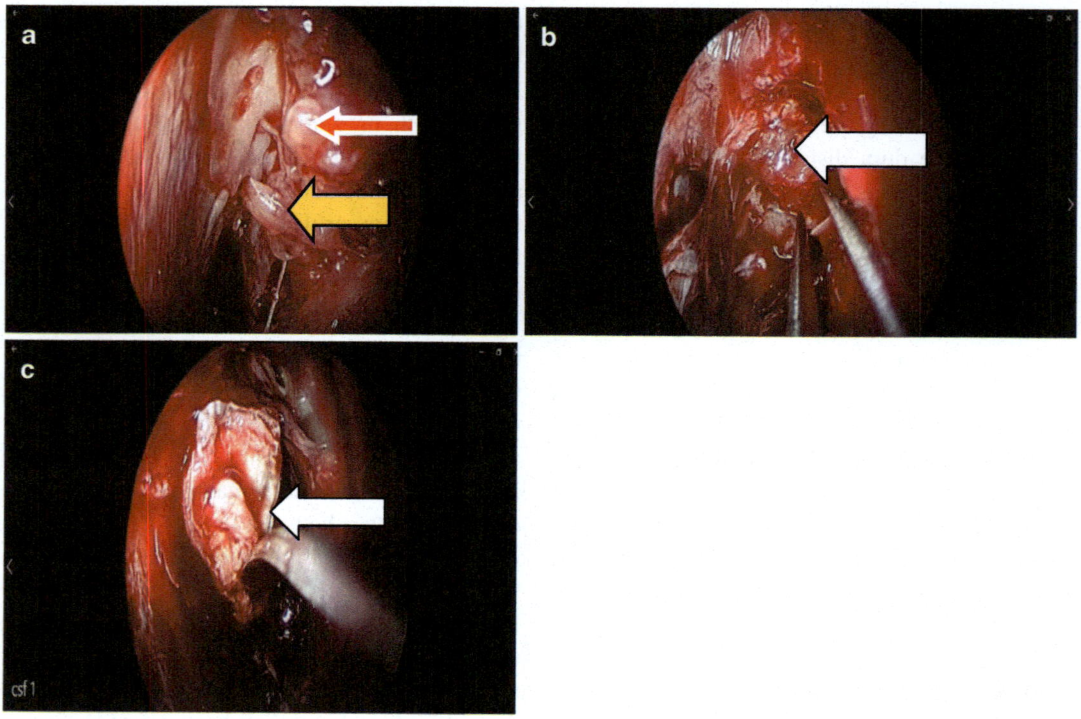

Fig. 29.2 (**a**) Cribriform plate with exit of olfactory fibers (yellow arrow), meningocele is seen at the level of fovea ethmoidalis (Red arrow). (**b**) Fat plug inserted into the defect. (**c**) Fascia lata placed as overlay graft

Take Home Messages
- Any unilateral nasal discharge should be investigated for CSF rhinorrhea.
- Beta-2 transferrin is the diagnostic lab test with high sensitivity and specificity.
- Endoscopic CSF rhinorrhea repair has high rate of success.
- Early diagnosis and localization of site of leak is key for successful management.

References

1. Han CY, Backous DD. Basic principles of cerebrospinal fluid metabolism and intracranial pressure homeostasis. Otolaryngol Clin N Am. 2005;38:569–76.
2. Har-El G. What is "spontaneous" cerebrospinal fluid rhinorrhea? Classification of cerebrospinal fluid leaks. Ann Otol Rhinol Laryngol. 1999;108:323–6.
3. Loew F, Pertuiset B, Chaumier EE, et al. Traumatic, spontaneous and postoperative CSF rhinorrhea. Adv Tech Stand Neurosurg. 1984;11:169–207.
4. Friedman JA, Ebersold MJ, Quast LM. Posttraumatic cerebrospinal fluid leakage. World J Surg. 2001;25:1062–6.
5. Kerman M, Cirak B, Dagtekin A. Management of skull base fractures. Neurosurg Q. 2002;12:23–41.
6. Friedman JA, Ebersold MJ, Quast LM. Post-traumatic cerebrospinal fluid leakage. World J Surg. 2001;25:1062–6.
7. Banks CA, Palmer JN, Chiu AG, et al. Endoscopic closure of CSF rhinorrhea: 193 cases over 21 years. Otolaryngol Head Neck Surg. 2009;140:826–33.
8. Kerr JT, Chu FW, Bayles SW. Cerebrospinal fluid rhinorrhea: diagnosis and management. Otolaryngol Clin N Am. 2005;38:597–611.
9. Schlosser RJ, Bolger WE. Significance of empty sella in cerebrospinal fluid leaks. Otolaryngol Head Neck Surg. 2003;128:32–8.
10. Reddy M, Baugnon K. Imaging of cerebrospinal fluid rhinorrhea and otorrhea. Radiol Clin N Am. 2017;55(1):167–87. https://doi.org/10.1016/j.rcl.2016.08.005. Review. PubMed PMID: 27890184.
11. Schlosser RJ, Wilensky EM, Grady MS, et al. Elevated intracranial pressures in spontaneous cerebrospinal fluid leaks. Am J Rhinol. 2003;17:191–5.

12. Eftekhar B, Ghodsi M, Nejat F, Ketabchi E, Esmaeeli B. Prophylactic administration of ceftriaxone for the prevention of meningitis after traumatic pneumocephalus: results of a clinical trial. J Neurosurg. 2004;101:757–61.
13. Eljamel MS, Foy PM. Acute traumatic CSF fistulae: he risk of intracranial infection. Br J Neurosurg. 1990;4:381–5.
14. Ohnishi T. Bony defects and dehiscences of the roof of the ethmoid cells. Rhinology. 1981;19(4):195–202.
15. Badia L, Loughran S, Lund V. Primary spontaneous cerebrospinal fluid rhinorrhea and obesity. Am J Rhinol. 2001;15:117–9.
16. El-Sayed IH, Roediger FC, Goldberg AN, et al. Endoscopic reconstruction of skull base defects with the nasal septal flap. Skull Base. 2008;18(6):385–94.
17. Normansell DE, Stacy EK, Booker CF, et al. Detection of beta-2 transferrin in otorrhea and rhinorrhea in a routine clinical laboratory setting. Clin Diagn Lab Immunol. 1994;1:68–70.
18. Yilmazlar S, Arslan E, Kocaeli H, et al. Cerebrospinal fluid leakage complicating skull base fractures: analysis of 81 cases. Neurosurg Rev. 2006;29:64–71.
19. Bell RB, Dierks EJ, Homer L, et al. Management of cerebrospinal fluid leak associated with craniomaxillofacial trauma. J Oral Maxillofac Surg. 2004;62(6):676–84.
20. Zagardo MT, Cail WS, Kelman SE, et al. Reversible empty sella in idiopathic intracranial hypertension: an indicator of successful therapy? AJNR Am J Neuroradiol. 1996;17(10):1953–6.
21. Dandy WE. Pneumocephalus (intracranial pneumocele or aerocele). Arch Surg. 1926;12:949–82.

30 Anterior and Midline Central Skull Base Tumors

Sara Ashkanani and Abhishek Menon

Key Points

- Mainstay of treatment for sinonasal squamous cell CA is surgical resection. Radiotherapy may be used as adjuvant therapy, except in nonresectable tumors, where they are used as mainstay.
- Perineural invasion is more common in adenocarcinoma.
- Clinical presentation and examination of olfactory neuroblastoma can mimic inflammatory polyps.
- Pituitary adenomas are usually seen in the third decade of life. MRI with gadolinium enhancement is the single best radiological test for midline central skul base tumor diagnosis. Treatment is usually surgical excision.
- Chordomas and chondrosarcomas are derived from embryonic remnants of the notochord.

30.1 Introduction

The skull base refers to the most inferior part of the neurocranium, on which the brain rests, and it is the major bony and soft tissue interface for the intracranial and extracranial compartments. Its anatomy is complex, containing multiple traversing foramina that act as conduits for various neurovascular structures. They are divided into anterior, central, and posterior parts (Fig. 30.1). In this chapter, we will be dealing with the anterior skull base and midline aspect of the central skull base and its pathologies. The various foramen and the structures passing through them are mentioned in Tables 30.1, 30.2, and 30.3.

30.2 Anatomy

The anterior skull base proper is formed medially by the cribriform plate, making up the roof of the nasal cavity, laterally by the orbital plates of the frontal bone which form the roof of the orbits and ethtmoid air cells and, posteriorly, by the planum sphenoidale and lesser wings of the sphenoid.

S. Ashkanani (✉)
Otolaryngology-Head and Neck Surgery Division, Department of Surgery, Hamad Medical Corporation, Doha, Qatar

Department of Otolaryngology-Head and Neck Surgery Division, Weill Cornell Medicine-Qatar, Doha, Qatar
e-mail: sashkanani@hamad.qa

A. Menon
Otolaryngology-Head and Neck Surgery Division, Department of Surgery, Hamad Medical Corporation, Doha, Qatar
e-mail: AMenon1@hamad.qa

A. Al-Qahtani et al. (eds.), *Textbook of Clinical Otolaryngology*,
https://doi.org/10.1007/978-3-030-54088-3_30

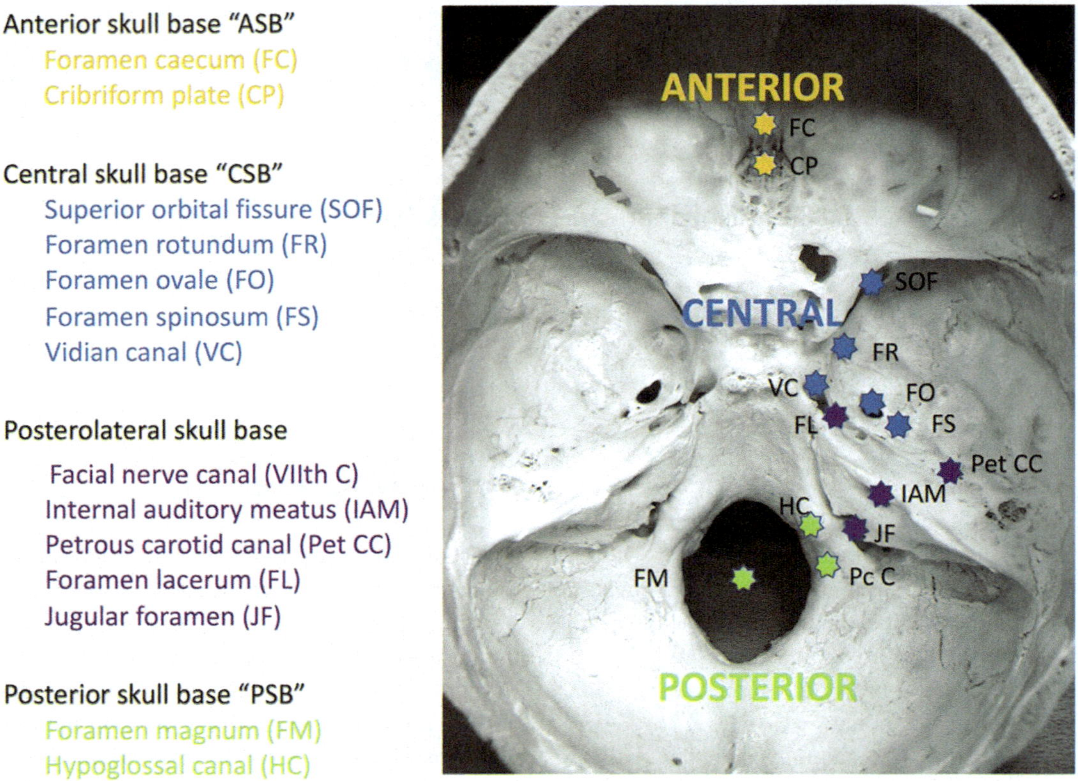

Fig. 30.1 Skull base showing the different parts and fissures within them

Table 30.1 The foramina of the anterior skull base and their traversing neurovascular structures

Foramen	Nerve	Vessel
Foramen caecum		Emissary vein to superior sagittal sinus
Cribriform plate	Olfactory nerve	
Optic canal	Optic nerve	Ophthalmic artery

The central skull base comprises the body and greater wing of sphenoid bone and squamous temporal bones, and is demarcated from the posterior skull base by the petrous temporal bone. They are divided into:

- *Midline Central Skull base Compartment*: Includes the pituitary (sella), sphenoid body, and clivus, and abuts the extracranial nasopharynx.
- *Paramidline Central Skull Base Compartment*: Includes a cluster of neurovascular foramina, the cavernous sinuses, and Meckel's caves.

This posterior skull base compartment includes the anatomical structures of the cerebellopontine angle, internal auditory meatus, petromastoid, jugular foramen, and hypoglossal canal.

Table 30.2 The foramina of the central skull base and their traversing neurovascular structures

Foramen	Nerve	Vessel
Superior orbital fissure	CN III, IV, V_1, VI	Superior and inferior ophthalmic vein
Foramen rotundum	Maxillary nerve (CN V2)	
Foramen ovale	Mandibular nerve (CN V3)	Accessory meningeal artery
Foramen spinosum	Meningeal branch of mandibular nerve	Middle meningeal artery
Vidian (pterygoid) canal	Vidian nerve	Vidian artery/vein
Meckel's canal	Trigeminal nerve ganglion	

The dura is particularly closely attached to the anterior skull base and so is prone to injury following a skull base fracture, potentially with pneumocephalus or cerebrospinal fluid (CSF)

Table 30.3 The foramina of the posterior skull base and their traversing neurovascular structures

Foramen	Nerve	Vessel
Facial nerve canal	Facial nerve (CN VII)	
Internal auditory meatus	Facial (CN VII) and vestibulocochlear (CN VIII) nerves	Labyrinthine artery
Petrous carotid canal		Petrous segment of the internal carotid artery
Foramen lacerum	Vidian nerve leaves its anterior aspect	Artery of pterygoid canal Emissary veins (carotid artery is immediately superior)
Jugular foramen	Glossopharyngeal (CN IX) Vagus (CN X) Spinal accessory nerve (CN XI)	Inferior petrosal sinus Jugular bulb
Foramen magnum	Medulla oblongata	Vertebral artery Anterior and posterior spinal arteries
Hypoglossal canal	Hypoglossal nerve	

rhinorrhoea. The anterior skull base also has a rich plexus of valveless venous perforations (e.g., the vein of Breschet) and so paranasal sinus infection can spread either into the frontal bones as osteomyelitis or traverse the anterior skull base giving intracranial sepsis.

MRI can clearly delineate the olfactory bulbs, which may have reduced volume in some neurodegenerative processes. The foramen caecum is generally blind ended or transmits an emissary vein in adulthood, but is also the site of a dural diverticulum in early life. If this diverticulum persists in the context of midline nasal developmental anomalies such as dermoid cysts, then it may predispose to ascending meningitis.

30.3 Tumors of the Anterior Skull Base

Pathologic processes affecting the anterior skull base may arise from the bones of the skull base proper, intracranially from the meningeal coverings, or exocranially from the sinonasal mucosa investing the nasal cavity, ethmoid and frontal sinuses, from the olfactory mucosa covering the roof of the nasal cavity, from the orbit, from cranial nerves and vessels, from the chondro-vomerian synchondrosis, or from embryonic remnants.

30.3.1 Sinonasal Neoplasms

Most sinonasal neoplasms are epithelial in origin and include, in decreasing order of frequency, squamous cell carcinoma, intestinal type adenocarcinoma, and minor salivary gland neoplasms. The remainder comprise neoplasms arising from the olfactory mucosa, (esthesioneuroblastomas), nasal lymphoma, melanoma, and a variety of mesenchymal tumors including rhabdomyossarcoma, the most common in the pediatric age group.

30.3.1.1 Squamous Cell Carcinoma

- Most common sinonasal tumor.
- Constitute 70% of all malignancies.
- Presents with nasal congestion, blockage, frequent epistaxis, headache.
- Imaging features are non-specific and include intermediate signal intensity on T2W images reflecting high cellularity and aggressive bone destruction occasionally with small bony fragments engulfed within the lesion [1, 2].
- Mainstay of treatment is surgical resection.
- Radiotherapy may be used as adjuvant therapy, except in nonresectable tumors, where they are used as mainstay.

30.3.1.2 Adenocarcinoma

- Comprises 10% of all sinonasal neoplasms.
- Perineural invasion more common.
- Three types:
  - Minor salivary gland tumors
  - Intestinal type adenocarcinoma
  - Neuroendocrine neoplasms
- Distinctive imaging features include T2W prolongation [3–5] and, in low-grade tumors, a less aggressive pattern of bone involvement, usually with remodelling and thinning rather than permeative destruction of surrounding bone (Fig. 30.2).
- Treatment is surgical resection.

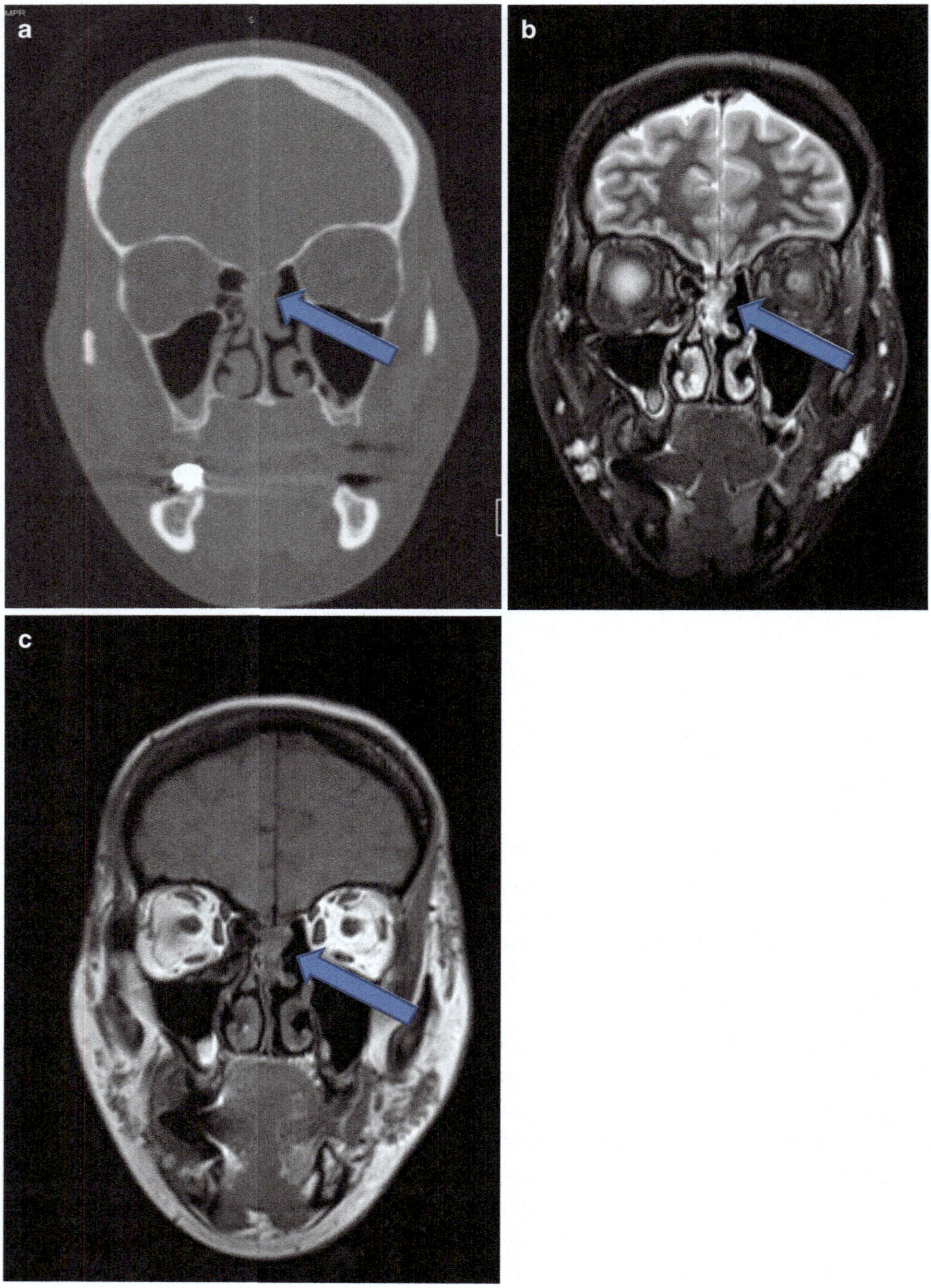

Fig. 30.2 (**a**) Coronal CT sinus showing adenocarcinoma extending from the roof of the left ethmoid sinus distally and medially through the olfactory recess eroding the nasal septum crossing into the contralateral side. (**b**) Coronal T1W MRI sinus showing intermediate signal intensity lesion mildly expanding predominantly left nasal roof and olfactory recess mass lesion inseparable from medial lamella of left middle turbinate, and infiltrating the nasal septum crossing to and expanding contralateral olfactory recess, with remodelling of cribriform plate with no definite intracranial extension. (**c**) Coronal T2W MRI sinus showing inhomogeneous mixed signal intensity lesion mildly expanding predominantly left nasal roof and olfactory recess mass lesion inseparable from medial lamella of left middle turbinate, and infiltrating the nasal septum crossing to and expanding contralateral olfactory recess, with remodelling of cribriform plate with no definite intracranial extension

30.3.1.3 Olfactory Neuroblastoma

- Also known as *esthesioneuroblastoma.*
- It is a rare tumor of neural crest origin which arises from the olfactory mucosa lining the nasal vault and cribiform plate and therefore is a site specific neoplasm.
- Clinical presentation and examination mimics inflammatory polyps.
- Intracranial extension through cribriform plate and orbital invasion through lamina papyracea are common.
- Meningeal spread and parenchymal invasion of the olfactory bulbs and inferior frontal lobes are often seen in advanced tumors.
- Typical imaging presentation is that of a solitary, polypoid, expansile soft tissue mass centered in the nasal vault and cribiform plate.
- This radiographic grading scale is as follows:
  - A—limited to nasal cavity.
  - B—nasal and paranasal cavity.
  - C—beyond nasal and paranasal cavity (invades cribriform plate, anterior cranial base or orbit, intracranial, and maxillary sinus).
- They tend to be slightly hyperdense on CT and of intermediate signal intensity on both T1W and T2W MR images (Fig. 30.3) [6, 7].
- Treatment is surgical enbloc resection.

30.3.1.4 Others

- Less common tumors include:
  - Malignant melanoma
  - B Cell lymphoma
  - T Cell lymphoma

30.3.2 Orbital Tumors

- Although less commonly, a variety of neoplasms arising from the orbital contents may affect the anterior skull base from below. These include lacrimal gland neoplasms, neurogenic tumors, lymphoma, rhadomyosarcoma, chloroma, and metastasis to name the most common.
- Benign lacrimal gland tumors manifest as mass lesions originating in the superior and outer aspect of the orbit, the normal anatomic location of the lacrimal gland. When large enough, they displace the globe and extraocular muscles inferiorly and medially and remodel and erode the orbital roof.

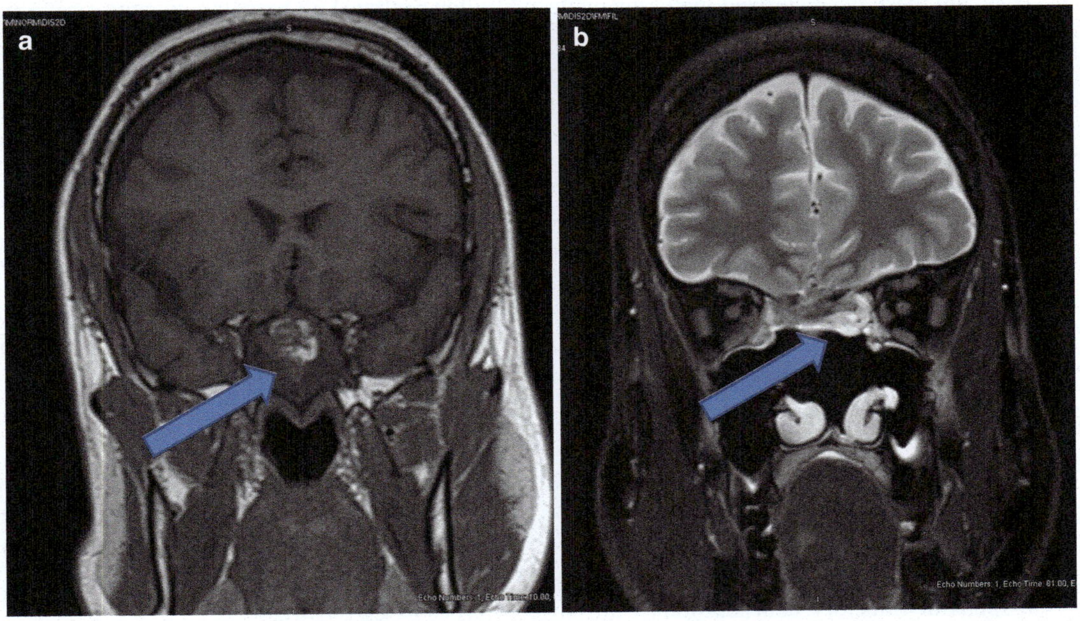

Fig. 30.3 (**a**) T1W MRI showing low T1 lesion with small bright patches in a post-op patient. (**b**) T2W MRI showing mixed signal, heterogenously enhancong lesion in a post-op patient

- Malignant neoplasms arising in the orbital compartment show aggressive features and may extend posteriorly through the orbital apex and orbital fissures into the medial cranial fossa.

30.4 Tumors Arising from Above the Anterior Skull Base

Besides meningiomas and their malignant counterparts, the skull base is rarely affected by other tumors arising from the intracranial compartment. Only rarely do primary CNS tumors grow outside the brain and when this occurs it is often along the path of a surgical defect.

30.4.1 Olfactory Groove Meningioma

- Most common intracranial lesion affecting the anterior skull base from above.
- Does not cause symptoms until tumor has grown to large size.
- Symptoms include anosmia, blurred vision, loss of memory, headache, nausea, vomiting, and personality changes.
- They are best characterized with magnetic resonance imaging.
- They are usually isointense to brain on both T1W and T2W images, well-circumscribed and show intense and homogeneous gadolinium enhancement.
- Treatment is usually surgical resection.

30.4.2 Subfrontal Schwannomas

- Rare neoplasms of unclear origin, thought to arise from the olfactory nerve or from a meningeal branch of cranial nerve V.
- Benign slow-growing lesions which tend to remodel adjacent bone and may be associated to bone sclerosis and intratumoral calcifications.
- Often misdiagnosed for olfactory groove meningomas or olfactory neuroblastomas due to their particular location imaging features.
- Treatment is surgical excision.

30.5 Pseudotumors

Many infectious inflammatory conditions such as mucoceles, sinonasal polyposis, abscesses, fungal infection, osteomyelitis and several granulomatous diseases including Wegener's can affect the skull base and even grow intracranially mimicking tumoral lesions. Correlation with clinical history and laboratory findings is mandatory to reach the diagnosis. Imaging features that might suggest inflammatory pseudotumor include the presence of MR signal changes, particularly on long TR images, in excess to the amount of soft tissue mass seen on CT and the presence of vessel occlusion. Whereas neoplasms invading the cavernous sinus tend to narrow or compress the internal carotid artery, rarely leading to a complete occlusion, infection and inflammation reaching the skull base may rapidly extend to the petrous or cavernous segments of the carotid artery, leading to inflammation of the vessel wall (endarteritis) and occlusion.

30.6 Tumors of the Midline Central Skull Base

Midline central skull base tumors may arise from the sphenoid sinus and clivus, sella or the extracranial tissues (nasopharynx). Most (>90%) sellar lesions are pituitary in origin, and the remaining can be meningiomas and craniopharyngiomas.

30.6.1 Pituitary Adenomas

- They are the most common causes of midline central skull base tumors [8].
- Pituitary adenomas are benign tumors of the adenohypophysis.
- Usually seen in the third decade of life.
- MEN1, Gs-alpha and AIP mutations have been shown to play a role in the development of the tumor.
- Types based on size:
  - *Microadenoma*: less than 1 cm
  - *Macroadenoma*: more than 1 cm

- Types based on cell type:
  - *Gonadotroph adenomas:* Clinically nonfuctioning
  - *Thyrotroph adenomas:* Clinically nonfunctioning, but can cause hyperthyroidism
  - *Corticotroph adenomas:* Can cause Cushing's disease
  - *Lactotroph adenomas:* Causes hyperprolactinemia
  - *Somatotroph adenomas:* Causes increased GH
- Symptoms include visual defects, diplopia, headches, and symptoms assoicated with hormonal imbalance.
- MRI with gadolinium enhancement is the single best radiological test for midline central skul base tumor diagnosis. Other test include CT.
- Hormanal studies are also recommended.
- Treatment is surgical excision or debulking (transnasal or open cranial approach), except in the case of pituitary incidentaloma where the patient has an incidental finding of pituitary tumor >1 cm on radiography, but no symptoms (Fig. 30.4).

30.6.2 Chordomas and Chondrosarcomas

- Chondromas are rare, locally aggressive, slow-growing neoplasms.
- Derived from embryonic remnants of the notochord.
- Can involve parts of the body other than skull base such as sacrococcygeal region, and vertebral column.
- Three types of chordomas:
  - *Conventional:* Absent cartilaginous or mesenchymal components.
  - *Chondroid:* Contains both chordomatous and cartilaginous features. Usually seen in sphenooccipital region.
  - *Dedifferentialted or sarcomatous type.*
- *Grossly they appear as gelatinous pink or gray masses with solid and cystic areas.*
- Whereas chondrosarcomas are rare malignant cartilaginous tumors.
- Chondrosarcomas grossly appear as smooth, lobulated, hard tumors.
- Microscopically chondrosarcomas are three types:
  - *Well differentiated*
  - *Moderately differntiated*
  - *Poorly differntiated*
- Surgical excision is preferred for both chordomas and chondrosarcomas (transnasal or transfacial approach).
- Radiotherapy/adjuavant radiotherapy is also used in treatment of chordomas and chondrosarcomas.

30.6.3 Craniopharyngomas

- Craniopharyngiomas are benign epithelial tumors that usually arise in the pituitary stalk in the suprasellar region, adjacent to the optic chiasm. A small percentage arise within the sella, and a few tumors have been described within the optic system or the third ventricle.
- Slow growing.
- Symptoms include headache, visual symptoms, hormonal deficiencies, growth failure, nausea, and vomiting.
- MRI and CT are used for radiography.
- Characteristic finiding is a cystic, calcified suprasellar mass.
- Pretreatment requisites include adrenal, thyroid function and neuroopthalmic evaluation.
- Treatment needs multidisciplinary team with surgical resection and radiotherapy followed by post-op hormonal therapy if required.

30.6.4 Others

- Meningioma: Benign tumor arising from the meninges.
- Pituicytoma: Uncommon, low-grade, indolent glioma arising from the pituicytes of the posterior pituitary. It presents as a sellar mass, which is usually mistaken for a pituitary adenoma, and has no known hormonal secretory function.

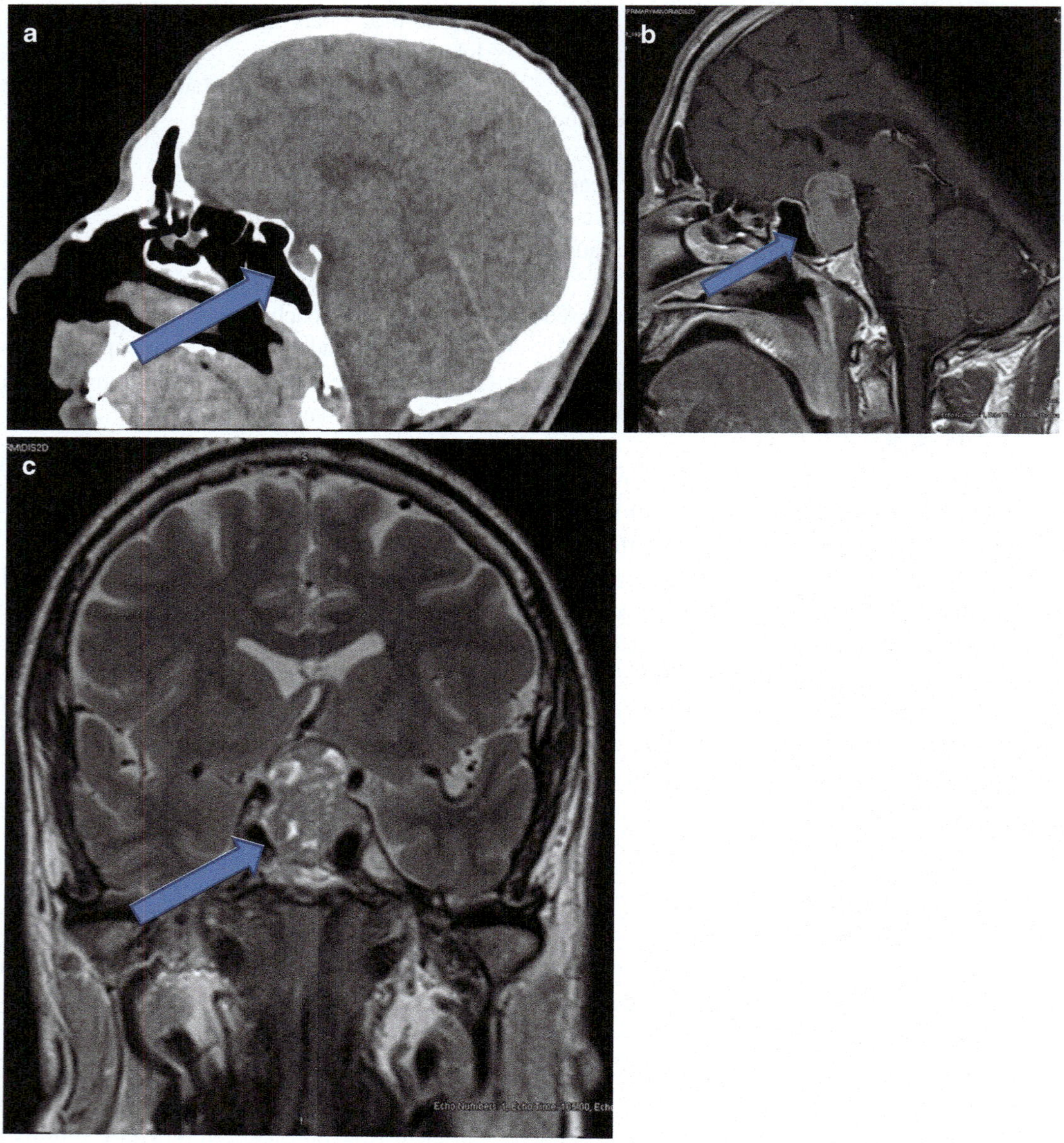

Fig. 30.4 (**a**) Ct head sagittal view showing sellar mass. (**b**) T1W MRI showing enhancing suprasellar lesion encroaching the cavernous sinus. (**c**) T2W MRI showing intensely enhancing suprasellar lesion encroaching the cavernous sinus

30.7 Tumors of Posterior Skull Base

- Cerebellopontine tumors
  - Vestibular schwannomas
  - Meningioma
  - Epidermoid schwannomas
  - Non-vestibular schwannoma
  - Arachnoid cyst (Table 30.4)

Take Home Messages

- The skull base is a highly complex region that includes multiple bones. Eleven pairs of cranial nerves and the olfactory nerves (CN I) pass through the inner table of the skull via seven pairs of bony foramina and the cribriform plate (CN I).
- Lesions and tumors can pose a challenge due to its location. Hence, apt knowledge of anatomy is necessary.

Table 30.4 CT vs. MRI for skull base imaging

	CT	MRI
Advantages	Good for spatial resolution	Good for soft tissue resolution
Bone imaging	Cortical bone well imaged	Medullary bone is well imaged (central skull base)
Used specifically for	Fractures, sinonasal disease, middle ear and mastoid disease	Extracranial, central skull base or intracranial extension of disease, cranial nerve pathology
Cuts	Submillimetric (mm) with multiplanar reformats	3 mm sections in at least two planes (including coronal) or increasingly volumetric. STIR (short tau inversion recovery), T1-weighted precontrast and T1-weighted fat-saturated post gadolinium

References

1. Atlas SW. Magnetic resonance imaging of the brain and spine. 3rd ed. Philadelphia: Lippincott Williams & Wilkins; 2002.
2. Quirk B, Connor S. Pract Neurol. 2019;1–11. https://doi.org/10.1136/practneurol-2019-002383.
3. Durden DD, Williams DW III. Radiology of skull base neoplasms. Otolaryngol Clin N Am. 2001;34(6):1043–64.
4. Borges A. Skull base tumours part I: Imaging technique, anatomy and anterior skull base tumours. Eur J Radiol. 2008;66:338–47.
5. Uptodate.
6. Som PM, Curtin HD. Head and neck imaging, skull base. 4th ed. St. Louis: Mosby Year Book; 2003. p. 261–373; 783–863.
7. Curtin HD, Chavali R. Imaging the skull base. Radiol Clin North Am. 1998;36(5):801–17.
8. Flint PW, Haughey BH, Lund VJ, Niparko JK, Robbins KT, Thomas JR, Lesperance MM. Cummings otolaryngology: head and neck surgery. 6th ed.

31 Epistaxis

Ahmed Shaikh, Hamad Al Saey, Sara Ashkanani, Mashael Alhail, Mansour Al Sulaiti, Maryam Abdulraheem, Emad Al Duhirat, and Shanmugam Ganesan

31.1 Introduction

Epistaxis is a common ENT emergency. The estimated lifetime incidence of epistaxis is approximately 60% [1]. Most episodes are minor in nature, self-limiting and do not require intervention. Minor bleeding episodes occur more frequently in children and adolescents, whereas severe bleeds requiring intervention often occur in individuals older than 50 years. Peaks in incidence are seen in those less than 10 years of age and aged over 40 years [2].

For management of epistaxis, it is imperative to learn about the vascular supply to the nose.

Blood supply to the nose:

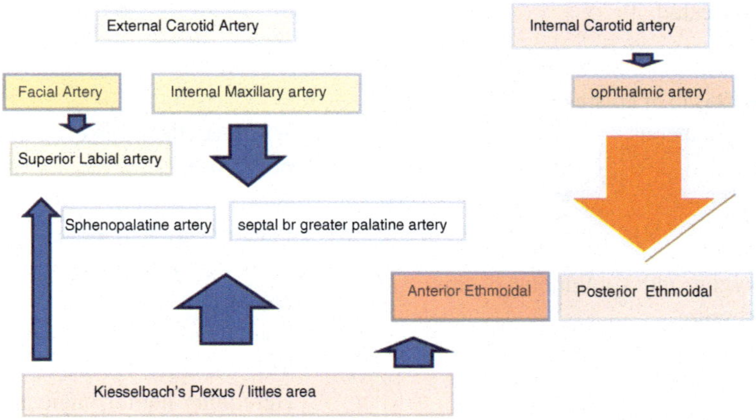

Nasal Septum

A. Shaikh (✉) · H. Al Saey · S. Ashkanani
M. Al Sulaiti · S. Ganesan
Otolaryngology-Head and Neck Surgery Division, Department of Surgery, Hamad Medical Corporation, Doha, Qatar

Department of Otolaryngology-Head and Neck Surgery Division, Weill Cornell Medicine-Qatar, Doha, Qatar
e-mail: Halsaey@hamad.qa; unknown_user_499795@meteor.springer.com; Malsulaiti1@hamad.qa; sganesan@hamad.qa

M. Alhail · M. Abdulraheem · E. Al Duhirat
Otolaryngology-Head and Neck Surgery Division, Department of Surgery, Hamad Medical Corporation, Doha, Qatar
e-mail: malhail@hamad.qa; Ashaikh4@hamad.qa; EAlDuhirat@hamad.qa

A. Al-Qahtani et al. (eds.), *Textbook of Clinical Otolaryngology*,
https://doi.org/10.1007/978-3-030-54088-3_31

31.2 Woodruffs Plexus

Mainly a venous plexus situated at the posterior and inferior end of the inferior turbinate.

31.3 Classification of Epistaxis [3–5]

Anterior epistaxis: anterior to pyriform aperture which can be visualised by head light.

Posterior epistaxis: posterior to pyriform aperture the source of which cannot be visualised by head lamp. Some authors [6] describe the maxillary ostium as landmark to differentiate anterior from posterior nasal bleeding.

31.3.1 Causes of Nasal Bleeding

Epistaxis can result from multiple causes both local and systemic, most of the time epistaxis is a manifestation of underlying disease, hence in all cases of epistaxis underlying cause should be investigated and treated.

Local Causes (Nasal) of Epistaxis

Idiopathic/spontaneous

Trauma

- Nose picking
- Foreign body
- Nasal oxygen and continuous positive airway pressure
- Nasal fracture

Inflammatory/infectious

- Common cold, viral rhinosinusitis
- Allergic rhinosinusitis
- Bacterial rhinosinusitis
- Granulomatous diseases
- Wegener granulomatosis
- Sarcoid
- Tuberculosis

Environmental irritants

- Smoke
- Chemicals
- Pollution
- Altitude

Postoperative/iatrogenic

- Nasal surgery
- Nasal crustations

Primary neoplasm

- Haemangioma of the septum, turbinates
- Haemangiopericytoma (glomangiopericytoma)
- Nasal papilloma
- Pyogenic granuloma
- Angiofibroma
- Carcinoma and other nasal malignancies

Structural

- Septal deformity, spurs
- Septal perforation

Drugs

- Topical nasal steroids
- Cocaine abuse occupational substances

General Disorders, Systemic Causes

Hypertension

Arteriosclerosis

Platelet deficiencies or dysfunction

Coagulopathies (e.g. warfarin, liver disease)

Leukaemia

Von Willebrand disease

Hereditary hemorrhagic telangiectasia

Organ failure (e.g. liver, kidney)

31.3.2 Management

31.3.2.1 General Management

ABC: Airway Breathing and Circulation Assessment

Patient should be quickly assessed for any hypovolemic shock; the signs include tachycardia, pale, cold extremities, sweating and hypotension.

Blood should be collected for haemoglobin, coagulation, cross matching and platelet function test and peripheral line should be secured.

After stabilisation of vitals, assessment includes

1. History taking: includes the history of onset, amount of blood loss, laterality and any systemic or family diseases.
2. Examination: examination of nasal septum should be done to visualise the little area which is commonest site of nasal bleeding; nasal septal deviation and nasal turbinates should be inspected, if the source of bleeding is not visualised by the head light, then nose should be decongested and nasal endoscopy should be done for visualisation of posterior aspect of nasal cavity.

31.3.3 Specific Management

Trotter's manoeuvre: cartilaginous part of the nose should be compressed for at least 15–20 min most of the time the anterior pressure stops the nasal bleeding.

Cauterisation of anterior nasal bleeding [7]: if the source of the bleeding can be seen, attempt should be made to cauterise it after local anaesthesia; silver nitrate cautery and the bipolar cautery are effective to control the bleeding from the anterior nasal septum.

Failure of cauterisation or medical management leads a clinician to consider packing as the next treatment option. Many different types of packs have been developed over the years, including no absorbable, anterior, and posterior packs.

31.4 Nasal Packing

31.4.1 Anterior Nasal Packs

31.4.1.1 Absorbable [8]

Oxidised cellulose (e.g. Surgicel): it is local hemostatic agent which acts by pressure compression and promotes the coagulation at the bleeding site.

Absorbable gelatin foams (Gelfoam): act by temponade effect and promote the platelet aggregation (Fig. 31.1).

Floseal: combination of thrombin with gelatin to promote the coagulation, it is easier to use with least patient discomfort, drawback is floseal and more expensive than other traditional packing materials.

31.4.1.2 Non-absorbable Packs

Carboxymethylcellulose Sponge (Merocel)

Usually used as first-line anterior nasal packs, they act by mechanical compression of the bleeding point, usually they are lubricated with antiseptic ointment for easy insertion and preventing the secondary infection. Once inserted they are left for 24–48 h. They are inserted along the floor of the nose. Side effects include patient discomfort at the time of insertion and removal of pack. They can act as focus of infection and can cause toxic shock syndrome, hence patient with nasal packs should be covered with antibiotics and Staphylococcus aureus.

Inflatable balloons: Rapid rhino they are inserted along the floor of the nose and inflated with normal saline. They also act by direct compression of bleeding site and promote the coagulation.

Impregnated gauze packing: This is a traditional way of nasal packing where impregnated gauze is used as layers for packing the nasal cavity; it caused significant pain to the patient and needs expertise for packing. They have fallen out

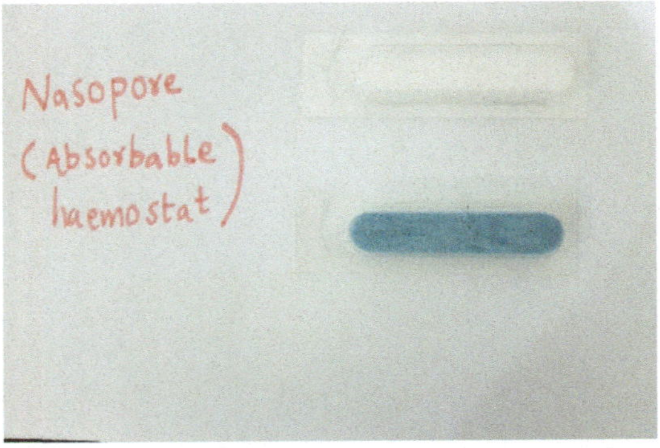

Fig. 31.1 Nasopore (absorbable haemostat)

of favour as more easy methods of anterior packing like merocel is available. One of the packs which is used for long-term packing is gauze impregnated with BIPP (Bismuth Iodine Paraffin Paste); BIPP is an antiseptic pack and can be left upto 7 days inside the nasal cavity (Fig. 31.2).

Posterior nasal packing: posterior packing is not as commonly used; it is used with anterior packing when anterior packing alone fails to stop the bleeding.

A Foleys catheter of size 14 or 12 is used, catheter is inserted along the nasal floor into the choana, the position is confirmed after visualisation of the tip in the posterior pharyngeal wall through the oral cavity, 5 to 10 ml of saline is used to fully inflate the balloon and catheter is pulled to hinge over the choana there by occupying the nasopharynx and putting a tamponade effect on posterior end of the nasal cavity. An artery forceps or vascular clip is used to keep the traction. The nasal cavity around the catheter is packed with impregnated gauze strips.

The side effects of posterior nasal packing are severe nasal pain, necrosis of columella and necrosis of posterior part of nasal septum by pressure effect. Posterior packs also lead to obstructive sleep apnoea and arrhythmia in some patients; the patients with posterior packs should be admitted and regular monitoring is needed for oxygen saturation.

Documented success rate of posterior packing is around 75%. Failure of posterior packing warrants surgical management of epistaxis.

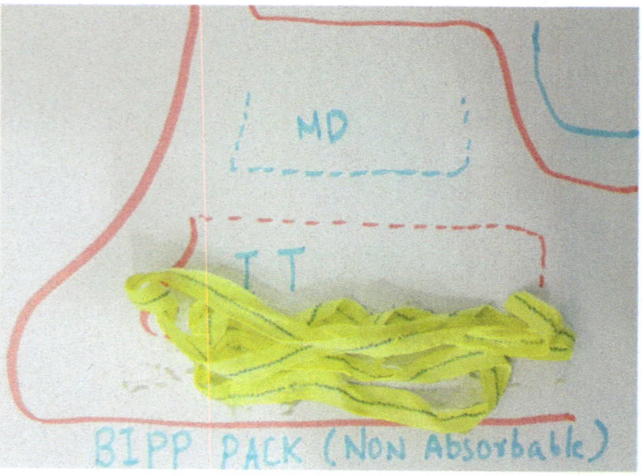

Fig. 31.2 BIPP (Bismuth Iodine Paraffin Paste) Pack

31.4.2 Surgical Management of Epistaxis [9–13]

Surgical management includes the cauterisation or ligation of major vessels in the nose, as discussed earlier nose is mainly supplied by anterior ethmoidal artery, posterior ethmoidal artery and sphenopalatine branch of internal maxillary artery.

31.5 Anterior Ethmoid Artery Ligation

Anterior ethmoidal artery [14] is a branch of ophthalmic artery which is branch of internal carotid artery; the course of AEA is described in three parts intraorbital, intranasal and intracranial.

The artery pierces the periorbital and enters the nose through anterior ethmoidal foramen. Anterior ethmoidal foramen is located at 24 mm distance from the lacrimal crest. The artery exits the orbit between medial rectus and superior oblique muscles; at the level of ethmoidal foramen lamina papyracea is dehiscent with projection that can be appreciated on CT sinus. The level of artery in relation to the skull base in the ethmoidal sinus is variable; the artery is covered with a thin bony canal which also contains the anterior ethmoidal nerve. Artery enters the cranium through lateral lamella of cribriform plate. Anterior ethmoidal artery supplies the nasal septum. Intracranial part of anterior ethmoidal artery gives anterior meningeal and anterior falcine artery which supplies the falx cerebri (Fig. 31.3).

The anterior ethmoidal artery ligation is considered in cases of refractory epistaxis when either the bleeding is seen coming from AEA or sphenopalatine artery ligation does not control the nasal bleeding. Embolization is not an option for AES bleed as there is high risk of blindness.

Traditionally ligation has been performed via an open approach using a Lynch-type incision [15] with the placement of the vascular clip on the AEA between the periorbital fascia and its entrance into the lamina papyracea. Now many endoscopic approaches have been described for ligation of AEA avoiding external scar.

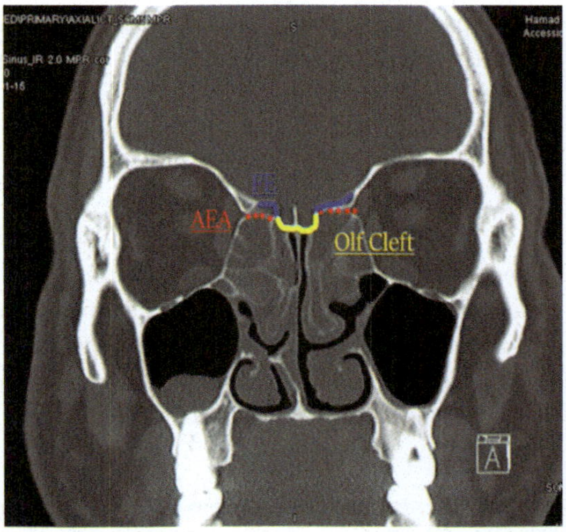

Fig. 31.3 Anterior ethmoidal artery (AEA, red), Olfactory Cleft (yellow Olf Cleft) and Fovea Ethmoidalis (Blue FE)

Retraction of the AEA into the orbit can lead to permanent vision loss, hence in case of failed endoscopic approach external approach is used (Figs. 31.4 and 31.5).

The posterior ethmoidal [16] artery which is a branch of ophthalmic artery passes through the posterior ethmoidal canal and enters the dura at the posterior margin of the cribriform plate and supplies the dura of the medial third of the floor of the anterior cranial fossa; PEA is seen at the roof of posterior ethmoidal cells and most of the time is covered with bone; the bleeding from posterior ethmoidal artery is rare and usually iatrogenic as PEA is a small artery as compared to AEA (Fig. 31.6).

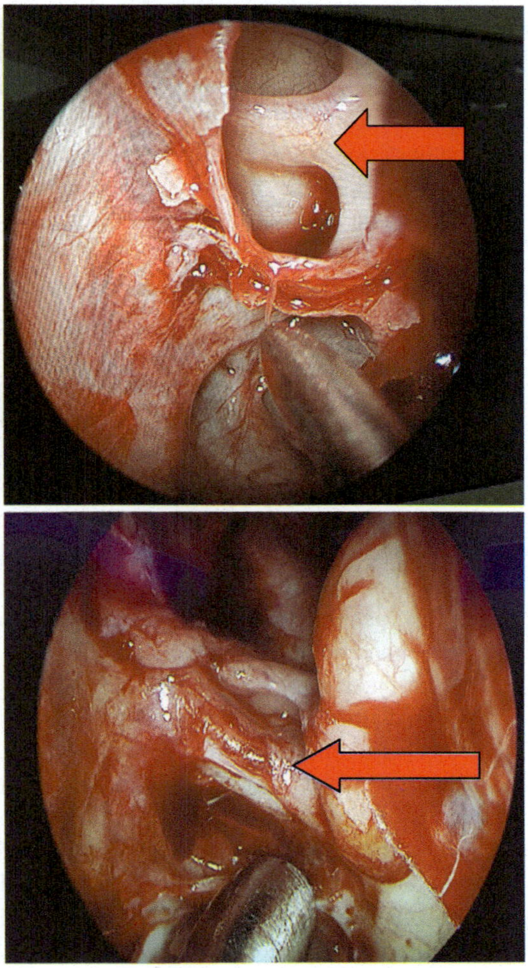

Figs. 31.4 and 31.5 Anterior ethmoidal artery at the skull base with anterior ethmoidal nerve with dehiscent lamina (RED ARROW)

31.6 Endoscopic Sphenopalatine Artery Ligation

31.6.1 Anatomy of Sphenopalatine Artery

Sphenopalatine artery is [17, 18] a terminal branch of the internal maxillary artery originating from the external carotid artery system. The SPA is the major blood vessel to the nasal cavity mucosa: supplying the superior, middle, and inferior turbinate; lateral nasal wall; and nasal

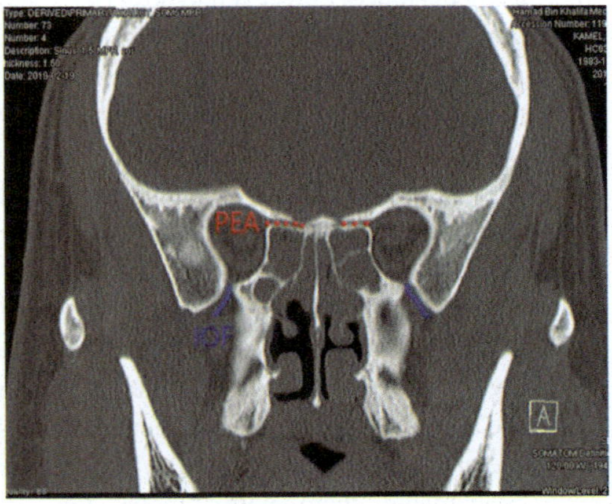

Fig. 31.6 Posterior ethmoidal artery (PEA red)

septum. The sphenopalatine artery travels within the pterygopalatine fossa and enters the nasal cavity through the sphenopalatine foramen within the superior meatus between the middle turbinate and the posterior end of the superior turbinate on the lateral nasal wall; the shape of the sphenopalatine foramen predicts the size of the sphenopalatine artery and branches. The SPA branches into two major vessels, the septal artery and posterior lateral nasal artery, before exiting the sphenopalatine foramen. The septal artery exits the sphenopalatine foramen, courses through the anterior inferior wall of the sphenoid sinus and distributes on the nasal septum. The posterior lateral nasal artery exits the sphenopalatine foramen, courses downward anteriorly to the posterior end of the middle turbinate along the lateral nasal wall, and runs inferiorly on the perpendicular plate of the palatine bone giving off branches to the inferior and middle turbinate.

Surgical management [19, 20] of epistaxis is typically only for those patients whose bleeding is refractory to more conservative therapies. Knowledge of the vascular anatomy and important landmarks is necessary to avoid intraoperative bleeding and to lower the risk of postoperative bleeding. The sphenopalatine artery can be exposed endoscopically by raising a posterolateral mucosal flap over the orbital process of the palatine bone. A maxillary antrostomy is done to visualise the posterior maxillary wall and palatine bone. A vertical incision is made inferior to the posterior portion of the middle turbinate, 1 cm anterior to its posterior tip. Raising the mucoperiosteal flap posteriorly and superiorly will expose the ethmoid crest [21]. The ethmoid crest represents a significant landmark for locating the position of the sphenopalatine artery and is consistently anteromedial to the sphenopalatine foramen. Resection of the ethmoid crest enhances exposure of the sphenopalatine artery and helps identify its branches to ensure appropriate vessel ligation. As the flap is raised and ethmoid crest resected, the fibroneurovascular bundle including the SPA and nasopalatine nerve will be reachable at the sphenopalatine foramen. After isolating the artery and its branches, the next step is either cauterising them with bipolar forceps, occluding with clips, or using a combination of both. Upon attaining bleeding control, the mucoperiosteal flap is put back in place and covered with surgicel (Figs. 31.7 and 31.8).

31.6.2 Embolization

Embolization for epistaxis was first performed by Sokoloff in 1974 [22]. Since then, embolization has become an accepted treatment for posterior epistaxis, where available. Common embolization targets include the IMA and facial artery. These

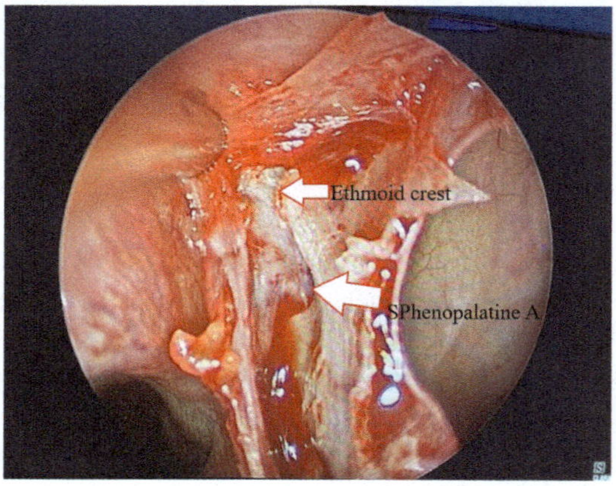

Fig. 31.7 Sphenopalatine artery and ethmoidal crest

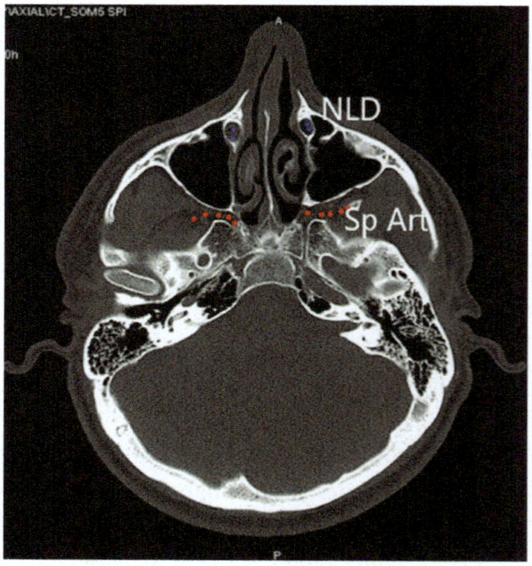

Fig. 31.8 Sphenopalatine artery exiting from the phenopalatine foramen (red) NLD: Nasolacrimal Duct

vessels can be embolised with various materials, including cyanoacrylate glue, polyvinyl alcohol sponges, metal coils, or gelatin foam. Bilateral IMA ligation is often used for cases in which the exact source is unidentifiable. Success rates have ranged from 79 to 96% in multiple studies. However, complication rates as high as 24% have been reported. Complications from embolization include rebleeding, stroke, blindness, facial numbness, skin sloughing, carotid artery dissection, and groin haematoma. Embolization is expensive. Miller and colleagues showed that embolization was twice as costly as modern surgical treatment for recurrent epistaxis. Another drawback for embolization is its inability to control bleeding from the ethmoidal arteries. Embolization needs expertised and trained intervention radiologists are not available at many centres. In this situation, if packing fails to control the bleeding, surgical treatment may become necessary [23].

Take Home Messages

- The estimated lifetime incidence of epistaxis is approximately 60%.
- All cases of epistaxis should be investigated and treated for underlying cause.
- Otolaryngologist should be well aware about the anatomy of major vessels in the nose.

References

1. Weiss NS. Relation of high blood pressure to headache, epistaxis, and selected other symptoms. The United States Health Examination Survey of Adults. N Engl J Med. 1972;287:631–3.
2. Massick D, Tobin EJ. Epistaxis. In: Cummings CW, Haughey BH, Thomas JR, et al., editors. Cummings otolaryngology: head and neck surgery. Philadelphia: Mosby; 2005. p. 942–61.
3. Tan LK, Calhoun KH. Epistaxis. Med Clin North Am. 1999;83:43–56.
4. Wormald PJ. Epistaxis. In: Bailey BJ, Calhoun KH, Derkay C, et al., editors. Head and neck surgery - otolaryngology. Philadelphia: Lippincott Williams & Wilkins; 2006. p. 505–14.
5. Orlandi RR, Lanza DC. Is nasal packing necessary following endoscopic sinus surgery? Laryngoscope. 2004;114(9):1541–4.
6. Floreani SR, Nair SB, Switajewski MC, et al. Endoscopic anterior ethmoidal artery ligation: a cadaver study. Laryngoscope. 2006;116:1263–7.
7. Douglas R, Wormald PJ. Pterygopalatine fossa infiltration through the greater palatine foramen: where to bend the needle. Laryngoscope. 2006;116(7):1255–7.
8. Hanif J, Tasca RA, Frosh A, et al. Silver nitrate: histological effects of cautery on epithelial surfaces with varying contact times. Clin Otolaryngol Allied Sci. 2003;28(4):368–70.
9. Brouz D, Charakidas A, Androulakis M, et al. Traumatic optic neuropathy after posterior ethmoidal artery ligation for epistaxis. Otolaryngol Head Neck Surg. 2002;126(3):323–5.
10. Thornton MA, Mahesh BN, Lang J. Posterior epistaxis: identification of common bleeding sites. Laryngoscope. 2005;115(4):588–90.
11. Pope LE, Hobbs CG. Epistaxis: an update on current management. Postgrad Med J. 2005;81:309–14.
12. Srinivasan V, Sherman IW, O'Sullivan G. Surgical management of intractable epistaxis: audit of results. J Laryngol Otol. 2000;114(9):697–700.
13. Klotz DA, Winkle MR, Richmon J, et al. Surgical management of posterior epistaxis: a changing paradigm. Laryngoscope. 2002;112:1577–82.
14. Mathiasen RA, Cruz R. Prospective, randomized, controlled clinical trial of a novel matrix hemostatic sealant in patients with acute anterior epistaxis. Laryngoscope. 2005;115(5):899–902.
15. Pletcher SD, Metson R. Endoscopic ligation of the anterior ethmoid artery. Laryngoscope. 2007;117(2):378–81.
16. Douglas SA, Gupta D. Endoscopic assisted external approach anterior ethmoidal artery ligation for the management of epistaxis. J Laryngol Otol. 2003;117(2):132–3.
17. Smith TP. Embolization in the external carotid artery. J Vasc Interv Radiol. 2006;17(12):1897–912.
18. Miller TR, Stevens ES, Orlandi RR. Economic analysis of the treatment of posterior epitaxis. Am J Rhinol. 2005;19:79–82.
19. Kumar S, Shetty A, Rockey J, et al. Contemporary surgical treatment of epistaxis. What is the evidence for sphenopalatine artery ligation? Clin Otolaryngol Allied Sci. 2003;28(4):360–3.
20. Budrovich R, Saetti R. Microscopic and endoscopic ligature of the sphenopalatine artery. Laryngoscope. 1992;102(12):1391–4.
21. Orlandi RR. Endoscopic sphenopalatine artery ligation. Op Tech Otolaryngol Head Neck Surg. 2001;12(2):98–100.
22. Morgan MK, Aldren CP. Oroantral fistula: a complication of transantral ligation of the internal maxillary artery for epistaxis. J Laryngol Otol. 1997;111(5):468–70.
23. Bolger WE, Borgie RC, Melder P. The role of the crista ethmoidalis in endoscopic sphenopalatine artery ligation. Am J Rhinol. 1999;13(2):81–6.

32 The Nasal Septum and Turbinates

Mansour Al Sulaiti, Emad Al Duhirat,
Hamad Al Saey, Shanmugam Ganesan,
and Abdulaziz Al Jufairi

32.1 Introduction

The sensation of normal nasal flow happens when the flow receptors in the nasal valve area are stimulated. The normal perception of flow requires a background level of resistance with the presence of a laminar air flow pattern.

Nasal resistance is the difference between air pressure at the nasal vestibule and air pressure in the nasopharynx, which is normally between 8 and 20 mm H_2O. This is why conditions with low resistance like "empty nose syndrome" are associated with the sensation of nasal obstruction, because a minimum level of resistance (normally greater than 6–8 mm H_2O) is needed for the normal perception of flow.

The internal nasal valve plays a major role in the resistance of the airways as it is the narrowest portion of the nasal cavity and, therefore, any compromise of the components of the valve creates symptoms of nasal obstruction. The angle is bound medially by the septum and laterally by the inferior edge of the upper lateral cartilages and the anterior aspect of the inferior turbinate.

Another factor affecting the physiological air flow is the nasal cycle, during which each side of the nasal airway undergoes an alternating cycle of congestion and decongestion. Normally, this cycle is not noticeable, but when accompanied by disorders affecting the nasal airway, cyclical alternating nasal obstruction may become apparent. The regulation of the nasal cycle is by the parasympathetic and sympathetic nervous systems on vascularity of the erectile tissue of the inferior turbinate and septum, causing a variation in the respective nasal resistance of each nasal airway. This explains the positive influence of exercise, during which increased sympathetic nervous system tone enables vasoconstriction via stimulation of nasal mucosal vascular α-adrenergic receptors. Adrenaline analogue drugs such as xylometazoline work in the same way. This demonstrates why intranasal vasoconstrictors may relieve nasal obstruction by causing mucosal decongestion. The turbinates in the dependent nasal fossa become congested when the patient is in the lateral decubitus position. The nasal cycle is an alternating one, with the total resistance in the nose remaining constant. In patients with a fixed septal deviation and intermittent nasal obstruction, the interplay of the

M. Al Sulaiti · H. Al Saey · S. Ganesan
Otolaryngology-Head and Neck Surgery Division, Department of Surgery, Hamad Medical Corporation, Doha, Qatar

Department of Otolaryngology-Head and Neck Surgery Division, Weill Cornell Medicine-Qatar, Doha, Qatar
e-mail: Malsulaiti1@hamad.qa; Halsaey@hamad.qa; sganesan@hamad.qa

E. Al Duhirat (✉) · A. Al Jufairi
Otolaryngology-Head and Neck Surgery Division, Department of Surgery, Hamad Medical Corporation, Doha, Qatar
e-mail: EAlDuhirat@hamad.qa; aaljufairi@hamad.qa

A. Al-Qahtani et al. (eds.), *Textbook of Clinical Otolaryngology*,
https://doi.org/10.1007/978-3-030-54088-3_32

nasal cycle becomes evident; the sensation of obstruction frequently mirrors the congestion phase [1–6].

32.2 The Nasal Septum

The nasal septum functions include separation of the nasal two nasal cavities, support of the nasal framework including the nasal tip and formation of part of the nasal valves.

The nasal septum consists [7] of (Fig. 32.1):

- Bony part:
  - The perpendicular plate of the ethmoid bone forms the upper one third of the nasal septum. Attached to the cribriform plate superiorly and posteriorly attached to the sphenoid rostrum, posteroinferiorly with the vomer, and anteroinferiorly with the septal cartilage.
  - The Vomer: forms the posterior and inferior nasal septum and articulates with the sphenoid rostrum, articulates with the nasal crest (the maxillary and palatine bones) and anteriorly articulates with the septal cartilage, and the posterior edge forms the posterior free edge of the septum.
  - Maxillary crest and palatine bone.
- Cartilaginous part: the septal or quadrilateral cartilage attached firmly to the nasal bones, perpendicular plate of the ethmoid and vomer. Inferiorly seated within the nasal crest of the maxilla.
- Membranous portion: the connective tissue between the caudal portion of the septal cartilage and columella.

32.3 Embryology

The nasal septum grows inferiorly from the nasofrontal prominence to the level of the palatal shelves following fusion to form the secondary palate. Anteriorly, the septum is contiguous with the primary palate originating from the nasomedial processes. At the end of its development, the nasal septum divides the nasal cavity into two separate chambers [8].

32.4 Blood Supply

- The external carotid artery:
  - The sphenopalatine: supplies the posteroinferior septum by a branch called the posterior septal artery (the base of the nasoseptal flap).

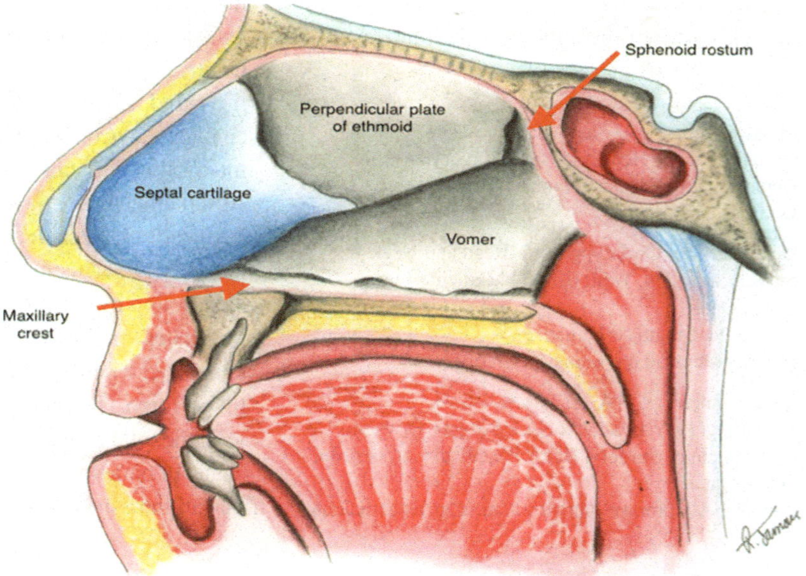

Fig. 32.1 Anatomy of the nasal septum

- The greater palatine arteries supply the anteroinferior portion of the septum.
- The superior labial artery (facial artery): supplies the caudal septum and columella.
- The internal carotid artery:
  - The anterior ethmoid artery (branch of the ophthalmic artery)
  - The posterior ethmoid artery (branch of the ophthalmic artery)

Kiesselbach's plexus (Little's area): The anterior ethmoid artery, posterior septal artery, greater palatine artery, and septal branch of superior labial artery.

32.5 Venous Drainage

The venous system drainage:

- The sphenopalatine vessels into the pterygoid plexus posteriorly and into the facial veins anteriorly.
- The ethmoidal veins communicate with the superior ophthalmic system and there are some direct intracranial connections through the foramen caecum into the superior sagittal sinus.

32.6 Nasal Valves (Table 32.1)

32.7 Nasal Septal Deviation

A physiological septum deviation is defined as a deviation without subjective or objective reduction of the nasal breathing (Fig. 32.2). A pathological septum deviation has to be defined as a septum deviation with subjective reduction of nasal breathing [2] (Table 32.2).

Table 32.1 Comparison between the internal nasal valve and the external nasal valve [1, 9]

Internal nasal valve	External nasal valve
Medial wall: septum Lateral wall: anterior part of the inferior turbinate Nasal floor: floor of the bony aperture	Medial wall: septum Lateral wall: lateral crus of the lower lateral cartilage (LLC) Nasal floor: Floor of the nasal vestibule

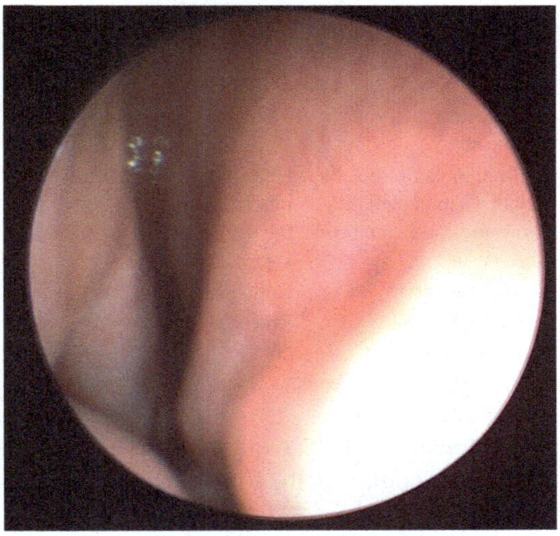

Fig. 32.2 Image of a deviated nasal septum to the right side

Table 32.2 Mladina classification of the nasal septal deviation [10]

Mladina classification for nasal septal deviation	
Type 1	Unilateral vertical ridge in the valve region
Type 2	Similar to type 1 but more severe obstruction and disturbance of nasal valve
Type 3	Unilateral vertical ridge at the level of the head of the middle turbinate
Type 4	Combination of type 3 with either type 1 or 2
Type 5	Prominent maxillary crest contralateral to the deviation with a septal crest on the deviated side
Type 6	Combination of previously described septal deformity types

32.8 Nasal Septal Surgeries (Table 32.3)

32.9 Indications for Septoplasty

The nasal septum very rarely lies absolutely straight within the skull but usually shows a more or less pronounced deviation that can be found in up to 90% of cases investigated [10, 12].

Table 32.3 Comparison between SMR and septoplasty [9, 11]

Submucosal resection	Septoplasty
The L-strut is *not* addressed	The L-strut is addressed
Killian incision: placed about 1 cm cephalad from the caudal end of the septum	Hemitransfixation incision: placed at the caudal edge of the septum and exposes the L-strut.
Radical surgery	Conservative surgery
Higher probability of complications	Lower probability of complications

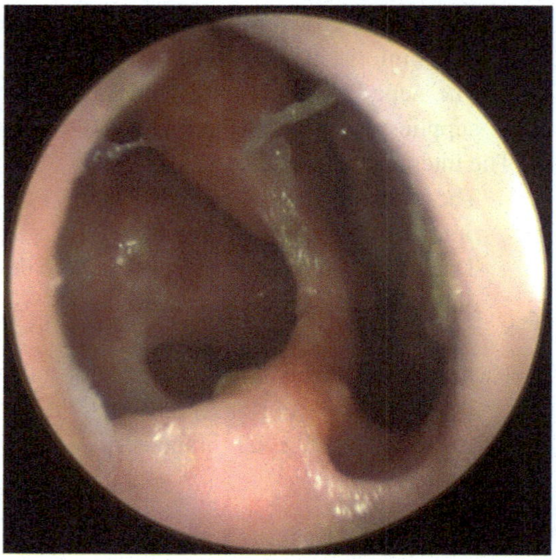

Fig. 32.3 Nasal septal perforation

Septoplasty may be required to correct a deviated nasal septum for the following:

- Irreversible symptomatic nasal obstruction
- Improving access for endoscopic sinus or skull base surgery
- Septal spurs causing epistaxis

32.10 Complications of Septoplasty

- Septal hematoma.
- Epistaxis from raw mucosal edges.
- Septal perforation: Bilateral opposing mucosal tears, excessive packing and septal hematoma.
- Nasal obstruction can be caused due to inadequate correction of septal deformity and synechiae from opposing, traumatized septal and inferior turbinate mucosal surfaces.
- Nasal deformity occurs from excessive removal of cartilage and preserving too little dorsal or caudal cartilage struts.

32.11 Nasal Septal Perforation

The most common causes of nasal septal perforations are trauma, iatrogenic, e.g., septoplasty, and pharmacologic, e.g., intranasal corticosteroids and cocaine abuse. Other etiologies such as vasculitis, malignancy, and infection should be considered when investigating a patient when a cause is not apparent (Fig. 32.3).

The majority of septal perforations are asymptomatic. Some of the most troublesome signs and symptoms include a whistling sound, crusting, and epistaxis; these are consequences of disruption of laminar airflow and its destructive effect on the nasal tissues.

The usual mechanism for developing a septal perforation is disruption of blood flow and ischemia of the septum. Despite its rich blood supply; perforations most commonly involve the anterior septum.

Treatment is mainly conservative by moisturizing the nasal mucosa with saline irrigation and topical ointments. Surgery is necessary only for patients who fail conservative treatment and are symptomatic. When septal perforations are related to an active disease, e.g., vasculitis, malignancy, or infection, treatment should be directed at the underlying disease process. Only once the etiology is controlled the treatment can be tailored to the extent of the symptomatology.

32.12 Indications for Surgery Include

Symptomatic perforations

- Crusting
- Whistling
- Nasal congestion
- Recurrent epistaxis

Perforations refractory to conservative management:

- Nasal moisturizers
- Septal button

32.13 Contraindications to Surgery Include

An active underlying cause such as:

- Vasculitis
- Malignancy
- Infection
- Diameter/location precluding harvesting of adequate tissue for reconstruction (approximately >3 cm)

32.14 The Turbinates

The inferior turbinate is an embryologically independent structure.

The inferior turbinate consists of a supporting cancellous conchal bone which is attached along the inferolateral aspect of the nasal cavity and extending from the interior nasal valve to just anterior to the Eustachian tube. The turbinate is covered by a ciliated pseudostratified respiratory mucosa that is supported by a lamina propria and specialized erectile mucosa with vascular channels and venous sinusoids which serve to warm and humidify air, modify nasal airflow resistance and maintain linear rather than turbulent air flow within the nose.

The blood supply to the inferior turbinates is from the lateral branch of the sphenopalatine artery that enters the posterior aspect of the turbinate. Sensation is supplied by the trigeminal nerve; sympathetic nerves travel along the feeding arterial blood vessels; the parasympathetic supply also travels along the vascular supply but travels along the vidian nerve before entering the nose through the sphenopalatine foramen.

The normal inferior turbinate is a dynamic structure that varies in size according to the degree of congestion. Congestion is determined by the control of blood flowing through the specialized erectile tissue. This change is governed by the autonomic neural supply:

- The sympathetic nerves induce reduction of blood flow and a decrease in volume.
- The parasympathetic supply congests the erectile tissue of the turbinate.

The degree of congestion varies in a cyclical manner in a healthy nose every few hours and is coordinated so that when one side is congested the other is constricted. This phenomenon is known as the nasal cycle.

The septum deviation itself gives rise for compensatory changes in the nose; an atrophy of the nasal turbinate on the convex side while the nasal turbinates on the concave side enlarge. The turbinates regulate the nasal air stream in a way that further functions like warming up and moistening are fulfilled even in the deviated nose.

Three different variations of inferior turbinates are often encountered; these include [13]:

- Bony: Bony turbinate hypertrophy is usually caused by a prominent (broad) inferolateral turn of the turbinate; it is very large but normally shaped obstructing inferior turbinates are also described.
- Soft tissue: very common and represents the majority of cases of inferior turbinate hypertrophy. The common underlying pathophysiology in soft tissue hypertrophy is chronic rhinitis and other conditions that cause chronic mucosal inflammation.
- Mixed hypertrophy: involves anatomic bony hypertrophy in the setting of chronic rhinitis.

Pneumatization of the inferior turbinate may cause inferior turbinate hypertrophy, which leads to nasal obstruction.

32.15 Management of the Hypertrophy of the Inferior Turbinates (Table 32.4)

Table 32.4 Methods of treatment of the inferior turbinates hypertrophy [14–16]

Method	
Turbinates lateralization	Not sufficient as a stand-alone procedure for the management of significant turbinate hypertrophy
Turbinates soft tissue reduction	The creation of an area of submucosal thermal injury, which ultimately heals by fibrosis and scar contracture • Monopolar • Bipolar • Radiofrequency: – The temperature generated is significantly lower than electrocautery – The distribution of the heat is limited, allowing for a more focused reduction of the deeper components of the inferior turbinate tissue
Soft tissue resection of the turbinates	Can be done using specialized microdebrider blades • Allows for precise and targeted removal which aims to reduce the bulk of the submucosal erectile tissue of the turbinate without injury to the epithelium • Reduction focused on the anterior half of the turbinates (nasal valve) which contributes mostly to the air flow resistance • Resection of the posterior part associated with higher risks of bleeding due to the arterial supply by the sphenopalatine artery
Bone resection of the turbinates	• Indicated when the bony component is the major contributor to the patient's turbinate hypertrophy • Submucosal resection of the bone
Turbinates resection	• Ranges from limited resection of the anterior aspect of the turbinate to total resections • Extensive subtotal or total resections have been suspected to predispose one to a paradoxic nasal obstruction or atrophic rhinitis

Take Home Messages

- The nasal cavity is highly vascular, and this serves multiple functions.
- A nasal septal deviation is considered pathological once it has subjective reduction of the nasal breathing, so not all deviations need to be assessed surgically.
- Multiple approaches can be used to address nasal blockage and it is different from one patient to another.
- Nasal septal and turbinates surgeries are simple procedures but can carry devastating complications.

References

1. Bridger GP. Physiology of the nasal valve. Arch Otolaryngol. 1970;92:543–53.
2. Kern EB, Arbour P. The phenomenon of paradoxical nasal obstruction. Arch Otolaryngol. 1976;102:669.
3. Proetz A. Applied physiology of the nose. St Louis: Annals Publishing; 1941.
4. Sheen JH. Spreader graft: a method of reconstructing the roof of the middle nasal vault following rhinoplasty. Plast Reconstr Surg. 1984; 73:230.
5. Glam T, Ahmad SK. Physiology of the nose and paranasal sinuses. In: Scott Brown Otorhinolaryngology head and neck surgery. 8th ed. Boca Raton: CRC Press; 2018. p. 1025–34.
6. Yigit O, Akgul G, Alkan S, Uslu B, Dadas B. Changes occurring in the nasal mucociliary transport in patients with one-sided septum deviation. Rhinology. 2005;43:257–60.
7. Maran AGD, Lund VJ. Nasal anatomy. In: Maran AGD, Lund VJ, editors. Clinical rhinology. Stuttgart: Thieme; 1990. p. 5.
8. Moore KL, Persaud TVN. The developing human. Clinically oriented embryology. 6th ed. Philadelphia: WB Saunders; 1998.
9. Dalgorf DM, Harvey RJ. Anatomy of the nose and paranasal sinuses. In: Scott Brown otorhinolaryngology head and neck surgery. 8th ed. Boca Raton: CRC Press; 2018. p. 1025–34.
10. Mladina R, Čujić E, Šubarić M, et al. Nasal septal deformities in ear, nose, and throat patients: an international study. Am J Otol. 2008;29(2):75–82.

11. Iqbal K, Khan MI, Amanullah A. Submucous resection versus septoplasty: complications and functional outcome in adult patients. Gomal J Med Sci. 2011;9(1):23–7.
12. Gray LP. Deviated nasal septum. Incidence and etiology. Ann Otol Rhinol Laryngol. 1978;87(3 Pt 3 Suppl 50):3–20.
13. Neskey D, Eloy J, Casiano R. Nasal, septal, and turbinate anatomy and embryology. Otolaryngol Clin N Am. 2009;42:193–205, vii. https://doi.org/10.1016/j.otc.2009.01.008.1.
14. Cavaliere M, Mottola G, Iemma M. Comparison of the effectiveness and safety of radiofrequency turbinoplasty and traditional surgical technique in treatment of inferior turbinate hypertrophy. Otolaryngol Head Neck Surg. 2005;133(6):972–8.
15. Swift AC, Leong SC. Management of enlarged turbinates. In: Scott Brown otorhinolaryngology head and neck surgery. 8th ed. Boca Raton: CRC Press; 2018. p. 1025–34.
16. Hol M, Huizing E. Treatment of inferior turbinate pathology: a review and critical evaluation of the different techniques. Rhinology. 2001;38:157–66.

33 Pitfalls and Pearls in Endoscopic Sinus Surgery

Omar M. Bargas and Ahmad AbuAlsoud

33.1 Introduction

The history of endoscopic sinus surgery return to early 1901 when HIRSCHMANN started using a modified cystoscope after that Maltz bring the name of the sinocopy to the world. The surgery started to improve and clarify year by year with the appearance of many interested rhinologist in the USA and Europe like Messerklinger, Stammberger, and Kennedy. Most of them assume that the endoscopic sinus surgery should be directed toward dealing with the diseased mucosa and preserving the normal tissue as much as possible. With further advancement of technology and continuous study of the anatomy and physiology of sinonasal region, the surgery started to be tailored according to the site of disease. Many nomenclatures then appear like MIST (minimal invasive sinus technique) and FESS (functional endoscopic sinus surgery), all of which directed toward mucosal preservation and avoidance of any unwanted mucosal stripping. Anteroposterior and posteroanterior dissection are the most followed technique in endoscopic sinus surgery. The presence of new instruments, powered devices like microdebrider, various angled telescopes, and navigation system make the surgery more interesting and challenging, with the proximity of vital structures like skull base, optic nerve, and carotid artery. It is now necessary for the surgeon to be familiar with anatomical variations and instrumentation to avoid injury to these vital structures.

33.2 Position of the Patient and the Surgeon

Each step in the patient and surgeon positioning is important and designed to make the surgery smooth. First of all, the surgeon has to sit or stand at the right side of the patient. The surgeon can use a mayo stand to rest his arm. The patient should be laying on a supine position while the operating table is tilted 30° anti-Trendelenburg. Patient's head has to be in a neutral position. The monitor, patient's head, and the surgeon have to be in a straight line. It is not a routine to sterilize the nose before the ESS; however, sterile drape is recommended with leaving the eyes exposed (it's advisable to use topical eye ointment to avoid dryness during surgery). The surgeon can turn the head of the patient to either direction for better angle and field. The scrub nurse should position their instrument table parallel to the head.

O. M. Bargas
Anbar College of Medicine, Ramadi, Iraq

A. AbuAlsoud (✉)
Union Memorial Hospital, Baltimore, MD, USA

A. Al-Qahtani et al. (eds.), *Textbook of Clinical Otolaryngology*,
https://doi.org/10.1007/978-3-030-54088-3_33

33.3 Nasal Preparation and Vasoconstriction

There are different materials and medications used in nasal preparation. The choice depends on the surgeon preference, patient's allergic history or comorbidities, and medications availability. For the nasal preparation, different packing can be used, e.g., neurosurgical patties or cotton ball. The communication with the anesthetist about the medications is the most important thing to do prior to the packing. Nasal preparation can be started by using a counted number of packs soaked with 1% oxymetazoline or cocaine in the nose for few minutes. If no contraindications, the lidocaine-adrenaline combination is drug of choice for infiltration; however, the concentration will be adjusted according to the patient. The area above the anterior end of the middle turbinate and the back end of the middle turbinate in the region of the sphenopalatine artery are injected. Another injections can be done in the anterior wall of the bulla, greater palatine foramen, and even the polyps itself.

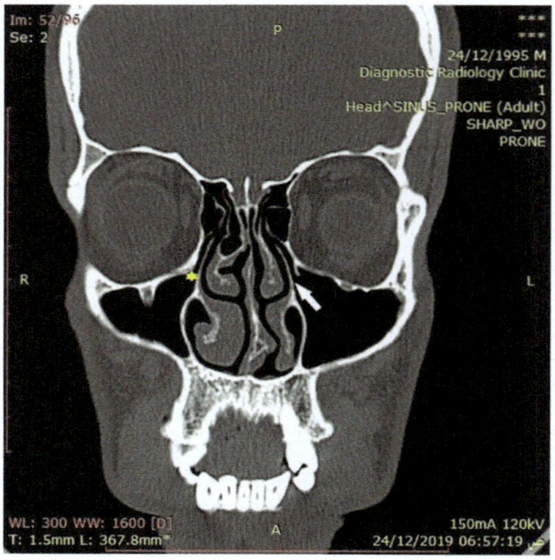

Fig. 33.1 CT scan of paranasal sinuses demonstrate the uncinate process (white arrow) and the Maxillary ostium (yellow asterisk)

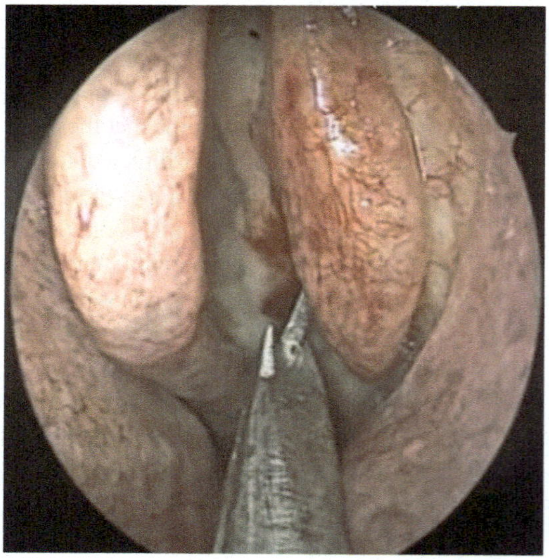

Fig. 33.2 Endoscopic picture explaining how the backbitter engage the posterior border of the uncinate process

33.4 Surgical Steps

33.4.1 Uncinectomy

The entrance to the endoscopic sinus surgery usually occurs from the uncinate door. Uncinectomy (aka infundibulotomy) usually began with identification of the posterior free border of this sickle shaped structure by an angled ball probe or curette at the same time the probe is advanced superiorly to identify the variable attachment of the superior end of the uncinate. The whole uncinate (Fig. 33.1 white arrow) should be removed otherwise there is risk of ESS failure and orbital injury. The techniques of uncinate removal are variable, all of them are aimed to complete excision of the uncinate and identification of the natural maxillary ostium. Swing door technique is our favorable technique [1] which began with making a cut in the middle 1/3 of the anterior attachment of the uncinate by the sickle knife or by size 11 blade, then it is advanced superiorly and inferiorly to free the attachment of uncinate, by the sickle itself or by freer's dissector; the uncinate slightly moved medially away from the lamina papyracea; here a pediatric (or adult size) backbiter introduced in the middle meatus and opened to engage the free posterior border of the uncinate (Fig. 33.2) and remove part of the uncinate to free it from the horizontal part and again make another cut near its superior attachment; here the orbit is guarded by the frontal process of maxilla [2] which is a hard bone, then remove the remaining part of the uncinate between the two cuts by straight Blakesley forceps. The bone of the horizontal part of the uncinate which passes inferiorly to natural maxillary ostium is dissected free from the mucosa. Now the natural maxillary ostium (Fig. 33.1 yellow asterisk) can be easily identified by angled degree or even by zero degree endoscope. Another technique to remove the uncinate is by removing a small portion of the uncinate by through-cutting backbiter to create a raw edge, then completely removing the bone either by microdebrider or upward and downward angled through-cutting Blakesley forceps. Using microdebrider allows trimming these edges without exposing the bone and thus allows healing by primary intention without scaring.

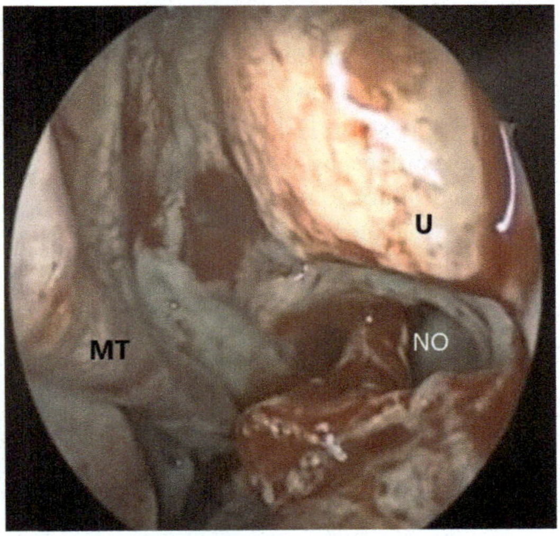

Fig. 33.3 Endoscopic picture after performing infundibulotomy showing the natural maxillary ostium (NO), uncinate (U) and middle turbinate (MT)

Pitfalls in Uncinectomy

- Take care of the variable attachment of superior end of the uncinate.
- Be aware of the atelectatic uncinate as in case of silent maxillary syndrome where the risk of orbital injury is high, so try retrograde excision rather than anterior one.
- Palpate the lateral nasal wall to identify the uncinate which considered a slightly mobile bone unlike the frontal process of maxilla to avoid injury to nasolacrimal duct.

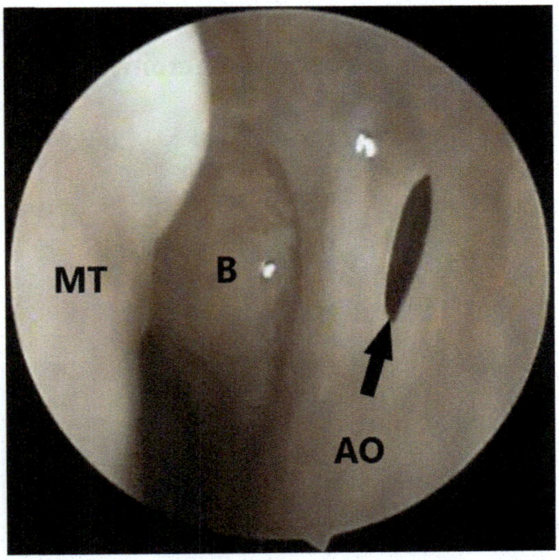

Fig. 33.4 Endoscopic picture of the nose showing the accessory ostium (AO), bulla ethmoidalis (B) and the middle turbinate (MT)

33.4.2 Middle Meatal Antrostomy

After completing dissection of the horizontal part of the uncinate process, the natural maxillary ostium can now be easily visualized in the opened infundibulum (Fig. 33.3); it is an oval shaped mucosal opening with oblique orientation; its superior margin marks the junction between orbital floor and the lamina papyracea. In case of minimal sinus disease, the natural ostium can be only stretched with ball probe of sucker without removing the mucosa while if there is extensive mucosal disease or in presence of accessory maxillary ostium (Fig. 33.4); here it should be enlarged and connected to the accessory ostium to avoid the chance of circular mucus flow. The optimal size of the enlarged ostium is variable and may be tailored to the severity of the disease. The enlargement can be started with using backbiter forceps which engage the anterior lip of the ostium and start cutting till fell a hard bone which represents the nasolacrimal duct system, then the ostium can be enlarged posteriorly but take care of the sphenopalatine artery which may be injured far posteriorly [3]. Inferior enlargement can also be done by down-biting forceps; here also avoid injury to superior surface of inferior turbinate which may lead to more bleeding. Now with angled endoscope the interior of the maxillary sinus can be visualized entirely.

Pitfalls on MMA

- Don't widen the maxillary ostium far posteriorly or far anteriorly.
- Keep the orbital floor your superior limit.
- Try to distinguish between accessory and the natural maxillary ostium.

33.4.3 Anterior Ethmoidectomy

Ethmoidal bulla (Figs. 33.5 and 33.6) is the largest and the most constant anterior ethmoidal cell. Its size and degree of pneumatization is variable so as its superior extension, its roof may be continuous with the skull base and may house the

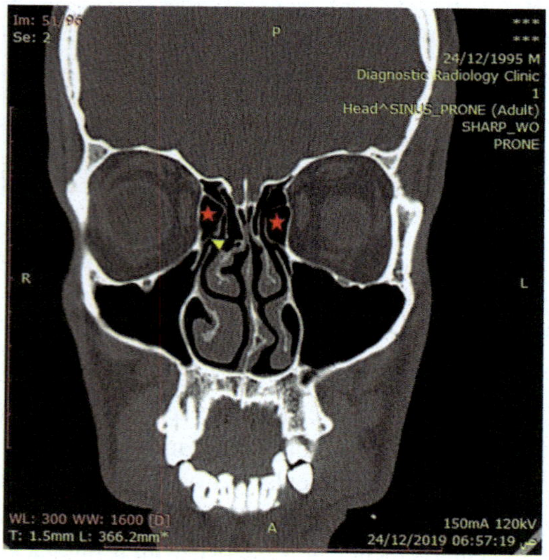

Fig. 33.5 Bulla red asterisk. Yellow arrow head: hiatus semilunaris inferior

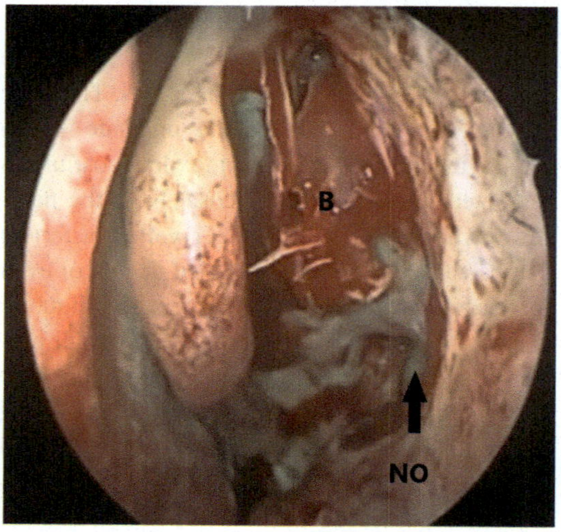

Fig. 33.6 Endoscopic picture of the nose after opening of the bulla (B) and the natural maxillary ostium (NO)

anterior ethmoidal artery or it may leave as a space above it known as suprabullar recess and here the anterior ethmoidal artery may run within the skull base or in isolated mesentery hanging downward. Rarely the anterior ethmoidal artery runs on the anterior surface of the bulla. Ethmoidal bulla located posterior to uncinate process and separated from it by hiatus semilunaris inferior (Fig. 33.5). Its natural ostium opens postero-medially [4] and it can be identified after excision of the anterior wall. Entrance to the bulla starts with puncturing it infero-medially to be away from the roof and the lateral wall which is represented by the lamina papyracea by using angled ball probe, angled curette, or even a suction tube. Then start removal of the remaining walls by either angled through-cutting Blakesley or shaver and try to stay away from the lamina papyracea which marks the lateral limit of dissection. It is recommended to compress the eyeball gently and dissect the bulla to highlight the lamina papyracea and to be sure you are away from the eye. At the same time you may leave a thin rim on the antero-lateral junction which may be used as landmark for dissection if you lost during dissection as it represents second ethmoturbinals after the first one (uncinate process). After completing the excision of the uncinate and the bulla, now the natural maxillary ostium, the basal lamella, and the frontal recess will be demonstrated clearly.

Pitfalls on Anterior Ethmoidectomy

- Puncture the bulla infero-medially.
- Read the CT scan well before surgery to know the expected location of AEA.
- Take care of the haller cell.

33.4.4 Posterior Ethmoidectomy

The transition between anterior (frontal, maxillary, and anterior ethmoidal) sinuses to the posterior (posterior ethmoid and sphenoid) sinuses considered the cornerstone of endoscopic sinus surgery. The basal lamella or the ground lamella can be regarded as the second oblique part of the middle turbinate and represent the bridge between the anterior and posterior ethmoidal cells (Figs. 33.7 and 33.8). After dissecting the bulla, the basal lamella will be the next block to be dissected. The entrance to the posterior ethmoidal cells start with opening the basal lamella infero-medially just above the junction between the vertical and horizontal part of the lamella to achieve that the endoscope is passed under the middle turbinate till reaching its end, then it is brought anteriorly under the horizontal part till it turns vertically and just above this point and enters the sinus by angled curette or suction tube, then complete dissecting the posterior ethmoidal cells by using through-cutting Blakesley, mushroom forceps, or by microdebrider. Here also the

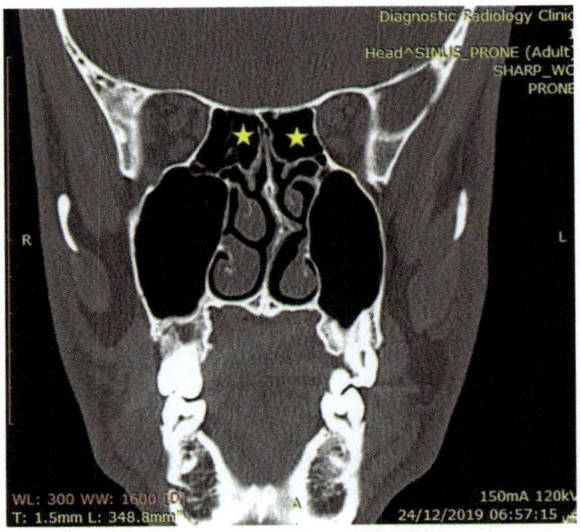

Fig. 33.7 The posterior ethmoidal cells (yellow asterisk)

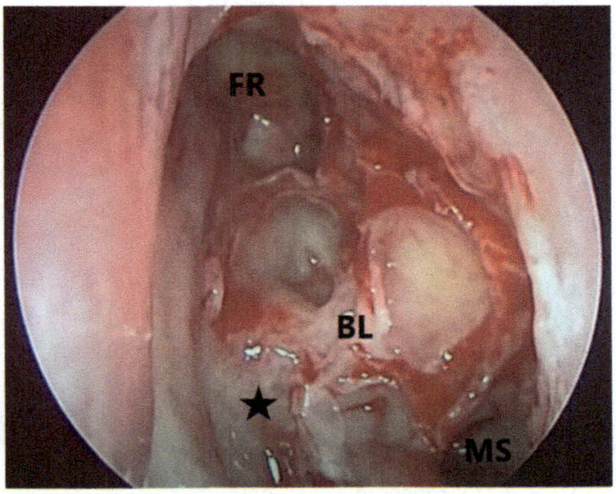

Fig. 33.8 Endoscopic Picture after completing anterior ethmoidectomy showing the basal lamina (BL), maxillary sinus (MS), Frontal recess (FR) and the asterisk refer to the site of penetration the posterior ethmoid aircells

lateral limit is represented by the lamina papyracea. Keeping dissection below the level of antral roof is a safe way to avoid the slopping skull base [5].

Pitfalls on Posterior Ethmoidectomy

- The posterior ethmoidal air cells are larger than the anterior ones.
- Look for onodi cells on CT to avoid injury of optic nerve and carotid artery.
- The PEA is larger than AEA and locate on the skull base just anterior to the sphenoid face.
- Entrance to posterior ethmoid via this way minimizes the risk of skull base injury, which may result if entrance occurs far above the point of junction between the horizontal and vertical part of ground lamella.

33.4.5 Sphenoidotomy

Sphenoid sinus (Figs. 33.9 and 33.10) represents the posterior room of the endoscopic sinus surgery; behind it the cranial cavity is located and the sphenoid ostium is located medial to superior turbinate in 83% of the patients [6]. Approach to sphenoid sinus is a step-up in endoscopic sinus surgery requiring good knowledge and excellent

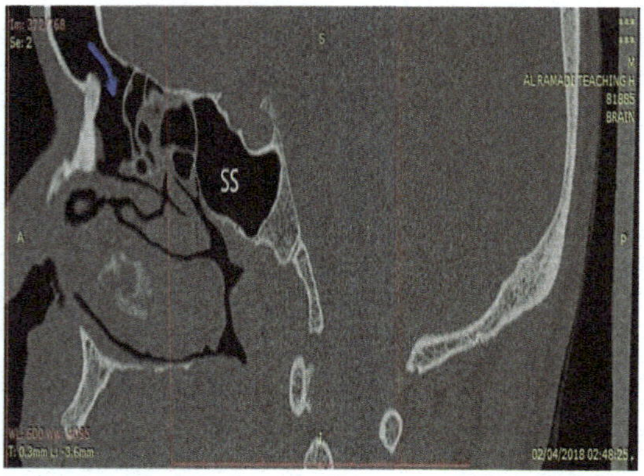

Fig. 33.9 *SS* sphenoid sinus, blue arrow represents the frontal recess

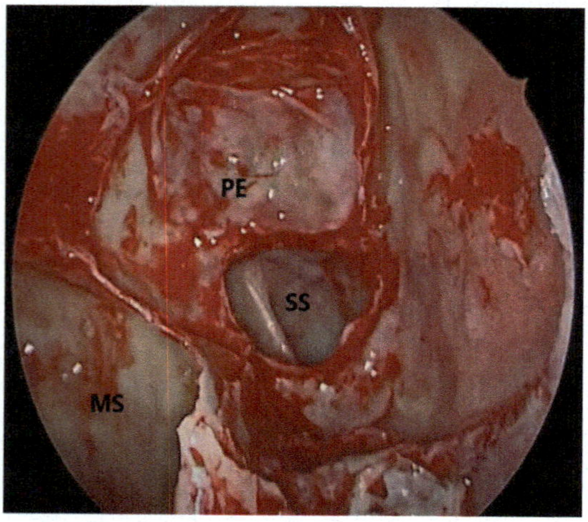

Fig. 33.10 Endoscopic picture after completing posterior ethmoidectomy showing the maxillary sinus posterior ethmoidal cell (PE), sphenoid sinus (SS) and the maxillary sinus (MS)

orientation of the normal anatomy and anatomical variation to avoid damage to nearby vital structures like optic nerve and carotid artery. Entry to sphenoid sinus can be done endoscopically by one of the following two techniques:

- *Transethmoidal*: After completing the dissection of the posterior ethmoidal cells, the ground lamella of the superior turbinate perforated infero-medially to avoid skull base superiorly and lamina papyracea laterally. Then this entry is widened medially to engage the natural ostium, superiorly and inferiorly.
- *Transnasal*: Sometimes approaching the sphenoid sinus can be done via nasal cavity rather than through ethmoidal sinuses and this is mostly chosen when the disease is isolated to sphenoid sinus like mycetoma, mucocele or even isolated sphenoiditis. To do this, the endoscope is passed medial to middle turbinate and this may require reduction in middle turbinate, then identify the sphenoethmoidal recess between the superior turbinate tail and the nasal septum; here the natural ostium can be visualized by careful palpation of the anterior sphenoidal wall by the suction tip or blunt instrument. The natural ostium looks like a slit, then start widening it in four directions. Another method for transnasal approaching of the sphenoid sinus is by locating the choana which considered a fixed and important landmark to reach the sphenoid sinus; here advance the endoscope toward the choana, then move it slightly upward on the anterior sphenoidal wall for 1–1.5 cm and start palpating with blunt instrument to reveal the natural ostium if failed to do so, then artificial opening can be done in this area then start widening. Widening of the sphenoidotomy can be done by mushroom forceps or the through-cutting forceps and try to avoid microdebrider in this area.

Pitfalls in Sphenoidotomy

- Sphenoid sinus opening considered advanced step in sinoscopic surgery.
- The sphenoid sinus can house multiple complete and incomplete septa which may be attached to carotid artery so take care in resecting it.
- Don't widen the ostium more inferiorly to avoid injury to a branch of sphenopalatine artery which may result in troublesome bleeding also don't go more laterally to avoid optic and carotid artery injury.
- Don't remove the mucosal lining of the sphenoid sinus; try just wash, suction, and leave it clean.
- Don't be deceived by onodi cell which may house the optic nerve.

33.4.6 Frontal Sinus (Figs. 33.11 and 33.12)

The frontal recess dissection is always a challenge to the surgeon [7–9] and it is considered as an advanced step in sinus surgery. In order to achieve the best outcome and avoid injury to the vital structures in the region "orbit and skull base" the surgeon has to be familiar with the frontal recess anatomical variation. Recurrence of diseases in the frontal sinus maybe due to either iatrogenic injury of the delicate frontal sinus pathway or incomplete excentration of the disease itself. The frontal recess is an hourglass shape pathway bounded anteriorly by posterior wall of agger nasi, posteriorly by bulla ethmoidalis, medially by middle turbinate, and laterally by lamina papyracea. Before starting the dissection of frontal recess, certain point should be accomplished which is to keep a well-mucosalized frontal recess to avoid postoperative scarring and neoosteogenesis. Angled instruments (like Hosemann, giraffe, Bachert, and mushroom forceps) and endoscopes are essential to success the surgery.

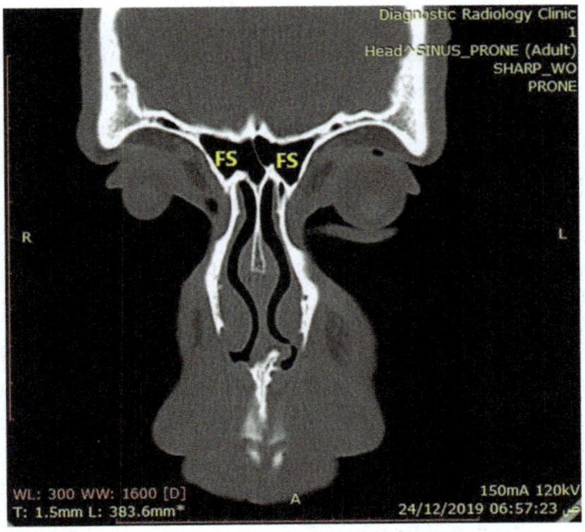

Fig. 33.11 CT scan of paranasal sinuses showing the frontal sinus (FS)

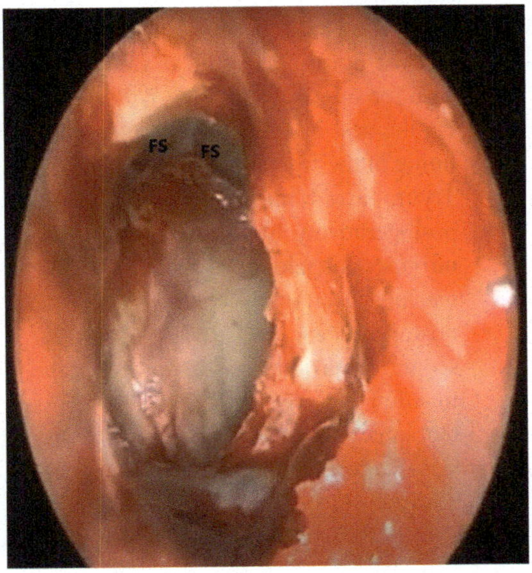

Fig. 33.12 Endoscopic picture after dissecting the frontal recess and the appearance of frontal sinus (FS)

Frontal sinus surgery can be classified according to Wolfgang Draf's into:

- *draf 1:* It comprises of anterior ethmoidectomy without touching the natural ostium.
- *draf 2a:* It is also called uncapping the egg. It comprises of removal of all ethmoidal cells that encroach the frontal recess like agger nasal and the other fronto-ethmoidal cells between the lamina papyracea laterally and middle turbinate medially.
- *draf 2b:* It comprises of removal of the frontal sinus floor between the lamina papyracea and nasal septum.
- *draf 3:* It comprises of drainage of both side through removal of the floor of frontal sinus from orbit to orbit with removal of part of the upper nasal septum (modified Lothrop procedure).

Choosing between these depends on the degree of disease extension. Approaching frontal recess can be done either after completing uncinectomy, MMA, (anterior and posterior) ethmoidectomy and sphenoidotomy or from the first remove the uncinate and identify the recess, then complete the remaining dissection. In the first approach, the aim is to identify the skull base at the level of sphenoid sinus, then follow it in post-ant direction till finding the anterior ethmoidal artery; this is done by using angled telescope (70° scope is highly useful in this step). An important landmark to locate the artery is the area of attachment of middle turbinate lamina to the skull base once the anterior ethmoidal artery identified the frontal recess is immediately anterior to it, then an angled probe (Bolger–Kuhn probe) is passed to the posterior frontal recess and start fracturing the posterior wall of the agger nasi cell and the other frontal recess cells in antero-inferior direction. Removal of the bony fragment and the mucosal pieces is better done by using through-cutting forceps and microdebrider rather than using standard punch forceps to avoid stripping of the mucosa. The movement of the instrument in the region of the frontal recess should be careful movement; it is better to move from posterior to anterior direction (to avoid the anterior ethmoidal artery, the skull base and due to the presence of the beak which is a thick bone anteriorly) and from medial to lateral direction (to be away from the lateral lamella). The other approach to the frontal recess is through what is called intact bulla technique in which the uncinate process is removed and start removing the agger nasi by passing above the bulla medial to middle turbinate. Once the agger posterior wall is removed, the anterior ethmoidal artery is identified and hence the skull base then the dissection continues the rest dissection. Another method of intact bulla technique is like what Wormald use in which a mucosal flap is elevated just anterior to the middle turbinate axilla and reflected posteriorly, then dissect the anterior wall of the agger nasi [10] to discover the frontal recess.

Various types of frontal cells are present which is best described in modified Kuhn classification as following:

- Type 1—Single cell above the agger nasi cell.
- Type 2—Tier of cells above agger nasi cell.
- Type 3—Single large cell extending to <50% of the vertical height of the frontal sinus.
- Type 4—Large cell extending to >50% of the vertical height of the frontal sinus or isolated cell within the sinus.

All these types of frontal cells should be removed in the same manner of removing agger nasi cell.

Other types of frontoethmoidal cells include:

- Suprabullar cells which present above the bulla and extend to skull base and may compress the frontal recess from behind.
- Supraorbital cell extends above the orbit and opens behind the frontal recess and anterior to anterior ethmoidal artery.
- interfrontal sinus septal cell a pneumatization of the interfrontal sinus septum with variable extension which may compress the frontal recess from medial to lateral.

These cells should be well studied on CT scan before working on the frontal sinus as it may require special instrument or even require combined approach to completely manage the disease and open the frontal recess correctly. Emerging of the navigation system in the endoscopic sinus surgery plays an important role in revision cases and in presence of anatomical variation especially in frontal recess region to avoid injury to the nearby vital structure and to achieve complete clearness of the recess.

Pitfall and Pearls of Frontal Sinus Surgery

- Endoscopic approach to frontal recess is the golden way to treat chronic frontal sinusitis.
- Good knowledge of the normal anatomy and the normal anatomical variation is vital for surgery success.
- Do the best in maintaining the mucosal lining of the frontal recess.
- Try to avoid middle meatal collapse postoperatively by maintaining middle turbinate attachment, use of middle meatal spacer, or even bolgerization.
- Postoperative care is crucial in endoscopic fontal surgery to maintain the function and avoid closure of the recess by blood clots and crust.
- CT scan coronal and sagittal cuts are necessary to study the frontal recess region.

Take Home Messages

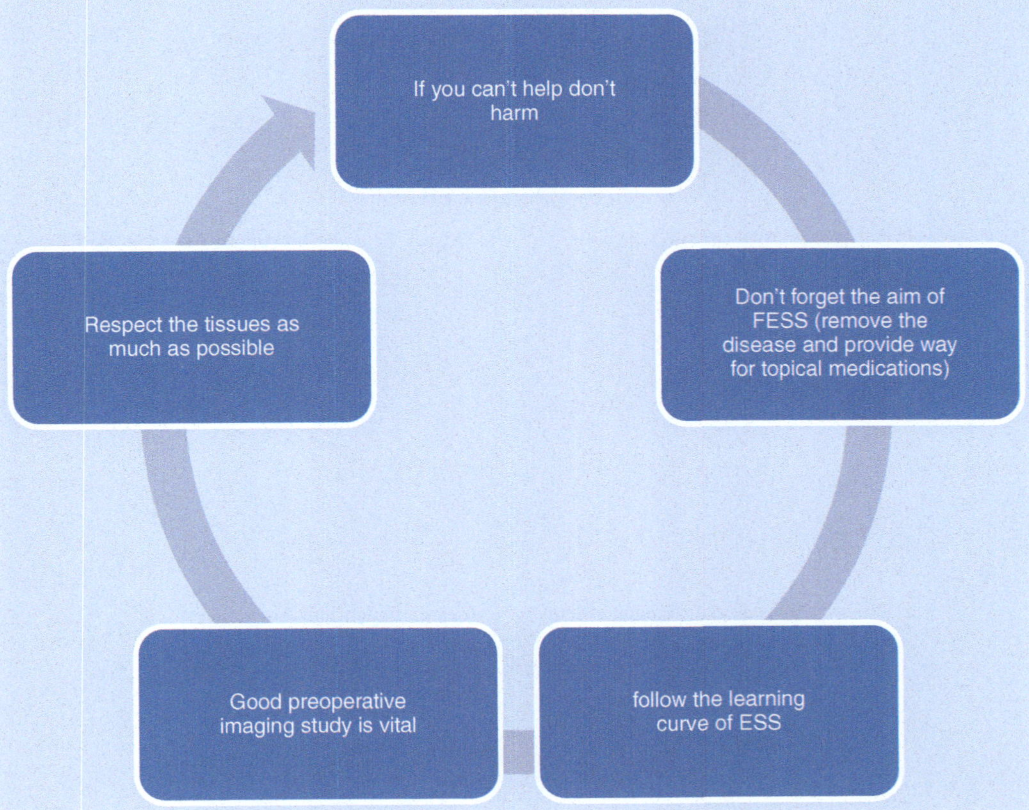

References

1. Wormald PJ, McDonogh M. The 'swing-door' technique for uncinectomy in endoscopic sinus surgery. J Laryngol Otol. 1998;112(6):547–51.
2. Wormald P-J. Endoscopic sinus surgery, vol. 5. Stuttgart: Thieme; 2013. p. 28–44.
3. Stammberger H. Endoscopic surgery for mycotic and chronic recurring sinusitis. Ann Otol Rhinol Laryngol. 1985;94(5_Suppl):1–11.
4. Yanagisawa E, Joe JK, Christmas DA. Where is the ostium of the ethmoid bulla? Ear Nose Throat J. 1999;78(12):886.
5. Schlosser RJ, Harvey RJ. Endoscopic sinus surgery: optimizing outcomes and avoiding failures. San Diego: Plural Publishing; 2012.
6. Kim H, Kim S, Kang SS, Chung IH, Lee J, Yoon J. Surgical anatomy of the natural ostium of the sphenoid sinus. Laryngoscope. 2001;111(9):1599–602.
7. Levine HL. Endoscopic sinus surgery: reasons for failure. Oper Tech Otolaryngol Neck Surg. 1995;6(3):176–9.
8. Kennedy DW, Senior BA. Endoscopic sinus surgery. A review. Otolaryngol Clin North Am. 1997;30(3):313–30.
9. Stammberger H, Kopp W, Dekornfeld TJ. Special endoscopic anatomy. In: Functional Endoscopic Sinus Surgery: The Messerklinger Technique. Philadelphia: Decker Publication; 1991. p. 61–90.
10. May M, Schaitkin B. Frontal sinus surgery: endonasal drainage instead of an external osteoplastic approach. Oper Tech Otolaryngol Neck Surg. 1995;6(3):184–92.

Part IV

Head and Neck

34 Thyroid and Parathyroid Glands

Hassan Haidar, Abdelrahman Alsaleh,
Waheed Rahman, and Hussein Enezi

34.1 Introduction

Thyroid gland comprises two types of cells: follicular cells (or thyrocytes) which produce and secrete thyroglobulin and thyroid hormones, and parafollicular cells (or C cells), which secrete calcitonin. Papillary Thyroid Carcinoma (PTC) and Follicular Thyroid Carcinoma (FTC) are tumors originating by thyrocytes and are referred as Differentiated Thyroid Carcinomas (DTCs). Anaplastic Thyroid Carcinoma (ATC) is the undifferentiated tumor which may arise from DTCs or may be undifferentiated to origin. Medullary Thyroid Carcinoma (MTC) is the tumor arising to C cell.

The four parathyroid glands, located posterior to the thyroid gland, regulate calcium homeostasis through release of parathyroid hormone (PTH). PTH increases serum calcium levels through direct action on bone and the kidneys. It stimulates osteoclasts to resorb bone and mobilize calcium into the blood.

H. Haidar (✉)
Hamad Medical Corporation, Doha, Qatar

A. Alsaleh · W. Rahman · H. Enezi
ENT Department, Hamad Medical Corporation, Doha, Qatar
e-mail: wrahman@hamad.qa; halenazi@hamad.qa

34.2 Thyroid Gland

34.2.1 Embryology

The thyroid gland develops from three pharyngeal bodies: the median anlage and two lateral bodies. Median anlage is derived as a ventral diverticulum at the foramen cecum. During the fourth to seventh week of gestation, the primitive thyroid tissue descends along the thyroglossal duct anterior to the hyoid bone and the laryngeal cartilages to reach its final position at the level of the second and fourth tracheal rings [1, 2].

Calcitonin-secreting parafollicular C cells arise within the ultimobranchial bodies from neural crest cells of the fourth pharyngeal pouch [3, 4].

The entire gland may lie close to its point of origin at the foramen cecum, giving rise to a lingual thyroid. About 70% of patients with lingual thyroid glands have no thyroid tissue in the neck. In many cases, the lingual thyroid does not function normally [3, 4].

The thyroglossal duct ultimately atrophies, but any portion of it may persist to become the site of a thyroglossal duct cyst.

34.2.2 Anatomy of the Thyroid Gland

The gland lies anterior to the second, third, and fourth tracheal rings. Posterolaterally, the gland overlaps the carotid sheath and its contents.

A. Al-Qahtani et al. (eds.), *Textbook of Clinical Otolaryngology*,
https://doi.org/10.1007/978-3-030-54088-3_34

A pyramidal lobe may be present in about 50% of patients [3, 4].

Arterial blood supply is derived from two pairs of arteries.

1. *The superior thyroid artery:* the first branch of the external carotid artery.
2. *The inferior thyroid artery:* a branch of the thyrocervical trunk of the subclavian artery. It courses behind the common carotid artery to enter the inferior thyroid pole.
3. *The thyroid ima artery:* inconsistently present (7%). Because of its relation to the anterior aspect of the trachea, the thyroid ima artery is in danger of injury during a tracheotomy.

34.2.2.1 Lymphatic Drainage of the Thyroid Gland

Dominant drainage to level VI known as precricoid, Delphian, paratracheal lymph node.

Anatomy of the Recurrent Laryngeal Nerve

The right recurrent laryngeal nerve arises from the vagus as this nerve crosses anterior to the right subclavian artery. It then loops around the artery and ascends in the tracheoesophageal groove, posterior to the thyroid gland, to enter the larynx behind the cricothyroid articulation [5].

The nerve on the left arises from the vagus where it crosses the arch of aorta. It then loops around the aorta to ascend in the tracheoesophageal. The left recurrent nerve is generally more closely applied to the trachea in the lower part of its ascending course than is the right nerve.

As the recurrent laryngeal nerves ascend toward the middle of the thyroid gland, they are intimately associated with the inferior thyroid artery [5, 6].

Classically, the recurrent laryngeal nerve is found intraoperatively in Simon's triangle, which is formed by the common carotid artery laterally, the esophagus medially, and the inferior thyroid artery superiorly. The nerve can also be reliably found where it enters the larynx just behind the inferior cornu of the thyroid cartilage.

Anatomy of the Superior Laryngeal Nerve

The superior laryngeal nerve originates at the inferior ganglion of the vagus nerve near the jugular foramen.

It has two branches; the internal branch pierces the thyrohyoid membrane and supplies sensation to the supraglottic and pyriform sinus [7] and the external branch which supplies the cricothyroid muscle.

The nerve is variable in its relationship to the highest point of the superior pole of the thyroid gland and is at risk of injury during thyroid surgery [8].

34.2.3 Benign Thyroid Disease

34.2.3.1 Graves' Disease

- *Pathophysiology:* Autoimmune, TSH receptor antibody → stimulation→ goiter and elevated levels of T3 and T4 secretion [9]. Associated with exophthalmos and dermatopathy.
- *Risk factors:* exposure to radiation, females more than males (adolescence or 30–40) and genetic predisposition.
- *Histopathology:* Shows scattered lymphocytic infiltration.
- *Investigations:* Thyroid-stimulating immunoglobulin levels (TSIs); Iodine-123 (I123) scanning shows a diffuse increased gland uptake [10].
- *Radioactive Iodine (131I):* the most common therapy used.
- *Subtotal Thyroidectomy:* indicated when medical therapy fails [11].
  - *Exophthalmos and optic neuropathy* If optic neuropathy persists despite medical therapy, corticosteroids for 2 weeks; if no improvement, then surgical decompression is needed which includes trans-nasal endoscopic approaches to the medial and inferior orbital wall [12].

34.2.3.2 Toxic Nodular Goiter

No eye or skin findings as in Graves' disease.

Evolution of hyperfunctional regions, which results in excess thyroid hormone that causes the suppression of TSH resulting in the adjoining normal gland becoming less active on I123 scans, with hyperfunctional areas being hot [13].

Hyperthyroidism typically does not occur, until the nodule is 3 cm or larger or multiple toxic nodules.

Treatment is either surgery or radioactive iodine, antithyroid medications might be considered prior to more definitive surgical or radio ablative treatment.

34.2.3.3 Hashimoto's Thyroiditis

- *Physiopathology:* Antithyroglobulin antibody →chronic lymphocytic inflammation →Transient hyperthyroidism followed by hypothyroidism [14].
- *Risk factors:* More common in females in third to fifth decade, genetic susceptibility (HLA-DR3). Can be associated with lymphoma, neoplasms, or other autoimmune disease such as SLE, Sjogren syndrome, and scleroderma.
- *Histopathology:* Lymphocytic infiltration with germinal center formation.
- *Investigations:* Antithyroid peroxidase (anti-TPO) [15].
- *Treatment:* thyroxin therapy; surgical excision for compressive symptoms or suspicious nodule.
- *Complications:* Rarely, progress into thyroid lymphoma. A rapidly enlarging mass within a Hashimoto's gland should always raise concern regarding lymphoma and warrants FNA or biopsy.

34.2.3.4 Subacute Granulomatous (De Quervain's) Thyroiditis

Typically, presents as enlarged, painful thyroid, after upper respiratory tract infection, fever and malaise are also common. Half of patients may show hyperthyroidism, then patients will enter a several-month hypothyroid period. Eventually, most patients return to euthyroidism.

I123 scanning usually shows less than 2% uptake.

It is a self-limiting disease that can be treated with anti-inflammatory drugs and rarely steroids [16].

34.2.3.5 Riedel's Thyroiditis

Fibrosis of thyroid gland of unknown cause that manifests as "rock-hard" thyroid produces local pressure and hypothyroidism. Histologically, it is characterized by widespread fibrotic process.

34.2.4 Thyroid Nodules

- The prevalence of palpable nodules is only 4–7% while high resolution ultrasound can detect 19–68% of individuals selected randomly with higher frequencies in women and the elderly [17].
- Only 5–10% of nodules being malignant [18]. A single dominant or solitary nodule is more likely to represent carcinoma than a single nodule within a multinodular gland, with an incidence of malignancy from 2.7 to 30% and 1.4 to 10%, respectively [19, 20].
- Important elements in patients' history that increase the likelihood of malignancy include prior head and neck irradiation, reports of rapid growth, dysphagia, dysphonia, male gender, and presentation at extremes of age.
- Physical examination findings that increase the concern for malignancy include: nodules larger than 4 cm in size (19.3% risk of malignancy), firmness, fixation to adjacent tissues, cervical lymphadenopathy. Vocal cord immobility [21].
- Ultrasound imaging studies and FNA are the main tools used to decide whether surgical excision of a thyroid nodule is warranted.
- Molecular genetic biomarker analyses are now being used to increase the accuracy of FNAB.

34.2.4.1 Ultrasonography

Solid appearance (or hypoechogenicity); increased vascularity; microcalcifications; irregular margins; and the absence of a halo are features that have been consistently associated with malignancy (Table 34.1).

34.2.4.2 Radioisotope Imaging

About 80–85% of thyroid nodules are cold and about 10% of these nodules represent a malignancy. While hot nodules account for 5% of all nodules and the likelihood of malignancy is less than 1% for these nodules.

Except for obviating the need to perform an FNAB on a hyperfunctioning nodule in patients who are thyrotoxic, the use of radioisotope scanning has been abandoned.

Table 34.1 The sensitivity and specificity of various sonographic characteristics

Sonographic characteristic	Sensitivity (%)	Specificity (%)
Microclassifications	52	83
Absence of halo	66	54
Irregular margins	55	79
Hypoechoic	81	53
Increased intranodular flow	67	81

Data from Fish SA, Langer JE, Mandel SJ. Sonographic imaging of thyroid nodules & cervical lymph nodes. Endocrinol Metab Clin North Am 2008;37(2):401–17

34.2.4.3 Fine Needle Aspiration Cytology

- Nodules 1 cm or larger or sonographically suspicious sub-centimeter nodules warrant cytologic analysis through FNAB to determine the risk for malignancy [22–24].

The pathology report from FNAB may be read as benign, malignant, indeterminate, or nondiagnostic.

The only malignant pathology reliably diagnosed through FNA is papillary thyroid carcinoma because features, such as Orphan Annie nuclei, nuclear grooves, intranuclear inclusions, and psammoma bodies, can be sufficient for a diagnosis.

Medullary carcinoma, anaplastic carcinoma, lymphoma, poorly differentiated carcinoma, and metastatic disease can also be classified on the basis of cytology.

Benign and malignant follicular neoplasms and oncocytic adenomas and carcinomas cannot be distinguished on the basis of cytology alone, because tissue architecture is required to make the diagnosis of malignancy through observation of capsular or angiolymphatic invasion. Patients with lesions classified as follicular or oncocytic neoplasm, or suspicious for malignancy should be offered a diagnostic lobectomy.

FNAB specimens read as unsatisfactory should be sent for a repeat biopsy while samples read as follicular lesions with unknown significance or "FLUS". FLUS are generally sent for repeat FNAB, as the risk for malignancy is only 5–10%. FNA that showed follicular neoplasm or suspicious for follicular neoplasm has a 15–30% risk of malignancy and diagnostic thyroidectomy should be discussed with the patient vs. radiological surveillance (see algorithm).

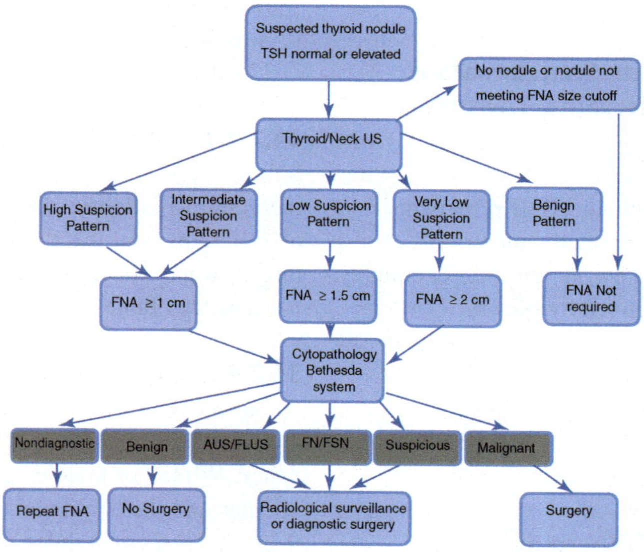

AUS/FLUS: Atypia of undetermined significance or follicular lesion of undetermined.

FN/FSN: Follicular neoplasm or suspicious for a follicular neoplasm [25].

34.2.5 Malignant Thyroid Disease

34.2.5.1 Papillary Thyroid Carcinoma

The most common type of thyroid cancer represents 75–85% of all thyroid cancer cases. More frequently in women and presents in the 20–55 years of age [26].

Features include:

- Characteristics: Orphan Annie eye nucleus and psammoma bodies on light microscopy.
- Lymphatic spread is more common than hematogenous spread.
- Multifocality is common.
- The so-called "Lateral Aberrant Thyroid" is actually a lymph node metastasis from papillary thyroid carcinoma.
- Papillary microcarcinoma is a subset of papillary thyroid cancer defined as measuring less than or equal to 1 cm and the management strategies for incidental papillary microcarcinoma on ultrasound (and confirmed on FNAB) range from total thyroidectomy with radioactive iodine ablation to observation alone.

Staging (AJCC staging)

- *T1*: ≤2 cm tumor confined to thyroid (*T1a* ≤ 1 cm tumor, *T1b* > 1 cm but ≤2 cm).
- *T2*: >2 cm but ≤4 cm tumor limited to thyroid gland.
- *T3*: >4 cm tumor *or* gross extrathyroidal extension invading strap muscles only (*T3a* > 4 cm tumor limited to thyroid, *T3b* gross extrathyroidal extension invading only strap muscles of any size).
- *T4*: includes gross extrathyroidal extension (*T4a* invades subcutaneous soft tissue, larynx, trachea, esophagus, or recurrent laryngeal nerve; *T4b* invades prevertebral fascia or encasing carotid or mediastinal vessels).

Management

- Thyroid lobectomy alone may be sufficient treatment for small (<1 cm), low-risk, unifocal, intrathyroidal papillary carcinomas.
- Gross disease (diameter over 1.0 cm)—total thyroidectomy, and central compartment lymph node removal is the therapy of choice.
- Central compartment neck dissection for patients with nodal disease or in high-risk patients (advanced papillary thyroid carcinoma (T3–T4).
- Lateral neck dissection is indicated for biopsy-proven metastatic lateral neck nodes.

Postoperative management

- For low-risk Well-Differentiated Thyroid Carcinoma (WDTC), radioactive iodine adjuvant therapy is not routinely recommended after thyroidectomy but should be considered in intermediate- and low-risk WDTC with other risk factors.
- Radioactive iodine adjuvant therapy is usually recommended after total thyroidectomy for high-risk WDTC.

Patient is considered high risk if any of the following present [27]:

- Macroscopic tumor invasion.
- Incomplete tumor resection with gross residual disease.
- Distant metastases.
- Postoperative serum thyroglobulin suggestive of distant metastases.
- Pathologic N1 with any metastatic lymph node ≥3 cm in largest dimension.
- Follicular thyroid cancer with extensive vascular invasion (>4 foci of vascular invasion).

- *Follow-up:* thyroglobulin measurement and diagnostic radioactive iodine scanning 2–8 days after radioiodine treatment.
  - Radioiodine scan is usually repeated 6–12 months after treatment with 131-I in moderate- to high-risk patients and in lower-risk patients who have detectable Tg

levels during follow-up that are not declining.

- *Prognosis:* 95% 5-year survival; poor prognostic indicators include tumors >1.5 cm or extracapsular spread (cervical metastases have increased cervical recurrence rates without affecting survival).

34.2.5.2 Follicular Carcinoma

The second most common thyroid carcinoma representing about 10% of thyroid cancers [28].

It is more common in female with median age around the sixth decade.

Twenty to 50% spread *hematogenously* with distant metastasis (lymphatic spread is rare).

- *Diagnosis*: Requires open biopsy in order to distinguish adenoma from carcinoma.
- *Histopathology*: It has a sub-stational morphologic overlap with the benign follicular adenoma. Typically, it shows unifocal neoplastic follicular cells that is less distinct from malignant papillary cells; malignancy can be determined if extracapsular spread is noted.
- *Staging*: is similar to that of PTC.
- *Treatment*: Total thyroidectomy ± neck dissection. Radioactive iodine adjuvant therapy is usually recommended after total thyroidectomy for high-risk WDTC *(see papillary thyroid cancer).*
- *Prognosis*: *70–85%* 5-year survival and reaches to about 20% with distant metastasis. Angioinvasion, extracapsular spread denotes worse prognosis.

34.2.5.3 Hurthle Cell Carcinoma

Occurs mostly in older patients (60s).

Can be considered a variant of follicular carcinoma, oxyphilic cells noted.

Believed to be more aggressive in nature, spread can occur via lymphatic or hematogenous pathways.

Distant metastasis can reach up to 30%, with 40% bone followed by 30% lung.

- *Management:* While the staging is similar to that of the PTC, radiouptake is poor in such cancers; aggressive surgery is the mainstay in treatment.
- *Prognosis:* about 50% 5-year survivals [29, 30].

34.2.5.4 Medullary Thyroid Carcinoma

The third most common of all thyroid cancers (3%), it originates from the parafollicular cells (C cells), which produce the hormone calcitonin [31, 32].

- 25% of medullary thyroid cancer cases are genetic in nature, caused by a mutation in the RET proto-oncogene and inherited as an autosomal dominant trait. This form is identified as *familial medullary thyroid cancer* (FMTC). When it coexists with tumors of the parathyroid gland and medullary component of the adrenal glands (pheochromocytoma), it is called multiple endocrine neoplasia type 2 (MEN2).
- Surgical removal of the thyroid in children who carry the mutant gene is curative if the entire thyroid gland is removed at an early age, before there is spread of the tumor.
- The parathyroid tumors and pheochromocytomas are removed when they cause clinical symptomatology.
- 75% of medullary thyroid carcinoma occurs in *"sporadic" fashion.*

Markers: Calcitonin is useful as a marker which can be tested in blood for detecting the presence of a tumor, and is an indicator of tumor mass.

Treatment: A plasma level of metanephrines should be checked before surgical thyroidectomy to evaluate for the presence of pheochromocytoma as 25% of people found to have medullary thyroid cancer and have the inherited form of the MEN2A syndrome. Undiagnosed pheochromocytoma leads to a very high intraoperative risk of hypertensive crisis and, potentially, death.

34.2.5.5 Surgery

- A total thyroidectomy with bilateral neck dissection is the gold standard for treating medullary thyroid cancer.
- About 50% of patients have metastasis to regional lymph nodes at the time of diagnosis.
- In gene carriers: The timing of surgery depends on the type of mutation present. For those in the highest risk group, surgery is recommended in the first year of life. In lower-risk cases, surgery may be delayed up to the age of 10 years, the precise timing depending on the mutation and other factors.

Unlike other differentiated thyroid carcinoma, there is no role for radioiodine treatment in medullary-type disease [33].

34.2.5.6 Protein Kinase Inhibitors

Protein kinase inhibitors (vandetanib, cabozantinib) which block the abnormal kinase proteins involved in the development and growth of medullary cancer cells, showed clear evidence of response in 10–30% of patients for treatment of late-stage (metastatic) medullary thyroid cancer in adult patients who are ineligible for surgery [34, 35].

34.2.5.7 Prognosis

- 5-year survival rate is 100% at stage I, 98% at stage II, 81% at stage III, and 28% at stage IV [36]. The prognosis of MTC is poorer than that of follicular and papillary thyroid cancer when it has metastasized (spread) beyond the thyroid gland.
- The prognosis correlated with the rate at which the postoperative calcitonin concentration doubles, termed the calcitonin doubling time (CDT), rather than the pre- or postoperative absolute calcitonin level.
- The calcitonin doubling time was a better predictor of MTC survival than *CEA* [21] but following both tests is recommended [37].

MEN1 (Werner's syndrome)	MEN2 (Sipple syndrome)	MEN2B
Parathyroid adenoma or hyperplasia	Medullary thyroid carcinoma	Medullary thyroid carcinoma
Pancreatic Islet cell tumors (insulinoma, gastrinoma)	Pheochromocytoma	Pheochromocytoma
Pituitary adenoma	Parathyroid hyperplasia	Mucosal neuroma Marfanoid habitus

34.2.5.8 Anaplastic Thyroid Carcinoma

Two percent of all thyroid carcinomas, but 15–39% of all deaths. Tend to be older patients (50–60s).

- *Aggressive:* rapidly growing infiltrative thyroid mass, vocal cord paralysis.
- *Metastasis* possible to lungs, liver, bones within weeks.
- FNA typically shows necrosis and degeneration.
- *Prognosis:* survival rates low (20%) at 1 year.
- *Management*: Aggressive multimodal therapy in early stage: total thyroidectomy, intensity-modulated radiation therapy (IMRT), and adjuvant chemotherapy [28, 38, 39].
- *Palliative therapy*: (tracheostomy controversial due to poor prognosis) for advanced lesions.

34.2.6 Thyroidectomy and Its Complications

34.2.6.1 Thyroidectomy Types

(a) Hemithyroidectomy: It involves removal of one lobe plus entire isthmus is removed. It is performed in benign disease involving one lobe (benign nodule or cyst).

(b) Subtotal thyroidectomy: Here about 8 g, or tissue size of pulp of finger is retained on lower pole of thyroid on both sides, and rest of gland is removed. Indications: Toxic thyroid, non-toxic multinodular goiter.

(c) Near-total thyroidectomy: Here both lobes except less than 2 g of thyroid tissue on the lower pole, near to the recurrent laryngeal nerve and parathyroid, are removed to retain blood supply to parathyroid gland. Indication: mostly done in papillary thyroid carcinoma.

(d) Total thyroidectomy: Here entire gland is removed. Indication: thyroid cancer. Total thyroidectomy provides the advantages of eliminating the risk of recurrence and hence an increasing number of total thyroidectomies are currently being performed for benign cases.

34.2.6.2 Complications

(a) *Hematoma*: Hematoma can usually be differentiated from seroma by the presence of skin ecchymosis, firmness to palpation, or clotted drain output. Two types of hematoma:
   - Deep to deep fascia: A deep bleeding produces tension hematoma. Usually due to slipping of the ligature of the superior thyroid artery, though it can also be from a thyroid remnant or a thyroid vein. This compresses on the airway and potentially life threatening unlike the subcutaneous bleeding. A tension hematoma requires opening of the wound, evacuation of hematoma, and ligature of the bleeding vessels.
   - Subcutaneous. A subcutaneous hematoma is most likely due to slipping of the ligature of the anterior jugular vein and can be aspirated.

(b) *Recurrent Laryngeal Nerve Injury*:
   - Temporary dysfunction because of nerve traction occurs in 2.5–5% of patients. —Return of normal vocal cord function occurs 6–12 months after temporary RLN injury occurs.
   - The incidence of permanent RLN paralysis is approximately 1–1.5% for total thyroidectomy and less for near-total procedures.
     – Unilateral RLN paralysis: 1/3rd are asymptomatic, 2/3 change in voice which improves within 6 months due to compensation by the healthy cord. —Concurrent injury of the SLN results in a more laterally positioned vocal cord and worsens voice quality and glottic competence. Patients may have difficulty with aspiration and pneumonia.
     – Bilateral RLN paralysis: dyspnea and biphasic stridor. Tracheostomy may be needed. Posterior cordectomy when bilateral nerve transaction was certain or after 6 months of injury.

(c) *Superior Laryngeal Nerve Injury:* Injury to the SLN alters function of the cricothyroid muscle. Often disturbance of SLN function is temporary and unrecognized by the patient and the surgeon. Patients may have difficulty shouting, and singers find difficulty with pitch variation, especially in the higher frequencies. The external branch of the SLN is not often visualized and lies near the superior pole vessels. Safest approach is to identify the branches of superior thyroid artery and avoid ligating the main trunk as in majority of cases superior laryngeal nerve lies close to the main trunk. Adequate exposure of the superior thyroid pole and close ligation of the superior thyroid artery close to the superior pole of thyroid gland is considered safe.

(d) *Hypoparathyroidism:*
   - Transient symptomatic hypocalcemia after total thyroidectomy occurs in approximately 7–25% of cases and may be related to parathyroid gland trauma or vascular compromise.
   - Permanent hypocalcemia is less common (1–3%). Due to removal of parathyroids or the parathyroid end artery.
   - Hypocalcemia: patients may experience paresthesias, tetany, bronchospasm, mental status changes, seizures, laryngospasm, and cardiac arrhythmias. Chvostek sign and Trousseau sign may develop with increased neuromuscular irritability as serum calcium levels drop.
   - Treatment for hypocalcemia is typically initiated if the patient is symptomatic or

serum calcium levels decrease to less than 7 mg/dL.

(e) *Postoperative infections*: are very unusual because of the abundant blood supply in the thyroid bed.

34.3 Parathyroid Glands

34.3.1 Embryology and Anatomy of the Parathyroid Glands

- Two pairs of glands: Superior and inferior.
- The inferior parathyroid glands arise from the 3rd pharyngeal pouch endoderm and have a common origin and migration with the thymus.
- They migrate inferiorly in a long course of descent that can lead to a large area of possible ectopic inferior parathyroid glands; can be found anywhere from the level of the mandibular angle to the pericardium.
- The most common ectopic location for an inferior gland is in the anterior mediastinum; this is found in 5% of ectopic cases.
- Typically, inferior glands can be found anterior to a plane drawn along the course of the recurrent laryngeal nerve.
- The fourth pharyngeal pouch gives rise to the superior parathyroid glands which has a shorter embryologic descent than their inferior counterparts.
- Symmetry in the approximate location of the glands when comparing right with left has been reported at 80% for the superior and 70% for the inferior glands [40, 41].

34.3.2 Primary Hyperparathyroidism

- Increased calcium levels with elevated PTH levels.
- Might be spontaneous, familial, or associated with multiple endocrine neoplasia (MEN) syndromes.
- Caused by *parathyroid adenoma* in 80–85%, by *hyperplasia* in all four glands in about 15% of cases and very rarely by parathyroid cancer [42, 43].
- Clinical manifestations: 80% asymptomatic; 20% symptomatic (fatigue, nephrolithiasis, hypercalciuria, bony pain, muscle weakness).

34.3.2.1 Indications for Treatment

Indications for treatment (parathyroidectomy) are:

- Symptomatic hyperparathyroidism.
- Asymptomatic hyperparathyroidism with any of the following:
  - serum calcium >1 mg/dl above upper limit of normal
  - objective evidence of renal involvement, including silent nephrolithiasis, nephrocalcinosis, hypercalciuria with increased stone risk, or impaired renal function
  - osteoporosis
  - People age < 50
- For asymptomatic individuals who do not fulfill the surgical criteria, serum calcium and creatinine monitoring along with bone density every year are recommended. If disease progression occurs, treatment is indicated.

34.3.2.2 Parathyroidectomy

Parathyroidectomy is the only definitive treatment of pHPT and it aims to remove the adenoma(s).

- Preoperative localization studies: The best imaging modality for preoperative localization of parathyroid adenomas is parathyroid scintigraphy (Sestamibi scanning). Technetium 99m methoxyisobutyl isonitrile (Tc99MIBI) is first absorbed by both thyroid and parathyroids. The thyroid uptake is, however washed out over time while sestamibi is retained by adenomatous parathyroid glands.
- Radioguided Parathyroidectomy: may be considered for an adenoma identified on a Sestamibi scan; a tracer is injected 1.5–3 hours prior to surgery, then a gamma probe could be utilized intraoperatively to identify abnormal gland.

- Obtaining intraoperative PTH before incision, then to proceed by removing presumed pathologic gland, then PTH 10 min later should be checked for reduction >50% and/or into the normal range. If persistently elevated, four gland exploration with subtotal (three glands) parathyroidectomy can be performed.
- Complications:
- Persistent hyperparathyroidism.
- Recurrent laryngeal nerve injury.
- Transient postoperative hypocalcemia.

34.3.2.3 Medical Treatment

A calcimimetic (such as cinacalcet) is a potential therapy for patients who are unable to have surgery and whose primary indication for surgery is symptomatic and/or severe hypercalcemia.

34.3.3 Secondary Hyperparathyroidism

Secondary hyperparathyroidism is due to physiological secretion of PTH by the parathyroid glands in response to hypocalcemia. The most common causes are vitamin D deficiency and chronic kidney failure.

In chronic kidney failure, there is a problem converting vitamin D to its active form in the kidney. Lack of vitamin D leads to reduced calcium absorption by the intestine leading to hypocalcemia and increased parathyroid hormone secretion. This increases bone resorption and leads to renal osteodystrophy.

Treatment of secondary hyperparathyroidism is with calcimimetic.

34.3.4 Tertiary Hyperparathyroidism

Tertiary hyperparathyroidism is seen in those with long-term secondary hyperparathyroidism, which eventually leads to hyperplasia of the parathyroid glands and a loss of response to serum calcium levels. Parathyroid response becomes autonomous and it persists even after correction of the primary metabolic derangement with increased PTH levels despite correction of calcium.

This disorder is most often seen in patients with end-stage kidney disease. Treatment is by subtotal parathyroidectomy.

34.3.5 Parathyroid Carcinoma

- Parathyroid carcinoma occurs rarely and accounts for approximately 1% of cases of HPT.
- Elevated calcium and PTH levels markedly elevated compared to adenomas.
- Intraoperative appearance is typically a hard lobulated fibrous mass.
- En bloc resection is key with resection of ipsilateral thyroid lobe with isthmus, and paratracheal and central neck dissection, as adjuvant therapy has been disappointing.
- Tendency for spread to local lymph nodes but can also metastasize to lung, liver, and bone.
- 5- and 10-year survival is 85 and 50–75%, respectively.

Take Home Messages

- The procedure of choice in the evaluation of thyroid nodules is FNAC which is increasingly being performed with ultrasound guidance to improve diagnostic outcomes.
- Management of well-differentiated thyroid carcinoma generally consists of total thyroidectomy, excision of pathologic lymph nodes, and is followed by radioactive iodine only in high-risk patients.
- Thyroglobulin measurement is of great value in the follow-up of patients with differentiated thyroid cancer.
- Parathyroid adenoma accounts for 80–85% of primary hyperparathyroidism.
- Localization of hyperfunctional parathyroid glands may be accomplished using functional nuclear uptake studies which allow a mini-invasive approach for resection of the pathologic gland.

References

1. Gray SW, Skandalakis JE, Akin JT. Embryological considerations of thyroid surgery: developmental anatomy of the thyroid, parathyroids and the recurrent laryngeal nerve. Am Surg. 1976;42(9):621–8.
2. Moore KL, TVN P. The pharyngeal (branchial apparatus). In: The developing human: clinically oriented embryology. 6th ed. Philadelphia: WB Saunders; 1998. p. 230–8.
3. Hoyes AD, Kershaw DR. Anatomy and development of the thyroid gland. Ear Nose Throat J. 1985;64(10):318–32.
4. Hollinshead WH. Anatomy of the endocrine glands. Surg Clin North Am. 1958;39:1115–40.
5. Skandalakis JE, Droulias C, Harlaftis N, et al. The recurrent laryngeal nerve. Am Surg. 1976;42(9):629–34.
6. Henry J, Audiffret J, Denizot A, et al. The nonrecurrent inferior laryngeal nerve: review of 33 cases, including two on the left side. Surgery. 1988;104:977–84.
7. Janfaza P, Nadol JB, Fabian RL, et al. Surgical anatomy of the head and neck. Philadelphia: Lippincott Williams & Wilkins; 2001.
8. Cernea C, Ferraz A, Nishio S, et al. Surgical anatomy of the external branch of the superior laryngeal nerve. Head Neck. 1992;14:380–3.
9. Di Cerbo A, Di Paola R, Menzaghi C, et al. Graves' immunoglobulins activate phospholipase A2 by recognizing specific Epitopes on Thyrotropin Receptor 1. J Clin Endocrinol Metab.1999;84:3283–92. https://doi.org/10.1210/jcem.84.9.5967.
10. Fatourechi V. Medical management of extrathyroidal manifestation of Graves disease. Endocr Pract. 2014;20(12):1333–44.
11. Matthews DC, Syed AA. The role of TSH receptor antibodies in the management of Graves' disease. Eur J Intern Med. 2011;22:213–6.
12. Eckstein AK, Plicht M, Lax H, et al. Thyrotropin receptor autoantibodies are independent risk factors for Graves' ophthalmopathy and help to predict severity and outcome of the disease. J Clin Endocrinol Metab. 2006;91:3464–70.
13. Vitti P, Rago T, Tonacchera M, Pinchera A. Toxic multinodular goiter in the elderly. J Endocrinol Invest. 2002;25(10 Suppl):16–8.
14. Neufeld M, Maclaren NK, Blizzard RM. Two types of autoimmune Addison's disease associated with different polyglandular autoimmune (PGA) syndromes. Medicine (Baltimore). 1981;60(5):355–62.
15. Caturegli P, De Remigis A, Rose NR. Hashimoto thyroiditis: clinical and diagnostic criteria. Autoimmun Rev. 2014;13(4–5):391–7.
16. Fatourechi V, Aniszewski JP, Fatourechi GZE, et al. Clinical features and outcome of subacute thyroiditis in an incidence cohort: Olmsted County, Minnesota, study. J Clin Endocrinol Metab. 2003;88(5):2100–5.
17. Tan GH, Gharib H. Thyroid incidentalomas: management approaches to nonpalpable nodules discovered incidentally on thyroid imaging. Ann Intern Med. 1997;126(3):226–31.
18. Mandel SJ. A 64-year-old woman with a thyroid nodule. JAMA. 2004;292(21):2632–42.
19. Molina PE. Endocrine physiology. Lange physiology series. New York: McGraw-Hill; 2004.
20. Barroeta JE, Wang H, Shiina N, et al. Is fine-needle aspiration (FNA) of multiple thyroid nodules justified? Endocr Pathol. 2006;17(1):61–5.
21. McCoy KL, Jabbour N, Ogilvie JB, et al. The incidence of cancer and rate of false-negative cytology in thyroid nodules greater than or equal to 4 cm in size. Surgery. 2007;142(6):837–44; discussion 844.e1–3.
22. Baloch ZW, Sack MJ, Yu GH, et al. Fine-needle aspiration ofthyroid: an institutional experience. Thyroid. 1998;8:565–9.
23. Hamburger JI. Consistency of sequential needle biopsy findings for thyroid nodules: management implications. Arch Intern Med. 1987;147:97–9, 198.
24. Bisi H, de Camargo RY, Longatto Filho A. Role of fine-needle aspiration cytology in the management of thyroid nodules: review of experience with 1,925 cases. Diagn Cytopathol. 1992;8:504–10.
25. Hu MI, Vassilopoulou-Sellin R, Lustig R, Lamont JP. Thyroid and parathyroid cancers. In: Pazdur R, Wagman LD, Camphausen KA, Hoskins WJ, editors. Cancer management: a multidisciplinary approach. 11th ed. Manhasset, NY: CMP Medica; 2008.
26. Mazzaferri EL, Young RL. Papillary thyroid carcinoma: a ten-year follow-up report on the impact of treatment in 576 patients. Am Med. 1981;70:511–8.
27. Haugen BR, Alexander EK, Bible KC, Doherty GM, Mandel SJ, Nikiforov YE, Pacini F, Randolph GW, Sawka AM, Schlumberger M, Schuff KG, Sherman SI, Sosa JA, Steward DL, Tuttle RM, Wartofsky L. American Thyroid Association Management guidelines for adult patients with thyroid nodules and differentiated thyroid cancer: The American Thyroid Association guidelines task force on thyroid nodules and differentiated thyroid cancer. Thyroid. 2016;26(1):1.
28. Rosai J, Carcangiu ML, DeLellis RA. Atlas of thyroid pathology. tumors of the thyroid gland. Washington, DC: Armed Forces Institute of Pathology; 1992.
29. Evans HL, Vassilopoulou-Sellin R. Follicular and Hurthle cell carcinomas of the thyroid: a comparative study. Am J Surg Pathol. 1998;22:1512–20.
30. Thompson NW, Dunn EL, Batsakis JG, et al. Hurthle cell lesions of the thyroid gland. Surg Gynecol Obstet. 1974;139:555–60.
31. Hu MI, Vassilopoulou-Sellin R, Lustig R, Lamont JP. Thyroid and parathyroid cancers. In: Pazdur R, Wagman LD, Camphausen KA, Hoskins WJ, editors. Cancer management: a multidisciplinary approach. 11th ed; 2008.
32. Stamatakos M, Paraskeva P, Stefanaki C, Katsaronis P, Lazaris A, Safioleas K, Kontzoglou K. Medullary thyroid carcinoma: the third most common thyroid cancer reviewed. Oncol Lett. 2011;2(1):49–53. https://doi.org/10.3892/ol.2010.223. PMC 3412473. PMID 22870127.

33. Quayle FJ, Moley JF. Medullary thyroid carcinoma: including MEN 2A and MEN 2B syndromes. J Surg Oncol. 2005;89(3):122–9. https://doi.org/10.1002/jso.20184. PMID 15719378.
34. American Thyroid Association - Thyroid Clinical Trials. Archived from the original on 2007-12-12. Accessed 21 Dec 2007.
35. FDA approves new treatment for rare form of thyroid cancer. Accessed 7 April 2011.
36. cancer.org > Thyroid Cancer Archived October 18, 2013, at the Wayback Machine By the American Cancer Society. In turn citing: AJCC Cancer Staging Manual. 7th ed.
37. Randolph GW, editor. Surgery of the thyroid and parathyroid glands. ASCO SEP 3rd edition. Philadelphia: Saunders; 2003.
38. LiVolsi VA, Merino M. Pathology of thyroid tumors. Philadelphia: Saunders; 1987.
39. Leeper RD. Thyroid cancer. Med Clin North Am. 1985;69:1079–96.
40. Moore K, Persaud T. The developing human. 6th ed. Philadelphia: WB Saunders; 1998.
41. Akerström G, Malmaeus J, Bergström R. Surgical anatomy of human parathyroid glands. Surgery. 1984;95(1):14–21.
42. Fraser WD. Hyperparathyroidism. Lancet. 2009;374(9684):145–58. https://doi.org/10.1016/S0140-6736(09)60507-9. PMID 19595349.
43. Primary hyperparathyroidism. NIDDK. August 2012. Archived from the original on 4 October 2016. Accessed 27 Sept 2016.

35 Diseases of the Salivary Glands

Hassan Haidar, Abhishek Menon, and Emad Al Duhirat

35.1 Introduction

There are essentially three-paired salivary glands: the parotid glands, submandibular glands, and the sublingual glands. In addition, the minor salivary glands, or accessory glands are present in the oral cavity. They can be split into three main categories: the anterolingual glands, the serous glands of Von Ebner, the lingual buccolabial and palatal glands.

35.1.1 Saliva

- Lubricates and moistens food.
- Protects mucosa from desiccation and chemical irritation.
- It has antibacterial action via secretory IgA, lactoferrin, salivary peroxidase, and lysozymes. Prevention of dental caries.

H. Haidar (✉)
Hamad Medical Corporation, Doha, Qatar

A. Menon · E. Al Duhirat
Otolaryngology-Head and Neck Surgery Division, Department of Surgery, Hamad Medical Corporation, Doha, Qatar

35.1.2 Saliva Secretion

- 1–1.5 L in 24 h, contains electrolytes.
- Non-stimulated flow primarily from submandibular gland.
  Mixed serous and mucinous saliva.
- Parotid gland supplies the majority of stimulated salivary flow.
  Serous saliva.

35.2 Anatomy

35.2.1 Parotid Gland

- Derived from first pharyngeal pouch.
- Situated between the external auditory canal, mastoid tip, and the ramus of the mandible. Anteriorly, it lies above the masseter muscle and sternocleidomastoid muscle posteriorly.
- The superficial layer of the deep cervical fascia forms the parotid gland fascia which incompletely surrounds the gland.
- The facial nerve divides the gland into a deep lobe and a superficial lobe.
- Lymphoid tissue makes up the gland. Histologically, it consists of basophilic and serous cells.
- Stensen's duct runs 1 cm inferior to the zygoma and opens opposite to the upper second molar.

A. Al-Qahtani et al. (eds.), *Textbook of Clinical Otolaryngology*,
https://doi.org/10.1007/978-3-030-54088-3_35

- Stylomandibular ligament, separates the parotid gland from the submandibular gland.
- Parasympathetics innervation: Mediate secretion of saliva. Inferior salivatory nucleus in brain stem → CN IX, Jacobsen's nerve → lesser superficial petrosal nerve → Otic Ganglion → auriculotemporal nerve (V3).
- Blood Supply: Posterior auricular and superficial temporal arteries, branch of external carotid Artery.

35.2.2 Submandibular Gland

- Second largest salivary gland, lies in the submandibular triangle.
- Enveloped by the superficial layer of the deep cervical fascia which contains the marginal mandibular nerve.
- The facial artery hooks over the posterior belly of the digastric to enter the gland. It runs medial to the digastric muscle.
- Hypoglossal nerve runs deep to the digastric tendon and medial to the deep layer of the deep cervical fascia,
- CN XII runs deep into the digastric tendon and the mylohyoid along the hyoglossus.
- Consists of serous and mucinous cells (mixed).
- Histologic cell type: mixed cells (serous and mucinous).
- Wharton's duct: opens lateral to frenulum in the anterior portion of the floor of mouth, behind the incisors.
- Parasympathetics innervation: superior salivatory nucleus → nervus intermedius → chorda tympani → submandibular ganglion→ lingual nerve.

35.2.3 Sublingual Gland

- Mucinous cell type.
- Opens into ducts of Rivinus.

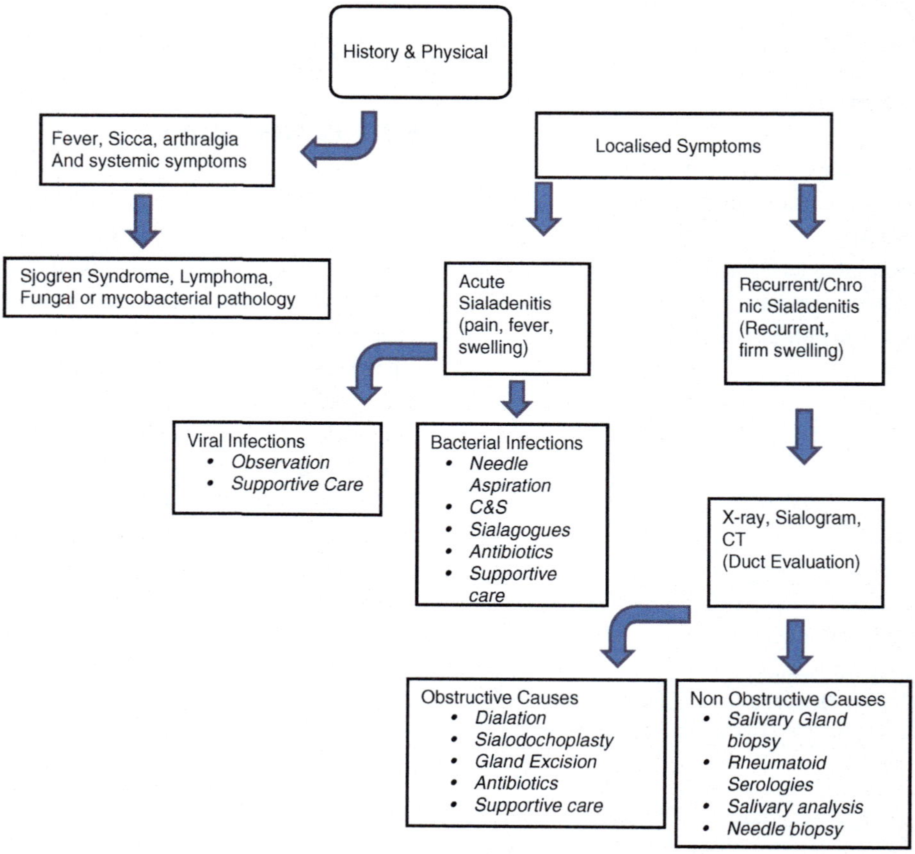

35.3 Salivary Gland Inflammatory Process

35.3.1 Acute Sialadenitis

35.3.1.1 Viral

- Mumps virus is the most common cause of acute parotid enlargement. Other causes include HIV, coxsackie, and influenza.
- Peak incidence at 4–6 years.
- Associated sudden sensorineural hearing loss, pancreatitis, meningitis, and orchitis.
- Secondary to salivary obstruction or stasis.
- Symptoms include trismus, warmth, erythema and tenderness over gland, purulence at ductal orifice, auricle may protrude (parotitis).
- Treatment similar to bacterial except for the use of antibiotics.

35.3.1.2 Bacterial

- Ascendant ductal infection.
- Dehydration, diabetes, renal diseases, wrong dental hygiene.
- S. aureus most common bacterial cause. Followed by Streptococcus viridans, H. influenzae, S. pyogenes, and E. coli.
- Diagnosed by clinical history and examination, cultures (FNA usually not required).
- Parotid most commonly infected due to stasis in serous secretions which are less.
- Bacteriostatic than mucinous secretion.
- Treatment: rehydration, warm compresses, antibiotics, sialogogues. If no resolution after 2–3 days, then consider CT or U/S to evaluate for abscess (may require I&D).
- Complications include deep neck space invasion (Ludwig's angina), ductal fistula (cutaneous), abscess (toxemia).

35.3.2 Sialolithiasis (Figs. 35.1 and 35.2)

- More common in *submandibular gland* (high mucin content, high PH, long duct with small orifice, and antigravity flow).
- *90% of submandibular calculi are radiopaque.*
- *90% of parotid calculi are radiolucent.*
- Symptoms include swelling and recurrent pain, worse with meals (salivary colic).
- Recurrent painful swelling at mealtime.
- Diagnosed by palpating the stone, sialography, CT, US.
- Treatment—gland massage, gland excision, sialoendoscopy.
- Complications include fistula, acute suppurative sialadenitis, ductal stricture.

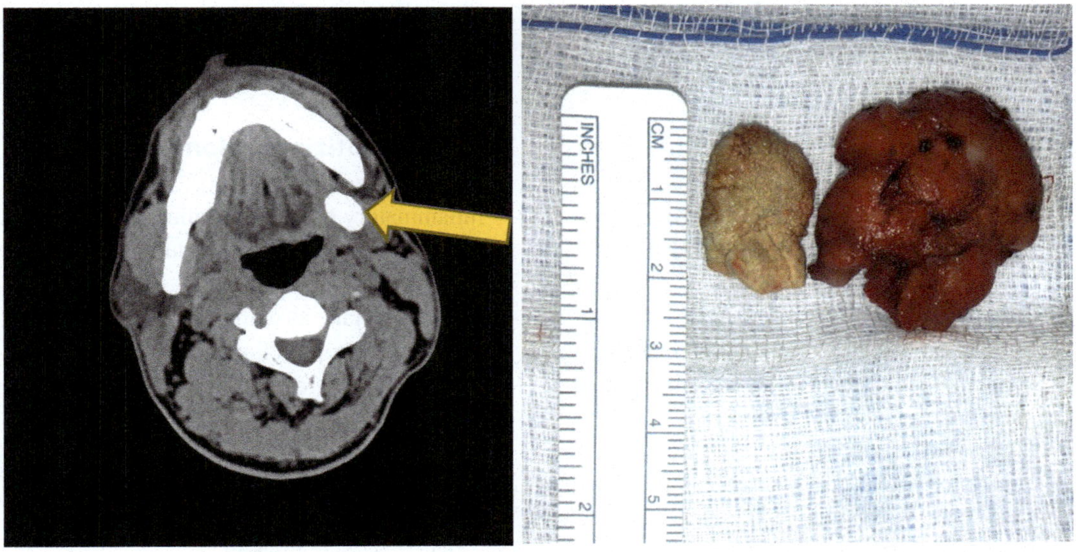

Fig. 35.1 Left submandibular gland stone (yellow arrow)

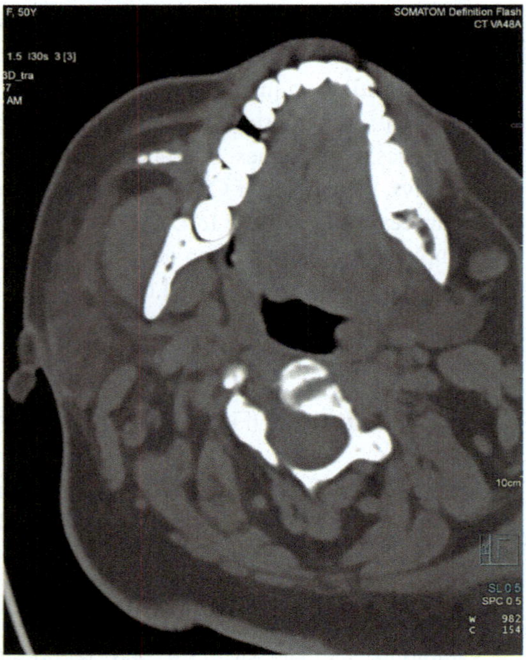

Fig. 35.2 Right parotid duct stone

35.3.3 Uveoparotid Fever (Heerfordt's Disease)

- Variant of sarcoidosis (seen in third to fourth decade).
- More common among women.
- Symptoms include parotitis, uveitis, CN VII paralysis in 50% of patients, sensorineural hearing loss, fever.
- Diagnosis confirmed with ACE levels.
- Treatment—steroids and ocular care.

35.3.4 Kuttner's Tumor (Chronic Sclerosing Sialadenitis)

- Autoimmune disease.
- Symptoms include firm, enlargement of the submandibular gland (can be mistaken as a malignancy), may be painful.
- Diagnosed on biopsy.
- Histopathology shows chronic inflammatory changes with destruction of acinar cells, sclerosis, and "cirrhotic" changes.
- Treatment is submandibular excision for diagnosis and treatment.

35.3.5 Sjogren's Syndrome

- Triad of symptoms: xerostomia, keratoconjunctivitis sicca, and a connective tissue disorder (rheumatoid arthritis in over 50% of the cases).
- Women are affected by Sjogren's syndrome more frequently than men.
- The parotid glands generally are enlarged bilaterally and the patient may have noticed a chronic progressive enlargement.
- Major histopathologic features are atrophy and loss of acinar tissue, with distortion of lobular architecture. Lymphoid infiltration occurs.

35.3.6 Recurrent Parotitis

Secondary to sialectasis, autoimmune disease (Mikulicz's disease, Sjogren's) or nonautoimmune (Mikulicz's syndrome—recurrent sialoadenitis, sialosis, multi-nodular gland).

35.3.7 Benign Lymphoepithelial Cysts

- Associated with HIV.
- Differential diagnosis—branchial cleft cyst, epidermoid cyst, dermoid cyst, mucocele, sialocele (pseudocyst).
- Treatment: aspiration or excision.

35.3.8 Necrotizing Sialometaplasia

- Inflammatory process that mimics malignancy.
- Presents as ulceration or nodular lesion of the minor salivary glands.
- Easy to mistake as malignancy histopathologically (pseudoepitheliomatous hyperplasia).
- Treatment: self-resolution.

35.4 Salivary Gland Neoplasms

Less than 2% are malignant.

Most neoplasms are in parotid 75%, most of them are benign.

	Frequency (%)	Malignant (%)
Parotid glands	65	25
Submandibular gl.	10	40
Sublingual gl.	< 1	90
Minor Salivary gl.	25	50

Fig. 35.3 Incidence of salivary gland tumors and percentage of malignancy according to localization

Rest equally distributed between submandibular gland (50% benign, 50% malignant) and minor salivary glands (most are malignant) (Fig. 35.3).

Tumors of the salivary gland

Benign	Malignant
Epithelial	
• Adenolymphoma (Warthin tumor)	• Mucoepidermoid carcinoma (low grade, high grade)
• Pleomorphic adenoma	• Cylindroma
• Oncocytoma	• Acinic cell carcinoma
• Other adenomas	• Adenocarcinoma
	• Malignant mixed tumor
	• Squamous cell carcinoma
	• Undifferentiated carcinoma
Mesenchymal	
• Hemangioma	• Lymphoma
• Lymphangioma	• Sarcoma
• Lipoma	
• Neurofibroma	

35.4.1 Benign Masses

35.4.1.1 Common Salivary Gland Tumors in Children

- Hemangioma.
- Pleomorphic adenoma (most common).
- Lymphangioma.
- Neurogenic.

35.4.1.2 Pleomorphic Adenoma

- Most common salivary gland tumor.
- Most common in parotid gland, 90% in superficial lobe.
- Slow growing tumor, usually unilateral, painless, firm mass, may progress rarely to cause dysphagia, dyspnea, hoarseness, facial nerve involvement.

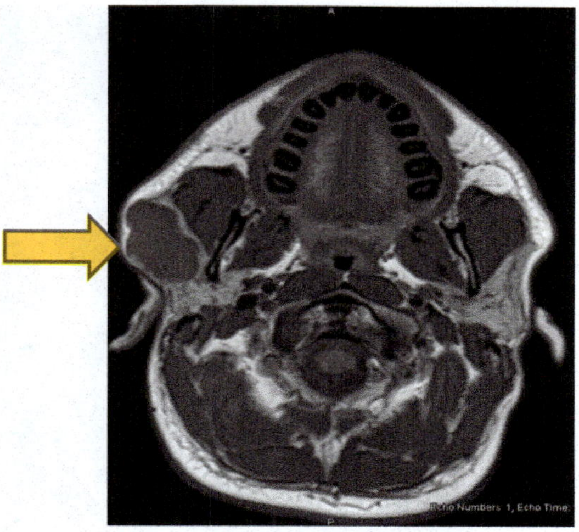

Fig. 35.4 T1 weighed MRI axial view of a case of right pleomorphic adenoma in an adult male

- Deep lobe involvement presents as intraoral swelling.
- Solitary vs. synchronous/metachronous neoplasms.
- Histopathology includes epithelial (varied growth patterns), mesenchymal (spindle-shaped nuclei) components and stromal component (myxoid, chondroid, fibroid, or osteoid components).
- Ten percent risk of malignancy after 15 years.
- Diagnosed by clinical presentation, MRI, FNA (Fig. 35.4 and 35.5).
- Treatment: complete surgical excision, avoid enucleation and tumor spill.

35.4.1.3 Warthin's Tumor (Papillary Cystadenoma Lymphomatosum)

Seen ONLY in the parotid gland.

Parotid is the last gland embryologically to be encapsulated.

The development of ectopic ductal epithelium within intraparotid lymph nodes, or hypersensitivity disease results in metaplasia of the duct.

Second most common tumor in the salivary gland.

- Risk factors: male sex, smoking.
- Ten percent bilateral, 10% multicentric.

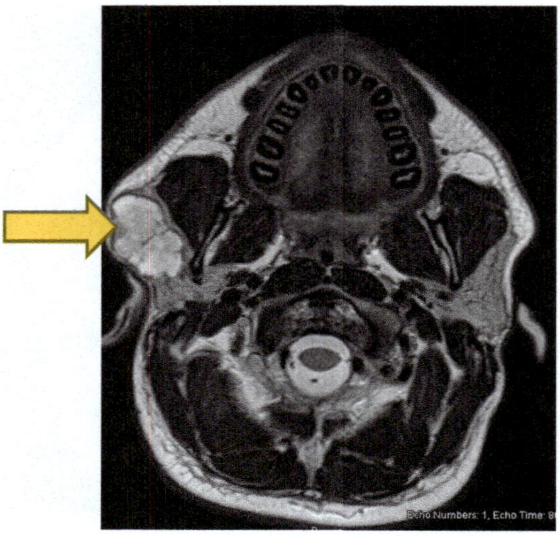

Fig. 35.5 T2 weighed MRI axial view of a case of right pleomorphic adenoma in an adult male

- Clinically presents as slow growing, painless, cystic, compressible mass.
- Biphasic composition (abundant lymphoid sheets and lining epithelium with bilayer of oncocytic papillary cells).
- No risk of malignancy.
- Diagnosed by biopsy, FNA, radiosialography.
- Treatment: surgical resection (superficial or deep parotidectomy).

35.4.1.4 Oncocytoma

- Most commonly in the parotid gland.
- Also known as oxyphilic adenoma.
- Slow growing, well circumscribed, but not encapsulated.
- High density of mitochondria with sheets of oncocytic cells (Technetium-99m scintigraphy).
- Treatment—surgical resection.

35.4.1.5 Monomorphic Adenoma

- Most commonly in minor salivary glands.
- No mesenchymal stromal component (unlike pleomorphic adenomas).
- Basal cell is the most common type.
- Other types: Clear cell, membranous, canalicular, myoepithelioma adenoma, glycogen-rich.

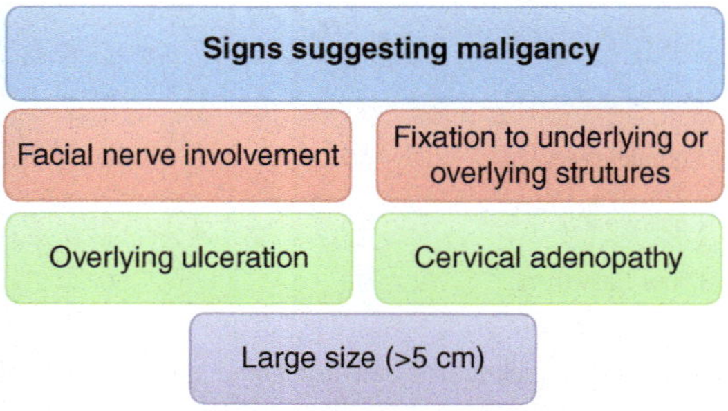

Fig. 35.6 Features suggesting malignancy

35.4.1.6 Hemangioma

- Benign.
- Usually discovered a few weeks after birth, enlarges for 6–12 months.
- But typically regress by second year of life.
- Fifty percent parotid hemangiomas are associated with cutaneous hemangiomas.
- two types—capillary and cavernous, capillary is more common, cavernous enlarges quickly and less chance of regression compared to capillary.

35.4.2 Salivary Gland Malignancies (Fig. 35.6)

35.4.2.1 Mucoepidermoid Carcinoma

- Most common salivary gland malignancy.
- Parotid most commonly, then minor salivary gland (palate), and submandibular gland.
- Low grade vs. high grade depends on mucinous-to-epidermoid cell ratio.
- Low grade: Higher amount of mucinous cells.
  - Similar to benign lesion but capable of local invasion and metastasis.
  - Seventy percent 5-year survival rate.
  - Treatment—surgical excision.
- High grade.
  - Low ratio of mucinous-to-epidermoid cells with high content of solid nests of cells.
  - Behaves similar to squamous cell carcinoma. Fifty percent 5-year survival rate.
  - Treatment—surgical excision with elective neck dissection (possible adjuvant radiation) (Fig.35.7).

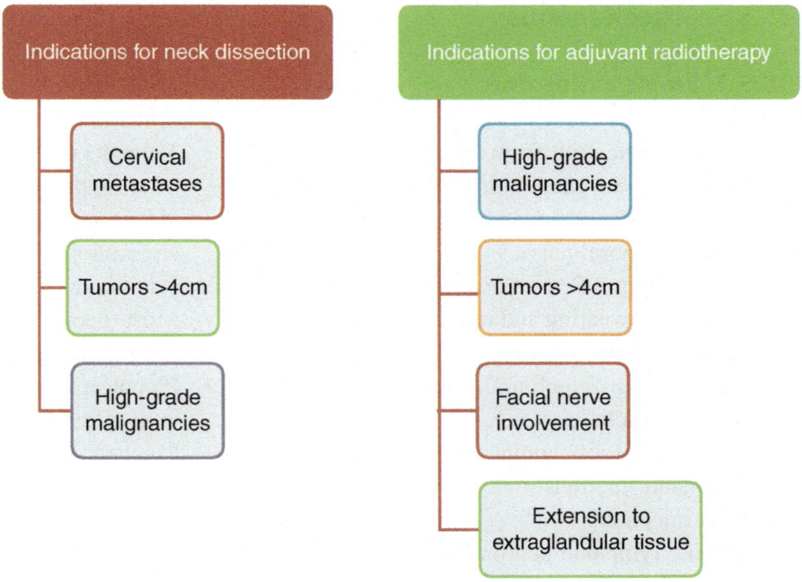

Fig. 35.7 Indications for neck dissection and for adjuvant radiotherapy in mucoepidermoid carcinoma

35.4.2.2 Adenoid Cystic Carcinoma

- Most common malignancy of submandibular gland and minor salivary glands.
- Also known as cylindroma.
- High-grade tumor with perineural spread.
- Three types:
  Solid: worst prognosis.
  Tubular: best prognosis.
  Cribriform: most common subtype and intermediate prognosis (swiss cheese appearance).
- Treatment: surgical resection. ± postoperative XRT.
- Prognosis: good 5-year survival, poor 10–15-year survival due to late metastasis to lungs.

35.4.2.3 Acinic Cell Carcinoma

- Second most common parotid and pediatric malignancy, low grade, better prognosis compared to adenoid cystic.
- Bilateral parotid disease in 3%.
- Derived from serous cells.
- Low-grade tumor.
- Treatment—surgical resection ± postoperative XRT.

35.4.2.4 Adenocarcinoma

- Most commonly in minor salivary glands.
- High grade and aggressive.
- Treatment—surgical resection with elective neck dissection (possible adjuvant radiation).

35.4.2.5 Polymorphous Low-Grade Adenocarcinoma

- Low grade.
- Second most common malignancy of the minor salivary gland (palate and buccal mucosa).
- Treatment—surgical resection.

35.4.2.6 Malignant Mixed Tumors

- High grade, aggressive, poor prognosis.
- Treatment is usually Resection + Post Op Radiotherapy ± Selective Neck Dissection.
- Types:
- Metastasizing Mixed Tumor: distinct from carcinoma ex-pleomorphic, remains histologically benign.
- Carcinosarcoma: contains components of both carcinomas and sarcomas.
- Noninvasive Carcinoma: carcinoma in situ within a pleomorphic adenoma.

35.4.2.7 Other Salivary Gland Malignancy Types

Squamous cell carcinoma, lymphomas, malignant oncocytoma, epithelial-myoepithelial carcinoma, salivary duct carcinoma.

35.5 Miscellaneous

35.5.1 Frey's Syndrome

- Gustatory sweating from aberrant reinnervation of post-ganglionic parasympathetic nerves to the sweat glands after injury to the auriculotemporal nerve.
- May occur upto 5 years post op.
- Presents as sweating and redness of the preauricular area during meals.
- Diagnosis with starch iodine test.
- Treatment includes:

  Medical: scopolamine, glycopyrrolate, diphemanil methylsulfate (anticholinergics), Botox injections

  Surgical: tympanic neuronectomy (controversial with high recurrence rates)

  Radiation therapy: for severe symptoms

35.5.2 Mucous Retention Cysts, Mucoceles, and Ranulas

- Pathophysiology: obstruction of minor salivatory glands (may be from trauma).
- *Mucous Retention Cyst:* it is a true cyst of the minor salivary glands (lined with epithelial layer).
- *Ranula:* mucous retention cyst of the floor of mouth, usually from the sublingual gland.
- *Plunging Ranula:* ranula that extends into the cervical tissues.
- *Mucocele:* not a true cyst, extravasation of mucus into soft tissue.
- Clinically presents as a cystic mass on floor of mouth, lip, buccal mucosa, or minor salivary gland.
- Diagnosed through clinical history and exam, excisional biopsy.
- Treatment is excision or marsupialization.
- *Benign Lymphoepithelial Cysts:* Presents as asymptomatic, multiple parotid cysts, can be bilateral, mostly in HIV patients.
- Diagnosed by clinical exam, FNA.
- Treatment can be aspiration or excision, antiviral therapy in HIV may cause regression, doxycycline can also be used (limited).

Take Home Messages

- Most salivary glands lesions are of an inflammatory origin.
- Mumps virus is the most common cause of acute parotid enlargement.
- Ninety percent of submandibular calculi are radiopaque while 90% of parotid calculi are radiolucent.
- Most neoplasms are in parotid 75%, most of them are benign.
- Pleomorphic adenoma is the most common salivary gland tumor.
- Mucoepidermoid carcinoma is the most common salivary gland malignancy.
- Adenoid cystic carcinoma is the most common malignancy of submandibular gland and minor salivary glands.
- Epithelial tumors are the most frequently encountered (>80%) salivary glands tumor, mesenchymal tumors which are a very mixed group (<20%), and hematolymphoid tumors (lymphoma and plasmacytoma) making up the rest.

Further Reading

1. Flint PW, Cummings CW. Cummings otolaryngology head & neck surgery. Maryland Heights: Mosby/Elsevier; 2010.
2. Parkin DM, Ferlay J, Curado MP, et al. Fifty years of cancer incidence: CI5 I-IX. Int J Cancer. 2010;127(12):2918–27.
3. Carvalho AL, Nishimoto IN, Califano JA, Kowalski LP. Trends in incidence and prognosis for head and neck cancer in the United States: a site-specific analysis of the SEER database. Int J Cancer. 2005;114(5):806–16.
4. Barnes EL, Eveson JW, Reichart P, Sidransky D. Pathology and genetics of head and neck tumours. In: Kleihues P, Sobin LH, editors. World Health Organization classification of tumours. Lyon: IARC Press; 2005.
5. Barnes L, Eveson JW, Reichart P, Sidransky D. Pathology and genetics of head and neck Tumours. Lyon: IARC Press; 2005.
6. Saunders JR Jr, Hirata RM, Jaques DA. Salivary glands. Surg Clin North Am. 1986;66(1):59–81.

7. Zou ZJ, Wang SL, Zhu JR, Wu QG, Yu SF. Chronic obstructive parotitis. Report of ninety-two cases. Oral Surg Oral Med Oral Pathol. 1992;73(4):434–40.
8. O'Brien CJ, Murrant NJ. Surgical management of chronic parotitis. Head Neck. 1993;15(5):445–9.
9. Levy DM, Remine WH, Devine KD. Salivary gland calculi. Pain, swelling associated with eating. JAMA. 1962;181:1115–9.
10. Epker BN. Obstructive and inflammatory diseases of the major salivary glands. Oral Surg Oral Med Oral Pathol. 1972;33(1):2–27.
11. Stenner M, Klussmann JP. Current update on established and novel biomarkers in salivary gland carcinoma pathology and the molecular pathways involved. Eur Arch Otorhinolaryngol. 2009;266(3):333–41.
12. Rogers J, McCaffrey TV. Inflammatory disorders of the salivary glands. In: Flint PW, Haughey BH, Lund VJ, et al., editors. Cummings otolaryngology head and neck surgery. 5th ed. Philadelphia: Mosby Elsevier; 2010. p. 1151–61.

An Approach to Neck Masses

36

Suzan Saeed Mohamed, Abhishek Menon, and Waheed Rahman

Key Points

- Ultrasonography is used in all cases of thyroid enlargement and in differentiating solid from cystic masses.
- Branchial cleft cysts most commonly occur in the second or third decades.
- Thyroglossal duct cysts elevate on protrusion of the tongue.
- Biopsy is contraindicated in carotid body tumors. MRI angiography is the investigation of choice.
- *Superficial parotidectomy* is considered as a diagnostic and therapeutic for most benign tumors of the parotid gland.

36.1 Introduction

The neck is the transitional area, the clavicles inferiorly and the base of the skull superiorly. It serves as a major conduit for the various vascular, neurological, and musculoskeletal structures between the head, trunk, and limbs and also the aerodigestive tract. The neck can be subdivided into various triangles and its subdivisions; it can be divided into zones/levels, all based on multiple landmarks, some of which will be discussed in this chapter.

S. S. Mohamed · A. Menon · W. Rahman (✉)
Hamad Medical Corporation, Doha, Qatar
e-mail: mohamed50@hamad.qa;
AMenon1@hamad.qa; wrahman@hamad.qa

36.2 An Approach to the Neck Mass

Our approach involves an understanding of two basic factors:

1. *Anatomy*—major structures of the neck and lymph nodes of the neck.
2. *Pathology* that may arise in the above structures, i.e., the differential diagnosis.

36.2.1 Prominent Landmarks

1. Hyoid bone
2. Thyroid cartilage
3. Cricoid cartilage
4. Trachea
5. Sternocleidomastoid muscle
6. Clavicle

A. Al-Qahtani et al. (eds.), *Textbook of Clinical Otolaryngology*,
https://doi.org/10.1007/978-3-030-54088-3_36

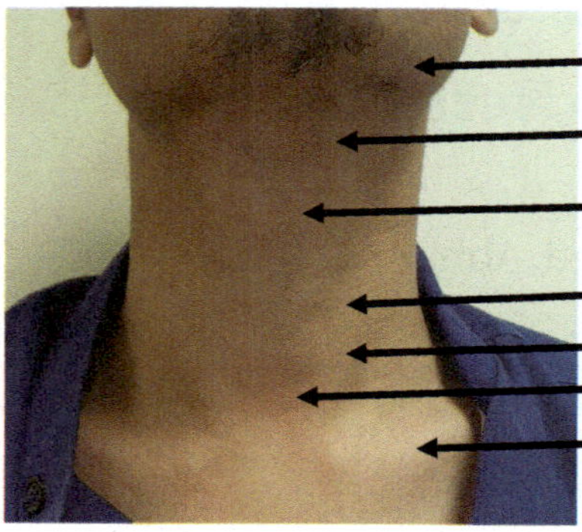

36.2.2 Triangles of the Neck

Anterior

1. Anterior border of the SCM, midline, lower border of the mandible
2. Subdivisions: submandibular, submental, carotid, muscular

Posterior

1. Posterior border of SCM, clavicle, anterior border of trapezius
2. Subdivisions: subclavian, occipital

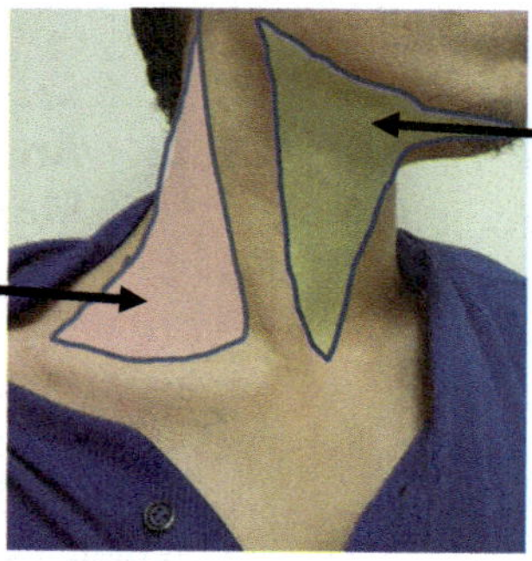

36.2.3 Lymph Node Levels of the Neck

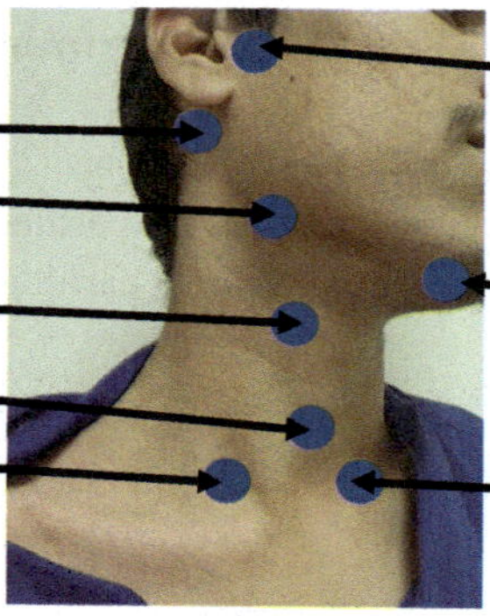

36.3 Differential Diagnosis

- Congenital (developmental), inflammatory or neoplastic.
- 2–9% of head and neck cancers present as cervical masses without a known primary.
- Up to 80% of neck masses that occur outside the thyroid are neoplastic in adults over the age of 40 years.

Differential diagnosis of neck masses

Development	Infectious	Benign neoplasm	Malignancies	Other
– Thyroglossal cyst – Branchial cleft cyst – Inclusion cyst – Congenital vascular malformation – Cystic hygroma – Laryngocele – Bronchogenic cyst – Teratoma	– Viral (EBV, CMV, HIV) – Bacterial (strep. pyogenes, staph. aureus) – Fungal (histoplasmosis) – Protozoal (toxoplasmosis)	– Thyroid nodule – Lipoma – Fibroma – Parathyroid adenoma – Sebaceous cyst – Neurofibroma – Benign salivary tumor (pleomorphic adenoma, Warthin's tumors)	– Thyroid cancer – Lymphoma – Carotid body tumor – Parathyroid carcinoma – Malignant salivary gland (mucoepidermoid)	– Sjogren syndrome – Sarcoidosis – Sialolithiasis

36.4 The Patient Presented with Neck Lump, Swelling, or Mass, What Is Your Workup?

- *History Age:*

Neck masses in children and young adults are more commonly inflammatory than congenital, and rarely neoplastic. In adults always there is suspicion to be neoplastic.

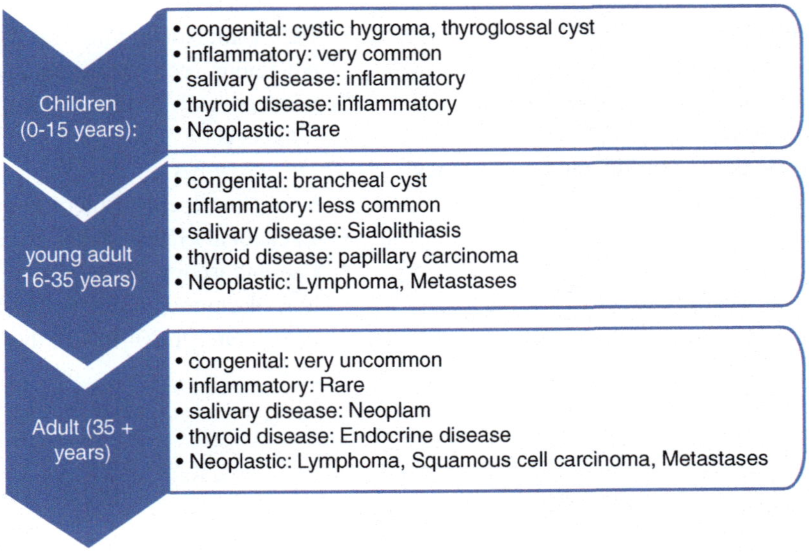

36.4.1 Duration

- Inflammatory disorders are usually acute in onset and resolve within 6 weeks.
- Cervical lymphadenitis is often associated with recent upper tract infection.
- Congenital masses are often present from birth as small masses, which enlarge rapidly after mild upper respiratory tract infection.
- Metastatic carcinoma tends to have a short history of progressive enlargement.

36.4.2 Others

- Family Hx: cancer, TB, etc.
- Social Hx: smoking, alcohol, and history of travel and contact.

36.5 Examination

- *Physical examination*
  - General examination: vital sign, the general condition of the patient
  - Full head and neck examination include:
    The oral cavity, oropharynx, hypopharynx and nasopharynx
    Palpation of the neck (all levels and thyroid gland)
    Laryngeal examination: fibro-optic.
    Cranial nerves.
    Assessment of the swelling, mass or lumps: relation to muscles, trachea, and hyoid bone.
    The location, mobility, and consistency of a neck mass.

36.6 Some of the Features Raise Suspicion of Malignancy

1. Voice change
2. Odynophagia
3. Dysphagia
4. Hemoptysis
5. Previous radiation
6. Oral lesions, recent trauma, globus sensation
7. Constitutional symptoms (e.g., night sweats, anorexia, weight loss)
8. Unilateral nasal discharge or epistaxis
9. Family history of cancer and previous tumors

36.7 Diagnostic Tools

1. *Blood Investigations*:
   - Full blood count
   - Throat swab: occasionally helpful but must be sent immediately in the proper medium
   - Viral serology: Epstein–Barr virus, HPV, cytomegalovirus, and toxoplasmosis
   - Thyroid function tests
2. *Images:*
   - Ultrasonography is used in all cases of thyroid enlargement and in differentiating solid from cystic masses.
   - Chest X-ray in smokers with a persistent neck lump.
   - CT scan and MRI to determine the extent of the masses.
   - PET scan: Not first line, used for metastatic squamous cell carcinoma of unknown primary and further workup for known diagnosis.
3. *Tissue diagnosis*
   - FNA (fine needle aspieration)
   - Excisional / incisional biopsy
   - Pan-endoscopy and biopsy
   - Tonsillectomy (tonsils are found to be the primary source in 20–40% of these patients)

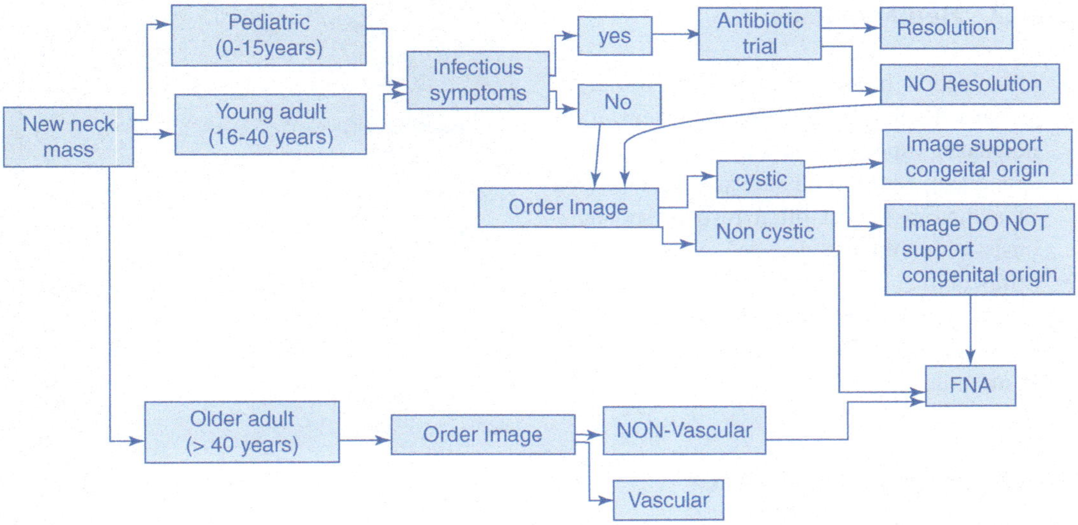

36.8 Treatment Differs According to the Diagnosis

36.8.1 Cystic Hygroma (Lymphangiomas)

- It is a congenital lesion usually present within the first year of life (posterior triangle).
- Usually, remain unchanged into adulthood.
- Is soft, cystic, multilocular, partially compressible, and brilliantly transilluminate and may present with pressure effects.
- CT or MRI may help define the extent of the neoplasm.
- Treatment includes injection with picibanil or excision of easily accessible lesions or those affecting vital functions.

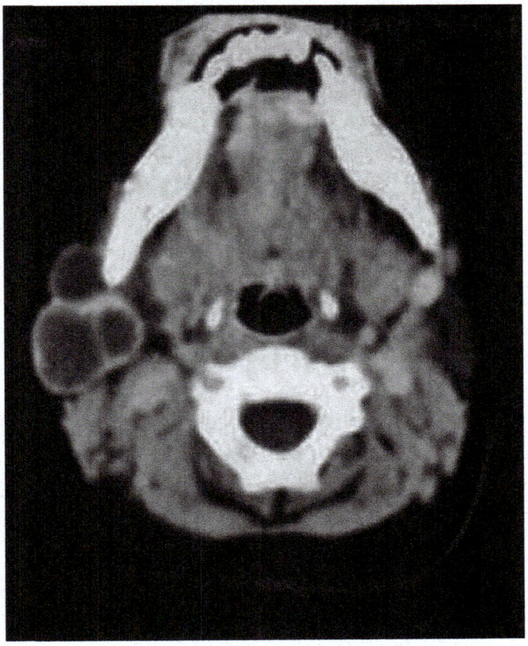

36.8.2 Hemangiomas

- Often appear bluish and are compressible.
- CT or MRI may help define the extent of the neoplasm, especially intrathoracic.
- Treatment: (depend on site, size, and severity of symptoms) most often resolve spontaneously within the first decade.
- Surgical treatment is reserved for lesions with rapid growth involving vital structures, which fail medical therapy (laser or oral propranolol in infantile type).

36.8.3 Branchial Cleft Cysts

- Remnant of branchial cleft (second).
- Most commonly occur in the second or third decades.
- Pain +/- (severe throbbing pain, can be painless).
- Usually presents as a smooth, fluctuant non-tender (or tender), non-transluminal mass mobile forwards and downwards, underlying the anterior border of the SCM muscle.
- Branchial fistula or sinus.
- Primary treatment is with control of infection by antibiotics, followed by surgical excision.

36.8.4 Thyroglossal Duct Cyst

- This is a common congenital midline neck mass.
- Can present as a mass in the lateral edge of the thyroid cartilage.
- Pain and tenderness +/-.
- During clinical examintion, swelling can be moved transversally but cannot be moved vertically.
- Elevates on protrusion of the tongue.
- Treatment is with initial control of infection with antibiotics, followed by surgical excision, including the mid-portion of the body of the hyoid bone (Sistrunk's procedure). Occasionally, these lesions become infected and resolve or persist following surgery as a thyroglossal fistula.

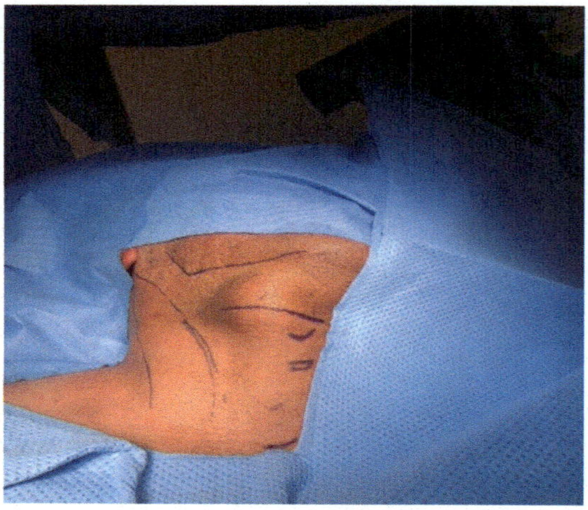

36.8.5 Sebaceous Cysts

- These are common masses often occurring in older people but can occur at any age.
- They are slow-growing, but sometimes fluctuant and painful when infected.
- Diagnosis is made clinically; the skin overlying the mass is adherent, and a punctum is often identified.
- Excisional biopsy confirms the diagnosis.

36.8.6 Cervical Lymphadenopathy

- Acute lymphadenitis present as tender swelling
- Antibiotic trial, less acute inflammatory nodes generally regress in size over 2–6 weeks. If lymph node did not subside then biopsy of the lymph node is advised.

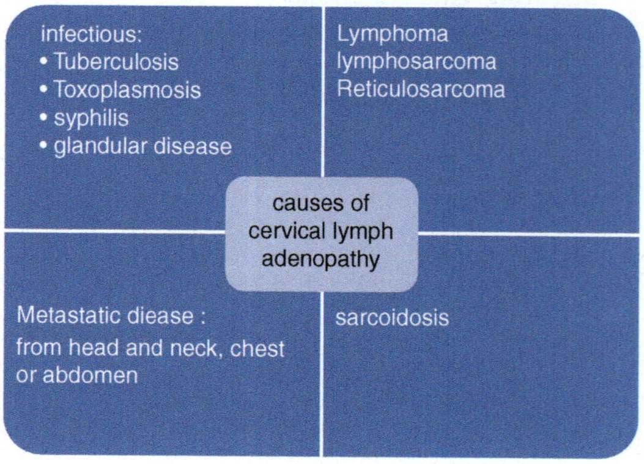

36.8.6.1 TB Cervical Lymphadenitis

- Upper and middle deep cervical LN
- Onset: gradually
- Pain: +/-
- Systemic symptoms unusual in young (patients with abscess (painful, increase size, and skin discoloration))
- Mass: indistinct, firm, matted, fluctuate in case of abcess collection
- Treatment with anti-TB (6–9 months)
  - Rifampicin
  - Ethambutol
  - INH
  - Pyrazinamide

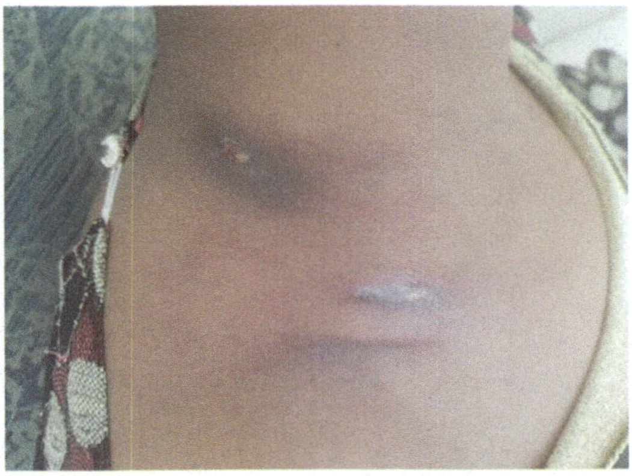

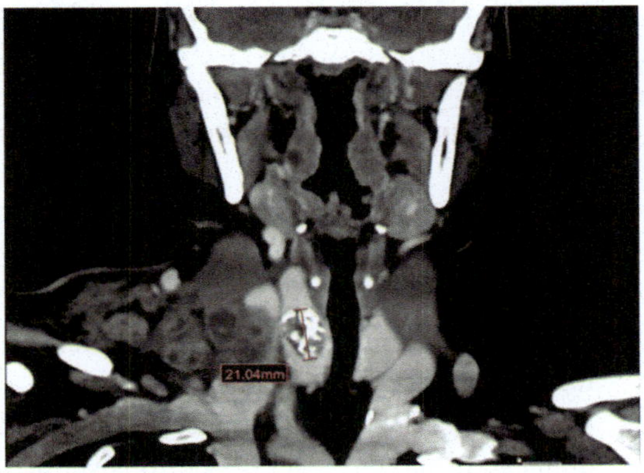

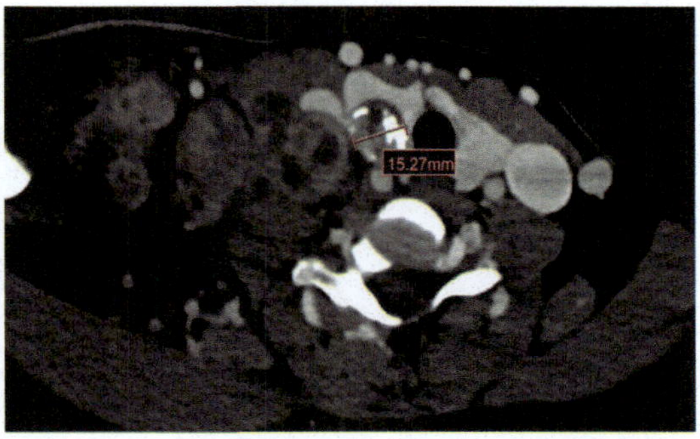

Coronal and axial CT neck with contrast for a patient with TB lymphadenitis

36.8.7 Carotid Body Tumor

- Rare tumor of chemoreceptors (age of presentation: 40–60 years).
- Slow-growing painless sometimes pulsating lump, may be bilateral.
- During examination: mass can be moved side to side.
- Symptoms of transient cerebral ischemia
- Potato tumors (hard, non-tender)
- Palpation may induce a vasovagal attack.
- Biopsy is contraindicated: MRI angiography is the investigation of choice.
- Surgical removal is based on patient presenting symptoms.

36.8.8 Pharyngeal Pouch

- Diverticulum of the pharynx through the gap between the horizontal fibers of the cricopharyngeus muscle inferiorly and the lowermost oblique fibers of the inferior constrictor muscle superiorly.
- History of halitosis regurgitation of froth and food. There is no bile or acid taste to it.
- Pressure on the swelling causes gurgling sounds and regurgitation.
- Treatment: cricopharyngeal myotomy.

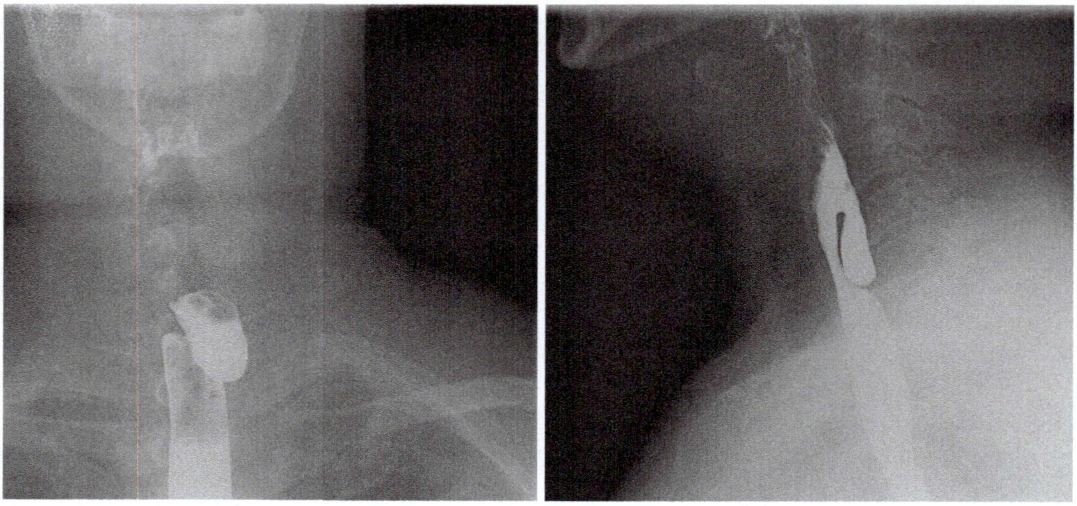

Anteroposterior and lateral view of barium swallow in a pharyngeal pouch

36.8.9 Thyroid Masses

- Thyroid neoplasms are a common cause of anterior compartment neck masses in all age groups, with a female predominance and are mostly benign.
- Ultrasound and fine needle aspiration of thyroid masses have become the standard of care.
- Unsatisfactory aspirates should be repeated, and negative aspirates should be followed up with a repeat FNAC and examination in 3 months time.

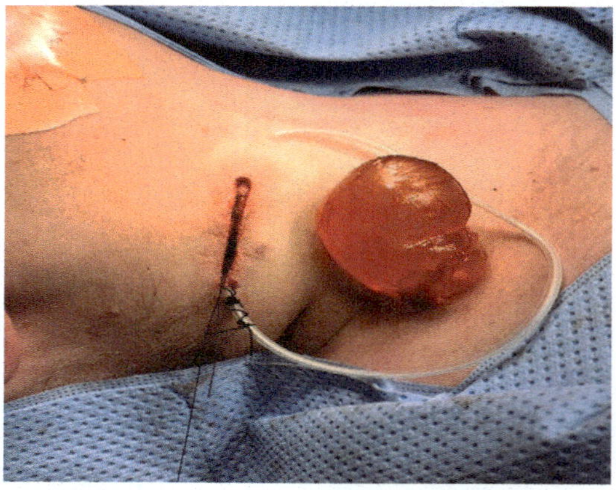

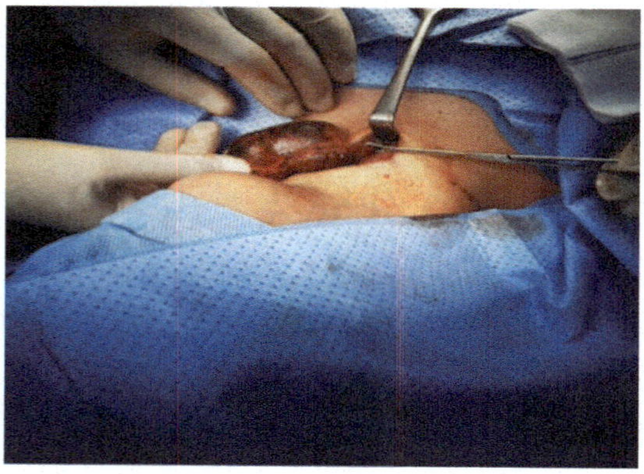

36.8.10 Ludwig's Angina

- Rare but serious connective tissue infection of the floor of the mouth
- Mostly due to dental infections
- Signs of inflammation present (pain, swelling, redness, tendrenss and fluctuation)
- Treatment: priority to protect the airway, drainage of the pus + antibiotic to cover aerobes and anaerobe

36.8.11 Salivary Gland Neoplasm

1. Major salivary gland
   (a) Parotid gland
   (b) Submandibular gland
   (c) Sublingual gland
2. Minor salivary gland
   - 600–1000 minor salivary glands distributed throughout the mucosa of the upper aerodigestive tract (more common in the soft and hard palate).
   - 80% of salivary gland tumors occur in the parotid.
   - 10–15% in the minor salivary gland.
   - 5–10% in the submandibular gland.
   - 80% of the parotid tumors are benign.
   - The most common benign parotid neoplasm is pleomorphic adenoma.
   - 50% of the submandibular gland tumors are benign.
   - 30% of the minor salivary gland tumors are benign.

36.8.11.1 The Most Common Benign Tumor of the Parotid

- Pleomorphic adenoma (benign mixed tumor)
- Warthin's tumor (papillary cyst adenoma lymphomatosum)
- Monomorphic adenoma
  – Basal cell adenoma
  – Canalicular adenomas
  – Oncocytoma
  – Myoepitheliomas
- Granular cell tumor
- Hemangioma
- *FNA* (fine needle aspiration) The accuracy is around 90% depending on the techniques of aspirate and the cytopathologist.
- *Superficial parotidectomy* is considered as a diagnostic and therapeutic for most benign tumors.

36.8.11.2 The Most Common Malignant Neoplasm of the Parotid Gland

1. Mucoepidermoid carcinoma—40%
2. Adenoid cystic carcinoma—10%
3. Acinic cell carcinoma—10–15%
   It is considered a low-grade tumor.
4. Malignant mixed tumor—7%
   It is considered a high-grade malignancy.
5. Polymorphous low-grade adenocarcinoma—10%
   It is a low-grade variant of adenocarcinoma.
6. Adenocarcinoma—10%
   It is a high-grade with poor prognosis.
7. Squamous cell carcinoma—4%
   It is high-grade, more common in elderly patients

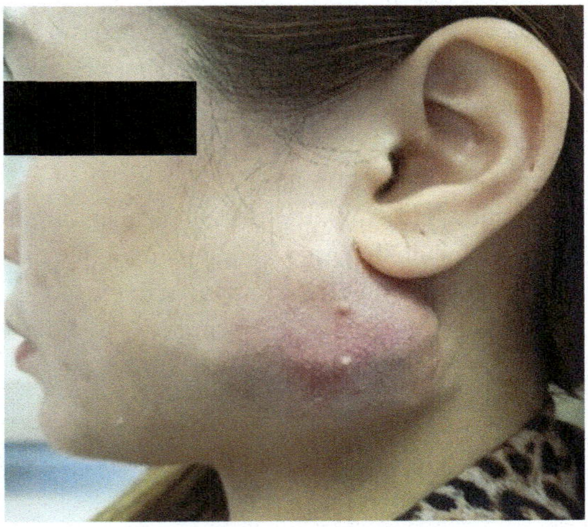

*A case of pleomorphic carcinoma invading the skin

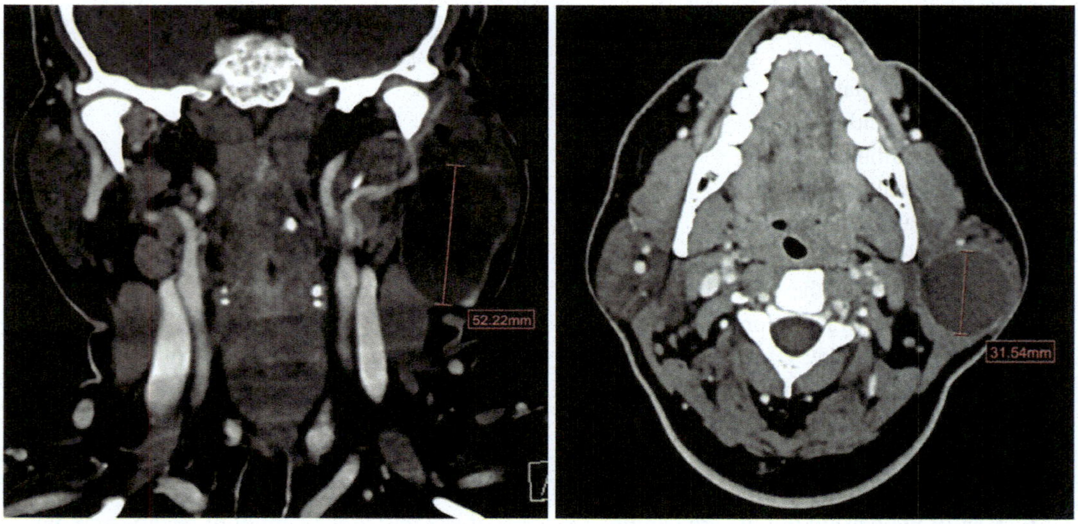

Coronal and axial CT with contrast for left parotid mass

36.8.12 Metastatic Lymph Nodes

- Upper cervical lymph nodes (upper aerodigestive tract).
- Accessory chain of nodes in the posterior triangle (nasopharyngeal malignancies).
- In many cases (occult primary), most common sites are tonsil, base of the tongue, nasopharynx, and pyriform sinus.
- Virchow's LN (left supraclavicular lymph node): abdomen and thoracic malignancies painless, non-tender, and hard masses.
- Workup: Search for primary, treatment according to the primary disease.

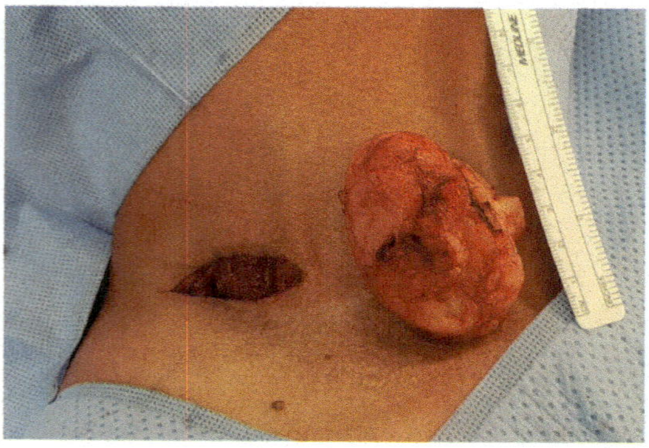

36.8.12.1 Characteristics of Malignant Neck Lumps

Lymphomas

- Painless lump, non-tender, smooth, and discrete slow growing.
- Patient presented with malaise, weight loss, pallor, fever, rigor, and hepatosplenomegaly.
- Abdomen pressure on IVC (inferior venacava) may cause bilateral leg edema, other lymph nodes in the axilla, groin, and abdomen should be examined.
- Treatment: according to the stage:
  - Chemotherapy.
  - Radiation therapy.
  - Immunotherapy.

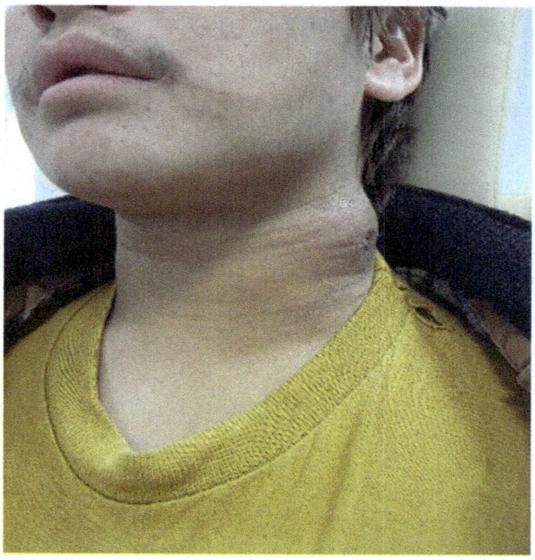

Take-Home Messages

- Neck masses are common and most often due to lymphadenopathy secondary to a self-limited infection or inflammation.
- Basic knowledge of neck anatomy and structures is required.
- Thorough history and examination usually suggest a diagnosis.
- In the differential diagnosis, the three most important categories to distinguish are: infective/inflammatory, congenital, and neoplastic masses.
- Appropriate investigations may be performed at a GP (General practitioner) or specialist level.
- Reasonable first-line management for a suspected infective/inflammatory mass is a course of a broad-spectrum antibiotic with referral to a specialist if the mass does not resolve within 2–4 weeks.
- All suspected neoplastic and congenital masses should be referred for specialist attention.

Further Reading

1. Flint PW, Haughey BH, Robbins KT, Thomas JR, Niparko JK, Lund VJ, Lesperance MM Cummings otolaryngology - head and neck surgery E-Book: head and neck surgery.
2. National Comprehensive Cancer Network clinical practice guidelines in oncology: thyroid carcinoma version 2.2013
3. Cooper DS, et al. Revised American Thyroid Association management guidelines for patients with thyroid nodules and differentiated thyroid cancer: the American Thyroid Association (ATA) guidelines taskforce on thyroid nodules and differentiated thyroid cancer. Thyroid. 2009;19(11):1167–214.
4. Current surgical therapy: management of thyroid nodules
5. Philip S, et al. Current surgical therapy: evaluation of the isolated neck mass.
6. Pierce, Niel. Surgery at a glance. 5th ed.

Principles of Management of Head and Neck Cancers

37

Anil K. D'Cruz, Richa Vaish, and Harsh Dhar

37.1 Introduction

Head and neck cancers is a term synonymous with the squamous cell carcinomas arising from the mucosal surfaces of the oral cavity, pharynx (oropharynx, hypopharynx), larynx and nasal cavity/paranasal sinuses. They are the seventh leading cause of cancer worldwide accounting for nearly 900,000 new cases and 450,000 deaths annually [1]. The majority of these cancers are a result of tobacco and alcohol abuse. With their decreasing consumption in parts of the developed world, there is lowering in the incidence of these cancers. Parallel to this, the last decade has witnessed a rise in the incidence of oropharyngeal cancers attributed to infection with human papillomavirus (HPV) type 16 and 18 [2]. HPV-related cancers are the cause of 60–70% of oropharyngeal cancers in the developed world. This change is not apparent in low- and middle-income countries where oropharyngeal cancers are still primarily tobacco related [3]. HPV-related cancers are recognized as a distinct biological entity with differences in epidemiology, pathophysiology and responses to treatment (discussed in Chap. 38). This chapter aims to conceptualize the overall principles of management of head and neck cancers in light of recent developments. Because of their unique characteristics, nasopharyngeal cancers are distinct and are covered in detail in a separate section.

- Natural history of the disease
- Evaluation and diagnosis
- Treatment philosophy
- Principles of management of head and neck cancers
- Management of recurrent/metastatic cancers
- Recent advances

A. K. D'Cruz (✉)
Apollo Group of Hospitals,
Mumbai, Delhi, Chennai, India

Department of Oncology, Apollo Hospital,
Navi Mumbai, Maharashtra, India

R. Vaish
Department of Head and Neck Oncology, Tata Memorial Hospital, Mumbai, Maharashtra, India

Department of Head and Neck Oncology, Homi Bhabha National Institute,
Mumbai, Maharashtra, India

H. Dhar
Department of Head and Neck Oncology, Narayana Superspeciality Hospitals,
Howrah, West Bengal, India

A. Al-Qahtani et al. (eds.), *Textbook of Clinical Otolaryngology*,
https://doi.org/10.1007/978-3-030-54088-3_37

37.2 Natural History of the Disease

Tobacco-related head and neck cancers develop after years of substance abuse through a well-defined tumour progression model [4]. Dysplastic and molecularly altered changes occur in the entire upper aerodigestive tract exposed to the carcinogenic effects of tobacco. This phenomenon, termed as field cancerization proposed initially by Slaughter [5], predisposes patients to the development of second primary cancers. In contrast, HPV-related oropharyngeal cancers occur de novo in normal mucosa and therefore do not have the increased risk of second primary cancers.

Second primary cancers occur following treatment of the index cancer at the rate of 1–5% per year [6]. The cumulative risk at 20 years varies to as high as 25–40% and more so if patients persist with their addictions [7–9]. These tumours occur in the head and neck region, oesophagus or lung. They could be simultaneous (diagnosed at the time of index cancers), synchronous (within 6 months of diagnosis of index cancers) or metachronous (6 months after diagnosis of index cancers). This must be kept in mind during workup and follow-up.

37.3 Diagnostic Workup

Treatment is primarily influenced by a) patient-related factors—comorbidities, performance status, medical/family history; b) tumour factors—tumour characteristics (HPV status) and extent of disease. Diagnostic workup is therefore directed towards these two areas to help glean maximum information in an attempt to select the best treatment, improve outcomes and limit morbidity.

(a) *Patient-related factors*: A thorough history of disease-related information and addictions/substance abuse is elicited. Associated comorbidities which occur in as high as 20–50% of patients must be sought for as it has a bearing on treatment decisions [10, 11]. Fanconi's anaemia, ataxia telangiectasia, xeroderma pigmentosa and immunosuppressive states are known to predispose to head and neck cancers and appropriate history must be elucidated. Dental history and examination of dental hygiene such as sharp teeth, ill-fitting dentures and dental caries are important.

(b) *Tumour factors*: Diagnosis is established by a punch biopsy avoiding obviously necrotic areas in the majority of head and neck tumours. Imaging is preferably performed prior to biopsy in obvious cases to avoid biopsy-induced artefacts. This is particularly important before positron emission tomography (PET) imaging to avoid false positives as the consequence of inflammation. Fine needle aspiration biopsy is a useful alternative in deep-seated inaccessible lesions and for neck nodes. Open node biopsy is to be avoided as it violates tissue planes and may cause tumour spillage. Excisional biopsy of nodes is done only when more material is needed for further studies (immunohistochemistry (IHC), microbiology, etc.).

Assessment of HPV status is particularly important for oropharyngeal cancers and patients who present with unknown primary. p16 IHC staining because of its simplicity and easy availability is recommended to establish HPV infection. The expression should be present both at the cytoplasmic and nuclear level with an intensity of +2/3 and a diffuse overexpression of 75% to be considered as positive. HPV DNA (deoxyribonucleic acid) in situ hybridization (ISH) and polymerase chain reaction (PCR) tests have a greater specificity but are not routinely used due to cost, the complexity of the procedure and the need for the fresh tissue [12].

Assessment of the extent of disease is important to stage and plan treatment. The mucosal spread is best evaluated endoscopically, usually an office procedure. Direct/microlaryngoscopic evaluation is required for glottic cancers and to evaluate blind spots, e.g. post cricoid region and apex of the pyriform fossa. Evaluation under anaesthesia is useful when flexible endoscopy and imaging are incongruous with clinical findings, e.g. root of tongue involvement. Imaging gives the true deep extent of disease. Contrast enhanced computed tomography (CECT) is the workhorse and is the investigation of choice in the majority of head and neck tumours. It is excellent for assessment of cortical bone and cartilage involvement and also has a high sensitivity for neck nodes. Magnetic resonance imaging (MRI) with its better soft tissue delineation is usually preferred for the tongue, floor of the mouth and oropharyngeal cancers. It is ideal for perineural spread, dural/intraorbital involvement and marrow infiltration. Its limitation is that early cartilage and bone erosion may be overestimated. Involvement of skull base, encasement of the internal carotid artery, infiltration of prevertebral fascia and mediastinal extension of the disease are definite signs of inoperability [13].

PET scan is indicated when there is a high likelihood of distant metastasis (locally advanced disease (T4), large bulky nodes (N2/N3), lower level nodes (levels III/IV), hypopharyngeal cancers and recurrent tumours) [14]. In cost constraint settings, a CECT thorax is a suitable replacement given that the lung is the most common site of distant metastasis. Kim et al. demonstrated that the detection rates for pulmonary metastasis between PET CT and CECT thorax were essentially the same [15]. PET CT scan is also indicated for response assessment following chemoradiotherapy (CRT) which is ideally performed 12 weeks after completion of treatment to avoid false positive finding [16]. Given its very high negative predictive value in this setting, a negative PET can be interpreted as the absence of disease with upwards of 90% surety [17].

PET scan is also the imaging modality of choice for an unknown primary and helps identify the site of origin in 25–50% of cases [18, 19]. Blind biopsies which were in vogue in the past are to be deprecated and should be directed based on imaging findings. With changing epidemiology, 90% of patients presenting with an unknown primary are HPV associated of oropharyngeal origin [12] and establishing HPV status is useful. Some authors recommend a routine tonsillectomy (unilateral/bilateral) and carpet excision of the ipsilateral base of tongue which can locate the primary in as high as 90% of cases [20]. Another site commonly associated with the unknown primary is the nasopharynx which is often Epstein–Barr Virus (EBV) associated. Detecting EBV encoded RNA (EBER) with ISH helps establish a nasopharyngeal primary [12].

37.4 Pathology

World health organization (WHO) describes various histological variants of SCC, namely acantholytic, adenosquamous, basaloid, cuniculatum, papillary, spindle cell or sarcomatoid and verrucous carcinoma. Although having specific pathological characteristics and disease biology, these variants are all essentially treated similarly [21]. Verrucous cancers are unique in that differentiating them from verrucous hyperplasia is often difficult and deep biopsies may need to be performed to obtain representative sections demonstrating invasion of the basement membrane (essential prerequisite to establish cancer). Up to 10–20% of verrucous carcinoma may be hybrid and reveal foci of SCC on final histology.

Histopathology is preferably reported by dedicated pathologists and captured in a synoptic reporting proforma to ensure recording of essential parameters to prognosticate and plan treatment. Histological parameters are best captured under the headings of essential, desirable and optional (Table 37.1).

37.5 Current American Joint Committee on Cancer (AJCC) Staging Eighth Edition Highlighting Major Stages

The current staging system followed is the eighth edition AJCC TNM staging system [22]. This replaced the seventh edition from 2018 [23]. The major changes are in the T stage of oral cancers

Table 37.1 Synoptic pathology report of head and neck tumours

Essential	Desirable	Optional
• T stage – Size (bidimensional) – Depth of invasion • Contiguous structure involvement – Skin – Muscle – Bone – Cartilage • Nodes – Size – Number (positive/total nodes harvested) – Level – Extra nodal extension • p16 IHC for HPV status in oropharyngeal cancer	• Tumour morphology – Endophytic – Exophytic – Ulcerative – Infiltrative • Grade • Lymphovascular invasion • Perineural invasion/spread • Extra nodal extension – Microscopic (≤2 mm) – Macroscopic (>2 mm) • Worst pattern of invasion (WPOI) • Histological variants of SCC	• EGFR expression • Markers of immunotherapy when relevant (e.g. PDL1, PD1)

and N stage of head and neck cancers. In addition, HPV-related oropharyngeal cancer is recognized as a separate entity with a dedicated staging.

Depth of invasion (DOI) has been incorporated into the T stage of oral cancers. DOI is different from tumour thickness and is measured as the perpendicular line dropped from the basement membrane of the most adjacent normal mucosa to the deepest point of invasion. This line is also referred to as the 'plumb line'. The restaging defines the tumours which are ≤2 cm in greatest dimension with DOI ≤5 mm as T1; tumours >2 cm and ≤4 cm in the greatest dimension with DOI ≤10 mm and ≤2 cm in greatest dimension with DOI >5 mm and ≤10 mm as T2; tumours >4 cm in greatest dimension with DOI ≤10 mm and ≤4 cm in the greatest dimension with DOI >10 mm as T3; and tumours >4 cm in greatest dimension with DOI >10 mm considered now as T4 [22].

The other important change is in the N stage with the incorporation of extranodal extension (ENE). ENE is defined as the extension of the carcinoma through the fibrous capsule of the node into the surrounding tissue. Presence of ENE upstages nodal disease to N2 if the size is ≤3 cm and to N3 if nodal size >3 cm. Both minor and major ENE are at present given similar importance but the AJCC task force recommends capture and documentation of ENE as minor <2 mm and major >2 mm from the capsule. Studies have shown a difference in outcomes with minor and major ENE and hence the need to capture this data which might be of help to modify staging subsequently [24]. ENE places the patients into a high-risk group and warrants adjuvant chemoradiotherapy.

With the growing evidence that HPV-related oropharyngeal cancers are a biologically different disease with better prognosis, the new staging system identifies these tumours as distinct and accords a separate staging system. Carcinoma in situ (Tis) and subdivision of T4a and T4b have been removed from HPV positive cancer. N staging for HPV cancers has undergone significant change with separate clinical and pathological N staging. Metastatic neck nodes ipsilateral single or multiple ≤6 cm is classified as N1 while bilateral/contralateral nodes ≤6 cm are staged as N2. Any node >6 cm in size is staged as N3. Pathological N stage is applicable to the group of patients undergoing surgery. The size of the node and laterality did not impact the outcome in patients treated with surgery. The N staging is done based on positive neck nodes: N1 being ≤4 and N2 being >4 metastatic lymph nodes.

Another minor change is the elimination of the stage T0 category from the staging of unknown primary for all subsites of head and neck except HPV-related oropharyngeal and nasopharyngeal cancers, where a diagnosis can be established with HPV ISH and EBER ISH in the absence of demonstratable structural disease in these subsites.

- Heterogeneous group of cancer arising from the mucosa of the head and neck.
- Tobacco and alcohol abuse continue to be the major etiological factors globally.
- Increase in the incidence of HPV-related oropharyngeal cancers which are biologically distinct and seen more in the developed world.
- Significant modification in the current eighth edition AJCC staging system.
- Field cancerization resulting in second primary cancers is common in tobacco-induced cancers.
- History and clinical evaluation are important to supplement imaging and help plan appropriate treatment.

37.6 Treatment Philosophy (Fig. 37.1)

Multidisciplinary care by a specialized team results in best outcomes. The core team responsible for planning and executing treatment must include head and neck surgeons, radiation oncologists, medical oncologists with inputs from dedicated pathologists and radiologists. Given that the goals of treatment are mitigating morbidity in addition to achieving best outcomes, ancillary support is imperative. Good plastic and reconstructive team, dentist, occupational therapist, physiotherapist, nutritionist and speech and language pathologist should form an integral part of the team. Given that a significant number of patients have a history of substance abuse, psychosocial support is important. So also, palliative care specialists should be integrated early in treatment plans in advanced disease.

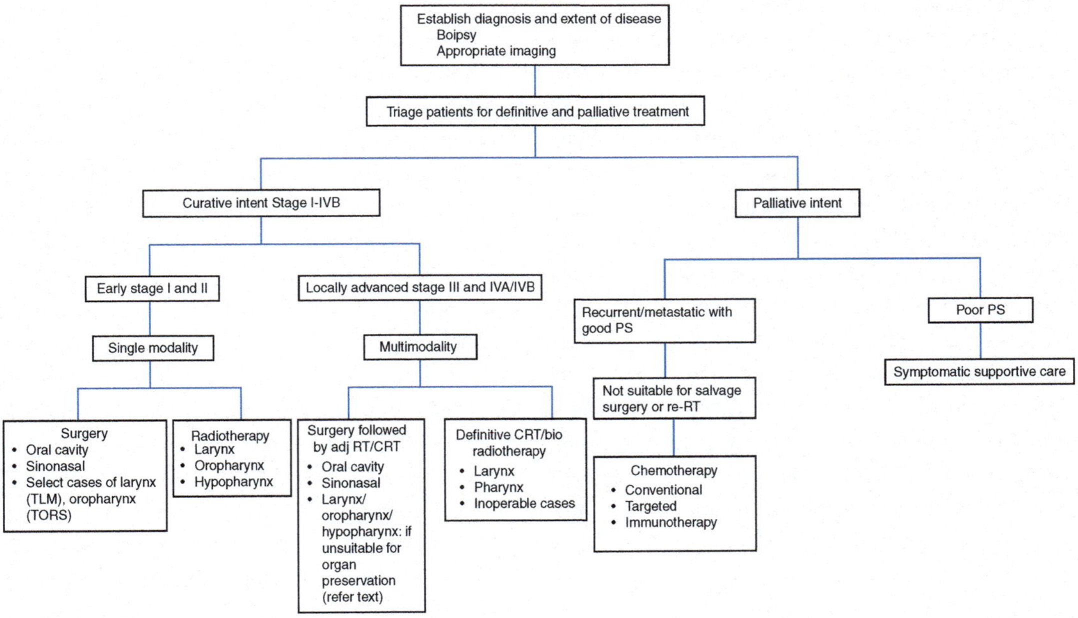

Fig. 37.1 Treatment algorithm for head and neck cancers. *TLM* transoral laser microsurgery, *TORS* transoral robotic surgery, *PS* performance status, *RT* radiotherapy, *CRT* chemoradiotherapy. Neoadjuvant chemotherapy usually not standard of care however considered in certain indications, refer text

Surgery and radiotherapy (RT) are definitive treatments for head and neck cancers. Chemotherapy is not curative by itself and is of maximum benefit only when used concurrently with radiotherapy. It does not have an established role in the neoadjuvant and adjuvant setting [25].

37.7 Stage I and II

Early stage (I and II) cancers are treated with single modality therapy either surgery or radiotherapy (RT) with similar outcomes and good control rates ranging from 70 to 90% [26]. Site of disease, accessibility, ease of treatment and morbidity of treatment are factors that help choose between the modalities. Patients' preference, availability of required infrastructure and expertise are other factors that influence the decision. Surgery is the preferred modality for oral cavity and sinonasal tumours as lesions involve or are in proximity to bone [14]. In addition, surgery is simple, quick, can be repeated and does not result in severe functional and cosmetic disability. Radiotherapy (brachytherapy± external beam) is preferred for superficial lip lesions particularly with commissure involvement and/or palatal lesions where surface mould brachytherapy avoids morbidity of surgery [27]. Cancers of the larynx and pharynx (oropharynx and hypopharynx) are usually treated with radiotherapy given the functional morbidity and/or technical difficulty associated with surgery at these sites. The advent of transoral laser microsurgery (TLM) and transoral robotic surgery (TORS) made the larynx and oropharynx accessible enabling a select subset of patients to be brought into the realm of surgery [14]. These approaches avoid the morbidity associated with open surgery and had the added advantage of overcoming the sequelae and duration of radiotherapy. TLM could also be performed as a day care surgery making it cost-effective [28].

37.8 Stage III and IVA

Given the advanced nature of these tumours, treatment consists of a multimodality approach [14]. Options include surgery followed by adjuvant treatment (radiotherapy/chemoradiotherapy) or platinum-based concurrent chemoradiotherapy (platinum occasionally replaced by biologicals) with surgery as salvage. As with early lesions, primary surgery is preferred for oral and paranasal sinus tumours.

There was a paradigm shift from surgical to non-surgical approaches for oropharyngeal, laryngeal and hypopharyngeal cancers. Until the 1990s, the treatment of stage III and IV cancers in these subsites was primarily surgery followed by adjuvant treatment [29]. The philosophy changed with the publication of the results of the Veterans affairs laryngeal cancer study group randomized controlled trial (RCT) in which induction chemotherapy followed by radiotherapy in responders was comparable to surgery and radiotherapy for outcomes with larynx preservation in two-third of patients who received non-surgical treatment [30]. Simultaneously a trial designed on similar lines showed success for hypopharyngeal tumours with this approach [31]. These two trials provided proof of principle that surgery could be replaced by non-surgical organ preservation strategies.

The landmark trial which established the role of concomitant chemoradiotherapy (CRT) as practised today was the Radiation Therapy Oncology Group and the Head and Neck Intergroup (RTOG 91-11) trial. Chemotherapy followed by radiotherapy (I + RT), CRT and RT alone were compared in a randomized setting. The primary endpoint was larynx preservation rate. Stage III and IV carcinoma larynx were included in the study excluding small T1 and large volume T4 disease (frank cartilage erosion and disease extending >1 cm in the base of tongue). At a median follow-up of 3.8 years, larynx preservation was 88% vs. 75% vs. 70% with CRT compared to I + RT and RT alone respectively establishing CRT as the standard of care [32]. Long-term follow-up (median follow-up 10.8 years) of the RTOG 91-11 trial continued to show the benefit of this approach with the larynx preservation rates highest in the CRT arm [33]. The concomitant use of cisplatin RT was corroborated by MACH-NC meta-analysis [34].

The non-surgical approach was also found to be successful for oropharyngeal cancers. The

GORTEC group compared RT vs. concomitant CRT for the treatment of locally advanced oropharyngeal cancers. Patients received conventional RT in both the arms with the addition of carboplatin (70 mg/m^2 per day) and 5 FU (600 mg/m^2 per day) by continuous infusion in concomitant CRT arm. There was an improved locoregional control, 3-year actuarial OS and DFS with CRT compared to RT alone arm [35].

Lesions not suitable for organ preservation are those with bone or cartilage erosion (excluding early perichondrial invasion), gross exolaryngeal spread or a dysfunctional larynx when primary surgery is offered.

37.9 Stage IVB

Stage IVB tumours technically constitute an unresectable group and primary CRT (if patients' performance status permits) is the treatment of choice [36]. However, in certain select situations, surgery may be offered when there is a possibility of total tumour extirpation, e.g. low infratemporal fossa disease in oral cancers (refer Chap. 38). The other option is the use of neoadjuvant chemotherapy (NACT) with an aim to downstage tumour and offer surgery to responders [37]. NACT approach is usually applied to oral and sinonasal tumours where the choice of primary treatment is surgery.

37.10 Stage IVC

The goal of treatment is usually palliative with chemotherapy. There are various regimes that use a combination of conventional chemotherapy with or without the addition of biologicals [38]. There is emerging data with exciting results of immunotherapy in this group but the majority of these publications explore its role as second-line therapy [39–42]. Radiotherapy is offered to metastatic disease most commonly for painful bony metastasis. In the rare instance of oligometastasis with a good disease-free interval, surgery may be offered in highly selected patients [43].

37.11 Principles of Treatment

37.11.1 Surgery

The goal of primary surgery is en bloc excision of the tumour with clear margins. There is no role for palliative excisions with partial removal of the tumour. Squamous cell carcinoma is biologically aggressive and resection of structures such as an internal carotid artery, prevertebral muscles/fascia is associated with significant morbidity and poor outcomes and hence are signs of inoperability [14, 44]. Sinonasal tumours have diverse histology and the grade of the tumour guides treatment philosophy [21]. En bloc resection is not always possible because of technical and anatomical constraints. Piecemeal resection which is at variance with the en bloc concept has been accepted for laser excision and sinonasal tumours. In these situations, adequacy of resection is confirmed by frozen section control under magnification [45].

What constitutes an adequate margin varies with the subsite of head and neck cancer. Margin positivity is seen to be higher for oral and oropharyngeal cancers as opposed to larynx primary [46]. Similarly, recurrent tumours have a higher likelihood of having close or positive margins [47]. The currently accepted norm for adequate margins is considered to be 5 mm [48]. Revising the margin based on the frozen section is not shown to offer benefit and adequacy of resection should be ensured at primary surgery [49]. Some authors have suggested a lesser margin for oral cancers but these findings are not validated by others and hence not standard of care [50]. Margins are known to shrink due to elasticity of tissue post excision and subsequent to fixation and this should be factored in, at the time of excision [51]. Hypopharyngeal cancers are known to have submucosal spread and margins wider than 5 mm may be indicated [52]. For glottic larynx, HPV-related TORS and sinonasal cancers lesser margins are acceptable, considering the biology and the anatomical constraints [53]. Margin sampling in these situations is patient-directed which is at variance with specimen directed sampling used otherwise [54–56].

TLM, TORS and endoscopic sinonasal surgery are now a part of the treatment armamentarium of the head and neck oncologists. TLM is used for early glottic (T1) cancers and shown to have similar control rates to RT, superior voice outcomes in select cases, is cost-effective and with the added advantage of being possible as a day care procedure [28, 57]. Moreover, salvage by way of conservative procedures is still possible should recurrence occur as opposed to those following radiotherapy where up to two-third of patients need to have a total laryngectomy [58, 59]. It is widely recommended to be considered as a suitable option across various guidelines. The ideal case is a superficial mid cord lesion. Laser excision has also been advocated for more extensive glottic (T2/T3), supraglottic and hypopharynx tumours but has not gained universal acceptance given the complexity of anatomy, the technical difficulty as well as the increased risk to nodal metastasis in these patients. The general dictum is that should the laser be chosen as treatment modality there should be no need for adjuvant therapy. Mopping up close or positive margins following laser using adjuvant radiotherapy results in poor oncological and functional outcomes. This dictum applies to the use of TORS as well.

TORS is evolving as the treatment strategy for early HPV positive oropharyngeal cancers though current literature is not robust enough to justify its use as the preferred modality (details in Chap. 38). Endoscopic sinus surgery has proven to have excellent outcomes in terms of local control, function and cosmesis. It has practically replaced open surgery in suitable cases. Even with extensive spread, it is used in combination with the open procedure (endoscopic assisted). Endoscopic resection is contraindicated in cases with macroscopic dural involvement, the lateral extension of the disease over the orbital roof, the involvement of anterior and lateral portion of the frontal sinus, invasion of the bony wall of the maxillary sinus except for the medial wall, hard palate involvement, erosion of the nasal bones, extensive lacrimal pathway infiltration and frank orbital invasion [60, 61].

37.11.2 Reconstruction

Microvascular flaps have replaced conventional axial/pedicled flaps for the majority of head and neck reconstructions. These flaps are associated with high success (upwards of 90%) and better cosmetic and functional outcomes [62, 63]. Use of microvascular flaps has enabled larger resections as there is a lesser limitation on flap size and earlier rehabilitation with lesser dependence on tube feeding and tracheostomies. Commonly used microvascular flaps are the radial forearm flap for skin and mucosa, anterolateral thigh flap for skin and soft tissue and the free fibula flap for bone replacement. Other flaps like lateral forearm, scapular, iliac crest have been described and used. The merits and technicalities of each of these flaps are out of the scope of this chapter. Pedicled axial flaps such as pectoralis major myocutaneous (PMMC), forehead and deltopectoral flaps which were once considered the workhorse of reconstruction have largely been relegated to history. However, these flaps are sometimes very useful particularly in elderly patients, those unfit for long procedures, for recurrent cases and as salvage in the event of microvascular flap failure. Local flaps are also useful for smaller defects. The general dictum for reconstruction is like for like-bone replaced by bone, soft tissue replaced by soft tissue, mucosa replaced by mucosa or skin.

37.11.3 Principles of Treatment of Neck

Cervical node metastasis is one of the most important factors that influences outcomes in head and neck cancers. Even a tiny metastatic deposit irrespective of the size of the primary upstages cancer to stage III. Appropriate management of the neck is therefore paramount in the treatment of head and neck cancers. The modality of choice (surgery or RT) for treatment of the neck is dictated by the modality chosen for treatment of the primary.

Selective neck dissection (SND) that samples nodes at the highest risk of metastasis is largely a staging procedure and usually done for a node negative neck [64]. The levels of nodes sampled are dependent on the site of the primary tumour. Supraomohyoid neck dissection (level I–III) is indicated for oral cavity and anterolateral neck dissection (levels II–IV) for oropharynx, larynx and hypopharynx cancers [65, 66]. There is data to suggest the adequacy of SND (I–IV) for small volume single node N1 in oral cavity cancers given the low propensity to involve level V. Modified neck dissection clearing levels I–V saving all three non-lymphatic structures (sternocleidomastoid (SCM), internal jugular vein (IJV), spinal accessory nerve (SAN)) is indicated for all node positive cases [67, 68]. The larynx and hypopharynx rarely involve level I and this area is not treated for cancer at these sites. Radical neck dissection is condemned in today's day and age. The IJV, SCM or SAN is sacrificed on a case to case basis only if directly involved by tumour. In larynx and hypopharynx cancers, the contralateral neck is always addressed given the high incidence of crossover lymphatics. For cancers of the oral cavity and oropharynx, the contralateral neck is addressed when the lesion reaches/crosses the midline [69].

The clinicoradiological node negative neck is electively treated even for small primaries of the oral cavity which are excised per orally. There is a level I evidence to show that this approach decreases recurrences and improves survival [70, 71]. While anatomical boundaries should be followed to ensure the adequacy of neck dissection, the numerical number of 18 has been suggested as an indicator of adequacy for cancers of the oral cavity/oropharynx [66]. The sentinel node biopsy has been advocated for cancers of the oral cavity and oropharynx. It is shown to have high diagnostic accuracy as well as a negative predictive value to the tune of 95% [72, 73]. However, given the cost, steep learning curve, two-staged procedure, cumbersome pathology (serial step sectioning and IHC) and no real benefit over a well-performed SND, the procedure has not gained universal acceptance.

Sinonasal tumours have a low propensity to neck node metastasis given that this area is sparse in lymphatics. The neck is usually not addressed if clinicoradiologically negative. Extensive buccal mucosa or skin subcutaneous involvement and high-grade histology are associated with a higher incidence of neck node metastasis and elective treatment of the neck should be considered. Glottic cancers similarly are sparse in lymphatics and the early glottic tumours do not need the neck addressed.

37.11.4 Principles of Radiotherapy

37.11.4.1 Definitive Radiotherapy

Radiotherapy, as mentioned earlier, is used as a definitive treatment when surgical excision would result in severe functional and cosmetic morbidity. It is used alone for early cancers stage I and II of the oropharynx, larynx and hypopharynx. Interstitial brachytherapy either alone or in combination with external beam RT is sometimes used in select head and neck cancers (oral and base of tongue). It is used alone for very early lesions at these sites. An ideal case for interstitial brachytherapy is a small lesion <3 cm, superficial, away from the bone, accessible and node negative [27]. Brachytherapy is also considered at times in clinical practice following surgery as a local boost to the tumour bed particularly for localized, recurrent or persistent disease. For locally advanced disease stage III and IV, current standard of care is to combine RT with chemotherapy (chemorads) with better outcomes compared to RT alone [32, 35]. The recommended chemotherapy is platinum-based cisplatin given at the dose of 100 mg/m^2 on day 1, 22 and 43 or 40 mg/m^2 weekly [74, 75]. These are toxic regimes with known complications and good supportive care is essential. A cumulative dose of cisplatin equivalent to 200 mg^2 should be aimed for, proven to have better control rates.

At times patients are platinum unsuitable due to advanced age, impaired renal function, impaired hearing, pre-existing neuropathies, compromised hepatic and cardiac function, poor performance status, etc. Prior receipt of platinum-based neoadjuvant chemotherapy may also restrict the subsequent use of platinum chemoradiotherapy [76]. Replacing cisplatin with biologicals (cetuximab), carboplatin alone or in combination with other chemotherapeutic agents and altered fractionation are suggested alternatives [77]. However, these approaches have their limitations. A meta-analysis specifically comparing carboplatin to cisplatin RT while showing no benefit in terms of locoregional control was inferior in terms of overall survival (OS) in carboplatin RT arm [78]. Cetuximab RT does have randomized evidence to show benefit over RT alone. However, this is a single trial with the majority of oropharyngeal primaries and a significant number of patients receiving altered fractionation RT which could be a confounding variable [79]. In a subsequent systematic review and meta-analysis comparing concomitant platinum-based chemotherapy or cetuximab with radiotherapy for locally advanced head and neck cancer, platinum-based CRT was associated with better progression-free survival (PFS) and OS [80]. Two RCTs since then, comparing cisplatin RT vs. cetuximab RT in HPV-related oropharyngeal cancer showed that cetuximab RT was inferior in terms of tumour control, PFS and OS [81, 82]. Altered fractionation has shown to have a similar 8% survival benefit comparable to that with chemoradiotherapy [83]. However, this is rarely practised in most oncological units on a daily basis for logistical reasons and toxicity. Cisplatin RT, therefore, is the gold standard and remains the first choice when chemoradiotherapy is considered.

Radio curable doses are aimed between 6600 and 7000 cGy. Intensity modulated radiotherapy is preferred to conformal radiotherapy and is shown to have lesser treatment related side effect particularly xerostomia [84]. There are different dose and fractionation schedules applied in different situations and details of which are out of the scope of this chapter.

37.11.4.2 Adjuvant Therapy

Adjuvant therapy is indicated for all stage III and IV head and neck cancers. In addition, certain stage I and II tumours may require postoperative RT based on histopathological features that place them at a higher risk for recurrence. Definite indications for RT are T3/T4 tumours, close resection margins and node positivity [14].

Literature is divided on whether the benefits of adjuvant RT outweigh the morbidity in the presence of other prognostic factors, namely perineural invasion, lymphovascular invasion, the grade of differentiation, DOI, single node positive and worst pattern of invasion, known to be associated with poorer prognosis. Commonly used guidelines such as NCCN place the onus on the treating clinician to consider RT in these settings. The general consensus is to assess the need on a case to case basis. In the absence of clear-cut guidelines, a commonly used thumb rule is to recommend adjuvant treatment in the presence of two or more of these factors [85, 86].

Recently, depth of invasion has been incorporated in the AJCC eighth edition staging for oral cancers placing tumours >10 mm DOI as T3/T4 making this an independent indication of adjuvant RT. However, depth of invasion is strongly associated with other adverse factors including primary tumour size, pN category, ECS, and close or involved margins. There was no benefit of PORT on disease-specific survival (DSS) based on depth as an isolated factor in the absence of other high-risk features in a multi-institutional collaborative study. This study concluded that the impact of DOI on DSS is through other adverse factors and the decision regarding adjuvant RT should not be based on DOI in the absence of these features [87]. This lends credence to the fact that the combination of prognostic factors may be the logical way to decide with regard to the need for adjuvant RT.

Extracapsular spread or positive margins are indications for postoperative CRT. Benefits are seen for this group of patients from the pooled results of the two RCTs, Radiation Therapy Oncology Group (RTOG) 9501 and European Organization for Research and Treatment of Cancer (EORTC) 22931 [88–90]. The recommended dose of chemotherapy is 100 mg/m^2 cisplatin once every 3 weeks (day 1, 22 and 43) or 40 mg/m^2 weekly. A lesser dose is associated with poorer locoregional control as shown in an

RCT comparing 100 mg/m^2 3 weekly vs. 30 mg/m^2 weekly [74, 75].

Postoperatively a dose of 5700–5800 cGy for low-risk patients and 6300–6400 cGy for high-risk patients is recommended. There is no benefit with escalation above these doses. Factors considered for risk categorization are close or positive margins, nerve invasion, >2 positive nodes, node >3 cm in size, treatment delay >6 weeks and performance status zubrod score ≥ 2, oral cavity primary and extracapsular extension of nodal disease. Early initiation and completion of adjuvant treatment are associated with better outcomes. Patients who start RT within 6 weeks of surgery or those who have a total package time (TPT) defined as the time from the date of surgery to completion of radiotherapy ≤ 85 days are associated with favourable outcomes [91–93].

37.11.5 Principles of Chemotherapy

As mentioned earlier, chemotherapy is not definitive treatment by itself in the management of head and neck cancers. The evidence in support of chemotherapy emerges from meta-analyses using individual patient data from 63 trials (10,741 patients) published by the Meta-Analysis of Chemotherapy on Head and Neck Cancer (MACH-NC) collaborative group. The benefit was highest (8%) for concomitant chemoradiotherapy [25]. Updated results of 87 trials (16,665 patients) confirmed the highest benefit of chemotherapy concomitant with RT [94]. These findings were reconfirmed by two further updates from the same group with a larger number of patients [95, 96]. When looking at benefit across the different subsites of head and neck cancers, maximum benefit was observed for the cancers of the oropharynx and larynx [34]. Platinum chemotherapy was superior compared to other chemotherapeutic agents.

The role of chemotherapy in the neoadjuvant setting has been explored on many occasions in an attempt to improve outcomes. There has been no significant survival benefit with the use of chemotherapy in this setting [97]. However, neoadjuvant chemotherapy (NACT) may have a potential role to help bio-select favourable patients. Licitra et al. showed that NACT downsized tumours making them more amenable to smaller surgeries as well as a decreased need for adjuvant RT [98]. Similarly, Urba et al. used this approach to bio-select patients for chemoradiotherapy and laryngeal preservation [99]. Patil et al. likewise used NACT to downstage oral cancers not considered suitable for primary surgery and brought 43% of patients into the realm of curative surgery [37]. While NACT continues to be used in the clinic at the time of difficult decisions for indications enumerated above it is not a routine standard of care. If NACT is administered, the ideal combination is the 3-drug regime of a taxane added to cisplatin and 5-fluorouracil (5-FU) which has been shown to have superior results over a 2-drug regime [100, 101].

37.12 Treatment of Recurrent and Metastatic Cancers

Recurrence is not uncommon in head and neck cancers and can occur in up to half the patients and depends on the initial stage and site of presentation. Salvage is possible in about fifth of these patients [102]. Recurrences may be difficult to detect given post treatment alterations in anatomy and sequelae. Salvage surgery offers the best chance at the cure [103]. It is prudent to excise with wider margins than usual as it is often difficult to distinguish between tumour and post treatment induration. Adjuvant treatment if feasible offers a survival benefit [104]. Re-radiotherapy is recommended if surgery is not possible [105]. The success of salvage depends on various factors that include the general condition of the patient, presence of comorbidities, the initial and current stage of the disease, the receipt of prior adjuvant treatment and most importantly the disease-free interval (DFI). The longer the DFI, the more the likelihood of salvage being successful.

If surgery or re-radiotherapy is not possible, palliative chemotherapy is the recommended option. Doublet chemotherapy of cisplatin plus

5-FU was the standard of care for a long time [106]. The practice changed with data supporting the addition of cetuximab resulting in improvement in OS [38]. Recently, immunotherapy targeting checkpoint inhibitors have shown promising results. Both programmed cell death ligand 1 (PD-L1) and programmed cell death (PD-1) factor have been targeted in platinum refractory recurrent and metastatic head and neck cancers. Nivolumab and pembrolizumab have shown survival benefit as second-line therapy [39–42]. These drugs along with other immunotherapeutic agents are currently being explored as first-line treatment. When the performance status is poor precluding chemotherapy, patients are offered the best supportive and symptomatic care.

37.13 Follow-Up

The majority of recurrences (≈90%) occur in the first 24 months following treatment and recommendations are for more frequent follow-up during this period [107]. Moreover, patients need care and rehabilitation from the morbidity of treatment, which is most required during this period. Recommendations for frequency of follow-up are every 2–3 months for the first 2 years, every 4–6 months for the third year, 6 monthly till fifth year and annually thereafter. The frequency of follow-up may need to be varied on a case to case basis and on patients' symptomatology [14].

At each follow-up, a thorough locoregional examination is performed to assess disease control. Second primary cancers are known to occur (described in the section on natural history) and a thorough examination of the entire upper aerodigestive tract should be performed in addition. Late sequelae of treatment are also enquired for, examined and addressed. The decision to image at each follow-up is individualized depending on the case and accessibility to the examination but it is prudent to have a baseline imaging at 12 weeks following completion of cancer treatment that serves as a baseline for comparison with subsequent imaging. Given that at least half the patients who have received RT have hypothyroidism, thyroid function tests are ordered yearly [108]. The peak incidence of hypothyroidism is 3 years post-treatment and plateaus thereafter [109]. Dental examination and fluoride prophylaxis are recommended at each follow-up to prevent radiation-induced caries. An annual chest X-ray is advised across many guidelines particularly in smokers to rule out the possibility of the second primary. A non-contrast CT scan serves as a useful alternative in high-risk patients prone to lung cancers as its ability to detect smaller lesions is superior. Specific consultations with ancillary departments (e.g. physiotherapy, speech and swallowing, audiologist) are recommended based on symptoms and sequelae of treatment.

- Surgery and RT are definitive treatments for head and neck cancers.
- Chemotherapy has no role by itself except in the recurrent/metastatic setting. Its benefit in the curative setting is when combined with RT (chemorads).
- Early stage cancers warrant single modality and advanced cancers multimodality treatment.
- Surgery should be performed en bloc with adequate margins. A 5 mm margin is usually considered adequate. Lesser margins are accepted for early glottic cancers, HPV-associated oropharyngeal cancers and low-grade paranasal sinus tumours.
- Concomitant chemoradiotherapy is now standard of care with an aim at organ preservation for cancers of the oropharynx, hypopharynx and larynx.

Take Home Messages

- HPV infection is now recognized as an etiological factor responsible for biologically different cancer from those traditionally caused by tobacco and alcohol abuse.
- There has been the emergence of new robust data (large pooled multi-institutional databases, RCT and meta-analysis) which has resulted in paradigm changes in staging, philosophy of treatment and management protocols.
- Oral and sinonasal tumours are primarily surgically treated while the pharynx and larynx are primarily treated non-surgically.
- Microvascular surgery, TORS, IMRT, monoclonal antibodies and immunotherapy have expanded the scope of treatment and also helped mitigate morbidity of treatment.
- Continued care during follow-up is important for rehabilitation as well as detection of recurrences/second primary cancers.

Conflicts of Interest None of the authors have any conflict of interest with respect to the manuscript.

References

1. Bray F, Ferlay J, Soerjomataram I, Siegel RL, Torre LA, Jemal A. Global cancer statistics 2018: GLOBOCAN estimates of incidence and mortality worldwide for 36 cancers in 185 countries. CA Cancer J Clin. 2018;68(6):394–424.
2. Fakhry C, Gillison ML. Clinical implications of human papillomavirus in head and neck cancers. J Clin Oncol. 2006;24(17):2606–11.
3. Chaturvedi AK, Anderson WF, Lortet-Tieulent J, et al. Worldwide trends in incidence rates for oral cavity and oropharyngeal cancers. J Clin Oncol. 2013;31(36):4550–9.
4. Califano J, van der Riet P, Westra W, et al. Genetic progression model for head and neck cancer: implications for field cancerization. Cancer Res. 1996;56(11):2488–92.
5. Slaughter DP, Southwick HW, Smejkal W. Field cancerization in oral stratified squamous epithelium; clinical implications of multicentric origin. Cancer. 1953;6(5):963–8.
6. León X, Ferlito A, Myer CM III, et al. Second primary tumors in head and neck cancer patients. Acta Otolaryngol. 2002;122(7):765–78.
7. Priante AV, Castilho EC, Kowalski LP. Second primary tumors in patients with head and neck cancer. Curr Oncol Rep. 2011;13(2):132–7.
8. Chuang SC, Scelo G, Tonita JM, et al. Risk of second primary cancer among patients with head and neck cancers: a pooled analysis of 13 cancer registries. Int J Cancer. 2008;123(10):2390–6.
9. Heroiu Cataloiu AD, Danciu CE, Popescu CR. Multiple cancers of the head and neck. Maedica (Buchar). 2013;8(1):80–5.
10. Yang Y-H, Warnakulasuriya S. Effect of comorbidities on the management and prognosis in patients with oral cancer. Transl Res Oral Oncol. https://doi.org/10.1177/2057178X16669961.
11. Ribeiro KC, Kowalski LP, Latorre MR. Impact of comorbidity, symptoms, and patients' characteristics on the prognosis of oral carcinomas. Arch Otolaryngol Head Neck Surg. 2000;126(9):1079–85. https://doi.org/10.1001/archotol.126.9.1079.
12. Lydiatt WM, Patel SG, O'Sullivan B, Brandwein MS, Ridge JA, Migliacci JC, et al. Head and Neck cancers-major changes in the American Joint Committee on cancer eighth edition cancer staging manual. CA Cancer J Clin. 2017;67(2):122–37.
13. Yousem DM, Gad K, Tufano RP. Resectability issues with head and neck cancer. AJNR Am J Neuroradiol. 2006;27(10):2024–36.
14. National Comprehensive Cancer Network clinical practice guidelines in oncology (NCCN guidelines): cancer of the oral cavity, version 1. 2020. http://www.nccn.org/professionals/physician_gls/pdf/head-and-neck.pdf.
15. Kim Y, Roh J-L, Kim JS, Lee JH, Choi S-H, Nam SY, et al. Chest radiography or chest CT plus head and neck CT versus 18F-FDG PET/CT for detection of distant metastasis and synchronous cancer in patients with head and neck cancer. Oral Oncol. 2019;1(88):109–14.
16. Goel R, Moore W, Sumer B, Khan S, Sher D, Subramaniam RM. Clinical Practice in PET/CT for the Management of Head and Neck Squamous Cell Cancer. AJR Am J Roentgenol. 2017;209(2):289–303. https://doi.org/10.2214/AJR.17.18301.
17. Isles MG, McConkey C, Mehanna HM. A systematic review and meta-analysis of the role of positron emission tomography in the follow up of head and neck squamous cell carcinoma following radiotherapy or chemoradiotherapy. Clin Otolaryngol. 2008;33(3):210–22.
18. Rusthoven KE, Koshy M, Paulino AC. The role of fluorodeoxyglucose positron emission tomography in cervical lymph node metastases from an unknown primary tumor. Cancer. 2004;101(11):2641–9.
19. Zhu L, Wang N. 18F-fluorodeoxyglucose positron emission tomography-computed tomography as a

diagnostic tool in patients with cervical nodal metastases of unknown primary site: a meta-analysis. Surg Oncol. 2013;22(3):190–4.
20. Graboyes EM, Sinha P, Thorstad WL, Rich JT, Haughey BH. Management of human papillomavirus-related unknown primaries of the head and neck with a transoral surgical approach. Head Neck. 2015;37(11):1603–11.
21. Barnes L, Eveson JW, Reichart P, Sidransky D. WHO classification of tumors: pathology and genetics of head and neck tumours. Lyon: IARC; 2005.
22. Amin MB, Edge SB, Greene FL, et al., editors. AJCC cancer staging manual. 8th ed. New York: Springer; 2017.
23. Edge SB, Byrd DR, Compton CC, Fritz AG, Greene FL, Trotti A, editors. AJCC cancer staging manual. 7th ed. New York: Springer; 2010.
24. Wreesmann VB, Katabi N, Palmer FL, et al. Influence of extracapsular nodal spread extent on prognosis of oral squamous cell carcinoma. Head Neck. 2016;38(Suppl 1):E1192–9.
25. Pignon JP, Bourhis J, Domenge C, Designé L. Chemotherapy added to locoregional treatment for head and neck squamous-cell carcinoma: three meta-analyses of updated individual data. MACH-NC Collaborative Group. Meta-Analysis of Chemotherapy on Head and Neck Cancer. Lancet. 2000;355(9208):949–55.
26. Chow LQM. Head and neck cancer. N Engl J Med. 2020;382(1):60–72.
27. Kovács G, Martinez-Monge R, Budrukkar A, et al. GEC-ESTRO ACROP recommendations for head & neck brachytherapy in squamous cell carcinomas: 1st update – improvement by cross sectional imaging based treatment planning and stepping source technology. Radiother Oncol. 2017;122(2): 248–54.
28. Feng Y, Wang B, Wen S. Laser surgery versus radiotherapy for T1-T2N0 glottic cancer: a meta-analysis. ORL J Otorhinolaryngol Relat Spec. 2011;73(6):336–42.
29. Tupchong L, Scott CB, Blitzer PH, et al. Randomized study of preoperative versus postoperative radiation therapy in advanced head and neck carcinoma: long-term follow-up of RTOG study 73-03. Int J Radiat Oncol Biol Phys. 1991;20(1):21–8.
30. Department of Veterans Affairs Laryngeal Cancer Study Group. Induction chemotherapy plus radiation compared with surgery plus radiation in patients with advanced laryngeal cancer. N Engl J Med. 1991;324(24):1685–90.
31. Lefebvre JL, Chevalier D, Luboinski B, Kirkpatrick A, Collette L, Sahmoud T. *Larynx* preservation in pyriform sinus cancer: preliminary results of a European Organization for Research and Treatment of Cancer phase III trial. EORTC Head and Neck Cancer Cooperative Group. J Natl Cancer Inst. 1996;88(13):890–9.
32. Forastiere AA, Goepfert H, Maor M, et al. Concurrent chemotherapy and radiotherapy for organ preservation in advanced laryngeal cancer. N Engl J Med. 2003;349(22):2091–8.
33. Forastiere AA, Zhang Q, Weber RS, Pajak TF, et al. Long-term results of RTOG 91-11: a comparison of three nonsurgical treatment strategies to preserve the larynx in patients with locally advanced larynx cancer. J Clin Oncol. 2013;31(7):845–52.
34. Blanchard P, Baujat B, Holostenco V, et al. Meta-analysis of chemotherapy in head and neck cancer (MACH-NC): a comprehensive analysis by tumour site. Radiother Oncol. 2011;100(1):33–40.
35. Calais G, Alfonsi M, Bardet E, et al. Randomized trial of radiation therapy versus concomitant chemotherapy and radiation therapy for advanced-stage oropharynx carcinoma. J Natl Cancer Inst. 1999;91(24):2081–6.
36. Adelstein DJ, Li Y, Adams GL, et al. An intergroup phase III comparison of standard radiation therapy and two schedules of concurrent chemoradiotherapy in patients with unresectable squamous cell head and neck cancer. J Clin Oncol. 2003;21(1):92–8.
37. Patil VM, Prabhash K, Noronha V, et al. Neoadjuvant chemotherapy followed by surgery in very locally advanced technically unresectable oral cavity cancers. Oral Oncol. 2014;50(10):1000–4.
38. Vermorken JB, Mesia R, Rivera F, et al. Platinum-based chemotherapy plus cetuximab in head and neck cancer. N Engl J Med. 2008;359(11):1116–27.
39. Ferris RL, Blumenschein G Jr, Fayette J, et al. Nivolumab for recurrent squamous-cell carcinoma of the head and neck. N Engl J Med. 2016;375(19):1856–67.
40. Ferris RL, Blumenschein G Jr, Fayette J, et al. Nivolumab vs investigator's choice in recurrent or metastatic squamous cell carcinoma of the head and neck: 2-year long-term survival update of CheckMate 141 with analyses by tumor PD-L1 expression. Oral Oncol. 2018;81:45–51.
41. Cohen EEW, Soulières D, Le Tourneau C, et al. Pembrolizumab versus methotrexate, docetaxel, or cetuximab for recurrent or metastatic head-and-neck squamous cell carcinoma (KEYNOTE-040): a randomised, open-label, phase 3 study. Lancet. 2019;393(10167):156–67.
42. Burtness B, Harrington KJ, Greil R, et al. Pembrolizumab alone or with chemotherapy versus cetuximab with chemotherapy for recurrent or metastatic squamous cell carcinoma of the head and neck (KEYNOTE-048): a randomised, open-label, phase 3 study. Lancet. 2019;394(10212):1915–28.
43. Sun XS, Michel C, Babin E, et al. Approach to oligometastatic disease in head and neck cancer, on behalf of the GORTEC. Future Oncol. 2018;14(9):877–89.
44. Kroeker TR, O'Brien JC. Carotid resection and reconstruction associated with treatment of head and neck cancer. Proc (Bayl Univ Med Cent). 2011;24(4):295–8.
45. Hinni ML, Ferlito A, Brandwein-Gensler MS, et al. Surgical margins in head and neck cancer: a contemporary review. Head Neck. 2013;35(9):1362–70.

46. Jacobs JR, Ahmad K, Casiano R, et al. Implications of positive surgical margins. Laryngoscope. 1993;103(1 Pt 1):64–8.
47. Jones AS, Bin Hanafi Z, Nadapalan V, Roland NJ, Kinsella A, Helliwell TR. Do positive resection margins after ablative surgery for head and neck cancer adversely affect prognosis? A study of 352 patients with recurrent carcinoma following radiotherapy treated by salvage surgery. Br J Cancer. 1996;74(1):128–32.
48. Anderson CR, Sisson K, Moncrieff M. A meta-analysis of margin size and local recurrence in oral squamous cell carcinoma. Oral Oncol. 2015;51(5):464–9.
49. Bulbul MG, Tarabichi O, Sethi RK, Parikh AS, Varvares MA. Does clearance of positive margins improve local control in oral cavity cancer? A meta-analysis. Otolaryngol Neck Surg Otolaryngol Head Neck Surg. 2019;161(2):235–44.
50. Zanoni DK, Migliacci JC, Xu B, et al. A proposal to redefine close surgical margins in squamous cell carcinoma of the oral tongue. JAMA Otolaryngol Head Neck Surg. 2017;143(6):555–60.
51. Mistry RC, Qureshi SS, Kumaran C. Post-resection mucosal margin shrinkage in oral cancer: quantification and significance. J Surg Oncol. 2005;91(2):131–3.
52. Harrison DF. Pathology of hypopharyngeal cancer in relation to surgical management. J Laryngol Otol. 1970;84(4):349–67.
53. Weinstein GS, O'Malley BW Jr, Magnuson JS, et al. Transoral robotic surgery: multicenter study to assess feasibility, safety, and surgical margins. Laryngoscope. 2012;122(8):1701–7.
54. Hamzany Y, Brasnu D, Shpitzer T, Shvero J. Assessment of margins in transoral laser and robotic surgery. Rambam Maimonides Med J. 2014;5(2):e0016.
55. Ambrosch P, Fazel A. Functional organ preservation in laryngeal and hypopharyngeal cancer. GMS Curr Top Otorhinolaryngol Head Neck Surg. 2011;10:Doc02.
56. Maxwell JH, Thompson LD, Brandwein-Gensler MS, et al. Early oral tongue squamous cell carcinoma: sampling of margins from tumor bed and worse local control. JAMA Otolaryngol Head Neck Surg. 2015;141(12):1104–10.
57. Higgins KM, Shah MD, Ogaick MJ, Enepekides D. Treatment of early-stage glottic cancer: meta-analysis comparison of laser excision versus radiotherapy. J Otolaryngol Head Neck Surg. 2009;38(6):603–12.
58. Holsinger FC, Funk E, Roberts DB, Diaz EM Jr. Conservation laryngeal surgery versus total laryngectomy for radiation failure in laryngeal cancer. Head Neck. 2006;28(9):779–84.
59. Canis M, Ihler F, Martin A, Matthias C, Steiner W. Transoral laser microsurgery for T1a glottic cancer: review of 404 cases. Head Neck. 2015;37(6):889–95.
60. Nicolai P, Battaglia P, Bignami M, et al. Endoscopic surgery for malignant tumors of the sinonasal tract and adjacent skull base: a 10-year experience. Am J Rhinol. 2008;22(3):308–16.
61. Hanna E, DeMonte F, Ibrahim S, Roberts D, Levine N, Kupferman M. Endoscopic resection of sinonasal cancers with and without craniotomy: oncologic results. Arch Otolaryngol Head Neck Surg. 2009;135(12):1219–24.
62. Suh JD, Sercarz JA, Abemayor E, et al. Analysis of outcome and complications in 400 cases of microvascular head and neck reconstruction. Arch Otolaryngol Head Neck Surg. 2004;130(8):962–6.
63. de Bree R, Reith R, Quak JJ, Uyl-de Groot CA, van Agthoven M, Leemans CR. Free radial forearm flap versus pectoralis major myocutaneous flap reconstruction of oral and oropharyngeal defects: a cost analysis. Clin Otolaryngol. 2007;32(4):275–82.
64. Brazilian Head and Neck Cancer Study Group. Results of a prospective trial on elective modified radical classical versus supraomohyoid neck dissection in the management of oral squamous carcinoma. Am J Surg. 1998;176(5):422–7.
65. Brazilian Head and Neck Cancer Study Group. End results of a prospective trial on elective lateral neck dissection vs type III modified radical neck dissection in the management of supraglottic and transglottic carcinomas. Head Neck. 1999;21(8):694–702.
66. Koyfman SA, Ismaila N, Crook D, et al. Management of the neck in squamous cell carcinoma of the oral cavity and oropharynx: ASCO Clinical Practice Guideline. J Clin Oncol. 2019;37(20):1753–74.
67. Liang L, Zhang T, Kong Q, Liang J, Liao G. A meta-analysis on selective versus comprehensive neck dissection in oral squamous cell carcinoma patients with clinically node positive neck. Oral Oncol. 2015;51(12):1076–81.
68. Rodrigo JP, Grilli G, Shah JP, et al. Selective neck dissection in surgically treated head and neck squamous cell carcinoma patients with a clinically positive neck: systematic review. Eur J Surg Oncol. 2018;44(4):395–403.
69. Singh B, Nair S, Nair D, Patil A, Chaturvedi P, D'Cruz AK. Ipsilateral neck nodal status as predictor of contralateral nodal metastasis in carcinoma of tongue crossing the midline. Head Neck. 2013;35(5):649–52.
70. D'Cruz AK, Vaish R, Kapre N, et al. Elective versus therapeutic neck dissection in node-negative oral cancer. N Engl J Med. 2015;373(6):521–9.
71. Hutchison IL, Ridout F, Cheung SMY, et al. Nationwide randomised trial evaluating elective neck dissection for early stage oral cancer (SEND study) with meta-analysis and concurrent real-world cohort. Br J Cancer. 2019;121(10):827–36.
72. Thompson CF, St John MA, Lawson G, Grogan T, Elashoff D, Mendelsohn AH. Diagnostic value of sentinel lymph node biopsy in head and neck cancer: a meta-analysis. Eur Arch Otorhinolaryngol. 2013;270(7):2115–22.

73. Schilling C, Stoeckli SJ, Haerle SK, et al. Sentinel European Node Trial (SENT): 3-year results of sentinel node biopsy in oral cancer. Eur J Cancer. 2015;51(18):2777–84.
74. Noronha V, Joshi A, Patil VM, Agarwal J, Ghosh-Laskar S, Budrukkar A, et al. Once-a-week versus once-every-3-weeks cisplatin chemoradiation for locally advanced head and neck cancer: a phase III randomized noninferiority trial. J Clin Oncol. 2018;36(11):1064–72.
75. Hu L, Xia W-X, Xing LV, et al. Concurrent chemoradiotherapy with 3-weekly versus weekly cisplatin in patients with locoregionally advanced nasopharyngeal carcinoma: a phase 3 multicentre randomised controlled trial (ChiCTR-TRC-12001979). J Clin Oncol. 2017;35(15_suppl):6006.
76. Ahn MJ, D'Cruz A, Vermorken JB, et al. Clinical recommendations for defining platinum unsuitable head and neck cancer patient populations on chemoradiotherapy: a literature review. Oral Oncol. 2016;53:10–6.
77. Szturz P, Cristina V, Herrera Gómez RG, Bourhis J, Simon C, Vermorken JB. Cisplatin eligibility issues and alternative regimens in locoregionally advanced head and neck cancer: recommendations for clinical practice. Front Oncol. 2019;9:464.
78. Guan J, Li Q, Zhang Y, et al. A meta-analysis comparing cisplatin-based to carboplatin-based chemotherapy in moderate to advanced squamous cell carcinoma of head and neck (SCCHN). Oncotarget. 2016;7(6):7110–9.
79. Bonner JA, Harari PM, Giralt J, et al. Radiotherapy plus cetuximab for squamous-cell carcinoma of the head and neck. N Engl J Med. 2006;354(6):567–78.
80. Petrelli F, Coinu A, Riboldi VM, et al. Concomitant platinum-based chemotherapy or cetuximab with radiotherapy for locally advanced head and neck cancer: a systematic review and meta-analysis of published studies. Oral Oncol. 2014;50(11):1041–8.
81. Mehanna H, Robinson M, Hartley A, et al. Radiotherapy plus cisplatin or cetuximab in low-risk human papillomavirus-positive oropharyngeal cancer (De-ESCALaTE HPV): an open-label randomised controlled phase 3 trial. Lancet. 2019;393(10166):51–60.
82. Gillison ML, Trotti AM, Harris J, et al. Radiotherapy plus cetuximab or cisplatin in human papillomavirus-positive oropharyngeal cancer (NRG Oncology RTOG 1016): a randomised, multicentre, non-inferiority trial. Lancet. 2019;393(10166):40–50.
83. Bourhis J, Overgaard J, Audry H, et al. Hyperfractionated or accelerated radiotherapy in head and neck cancer: a meta-analysis. Lancet. 2006;368(9538):843–54.
84. Nutting CM, Morden JP, Harrington KJC, et al. Parotid-sparing intensity modulated versus conventional radiotherapy in head and neck cancer (PARSPORT): a phase 3 multicentre randomised controlled trial. Lancet Oncol. 2011;12(2):127–36.
85. Chen WC, Lai CH, Fang CC, et al. Identification of high-risk subgroups of patients with oral cavity cancer in need of postoperative adjuvant radiotherapy or chemoradiotherapy. Medicine (Baltimore). 2016;95(22):e3770.
86. Fan KH, Wang HM, Kang CJ, et al. Treatment results of postoperative radiotherapy on squamous cell carcinoma of the oral cavity: coexistence of multiple minor risk factors results in higher recurrence rates. Int J Radiat Oncol Biol Phys. 2010;77(4):1024–9.
87. Ebrahimi A, Gil Z, Amit M, et al. Depth of invasion alone as an indication for postoperative radiotherapy in small oral squamous cell carcinomas: an international collaborative study. Head Neck. 2019;41(6):1935–42.
88. Bernier J, Domenge C, Ozsahin M, et al. Postoperative irradiation with or without concomitant chemotherapy for locally advanced head and neck cancer. N Engl J Med. 2004;350(19):1945–52.
89. Cooper JS, Pajak TF, Forastiere AA, et al. Postoperative concurrent radiotherapy and chemotherapy for high-risk squamous-cell carcinoma of the head and neck. N Engl J Med. 2004;350:1937–44.
90. Bernier J, Cooper JS, Pajak TF, et al. Defining risk levels in locally advanced head and neck cancers: a comparative analysis of concurrent postoperative radiation plus chemotherapy trials of the EORTC (#22931) and RTOG (# 9501). Head Neck. 2005;27(10):843–50.
91. Peters LJ, Goepfert H, Ang KK, Byers RM, Maor MH, Guillamondegui O, et al. Evaluation of the dose for postoperative radiation therapy of head and neck cancer: first report of a prospective randomized trial. Int J Radiat Oncol Biol Phys. 1993;26(1):3–11.
92. Rosenthal DI, Mohamed ASR, Garden AS, Morrison WH, El-Naggar AK, Kamal M, et al. Final report of a prospective randomized trial to evaluate the dose-response relationship for postoperative radiation therapy and pathologic risk groups in patients with head and neck cancer. Int J Radiat Oncol Biol Phys. 2017;98(5):1002–11.
93. Ang KK, Trotti A, Brown BW, et al. Randomized trial addressing risk features and time factors of surgery plus radiotherapy in advanced head-and-neck cancer. Int J Radiat Oncol Biol Phys. 2001;51(3):571–8.
94. Pignon JP, le Maître A, Bourhis J, MACH-NC Collaborative Group. Meta-Analyses of Chemotherapy in Head and Neck Cancer (MACH-NC): an update. Int J Radiat Oncol Biol Phys. 2007;69(2 Suppl):S112–4.
95. Pignon JP, le Maître A, Maillard E, Bourhis J, MACH-NC Collaborative Group. Meta-analysis of chemotherapy in head and neck cancer (MACH-NC): an update on 93 randomised trials

and 17,346 patients. Radiother Oncol. 2009;92(1): 4–14.
96. Blanchard P, Landais C, Petit C, et al. Meta-analysis of chemotherapy in head and neck cancer (MACH-NC): an update on 100 randomized trials and 19,248 patients, on behalf of MACH-NC group. Ann Oncol. 2016;27:vi328. https://doi.org/10.1093/annonc/mdw376.02.
97. Zhang L, Jiang N, Shi Y, Li S, Wang P, Zhao Y. Induction chemotherapy with concurrent chemoradiotherapy versus concurrent chemoradiotherapy for locally advanced squamous cell carcinoma of head and neck: a meta-analysis. Sci Rep. 2015;5:10798.
98. Licitra L, Grandi C, Guzzo M, et al. Primary chemotherapy in resectable oral cavity squamous cell cancer: a randomized controlled trial. J Clin Oncol. 2003;21(2):327–33.
99. Urba S, Wolf G, Eisbruch A, et al. Single-cycle induction chemotherapy selects patients with advanced laryngeal cancer for combined chemoradiation: a new treatment paradigm. J Clin Oncol. 2006;24(4):593–8.
100. Vermorken JB, Remenar E, van Herpen C, et al. Cisplatin, fluorouracil, and docetaxel in unresectable head and neck cancer. N Engl J Med. 2007;357(17):1695–704.
101. Posner MR, Hershock DM, Blajman CR, et al. Cisplatin and fluorouracil alone or with docetaxel in head and neck cancer. N Engl J Med. 2007;357(17):1705–15.
102. Ho AS, Kraus DH, Ganly I, Lee NY, Shah JP, Morris LG. Decision making in the management of recurrent head and neck cancer. Head Neck. 2014;36(1):144–51.
103. Wong LY, Wei WI, Lam LK, Yuen AP. Salvage of recurrent head and neck squamous cell carcinoma after primary curative surgery. Head Neck. 2003;25(11):953–9.
104. Janot F, de Raucourt D, Benhamou E, Ferron C, Dolivet G, Bensadoun RJ, et al. Randomized trial of postoperative reirradiation combined with chemotherapy after salvage surgery compared with salvage surgery alone in head and neck carcinoma. J Clin Oncol. 2008;26(34):5518–23.
105. Spencer SA, Harris J, Wheeler RH, Machtay M, Schultz C, Spanos W, et al. Final report of RTOG 9610, a multi-institutional trial of reirradiation and chemotherapy for unresectable recurrent squamous cell carcinoma of the head and neck. Head Neck. 2008;30(3):281–8.
106. Jacobs C, Lyman G, Velez-García E, et al. A phase III randomized study comparing cisplatin and fluorouracil as single agents and in combination for advanced squamous cell carcinoma of the head and neck. J Clin Oncol. 1992;10(2):257–63.
107. Oksuz DC, Prestwich RJ, Carey B, et al. Recurrence patterns of locally advanced head and neck squamous cell carcinoma after 3D conformal (chemo)-radiotherapy. Radiat Oncol. 2011;6:54.
108. Boomsma MJ, Bijl HP, Langendijk JA. Radiation-induced hypothyroidism in head and neck cancer patients: a systematic review. Radiother Oncol. 2011;99(1):1–5.
109. Lin Z, Yang Z, He B, Wang D, Gao X, Tam SY, et al. Pattern of radiation-induced thyroid gland changes in nasopharyngeal carcinoma patients in 48 months after radiotherapy. PLoS One. 2018;13(7): e0200310.

38 Neoplasms of the Oral Cavity and Oropharynx

Anil K. D'Cruz, Harsh Dhar,
Khuzema Fatehi, and Richa Vaish

38.1 Introduction

Oral and oropharyngeal cancers (OPC) together constitute a major global public health problem with an estimated annual incidence of 354,864 and 92,887 cases worldwide, respectively [1]. Although these two sites are in close anatomical proximity and often considered a single entity, cancers affecting these areas are distinct with significant differences in disease biology as well as management protocols [2, 3].

There have been significant new data resulting in a shift in management protocols of both these cancers. This chapter attempts to highlight these details in light of the current evidence. Benign tumours of the oral cavity and oropharynx are beyond the scope of this chapter.

- Changing epidemiology, recognition of new prognostic factors and different biology of oral and oropharyngeal cancers.
- Salient clinical features, relevant diagnostic workup, and recent staging system.
- Principles of management with incorporation of new data.

38.2 Oral Cancers

Oral cavity squamous carcinomas (OSCC) are a global problem, with approximately 354,864 cases and 177,384 deaths occurring annually. The disease predominantly affects males and is strongly linked to the habits of tobacco and alcohol consumption. Two-thirds of cases occur in the developing world [1]. In India alone, there are 119,992 new cases and 72,616 deaths yearly [4]. This is primarily due to the fact that tobacco is a socially accepted custom with nearly a third of all adults and 42.4% of males addicted to this habit [5]. Moreover, there is a

A. K. D'Cruz (✉)
Apollo Group of Hospitals,
Navi Mumbai, Maharashtra, India

Department of Oncology, Apollo Hospital,
Navi Mumbai, Maharashtra, India

H. Dhar
Department of Head and Neck Oncology, Narayana Superspeciality Hospitals,
Howrah, West Bengal, India

K. Fatehi
Department of Head Neck Oncology, Apollo Hospital, Navi Mumbai, Maharashtra, India
e-mail: drkhuzema_f@apollohospitals.com

R. Vaish
Department of Head and Neck Oncology, Tata Memorial Hospital, Mumbai, Maharashtra, India

Department of Head and Neck Oncology, Homi Bhabha National Institute,
Mumbai, Maharashtra, India

A. Al-Qahtani et al. (eds.), *Textbook of Clinical Otolaryngology*,
https://doi.org/10.1007/978-3-030-54088-3_38

widespread use of the areca nut, and two-thirds of the tobacco consumed is in the smokeless form with its carcinogenic effects occurring locally. These habits are popular in the entire Indian subcontinent, Taiwan as well as part of Saudi Arabia and Yemen [6].

The oral cavity includes the lip, buccal mucosa, alveolus (including upper and lower gums), hard palate, retromolar trigone, anterior two-thirds of the tongue and floor of the mouth (Fig. 38.1). While each of these subsites does have variations in incidence, patterns of spread and prognosis, the general principle governing the management of these cancers is essentially the same.

38.2.1 Presentation

Despite a well-defined tumour progression model, well-established premalignant lesions (leukoplakia/erythroplakia) and ease at examination, the majority of oral cancers present at a locally advanced stage. This is due to the fact that patients are from a lower socio-economic background with a heavy dependence on tobacco and alcohol and early signs and symptoms are subtle. Locally advanced presentation is not restricted to just developing countries but is seen in the developed world as well, 55% present in the USA with locally advanced stages as seen in a large national cancer database (NCDB) study [7]. In addition prevalence of co-morbidities, which could be in as high as half the patients, compounds problems posing a challenge to appropriate treatment and compliance [8].

Attempts at early detection through population screening or the use of adjunctive aids (toluidine blue, brush cytology, fluorescent imaging, etc.) have not proven to be beneficial [9]. Three rounds of oral examination by a trained health worker every 3 years in addition to health education did not show mortality reduction in a randomized control trial (RCT) [10]. However, benefit was seen in high-risk individuals (tobacco/alcohol users). Extrapolating these findings to clinical practice there is a strong case for opportunistic screening of such high-risk populations by dentists/medical professionals during examination.

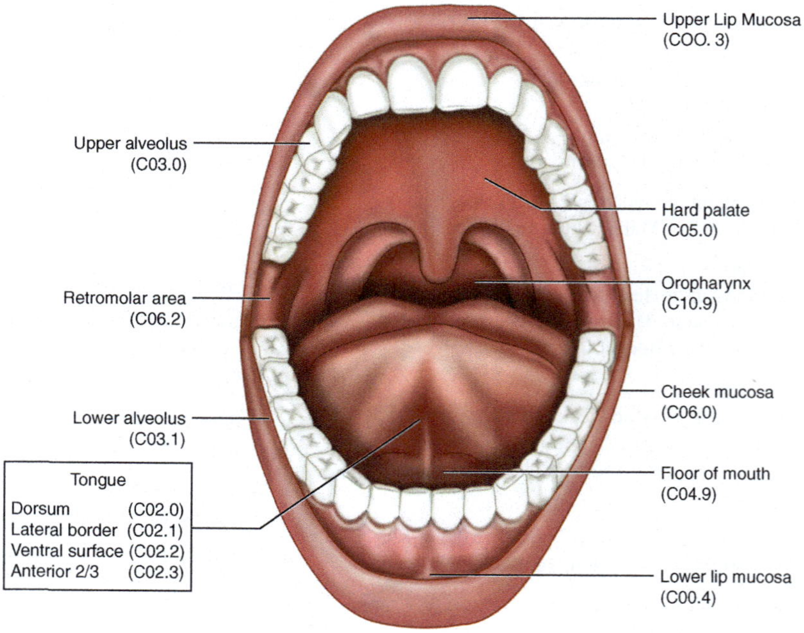

Fig. 38.1 Subsites of the oral cavity [ICD codes mentioned against each subsite in parenthesis]

38.2.2 Workup

Appropriate treatment is planned based on the clinical workup and staging of disease influenced by both patient-related and disease-related factors.

Patient-related factors include the performance status and general condition.

In addition, the presence of any co-morbidities also bears an impact on treatment planning. Disease-related factors include the tumour extent, involvement of vital structures (which may reflect inoperability) and presence of distant metastasis. This is assessed clinically as well as by appropriate imaging.

38.2.2.1 Clinical Assessment

Presentation depends on the subsite involved, classical features being a non-healing ulcer or growth, with or without pain. Pain is a feature more commonly associated with tongue lesions and hence patients present earlier than other subsites of the oral cavity. Similarly, lip cancers where the growth is readily visible, present early. Gingivo-buccal cancers present with locally advanced disease in contrast. Advanced lesions can present with pain, bleeding, or fixity to surrounding structures. Advanced tongue and floor of mouth cancers are associated with hypoglossal palsy, ankyloglossia, progressive difficulty in mastication and speech, pooling of saliva and surface bleeding. Cervical adenopathy is common given the propensity to neck node metastasis. Advanced gingivo-buccal cancers in contrast present with a large growth which may lead to subcutaneous and skin involvement, manifested by erythema, puckering or frank ulceration. In addition, there could be spontaneous loosening of teeth. Clinical signs of inoperability of tongue cancers are root of tongue involvement manifested by ankyloglossia and induration of suprahyoid musculature, while in buccal cancer, high infratemporal fossa (ITF) involvement manifested clinically with progressive trismus. Other signs of inoperability are extensive skin and subcutaneous involvement, presence of dermal skin nodules and a hard-fixed nodal mass.

38.2.2.2 Biopsy

A biopsy is required to establish the histological confirmation of malignancy. The majority of oral cancers are amenable to punch biopsy, easily performed as an office procedure. Biopsy should be performed from representative tissue avoiding obvious necrotic areas. Occasionally lesions are submucosal or infiltrative when an incisional biopsy is warranted. Similarly, for verrucous lesions, an incisional biopsy that includes deeper tissues helps the pathologist in differentiating a carcinoma from hyperplasia. Scrape cytology is not routinely used for oral lesions given the ease of a punch biopsy and lower sensitivity of this procedure.

38.2.2.3 Imaging

Imaging is important to ascertain the locoregional spread and help plan treatment. Contrast-enhanced computed tomography (CECT) scan is the workhorse and imaging modality of choice for the majority of oral cancers. It is accurate to assess the extent of disease as well as mandibular involvement. Similar diagnostic accuracy between a CECT and magnetic resonance imaging (MRI) for mandibular involvement was shown in a meta-analysis of 477 patients from 11 studies [11]. Cone-beam CT (CBCT) and single-photon emission computed tomography (SPECT) have also a high diagnostic accuracy for mandibular involvement but given the inadequate soft tissue delineation of both these modalities, they are not routinely preferred for imaging of oral malignancies [12].

Given its better soft tissue delineation, MRI is the preferred imaging modality for tongue and floor of mouth lesions. MRI has also been validated in recent studies to assess the depth of invasion (DOI) with acceptable accuracy [13, 14]. Intraoral ultrasonography (US) has also been evaluated for the assessment of DOI with similar accuracy to that of MRI [15]. However, given that it is highly operator dependent, cumbersome and could be painful, it is not used in routine practice.

Distant metastatic workup is not routinely indicated given that these cancers even in advanced stages are largely confined locoregionally. However, in patients with large bulky adenopathy (N2/N3), nodal involvement in the lower reaches of the neck (level IV and V), or large primary T4 tumours, it is prudent to investigate for the same. Positron emission technology (PET) scan is the investigation of choice in such situations [16]. Given that the lung is the most common site of distant spread, CT thorax is a useful alternative, especially in a cost constraint setting. It has a similar diagnostic accuracy for the detection of lung metastasis when compared to PET scan as shown in a large study [17].

All commonly used imaging modalities (CT, US, MRI, PET) have been studied for evaluating the neck. CECT and MRI have both shown comparable sensitivity to detect neck node metastasis with some studies suggesting that the CECT may have higher sensitivity [18]. Liao et al, in a meta-analysis specific to the node-negative neck, similarly showed a higher specificity of the CT scan. PET CT scan has limited application in detecting neck node metastasis especially in the node-negative setting [19]. US-guided fine-needle aspiration had the highest diagnostic odds ratio in a meta-analysis [20]. However, this modality is not extensively used given the fact that cross-sectional imaging needs to be performed in every case. The general dictum is to utilize the modality chosen for imaging of the primary tumour to image the neck as well. There is emerging data on the potential role of diffusion-weighted imaging sequences of MRI in increasing the accuracy of neck imaging [21].

38.2.3 Staging of Oral Cancers

The commonly used staging system for oral cancer is the American Joint Committee on Cancer (AJCC)/Union for International Cancer Control (UICC) TNM system 8th edition implemented from 2018 (Fig. 38.2). Amongst the benefits of staging, the most important from a clinical standpoint is the planning of appropriate treatment and prognostication. The two main modifications for oral cancers in the current edition are the addition of depth of invasion (DOI) of the primary tumour in the T category and extranodal extension (ENE) in the N category [22]. Changes in DOI were based on the results of the International

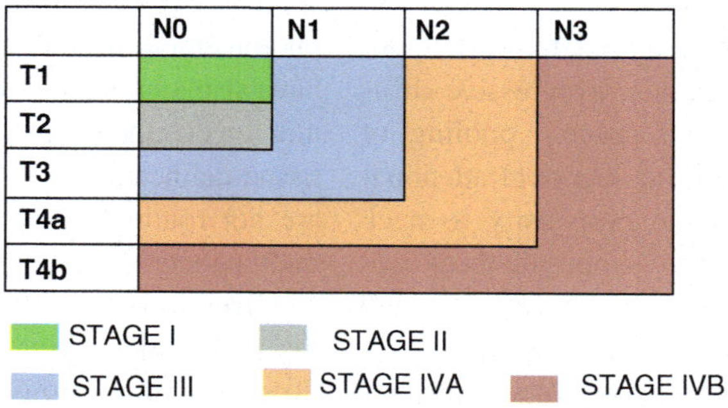

T staging *
T1: T≤ 2 cm, DOI ≤ 5 mm
T2: Tumour ≤ 2 cm, DOI > 5 mm and ≤10 mm OR
Tumour > 2 cm but ≤ 4cm, and DOI ≤10 mm
T3: Tumour > 4 cm & DOI ≤ 10 mm OR
Tumour ≤ 4 cm and DOI >10 mm
T4a: tumour > 4 cm and DOI >10 mm OR any T with DOI > 20 mm
Local invasion into the mandible, maxilla, skin, inferior alveolar nerve
T4b: Involvement of masticator space, pterygoid plates, skull base, encasement of the ICA

N staging *
N1: Single node ≤ 3 cm, ENE negative
N2: Single node ≤ 3 cm with ENE positive OR multiple ipsilateral, bilateral and contralateral nodes, none > 6 cm and ENE negative
N3: Any node > 6 cm or any node(s) >3 cm with ENE positive

Fig. 38.2 TNM group staging for oral cancers. *For detailed TNM staging, refer to the AJCC TNM 8th edition. *DOI* depth of invasion, *ENE* extranodal extension consortium for outcomes research (ICOR) study, which used data from 11 institutions worldwide (3149 patients). The study showed a significant difference in outcomes when DOI was incorporated into prognostication models with an incremental increase of every 5 mm translating into a higher T stage (≤5 mm as T1, 5–10 mm as T2 and >10 mm as T3/T4) [23]. For the N category, while size, number and location of lymph nodes were already part of the staging system, ENE was in addition incorporated as a prognostic factor [24–26]. Presence of ENE upstages to N2 for nodes ≤3 cm while ENE in a node >3 cm or the presence of ENE in more than one node upstages disease to N3. The relevance of the extent of ENE (microscopic vs. macroscopic) is uncertain. Wreesman et al. showed 1.7 mm to be the critical cutoff value of prognostic relevance (ENE <1.7 mm to be labelled as minor and >1.7 mm as major) [25]. While current practice necessitates both (microscopic and macroscopic) be treated similarly, it is recommended by the TNM task force that the extent of ENE be recorded (microscopic <2 mm) for subsequent modifications, should the need arise.

It should be borne in mind that the suggested changes are based primarily on pathological findings across the various studies [22, 23]. Moreover, assessment of both DOI and ENE could be subjective and difficult to evaluate clinicoradiologically. The AJCC 8th edition explicitly states that in the case of uncertainty, the lower staged group should be considered. It is important to corroborate both these findings with final histopathology for accurate assessment of prognosis and appropriate adjuvant treatment [27].

- Tobacco and alcohol are major risk factors for oral cancers.
- Majority present with locally advanced disease.
- Early detection methods and routine public screening lack evidence.
- Current staging system (8th Edition) has incorporated DOI for T Stage and ENE for N stage.

- CT is the preferred modality of imaging; MRI is the modality of choice for tongue, floor of mouth, recurrent cases and base of skull involvement.
- Definite signs for inoperability are involvement of high ITF and skull base, prevertebral fascia, carotid sheath, root of tongue with indistinct planes near the hyoid, extensive skin and soft tissue infiltration with dermal nodules.

38.2.4 Principles of Management of Oral Cancers

Management of oral cancers presents a unique challenge given that patients present late and treatment has implications on both function and cosmesis. Care of patients must be multidisciplinary with a team comprising of oncologists (surgery, radiation and medical), ancillary specialties (radiology, pathology) and reconstructive and rehabilitative services (dental, plastic reconstructive, physiotherapy, speech and swallowing) for best results. Treatment depends on the stage of cancer at presentation and broad treatment guidelines are: early-stage disease (stage I, II)-single modality therapy which could be either surgery or radiotherapy; locally advanced cancers should be triaged into those that are operable and those that are very advanced and inoperable. Locally advanced operable lesions (stage III, IVA and select IVB) are treated with combined modality treatment, surgery being the primary modality. Locally advanced inoperable tumours (Stage IVB) are treated with either radiation (RT) or chemoradiotherapy (CRT). Some of these patients can be brought into the realm of curative treatment with salvage surgery following initial treatment. Neoadjuvant chemotherapy (NACT) has also been explored in this setting with some encouraging results (discussed later). Patients with metastatic disease are treated primarily with chemotherapy. Patients with advanced/metastatic disease with a poor performance status are treated symptomatically

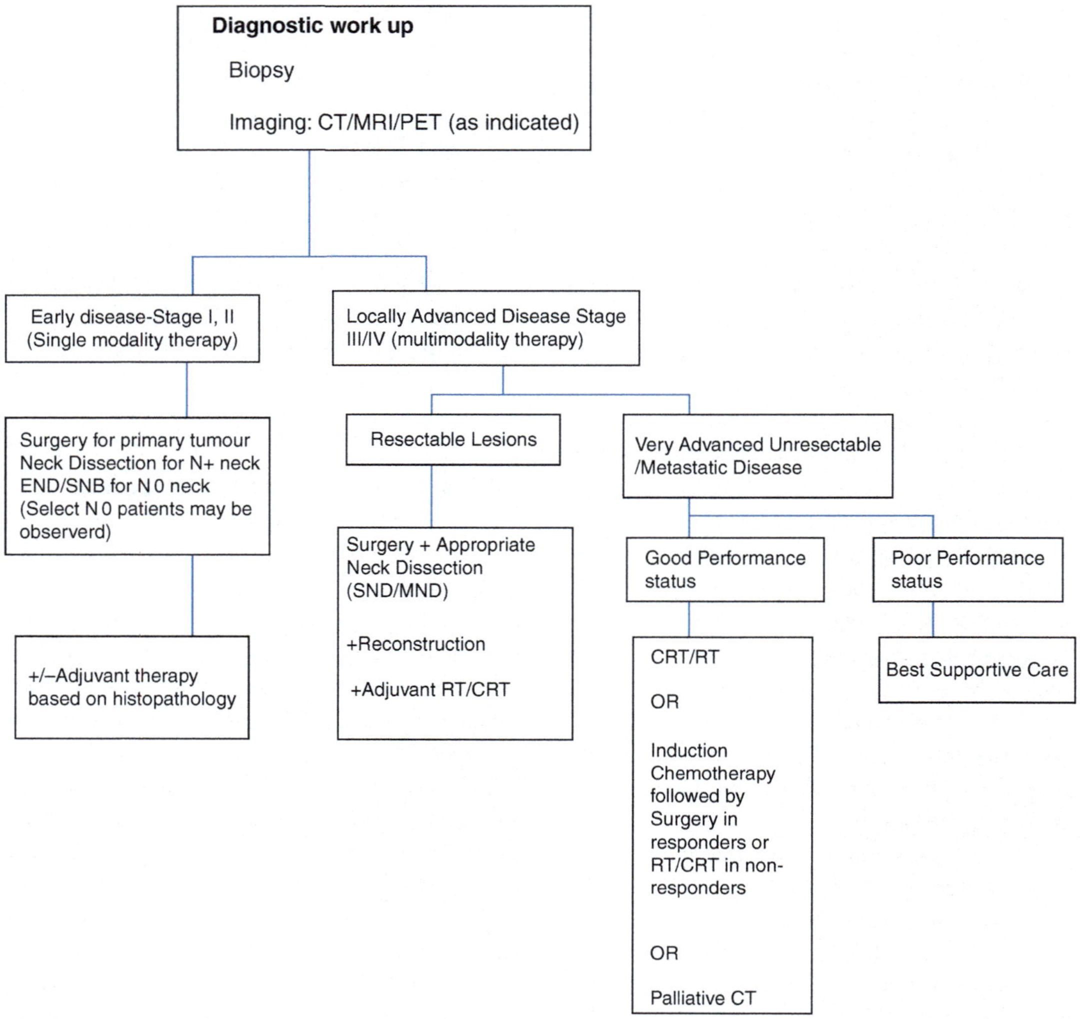

Fig. 38.3 Algorithm for oral cancer management

[16]. (Algorithm detailing the broad principles is provided in Fig. 38.3.)

38.2.4.1 Early-Stage Disease (Stage I, II)

Outcomes are essentially similar for surgery and radiotherapy for early-stage disease. While surgery has the advantage of being simple, quick, with no significant cosmetic and functional morbidity and therefore cost-effective, radiotherapy requires specialized centres and expertise, is prolonged (4–6 weeks) and with side effects of xerostomia, radiation-induced caries and occasionally osteoradionecrosis. Most importantly, radiation usually can only be given once, whereas repeated surgical procedures are possible both for recurrence and the development of a second primary. A recently published NCDB study from the USA revealed that clinicians preferred surgery over the radiotherapy in early oral cancers in 95% of cases. There was also a survival advantage in favour of surgery [28]. Brachytherapy is preferred when surgery would result in functional or cosmetic morbidity, e.g. superficially large lesions of the lip particularly with commissure involvement or superficial spreading lesions of the hard palate without bone involvement (surface mould brachytherapy) [29]. The ideal lesion suitable for interstitial brachytherapy should be superficial, accessible, and away from bone where placement of interstitial brachytherapy catheters is possible.

38.2.4.2 Locally Advanced Operable Lesions (Stage III, IVA and Select IVB)

Surgery is the mainstay of treatment and primary modality of choice for locally advanced operable oral cancers (stage III, IVA). Results with primary surgery are better than in the salvage setting in this group of patients. There have been two randomized trials to date attempting to address this issue, one of which had to be prematurely terminated while the other was overwhelmingly in favour of surgery [30, 31]. A recent NCDB study including 6900 patients of oral cancer demonstrated that surgery followed by adjuvant RT had better overall outcomes as compared to upfront chemoradiation when analysed for the entire cohort as well as for T3, T4a tumours [32]. Stage T4b cancers (masticator space-ITF complex involvement), considered inoperable earlier, could benefit from surgery in a select subset of patients. Studies have demonstrated that low ITF involvement—described as the area below an imaginary line drawn through the sigmoid notch—could be offered surgery with acceptable outcomes [33–35]. It should be noted, however, that these studies are all focused on gingivo-buccal cancers and extrapolating this concept to other subsites of the oral cavity is without scientific justification. RT/CRT with a goal at organ preservation is inadequate because of the aggressive nature of oral cancers as well as the close proximity to the mandible. There have been few reports suggesting the possibility of its use in a select subset of patients with an unacceptably high rate of complications [36].

38.2.5 Principles of Surgery

Oral cancers are a surgical disease when feasible for reasons alluded to. The aim at surgery is wide excision of the tumour, radical enough for gross tumour excision with margins, but conservative enough to preserve function and cosmesis. The broad surgical principles are as follows:

38.2.5.1 Margins

Achieving tumour free margins is of paramount importance. Clear margins have consistently shown better overall survival as compared with close or involved margins [37]. Although there have been various cut-offs proposed as the ideal tumour free margin, the consensus is in favour of 5 mm as the gold standard. A MEDLINE and EMBASE search for local recurrence following excision for oral cancer, without receipt of adjuvant therapy identified five studies. The pooled recurrence rates demonstrated a 21% absolute risk reduction when margins were more than 5 mm [38]. It should be borne in mind that there is a 20–30% shrinkage of margins after excision and fixation of the specimen and hence one should aim at placing the incision 1 cm away at surgery [39].

Tumour free margins must be achieved three-dimensionally and should be adequate for mucosa, bone and soft tissue. There have been recent reports of similar outcomes with <5 mm margin but these are retrospective single institutional studies, and therefore should not be considered as the standard of care till ratified by others [40].

The role of frozen section (FS) to guide adequacy of margin is contentious. A meta-analysis of eight studies showed that revision of positive margins to clear margins based on FS guidance does not equate to the local control achieved by adequate margins in the first instance. However, it is prudent at times to use FS control especially in complex resections and for the deep margins of excision. Analysis of margins, if done, is more accurate from the tumour specimen rather than the tumour bed [41].

38.2.5.2 Establishing Operability

There is a grey area occasionally between operability and inoperability. The decision is often subjective and based primarily on the philosophy of the treating surgeon and centre. The ability to achieve oncologically safe margins and ensure appropriate reconstruction with early institution of adjuvant therapy is a useful guide to establish operability. While involvement of the prevertebral fascia, carotid sheath, high ITF/skull base and mediastinum are definite signs of inoperability, features such as extensive skin and subcutaneous involvement, extensive lymphoedema with dermal nodules, high-grade tumours and multiple large bilateral nodes signify aggressive tumour biology and one should be cautious to recommend surgery.

38.2.5.3 Addressing the Mandible

Gross involvement of the mandible necessitates segmental resection. For tumours close to the mandible, rim resection (marginal mandibulectomy) may be performed to achieve adequate clearance. This procedure can also be performed for superficial erosion of the bone, selecting cases judiciously. A margin of 0.5–1 cm should be achieved on bone with a minimum of 1 cm of residual mandibular height preserved to prevent postoperative fracture. Edentulous mandibles, where the vertical height is reduced (pipe stem), gross paramandibular disease (point of abutment is the site of potential spread to the mandible) [42] and the post-radiation setting (due to compromised periosteal integrity and multiple routes of tumour entry to the mandible) preclude the use of this procedure. Marginal mandibulectomy is performed in the horizontal plane for gingivobuccal cancers (horizontal mandibulectomy) or the vertical plane for tongue and floor of mouth cancers (lingual plate marginal mandibulectomy). However, performing a pure lingual plate excision is technically difficult and an oblique marginal mandibulectomy is recommended. A marginal mandibulectomy should be canoe-shaped to prevent sharp angles which predispose to fracture caused by forces of mastication.

38.2.5.4 Approaches

To ensure adequate three-dimensional clearance, there should be due diligence to the approach at the time of surgery. Peroral excision is recommended for small lesions that are anteriorly placed with ease of accessibility around its entirety. Posteriorly placed lesions or lesions requiring mandibular resection are usually approached via a lip-split incision. A pull-through approach dividing muscles in the floor of the mouth is useful for tongue and floor of mouth lesions which necessitate deep excision. Occasionally, posteriorly based tongue and floor of mouth lesions are approached by a mandibulotomy which could be median or paramedian. The paramedian position is preferred as it does not disrupt the geniohyoid complex and there is maximum divergence of roots between the canine and incisors, which helps preserve the integrity of these teeth.

38.2.5.5 Management of the Neck

Consensus today is in favour of operating the neck electively, for clinicoradiologically node-negative early oral cancers amenable to peroral excision. This is based on the results of two large randomized trials as well as numerous other meta-analyses to show the benefit of this approach [43–46]. There may be a limited role of observation in small superficial lesions in highly reliable patients willing for close surveillance though the quality of evidence to support that this recommendation is intermediate [47].

A selective neck dissection clearing levels I, II and III is adequate in the N zero setting. A minimum of 18 nodes harvested and studied ensures the adequacy and appropriateness of the procedure [47]. A modified neck dissection clearing levels I through V is recommended for node-positive cases. However, there is evidence that a selective neck dissection is a valid option in this setting when nodes are not fixed, there is an absence of metastasis in levels IV and V, nodal volume <3 cm, absence of multiple nodes or nodal involvement at multiple levels [48]. The overall incidence of metastasis to level V in oral cavity cancers is very low. Presence of metastatic nodes at the jugulodigastric area (level IIA) and retromolar trigone disease predispose to metastasis at level V [49].

38.2.6 Adjuvant Treatment

Radiotherapy is indicated as an adjuvant for all stage III/IV cancers. Definite indications are T3/T4 tumours, N2/N3 neck status, and close margins. Literature is divided on the role of adjuvant radiotherapy for intermediate-risk factors, namely high grade, lymphovascular invasion (LVI), perineural invasion (PNI), single node-positive (without ENE) and worst pattern of invasion (WPOI). While their presence does indicate an aggressive biology, the commonly followed practice is to recommend radiotherapy when a combination of two or more of these factors are present [50, 51]. Chemotherapy is added to radiotherapy for high-risk disease, namely ENE and positive margins ≤1 mm [24].

The recommended doses of radiotherapy are 5600–6000 cGy for low-risk areas and 6000–6400 cGy for high-risk areas [52]. Early initiation of RT following surgery is beneficial. Starting within 6 weeks of surgery or a treatment package time (defined as the duration from the date of surgery till the conclusion of adjuvant therapy) <85–100 days are associated with better outcomes [50].

38.2.7 Role of Neoadjuvant Chemotherapy

Traditionally, it is believed that there is no role for chemotherapy in oral cancers except in combination with radiotherapy. However, there have been attempts to explore its role in the neoadjuvant setting. There have been two randomized trials to date addressing this question, both did not show an improvement in overall survival [53, 54]. However, the Licitra trial [53] did demonstrate the potential benefit of NACT in downsizing tumours necessitating smaller and more conservative surgeries and a decreased need for adjuvant radiotherapy. While exciting, this approach has not been ratified as others and still remains largely investigational. Patil et al. explored NACT with a similar aim of tumour downsizing but applied it to the setting of borderline operable lesions. In a large single-institution series ($n = 721$), 43% of patients could be brought into the realm of curative treatment. Median survival was 19.6 months in responders as compared to 8.16 months in non-responders [55]. While there seems to be a potential role of NACT in borderline operable tumours, its potential role in operable oral cancers needs to be established in further well-designed trials.

38.2.8 Management of Recurrent and Metastatic Disease

Oral cancer is an aggressive disease and coupled with the fact that patients present late, as high as 2/3rd of patients develop recurrences. Salvage surgery if feasible is the treatment of choice and is guided by factors such as the stage of presentation, disease-free interval (preferably >6–12 months), feasibility of achieving tumour-free margins, and performance status of the patient. These recurrent lesions are difficult to diagnose and tend to be missed out in a background of post-treatment fibrosis and distorted anatomy [56, 57]. Adjuvant re-radiotherapy, whenever feasible, is warranted as it is known to result in superior outcomes [58].

Re-irradiation should be offered to patients who are not candidates for surgery. It has been shown to have superior outcomes in a multi-institutional prospective trial (RTOG 9610) [59]. For those who are not suitable for surgery or re-radiotherapy, palliative chemotherapy should be offered to those with good performance status and symptomatic therapy for the rest. Platinum agents with 5 Fluorouracil combined with epidermal growth factor receptor (EGFR) antagonist cetuximab are considered the standard of care in this setting [60]. Recent evidence has emerged supporting the role of programmed-death-ligand

1(PD-L1) immunotherapy in platinum-resistant patients [61, 62]. However, cost constraints and lack of evidence on its role in platinum naïve patients limit its use.

- Surgery is the primary treatment modality. Patients should be triaged into operable and inoperable based on imaging and clinical assessment.
- Establishing tumour free margins in all three dimensions (minimum of 5 mm clear margins) is to be aimed for ensuring disease control.
- Elective neck dissection is recommended for clinically node-negative early oral cancers. Selective neck dissection may apply to certain node-positive patients.
- Advanced T stage, N2/N3 nodal status and close margins are definite indications for adjuvant RT. Positive margins and ENE warrant adjuvant CRT. The need for adjuvant treatment with other factors (PNI, LVE, single node-positive, WPOI) is contentious. The presence of more than one of these signifies aggressive disease and adjuvant treatment may be recommended.
- There is a potential role of NACT to downsize tumours with the role of increasing operability and organ preservation.
- Inoperable tumours are treated with radiation/chemoradiation. Salvage surgery offers the best outcomes for recurrent tumours. Chemotherapy, biologicals and immunotherapy are treatment options for other recurrent/metastatic diseases.

38.3 Oropharyngeal Cancers

38.3.1 Introduction

The oropharynx is the area bounded superiorly by an arbitrary line drawn from the soft palate to the posterior pharyngeal wall and inferiorly by a line from the hyoid to the posterior pharyngeal wall. Anteriorly it is bounded by the circumvallate papillae and the anterior tonsillar pillars, separating it from the oral cavity. It comprises four subsites: (1) base of tongue and vallecula, (2) tonsil, (3) pharyngeal wall-lateral and posterior and (4) soft palate and uvula. Tumours that arise from these subsites are predominantly squamous cell carcinomas.

Traditionally oropharyngeal cancers like other cancers of the upper aerodigestive tract were predominantly tobacco related. With a decreasing consumption of tobacco, particularly in the developed world, a paradigm shift has occurred in the etiopathogenesis of cancers affecting this subsite. Human Papilloma Virus (HPV) is now the major causative agent for the majority of cancers of the tonsil and base of tongue [63]. This has resulted in an exponential increase in the incidence of OPC. HPV-related cancers are now recognized as a distinct biological entity (reasons discussed later), with a better prognosis and are therefore currently a topic of extensive research for different and less intensive management protocols [64]. One must, therefore, establish the HPV status before counselling and initiation of treatment. This section deals with the changing epidemiology, biology of HPV tumours and principles of management of OPCs, highlighting recent advances.

38.3.2 HPV Positive OPC

38.3.2.1 Epidemiology

A sharp increase in the incidence of OPC was observed from the late 1990s in North America and Western Europe [65]. Surveillance, epidemiology and end results (SEER) database analysis demonstrated an increase in HPV prevalence in patients with OPC, from 16.3% during 1984–1989 to 71.7% in 2000–2004 with a concomitant fall in HPV negative OPC by 50% [66]. In a similar analysis of 69,592 OPCs and 113,144 OCCs across 23 countries from 1983 to 2002, a significant rise in HPV-related OPCs was seen in developed countries, mainly among young males [67].

Table 38.1 Characteristics of HPV-RELATED and HPV-unrelated tumours

	HPV positive	HPV negative
Incidence	Increasing	Declining
Age	Younger	Older
Sex ratio	3:1(Males)	3:1(Males)
Predisposing factors	High-risk sexual behaviour	Substance abuse: tobacco, alcohol
	Ethnicity—Caucasian	
Head neck sites affected	Base tongue, tonsil	All subsites
Histological features	Non-keratinizing Poorly differentiated with basaloid features	Keratinizing—Well to moderately differentiated
Tumour biology	Wild type p53	Mutated p 53
	P 16 Elevated	P 16 suppressed
	EGFR downregulation	EGFR upregulation
	Lesser hypoxic areas	More hypoxic areas
Tumour presentation	Early T stages, advanced nodal stage (cystic nodes)	Variable Nodes are likely to be necrotic, less likely to be cystic
Response to treatment	Superior outcomes	Variable
Second primaries	Lower incidence of second primaries	Higher incidence of second primaries due to field cancerization
Metastasis	Metastasis can occur late	Metastasis occur earlier
	Disseminated—more than 1 site	Commonly to the lungs
	Associated with longer survival in some patients	Shorter median survival

HPV positive OPCs are seen to be a different disease entity (Table 38.1) [68]. A typical patient is a young Caucasian male with a history of high-risk sexual behaviour (high number of lifetime oral sex partners, vaginal sexual partners). There may be an associated history of marijuana abuse. Tumours have a non-keratinizing morphology and are poorly differentiated/undifferentiated with basaloid characteristics as opposed to HPV negative tumours. The primary tumour shows smaller T sage but a higher N stage. Nodal metastasis is often associated with a cystic component. There is an absence of field cancerization and a lower incidence of second primaries. Distant metastases occur in the same frequency as for HPV negative tumours, may occur after a longer interval and are of the disseminating type (more than one organ affected) with some patients having prolonged survival after treatment [69].

38.3.2.2 Etiopathogenesis

HPV subtypes 16 and 18 are the common strains related to cancers of the oropharynx [70]. The infection affects the palatine or lingual crypts from where the tumours arise de novo in the absence of pre-existing epithelial dysplasia. The malignant potential is attributed to the presence of two important viral oncoproteins—E 6 and E 7 which inactivate major tumour suppressor genes—p 53 and retinoblastoma (Rb), respectively. This results in an environment of uncontrolled cellular proliferation, reduced apoptosis and an increase in spontaneous and mutagen induced genomic mutations [71]. An important member of the cyclin-dependent kinase 4 (CDK4) inhibitors, the p16 molecule promotes Rb activation and subsequent G1 cell cycle arrest. The p16 and Rb molecules are known to share a reciprocal relationship and inactivation of Rb by E7 oncoprotein results in an elevation of p16 levels, which is considered as a surrogate marker for HPV infection.

38.3.2.3 Improved Outcomes

HPV positive OPCs are associated with better outcomes [64, 72, 73]. In a seminal publication looking at the association between HPV and outcomes, Ang et al. retrospectively analysed data from the RTOG 0129 [74] in which 63.8% were HPV positive. On comparing survival outcomes, HPV positive showed a significantly higher overall survival (OS) (82.4% vs. 57.1%, $p < 0.001$).When adjusted for age, race, tumour and nodal stage, tobacco exposure and treatment assignment, these tumours demonstrated a 58% reduction in risk of death (hazard ratio, 0.42; 95% CI, 0.27–0.66). Similar results were seen when survival analysis was done comparing p16 marker status (3-year OS being 83.6% [95% CI, 78.7–88.6] vs. 51.3% [95% CI, 41.5–61.0)] indicating that p 16 could be considered a reliable surrogate marker for HPV. Recursive partitioning analysis placed patients into three groups of increasing risk of death, based on HPV status, pack-years of smoking, tumour and nodal stage. Patients with HPV-related OPC, having ≤10 pack-years and limited nodal disease (N0–N2a) constituted the low-risk group, whereas those with non-HPV related tumours, having >10 pack-years of smoking and advanced T stage (T4) formed the high-risk group. A positive history of tobacco usage was seen to mitigate the protective effect conferred by HPV on these tumours. A subsequent meta-analysis of 34 studies worldwide confirmed the superior outcomes of HPV positive tumours with a 60% reduction in risk of death [75].

38.3.2.4 Biological Explanation for Improved Survival

Various theories have been postulated to explain the improved survival. These patients are known to be younger, without addictions and hence tolerate treatment better. The tumours are biologically different, possess p53 wild type [70] and thereby proposed to have intact apoptotic response to chemotherapy-induced stress. They are also known to be associated with a decreased EGFR expression [76], and with less hypoxic areas [77].

38.3.3 Staging of Oropharyngeal Cancers

The AJCC staging system 7th edition for OPC was primarily derived from data of tobacco-related cancers. With the identification of HPV tumours as a distinct entity, there was a consensus regarding the need for a different staging system for these cancers. The Princess Margaret Hospital (PMH) studying a cohort of 573 patients using regressive partitioning analysis (RPA) proposed a new TNM stage grouping—Stage I is T1–T3, N0–N2B, Stage II: T1–T3 N2C, Stage III: T4/N3 and stage IV is M1 disease [78]. These findings were validated by the International Collaboration on Oropharyngeal cancer Network for Staging (ICON-S) [79] which was a multicentric cohort study of 1907 patients with HPV positive OPC. This led to the incorporation of changes in the 8th edition of the AJCC TNM wherein two different staging systems were recommended for HPV positive and negative OPCs. T staging for the former did not differentiate between T4a and T4b. The clinical N staging was simplified, with N1 indicating one or more ipsilateral nodes (none >6 cm), contralateral or bilateral nodes (none >6 cm) as N2 and any node >6 cm as N3. Metastatic disease has been placed in stage IV, with stages I–III representing local and regional disease (Fig. 38.4).

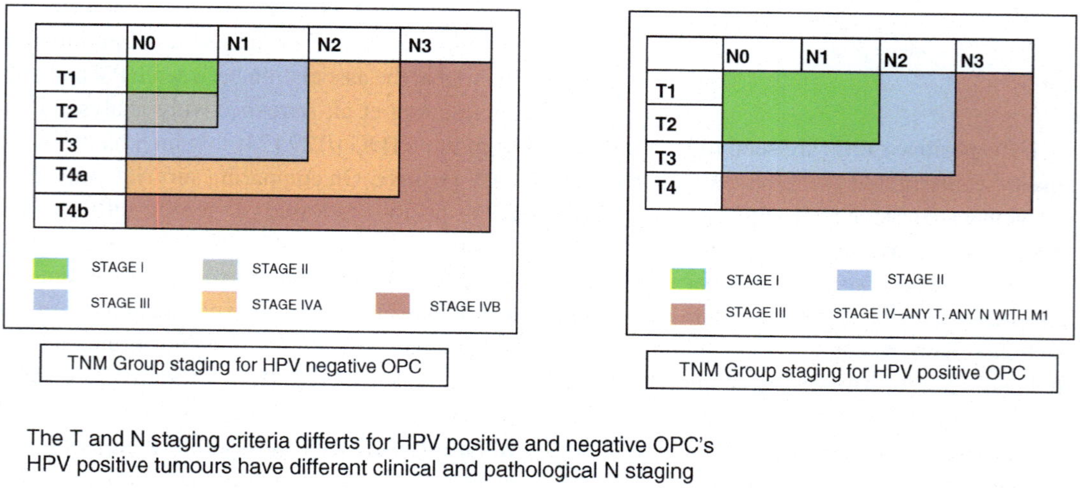

Fig. 38.4 TNM group staging for oropharyngeal cancers. *For detailed TNM staging, refer to the AJCC TNM 8th edition. *HPV* human papilloma virus, *OPC* oropharyngeal cancers

The T staging for HPV negative OPC has remained unchanged from the 7th AJCC TNM staging. The only change was the presence of ENE being incorporated into the nodal staging in keeping with other head and neck subsites.

38.3.4 Diagnostic Assessment of Oropharyngeal Cancers

Contrast-enhanced MRI is the preferred modality of imaging and has a high sensitivity for both the primary and neck. Distant metastasis are assessed with a whole-body PET CT. Chest CT may be performed for lung metastasis in the absence of the availability of PET scan. In patients who present with an unknown primary, a high index of suspicion must be maintained for an HPV related tonsil/base tongue tumour. These tumours are known to be small and within the crypts of the tonsil or the papillae of the base of tongue. Diligent, clinicoradiological evaluation must be performed. Many advocate a tonsillectomy (ipsilateral /bilateral) and surface excision of the base of tongue with a yield of the primary in as high as 89% of patients [80].

Current guidelines recommended checking the HPV status to help prognosticate and plan treatment [16, 81]. Immunohistochemistry (IHC) is widely accepted given its simplicity and ease of performance in addition to its high sensitivity (94%) [82] and cost-effectiveness. The presence of strong nuclear and cytoplasmic staining in more than 70% of malignant cells represents p16 positivity. If IHC is negative, the cancer is considered as HPV negative. The presence of HPV can be further confirmed by assessing for HPV DNA using in situ hybridization (ISH) given its higher specificity, when available. HPV DNA PCR has high specificity and along with p16 IHC has the highest sensitivity and specificity (94% and 96%), respectively [82].

HPV PCR tests on formalin-fixed tissue have their limitations and are better performed on fresh biopsy samples. DNA ISH and PCR though ideal, however, add to cost and time hence not routinely performed in clinical practice [81].

38.3.5 Principles of Management

Early-stage oropharyngeal tumours are treated with a single modality while locally advanced with combined modality therapy. Given the high rates of nodal metastasis (25–40%) [83, 84], difficulty in accessibility and functional morbidity, non-surgical treatment was the preferred option across all stages of OPC. Parsons et al. from data of 51 published series with 6400 patients showed similar control and survival rates for primary surgery compared to upfront RT [85]. Severe and fatal complications were significantly higher in the surgical group (32% vs. 3.8% for severe complications and 3.5% vs. 0.4% for fatal complications). Moreover, functional outcomes were also inferior in comparison to radiotherapy. Given the above, oropharyngeal cancers are traditionally treated with radiotherapy with surgery as salvage. The benefits of concurrent chemoradiotherapy were established through the Meta-analysis of Chemotherapy in Head Neck Cancer (MACH-NC), resulting in single modality radiotherapy being replaced by cisplatinum-radiotherapy for stage III/IV cancers [86, 87].

Radical radiotherapy prescribed in oropharyngeal cancers is 6600–7000 cGy, with or without chemotherapy, is delivered to the gross tumour volume with dose moderation to the remaining neck regions judged by the risk of disease. Intensity modulated radiotherapy (IMRT) is shown to have lesser side effects [88, 89]. Chemotherapy is administered as 100 mg/m^2 on days 1, 22 and 43 or weekly at 40 mg/m^2.

The alternate approach of cetuximab added to radiotherapy has shown to be of benefit in a trial of 424 patients, the majority of whom had oropharyngeal cancers (59.6%). The median OS was significantly in favour of cetuximab RT over RT alone [90]. The other approach is altered fractionation radiotherapy in lieu of conventional fractionation. Hyperfractionated radiotherapy was shown to have an absolute benefit of 8% over conventional RT [91], similar to the 8% benefit t of concurrent. Both these approaches of altered fractionation and adding biologicals are not standard of care at present. Cisplatinum-RT is the modality in widespread use and recommended in day to day clinical practice. The Bonner trial was a single study while Cisplatinum-RT has stood the test of time. Also, a systematic review did show the superiority of cisplatinum-RT over cetuximab RT [92]. Replacing cisplatinum by biologicals is only recommended for platinum unsuitable patients. Altered fractionation has not gained universal acceptance being logistically difficult.

38.3.6 Management of the Neck in OPC

Since OPC is treated non-surgically, nodal disease is addressed with appropriate fields of RT. In the post-RT/CRT setting, a response assessment PET CT is advised at 12 weeks from treatment conclusion. Given its high negative predictive value, the neck may be observed if PET negative, an approach shown to be safe in a RCT [93]. It prevents the morbidity of a routinely performed neck dissection and is also cost-effective. If PET is unavailable, cross-sectional imaging is recommended and in the absence of structural nodal disease, it is safe to keep patients on observation [47].

In patients offered primary TORS (discussed later) with lateralized lesions the ipsilateral neck should be addressed, given the high incidence of nodal metastasis. While neck dissection could be concurrent or interval, the majority preference is in favour of concurrent. Ligation of feeding blood vessels to decrease the incidence of postoperative haemorrhage is also advocated by some [47]. For tumours that extend to the midline (base tongue and palate), bilateral neck dissection should be performed.

38.3.7 Transoral Robotic Surgery: An Evolving Paradigm

Transoral Robotic Surgery (TORS) revolutionized the approach to the oropharynx enabling tumours to be accessed per orally, avoiding morbidity and complications, associated with open surgery. Added to this, there was better three-dimensional magnified vision, greater dexterity of movement assuring greater precision. Node-negative T1–T2 tumours are ideal indications for TORS, though some authors have extended the approach to select T3 lesions as well. Contraindications include: (1) T4b tumours, (2) large cervical adenopathy, (3) tumours warranting excision of >50% of the base tongue and posterior pharyngeal wall, (4) retropharyngeal carotid, (5) epicentre of tumour situated in the centre of base tongue placing bilateral lingual arteries at risk and (6) technical issues such as trismus or degenerative cervical spine precluding access to the lesion [94].

Adding adjuvant radiotherapy following TORS decreases functional outcome and the ideal case, therefore, is one that can be treated with single modality TORS. Favourable oncological and functional outcomes were demonstrated in two systemic reviews by Almeida and Yeh [95, 96] giving a boost to TORS in oropharyngeal cancers. It should be kept in mind that these were retrospective reviews with inherent limitations and the ORATOR trial (described below) did not confirm the benefit of TORS [97].

38.3.8 Deintensification Approaches for HPV-Related Oropharyngeal Cancers

Chemoradiotherapy, though the standard of care, was not without associated toxicity. One-third of patients with OPC are known to be affected by toxicity post-treatment [98]. Given that HPV-related OPC has an excellent prognosis, patients are younger with more survivors, attempts were made to de-intensify treatment to avoid long-term morbidity.

Deintensification strategies are largely focused on three approaches:

1. Reducing RT doses and volumes

Trials are on, to decrease radio-curative doses for HPV cancers. Approaches include reduced total doses in low-risk patients ranging from 5400–6000 cGy with or without cisplatinum, and induction chemotherapy with response adapted RT (5400 to 6600–7000 cGy) [99].

Strictures, feeding tube dependence, aspiration and dysphagia undergo an incremental increase with higher doses of radiotherapy. The alternate approach is to limit treatment volumes. The constrictors, glottis and supraglottic larynx have been identified as the dysphagia-aspiration related structures (DARS) and a novel approach limiting the radiation dose to these structures has been proposed as Dysphagia Optimized-IMRT (DO-IMRT) [100].

2. Omitting/reducing the dose/ and replacing chemotherapy with biologics:

   The addition of chemotherapy increases toxicity to the tune of 30% [101, 102]. Approaches include omitting chemotherapy, replacing high dose chemotherapy with biologicals or weekly cisplatinum or carboplatinum in an attempt to decrease toxicity.
3. *Integrating surgery in the management* with an attempt to triage patients based on pathological findings into low or high risk and adjust adjuvant treatment accordingly.

Initial results available of trials testing the deintensification approaches have not confirmed their safety or superiority in terms of functional outcome.

1. The *ORATOR* phase II randomized trial comparing TORS with IMRT for T1–T2, N0–2 OPC demonstrated similar oncological outcomes with functional in favour of IMRT [97]. The study had limitations and further studies are needed to address this issue [103].
2. Replacing cisplatinum by cetuximab in CRT regimens explored in two trials—the *RTOG 1016* [104] and the *De-ESCALaTE* [105]. Both studies showed significantly inferior outcomes within the cetuximab arm compared to cisplatinum-RT. Postulated explanations for these results are a reduced expression of EGFR in HPV positive tumours as well as inappropriate patient selection [106].

Given these initial trial results, conventional cisplatinum-RT as in HPV negative OPC remains the standard of care in routine practice. Patients should, therefore, be treated with deintensification strategies only in the trial settings. The only accepted difference between the two groups of oropharyngeal cancers is the changes in the staging system recategorizing various TNM classifications into the different stage groupings for HPV-related tumours.

38.3.9 Management of Recurrent/Metastatic Oropharyngeal Cancers

Recurrent oropharyngeal tumours show best outcomes with surgical salvage followed by adjuvant radiotherapy (refer to Chap. 37) [56, 58] or re-irradiation, depending on the time since earlier radiation as well as sequelae of prior treatment.

Patients with metastatic disease and recurrent tumours not feasible to surgery or re-irradiation are treated with palliative intent. Those with good functional status are offered chemotherapy/palliative RT. Triplet therapy with cetuximab, 5 FU and platinum agents is the standard regimen of choice [60]. Those with poor performance status are offered symptomatic care. Recent exciting literature supporting the use of PD-L1 immunotherapy has led to the incorporation of this approach in cisplatinum resistant recurrent/metastatic patients [61, 62]. (Algorithm detailing the broad principles is provided in Fig. 38.5.)

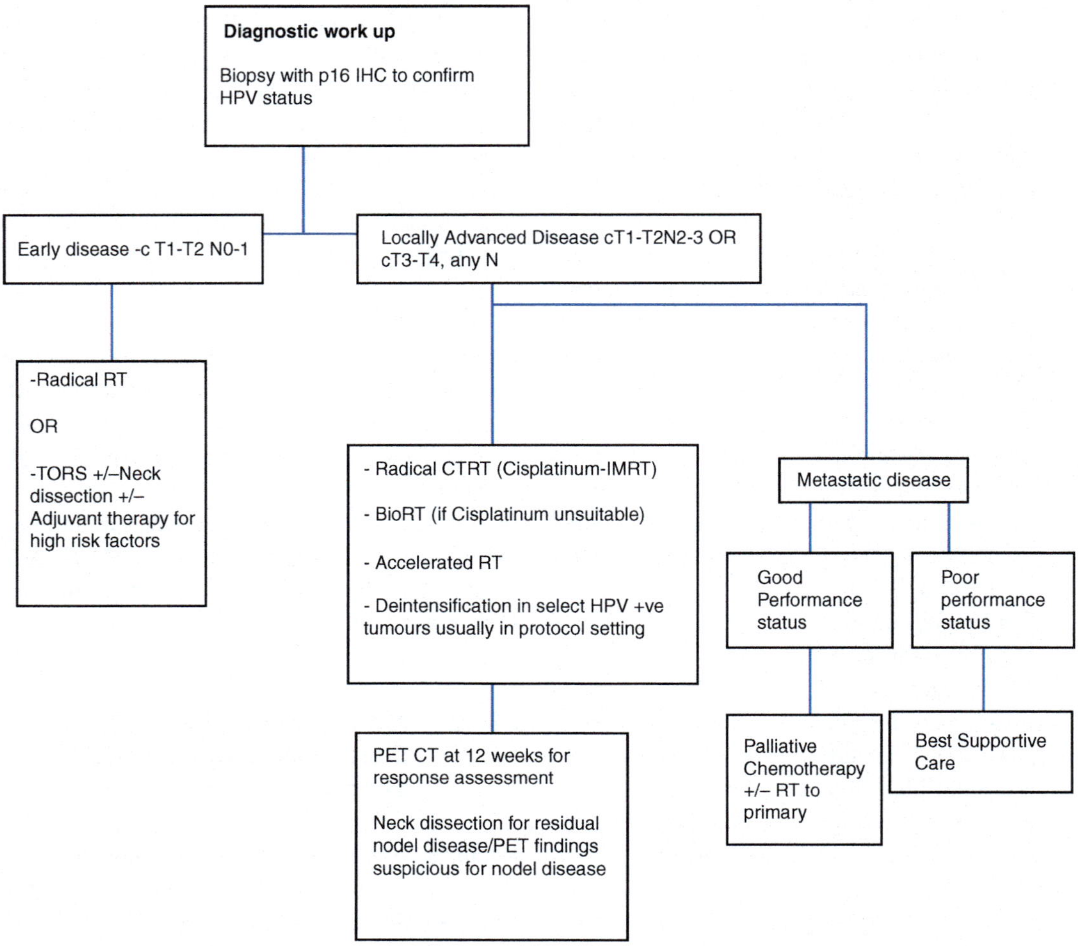

Fig. 38.5 Algorithm for oropharyngeal cancer management

38.3.10 Follow-Up of Patients with Oral and Oropharyngeal Cancer

Guidelines recommend that patients should be followed up at intervals of 1–3 months in the first year, 2–6 months in the second year, 4–8 months during the third to fifth year and annually thereafter [16, 81]. A detailed history and clinical examination of the head and neck including office-based endoscopy is warranted in all patients to rule out recurrence as well as second primary tumour. While many centres routinely perform imaging-based surveillance, others follow the practice of symptom-based imaging.

- OPC are HPV positive and negative-both being distinct entities with different etiopathogenesis, biology, staging systems and outcomes.
- Establishing HPV status is mandatory, p16 IHC is the recommended clinical test for the same.
- MRI with its better soft tissue delineation is the imaging of choice.
- Given morbidity and accessibility, treatment primarily revolves around non-surgical modalities (RT/CRT).

- TORS is emerging as an alternative for early-stage disease in an attempt to avoid the morbidity of radiotherapy.
- Given the better prognosis of HPV-related tumours, deintensification of treatment with strategies that include alterations with radiotherapy, use of biologicals, avoidance of chemotherapy and TORS are being explored.

Take-Home Messages

- Oral and oropharyngeal cancers are different disease entities.
- Oropharyngeal cancers are HPV positive and negative both being distinct.
- Oral cancers are surgically treated while oropharyngeal cancers are treated with predominantly non-surgical protocols.
- The aim of treatment is improving surgical outcomes while mitigating morbidity and maintaining the quality of life of patients.

Conflicts of Interest None of the authors have any conflict of interest with respect to the manuscript

References

1. Bray F, Ferlay J, Soerjomataram I, Siegel RL, Torre LA, Jemal A. Global cancer statistics 2018: GLOBOCAN estimates of incidence and mortality worldwide for 36 cancers in 185 countries. CA Cancer J Clin. 2018;68(6):394–424.
2. Chi AC, Day TA, Neville BW. Oral cavity and oropharyngeal squamous cell carcinoma-an update: oral & oropharyngeal cancer update. CA Cancer J Clin. 2015;65(5):401–21.
3. Weatherspoon DJ, Chattopadhyay A, Boroumand S, Garcia AI. Oral cavity and oropharyngeal cancer incidence trends and disparities in the United States: 2000–2010. Cancer Epidemiol. 2015;39(4):497–504.
4. Globocan 2018: India factsheet. India Against Cancer. 2018. Available from: https://gco.iarc.fr/today/data/factsheets/populations/356-india-fact-sheets.pdf. Accessed 14 April 2020.
5. GATS2 (Global Adult Tobacco Survey) fact sheet, India, 2016-17. https://www.who.int/tobacco/surveillance/survey/gats/GATS_India_2016-17_FactSheet.pdf. Accessed 14 April 2020.
6. Kujan O, Farah CS, Johnson NW. Oral and oropharyngeal cancer in the Middle East and North Africa: incidence, mortality, trends, and gaps in public databases as presented to the Global Oral Cancer Forum. Transl Res Oral Oncol. 2017;2:1–9.
7. Patel UA, Lynn-Macrae A, Rosen F, Holloway N, Kern R. Advanced stage of head and neck cancer at a Tertiary-Care County Hospital. Laryngoscope. 2006;116(8):1473–7.
8. Ribeiro KC, Kowalski LP, Latorre MR. Impact of comorbidity, symptoms, and patients' characteristics on the prognosis of oral carcinomas. Arch Otolaryngol Head Neck Surg. 2000;126(9):1079–85.
9. Macey R, Walsh T, Brocklehurst P, Kerr AR, Liu JL, Lingen MW. et al, Diagnostic tests for oral cancer and potentially malignant disorders in patients presenting with clinically evident lesions. Cochrane Database Syst Rev. 2015;(5):CD010276.
10. Sankaranarayanan R, Ramadas K, Thara S, Muwonge R, Thomas G, Anju G, et al. Long term effect of visual screening on oral cancer incidence and mortality in a randomized trial in Kerala, India. Oral Oncol. 2013;49(4):314–21.
11. de Souza Brandão Neto J, Aires FT, Dedivitis RA, Matos LL, Cernea CR. Comparison between magnetic resonance and computed tomography in detecting mandibular invasion in oral cancer: a systematic review and diagnostic meta-analysis: MRI x CT in mandibular invasion. Oral Oncol. 2018;78:114–8.
12. Qiao X, Liu W, Cao Y, Miao C, Yang W, Su N, et al. Performance of different imaging techniques in the diagnosis of head and neck cancer mandibular invasion: a systematic review and meta-analysis. Oral Oncol. 2018;86:150–64.
13. Alsaffar HA, Goldstein DP, King EV, de Almeida JR, Brown DH, Gilbert RW, et al. Correlation between clinical and MRI assessment of depth of invasion in oral tongue squamous cell carcinoma. J Otolaryngol Head Neck Surg. 2016;45(1):61.
14. Weimar EAM, Huang SH, Lu L, O'Sullivan B, Perez-Ordonez B, Weinreb I, et al. Radiologic-pathologic correlation of tumor thickness and its prognostic importance in squamous cell carcinoma of the oral cavity: implications for the eighth edition tumor, node, metastasis classification. AJNR Am J Neuroradiol. 2018;39(10):1896–902.
15. Marchi F, Filauro M, Iandelli A, Carobbio ALC, Mazzola F, Santori G, et al. Magnetic resonance vs. intraoral ultrasonography in the preoperative assessment of oral squamous cell carcinoma: a systematic review and meta-analysis. Front Oncol. 2019;9:1571.
16. National Comprehensive Cancer Network clinical practice guidelines in oncology (NCCN guidelines): cancer of the oral cavity, version 1. 2020 http://www.nccn.org/professionals/physician_gls/pdf/head-and-neck.pdf.

17. Kim Y, Roh J-L, Kim JS, Lee JH, Choi S-H, Nam SY, et al. Chest radiography or chest CT plus head and neck CT versus 18F-FDG PET/CT for detection of distant metastasis and synchronous cancer in patients with head and neck cancer. Oral Oncol. 2019;88:109–14.
18. Sun J, Li B, Li C, Li Y, Su F, Gao Q, et al. Computed tomography versus magnetic resonance imaging for diagnosing cervical lymph node metastasis of head and neck cancer: a systematic review and meta-analysis. OncoTargets Ther. 2015;8:1291–313.
19. Liao L-J, Lo W-C, Hsu W-L, Wang C-T, Lai M-S. Detection of cervical lymph node metastasis in head and neck cancer patients with clinically N0 neck—a meta-analysis comparing different imaging modalities. BMC Cancer. 2012;12(1):236.
20. de Bondt RBJ, Nelemans PJ, Hofman PAM, Casselman JW, Kremer B, van Engelshoven JMA, et al. Detection of lymph node metastases in head and neck cancer: a meta-analysis comparing US, USgFNAC, CT and MR imaging. Eur J Radiol. 2007;64(2):266–72.
21. Wu L-M, Xu J-R, Hua J, Gu H-Y, Zhu J, Hu J. Value of diffusion-weighted MR imaging performed with quantitative apparent diffusion coefficient values for cervical lymphadenopathy. J Magn Reson Imaging. 2013;38(3):663–70.
22. Lydiatt WM, Patel SG, O'Sullivan B, Brandwein MS, Ridge JA, Migliacci JC, et al. Head and neck cancers-major changes in the American Joint Committee on cancer eighth edition cancer staging manual. CA Cancer J Clin. 2017;67(2):122–37.
23. Ebrahimi A, Gil Z, Amit M, Yen T-C, Liao C-T, Chaturvedi P, et al. Primary tumor staging for oral cancer and a proposed modification incorporating depth of invasion: an international multicenter retrospective study. JAMA Otolaryngol Neck Surg. 2014;140(12):1138.
24. Bernier J, Cooper JS, Pajak TF, van Glabbeke M, Bourhis J, Forastiere A, et al. Defining risk levels in locally advanced head and neck cancers: a comparative analysis of concurrent postoperative radiation plus chemotherapy trials of the EORTC (#22931) and RTOG (# 9501). Head Neck. 2005;27(10):843–50.
25. Wreesmann VB, Katabi N, Palmer FL, Montero PH, Migliacci JC, Gönen M, et al. Influence of extracapsular nodal spread extent on prognosis of oral squamous cell carcinoma. Head Neck. 2016;38(Suppl 1):E1192–9.
26. Agarwal JP, Kane S, Ghosh-Laskar S, Pilar A, Manik V, Oza N, et al. Extranodal extension in resected oral cavity squamous cell carcinoma: more to it than meets the eye. Laryngoscope. 2019;129(5):1130–6.
27. Amin MB, American Joint Committee on Cancer, American Cancer Society, editors. AJCC cancer staging manual. 8th ed. Berlin: Springer; 2017. 1024p.
28. Ellis MA, Graboyes EM, Wahlquist AE, Neskey DM, Kaczmar JM, Schopper HK, et al. Primary surgery vs radiotherapy for early stage oral cavity cancer. Otolaryngol Head Neck Surg. 2018;158(4):649–59.
29. Kovács G, Martinez-Monge R, Budrukkar A, Guinot JL, Johansson B, Strnad V, et al. GEC-ESTRO ACROP recommendations for head & neck brachytherapy in squamous cell carcinomas: 1st update – improvement by cross sectional imaging based treatment planning and stepping source technology. Radiother Oncol. 2017;122(2):248–54.
30. Iyer NG, Tan DSW, Tan VK, Wang W, Hwang J, Tan N-C, et al. Randomized trial comparing surgery and adjuvant radiotherapy versus concurrent chemoradiotherapy in patients with advanced, nonmetastatic squamous cell carcinoma of the head and neck: 10-year update and subset analysis: surgery plus RT versus ChemoRT in HNSCC. Cancer. 2015;121(10):1599–607.
31. Robertson AG, Soutar DS, Paul J, Webster M, Leonard AG, Moore KP, et al. Early closure of a randomized trial: surgery and postoperative radiotherapy versus radiotherapy in the management of intra-oral tumours. Clin Oncol (R Coll Radiol). 1998;10(3):155–60.
32. Spiotto MT, Jefferson G, Wenig B, Markiewicz M, Weichselbaum RR, Koshy M. Differences in survival with surgery and postoperative radiotherapy compared with definitive chemoradiotherapy for oral cavity cancer: a national cancer database analysis. JAMA Otolaryngol Head Neck Surg. 2017;143(7):691–9.
33. Liao C-T, Ng S-H, Chang JT-C, Wang H-M, Hsueh C, Lee L-Y, et al. T4b oral cavity cancer below the mandibular notch is resectable with a favorable outcome. Oral Oncol. 2007;43(6):570–9.
34. Mair MD, Sawarkar N, Nikam S, Sarin R, Nair D, Gupta T, et al. Impact of radical treatments on survival in locally advanced T4a and T4b buccal mucosa cancers: selected surgically treated T4b cancers have similar control rates as T4a. Oral Oncol. 2018;82:17–22.
35. Pillai V, Yadav V, Kekatpure V, Trivedi N, Chandrashekar NH, Shetty V, et al. Prognostic determinants of locally advanced buccal mucosa cancer: do we need to relook the current staging criteria? Oral Oncol. 2019;95:43–51.
36. Foster CC, Melotek JM, Brisson RJ, Seiwert TY, Cohen EEW, Stenson KM, et al. Definitive chemoradiation for locally-advanced oral cavity cancer: a 20-year experience. Oral Oncol. 2018;80:16–22.
37. Looser KG, Shah JP, Strong EW. The significance of "positive" margins in surgically resected epidermoid carcinomas. Head Neck Surg. 1978;1(2):107–11.
38. Anderson CR, Sisson K, Moncrieff M. A meta-analysis of margin size and local recurrence in oral squamous cell carcinoma. Oral Oncol. 2015;51(5):464–9.
39. Mistry RC, Qureshi SS, Kumaran C. Post-resection mucosal margin shrinkage in oral cancer: quantification and significance. J Surg Oncol. 2005;91(2):131–3.

40. Zanoni DK, Migliacci JC, Xu B, Katabi N, Montero PH, Ganly I, et al. A proposal to redefine close surgical margins in squamous cell carcinoma of the oral tongue. JAMA Otolaryngol Neck Surg. 2017;143(6):555–60.
41. Maxwell JH, Thompson LDR, Brandwein-Gensler MS, Weiss BG, Canis M, Purgina B, et al. Early oral tongue squamous cell carcinoma: sampling of margins from tumor bed and worse local control. JAMA Otolaryngol Neck Surg. 2015;141(12):1104.
42. Brown JS, Lowe D, Kalavrezos N, D'Souza J, Magennis P, Woolgar J. Patterns of invasion and routes of tumor entry into the mandible by oral squamous cell carcinoma. Head Neck. 2002;24(4):370–83.
43. D'Cruz AK, Vaish R, Kapre N, Dandekar M, Gupta S, Hawaldar R, et al. Elective versus therapeutic neck dissection in node-negative oral cancer. N Engl J Med. 2015;373(6):521–9.
44. Hutchison IL, Ridout F, Cheung SMY, Shah N, Hardee P, Surwald C, et al. Nationwide randomised trial evaluating elective neck dissection for early stage oral cancer (SEND study) with meta-analysis and concurrent real-world cohort. Br J Cancer. 2019;121(10):827–36.
45. Abu-Ghanem S, Yehuda M, Carmel N-N, Leshno M, Abergel A, Gutfeld O, et al. Elective Neck dissection vs observation in early-stage squamous cell carcinoma of the oral tongue with no clinically apparent lymph node metastasis in the neck: a systematic review and meta-analysis. JAMA Otolaryngol Neck Surg. 2016;142(9):857.
46. Ren Z-H, Xu J-L, Li B, Fan T-F, Ji T, Zhang C-P. Elective versus therapeutic neck dissection in node-negative oral cancer: evidence from five randomized controlled trials. Oral Oncol. 2015;51(11):976–81.
47. Koyfman SA, Ismaila N, Crook D, D'Cruz A, Rodriguez CP, Sher DJ, et al. Management of the neck in squamous cell carcinoma of the oral cavity and oropharynx: ASCO clinical practice guideline. J Clin Oncol. 2019;37(20):1753–74.
48. Liang L, Zhang T, Kong Q, Liang J, Liao G. A meta-analysis on selective versus comprehensive neck dissection in oral squamous cell carcinoma patients with clinically node-positive neck. Oral Oncol. 2015;51(12):1076–81.
49. Pantvaidya GH, Pal P, Vaidya AD, Pai PS, D'Cruz AK. Prospective study of 583 neck dissections in oral cancers: implications for clinical practice. Head Neck. 2014;36(10):1503–7.
50. Ang KK, Trotti A, Brown BW, Garden AS, Foote RL, Morrison WH, et al. Randomized trial addressing risk features and time factors of surgery plus radiotherapy in advanced head-and-neck cancer. Int J Radiat Oncol. 2001;51(3):571–8.
51. Chen W-C, Lai C-H, Fang C-C, Yang Y-H, Chen P-C, Lee C-P, et al. Identification of high-risk subgroups of patients with oral cavity cancer in need of postoperative adjuvant radiotherapy or chemo-radiotherapy. Medicine (Baltimore). 2016;95(22):e3770.
52. Peters LJ, Goepfert H, Ang KK, Byers RM, Maor MH, Guillamondegui O, et al. Evaluation of the dose for postoperative radiation therapy of head and neck cancer: first report of a prospective randomized trial. Int J Radiat Oncol Biol Phys. 1993;26(1):3–11.
53. Licitra L, Grandi C, Guzzo M, Mariani L, Vullo SL, Valvo F, et al. Primary chemotherapy in resectable oral cavity squamous cell cancer: a randomized controlled trial. J Clin Oncol. 2003;21(2):327–33.
54. Zhong L, Zhang C, Ren G, Guo W, William WN, Sun J, et al. Randomized phase III trial of induction chemotherapy with docetaxel, cisplatin, and fluorouracil followed by surgery versus up-front surgery in locally advanced resectable oral squamous cell carcinoma. J Clin Oncol. 2013;31(6):744–51.
55. Patil VM, Prabhash K, Noronha V, Joshi A, Muddu V, Dhumal S, et al. Neoadjuvant chemotherapy followed by surgery in very locally advanced technically unresectable oral cavity cancers. Oral Oncol. 2014;50(10):1000–4.
56. Goodwin WJ. Salvage surgery for patients with recurrent squamous cell carcinoma of the upper aerodigestive tract: when do the ends justify the means? 2000;110(3 Pt 2 Suppl 93):1–18. https://doi.org/10.1097/00005537-200003001-00001.
57. Wong LY, Wei WI, Lam LK, Yuen APW. Salvage of recurrent head and neck squamous cell carcinoma after primary curative surgery. Head Neck. 2003;25(11):953–9.
58. Janot F, de Raucourt D, Benhamou E, Ferron C, Dolivet G, Bensadoun R-J, et al. Randomized trial of postoperative reirradiation combined with chemotherapy after salvage surgery compared with salvage surgery alone in head and neck carcinoma. J Clin Oncol. 2008;26(34):5518–23.
59. Spencer SA, Harris J, Wheeler RH, Machtay M, Schultz C, Spanos W, et al. Final report of RTOG 9610, a multi-institutional trial of reirradiation and chemotherapy for unresectable recurrent squamous cell carcinoma of the head and neck. Head Neck. 2008;30(3):281–8.
60. Vermorken JB, Mesia R, Rivera F, Remenar E, Kawecki A, Rottey S, et al. Platinum-based chemotherapy plus cetuximab in head and neck cancer. N Engl J Med. 2008;359(11):1116–27.
61. Ferris RL, Blumenschein G, Fayette J, Guigay J, Colevas AD, Licitra L, et al. Nivolumab for recurrent squamous-cell carcinoma of the head and neck. N Engl J Med. 2016;375(19):1856–67.
62. Burtness B, Harrington KJ, Greil R, Soulières D, Tahara M, de Castro G, et al. Pembrolizumab alone or with chemotherapy versus cetuximab with chemotherapy for recurrent or metastatic squamous cell carcinoma of the head and neck (KEYNOTE-048): a randomised, open-label, phase 3 study. Lancet. 2019;394(10212):1915–28.

63. Sturgis EM, Cinciripini PM. Trends in head and neck cancer incidence in relation to smoking prevalence. Cancer. 2007;110(7):1429–35.
64. Gillison ML. Human papillomavirus-associated head and neck cancer is a distinct epidemiologic, clinical, and molecular entity. Semin Oncol. 2004;31(6):744–54.
65. Gillison ML, Chaturvedi AK, Anderson WF, Fakhry C. Epidemiology of human papillomavirus–positive head and neck squamous cell carcinoma. J Clin Oncol. 2015;33(29):3235–42.
66. Chaturvedi AK, Engels EA, Pfeiffer RM, Hernandez BY, Xiao W, Kim E, et al. Human papillomavirus and rising oropharyngeal cancer incidence in the United States. J Clin Oncol. 2011;29(32):4294–301.
67. Chaturvedi AK, Anderson WF, Lortet-Tieulent J, Curado MP, Ferlay J, Franceschi S, et al. Worldwide trends in incidence rates for oral cavity and oropharyngeal cancers. J Clin Oncol. 2013;31(36):4550–9.
68. Gillison ML, D'Souza G, Westra W, Sugar E, Xiao W, Begum S, et al. Distinct risk factor profiles for human papillomavirus type 16–positive and human papillomavirus type 16–negative head and neck cancers. JNCI J Natl Cancer Inst. 2008;100(6):407–20.
69. Huang SH, Perez-Ordonez B, Weinreb I, Hope A, Massey C, Waldron JN, et al. Natural course of distant metastases following radiotherapy or chemoradiotherapy in HPV-related oropharyngeal cancer. Oral Oncol. 2013;49(1):79–85.
70. Gillison ML. Evidence for a causal association between human papillomavirus and a subset of head and neck cancers. J Natl Cancer Inst. 2000;92(9):709–20.
71. McDougall JK. Immortalization and transformation of human cells by human papillomavirus. Curr Top Microbiol Immunol. 1994;186:101–19. Review. PubMed PMID:8205836.
72. Weinberger PM, Yu Z, Haffty BG, Kowalski D, Harigopal M, Brandsma J, et al. Molecular classification identifies a subset of human papillomavirus--associated oropharyngeal cancers with favorable prognosis. J Clin Oncol. 2006;24(5):736–47.
73. Fakhry C, Westra WH, Li S, Cmelak A, Ridge JA, Pinto H, et al. Improved survival of patients with human papillomavirus-positive head and neck squamous cell carcinoma in a prospective clinical trial. JNCI J Natl Cancer Inst. 2008;100(4):261–9.
74. Ang KK, Harris J, Wheeler R, Weber R, Rosenthal DI, Nguyen-Tân PF, et al. Human papillomavirus and survival of patients with oropharyngeal cancer. N Engl J Med. 2010;363(1):24–35.
75. Dayyani F, Etzel CJ, Liu M, Ho C-H, Lippman SM, Tsao AS. Meta-analysis of the impact of human papillomavirus (HPV) on cancer risk and overall survival in head and neck squamous cell carcinomas (HNSCC). Head Neck Oncol. 2010;2:15.
76. Kim S-H, Koo B-S, Kang S, Park K, Kim H, Lee KR, et al. HPV integration begins in the tonsillar crypt and leads to the alteration of p16, EGFR and c-myc during tumor formation. Int J Cancer. 2007;120(7):1418–25.
77. Rischin D, Young RJ, Fisher R, Fox SB, Le Q-T, Peters LJ, et al. Prognostic significance of p16INK4A and human papillomavirus in patients with oropharyngeal cancer treated on TROG 02.02 Phase III trial. J Clin Oncol. 2010;28(27):4142–8.
78. Huang SH, Xu W, Waldron J, Siu L, Shen X, Tong L, et al. Refining American Joint Committee on Cancer/Union for International Cancer Control TNM stage and prognostic groups for human papillomavirus–related oropharyngeal carcinomas. J Clin Oncol. 2015;33(8):836–45.
79. O'Sullivan B, Huang SH, Su J, Garden AS, Sturgis EM, Dahlstrom K, et al. Development and validation of a staging system for HPV-related oropharyngeal cancer by the International Collaboration on Oropharyngeal cancer Network for Staging (ICON-S): a multicentre cohort study. Lancet Oncol. 2016;17(4):440–51.
80. Graboyes EM, Sinha P, Thorstad WL, Rich JT, Haughey BH. Management of human papillomavirus-related unknown primaries of the head and neck with a transoral surgical approach. Head Neck. 2015;37(11):1603–11.
81. Mehanna H, Evans M, Beasley M, Chatterjee S, Dilkes M, Homer J, et al. Oropharyngeal cancer: United Kingdom National Multidisciplinary Guidelines. J Laryngol Otol. 2016;130(S2):S90–6.
82. Prigge E-S, Arbyn M, von Knebel Doeberit M, Reuschenbach M. Diagnostic accuracy of p16INK4a immunohistochemistry in oropharyngeal squamous cell carcinomas: a systematic review and meta-analysis. Int J Cancer. 2017;140(5):1186–98.
83. Lindberg R. Distribution of cervical lymph node metastases from squamous cell carcinoma of the upper respiratory and digestive tracts. Cancer. 1972;29(6):1446–9. PubMed PMID: 5031238.
84. Van Abel KM, Moore EJ. Focus issue: neck dissection for oropharyngeal squamous cell carcinoma. ISRN Surg. 2012;2012:547017.
85. Parsons JT, Mendenhall WM, Stringer SP, Amdur RJ, Hinerman RW, Villaret DB, et al. Squamous cell carcinoma of the oropharynx: surgery, radiation therapy, or both. Cancer. 2002;94(11):2967–80.
86. Pignon J-P, le Maître A, Maillard E, Bourhis J. Meta-analysis of chemotherapy in head and neck cancer (MACH-NC): an update on 93 randomised trials and 17,346 patients. Radiother Oncol. 2009;92(1):4–14.
87. Blanchard P, Landais C, Petit C, Zhang Q, Grégoire V, Tobias J, et al. Meta-analysis of chemotherapy in head and neck cancer (MACH-NC): An update on 100 randomized trials and 19,248 patients, on behalf of MACH-NC group. Ann Oncol. 2016;27(6):328.
88. Nutting CM, Morden JP, Harrington KJ, Urbano TG, Bhide SA, Clark C, et al. Parotid-sparing intensity modulated versus conventional radiotherapy in head and neck cancer (PARSPORT): a phase 3 multicentre randomised controlled trial. Lancet Oncol. 2011;12(2):127–36.

89. Gupta T, Kannan S, Ghosh-Laskar S, Agarwal JP. Systematic review and meta-analyses of intensity-modulated radiation therapy versus conventional two-dimensional and/or or three-dimensional radiotherapy in curative-intent management of head and neck squamous cell carcinoma. PLoS One. 2018;13(7):e0200137.
90. Bonner JA, Harari PM, Giralt J, Azarnia N, Shin DM, Cohen RB, et al. Radiotherapy plus cetuximab for squamous-cell carcinoma of the head and neck. N Engl J Med. 2006;354(6):567–78.
91. Bourhis J, Overgaard J, Audry H, Ang KK, Saunders M, Bernier J, et al. Hyperfractionated or accelerated radiotherapy in head and neck cancer: a meta-analysis. Lancet Lond Engl. 2006;368(9538):843–54.
92. Petrelli F, Coinu A, Riboldi V, Borgonovo K, Ghilardi M, Cabiddu M, et al. Concomitant platinum-based chemotherapy or cetuximab with radiotherapy for locally advanced head and neck cancer: a systematic review and meta-analysis of published studies. Oral Oncol. 2014;50(11):1041–8.
93. Mehanna H, Wong W-L, McConkey CC, Rahman JK, Robinson M, Hartley AGJ, et al. PET-CT surveillance versus neck dissection in advanced head and neck cancer. N Engl J Med. 2016;374(15):1444–54.
94. Weinstein GS, O'Malley BW, Rinaldo A, Silver CE, Werner JA, Ferlito A. Understanding contraindications for transoral robotic surgery (TORS) for oropharyngeal cancer. Eur Arch Otorhinolaryngol. 2015;272(7):1551–2.
95. de Almeida JR, Li R, Magnuson JS, Smith RV, Moore E, Lawson G, et al. Oncologic outcomes after transoral robotic surgery: a multi-institutional study. JAMA Otolaryngol Neck Surg. 2015;141(12):1043.
96. Yeh DH, Tam S, Fung K, MacNeil SD, Yoo J, Winquist E, et al. Transoral robotic surgery vs. radiotherapy for management of oropharyngeal squamous cell carcinoma – a systematic review of the literature. Eur J Surg Oncol EJSO. 2015;41(12):1603–14.
97. Nichols AC, Theurer J, Prisman E, Read N, Berthelet E, Tran E, et al. Radiotherapy versus transoral robotic surgery and neck dissection for oropharyngeal squamous cell carcinoma (ORATOR): an open-label, phase 2, randomised trial. Lancet Oncol. 2019;20(10):1349–59.
98. Machtay M, Moughan J, Trotti A, Garden AS, Weber RS, Cooper JS, et al. Factors associated with severe late toxicity after concurrent chemoradiation for locally advanced head and neck cancer: an rtog analysis. J Clin Oncol. 2008;26(21):3582–9.
99. Mirghani H, Blanchard P. Treatment de-escalation for HPV-driven oropharyngeal cancer: where do we stand? Clin Transl Radiat Oncol. 2018;8:4–11.
100. Eisbruch A, Schwartz M, Rasch C, Vineberg K, Damen E, Van As CJ, et al. Dysphagia and aspiration after chemoradiotherapy for head-and-neck cancer: which anatomic structures are affected and can they be spared by IMRT? Int J Radiat Oncol Biol Phys. 2004;60(5):1425–39.
101. Adelstein DJ, Li Y, Adams GL, Wagner H, Kish JA, Ensley JF, et al. An intergroup phase III comparison of standard radiation therapy and two schedules of concurrent chemoradiotherapy in patients with unresectable squamous cell head and neck cancer. J Clin Oncol Off J Am Soc Clin Oncol. 2003;21(1):92–8.
102. Denis F, Garaud P, Bardet E, Alfonsi M, Sire C, Germain T, et al. Final results of the 94–01 French Head and Neck Oncology and Radiotherapy Group randomized trial comparing radiotherapy alone with concomitant radiochemotherapy in advanced-stage oropharynx carcinoma. J Clin Oncol. 2004;22(1):69–76.
103. Grégoire V, Nicolai P. Choosing surgery or radiotherapy for oropharyngeal squamous cell carcinoma: is the issue definitely settled? Lancet Oncol. 2019;20(10):1328–9.
104. Gillison ML, Trotti AM, Harris J, Eisbruch A, Harari PM, Adelstein DJ, et al. Radiotherapy plus cetuximab or cisplatin in human papillomavirus-positive oropharyngeal cancer (NRG Oncology RTOG 1016): a randomised, multicentre, non-inferiority trial. Lancet. 2019;393(10166):40–50.
105. Mehanna H, Robinson M, Hartley A, Kong A, Foran B, Fulton-Lieuw T, et al. Radiotherapy plus cisplatin or cetuximab in low-risk human papillomavirus-positive oropharyngeal cancer (De-ESCALaTE HPV): an open-label randomised controlled phase 3 trial. The Lancet. 2019;393(10166):51–60.
106. Orlandi E, Licitra L. The day after De-ESCALaTE and RTOG 1016 trials results. Future Oncol. 2019;15(18):2069–72.

39 Neoplasms of the Larynx and Laryngopharynx

Ismail Zohdi, Louay ElSharkawy, and Mahmoud ElBestar

39.1 Introduction

Benign neoplasms of the larynx and laryngopharynx are uncommon, and their symptoms vary from mild hoarseness to severe stridor. According to their site and clinical presentation, they are managed by follow-up or excision.

More than 95% of malignant laryngeal and laryngopharyngeal tumours are proven to be squamous cell carcinomas. Laryngeal cancers are the most common malignancy of the head and neck. Preoperative evaluation is essential for planning treatment. Most of the patients' laryngeal and laryngopharyngeal tumours are treatable apart from those with distant metastases or locally and regionally very advanced tumours.

39.2 Benign Neoplasms

Benign neoplasms constitute less than 5% of all laryngeal and laryngopharyngeal tumours. The most common benign tumour of the larynx is papilloma (85%), and other types include haemangioma, granular cell tumour, paraganglioma, chondroma, adenoma, leiomyoma, rhabdomyoma, fibroma, lipoma and schwannoma.

I. Zohdi (✉) · L. ElSharkawy · M. ElBestar
Cairo University, Cairo, Egypt
e-mail: louay.sharkawy@kasralainy.edu.eg

Single papilloma occurs in adults, and it usually arises from the anterior half of the vocal cord. The papilloma is excised by microlaryngeal surgery. It is liable to recurrence and malignant change. Recurrent respiratory papillomatosis is a benign lesion of the larynx and trachea. It is caused by the human papillomavirus types 6 and 11. Recurrent respiratory papillomatosis usually occurs before the age of 5 years, but can also occur less often in adults, thus there is a bimodal distribution, juvenile and adult onset types. Patients present with weak cry, hoarseness and later stridor. Papillomas are mostly seen on the true vocal cords, ventricular bands and epiglottis, but they may involve other sites in larynx, trachea and bronchi. They appear as pedunculated or sessile, glistening white, irregular growths. Papillomas tend to disappear spontaneously after puberty. Surgery by using cup forceps, CO2 laser or microdebrider aims to restore the airway and improve the voice. Papillomas frequently recur, therefore multiple laryngoscopies may be needed, increasing the risk of complications. Vocal cord scarring, web formation and laryngeal stenosis can be avoided by accurately using the CO2 laser, choosing the best spot-size and appropriate power setting, and wiping lased tissues with wet sponges. Medical therapies used as adjuvant therapy include interferon, cidofovir and ribavirin [1]. So it is recommended to avoid performing

A. Al-Qahtani et al. (eds.), *Textbook of Clinical Otolaryngology*,
https://doi.org/10.1007/978-3-030-54088-3_39

tracheostomy even if it means repetition of surgery every 2–4 weeks.

Subglottic haemangioma is a rare condition, with a female to male ratio of 2:1. Symptoms are similar to those of croup, manifesting with barking cough and biphasic stridor. Hoarse cry is not common. It may be associated with skin haemangiomas. Rigid bronchoscopy shows a pink-blue, sessile and compressible mass. Propranolol appears to be an effective treatment and should therefore be a first-line treatment for subglottic haemangioma [2]. Systemic administration of corticosteroids or intralesional steroid injection may lead to involution. Endoscopic laser resection carries the risk of scarring, so it is indicated in small noncircumferential lesions. Open surgery is recommended in patients with circumferential subglottic haemangioma.

Granular cell tumour is a rare soft tissue neoplasm derived from Schwann cells. It presents as a rounded lesion covered with whitish grey or yellow mucosa. These tumours usually involve the posterior third of the true vocal cords but are also found on the anterior commissure, ventricular bands, subglottis, and the postcricoid region [3]. Treatment is by complete local surgical excision with recurrence rates at only 2–3%. Less than 2% of granular cell tumours are malignant.

Paragangliomas of the larynx are rare benign slowly growing tumours. They are mostly derived from neuroendocrine cells associated with the internal branch of the superior laryngeal nerve. They present with foreign body sensation in the throat and hoarseness. The majority of laryngeal paragangliomas appear as supraglottic submucosal masses. Surgical excision after preoperative transarterial embolization leads to complete cure of the tumour [4].

Laryngeal chondroma, a rare benign tumour, affects men in age group 40–60 years. It commonly arises from the inner posterior plate of the cricoid cartilage presenting in the subglottic area as a rounded shape mass covered with normal mucous membrane, causing dyspnoea. Chondroma may arise from the posterior aspect of the cricoid and grow outwards to compress the laryngopharynx causing dysphagia. CT scanning is used to delineate the extent of the neoplasm. Surgical excision with a safety margin is the treatment of choice [5].

39.3 Malignant Neoplasms

39.3.1 Incidence and Pathogenesis

Laryngeal carcinoma, the most common site of malignancy in the head and neck, accounts for approximately 2.4% of new malignancies worldwide each year. Its incidence is 4–5 times that of laryngopharyngeal cancer. Squamous cell carcinomas comprise over 95% of all malignant neoplasms of the larynx, of these approximately 60% affect the glottic region [6]. It is four times commoner in males than in females, with the majority of patients presenting between ages 55 and 65. In laryngopharyngeal cancer, the male-to-female ratio is 3:1, the reverse is true in postcricoid cancers due to nutritional deficiencies.

Smoking is the most common aetiologic factor for laryngeal and laryngopharyngeal carcinoma with alcohol consumption being an independent and highly synergistic risk factor. Other possible risk factors include gastroesophageal reflux, laryngeal respiratory papillomatosis, exposure to asbestos, volatile chemicals, diesel fume and ionizing radiation [7].

Carcinomas of the laryngopharynx have a worse prognosis as they are usually poorly differentiated, patients present late and over 65% of them already have lymph node metastases at the time of diagnosis [8]. The primary sites of distant metastases are the lungs, liver and bone, and its incidence is among the highest of all head and neck cancers. There is frequent association with alcohol abuse, poor nutrition and immunologic depletion. Patients with head and neck cancer have approximately a 10% to 20% chance of developing a second primary, most commonly bronchogenic carcinoma, within 5 years of initial diagnosis [9].

39.3.2 Surgical Anatomy

Based on its embryologic development, the larynx can be divided into three regions: supraglottic, glottic and subglottic, with each region containing a number of subsites.

The supraglottic larynx is composed of the supra- and infrahyoid epiglottis, the preepiglottic space, the aryepiglottic folds, the arytenoids, the false vocal cords (ventricular bands) and the ventricles (Figs. 39.1 and 39.2). The vocal cords, the floor of the ventricle, anterior and posterior commissures comprise the glottis. The subglottic larynx has its superior border approximately 1 cm below the upper surface of true vocal cords extending inferiorly to the inferior aspect of the cricoid cartilage. The laryngopharynx is a muscle-lined tube linking the oropharynx to the cervical oesophagus. It extends from the superior border of the hyoid bone to the lower border of the cricoid cartilage, and is subdivided into the pyriform sinus on each side, posterior pharyngeal wall, and postcricoid area.

39.3.3 Pathology

Over 95% of laryngeal malignancies are squamous cell carcinoma, ranging from carcinoma in situ to poorly differentiated carcinoma. Rarer cell types include verrucous, adenoid cystic, and neuroendocrine carcinomas and sarcomas as chondrosarcoma, fibrosarcoma and liposarcoma. Laryngeal cancer arises in the glottis in 59%, in the supraglottis in 40%, while subglottic cancer accounts for 1% of all cancer larynx cases [7]. Lesions arising on the free edge and upper surface of the vocal cords may extend to the anterior commissure. The fibrous Broyles' ligament, a confluence of the vocal ligament, the thyroepiglottic ligament, the conus elasticus and the internal perichondrium of the thyroid ala, acts early as an effective barrier [10]. The tumour may extend inferiorly to reach the cricothyroid membrane or display superior surface invasion of the infrapetiole region of the supraglottis. With more spread of the tumour anteriorly the thyroid cartilage, devoid of inner perichondrium,

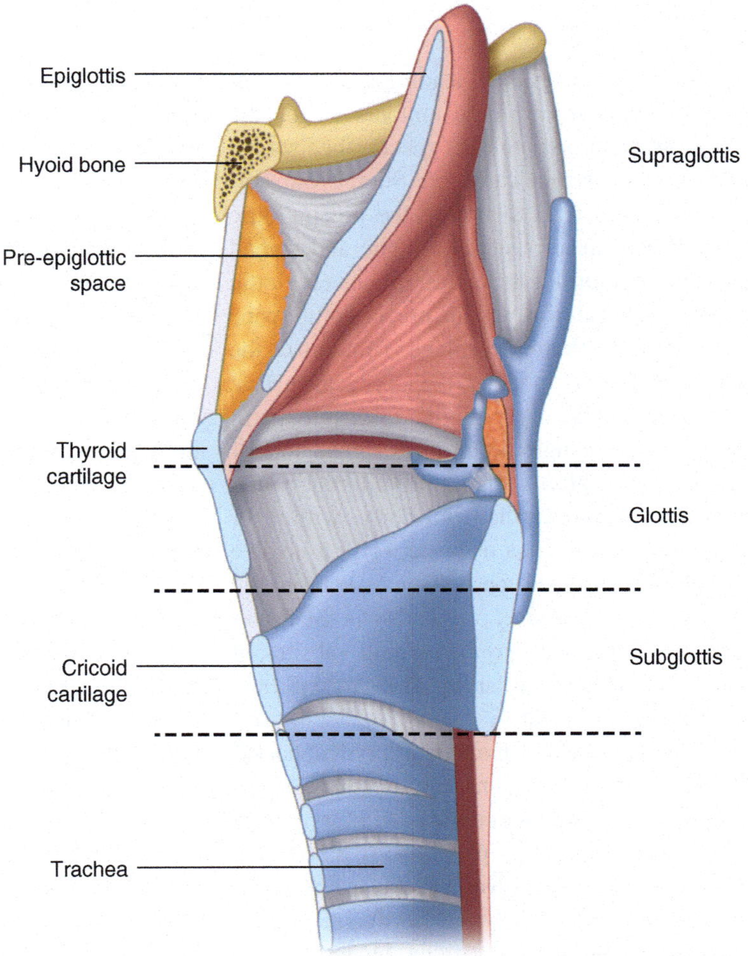

Fig. 39.1 Sagittal view of the larynx showing the preepiglottic space (bounded by hyoepiglottic ligament, epiglottis, thyrohyoid ligament, thyroid cartilage)

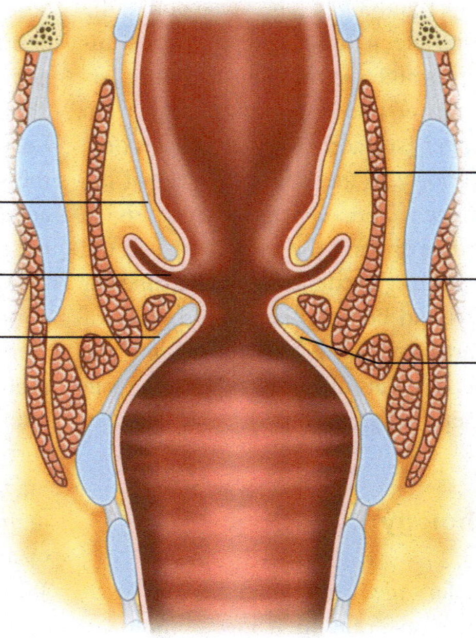

Fig. 39.2 Coronal view of the larynx showing the paraglottic space (bounded by thyroid ala, conus elasticus, quadrangular membrane and pyriform fossa mucosa)

is vulnerable for invasion leading to extralaryngeal spread. Larger glottic tumours invade the paraglottic and preepiglottic spaces, then spread through the thyroid cartilage. Suprahyoid epiglottic lesions tend to invade the preepiglottic space, deep muscles of the tongue and spread into the pyriform fossae. Infrahyoid epiglottic lesions grow anteriorly to the preepiglottic space and invade the thyroid cartilage. Tumours of the ventricular bands spread to the laryngeal surface of the epiglottis, aryepiglottic fold, into paraglottic space. Subglottic tumours spread superiorly to the glottis, anteriorly through the cricothyroid membrane, inferiorly within or external to the trachea or posteriorly to involve laryngopharynx and oesophagus. Transglottic tumours are aggressive, originating in the laryngeal ventricle, they may involve all subsites of the larynx, invade the laryngeal framework and spread extralaryngeal.

More than 95% of malignant laryngopharyngeal tumours are proven to be squamous cell carcinomas. The most common site of origin of these tumours is the pyriform fossa (60%). Postcricoid area is involved in 30% and posterior pharyngeal wall in 10% of laryngopharyngeal carcinomas. Postcricoid carcinoma lesions are typically ulcerated, tumours of the posterior pharyngeal wall and the pyriform fossa are usually exophytic. Tumours arising from the medial wall of the pyriform sinus and the postcricoid region extend early to the larynx. Tumours of the lateral wall of the pyriform fossa may invade the thyrohyoid membrane to present as a neck mass, and the inferior constrictor muscle limits the spread of these tumours to the carotid sheath and related neurovascular bundle. Tumours of the pyriform apex and postcricoid area tend to extend through the cricothyroid membrane to invade the thyroid gland. Postcricoid lesions extend inferiorly through the superior oesophageal sphincter. Posterior laryngopharyngeal wall tumours may deeply infiltrate the prevertebral fascia, prevertebral muscles and vertebral bodies [11].

Laryngeal carcinoma metastasizes to nodal levels II, III and IV in the neck. Early glottic lesions have a less than 7% incidence of occult metastasis, but T4 lesions can have up to a 40% incidence. Supraglottic tumours have the highest rates of occult cervical metastasis. Early supraglottic cancer has 20–30% incidence of occult metastasis, and T4 lesions may amount to 80% incidence. Patients with laryngopharyngeal carcinoma have a high incidence of occult nodal metastases. More

Table 39.1 T staging of supraglottic tumours

T1	Tumour is limited to one subsite of supraglottis with normal vocal cord mobility
T2	Tumour invades mucosa of more than one adjacent subsite of supraglottis or glottis or region outside the supraglottis (e.g. mucosa of base of tongue, vallecula, medial wall of pyriform sinus) without fixation of the larynx
T3	Tumour is limited to larynx with vocal cord fixation and/or invades any of the following: postcricoid area, preepiglottic tissues, paraglottic space, and/or minor thyroid cartilage erosion (e.g. inner cortex)
T4a	Tumour invades through the thyroid cartilage and/or invades tissues beyond the larynx (e.g. trachea, soft tissues of neck including deep extrinsic muscle of the tongue, strap muscles, thyroid or oesophagus)
T4b	Tumour invades prevertebral space, encases carotid artery or invades mediastinal structures

Table 39.2 T staging of glottic tumours

T1	Tumour is limited to the vocal cord or cords (may involve anterior or posterior commissure) with normal mobility
T1a	Tumour is limited to one vocal cord
T1b	Tumour involves both vocal cords
T2	Tumour extends to the supraglottis and/or subglottis, and/or with impaired vocal cord mobility
T3	Tumour is limited to the larynx with vocal cord fixation and/or invades paraglottic space, and or minor thyroid cartilage erosion (e.g. inner cortex)
T4a	Tumour invades through the thyroid cartilage and/or invades tissues beyond the larynx (e.g. trachea, soft tissues of the neck including deep extrinsic muscle of the tongue, strap muscles, thyroid, or oesophagus)
T4b	Tumour invades prevertebral space, encases carotid artery or invades mediastinal structures

Table 39.3 T staging of subglottic tumours

T1	Tumour is limited to the subglottis
T2	Tumour extends to the vocal cord(s), with normal or impaired mobility
T3	Tumour is limited to the larynx with vocal cord fixation
T4a	Tumour invades the cricoid or thyroid cartilage and/or invades tissues beyond the larynx (e.g. trachea, soft tissues of neck including deep extrinsic muscles of the tongue, strap muscles, thyroid, or oesophagus)
T4b	Tumour invades the prevertebral space, encases carotid artery or invades mediastinal structures

Table 39.4 T staging of laryngopharyngeal tumours

T1	Tumour is limited to one subsite of the hypopharynx and is 2 cm or less at its greatest dimension
T2	Tumour involves more than one subsite of the hypopharynx or an adjacent site or is larger than 2 cm but not larger than 4 cm at its greatest diameter without fixation of the hemilarynx
T3	Tumour is larger than 4 cm at its greatest dimension or involves fixation of the hemilarynx
T4a	Tumour invades the thyroid/cricoid cartilage, hyoid bone, thyroid gland, oesophagus or central compartment soft tissues, including prelaryngeal strap muscles and subcutaneous fat
T4b	Tumour invades the prevertebral fascia, encases the carotid artery or involves mediastinal structures

than 65% of them may present with lymph nodal metastases to levels II, III and IV. Lesions involving postcricoid or pyriform sinus apex metastasize to paratracheal and paraoesophageal nodes, and retropharyngeal nodes can be involved in posterior pharyngeal wall cancers [7].

The American Joint Committee on Cancer (AJCC), tumour, node, metastasis (TNM) tumour staging system was developed to guide treatment options and assist in estimating outcomes and prognosis (Tables 39.1, 39.2, 39.3, 39.4).

39.3.4 Evaluation

The evaluation of patients with laryngeal and laryngopharyngeal cancer begins with taking a detailed history including the chief complaints, past medical, personal and family history. Frequent symptoms are hoarseness, throat discomfort, neck mass, referred otalgia, dysphagia, odynophagia, dyspnea, stridor and haemoptysis.

Glottic tumours present early with voice changes, hoarseness or breathy voice. Patients with supraglottic tumours commonly present with a persistent sore throat, otalgia and a neck lump. Dysphagia and odynophagia suggest spread to the tongue base or to the laryngopharynx. Change of voice occurs late, and it is caused by direct extension to the vocal cords, cricoarytenoid joint or paraglottic space involvement. Subglottic tumours may progress with minimal symptoms. Patients with laryngopharyngeal tumours usually present late, 60–70% are diagnosed stage IV disease at initial presentation. The earliest symptom may be throat discomfort and otalgia. Cardinal symptoms include odynophagia, dysphagia at first for solids then for fluids, neck lump, halitosis and weight loss. Hoarseness may be caused by direct laryngeal invasion or involvement of the recurrent laryngeal nerve [9].

Careful palpation of all regions of the neck, for detection of direct extralaryngeal spread or metastatic disease, is carried out. All cervical lymph node levels are examined in a systematic pattern. Any detected lymph node should be thoroughly examined to assess location, size, consistency and mobility. Head and neck examination includes inspection of the oral cavity and oropharynx, for presence of leukoplakia or a second primary lesion, with dental evaluation and digital palpation of the tongue base. The larynx is palpated for tenderness and widening. Loss of the normal crepitus with side-to-side movement of the laryngeal framework may signify postcricoid involvement. Complete fixation of the larynx may denote prevertebral involvement [7].

Physical examination by mirror, flexible fiberoptic or rigid endoscopy evaluates the extent of tumour, vocal cord mobility and airway patency. Findings include nodular or fungating mass lesions, hyperkeratotic or erythematous mucosal lesions, ulcerations and vocal cord paralysis. To detect arytenoid mobility, ask the patient to vocalize a sustained e, to breathe gently and to vocalize at a higher pitch [11]. Endoscopy when combined with a stroboscopic light source allows for detection of changes in the character of the mucosal wave caused by early glottic lesions. It is sometimes difficult to view laryngopharyngeal lesions; phonation and modified Valsalva technique during flexible endoscopy help to reveal an obvious tumour, oedema of the arytenoids or pooling of saliva in the pyriform fossa. Recently, fiberoptic endoscopy is used for effective transnasal oesophageal examination in the clinic [12].

To prepare patients for surgery, it is essential to evaluate their medical condition, specially the cardiopulmonary and nutritional status. Patient's tolerance to general anaesthesia and any condition affecting wound healing has to be assessed. Ageing, chronic obstructive pulmonary disease and risk of post-operative aspiration with laryngeal conservation procedures increase the risk of post-operative complications. Pulmonary function tests are indicated, to determine patient's preoperative pulmonary reserve, if conservation surgery is planned. Routine laboratory tests are ordered including blood count, haemoglobin, albumin, calcium and creatinine levels, liver and thyroid function tests.

Imaging is helpful in evaluating spread of disease to the preepiglottic and paraglottic spaces, subglottic extent of tumour, cartilage invasion, extralaryngeal extension, nodal metastasis, and tumour volume (Fig. 39.3). It helps in determining resectability, and feasibility for organ preservation surgery. Computed tomography (CT) scan with intravenous contrast shows metastatic nodes as a rounded shape node measuring greater than 10 mm, containing central necrosis, with loss of fatty hilum, increased peripheral enhancement and possible extracapsular spread. CT scan is faster, cheaper and more available than magnetic resonance imaging (MRI). MRI is more accurate

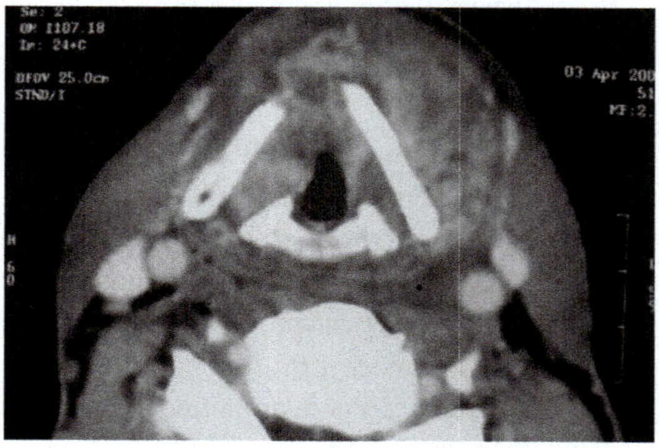

Fig. 39.3 CT scan showing extralaryngeal spread

in assessment of cartilage and tongue base involvement, paraglottic and preepiglottic space extension of tumour. MRI is also more useful in the detection of recurrent carcinoma [13].

A chest X-ray is done to screen for distant metastasis, while a CT chest is indicated in patients with advanced stage tumours to evaluate the mediastinum and detect second primary tumours. Positron emission tomography (PET) imaging is not routinely used in the evaluation and treatment planning of early cases, and its role is increased in the staging of more advanced cancers [14]. Surgery and radiation therapy change the normal laryngeal anatomy and may cause oedema, fibrosis and scarring making diagnosis of recurrent carcinoma with CT or MRI more difficult. PET scan is valuable in posttherapy monitoring, distinguishing recurrence from these alterations. It is done at least 3 months following completion of treatment. PET/CT combines PET and CT into one scanner, with fusion of anatomic and metabolic data higher diagnostic accuracy is provided [7].

Pretreatment endoscopy under anaesthesia, with the use of microscopic and endoscopic techniques, is recommended in all patients. Endoscopic evaluation with 0, 30, and 70° telescopes provide better inspection of the anterior commissure, ventricles and the subglottis. Paralysis of the cord is differentiated from arytenoids fixation by palpation and manipulation of the arytenoid cartilage. In laryngopharyngeal cancer bilateral pyriform fossae, lateral and posterior walls of the laryngopharynx, and the postcricoid region are examined. The distal extent of tumour should be determined, if the endoscope can be passed through the tumour; the rest of the oesophagus is examined to rule out the presence of synchronous tumours. Bronchoscopy may be performed to detect the presence of tracheal invasion [12].

Biopsy is needed to confirm the diagnosis because the gross appearance of sarcoidosis or Wegener granulomatosis can mimic advanced carcinoma. Deep biopsies obtained from the tumour should reach stroma or muscle to diagnose an invasive squamous cell carcinoma. Small lesions are completely excised with a small cuff of normal appearing submucosa to detect the depth of invasion. Biopsy is recommended for any other suspicious area discovered during endoscopy [7]. To avoid a tracheostomy, that could lead to tumour seeding and stomal recurrence, laser is used to debulk large tumours partially obstructing the airway.

39.4 Treatment of Early Cancer Larynx

Treatment of early cancer larynx should aim to completely remove the tumour, prevent recurrence and preserve laryngeal function by a single modality with the least morbidity. Treatment options include radiotherapy, transoral laser microsurgery or open surgery. The choice of treatment should be made depending on tumour primary site, extension and accessibility, surgeon's experience as well as patient's lifestyle and preference.

39.4.1 Treatment of Early Glottic Cancer

Early glottic cancer refers to tumours ranging from Tis to T2 lesions. Transoral laser microsurgery has become an established treatment modality for early glottic cancer larynx [15]. It is associated with minimal bleeding, absence of post-operative oedema, less patient morbidity, short hospital stay, high local control rates, preservation of function and excellent re-treatment options for local failure. Tracheostomy is rarely required. The tumour is transected and removed piecemeal; this allows for exposure of the dissection plane and precise visualization of the interface between tumour and the underlying normal tissue. Using the magnification and good illumination of the operating microscope makes this feasible. Obtaining an adequate surgical exposure of anterior commissure lesions in endoscopic laser surgery is difficult but not impossible [16]. In case of suspected cartilage involvement, endoscopic cartilage resection may be performed but is technically challenging. Combined laser endoscopic and open technique may be a better alternative treatment choice. Extent of voice affection after surgery depends on the depth of resection. If limited to the superficial layer of the lamina propria and the vocal ligament resection usually results in near normal voice production. Resections extending to the vocalis muscle can cause post-operative phonatory function deficits. After a post-operative period of total voice rest to facilitate healing, patients require voice therapy to maximize voice outcome. If needed reconstruction after endoscopic laser surgery is performed by augmentation using cordal injection or medialization thyroplasty [17].

Radiation therapy and conservation surgery are almost equally effective treatments for early glottic carcinoma. Endoscopic laser resection is recommended over radiation therapy for the well-defined superficial lesion located in the middle third of the vocal cord. Because the surgical management of larger lesions requires the removal of greater amounts of tissue, radiation is usually the preferred initial treatment for those tumours. Older patients with greater comorbidity are selected for radiation therapy. Primary standard radiation therapy is delivered at 2 Gy per fraction per day, 5 days a week over 7 weeks for a total dose of 70 Gy. It produces a control rate of 85–95% for T1 tumours, 70–80% for T2 tumours, and an ultimate local control rate including salvage laryngectomy of up to 100%. Radiotherapy, however, is a time-consuming procedure necessitating several weeks; there is also a risk of radiogenic carcinoma specially in younger patients. Because the amount of normal tissue in the treatment port for early T1 or T2 glottic carcinoma is small, radiation for these lesions is associated with mild side effects. Voice disturbance may be a result of radiation induced mucositis, atrophic changes and fibrosis [18]. Continued smoking during treatment increases tissue susceptibility to radiation injury.

Larger more infiltrating T2 tumours with posterior extension or anterior commissure involvement may require open procedures, vertical hemilaryngectomy or supracricoid resection, that have a greater local control rate. Patients usually need a temporary tracheostomy after open partial surgery. The vertical partial hemilaryngectomy includes resection of the corresponding thyroid ala along with tumour at the glottic level. Lesions involving the anterior commissure are treated with frontolateral hemilaryngectomy or supracricoid laryngectomy. Frontolateral partial laryngectomy removes a vocal fold, anterior commissure, anterior third of the contralateral vocal fold, and the overlying medial thyroid cartilage. Supracricoid laryngectomy involves resection of both true and false vocal folds, the thyroid cartilage, both paraglottic spaces, and one partial or full arytenoid, but preserves at least one crico-arytenoid unit (arytenoid associated musculature, plus the superior and recurrent laryngeal nerve) and cricoid cartilage. Contraindications to this surgical procedure include bilateral arytenoid involvement, posterior commissure disease, hyoid bone involvement, and subglottic extension beyond the upper margin of the cricoid ring. Reconstruction is performed with cricohyoido-epiglottopexy [19]. Supracricoid laryngectomy for T1b and T2 carcinomas results in high local control rates. It also plays an important role in the surgical salvage of selected radiation failures in patients in whom the recurrent tumour has not extended beyond its original site.

39.4.2 Treatment of Early Supraglottic Cancer

Early supraglottic cancer refers to tumours ranging from T1 to T2 lesions. The treatment options for early supraglottic lesions include radiotherapy, supraglottic laryngectomy (open or transoral laser microsurgery) or supracricoid laryngectomy. Patients with T1–2 lesions have a 20–30% incidence of occult nodal metastasis and a higher frank nodal disease at presentation. It carries therefore a somewhat poorer prognosis than glottic cancer. For early supraglottic tumours, the clinically N0 neck needs to be addressed due to the high risk of microscopic lymph node metastasis. Elective treatment of the neck is performed by either radiotherapy or selective neck dissection (unilateral or bilateral) depending on the initial line of treatment [20]. The general recommendation is to irradiate patients with T1 and small exophytic T2 lesions, as well as patients with poor pulmonary function, with poor access for surgery or high risk for general anaesthesia. The target volume for radiation treatment includes the primary tumour and lymph nodes bilaterally (Level II–IV).

In a supraglottic laryngectomy, the larynx is resected between the preepiglottic space and the ventricles, with preservation of both true vocal folds and both arytenoids. Tumour extension below the laryngeal ventricle and substantial cartilage involvement contraindicates this surgical procedure. Swallowing can be temporary affected with variable degrees of aspiration. Dietary modifications and compensatory techniques as Mendelsohn manoeuvre, supraglottic swallow and effortful swallow can be used to improve swallowing. Patients indicated for supraglottic partial laryngectomy require adequate pulmonary reserve. Advance aged patients are poor candidates for this procedure [21].

Endoscopic laser resection of supraglottic tumours is recently gaining more ground.

Patients complain of less post-operative dysphagia and rapidly recover normal swallowing. This improved outcome and better functional recovery of swallowing in contrast to open supraglottic laryngectomy are mostly due to the preservation of the superior laryngeal nerve [22]. Patients with trismus, projecting teeth or cervical spine deformity are not suitable for endoscopic laser resection. Inserting the largest possible laryngoscope or bivalved laryngoscope into the patient increases the visibility and accessibility of these tumours to transoral excision. The local control rates with laser excision appear to be equal to open procedures for T1 and T2 lesions. Extended procedures may include resection of the tongue base, arytenoid, aryepiglottic fold, or superior medial pyriform wall. Transoral robotic surgery has emerged as a new, safe, useful procedure in the management of supraglottic tumours [23]. Advantages of robotic surgery include improved optics, three-dimensional viewing, increased instrument freedom of motion and modulating tremor. A supraglottic partial laryngectomy is feasible in selected patients, with early supraglottic cancer, who have failed initial treatment with radiotherapy. Supracricoid laryngectomy with cricohyoidopexy is used for selected T2 supraglottic carcinomas that have extension from the supraglottis to the glottic level.

Key Points

- Early laryngeal cancer can be treated with single modality.
- Treatment options include radiotherapy, transoral laser microsurgery or open surgery.
- Endoscopic laser resection is recently gaining more ground.
- To maximize voice outcome, reconstruction may be needed.
- Treatment of the neck for occult metastatic disease must be considered for early supraglottic cancer.

39.5 Treatment of Subglottic Carcinoma

Early subglottic carcinoma is treated with radiation therapy. More advanced disease is treated by total laryngectomy with bilateral paratracheal node dissection, and ipsilateral or total thyroidectomy and adjuvant post-operative radiation or chemoradiation therapy if indicated.

39.6 Treatment of Advanced Cancer Larynx

Advanced laryngeal carcinoma (T3–4) carry long-term survival rates ranging from 30 to 60% depending on the site and stage of the tumour.

They were treated with total laryngectomy and adjuvant radiation or chemoradiation therapy. Some cases of T3 glottic or supraglottic cancers can be treated by endoscopic resection, but these patients need thorough preoperative evaluation and strict post-operative follow-up. Supraglottic cancers staged as T3 (invasion of the preepiglottic space with intact ventricles and vocal folds) can be treated by open supraglottic laryngectomy with resection of the hyoid bone. The supracricoid laryngectomy plays an important role in treatment of some selected advanced tumours (T3 or early T4) and early postradiotherapy failure. This is achieved with preserving physiologic speech, and respiration without the need for a permanent tracheostoma. In supraglottic tumours, with paraglottic space invasion causing vocal cord fixation, supracricoid laryngectomy with cricohyoidopexy may be the alternative to total laryngectomy. Glottic tumours with supraglottic extension can be treated by supracricoid laryngectomy with cricohyoidoepiglottopexy [19]. The high local control rate of this procedure is achieved by the wide resection of the paraglottic space, the thyroid cartilage and inferior portion of the preepiglottic space.

Radiation therapy alone is used if patients are medically unfit to undergo surgery. It results in lower local control rates, and many patients may need total laryngectomy for salvage. Side effects from radiation increase with larger fields, as in patients requiring extensive nodal irradiation. It may be associated with severe acute and long-term side effects, such as skin problems, dry mouth, mucositis, difficult swallowing, tooth decay, chondronecrosis, hypothyroidism, oesophageal stricture and oedema requiring tracheostomy in some cases. Using radiation therapy causes difficulty in detecting local recurrence due to laryngeal oedema, and increased post-operative complications if surgery is required for salvage. Radiation efficacy is improved with accelerated and hyperfractionated schemes. Intensity modulated radiation therapy uses advanced technology to provide higher target volume and to minimize the dose delivered to surrounding structures such as the spinal cord, salivary glands, and swallowing apparatus hence limiting the side effects of treatment [24].

Due to the discouraging outcomes of treating advanced laryngeal carcinoma with radiotherapy alone, chemoradiation began to be used. Organ preservation strategies using chemoradiation protocols is now the standard treatment option for most T3 and T4a tumours without extensive cartilage invasion. A major advantage of chemoradiation is the synergistic effect on the tumour and the eradication of micrometastases. Induction chemotherapy with cisplatin plus 5-fluorouracil is evaluated after 2 or 3 cycles by CT or MRI with contrast. In cases of complete response or partial response with tumour size reduction to 50% or more, definitive radiotherapy is given. Induction chemotherapy followed by radiation therapy allows preservation of the larynx in over 60% of patients. In case there is no response or insignificant reduction of tumour size the patient is subjected to surgery. Concurrent radiation therapy and cisplatin 100 mg/m^2 on days 1, 22 and 43 achieves higher rates of organ preservation and better loco-regional control compared to radiation therapy alone or induction chemotherapy followed by radiation therapy. Chemotherapy is better tolerated when given sequentially than concurrently with radiotherapy. Concurrent chemoradiation has been associated with acute and long-term toxicity [24].

Patients with more advanced laryngeal carcinoma, with bulky tumours, destruction of the thyroid or cricoid cartilage, penetration through the cartilage, extralaryngeal soft tissue spread and extension beyond the posterior third of the base of tongue are treated by total laryngectomy [25]. Indications for post-operative radiation or chemoradiation therapy include close or positive margins, extracapsular extension, multiple positive nodes, invasion of the soft tissues of the neck, perineural invasion and vascular spread. It should start within 6 weeks of surgery [26]. Using chemoradiation protocols alone in these more advanced cases results in poor functional preservation, high failure rates and increased post-operative complications if surgery is required for salvage.

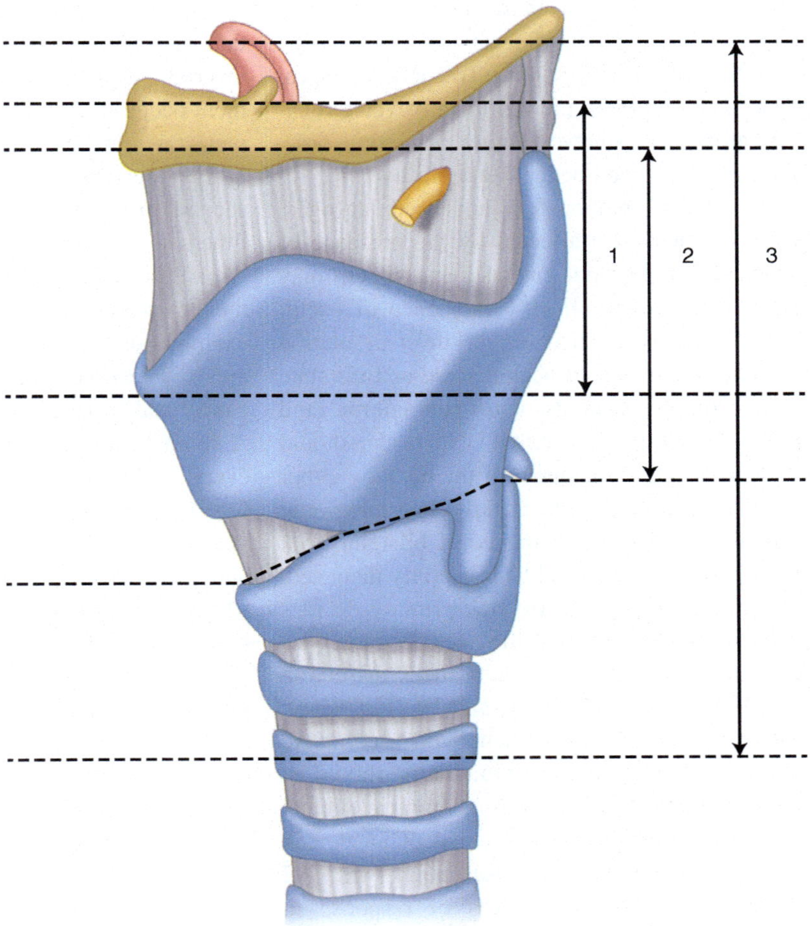

Fig. 39.4 Diagram showing the extent of resection in different types of laryngectomy. (1) Horizontal partial laryngectomy (supraglottic laryngectomy), (2) Supracricoid laryngectomy, (3) Total laryngectomy

In total laryngectomy the larynx is resected from the vallecula to the upper trachea, including the vocal folds, hyoid bone, epiglottis, thyroid and cricoid cartilages and a few tracheal cartilage rings (Figs. 39.4 and 39.5). Parts of the pharyngeal mucosa of pyriform sinus or lateral pharyngeal wall are resected ensuring adequate resection margins but enough mucosa should be preserved for later closure. The airway is interrupted, and patients respirate through a tracheal stoma. Post-laryngectomy rehabilitation is required to achieve intelligible speech and restore swallowing function and oral feeding. Post-laryngectomy patients communicate by oesophageal speech, artificial larynx, or creation of a tracheoesophageal fistula with insertion of vocal prosthesis. The voice

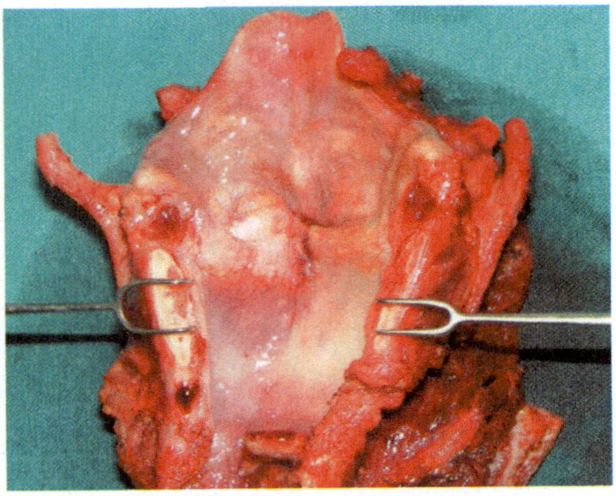

Fig. 39.5 Specimen of total laryngectomy (the cricoid lamina is incised showing advanced tumour in the left glottic area)

prosthesis allows air from the lungs to pass into a narrow pharyngoesophageal segment that vibrates to produce sound. Tracheoesophageal speech is now the preferred form of voice rehabilitation as it achieves longer phonation time, greater volume and better intelligibility [27].

Results of treatment in advanced laryngeal cancer patients are affected by the presence of cervical lymph node metastases, which may amount to an overall 30% incidence of occult neck metastasis. There is an inverse relation between the extent of neck disease and ultimate local control. Patients with supraglottic and advanced glottic cancer with N0 necks should undergo elective treatment of the neck by either neck dissection or radiotherapy. In supraglottic tumours, with more incidence of bilateral neck metastasis, necks should be bilaterally managed. The option of treatment of the primary decides the method used to treat the neck. If surgery is chosen for the primary tumour, neck dissection should include levels II, III and IV (Fig. 39.6). Patients with N1 involvement with a complete clinical response after chemoradiation should be closely observed. Those with incomplete clinical response require neck dissection. A planned neck dissection is recommended for patients with N2 disease or greater, regardless of response to chemoradiotherapy [28].

Treating patients with combined modalities have improved local-regional control, but overall survival has remained unchanged as result of distant metastases and second primary tumours. Overall, local and regional failures after treatment occur in about 30% of patients, and distant metastases in 10–30% of patients depending on cancer location. About 50% of patients die of second primary tumours or other intercurrent illness.

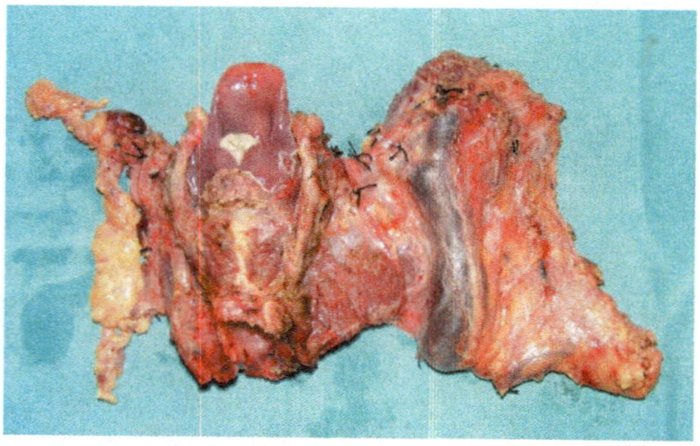

Fig. 39.6 Specimen of total laryngectomy with left selective and right radical neck dissection (back view)

Follow-up care after laryngeal cancer treatment is mandatory, it includes regular physical examinations and medical tests. Follow-up visits aim to detect recurring cancer or second primary cancer and manage late side effects of treatment. A common follow-up schedule after treatment is every 2 months for the first year, every 3 months for the second year, every 4 months for the third year, every 6 months for the fourth and fifth year, and once a year after that. It is important to identify early recurrence and start salvage treatment before the disease reaches more advanced stages. PET/CT scan may be used for surveillance purposes. It gained a role in the detection of local and regional recurrences, even if CT and MRI fail to diagnose them [7].

Surgery remains the gold standard treatment in loco-regional recurrence. Salvage surgery is mostly performed by total laryngectomy. Supracricoid laryngectomy is an appropriate treatment option in selected patients, in whom the recurrent tumour has not extended beyond its original site.

Patients radiologically staged N0 by CT imaging are not submitted to neck dissection, as they most probably are free from occult neck metastases. Post-operative complication rates reach more than 50%, pharyngocutaneous fistula being the most encountered local complication [29]. Chemotherapy or chemoradiation may be used, especially if surgery is not amenable, to help control local and distant disease. Immunotherapy is recently under trial among some cases. Palliative care is interdisciplinary care that provides support for the physical and psychological suffering of patients.

Key Points

- Advanced cancer larynx is treated with combined modality, either surgery with adjuvant radiotherapy or initial chemoradiation.
- Laryngeal cartilage penetration is an indication for laryngectomy.
- Tracheoesophageal speech is now the preferred form of voice rehabilitation.
- Treatment of the neck for palpable or occult metastatic disease is indicated for all advanced laryngeal cancer.

39.7 Treatment of Laryngopharyngeal Carcinoma

Early stage laryngopharyngeal cancer may be managed with either surgery or radiotherapy with equally good results. Choice of treatment depends on site, inferior and superior extent, circumferential involvement and laryngeal spread of the tumour [30]. Surgical procedures include open partial pharyngectomy or laryngopharyngectomy and transoral laser surgery in conjunction with staged or synchronous neck dissection. Transoral robotic surgery that aims at less invasiveness and functional preservation is becoming popular. Radiotherapy is usually the treatment of choice in patients who are medically unfit or cannot tolerate early post-operative aspiration and in early lesions involving pyriform sinus apex or postcricoid region.

Tumours of the laryngopharynx with gross thyroid cartilage destruction, advanced tumours of the postcricoid region or of the pharyngeal wall with circumferential involvement are managed with total pharyngolaryngectomy along with uni- or bilateral selective neck dissection with the removal of levels II–IV lymph nodes. The presence of cervical nodal metastasis requires modified radical neck dissection. Extension into the oesophagus necessitates pharyngo-oesophagectomy, paraesophageal and paratracheal lymph node dissection with hemithyroidectomy. Laryngopharyngeal cancer patients commonly suffer from malnutrition increasing the risk of post-operative complications. Complete resection of the tumour is followed by appropriate reconstruction and post-operative adjuvant treatment. Prevertebral musculature or cervical spine involvement, massive mediastinal nodal enlargement and carotid artery involvement are contraindications to surgery [31].

Reconstruction after resection of tumours ensures proper wound healing and recovery of swallowing function. After partial pharyngectomy for tumours limited to the pyriform fossa, the pectoralis major myocutaneous flap is applied as a patch repair to reconstruct the pharynx. For reconstruction of circumferential pharyngectomy defects free flap surgery, as tubed skin flaps and visceral flaps, is performed by microvascular surgical technique. The tubed radial forearm fasciocutaneous free flap is reliable due to the large vascular pedicle calibre. Microvascular anastomosis is performed under magnification to suitable recipient vessels in the neck. Ease of harvest, immediate reconstruction, limited donor site morbidity, radiation tolerance, high flap reliability and good swallowing outcome are all advantages of the radial forearm free flap [32]. The free jejunal flap is harvested through an upper midline laparotomy and transferred to the neck. The advantages of using visceral flaps include lower incidence of pharyngocutaneous fistula and stricture formation at the site of anastomosis [33]. After pharyngolaryngoesophagectomy the stomach, fashioned into tube-like configuration, is pulled up through the retrosternal plane to the neck and anastomosed to the oropharynx. Laparoscopic gastric pull-up is recently indicated to minimize the morbidity of the open technique. In cases when gastric pull-up is not feasible, pedicled jejunum or colonic interposition is used.

Combined chemoradiotherapy has become now the standard of care for a vast majority of patients with advanced laryngopharyngeal cancer, among them are also patients, who are unfit for or refuse surgery. This treatment modality achieves organ preservation without compromising survival. Surgery for laryngopharyngeal cancer is on the retreat. In very advanced lesions T4b, not amenable for resection, chemoradiation is the only option. Intention of this treatment is mostly palliative. Combined modality therapies include concurrent chemoradiotherapy, induction chemotherapy followed by radiotherapy and sequential therapy with induction chemotherapy followed by concurrent chemoradiotherapy [31].

Despite some improvement in local and functional outcomes with the advent of organ laryngeal preservation, overall survival for patients with laryngopharynx cancer remains poor. The average rates lies between 25 and 40% 5 years survival. Prognosis is considered to be the worst among all head and neck sites. Up to 95% of all recurrences occur in the first 36 months and over half of the first recurrences are distant metastases.

Key Points

- In early laryngopharyngeal cancer, transoral laser microsurgery and robotic surgery show good oncological benefits.
- In advanced cases, organ preservation by chemoradiation took ground from surgery and adjuvant chemoradiation.
- Radical surgery (pharyngolaryngectomy) has a role in the non-functioning larynx, in advanced volume disease and in salvage surgery.
- Treatment of the neck is determined according to tumour location and neck stage.

Take Home Messages

- True benign tumours constitute 5% or less of all laryngeal tumours. The most common benign tumour of the larynx is papilloma.
- Hoarseness lasting longer than 3 weeks and persistent odynophagia or dysphagia in elderly patients are warning symptoms suggesting cancer, and should be thoroughly investigated.
- Preoperative evaluation is essential for planning treatment; it includes history, examination, endoscopy and imaging.
- Early laryngeal and laryngopharyngeal cancer can be treated with single modality either conservation surgery or radiotherapy.
- Laryngopharyngeal carcinomas have a worse prognosis, as most of the patients have advanced stage disease when first diagnosed.
- Organ preservation strategies using chemoradiation protocols is now the standard treatment option for a vast majority of patients with advanced laryngeal and laryngopharyngeal cancer.
- Treatment of the neck for palpable or occult metastatic disease must be considered for all supraglottic, laryngopharyngeal and advanced laryngeal cancer.
- Follow-up care after cancer treatment is mandatory, salvage treatment is less successful once the disease reaches the advanced stages.
- Surgery remains the gold standard treatment in loco-regional recurrence.

References

1. Stamataki S, Nikolopoulos TP, Korres S, Felekis D, Tzangaroulakis A, Ferekidis E. Juvenile recurrent respiratory papillomatosis: still a mystery disease with difficult management. Head Neck. 2007;29(2):155–62.
2. Bajaj Y, Kapoor K, Ifeacho S, et al. Great Ormond Street Hospital treatment guidelines for use of propranolol in infantile isolated subglottic haemangioma. JLaryngolOtol. 2013;127(3):295–8.
3. Sataloff RT, Ressue JC, Portell M, Harris RM, Ossoff R, Merati AL, et al. Granular cell tumours of the larynx. J Voice. 2000;14(1):119–34.
4. Naik S, Shenoy A, Chavan P, Patil A, Gupta S. Laryngeal paraganglioma. Indian J Otolaryngol Head Neck Surg. 2013;65(Suppl 1):95–104.
5. Devaney K, Ferlito A, Silver CE. Cartilaginous tumours of the larynx. Ann Otorhinolaryngol. 1995;104:251.
6. Tibbetts K, Than M. Role of advanced laryngeal imaging in glottic cancer. Otolaryngol Clin N Am. 2015;48:565–84.
7. Chu E, Kim Y. Laryngeal cancer: diagnosis and preoperative work-up. Otolaryngol Clin N Am. 2008;41:673–95.
8. Hoffman H, Karnell L, Shah J, Ariyan S, Brown G, Fee W. Hypopharyngeal cancer patient care evaluation. Laryngoscope. 1997;107:1005–17.
9. Thekdi AA, Ferris RL. Diagnostic assessment of laryngeal cancer. Otolaryngol Clin North Am. 2002;35(5):953–69.
10. Mor N, Blitzer A. Functional anatomy and oncologic barriers of the larynx. Otolaryngol Clin North Am. 2015;48:533–45.
11. Tufano R, Stafford E. Organ preservation surgery for laryngeal cancer. Otolaryngol Clin North Am. 2008;41:953–69.
12. Piazza C, Paderno A, Ravanelli M, Pessina C. Clinical and radiological evaluation of hypopharyngeal carcinoma. Adv Otorhinolaryngol. 2019;83:35–46.
13. Blitz A, Aygun N. Radiologic evaluation of larynx cancer. Otolaryngol Clin N Am. 2008;41:697–713.
14. Isles MG, McConkey C, Mehanna HM. A systematic review and meta-analysis of the role of PET in the follow up of head and neck squamous cell carcinoma following radiotherapy or chemoradiotherapy. ClinOtolaryngol. 2008;33:210–22.
15. Gallo A, Vincentiis M, Manciocco V, Simonelli M, Fiorella M, Shah J. CO2 laser cordectomy for early-stage glottic carcinoma. Laryngoscope. 2002;112:370–4.
16. Steiner W, Ambrosch P, Rodel R, Kron M. Impact of anterior commissure involvement on local control of early glottic carcinoma treated by laser microresection. Laryngoscope. 2004;114:1485–91.
17. Zeitels S. Optimizing voice after endoscopic partial laryngectomy. Otolaryngol Clin North Am. 2004;37:627–36.
18. Wedman J, Heimdal JH, Elstad I, Olofsson J. Voice results in patients with T1a glottic cancer treated by radiotherapy or endoscopic measures. Eur Arch Otorhinolaryngol. 2002;259:547–50.
19. Laccourreye H, Laccourreye O, Weinstein G, Menard M, Brasnu D. Supracricoid laryngectomy with cricohyoidopexy: a partial laryngeal procedure for glottic carcinoma. Ann Otol Rhinol Laryngol. 1990;99:421–6.
20. Redaelli de Zinis LO, Nicolai P, Tomenzoli D, et al. The distribution of lymph node metastases in supraglottic squamous cell carcinoma: therapeutic implications. Head Neck. 2002;24(10):913–20.
21. Peretti G, Piazza C, Cattaneo A, et al. Comparison of functional outcomes after endoscopic versus open neck supraglottic laryngectomies. Ann Otol Rhinol Laryngol. 2006;115:827–32.
22. Sasaki CT, Leder SB, Acton LM, et al. Comparison of the glottic closure reflex in traditional "open" versus endoscopic laser supraglottic laryngectomy. Ann Otol Rhinol Laryngol. 2006;115:93–6.
23. Smith R. Transoral robotic surgery for larynx cancer. Otolaryngol Clin North Am. 2014;47:379–95.
24. Lee N, O'Meara W, Chan K, et al. Concurrent chemotherapy and intensity modulated radiotherapy for locoregionally advanced laryngeal and hypopharyngeal cancers. Int J Radiat Oncol Biol Phys. 2007;69:459–68.
25. Agrawal N, Goldenberg D. Primary and salvage total laryngectomy. Otolaryngol Clin N Am. 2008;41:771–80.
26. De Stefani A, Magnano M, Cavalot A, et al. Adjuvant radiotherapy influences the survival of patients with squamous carcinoma of the head and neck who have poor prognoses. Otolaryngol Head Neck Surg. 2000;123(5):630–6.
27. Kao WW, Mohr RM, Kimmel CA, et al. The outcome and techniques of primary and secondary tracheoesophageal puncture. Arch Otolaryngol Head Neck Surg. 1994;120(3):301–7.
28. Ferlito A, Silverb C, Rinaldoa A, Smith R. Surgical treatment of the neck in cancer of the larynx. ORL J Otorhinolaryngol Relat Spec. 2000;62:217–25.
29. Holsinger FC, Funk E, Roberts DB, et al. Conservation laryngeal surgery versus total laryngectomy for radiation failure in laryngeal cancer. Head Neck. 2006;28:779–84.
30. Eckel H, Bradley P. Treatment options for hypopharyngeal cancer. Adv Otorhinolaryngol. 2019;83:47–53.
31. Habib A. Management of advanced hypopharyngeal carcinoma: systematic review of survival following surgical and non-surgical treatments. J Laryngol Otol. 2018;132:385–400.
32. Scharpf J, Esclamado R. Reconstruction with radial forearm flaps after ablative surgery for hypopharyngeal cancer. Head Neck. 2003;3:261–6.
33. Wei W, Chan J. Surgical treatment of advanced staged hypopharyngeal cancer. Adv Otorhinolaryngol. 2019;83:66–75.

Cancer of the Nasal Cavity and Paranasal Sinuses

40

Ahmed Eldaly, Mohammed Hassab, and Ali Al Ansari

40.1 Introduction

Cancers of the nasal cavity and paranasal sinuses are rare. They comprise about 3% of head and neck malignancies and less than 1% of all human malignancies [1]. The estimated annual incidence is about 0.56–1:100,000 of population. The male–female ratio is about 2:1 with an average age at presentation between 50 to 60 years [2].

The maxillary sinus is the most common site of origin (55%) followed by the nasal cavity (23%) and the ethmoid sinus (20%) [3]. Primary tumors of the sphenoid and the frontal sinus are exceedingly rare. However, extension of paranasal sinus malignancies to involve the sphenoid and frontal sinuses occurs frequently because of the anatomic contiguity of the paranasal sinuses and because a significant number of tumors may involve more than one site at the time of initial diagnosis making it difficult to ascertain the primary site of origin.

A. Eldaly · M. Hassab (✉)
Otolaryngology-Head and Neck Surgery, University of Alexandria, Tharwat, Alexandria, Egypt

A. Al Ansari
Otolaryngology-Head and Neck Surgery, Hamad Medical Corporation, Doha, Qatar

A. Al-Qahtani et al. (eds.), *Textbook of Clinical Otolaryngology*, https://doi.org/10.1007/978-3-030-54088-3_40

40.2 Pathology and Biology

Paranasal sinus malignancies include a heterogeneous group of tumors with widely varying histology and prognosis. The World Health Organization classification of tumors includes more than 40 unique histopathological types for malignancies of the nasal cavity and paranasal sinuses [4].

These etiologies are broadly subclassified into epithelial or nonepithelial malignancies. Epithelial neoplasms constituted more than two-thirds of all malignant neoplasms in the sinonasal tract [5].

The distribution of those tumors varies from one geographical region to another however globally; Squamous cell carcinoma (SCC) and glandular malignancies are the most common epithelial tumors whereas rhabdomyosarcoma and lymphomas are well-known nonepithelial tumors that occur in this region.

Squamous cell carcinoma is the most common malignancy of the sinonasal tract occurring with a frequency between 36% and 58% of all paranasal sinus cancers. These tumors have a peak incidence between 60 to 70 years of age and occur more commonly in males [6].

The maxilla is the most common site of origin within the sinonasal region followed by the nasal cavity and the ethmoids [7, 8]. Associations between the development of paranasal SCC and working in nickel refining industry have been identified where workers are estimated to have 100 times more risk of developing paranasal SCC than the general population [9].

Human papillomavirus, specifically subtypes 6 and 11, also seems to play a role in development of SCC by promoting malignant transformation of sinonasal inverted papilloma [10].

Histologically 80% are keratinizing (containing areas of keratin formation, either as sheets or as epithelial pearls), while 20% are nonkeratinizing [11]. Transitional (Schneiderian) carcinoma is a special type of nonkeratinizing SCC that has no particular site of predilection. It is transitional only in that it tends toward squamous cell differentiation [12].

Non salivary gland Adenocarcinoma: Adenocarcinoma comprises about 15% of all sinonasal malignancies. Adenocarcinomas exhibit a striking male predominance (75–90%), with a peak age incidence between 55 and 60 years. The ethmoids are the most common site of origin for these tumors. Adenocarcinomas are divided into intestinal and nonintestinal types.

The intestinal-type adenocarcinoma (ITAC) is identical to those arising in the intestinal tract. It has been hypothesized that ITAC derives from a stem cell capable of undergoing differentiation into various type of epithelial cells [13]. Exposure to hard wood dust is a well-recognized risk factor since 1965 [14]. Acheson estimated that woodworkers in the furniture industry had an approximately 875-fold higher incidence in sinonasal adenocarcinoma when compared to the normal population [15]. Most series reveal a high rate of ethmoid adenocarcinoma (90%) linked to wood exposure and some European countries include it with occupational diseases [16]. ITAC histologically and immunohistochemically resembles intestinal neoplasms [17]. Barnes subdivided those neoplasms into five subtypes: papillary, colonic, solid, mucinous, and mixed. The papillary type shows the less aggressive course while mucinous adenocarcinomas have the highest mortality [18].

The nonintestinal adenocarcinomas are typically seromucinous adenocarcinoma lacking any histological or immunophenotypical features of ITACs or salivary type adenocarcinomas. There are no known occupational or environmental etiological factors.

Typically, they are characterized by a back-to-back proliferation of glands without intervening stroma. Based on the degree of cytomorphological characteristics, non-ITACs can be further divided into low-grade and high-grade tumors. Low-grade tumors commonly affect the ethmoids while the high-grade tumors are more common at the maxillary sinus [19]. Low-grade nonintestinal-type sinonasal adenocarcinomas have an excellent prognosis.

Adenoid cystic carcinoma (ACC) account for about 10% % of sinonasal malignancies. It is slightly more common among women and most commonly present in the fifth and sixth decades of life. Those tumors are characterized by slowly progressive relentless course. Late recurrence can occur 10–20 years after remission by initial treatment [20]. Perineural spread, the hallmark of adenoid cystic carcinoma, is usually evident and provides avenues of spread to the cranial base commonly through the maxillary division of trigeminal. Perineural invasion in ACC has been considered as one of the determining factors for locoregional recurrence or distant metastasis [21]. The tumor also has a propensity for bony invasion, which can lead to significant involvement of the skull base. Distant metastasis is more frequent than lymphatic metastasis, with an average incidence of 40%. The lungs and bones are the sites most frequently involved in systemic metastasis [22]. Adenoid cystic carcinoma exhibits three histologic subtypes based on tumor architecture: cribriform, tubular, and solid. The most common subtype is the cribriform, but the solid subtypes are known to have the worst prognosis among the three subtypes [23].

Esthesioneuroblastoma is a rare malignant tumor of neuroectodermal origin, arising from olfactory bipolar cells. The tumor was first recognized by Berger et al. in 1924, who coined the term "esthesioneuroepitheliome olfactif" [24]. It accounts for 3% of all intranasal malignancies. The tumor exhibits a bimodal age incidence showing peaks in age groups 11–20 years and 51–60 years [25]. The sex distribution is roughly equal. Most olfactory neuroblastomas arise in the superior nasal cavity and are intimately related to the cribriform plate through which they readily spread intracranially [26].

The incidence of metastasis is reportedly 10–33% at the time of diagnosis; cervical nodal metastasis is the most common occurring in 15.6–20.2% [27]. Hyams' developed a grading system, which assigns ENB tumors a grade of I to IV based on lobular architecture, mitosis, necrosis, nuclear pleomorphism, fibrillary matrix, and rosettes formation. Grades I and II may be placed together as low grade, and grades III and IV are considered high grade [28].

Sinonasal undifferentiated carcinoma (SNUC) was first described in 1986 by Frierson and colleagues as a distinct pathological entity arising in the nasal cavity and paranasal sinuses [29].

SNUC is a rapidly progressive epithelial malignancy with an incidence of about 0.02 per 100,000 individuals and a median age of diagnosis in the sixth decade of life. These high-grade neoplasms lack squamous or glandular differentiation and frequently arise from the ethmoid sinuses. Immunohistochemistry analysis is often required for diagnosis. Sinonasal undifferentiated carcinoma (SNUC) is composed of pleomorphic cells with a high nuclear-cytoplasmic ratio, arranged in nests, sheets, and trabeculae with central areas of central necrosis [30]. Most patients with SNUC are typically diagnosed with advanced disease extending beyond the paranasal sinuses to involve the orbit (53%) and skull base (41%). In addition, cervical nodal and distant metastasis to the lungs and liver commonly occur [31]. Although outcomes have improved substantially from the median survival of 4 months originally reported by Frierson and colleagues, the prognosis for SNUC remains poor [32].

Rhabdomyosarcoma is the most common sinonasal malignancy among children; it originates from primitive myogenic cells. Histologically, These tumors appear as small round blue cells and are further classified into four distinct histologic groups (embryonic, alveolar, anaplastic, and undifferentiated)with varying prognosis [33]. Embryonal histology has a favorable prognosis and 5-year survival rate of 80%, compared with a corresponding rate of only 52% for alveolar subtypes [34].

Malignant melanoma: The nasal cavity is the most common site for mucosal melanomas in the head and neck, it accounts for approximately 3% of sinonasal cancers. The peak age of incidence is between the fifth and eighth decades [35]. Mucosal melanomas are less commonly pigmented than are their cutaneous counterparts. Histologic appearance includes high mitotic rate and vascular invasion. Immunostaining and electron microscopy are frequently needed to establish the diagnosis. Mucosal melanomas of the paranasal sinuses are rapidly lethal neoplasms [36].

Other less common malignant tumors of the nasal cavity and paranasal sinuses are mucoepidermoid carcinoma, plasmacytoma, lymphoma, germ cell tumors, and various sarcomas.

Metastases to the sinonasal region are rare. Renal cell carcinoma is by far the most common source of metastases to this area, followed by lung and breast cancers [37].

40.3 Evaluation

40.3.1 Presentation

Because of the anatomical configuration of the paranasal sinuses as air containing spaces in the skull bones; early or small-sized sinus tumors will produce no or nonspecific symptoms. Clinician should have a high index of suspicion to diagnose such early lesions which will dramatically improve the prognosis and the chances of cure for such patients. It was estimated that between 9% and 12% of patients diagnosed with sinonasal malignancies are asymptomatic [38].

The presence of unilateral sinusitis associated with pain and sinus pressure that is not responding well to medical treatment should raise the suspicion for an early neoplasm involving that sinus and causing obstructive phenomenon. Unexplainable dental symptoms such as dental pain, loosening of teeth, ill-fitting denture or a non-healing oroantral fistula developing after tooth extraction are possible suspicious signs that warrant further workup with a high resolution CT scan.

The most common symptoms of sinonasal malignancies are unilateral nasal obstruction, nasal discharge that may be bloody, epistaxis, or anosmia. Such common complaints may be overlooked for a long time by patients and clinicians, causing a significant delay in the diagnosis.

It has been estimated that an average delay of 6–8 months occurs between the onset of symptoms and the definitive diagnosis and, at this time, more than half of the tumors have reached an advanced stage with a poor prognostic outcome [39, 40].

Many patients present with an advanced stage tumor that make the diagnosis very obvious. Maxillary tumors may extend inferiorly causing a submucosal bulge or ulceration involving the alveolar ridge or hard palate. Anterior extension will breach the anterior maxillary wall causing evident facial swelling. Medial extension to the nasal cavity producing nasal obstruction and intranasal mass. Extension to the orbit commonly occurs especially with ethmoid tumors producing ocular symptoms in about 50% of cases and is related to the site and degree of invasion [41]. The occurrence of proptosis, epiphora (that might be bloody), diplopia, limited ocular motility, blindness or even tumor fungation are all manifestations of orbital involvement by malignant sinonasal neoplasms. On the other hand, orbital involvement can be completely asymptomatic and discovered only on imaging.

Involvement of the infraorbital nerve commonly occurs with maxillary tumors leading to hypoesthesia overlying the cheek. Posterior extension will lead to trismus due to invasion of pterygoid muscles.

Extension to the cranial base may lead to blurred vision, diplopia, or in hypoesthesia along the branches of the trigeminal nerves.

Nasal examination might reveal an intranasal mass that is amenable to office examination using the nasal speculum, on the other hand suspicious cases not presenting with a frank nasal mass should have a meticulous endoscopic intranasal examination with the use of nasal decongestant and topical anesthetic. Endoscopic examination may reveal the presence of a small intranasal mass or a polyp (Fig. 40.1), an ulcerative bleeding area in the nasal mucosa. Tumors may also present as a submucosal mass without any mucosal changes or even a bulging lateral nasal wall with overlying intact mucosa.

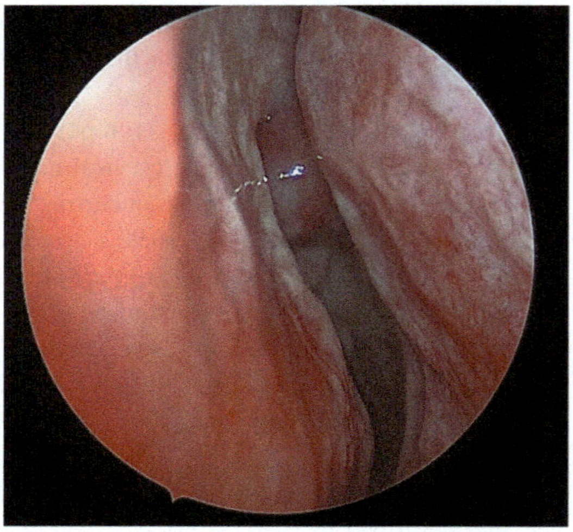

Fig. 40.1 Endoscopic view of an esthesioneuroblastoma

The presence of cervical adenopathy is not common at the time of diagnosis (less than 10%). Significant adenopathy at initial presentation should raise the suspicion of lymphoma.

40.3.2 Diagnostic Imaging

A non-contrast CT scan is the most commonly request imaging modality for patients presenting with nonspecific (suspicious) sinonasal symptoms. The presence of bone erosion or unilateral soft-tissue shadow is enough to raise the suspension of a sinonasal neoplasm that mandates full radiological evaluation. Contrast-enhanced CT and magnetic resonance imaging (MRI) of the paranasal sinuses are generally needed for the accurate assessment of sinonasal neoplasia. CT is better for evaluating bony changes, including expansion, remodeling, and erosion or destruction, while MRI is more useful in assessing soft tissues such as orbital invasion, intracranial extension, and perineural spread. The

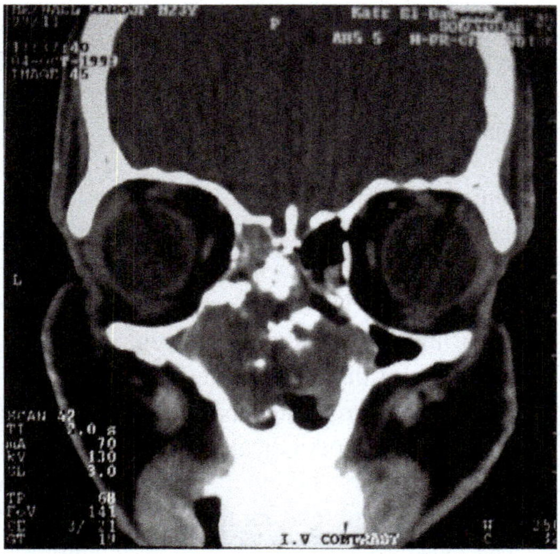

Fig. 40.2 CT scan of a chondrosarcoma of the septum

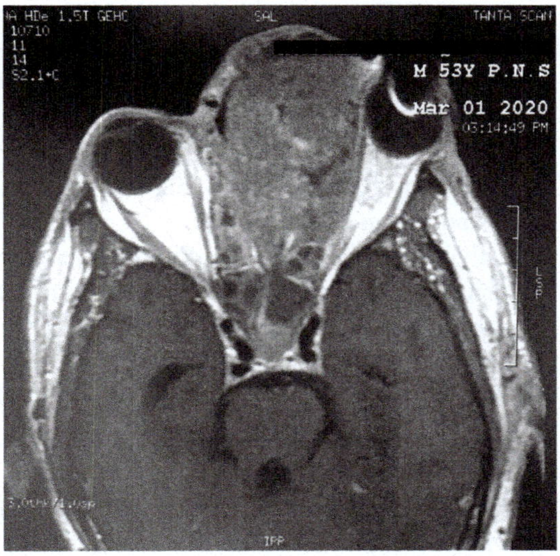

Fig. 40.3 MRI scan demonstrating orbital invasion by SCC of the ethmoid

information gained from both CT and MRI complement each other in defining the precise extent of the tumor.

Bone destruction is seen with aggressive malignant tumors. On the other hand, low-grade malignancies may produce bone remodeling. Tumors of cartilage and bone origin exhibit cartilaginous or bony matrix (Fig. 40.2). Calcification within the tumor mass is seen with esthesioneuroblastoma and chondrosarcoma. These radiographic features can help in narrowing the differential diagnosis of a tumor however, aggressive inflammatory lesions (Wegener's granulomatosis or granulomatous fungal sinusitis may mimic a malignancy).

MRI is the most sensitive imaging modality in assessment of orbital invasion (Fig. 40.3). The condition of the periorbita is a key element in assessment of early stages of orbital invasion. The periorbita appears as a hypointense line interspersed between the hyperintense extraconal fat and the tumor. The presence of unsharp or nodular tumor-fat interface predicts orbital invasion with high accuracy [42]. In cases with cranial base invasion; the condition of the dura is an important determining factor. Linear enhancement at the site of contact with the tumor is generally a reactive change while dural invasion appears as thickening (>5 mm) or nodular dural tumor interface with a sensitivity of 88% [43]. CT scans are much less sensitive in demonstration of such subtle changes.

Perineural tumor spread manifests as thickening or altered enhancement of a nerve segment, widening or erosion of skull base foramina and fissures, enlargement and bulging of the cavernous sinus.

Posterior extension to the pterygopalatine and infratemporal fossa is shown equally by both CT and MRI. Bone lysis and erosion are quite often associated with partial or complete effacement of fat pads in both fossae.

Functional imaging (PET-CT and the newly emerging PET-MRI) does not generally play an important role in the initial assessment of sinonasal tumors. However, they are particularly useful in post-treatment follow-up. The high negative predictive value of the technique allows recurrent tumors to be safely ruled out, whereas positive studies need to be viewed cautiously because of the high rate of false-positive results [44].

In the postoperative follow-up settings MRI has greater potential in the differentiation between scar tissue and recurrence. The wide array of pulse sequences available (including diffusion weighted imaging) allows collection of information quantitatively and qualitatively superior to that obtained with multislice CT [45].

40.3.3 Biopsy

Biopsy and histopathological examination are mandatory before embarking on any management of a malignant sinonasal mass. Biopsy should be obtained after full imaging evaluation of the case. An endoscopic transnasal biopsy is the preferred method. It offers excellent visualization and minimal alteration of the tumor and surrounding structures. However, the surgeon should avoid attempts at either debulking or an attempted resection of the tumor while taking the biopsy because the resulting anatomical alteration will make definitive surgery more difficult.

Open biopsy is generally not needed even with deeply located maxillary lesion can be reached by the creation an astronomy and the use of endoscopes with different viewing angles and curved instruments.

An adequate biopsy should be obtained avoiding the core of bulky tumors (least viable) and areas of inflammatory polypoid mucosal changes beside the tumor mass. The specimen should be handled carefully to avoid crush artifacts and a part of the specimen should be sent in saline especially if lymphoma is suspected.

Because of the rarity of sinonasal tumors, the diversity of the histological types, the high histological spectrum of differentiation among the same histological type and the presence of overlapping pathological features with other entities; reaching a correct histopathological diagnosis of malignant sinonasal tumors is often difficult.

The use of immunostaining is frequently needed to reach a definitive diagnosis which will have a great impact on the management decision. It is extremely important to have a skilled head and neck pathologist and to consider the need for a second opinion in many instances.

40.3.4 Staging

The extent of a cancer at time of diagnosis is an important factor used to define treatment and to assess the chance of successful outcome. Cancer staging systems were developed to code the extent of cancer. In addition to its prognostic value, it also allows homogeneous classification to compare groups of patients in clinical trials who receive standard care around the world facilitating communication and publication.

The most widely used staging system in the current clinical practice is the TNM system maintained by the American Joint Committee on Cancer (AJCC) and the International Union for Cancer Control (UICC). The system codes the extent of the primary tumor (T), regional lymph nodes (N), and distant metastases (M) and provides a "stage grouping" based on T, N, and M. The system is periodically updated based on advances in understanding of cancer prognosis to remain current and relevant to clinical practice.

The latest revision of TNM is the eighth edition that included many changes related to the classification on nasopharyngeal and oropharyngeal carcinoma, on the other hand the classification of sinonasal malignancies remained the same as the previous edition [46]. The seventh edition of this classification includes two different grouping systems, one for carcinoma of the maxillary sinus and one for malignant tumors of the ethmoid sinuses and the nasal cavity. This classification divides T4 lesions into T4a (moderately advanced local disease) and T4b (very advanced local disease), leading to the stratification of stage 4 into stage 4A (moderately advanced local/regional disease), stage 4B (very advanced local/regional disease), and stage 4C (distant metastatic disease) [47].

The TNM is essentially an anatomically based staging. However, the rapidly increasing knowledge of cancer biology provides prognostic information that is in many instances more relevant than anatomic extent. This information need to be incorporated into the TNM nomenclature.

A variety of alternative systems have been proposed for use with individual histopathological types, including esthesioneuroblastoma, SNUC, sinonasal mucosal melanoma and rhabdomyosarcoma. Many of these staging systems have been found to be of great utility and accurately predict patient survival.

Several staging systems have been proposed for esthesioneuroblastoma. The Kadish system [48] is the most commonly used, and it classified tumors into three categories (A–C) by location and extension; the system was later updated with redefined stage C and introducing a new stage D (for metastases) [49]. A third classification system proposed by Dulguerov and Calcaterra is based on the TNM system [50].

40.4 Treatment

The management of paranasal sinus tumors is a multidisciplinary endeavor that involves a team of specialists beside the head and neck surgeon such as pathology, radiation oncology, medical oncology, prosthodontists, neurosurgery, and plastic surgery. The prime parameters that drive management decisions are the tumor pathology, the ability to achieve a gross total resection, and the availability of adjunctive therapies.

Complete surgical resection (when feasible) followed by postoperative irradiation is considered the standard of care in most cases of malignant sinonasal tumors.

40.4.1 Surgical Treatment

Irrespective of the surgical technique used, the aim of curative surgery is to achieve complete tumor resection with microscopically negative resection margins. The extent of surgically resection is largely dependent on the extension of the tumor and to a lesser extent on the known biological behavior of a particular tumor e.g., biologically aggressive versus none.

40.4.1.1 Nasoethmoidal Tumors

Historically, those tumors were managed by a transfacial resection. The major surgical failure was an inadequate excision of the tumor, most commonly at the cribriform plate, with subsequent high local recurrence rates [51, 52] and very low cure rates of 27–35% of malignancies of the nasal vault and 9–10% for ethmoid tumors [53]. Radiation therapy was also associated with high failure rate and serious complications because of the limited tolerance of the visual pathway and other neuronal structures to the high doses required for primary irradiation [54, 55].

It was not possible until the early sixties that Mon bloc resection of the ethmoids was possible through a combined transcranial and facial approaches. In 1963, Ketcham and his colleagues reported the first series of 19 patients who had an anterior craniofacial resection, but 80% of his patients suffered some type of complications [56]. The technique fell in disfavor until the pericranial flap was described to protect dural closure after anterior craniofacial resection which has led to marked reduction of intracranial complication and the anterior craniofacial resection became a safe surgical procedure [57].

Anterior craniofacial resection is the standard procedure for surgical management of ethmoidal malignancies abutting or invading the anterior cranial base. Intracranial exposure is obtained through a bicoronal incision and bifrontal craniotomy. Cerebral dehydrating measures are administered and the dura is lifted off the anterior cranial base to expose the roof of the ethmoids (Fig. 40.4). An appropriate transfacial approach is combined (according to tumor extension). The ethmoid block is ostetomized and the ethmoid block is delivered through the facial approach (Fig. 40.5), dura is reconstructed and closed in a watertight manner and the pericranial flap is used to separate the intracranial contents from the nasal cavity. Transdural invasion into the brain parenchyma is not a contraindication to surgical resection, alternatively cavernous sinus or inter-

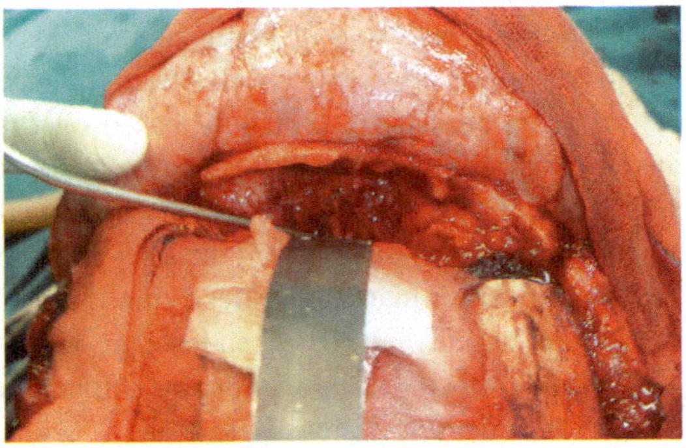

Fig. 40.4 Operative photograph demonstrating intracranial extension of ethmoid tumor through the ethmoid roof (viewed through a bifrontal craniotomy)

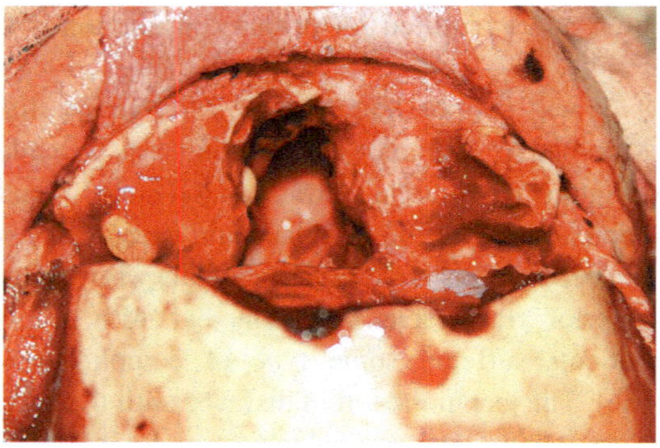

Fig. 40.5 The surgical defect of anterior craniofacial resection

nal carotid artery invasion are not amenable to curative aggressive resection especially with high-grade malignancies.

Endoscopic Resection of Nasoethmoidal Malignancies

Surgical treatment for nasoethmoidal malignancies has witnessed a dramatic change over the last two decades with a paradigm shift toward the application of transnasal endoscopic techniques. This was largely due to an increase in surgical expertise, advances in imaging techniques and surgical instrumentation.

Early reports on endoscopic resection of nasoethmoidal malignancies included only patients with centrally located lesions limited to their site of origin without involvement of the adjacent skull base. However, in the following years and with increasing experience skull base involvement was also deemed amenable to a purely endoscopic excision [58].

Endoscopic resection of malignant sinonasal neoplasms have been extensively debated since its introduction. This was mainly based on the inability to perform a monbloc resection and that a piece meal removal of tumor is not considered oncologically sound in that it predisposes the patient to positive margins postresection [59].

Theoretical advantages of endoscopic resection include superior illumination, magnification and visualization of the surgical field, wider angles of vision using angled endoscopes, avoidance of facial incisions, shorter hospital stays, and lower costs [60].

The limitations of endoscopic techniques include the lack of stereoscopic visualization and depth perception, the inability to repair or patch dural defects with suture techniques, which limits the reconstructive options after endoscopic resection of intradural tumors. Lund and coworkers do not recommend endoscopic resection in isolation if there is transdural extension—a craniofacial resection is typically recommended [61]. Also in cases with extensive invasion and perineural spread an open technique is usually recommended.

Many studies comparing endoscopic vs open techniques demonstrated that endoscopic resection of sinonasal malignancies have oncologic results equivalent to those of open surgery in selected cases however most of the cases who underwent endoscopic resection where of a lower grade tumors and none of them were T4 tumors [62–64]. Lu et al. in a recent meta-analysis concluded that "current pooled evidence suggested that when compared to open resection, endoscopic resection is a comparable surgical approach for sinonasal malignancies" and that it is likely that "particular patients and presentations will benefit more from one of the approaches versus the other." [65]

In experienced hands and in well-selected patient populations, endoscopic resection of sinonasal malignancies is safe, and survival and recurrence data seem to be comparable with those for open techniques.

40.4.1.2 Maxillary Tumors

Tumors originating in the maxillary sinus are removed by some form of maxillectomy. The maxillectomy operation represents one of the earliest attempts at oncological resection of head and neck cancer. The first report of maxillectomy appeared in 1826 by Lizars [66]. Arguably, the most famous of maxillectomies was that performed on President Grover Cleveland on board the yacht Oneida as it sailed up the East River on the morning of July 1, 1893. A verrucous squamous carcinoma was removed, the patient was fitted an obturator and he remained tumor-free until his death from cardiopulmonary disease 15 years later [67].

To avoid confusing terms like extended and radical maxillectomy, Spiro et al. developed a simple classification of maxillectomy. A limited maxillectomy indicated removal of one wall of the maxilla (e.g. medial, inferior or superior maxillectomy), total maxillectomy indicated removal of the entire maxilla while a subtotal maxillectomy describes removal of at least two walls of the maxilla. In all cases any additional resection of adjacent structures e.g., the orbit, facial skin, pterygopalatine, or infratemporal fossa must be identified [68].

Medial maxillectomy requires removal of the entire lateral nasal wall and the ethmoids on one side. This can be performed classically through a lateral rhinotomy. Alternatively the operation can be accomplished successfully through an endoscopic endonasal approach or through a transantral approach avoiding the facial incision. The operation is commonly performed for early or low-grade tumors involving the lateral nasal wall. Malignancies confined to the lower half of the maxilla are managed by limited (inferior) maxillectomy and this can be performed through a transoral route. In both medial and inferior maxillectomy the infraorbital nerve is preserved. Larger maxillary tumors would require a subtotal maxillectomy, a procedure that removes at least two walls of the sinus including a portion of the hard palate or the orbital floor. The extent of resection is dictated by the extent of the tumor.

More extensive tumors would require a total maxillectomy where the entire maxilla is removed, where tumors extend posteriorly to the pterygopalatine or infratemporal fossa; the pterygoid plates may be included with the maxillectomy (Fig. 40.6) or an infratemporal fossa dissection is required for complete tumor extirpation. Total maxillectomy is generally performed through a Weber-Ferguson incision with a subciliary or transconjunctival extension (Fig. 40.7).

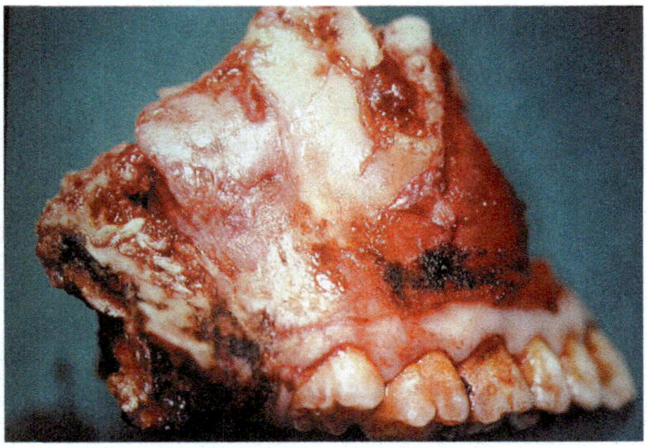

Fig. 40.6 The surgical specimen of total maxillectomy with the pterygoid plates

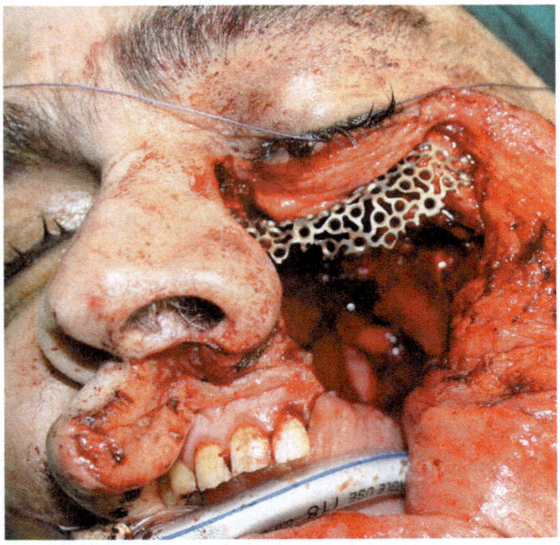

Fig. 40.7 The surgical defect of total maxillectomy after reconstruction of preserved orbit (medial palpebral ligament reattached and a titanium mesh is used to support the orbital floor)

Alternatively, the operation can be performed through a combined wide sublabial and subciliary incisions incision to minimize facial incisions.

Resection of the hard palate and alveolus requires reconstruction this is commonly performed using a dental obturator; some centers prefer the use of composite free flaps that are fashioned to replace missing bone.

40.4.2 Non-surgical Treatment

40.4.2.1 Radiation Therapy

Postoperative radiotherapy is generally indicated patients with high-grade tumors, microscopically positive resection margin or histopathological features of aggressive behavior such as lymphovascular, bone or perineural invasion. Postoperative radiotherapy is also indicated in cases where the surgeon is not confident about complete tumor resection (close surgical margin) or tumor spillage during surgery [69].

Postoperative doses typically range from 50 to 66 Gy, but doses of 70 to 74.4 Gy or higher may be necessary to control gross residual or unresectable disease. The necessity for high dose for disease control and the sensitivity of adjacent neural structures presents challenges to the treating radiation oncologist [70].

Historically, radiation therapy delivered via conventional techniques has been associated with significant complications. Severe visual toxicity has been observed with unilateral and bilateral blindness rates reported to be as high as 30% and 10%, respectively [71].

Subsequent improvements in three-dimensional conformal radiation therapy (3D-CRT) techniques allowed planning based on computed tomography anatomy and led to improvements in target coverage and normal tissue sparing appeared to reduce the risk on optical pathways [72].

Intensity-modulated radiation therapy (IMRT) was one of the most important advances in modern radiotherapy planning it allows for better sparing of optic and brain structures and improved coverage of tumor [73, 74].

Charged particle therapy using protons or carbon ions have garnered particular interesting the treatment of sinonasal cancer it have the potential to maintain target coverage and further lower dose to surrounding normal organs [75]. A recent meta-analyses showed an increase in disease control with charged particle therapy compared to photon radiation therapy [76].

40.4.2.2 Chemotherapy

Classically, the role of chemotherapy in the management of sinonasal malignancies has been limited to palliative treatment of locally advanced or metastatic cancers [77]. This role has recently expanded to be become a part of the multimodal management where systemic chemotherapy is administered in neoadjuvant, concurrent, or adjuvant settings.

Clinical studies have demonstrated a potential benefit of induction chemotherapy in the multimodal treatment of advanced cases [78]. The approach with induction chemotherapy aims to reduce the local burden of disease, with the two objectives of promoting a better approach with radical surgery or radiotherapy, and to reduce the risk of distant spread, for the most aggressive forms. Favorable response to induction chemotherapy is considered a strong prognostic factor [79, 80]. Induction chemotherapy has become key aspect of orbit-sparing protocols [81].

Concomitant chemotherapy and radiotherapy achieved promising survival and locoregional control rates in certain cases [82]. Chemotherapeutic agents may also be used as radiosensitizers, enhancing the effects of radiation on tumor cells [83]. Most accepted protocols currently used involve platinum-based agents [84].

Intra-arterial delivery of chemotherapeutic agents was developed in an effort to deliver higher concentrations to the tumor site while minimizing toxic reactions [85]. Despite exciting organ-preservation and local control rates, intra-arterial chemotherapy carries substantial risk of toxicity that was not justified, given that the efficacy was similar to that of evolving induction chemotherapy regimens [86]. And the technique remains largely an experimental option.

The development of many biologic agents over the past decade, including cetuximab and other monoclonal antibodies, harbors significant potential for targeted therapy [87].

40.4.3 Management of Orbital Invasion

The incidence of orbital invasion by malignancies of the sinonasal tract varies with the site of origin, histology, and aggressiveness of the tumor. Invasion of the orbital wall is present in 66–82% of the patients with ethmoidal malignancy, with involvement of the orbital periosteum in 30–50% of patients [88].

Till the early 1960s, orbital exenteration was required for any degree of orbital invasion [89]. During the early 1970s, an emerging consensus toward orbital preservation have emerged and the criteria defining the indications for orbital preservation versus exenteration have evolved. In 1970, Sisson introduced the concept of selective orbital preservation surgery following adjunctive preoperative radiation for paranasal sinus malignancy [90]. Conley had stated that "most patients are willing to take extra risks to save the eye" [91].

Several investigators like Perry et al. [92], McCarry et al. [93], and Sisson et al. [94] have demonstrated that the periorbita is an effective barrier to tumor invasion and they concluded that the orbit can be preserved if the full thickness of the periorbita is not breached by tumor. The results showed no significant adverse effect on local recurrence using this strategy pushing the limits of orbital preservation even further, Tiwari has noted that a thin fascial layer exists around the periorbital fat that is distinct from the periorbita and believes that invasion of this layer should determine the need for exenteration [95].

Reconstruction. Reconstruction of the orbit is frequently needed to maintain function of the preserved eye and avoid sequelae such as enophthalmos, hypotropia, and diplopia. Reconstructive goals include appropriate support and positioning of preserved orbital contents. Techniques and options for repairing orbital defects depend hon the extent of resection. Resected periorbita is reconstructed with a fascial graft, limited resection of the orbital floor requires no reconstruction. Larger defects involving the orbital floor must undergo immediate rigid reconstruction [96]. Titanium mesh and porous polyethylene implants are among the commonly used materials in this regard [97]. Larger tumor resection including maxillectomy, orbital exenteration, and facial soft-tissue sacrifice necessitate utilization of free tissue transfer. Complementary strategies, such as prosthetics, can be exceedingly helpful in restoring form.

Take Home Messages

- Cancer of the nasal cavity and paranasal sinuses is rare, representing less than 1% of all human malignancies.
- Sinonasal malignancies comprise a wide variety of neoplasms with different biologic behavior, ranging from slow-growing and indolent to highly aggressive and lethal.
- Understanding the biologic behavior of these tumors is of paramount importance in selecting the optimal treatment strategy.
- The signs and symptoms of early stage sinonasal malignancy are similar to those of benign conditions and a high index of suspicion is required for their diagnosis.
- Both CT and MRI are complimentary in the evaluation of patients with sinonasal malignancies.
- Surgery plays an important role in the management of most patients with sinonasal malignancies.
- Treatment of sinonasal tumors is frequently multimodal and requires close ongoing multidisciplinary cooperation.

References

1. Youlden DR, Cramb SM, Peters S, Porceddu SV, Moller H, et al. International comparisons of the incidence and mortality of sinonasal cancer. Cancer Epidemiol. 2013;3786:770–9.
2. Turner JH, Reh DD. Incidence and survival in patients with sinonasal cancer: a historical analysis of population-based data. Head Neck. 2012;34:877–85.
3. Muir CS, Nectoux J. Descriptive epidemiology of malignant neoplasms of nose, nasal cavities, middle ear and accessory sinuses. Clin Otolaryngol Allied Sci. 1980;5:195–211.
4. Barnes L, Eveson J, Reichart P. Pathology and genetics of head and neck tumors. Lyon, France: Oxford University Press; 2005.

5. Khademi B, Moradi A, Hoseini S, et al. Malignant neoplasms of the sinonasal tract: report of 71 patients and literature review and analysis. Oral Maxillofac Surg. 2009;13:191–9.
6. Myers LL, Oxford LE. Differential diagnosis and treatment options in paranasal sinus cancers. Surg Oncol Clin N Am. 2004;13:167–86.
7. Dulguerov P, Jacobsen MS, Allal AS, et al. Nasal and paranasal sinus carcinoma: are we making progress? Cancer. 2001;92(12):3012–29.
8. Turner JH, Reh DD. Incidence and survival in patients with sinonasal cancer: ahistorical analysis of population-based data. Head Neck. 2011;34(6):877–85.
9. Doll R, Morgan LG, Speizer FE. Cancers of the lung and nasal sinuses in nickel workers. Br J Cancer. 1970;24:623–32.
10. Syrjanen K, Syrjanen S. Detection of human papillomavirus in sinonasal carcinoma: systematic review and meta-analysis. Hum Pathol. 2013;44(6): 983–91.
11. Rosai J. Rosai and Ackerman's surgical pathology. Edinburgh: Mosby; 2004.
12. Batsakis J. Pathology of tumors of the nasal cavity and paranasal sinuses. In: Thawley SE, Panje WR, Batsakis JG, et al., editors. Comprehensive management of head and neck tumors, vol. 1. 2nd ed. Philadelphia: WB Saunders; 1999. p. 522–39.
13. Mills SE, Fechner RE, Cantrell RW. Aggressive sinonasal lesion resembling normal intestinal mucosa. Am J Surg Pathol. 1982;6:803–9.
14. Macbeth R. Malignant disease of the paranasal sinuses. J Laryngol Otol. 1965;79:592–612.
15. Acheson ED. Nasal cancer in the furniture and boot and shoe manufacturing industries. Prev Med. 1976;5:295–315.
16. Choussy O, Ferron C, Védrine P, et al. Adenocarcinoma of ethmoid: a GETTEC retrospective multicenter study of 418 cases. Laryngoscope. 2008;118: 437–4.
17. Thompson L. World Health Organization classification of tumors: pathology and genetics of head and neck tumors. Ear Nose Throat J. 2006;85(2):74.
18. Barnes L. Intestinal-type adenocarcinoma of the nasal cavity and paranasal sinuses. Am J Surg Pathol. 1986;10(3):192–202.
19. Heffner DK, Hyams VJ, Hauck KW, et al. Low-grade adenocarcinoma of the nasal cavity and paranasal sinuses. Cancer. 1982;50(2):312–22.
20. Lupinetti AD, Roberts DB, Williams MD, et al. Sinonasal adenoid cystic carcinoma: the M. D. Anderson Cancer Center experience. Cancer. 2007;110:2726–31.
21. Teymoortash A, Pientka A, Schrader C, et al. Expression of galectin-3 in adenoid cystic carcinoma of the head and neckand its relationship with distant metastasis. J Cancer Res Clin Oncol. 2005;24:1–6.
22. Haerle SK, Gullane PJ, Witterick IJ, et al. Sinonasal carcinomas: epidemiology, pathology, and management. Neurosurg Clin N Am. 2013;24:39–49.
23. Naficy S, Disher MJ, Esclamado RM. Adenoid cystic carcinoma of the paranasal sinuses. Am J Rhinol. 1999;13:311–4.
24. Berger L, Luc R, Richard D. L'esthesioneuroepitheliome olfactif. Bull Assoc Fr Etude Cancer. 1924;13:410–21.
25. Elkon D, Hightower SI, Linn ML, et al. Esthesioneuroblastoma. Cancer. 1979;44:1087–94.
26. Lund V, Howard D, Wie W, et al. Olfactory neuroblastoma: past, present, and future? Laryngoscope. 2003;113:502–7.
27. Nalavenkata SB, Sacks R, Adappa ND, et al. Olfactory neuroblastoma: fate of the neck—a long-term multicenter retrospective study. Otolaryngol Head Neck Surg. 2015;154(2):383–9.
28. Hyams V. Tumors of the upper respiratory tract and ear. In: Hyams V, Batsakis L, Michaels L, editors. Atlas of tumor pathology. Washington, DC: Armed Forces Institute of Pathology; 1988. p. 240–8.
29. Frierson HF, Mills S, Fechner R, et al. Sinonasal undifferentiated carcinoma: an aggressive neoplasm derived from schneiderian epithelium and distinct from olfactory neuroblastoma. Am J Surg Pathol. 1986;10(11):771–9.
30. Ejaz A, Wenig BM. Sinonasal undifferentiated carcinoma: clinical and pathologic features and a discussion on classification, cellular differentiation, and differential diagnosis. Adv Anat Pathol. 2005;12:134–43.
31. Reiersen DA, Pahilan ME, Devaiah AK. Meta-analysis of treatment outcomes for sinonasal undifferentiated carcinoma. Otolaryngol Head Neck Surg. 2012;147(1):7–14.
32. Kuan EC, Arshi A, Mallen-St Clair J, et al. Significance of tumor stage in sinonasal undifferentiated carcinoma survival: a population-based analysis. Otolaryngol Head Neck Surg. 2016;154(4):667–73.
33. Malempati S, Hawkins DS. Rhabdomyosarcoma: review of the children' s oncology group (COG) soft-tissue sarcoma committee experience and rationale for current COG studies. Pediatr Blood Cancer. 2012;59(1):5–10.
34. Radzikowska J, Kukwa W, Kukwa A, et al. Rhabdomyosarcoma of the head and neck in children. Contemp Oncol (Pozn). 2015;19(2):98–107.
35. Freedman HM, DeSanto LW, Devine KD, et al. Malignant melanoma of the nasal cavity and paranasal sinuses. Arch Otolaryngol. 1973;97:322–5.
36. Medina JE, Ferlito A, Pellitteri PK, et al. Current management of mucosal melanoma of the head and neck. J Surg Oncol. 2003;83:116–22.
37. Batsakis JG, Rice DH, Solomon AR. The pathology of head and neck tumors: squamous and mucous-gland carcinomas of the nasal cavity, paranasal sinuses, and larynx, part 6. Head Neck Surg. 1980;2:497–508.
38. Lewis JS, Castro EB. Cancer of the nasal cavity and paranasal sinuses. J Laryngol Otol. 1972;86: 255–62.
39. Bhattacharyya N. Cancer of the nasal cavity: survival and factors influencing prognosis. Arch Otolaryngol Head Neck Surg. 2002;128(9):1079–83.

40. Thorup C, Sebbesen L, Danø H, et al. Carcinoma of the nasal cavity and paranasal sinuses in Denmark 1995–2004. Acta Oncol. 2010;49(3):389–94.
41. Lund VJ. Malignant tumors of the nasal cavity and paranasal sinuses. ORL J Otorhinolaryngol Relat Spec. 1983;45:1–12.
42. Maroldi R, Farina D, Battaglia G, et al. MR of malignant nasosinusal neoplasms. Frequently asked questions. Eur J Radiol. 1997;24(3):181–90.
43. Yousem DM, Gad K, Tufano RP. Resectability issues with head and neck cancer. AJNR Am J Neuroradiol. 2006;27(10):2024–36.
44. Lamarre ED, Batra PS, Lorenz RR, et al. Role of positron emission tomography in management of sinonasalneoplasms—a single institution's experience. Am J Otolaryngol. 2012;33(3):289–95.
45. Farina D, Borghesi A, Botturi E, Ravanelli M, Maroldi R. Treatment monitoring of paranasal sinus tumors by magnetic resonance imaging. Cancer Imaging. 2010;10:183–93.
46. Amin MB, Edge S, Greene F, et al. AJCC cancer staging manual. 8th ed. New York: Springer International Publishing; 2017. p. 67–507.
47. Patel S, Shah JP. Part II. Head and neck sites. In: Edge SB, Byrd DR, Carducci MA, Compton CA, editors. AJCC cancer staging manual. 7th ed. New York: Springer; 2009.
48. Kadish S, Goodman M, Wang CC. Olfactory neuroblastoma. A clinical analysis of 17 cases. Cancer. 1976;37:1571–6.
49. Morita A, Ebersold MJ, Olsen KD, et al. Esthesioneuroblastoma. Neurosurgery. 1993;32(5):706–15.
50. Dulguerov P, Calcaterra. Esthesioneuroblastoma: the UCLA experience 1970–1990. Laryngoscope. 1992;102:843–9.
51. Cramer LR. Malignant neoplasms of the paranasal sinuses. Arch Otolaryngol. 1953;58:704–9.
52. Frazell EL, Lewis JS. Cancer of the nasal cavity and accessory sinuses. Cancer. 1963;16:1293–301.
53. Osguthorpe JD. Sinus neoplasia. Arch Otolaryngol Head Neck Surg. 1994;120:19–25.
54. Parsons JT, Mendenhall WM, Mancuso AA. Malignant tumors of the nasal cavity and ethmoid and sphenoid sinuses. Int J Radial Oncol Biol Phys. 1988;14:11–8.
55. Baron SH. Brain necrosis following treatment of esthesioneuroblastoma. Laryngoscope. 1979;89:214–23.
56. Ketcham AS, Wilkins RH, Van Buren JM. A combined intracranial facial approach to the paranasal sinuses. Am J Surg. 1963;106:986–703.
57. Johns ME, Winn HR, McLean WC, Cantrell RW. Pericranial flap for the closure of defects of the craniofacial resection. Laryngoscope. 1981;91:952–9.
58. Arnold A, Ziglinas P, Ochs K, et al. Therapy options and long-term results of sinonasal malignancies. Oral Oncol. 2012;48:1031–7.
59. Penel N, Mallet Y, Mirabel X, et al. Primary mucosal melanoma of head and neck: prognostic value of clear margins. Laryngoscope. 2006;116:993–5.
60. Kasemsiri P, Carrau RL, Ditzel Filho LF, et al. Advantages and limitations of endoscopic endonasal approaches to the skull base. World Neurosurg. 2014;82:S12–21.
61. Lund V, Howard DJ, Wei WI. Endoscopic resection of malignant tumors of the nose and sinuses. Am J Rhinol. 2007;21:89–94.
62. Hanna E, DeMonte F, Ibrahim S, et al. Endoscopic resection of sinonasal cancers with and without craniotomy: oncologic results. Arch Otolaryngol Head Neck Surg. 2009;135:1219–24.
63. Nicolai P, Battaglia P, Bignami M, et al. Endoscopic surgery for malignant tumors of the sinonasal tract and adjacent skull base: a 10-year experience. Am J Rhinol. 2008;22:308–16.
64. Bogaerts S, VanderPoorten V, Nuyts S, et al. Results of endoscopic resection followed by radiotherapy for primarily diagnosed adenocarcinomas of the paranasal sinuses. Head Neck. 2008;30:728–36.
65. Lu VM, Ravindran K, Phan K, et al. Surgical outcomes of endoscopic versus open resection for primary sinonasal malignancy: a meta-analysis. Am J Rhinol Allergy. 2019;33(5):608–16.
66. Stell PM. History of surgery of the upper jaw. In: Harrison DFN, Lund VJ, editors. Tumors of the upper jaw. Edinburgh: Churchill Livingstone; 1993. p. 4.
67. Morreels CL Jr. New historical information on the Cleveland operations. Surgery. 1967;62:542–51.
68. Spiro RH, Strong EW, Shah JP. Maxillectomy and its classification. Head Neck. 1997;19:309–14.
69. Seong SY, Hyun DW, Kim YS, et al. Treatment outcomes of sinonasal adenoid cystic carcinoma: 30 cases from asingle institution. J Craniomaxillofac Surg. 2014;42:171–5.
70. Ganly I, Patel SG, Singh B, et al. Complications of craniofacial resection for malignant tumors of the skull base: report of an International Collaborative Study. Head Neck. 2005;27(6):445–51.
71. Lindeman P, Eklund U, Petruson B. Survival after surgical treatment in maxillary neoplasms of epithelial origin. J Laryngol Otol. 1987;101(6):564–8.
72. Pommier P, Ginestet C, Sunyach M, et al. Conformal radiotherapy for paranasal sinus and nasal cavity tumors: three-dimensional treatment planning and preliminary results in 40 patients. Int J Radiat Oncol Biol Phys. 2000;48(2):485–93.
73. Duprez F, Madani I, Morbée L, et al. IMRT for sinonasal tumors minimizes severe late ocular toxicity and preserves disease control and survival. Int J Radiat Oncol Biol Phys. 2012;83:252–9.
74. Dirix P, Vanstraelen B, Jorissen M, et al. Intensity-modulated radiotherapy for sinonasal cancer: improved outcome compared to conventional radiotherapy. Int J Radiat Oncol Biol Phys. 2010;78:998–1004.
75. Chera BS, Malyapa R, Louis D, et al. Proton therapy for maxillary sinus carcinoma. Am J Clin Oncol. 2009;32:296–303.
76. Patel SH, Wang Z, Wong WW, et al. Charged particle therapy versus photon therapy for paranasal sinus andnasal cavity malignant diseases: a

systematic review and meta-analysis. Lancet Oncol. 2014;15(9):1027–38.
77. Bossi P, Saba NF, Vermorken JB, et al. The role of systemic therapy in the management of sinonasal cancer: a critical review. Cancer Treat Rev. 2015;41:836–43.
78. Hanna EY, Cardenas AD, DeMonte F, et al. Induction chemotherapy for advanced squamous cell carcinoma of the paranasal sinuses. Arch Otolaryngol Head Neck Surg. 2011;137:78–81.
79. Hanna EY, Cardenas AD, DeMonte F, Roberts D, Kupferman M, Weber R, et al. Induction chemotherapy for advanced squamous cell carcinoma of the paranasal sinuses. Arch Otolaryngol Head Neck Surg. 2011;137(1):78–81.
80. Björk-Eriksson T, Mercke C, Petruson B, et al. Potential impact on tumor control and organ preservation with cisplatin and 5-fluorouracil for patients with advanced tumors of the paranasal sinuses and nasal fossa. A prospective pilot study. Cancer. 1992;70(11):2615–20.
81. McCary WS, Levine PA, Cantrell RW. Preservation of the eye in the treatment of sinonasal malignant neoplasms with orbital involvement: a confirmation of the original treatise. Arch Otolaryngol Head Neck Surg. 1996;122:657–9.
82. Choi KN, Rotman M, Aziz H, et al. Concomitant infusion cisplatin and hyperfractionated radiotherapy for locally advanced nasopharyngeal and paranasal sinus tumors. Int J Radiat Oncol Biol Phys. 1997;39(4):823–9.
83. Choi KN, Rotman M, Aziz H, et al. Locally advanced paranasal sinus and nasopharynx tumors treated with hyperfractionated radiations and concomitant infusion cisplatin. Cancer. 1991;67:2748–52.
84. Rosen A, Vokes EE, Scher N, et al. Locoregionally advanced paranasal sinus carcinoma. Favorable survival with multimodality therapy. Arch Otolaryngol Head Neck Surg. 1993;119:743–6.
85. Homma A, Oridate N, Suzuki F, et al. Superselective high-dose cisplatin infusion with concomitant radiotherapy in patients with advanced cancer of the nasal cavity and paranasal sinuses: a single institution experience. Cancer. 2009;115:4705–14.
86. Lee YY, Dimery IW, Van Tassel P, et al. Superselective intra-arterial chemotherapy of advanced paranasal sinus tumors. Arch Otolaryngol Head Neck Surg. 1989;115:503–11.
87. Feldman R, Gatalica Z, Knezetic J, et al. Molecular profiling of head and neck squamous cell carcinoma. Head Neck. 2016;38(Suppl 1):E1625–38.
88. Ganly I, Patel SG, Singh B, et al. Craniofacial resection for malignant paranasal sinus tumors: report of an international collaborative study. Head Neck. 2005;27:575–84.
89. Ketcham AS, Chretien PB, Van Buren JM, et al. The ethmoid sinuses: a re-evaluation of surgical resection. Am J Surg. 1973;126:469–75.
90. Sisson GA. Symposium III: treatment of malignancies of paranasal sinuses—discussion and summary. Laryngoscope. 1970;80:945–53.
91. Conley J. The risk to the orbit in head and neck cancer. Laryngoscope. 1985;95:515–21.
92. Perry C, Levine PA, Williamson BR, Cantrell RW. Preservation of the eye in paranasal sinus cancer surgery. Arch Otolaryngol Head Neck Surg. 1988;114:632–4.
93. McCary WS, Levine PA, Cantrell RW. Preservation of the eye in the treatment of sinonasal malignant neoplasms with orbital involvement: a confirmation of the original treatise. Arch Otolaryngol. 1996;122:657–9.
94. Sisson GA, Toriumi DM, Atiyah RA. Paranasal sinus malignancy: a comprehensive update. Laryngoscope. 1989;99:143–50.
95. Tiwari R, van der Wal J, van der Waal I, Snow G. Studies of the anatomy and pathology of the orbit in carcinoma of the maxillary sinus and their impact on preservation of the eye in maxillectomy. Head Neck. 1998;20:193–6.
96. Lal D, Cain RB. Updates in reconstruction of skull base defects [review]. Curr Opin Otolaryngol Head Neck Surg. 2014;22(5):419–28.
97. Janecka IP. New reconstructive technologies in skull base surgery: role of titanium mesh and porous polyethylene. Arch Otolaryngol Head Neck Surg. 2000;126:396–401.

41 Nasopharyngeal Cancer

Aisha Larem, Emad Al Duhirat, and Hassan Omer

41.1 Introduction

The nasopharynx is the space behind the nasal cavity and above the oropharynx. As it is deep space, it makes it difficult to be examined during regular examination, the presentation of any pathology will be late due to this position, and the surgical excision of any pathology will be difficult and incomplete. The proximity of this space to multiple vital structures like the ear through the Eustachian tube, skull base, and cranial nerves gives it a crucial functional and pathological importance.

41.2 Anatomy

The nasopharynx is bounded.

- Inferiorly by the lower surface of the soft palate.
- Anteriorly by the choana (nasal cavity).
- Superiorly the floor of the sphenoid which slopes down to become the posterior wall formed by the clivus bone.
- Laterally by the opening of the Eustachian tubes superiorly and the upper part of the superior constrictor muscle inferiorly.

A. Larem (✉) · E. Al Duhirat · H. Omer
Hamad Medical Corporation, Doha, Qatar
e-mail: alarem@hamad.qa; EAIDuhirat@hamad.qa

The fossa of Rosenmuller (the most common area of nasopharyngeal carcinoma) [1]: Is a recess extends postero-laterally on both sides of the posterior wall of the nasopharynx to form the lateral recess which has variable depths and bounded anteriorly by the opening of the Eustachian tube (Fig. 41.1).

The nasopharynx is lined by pseudostratified squamous epithelium, the lymphatic drainage mainly to the lymph nodes in the retropharyngeal space (nodes of Rouvière) and into the deep cervical nodes. The cranial nerves IX, X, XI, and XII, the carotid sheath and the sympathetic trunk traverse the parapharyngeal space which is lateral to the superior constrictor muscle.

Blood supply to the nasopharynx is through branches of the internal maxillary artery while venous drainage is to the pterygoid plexus, then to the facial and internal jugular veins.

The area with the highest incidence of nasopharyngeal carcinoma (NPC) is in Southern China [2]. The male to female ratio of the disease is 3 to 1. The peak age group of presentations of NPC in endemic areas is 50–55 years old, and it decreases with increasing age.

41.3 Etiologies

– Genetic factors

A. Al-Qahtani et al. (eds.), *Textbook of Clinical Otolaryngology*,
https://doi.org/10.1007/978-3-030-54088-3_41

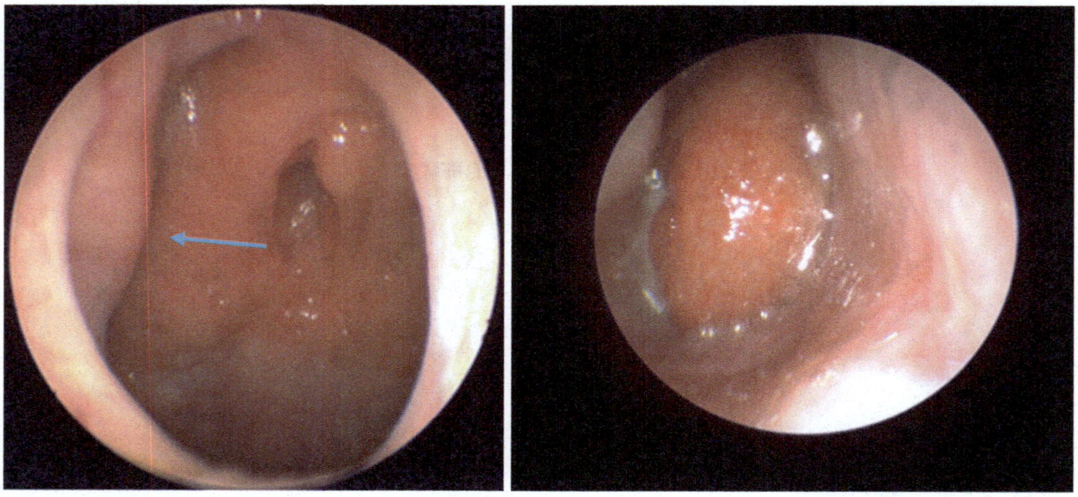

Fig. 41.1 Endoscopic view of normal postnasal space compared to nasopharyngeal tumor, Rosenmiller fossa (arrow)

- Environmental factors: salted fish, preserved foods may be due to the high nitrosamine content [3–6]
- Epstein-Barr virus in endemic areas

41.4 Pathology

Nasopharyngeal cancer is a squamous cell carcinoma which arises from the epithelium.

The World Health Organization (WHO) originally categorized the epithelial malignancies from the nasopharynx into three subtypes:

1. Well-differentiated keratinizing squamous cell carcinoma (WHO type 1)
2. Nonkeratinizing carcinoma (WHO type 2)
3. Undifferentiated carcinoma (WHO type 3) [7]

The classification was later revised to two subtypes:

- Keratinizing squamous cell carcinoma
- Combining type 2 and type 3 into nonkeratinizing carcinoma. The nonkeratinizing carcinoma can be further subclassified as differentiated and undifferentiated types [7].

Only the nonkeratinizing class is associated with Epstein-Barr virus (EBV) infection. This classification shows prognostic significance. The undifferentiated NPC have a higher local tumor control rate with therapy although the possibility of distant metastasis is also higher (Fig. 41.2) [8, 9].

41.5 Clinical Manifestations

- A painless mass in the neck: About 70% of patients have an enlarged lymph node in the neck on presentation. The most frequently involved nodes are level II (upper jugular) and upper level V (apex of posterior triangle) [10].
- Otological symptoms: Eustachian tube dysfunction secondary to tumor bulk and/or invasion. Unilateral secretory otitis media in an adult patient is an alarming symptom for nasopharyngeal cancer.
- Nasal symptoms: Blood-stained nasal discharge, postnasal drip and blockage.
- Neurological symptoms: Headache or presentation related to cranial nerve involvement. The prevalence of cranial nerve palsy on presentation is around 20% [11]. When the tumor extends superiorly to affect the lateral wall of the cavernous sinus, then the cranial nerves III to VI might be affected and with lateral extension of the tumor into the parapharyngeal space, cranial nerves IX–XII might be affected.

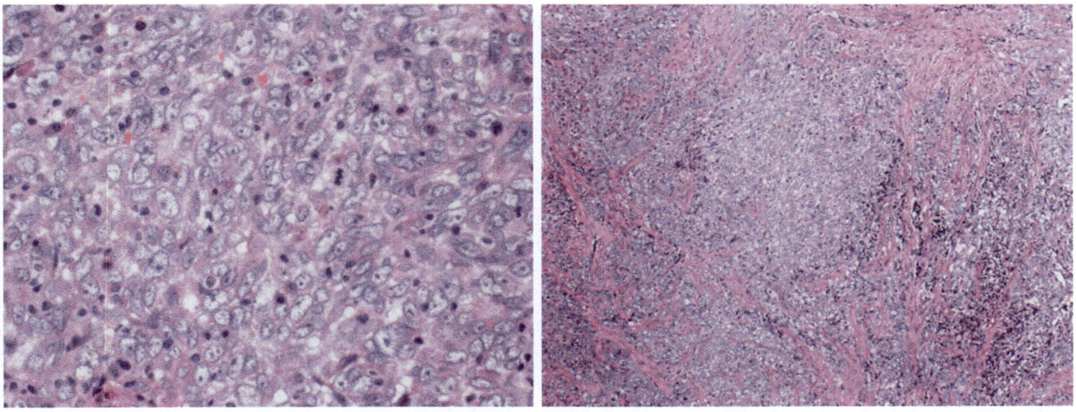

Fig. 41.2 Nonkeratinizing nasopharyngeal carcinoma, undifferentiated, high magnification and low magnification respectively. (Photo credits, Dr. Adham A. Ammar—Senior Consultant Pathology—HMC)

The cranial nerves most frequently affected are the third, fifth, sixth, and twelfth [12].

Common sites of distant metastases are liver, lung, and bone, with brain metastasis being rare.

41.5.1 Diagnosis

- Thorough history
- Physical exam

Full ENT exam concentrating on the following points:

- Endoscopy of the post nasal space, attention showed be made to the submucosal NPC
- Neck exam looking for lymph nodes
- Ears exam looking for secretory otitis media (Unilateral)
- Cranial nerves examination
- Fine needle biopsy: With the addition of immunohistochemical staining for EBV RNA (EBER), a definitive diagnosis of NPC with neck lymph node metastasis can be made
- Biopsy, Gold standard
- Blood tests

41.5.1.1 EBV Antibodies Serology

In NPC, the level of IgA in response to early intracellular antigen (EA) and viral capsid antigen (VGA) are much higher than those detected, in the general population [13].

The IgA anti-EA has been shown to be more specific while IgA anti-VCA is more sensitive for the diagnosis of NPC [14].

41.5.2 Imaging Studies

41.5.2.1 CT Scan

See Fig. 41.3.

41.5.2.2 MRI

MRI's superiority in soft tissue pathology detection makes it the preferred modality in nasopharyngeal cancer. For assessment of tumor extent, MRI can better delineate parapharyngeal extension of tumor, perineural spread and marrow infiltration. MRI can also differentiate between tumor infiltration from secretions in the paranasal sinuses, and can define better the limits of the optic chiasma, optic nerves, and brainstem (Fig. 41.4) [15].

41.5.2.3 Positron Emission Tomography (PET)

PET-CT can detect distant metastases in addition to locoregional disease extent. PET-CT is very useful in assessing residual and recurrent disease after treatment (Fig. 41.5).

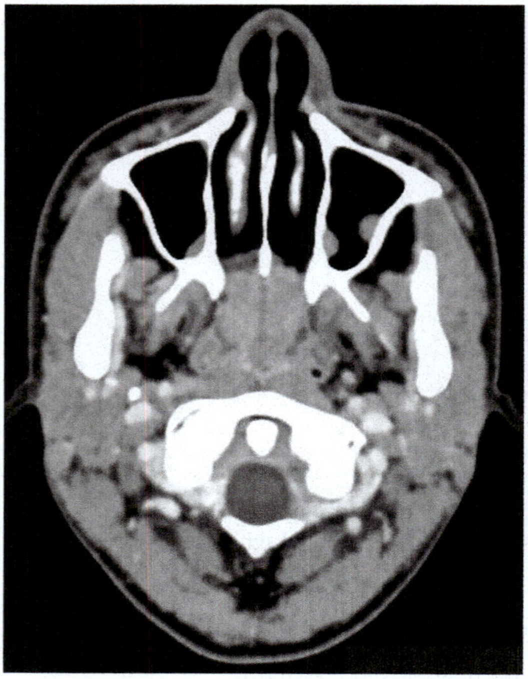

Fig. 41.3 Axial postnasal space CT scan shows a nasopharyngeal mass completely obstructing the post nasal space with features suspicious of malignancy

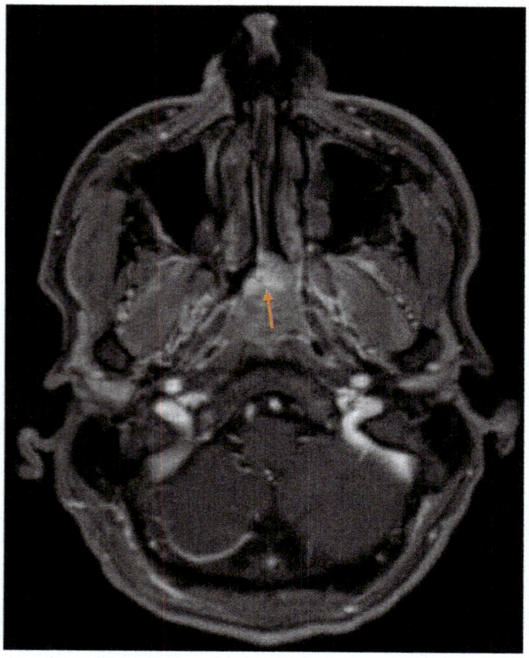

Fig. 41.4 T1 MRI scan with contrast showing a nasopharyngeal mass (arrow) with contrast enhancement

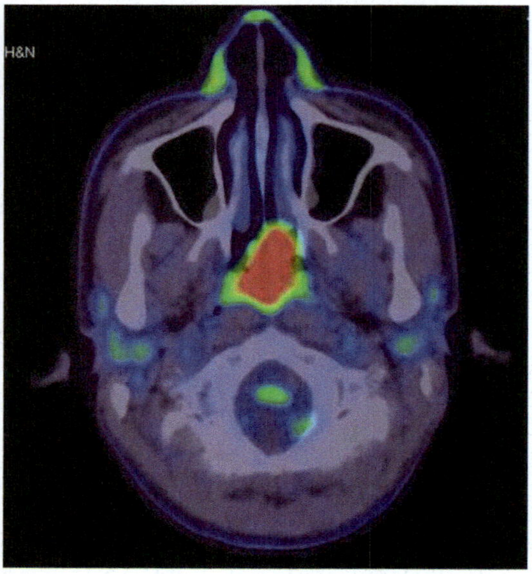

Fig. 41.5 FDG PET Axial CT scan, of patient with nasopharyngeal cancer noted by the increase uptake in the scan noted by increase uptake of glucose in affected areas

41.6 Staging and TNM Classification [16]

T Category	T Criteria
TX	Primary tumor cannot be assessed
T1	Tumor confined to nasopharynx, or extends to oropharynx and/or nasal cavity without parapharyngeal space involvement
T2	Tumor with extension to parapharyngeal space and/or infiltration of the medial pterygoid, lateral pterygoid, and/or prevertebral muscles
T3	Tumor invades bony structures of skull base cervical vertebra, pterygoid structures, and/or paranasal sinuses
T4	Tumor with intracranial extension and/or involvement of cranial nerves, hypopharynx, orbit, parotid gland and/or infiltration beyond the lateral surface of the lateral pterygoid muscle

N Category	N Criteria
Nx	Regional lymph nodes cannot be assessed
N0	No regional lymph node metastasis
N1	Unilateral metastasis, in cervical lymph node(s), and/or unilateral or bilateral metastasis in retropharyngeal lymph nodes, 6 cm or less, above the caudal border of cricoid cartilage

N Category	N Criteria
N2	Bilateral metastasis in cervical lymph node(s), 6 cm or less above the caudal border of cricoid cartilage
N3	Metastasis in cervical lymph node(s) greater than 6 cm in dimension and/or extension below the caudal border of cricoid cartilage

M category	M criteria
M0	No distant metastasis
M1	Distant metastasis

Stages			
I	T1	N0	M0
II	T1	N1	M0
	T2	N0, N1	M0
III	T1, T2	N2	M0
	T3	N0, N1, N2	M0
IVA	T4	N0, N1, N2	M0
	Any T	N3	M0
IVB	Any T	Any N	M1

41.7 Treatment

- Radiotherapy (primary treatment)
- Concurrent chemoradiotherapy (for advanced cases)
- Surgery (salvage surgery for failure of primary treatment)

Radiotherapy is the mainstay treatment for primary NPC (radiosensitive) and surgical treatment is reserved for salvage of radiation failures [15].

Intensity-modulated radiotherapy (IMRT) allows different dose levels to different regions to be applied in the same treatment.

Nasopharyngeal carcinoma has a tendency of early spread to paranasopharyngeal and cervical lymphatics, hence prophylactic nodal treatment is mandatory and radiotherapy can cover these areas adequately.

For effective treatment of nasopharyngeal carcinoma, the radiation target volume includes the nasopharynx and also the parapharyngeal space, oropharynx, base of skull, sphenoid sinus, posterior ethmoid sinus and posterior half of maxillary antrum. Cervical nodal irradiation is mandatory even in clinically node-negative patients due to the high incidence of neck relapse in the absence of prophylactic nodal irradiation [17].

A dose of 65–70 Gy is normally given to the primary tumor, 65–70 Gy to the involved neck nodes, and 50–60 Gy to the node-negative neck.

41.7.1 Chemotherapy

Current evidence indicates that concurrent chemoradiotherapy has a major role in advanced stage nasopharyngeal carcinoma. Combined induction and concurrent chemotherapy may have the added benefit of tumor shrinkage prior to radiotherapy, and excellent control can be achieved using this approach in advanced T stage NPC [18].

Stage I and low-risk stage II, can be treated with radical radiotherapy alone.

Stage II disease with higher tumor load and stage III, IV disease require combination chemotherapy and radiotherapy.

41.7.2 Surgery

Surgical resection of the nasopharynx, is only reserved for salvaging radiation failures. Neck dissection is considered as the standard of care for management of nodal failures [19].

41.7.3 Follow-up

Regular examination of the nasopharynx by endoscopy should be performed as part of follow-up.

- Every 3 months first year
- Every 6 months during the second and third years after treatment
- Follow-up is necessary every year afterward
- CT and/or MR imaging of the nasopharynx should also be performed every 6 months

Complications of radiotherapy:

Although radiotherapy is the main treatment of nasopharyngeal cancer, many complications can affect the quality of life of patients post radiotherapy.

1. Xerostomia is almost always present after conventional radiotherapy which causes dry mouth, poor oral hygiene, and dental caries (1).
2. Hearing impairment is also seen either due to direct radiation trauma to the hearing organs, Eustachian tube dysfunction or ototoxicity due to chemotherapy (2).
3. Radiotherapy may induce soft tissue fibrosis and rigidity that might affect the neck movement and mouth opening (3).
4. CN^{T} IX, X, XI, and XII) can also be damaged by radiation (4).
5. Cranial nerve palsies, dryness or pharyngeal stricture can contribute to the dysphagia (5).
6. Hormonal insufficiency and disturbance can develop due to damage to the hypothalamic-pituitary axis or organs like the thyroid gland (6).
7. Carotid artery stenosis is a possibility following neck irradiation and may cause cerebral ischemia (7).
8. Neurological sequelae like memory loss, cognitive dysfunction, and neuropsychological dysfunction can happen after radiotherapy (8–10).

The advent of conformal radiotherapy such as IMRT has the potential of reducing late radiation problems by reducing the dose delivered to critical structures.

41.8 Prognosis

Stage I and II disease treated with radiotherapy have a 5 years survival rate up to 80% and more, Stage III and IV with concurrent chemoradiation have 5 years survival around 70% [20].

Take Home Messages

- As an otolaryngologist a complete ENT exam involves the postnasal space.
- Any adult patient presenting with unilateral secretory otitis media should have his post nasal space examined with focus on the fossa of Rosenmuller.
- Radiotherapy is the main treatment modality for nasophargeal cancer, with less side effects when using the IMRT.
- Epstein-Barr virus is a main pathogen in nasopharyngeal cancer.

Acknowledgment Authors of this chapter appreciate the help of Dr. Adham A. Ammar—Senior Consultant Pathology, Dr. Khalid Murshed—Pathology Resident, HMC, Qatar, and the help of Dr. Adham Aljariri, an ENT resident in HMC of his effort in editing the chapter.

References

1. JKS W. Clinical diagnosis. In: van Hasselt CA, Gibb AG, editors. Nasopharyngeal carcinoma. 2nd ed. Hong Kong: The Chinese University Press; 1999. p. 337.
2. Wei KR, Zheng RS, Zhang SW, et al. Nasopharyngeal carcinoma incidence and mortality in China in 2010. Chin J Cancer. 2014;33(8):381–7. https://doi.org/10.5732/cjc.014.10086.
3. Yu MC, Ho JH, Lai SH, Henderson BE. Cantonese-style salted fish as a cause of nasopharyngeal carcinoma: report of a case-control study in Hong Kong. Cancer Res. 1986;46(2):956–61.
4. Huang DP, Ho JH, Saw D, Teoh TB. Carcinoma of the nasal and paranasal regions in rats fed Cantonese salted marine sh. IARC Sci Publ. 1978;20:315–28.
5. Gallicchio L, Matanoski G, Tao XG, et al. Adulthood consumption of preserved and nonpreserved vegetables and the risk of nasopharyngeal carcinoma: a systematic review. Int J Cancer. 2006;119(5):1125–35.
6. Zou XN, Lu SH, Liu B. Volatile N-nitrosamines and their precursors in Chinese salted fish: a possible etiological factor for NPC in China. Int J Cancer. 1994;59(2):155–8.
7. Shanmugaratnam K, Sobih LH. Histological typing of tumors of the upper respiratory tract and ear. In: International Histological Classification of Tumors:

No. 19. Geneva: World Health Organization; 1991. p. 32–3.
8. Reddy SP, Raslan WF, Gooneratne S, et al. Prognostic significance of keratinization in nasopharygeal carcinoma. Am J Otolaryngol. 1995;16:103–8.
9. Marks JE, Philips JL, Menck HR. The National Cancer Data Base report on the relationship of race and national origin to the histology of nasopharyngeal carcinoma. Cancer. 1998;83:582–8.
10. Sham J, Choy D, Wei W. Nasopharyngeal carcinoma: orderly neck node spread. Int J Radiat Oncol Biol Phys. 1990;19(4):929–33.
11. Lee AW, Foo W, Law SC, et al. Nasopharyngeal carcinoma: presenting symptoms and duration before diagnosis. Hong Kong Med J. 1997;3:355–61.
12. Ozyar E, Atahan IL, Akyol FH, et al. Cranial nerve involvement in nasopharyngeal carcinoma: its prognostic role and response to radiotherapy. Radiat Med. 1994;12:65–8.
13. Klein G, Giovanella BC, Lindahl T, et al. Direct evidence for the presence of Epstein-Barr virus DNA and nuclear antigen in malignant epithelial cells from patients with poorly differentiated carcinoma of the nasopharynx. Proc Natl Acad Sci U S A. 1974;71:4737–41.
14. Ho HC, Ng MH, Kwan HC, Chau JC. Epstein-Barr-virus- specific IgA and IgG serum antibodies in nasopharyngeal carcinoma. Br J Cancer. 1976;34:655–60.
15. King R, Tsang Y, Kwong DLW. Nasopharyngeal carcinoma. In: Brown S, editor. Otorhinolaryngology head and neck surgery. 8th ed. Boca Raton: CRC Press; 2018. p. 1025–34.
16. Amin MB, Edge SB, Greene FL, et al., editors. AJCC cancer staging manual. 8th ed. New York: Springer; 2017.
17. Lee AWM, Sham JS, Poon YF, Ho JH. Treatment of Stage I nasopharyngeal carcinoma: analysis of the patterns of relapse and the results of withholding elective neck irradiation. Int J Radiat Oncol Biol Phys. 1989;17:1183–90.
18. Rischin D, Corry J, Smith J, et al. Excellent disease control and survival in patients with advanced nasopharyngeal cancer treated with chemoradiation. J Clin Oncol. 2002;20:1845–52.
19. Wei W, Mok V. The management of neck metastases in nasopharyngeal cancer. Curr Opin Otolaryngol Head Neck Surg. 2007;15(2):99–102.
20. Flint PW, et al., editors. Cummings otolaryngology, head and neck surgery. 5th ed. Philadelphia, PA: Mosby Elsevier; 2010.

Difficult Airway Management for ENT Surgery for Non-anesthesiologists

42

Nabil A. Shallik, Odai Khamash, and Mohammad Al Nobani

42.1 Introduction and Facts

Maintaining airway patency and ensuring a proper gas exchange is a fundamental role of the anesthetist. Failure to secure the airway or achieve any of these goals may end up with catastrophic complications, including airway trauma, surgical airway, cardiopulmonary arrest, brain injury, and unfortunately, and possible death [1].

Difficulties in maintaining the airway can be related to a problem in mask ventilation, supraglottic airway device (SAD) insertion, laryngoscopy manipulation, or endotracheal tube insertion.

Many factors could contribute to this issue, including health provider's factors, patients' factors, equipment, and health facilities' factors. Proper airway assessment and difficulty prediction, well-trained health providers, well preparation, and situation optimization may help decrease the incidence of these events.

N. A. Shallik (✉)
Weill Cornell Medical College in Qatar, Doha, Qatar

O. Khamash · M. Al Nobani
Hamad Medical Corporation, Doha, Qatar

42.2 Definition of the Difficult Airway

As per the American Society of Anesthesiologists (ASA), a standard definition of the difficult airway cannot be identified in the available literature. However, they described difficult airway "as the clinical situation in which a conventionally trained anesthesiologist experiences difficulty with face mask ventilation of the upper airway, difficulty with tracheal intubation, or both" [2].

Therefore, it is a scenario that represents a complex interaction between patient factors, the clinical setting, and the skills of the practitioner. The difficult airway can be expressed according to the level we faced:

42.2.1 Difficult Face Mask Ventilation (DMV)

Mask ventilation is a basic, but a fundamental airway management skill. It can be a bridge to definitive airway placement or a temporary rescue maneuver in patients with an unanticipated difficult airway.

The definition of DMV has been described over the years through a lot of literature.

Langeron and colleagues defined DMV as "the inability of an unassisted anesthesiologist to maintain oxygen saturation >92%, as measured by pulse oximetry, or to prevent or reverse signs of

A. Al-Qahtani et al. (eds.), *Textbook of Clinical Otolaryngology*,
https://doi.org/10.1007/978-3-030-54088-3_42

inadequate ventilation during positive-pressure mask ventilation under general anesthesia." In their study, mask ventilation was considered difficult if one or more of six criteria were present [2]:

1. failure to maintain oxygen saturation >92% or performing adequate positive-pressure mask ventilation by an unassisted anesthesiologist,
2. significant leak during face mask ventilation,
3. the necessity to increase gas flow to >15 L/min or the need to use the oxygen flush valve more than twice,
4. inadequate chest movement,
5. reverting to the use of a two-handed mask ventilation technique,
6. the need to switch operators.

Other experts defined it as the "inability to obtain chest excursion sufficient to maintain a clinically acceptable capnogram waveform despite optimal head and neck positioning and use of muscle paralysis, use of an oral airway, and optimal application of a face mask by anesthesia personnel" [3].

In 2013, the American Society of Anesthesiologists (ASA) defined it as a situation in which it is not possible to provide adequate mask ventilation owing to either inadequate mask seal, excessive gas leak, or excessive resistance to the ingress or egress of gas.

42.2.1.1 Incidence of Difficult Mask Ventilation

Kheterpal and associates published two big studies on difficult and impossible mask ventilation, which showed that the incidence of DMV was 1.4% in 22,660 patients and 2.2% in a subsequent study of 50,000 patients. The incidence of impossible ventilation ranged from 0.15% to 0.16% in these two big studies [1].

42.2.1.2 Causes and Risk Factors of Difficult Mask Ventilation

There are two leading reasons of an inadequate face mask ventilation:

The first is inadequate seal between the face and the mask, which results in a leak of respiratory gas. The second is inadequate patency of the airway at the level of the nasopharynx, oropharynx, hypopharynx, larynx, or trachea. These conditions manifest as either inability to generate airway pressure that is adequate to drive gas into the lungs or failure to move gas into the lungs despite a sufficient driving pressure [3].

Langeron and colleagues described specific factors that may be related to DMV, including age older than 55 years, BMI > 26 kg/m^2, lack of teeth, history of snoring, and presence of a beard. In addition, Davide Cattano and colleagues listed seven risk criteria including age of 47 years or older, BMI of 35 kg/m^2 or greater, neck circumference of 40 cm or higher, history of difficult intubation, presence of facial hair, perceived short neck, and OSA. Mallampati class of 3 or 4 and previous neck radiation exposure again are important contributors to DMV [2].

42.2.1.3 Techniques of Mask Ventilation (MV)

Different methods can be used to ensure better MV, including head-tilt, jaw-thrust and chin-lift maneuvers, oral or nasal airways, choosing a different face mask and using a two-hand or two-person technique.

When two-persons are needed ideally, the primary intubator stands at the patient's head and initiates jaw thrust with the left hand at the angle of the left mandible and left-sided mask seal in contrast, the right hand compresses the reservoir bag. The secondary (helping) person stands at the patient's side, at the level of the patient's shoulder, facing the primary intubator. The right hand of the secondary intubator should cover the left hand of the primary intubator and contribute to left-sided jaw thrust and mask seal, and the left hand of the second person initiates right-sided jaw thrust and mask seal. In this way, all four hands are doing something important without interfering with one another, and there is almost no redundant effort. With this positioning, the secondary person can watch the monitors continuously, manipulate the larynx externally, and hand equipment to the primary intubator [3].

42.3 Difficult Supraglottic Airway Device (SAD) Insertion

Supraglottic airway device (SAD) or extraglottic airway device, is a medical device that maintains upper airway patency during anesthesia or unconscious situation. It also allows for limited intermittent positive-pressure ventilation (IPPV), offers some degree of protection against the aspiration of gastric contents, and can be used easily especially because it can be inserted atraumatically by a low-skilled practitioner [4].

Laryngeal mask (LMA) is an excellent example of the widely use of SADs. LMA was invented by Dr. Archibald ("Archie") Brain, a British anesthesiologist in the early 1980s and first came to market in the United Kingdom between 1987–1988, and currently, it is an integral part of difficult airway society guidelines and algorithms [5].

There are different types and shapes of LMAs; however, almost all of them are categorized as either first and second generation LMAs, and recently invented the third generation LMAs.

A significant difference exits between these generations.

42.3.1 SAD/LMA Generations [6] (Figs. 42.1 and 42.2)

- *First Generation SGA*: Simple breathing tube, usually with some form of mask or opening at the larynx. Examples: Classic LMA, LMA-Unique, SureSeal LM, Cobra PLA, Laryngeal Tube Airway.
- *Second Generation SGA*: In general, it has provision for gastric drainage, better sealing through a posterior inflatable cuff that improved protection against aspiration, in addition to integral bite block. Examples: Combi-tube, Pro-seal LMA, LMA-Supreme, I-Gel, LTS-D, Air-Q, Aura-Gain, Protector, LMA Gastro.
- *Third Generation SGA*: Has dynamic sealing mechanism plus double suction ports, in addition to the characteristic of the second Generation. Examples: Baska, Elisha, and 3G LM.

With all the development and growth in the field of supraglottic airway devices, still, we are facing difficulties when dealing with them; including failure of insertion, improper positioning inside the mouth, displacement after insertion, loss of air-

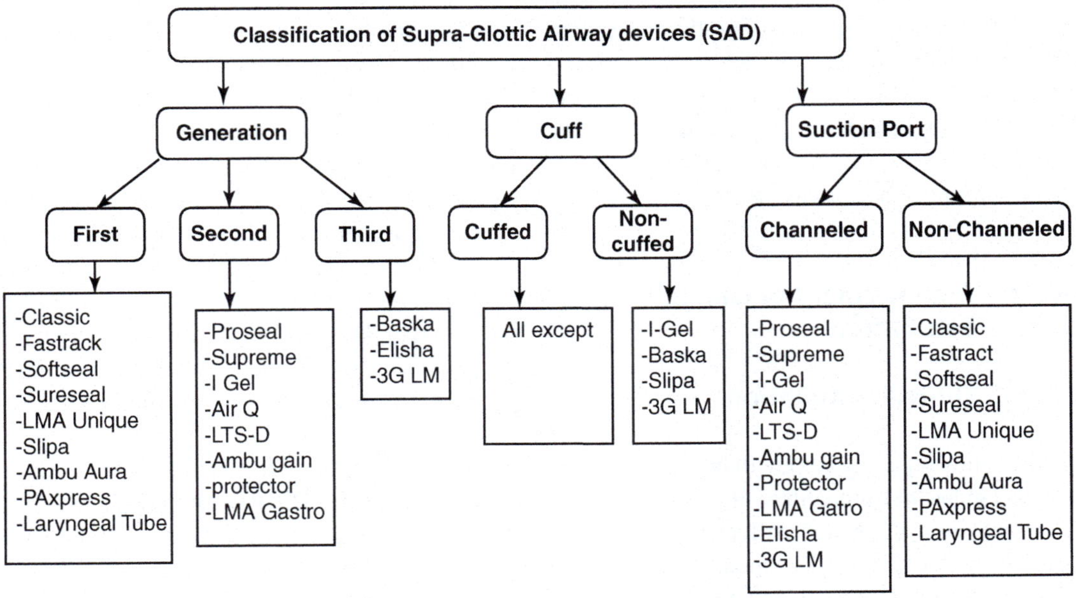

Fig. 42.1 Classification of supraglottic airway devices (SAD). (Image courtesy Dr. Nabil Shallik)

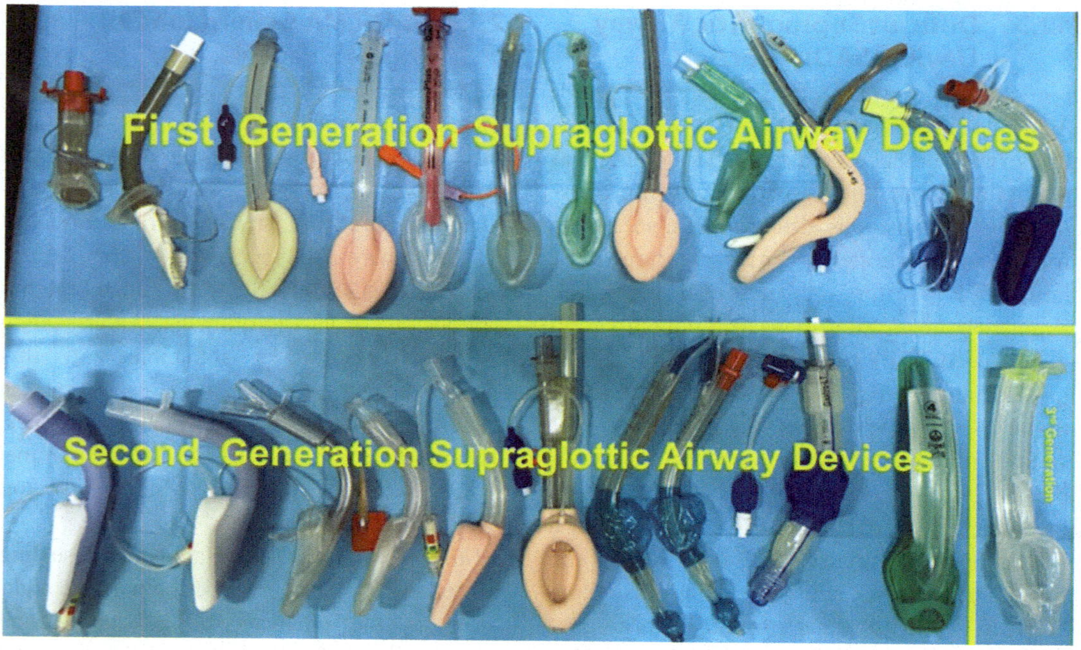

Fig. 42.2 The most common brands of Supraglottic Airway Device (SAD) in the market. (Image courtesy Dr. Nabil Shallik)

way during maintenance, failure to form an effective seal in the airway and risk of aspiration, airway trauma, and extubation-related problems [4, 5]. In most cases, multiple factors such as obesity with a BMI over 30, traumatic insertion, inappropriate use of the devices, low operator experience, non-standard patient positioning, or shallow anesthesia contributed significantly to these complications [6]. Other factors that may contribute to the failure of SADs to function correctly are male patients, aged 45 or older, having short thyromental distance, or limited neck movement [7].

42.4 Management of Difficult Intubation

42.4.1 Difficult Intubation

In the following section we will be discussing the management and guidelines of difficult intubation and extubation and different strategies to achieve a safe airway placement, as well as the common equipment needed to achieve it. Also, a discussion of some of the conditions associated with difficult intubation.

42.4.1.1 Management of Anticipated Difficult Airway

In 2013 the American Society of Anesthesiologists issued a practice guideline for the management of difficult airway focusing on essential preparation that includes [8]: (1) availability of equipment for the management of a difficult airway (i.e., airway trolley that contains specialized equipment), (2) informing the patient with a known or suspected difficult airway, (III) availability of assistance when a difficult airway is encountered, (IV) preoxygenation by face mask, and (V) oxygen supplementation throughout the process of airway management through a nasal cannula, facemask, LMA or insufflation, etc. [9]

42.4.1.2 Strategy for Intubation of the Difficult Airway

A clear and preplanned strategy is vital for the successful management of the difficult airway. The strategy should primarily include preparing the patient and optimizing head position, preparing appropriate equipment, medications and monitors; involvement of experienced assistants and availability of help by the senior provider is preferable. Following the difficult airway algorithm and formulating plans B and C in advance would help mitigate difficulties during the management of the airway [10].

Always remember that mask ventilation is considered a fundamental basic skill and life-saving technique for the patient who requires assisted ventilation during induction of anesthesia, post-extubation or during other critical conditions when the ventilatory support is required as in for example cardiac arrest.

Various interventions have been designed to facilitate intubation should a difficult airway occur, according to the situation, the experience of the provider and availability of equipment:

1. Awake intubation through flexible bronchoscope: studies showed a success rate might reach up to 88–100%, but it is expensive equipment that requires highly experienced providers.
2. Video-assisted laryngoscopy (VL): is promoted as a first choice in anticipated difficult airway where literature described that it improves laryngeal views, higher frequency of successful intubations, a higher chance for first-attempt intubation, with no differences in time to intubate, airway trauma, lip/gum trauma, dental trauma, or sore throat incidents.
3. Intubating stylets or tube exchangers: some observational studies showed successful intubation in 78–100% of the difficult airway using stylets, although associated with mild mucosal bleeding and sore throat. However, using tube-exchanger may end up with lung laceration and gastric perforation.
4. Supraglottic airway device (SAD) for ventilation (e.g., LMA, laryngeal tube): can be used as a temporary or permanent measure in patients who cannot be mask ventilated or intubated.
5. SAD for intubation (e.g., ILMA).
6. Rigid laryngoscopic blades: different designs and sizes should be available; they improve glottic visualization and help in intubation.
7. Fiber-optic-guided intubation.
8. Lighted stylets or light wands.

42.4.1.3 Common Equipment for Intubation

The tracheal intubation is the only definitive airway management type that, could be performed through the nose, the mouth or the trachea directly as in tracheostomy. The tracheal intubation could be done by the *Direct Laryngoscopy, Video-laryngoscopy, Flexible Bronchoscopy, and Rigid Bronchoscopy*.

1. *Direct Laryngoscopy (DL)*: is considered the most common intubating technique, and first choice in 50% of cases in current practice [11]. Using direct laryngoscopy blade, it allows for alignment of the oral, pharyngeal and laryngeal axis together by lifting the tongue and the jaw forward to expose the laryngeal inlet. It is a simple and easy technique using an age appropriate blade size but has been shown to have very high failure rate, especially in difficult cases with anatomical abnormalities that obscure the required alignment among the three axes. Given the high failure rate in difficult situation, the recommendation is once difficult airway is suspected, DL should not be the first choice, trials by DL should be limited to two, with immediate availability of more advanced techniques [12].
2. *Video-laryngoscopy (VL)*: is an indirect way for laryngeal visualization and intubation, by which the images are displayed, magnified, and recorded on a monitor. Different devices have shown variable performance in the airway management as shown in Table 42.1. Video-assisted visualization currently is promoted as a first choice in anticipated difficult airway. Glidescope and C-Mac VL (angulated VL) for example have shown a similar success rate for intubation at first attempt comparable with flexible bronchoscopic intubation, significantly higher success than the direct laryngoscopy technique. (for more

Table 42.1 Classification of different video-laryngoscopes (VL) from different manufactures

Rigid blades		Guided channels		Video stylets	
Standard blade (MAC)	Angled blade	Channeled blade	Channeled airway	Rigid stylet	Rigid stylet + Flexing tip
– Storz C-Mac – Storz V-Mac – Venner APA	– GlideScope – Storz D-Blade – King Vision – McGrath™ MAC – Venner APA	– AirTraq – Pentax-AWS – Res-Q-Scope II – Venner APA	– Total track Video-Laryngeal Mask (VLM)	– Bonfils	– Rigid Intubating Fiber-optic-Laryngoscope (RIFL) – Storz VS Video Stylet

detalis, Plesae refer to chapter Anesthetic considerations for Pediatric ENT surgeries for Non-anesthesiologists title under 3.4.)

3. *Bronchoscopic Intubation*: It is the gold standard in adult airway management. Both flexible and rigid bronchoscopies are available. The main indication for flexible bronchoscopic intubation in anesthesia is to secure the placement of endotracheal tube when there is anticipated airway difficulty and confirmation of tube position after intubation if necessary. It can be used as well in the management of abnormal airway anatomy, obstructive upper airway lesion, and unstable cervical spine to limit the cervical mobility, and the evaluation of airway obstruction is another anesthetic indication as a preoperative assessment (preoperative nasoendoscopy in pre-assessment anesthesia clinic (Sect. 42.4.2.3) or directly prior to intubation for patients with known anatomical abnormalities in the upper airway. Fiber-optic Intubation can be done through a Supraglottic Airway Device (SAD) in difficult cases as well [13].

The choice of the route has its indications as well, as nasal route is used in a case of limited mouth opening or a strong gag reflex, or if the surgery needs nasal intubation. Also, intubation can be done during sleep or awake intubation in special situations [14].

42.4.2 Causes of Difficult Intubation

Many pathological diseases are associated with difficulties when it comes to managing the airway, paying a particular attention to such conditions would make airway management planning and execution a lot safer and smoother.

Table 42.2 Congenital disorders associated with difficult airway

Syndrome	Anatomical site involved
Down syndrome	Oropharynx, larynx, trachea, cervical spine
Beckwith-Weidmann syndrome	Oropharynx, maxilla, diaphragm
Pierre Robin syndrome	Mandible, maxilla, oropharynx
Klippel–Feil syndrome	Cervical spine
Cri-Du-Chat syndrome	Mandible, larynx
Treacher Collins syndrome	Mandible, oral opening, zygomatic bone

Conditions associated with difficult airway can be divided into congenital and acquired disorders. Acquired disorders include inflammatory disorders, traumatic conditions, infections, metabolic disorders, obesity and obesity-related disorders, burns, and tumors.

42.4.2.1 Congenital Disorders Associated with Difficult Airway (Table 42.2)

There are many congenital disorders that are related to difficulties with managing the airway, but we will focus on some of the common congenital disorders. Although most of those patients present during their childhood years, but we still see syndromic patients present to the operating theaters during the adulthood period.

Down's Syndrome (Trisomy 21)

Down syndrome is the most common congenital anomaly, with incidence up to 1 in 600 live births. Multisystem involvements in those patients such as congenital heart disease, obesity, hypothyroidism, hematologic malignancies might complicate the perioperative period.

Airway management difficulties arise due to multiple anatomical abnormalities, including short neck, relative macroglossia, smaller tracheal diameter, subglottic stenosis, and atlanto-axial instability [15].

During the management of the airway, neck movements should be kept to a minimum since those patients have increased incidence of atlantoaxial instability. In symptomatic patients or patients with abnormal radiological findings, full cervical spine precautions should be implemented during the management of the airway [16].

Beckwith-Wiedemann Syndrome

Patients with Beckwith-Weidmann syndrome present a set of challenges for the health care provider during the perioperative period, such as the risk of hypoglycemia, diaphragmatic hernia-related respiratory complication, and airway management-related difficulties.

Mask ventilation might prove to be challenging in those patients due to the macroglossia. Direct laryngoscopy is also challenging due to the macroglossia and maxillary hypoplasia.

Pierre Robin Syndrome

Pierre Robin syndrome is characterized by a triad of micrognathia, retraction of the tongue (glossoptosis), and a cleft palate. Patients with Pierre Robin sequence (PRS) usually present with respiratory and feeding difficulties that is severed enough to require surgical interventions such as distraction osteogenesis of the mandible, glossopexy, or even tracheostomies. In a case series of 74 patients with PRS more than 50 percent of the patients required airway intervention, whereas one-third required surgical intervention to manage the airway [17]. Direct laryngoscopy and endotracheal intubation are usually very difficult in patients with PRS, which warrant proper preparation, and availability of experienced staff. Elective fiberoptic intubation is the preferred method in such patients.

42.4.2.2 Acquired Disorders Associated with Difficult Airway Management

Many pathological processes can complicate managing the airway, keeping that in mind of all cases that were reported to the NAP4 project (a national audit of major complications of airway management in the United Kingdom) 40% were associated with head and neck pathologies [18].

Diabetes Mellitus

Long-standing diabetes mellitus might result in glycosylation of the tendons which in turn might result into limited mobility of the cervical spine and limited mobility of the temporomandibular joint both of which can contribute to increased difficulty when it comes to managing the airway in those patients [19].

In a retrospective analysis over a 10-year period in patients undergoing renal and pancreatic transplant, the frequency of difficult laryngoscopy was reported to be as high as 32%, warranting proper assessment of the joint mobility before attempting laryngoscopy in diabetic patients [19]. Prayer sign can be used to assess the movement of the joint by asking the patient to approximate the palms as close as possible similar to a prayer position, inability to do so indicate limited phalangeal extension, which can be used as an indicator for stiff neck joints.

Rheumatoid Arthritis

Rheumatoid arthritis is an autoimmune disease that is characterized by widespread arthritis of the joints. Rheumatoid arthritis can also involve the larynx and the joints of the airway (vocal cords nodules, edema, and erythema of the vocal cords, cricoarytenoid arthritis, arthritis of the temporomandibular joint, cricothyroid joint involvement, as well as the involvement of the atlantoaxial and cervical spine joints). Radiological studies reported that up to 50% of patients with long-standing severe rheumatoid arthritis might have laryngeal involvement. Signs and symptoms of dysphonia, dysphagia, sore throat, hoarseness of voice, pain on swallowing, or stridor might indicate airway involvement. Mask ventilation and laryngoscopy might prove to be challenging in those patients due to the upper airway obstruction and the difficulties to visualize the glottic opening due to the edema, stiffness of the larynx, and involvement of the temporomandibular joint. Upper airway obstruction and exacerbation of laryngeal symptoms have been reported after endotracheal intubation or the use of supraglottic devices [20].

Obesity

Airway management in obese patients present a unique set of challenges, and obese patients tend to desaturate quickly due to the reduction in functional residual capacity and the increase in closing capacities, warranting proper preoxygenation and positioning before the induction of anesthesia.

Moreover, during emergency airway management, obese patients were more likely to have difficult intubations when compared to lean patients. Furthermore, obesity was also associated with difficulties in mask ventilation [21]. Body mass index above 30 kg/m^2 was associated with difficult mask ventilation [13, 14]. Besides that, obese patients are more likely to develop other disorders that might complicate airway management like obstructive sleep apnea and diabetes.

BMI of 40 kg/m^2 does not appear to be an independent predictor of difficult intubation, but a BMI of 50 kg/m^2 or higher and measuring the neck circumference might be of a greater predictive value, neck circumference more than 42 centimeters might predict difficult airway [22].

Obstructive Sleep Apnea

Obstructive sleep apnea (OSA) is a sleep disorder that is characterized by repetitive closure of the airway during sleep, resulting in repeated episodes of apnea and hypopnea.

Patients with obstructive sleep apnea were associated with a higher incidence of difficult tracheal intubation [23]. In a prospective observational study on 22,000 patients investigating mask ventilation difficulties among patients with confirmed OSA, mask ventilation was more difficult in OSA patients compared to non-OSA patients. Impossible to ventilate was also higher in a patient with OSA [24].

History of snoring, daytime fatigue, inability to concentrate, and observed apnea are suggestive of OSA. Preoperatively the physician should inquire about polysomnography results, use of home oxygen, continuous positive airway pressure (CPAP), or the presence of cardiopulmonary complications related to OSA.

42.4.2.3 Masses of the Head and Neck

Masses affecting the airway passages should have a thorough examination and appropriate imaging studies. Preoperative Nasopharyngeal endoscopy might be warranted as well.

They can affect multiple sites along the airway, including the nose, nasopharynx, oropharynx, tongue, larynx, vocal cords, or trachea, and they can be external to the airway passages like thyroid, esophageal or mediastinal masses.

The examination must be dynamic, assessing the patients in sitting position as well as in supine position, inquiring about changes in voice, difficulty breathing, or stridor with position change are of paramount importance (Table 42.3).

Pulmonary function testing can be helpful in a patient with masses affecting the airway passages. It should also be dynamic since static studies might be normal [25].

Supraglottic masses might not be visible during the regular physical exam and might present after anesthesia induction in the form of difficult ventilation or difficult intubation.

Masses at the base of the tongue can interfere with direct laryngoscopy and oral intubation, nasal video-laryngoscopy and intubation would be a better strategy to manage the airway.

Table 42.3 Summarizes the characteristic clinical findings and their implications on airway management

Clinical finding	Underlying changes
Voice change	Laryngeal involvement
Difficulty swallowing	Intrinsic or extrinsic mass effect
Difficulty with deep inspiration	Airway narrowing due to internal or external mass effect
Noisy breathing changes with body position	Tracheomalacia

Tonsillar masses like lingual tonsillar hypertrophy might result in an anticipated difficult airway, in a case series by Ovassapian and his colleagues that investigated 33 patients with unanticipated failed intubation and unremarkable routine physical examination found that all the patients had lingual tonsillar hypertrophy on postoperative fiber-optic pharyngoscopy [26].

Subglottic stenosis might present with the inability to pass the endotracheal tube. It could be caused by an intratracheal lesion or extratracheal masses. Thyroid tumors or goiter might invade the tracheal lumen leading to airway obstruction. Using smaller endotracheal tubes would be an appropriate option. The use of rigid or flexible bronchoscopy to assist the intubation might be needed in some cases.

42.4.2.4 Deep Neck Infections

Ludwig angina is potentially a fatal infection of the floor of the mouth, as well as other infections of the airway passages, like epiglottitis, managing the airway must be in a controlled setting like in the operating theater. Awake fiber-optic intubation or even tracheostomy might be appropriate in such cases. Due to the excessive salivation and in many cases inability to swallow it, managing the airway in a sitting position might be proper in such scenarios [27].

42.4.2.5 Burns

Inhalational injury is a significant cause of morbidity and mortality in burn victims. The prevalence of inhalational injury in burn patients is around 15%, with an in-hospital mortality rate of about 3% [28].

Swelling of the airway passages usually occurs within 24 h after the thermal injury but can occur as early as 2 h; in severe, erosion ulcers, and granulation formation might occur. Carbonaceous material around the mouth, pharynx, or nares should raise suspicion of inhalational injury. Other symptoms include stridor, hoarseness of voice, difficulty breathing, and respiratory distress. Difficult airway management and airway compromise are not uncommon. Prophylactic elective intubation is often needed.

Patient with history of inhalational injury might develop chronic airway problems, including stiff facial and neck scar tissues formation, limiting mouth opening and neck mobility which might lead to difficult airway management in the future.

42.4.3 Extubating Difficult Airway

If intubation is a skill, then tracheal extubation is the art of this skill. Most morbidity and mortality incidents that were described in general anesthesia happened at the time of extubation. In general, the majority of extubations are expected to be uneventful, but even these routine extubations may be associated with complications as described in Table 42.4.

Problems with extubation can be split into two categories:

1. Failure to extubate; when an attempt to remove a tracheal tube is unsuccessful.
2. Failure to reintubate; when extubation is followed by an immediate or delayed but unsuccessful attempt to reintubate the trachea.

Many factors are required for proper extubation that is subjective and objective such as improving or resolving the underlying disease, hemodynamic stability, regular breathing, normal respiratory and blood gases parameters, etc. However, extubating a difficult airway is always challenging. The accurate decision, proper timing, proper technique is always required [29].

Table 42.4 Complications of routine extubations

Accidental extubation
Fixation of the endotracheal tube
Increase of BP, increase heart rate
Coughing and/or breath-holding
Laryngeal trauma
Laryngospasm or vocal cord paralysis
Stridor, airway obstruction
Negative-pressure pulmonary edema
Laryngeal incompetence
Aspiration

Proper planning involves identification of high-risk patients who may develop a difficult airway, such as those with obesity, obstructive sleep apnea, major head/neck, and upper airway surgery, and obstetric and cervical spine.

Preemptive optimization of patients' conditions, careful timing of extubation, the presence of experienced personnel trained in advanced airway management, and the availability of the necessary equipment and appropriate post-extubation monitoring is an effective strategy to minimize post-extubation airway complications [30].

42.4.3.1 The Difficult Airway Society (DAS) Issued Guidelines for Management of Tracheal Extubation

The DAS guidelines describe a basic extubation algorithm consisting of four steps [31]:

1. Plan extubation.
2. Prepare for extubation (risk stratify to at-risk or low risk).
3. Perform extubation.
4. Post-extubation care and follow-up.

Step 1: consists of assessing airway risk factors (e.g., known difficult airway, obesity, obstructive sleep apnea, aspiration risk) and general risk factors (e.g., hemodynamic and neurological stability).

Step 2: includes optimizing patient factors (e.g., cardiovascular, respiratory, metabolic) and environmental factors (e.g., location, availability of skilled help, specialized equipment). Once optimized, patient risk stratification is categorized into "low-risk" and "at-risk" extubation groups.

Step 3: includes the act of extubation.

Awake extubation is preferable most of the time, although deep extubation can be considered in cases of low-risk patients.

When awake extubation is planned, remember to follow the appropriate steps that include; preoxygenation with 100% oxygen, proper positioning, suctioning if needed, insertion of a bite block (e.g., oral airway, rolled gauze), a reversal for a muscle relaxant, establishing regular breathing with good tidal volume, and monitoring patient until awake (eye-opening, obeying command).

For at-risk group, where the ability to oxygenate is uncertain or there exists a general and airway risk factor, it is recommended to perform awake extubation, keep intubated or tracheostomy insertion with help from ENT doctors.

Finally, in *step 4*: we do post-extubation care (e.g., proper monitoring, provision of oxygen, and safe transfer).

42.5 Prediction of Difficult Airway

42.5.1 Traditional Airway Assessment

Assessment of airway and prediction of difficulties is a crucial step in managing the airway to ensure adequate oxygenation and ventilation and avoiding respiratory complications that may end up with life-threatening situation.

The fourth National Audit Project (NAP4) found that failure to assess for and identify the potential difficulty, or the application of poor judgment in management planning, may contribute to a poor outcome [18].

A perfect airway assessment tool does not exist, and unanticipated difficulty will still occur; however, taking a comprehensive history, a proper physical examination, doing relative investigations, and using multiple tests to predict difficulty in airway management is a better predictor than any single test used in isolation.

42.5.1.1 Clinical History

Reviewing medical records and previous anesthesia notes would be of great help if available. Assessing medical, surgical, and anesthesia-related history is vital in the anticipated difficult airway.

42.5.1.2 Physical Examination

Clinical examination of the airway is critical; its purpose is to assess for difficult mask ventilation, laryngoscopic access, and ease of subsequent maneuvers. Any gross abnormality of the face, nose, mouth, and neck should be immediately apparent.

Patency of nares, polyps, or mass inside the nasal cavity, nasal septum deviation should be ruled out.

The adequate mouth opening of at least 2–3 large fingerbreadths between upper and lower incisors in adults is desirable, with distance varies from 4–6 cm and gives an indication of temporomandibular joint (TMJ) mobility, also assess TMJ for movement restriction as in ankylosis/fibrosis, tumors, etc. Examination of the ability to protrude the lower jaw beyond the upper incisors.

Teeth examination for prominent upper incisors, or overbite, can impose a limitation on the alignment of oral or pharyngeal axes during laryngoscopy, and especially in association with a large base of the tongue, they can compound the difficulty during the direct laryngoscopy or bag-mask ventilation.

Examination of the neck if it is short, wide, any deformity, or limitation in mobility (atlanto-occipital extension) [32].

Some mnemonics are helpful for remembering patient factors that are associated with a difficult airway, such as MMMMASK (Table 42.5): and OBESE for difficult mask ventilation (Table 42.6) or LEMON (Table 42.7).

Table 42.5 MMMMASK mnemonics difficult airway

MMMMASK	Description
M	Male gender
M	Mask seal which is affected by bread or being edentulous
M	Mallampati grade 3 or 4
M	Mandibular
A	Age
S	Snoring and OSA
K	Kilograms (weight)

Table 42.6 OBESE mnemonics for difficult mask ventilation

OBESE	Description
O	Obese (BMI >26 kg/m^2)
B	Bearded
E	Edentulous
S	Snoring
E	Elderly (>55 years)

Table 42.7 LEMON mnemonics for airway assessment

LEMON	Criterion	Score
L	Look externally:	(1–4)
	– Facial trauma	1
	– Large incisors	1
	– Beard or mustache	1
	– Large tongue	1
E	Evaluate:	(1–3)
	– Incisor distance	1
	– Hyoid-mental distance	1
	– thyroid-to-mouth distance	1
M	Mallampati	1
O	Obstruction	1
N	Neck mobility	1

42.5.1.3 Specific Tests and Scores for Airway Assessment

Anatomical Criteria

Mouth Opening and Inter-Incisor Gap (IIG)

The mouth opening is central to airway management and intubation. The reduced mouth opening is associated with difficult laryngoscopy, intubation, and LMA insertion. The difficulty lies in determining whether this is mechanical or functional as the latter may improve with general anesthesia and muscle relaxation.

One helpful way to quantify mouth opening is to ask the patient whether he/she can place three fingers between their upper and lower teeth. Whereas three fingerbreadths test is ideal, anything less than two (around 3 cm) predicts an increased risk of airway difficulties.

An inter-incisor distance of less than 5 cm or two to three fingerbreadths may make conventional laryngoscopy difficult.

The mouth opening of 1.5 cm or less than one fingerbreadth may impair the insertion of a supraglottic airway device or laryngoscope and an inter-incisor distance of 2 cm is needed to insert the intubating LMA (ILMA). At least 2.5 cm is required to insert an LMA. An IIG of 5 cm for intubation and 4 cm for the insertion of an LMA is a simple test with a relatively high predictive value [32, 33].

Mallampati Score

Described in Mallampati's original paper 1985, this is assessed by asking the patient (in a sitting or upright position) to open his/her mouth and protrude the tongue maximally. Visibility of faucial pillars, soft palate, and uvula inside the patient's mouth will result in a score of one to three. A Mallampati score of four was later added.

Original Mallampati Scoring

- Class 1: Faucial pillars, soft palate, and uvula could be visualized.
- Class 2: Faucial pillars and soft palate could be visualized, but uvula was masked by the base of the tongue.
- Class 3: Only soft palate visualized.

Modified Mallampati Scoring as in (Fig. 42.3)

- Class I: Soft palate, uvula, fauces, pillars visible.
- Class II: Soft palate, a major part of uvula, fauces visible.
- Class III: Soft palate, a base of uvula visible.
- Class IV: Only hard palate visible.

Upper Lip Bite Test (ULBT)/Mandible Protrusion Test

Described into three classes: (Fig. 42.4)

- Class I: Lower incisors biting the upper lip, making the mucosa of the upper lip totally invisible.
- Class II: The same biting maneuver revealing a partially visible mucosa.
- Class III: The lower incisors fail to bite the upper lip.
- (ULBT Class II and III considered as difficult intubation) [34].

Mandibular Space (Fig. 42.5)

As mentioned above, we can do some measurements to assess the airway [32]:

1. *Thyromental (TM) distance (Patil's test)*: It is defined as the distance from the mentum to the thyroid notch while the patient's neck is fully extended. This measurement helps in determining how readily the laryngeal axis will fall in line with the pharyngeal axis when the atlantooccipital joint is extended. Alignment of

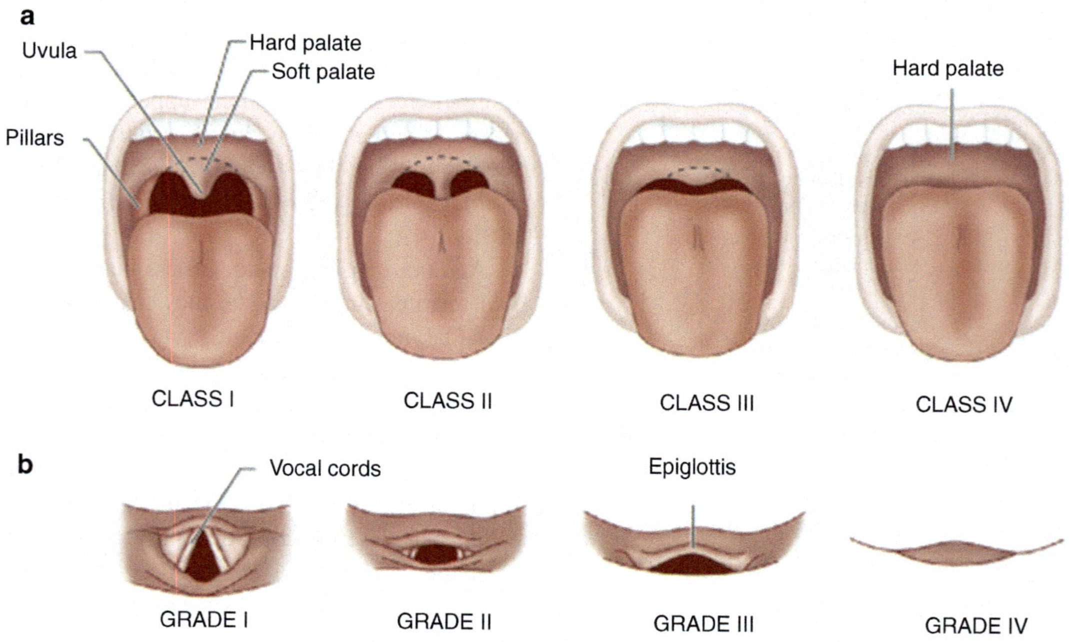

Fig. 42.3 Modified Mallampati Scoring (**a**) and Cormack and Lehane (CL) grades (**b**)

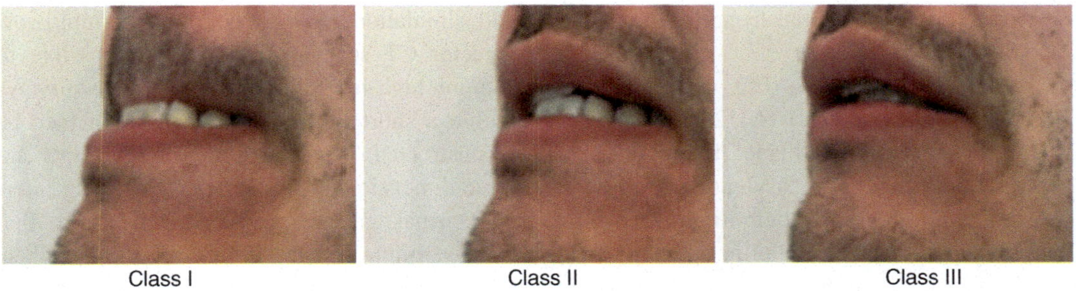

Fig. 42.4 Shows upper lip bite test (ULBT)/Mandible protrusion test

Fig. 42.5 Rule of 3-3-2 fingers

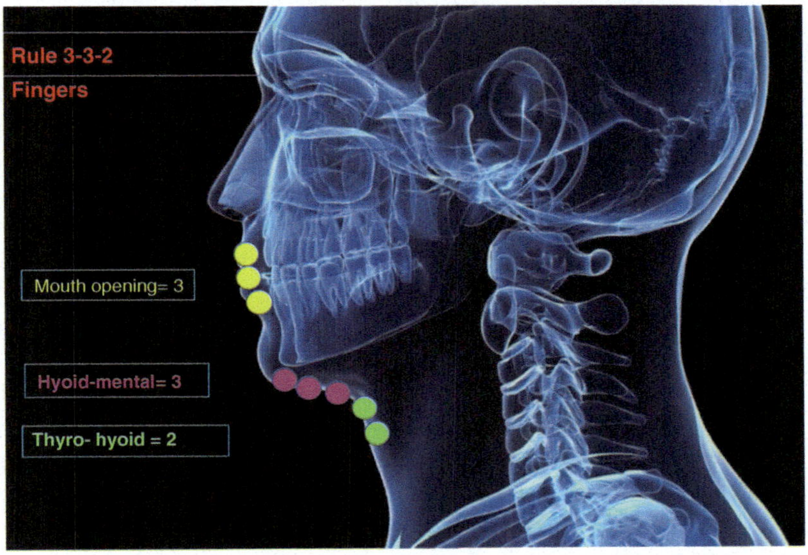

these two axes is difficult if the T-M distance is <3 fingerbreadths or <6 cm in adults; 6–6.5 cm is less difficult, while >6.5 cm is normal.

2. *Sterno-mental distance*: It was measured with the head fully extended on the neck with the mouth closed. A value of less than 12 cm is found to predict difficult intubation.
3. *Mandibulo-hyoid distance*: Measurement of mandibular length from chin (mental) to hyoid should be at least 4 cm or three fingerbreadths. It was found that laryngoscopy became more difficult as the vertical distance between the mandible and hyoid bone decreased.

The LEMON Score for Airway Assessment

Table 42.7

This score has a maximum of 10 points calculated by assigning 1 point for each of the following LEMON criteria:

L: Look externally for (facial trauma, large incisors, beard or mustache, large tongue).

E: Evaluate the 3–3-2 rule (incisor distance < 3 fingerbreadths, distance < 3 fingerbreadths, thyroid-to-mouth distance < 2 fingerbreadths) (Fig. 42.5).

M: Mallampati (Mallampati score ≥ 3).

O: Obstruction (presence of any condition like epiglottitis, peritonsillar abscess, trauma).

N: Neck mobility (limited neck mobility).

Patients in the difficult intubation group have higher LEMON scores.

Direct Laryngoscopy View and Fiber-Optic Bronchoscopy

In 1984, Cormack and Lehane described classification according to the views obtained by direct laryngoscopy based on the structures seen, as a way of simulating potential scenarios that trainee anesthetists might face.

As you can see in the (Fig. 42.3), Cormack and Lehane (CL) grades 1 (A), 2 (B), 3 (C), and 4 (D). (a) Laryngoscope blade; (b) epiglottis; (c) glottic opening; (d) arytenoid cartilages. According to the original definition by Cormack and Lehane, most of the glottic opening can be seen with grade 1. In grade 2, only the posterior portion of the glottis or only arytenoid cartilages are visible. In grade 3, only the epiglottis but no portion of the glottis is visible, whereas, in grade 4, neither the glottis nor the epiglottis can be seen [35].

Later on, a modified version that subdivided Grade 2 was described in 1998, dividing it into grade 2A and 2B, where is in 2A partial view of the glottis, and 2B only arytenoids can be seen [36].

42.5.1.4 Investigations

Routine imaging studies are not indicated for the assessment of the airway, nonetheless, diagnostic imaging studies provide valuable information when dealing with head and neck pathologies.

Even though plain X-ray has low predictive value for the prediction of a difficult airway, lateral flexion-extension neck. X-ray might be of help in patients with suspected atlantoaxial instability.

More specific tests like magnetic resonance images (MRI) and computed tomography (CT) scan can be of value in particular situations. Tumors with a mass effect that might compromise the airway passages invade the airway lumen or displace the larynx would be detected using MRI or CT scan.

Thyroid goiter or thyroid tumors with posterior extension can be evaluated with MRI scans. They can also be helpful in detecting cases with suspected tracheomalacia as well.

42.5.1.5 Nontraditional Airway Assessment

Virtual Endoscopy (VE)

Over the past few years, astonishing progress has been made in the field of noninvasive imaging and simulation. The introduction of multi-row detector CT scanners has made it possible to acquire high-resolution images of the airways within a short time. Those images can then be reconstructed into two-dimensional (2D) and three-dimensional (3D) images, including internal virtual endoscopic (VE) renderings that closely mimic images from conventional fiberoptic endoscopy. Using specialized VE software that process surface and volume-rendering data, the CT images can be reformatted into a 3D model that would make performing a virtual endoscopy possible.

Virtual endoscopy has many advantages over conventional endoscopy. Since the images are of equivalent quality to the live procedure, unnecessary patient's discomfort is avoided, the use of local anesthetics will not be needed avoiding the hazards associated with their use, procedure-related side effects like vomiting, coughing, sneezing, potential aspirations or laryngeal edema and spasm would be avoided as well. Other potential hazards of conventional endoscopy that can be omitted as well include bleeding, pneumothorax, hypoxemia, and aspiration.

Moreover, the use of virtual endoscopy (VE) can help in visualizing structures that cannot be duplicated by any other means, an example, visualization of the posterior nares, the Eustachian tube orifices, and the subglottic regions. Also, it can visualize areas that conventional endoscopy cannot reach, providing physicians with data that would ultimately alter airway management decisions.

However, physicians must take into advisement that virtual endoscopy (VE) has some limitations; airway diameter readings might not be accurate since it changes during the respiratory cycle. Furthermore, visualizing superficial lesions is less sensitive. Also, the presence of retained mucus or blood can falsely be interpreted as tracheobronchial stenosis or a foreign body [37].

3D Reconstruction and Decision-Making

3D reconstruction of cross-sectional images provides physicians with images that are far easier to comprehend, making the understanding of the extent of the pathological processes simpler that would ultimately result in better clinical outcome and better decision-making. Therefore, it is crucial that physicians from different specialties familiarize themselves with the use of such techniques.

Being familiar with the 3D reconstructed image anatomy would help reading the images faster and more precisely. This includes the evaluation of the airway proper using tissue transparent projection (TTP) and volume-rendering techniques (VRT) protocols.

The Benefits of VE and 3D Reconstructions in Airway Management

VE and 3D reconstructions are one-stop shop in the management of the difficult airway; After performing the MDCT examination as well as the post-processing methods, the following pearls would be addressed and thoroughly commented upon [38]:

1. Human airway canal (diameter, narrow segments including its sites, level, and quantitative assessment in mm regarding its caliber and length for those following the application of modified Valsalva maneuver).
2. Posterior choana/nares (in children assess choanal atresia) whether it is primarily bony or membranous.
3. Nasal septum, deviation, swellings, Concha Bullosa, or mucosal thickening, antro-choanal polyp, or inverted papilloma or other nasal pathologies, antro-choanal polyp, or inverted papilloma or other nasal pathologies.
4. Dental assessment (panoramic-like view) using curved multi-planar reconstruction to show orthopantomogram (OPG) missed teeth, loosening, or loss of the normal lamina dura. Denture artificial teeth or loose implant/prosthesis also can be seen.
5. Dislocation of Temporomandibular Joint (TMJ), dislocation, disorder, ankyloses, osteoarthrosis, osteomyelitis, or fractures).
6. Assessment of cervical spine in case of trauma to the cervical region.
7. Abnormal variants of blood vessels and tumor blood supply in the head and neck region.
8. Thyroid enlargement and retrosternal extension and its effect on the trachea, whether it is displaced or compressed from outside or invasion by the tumor.
9. Abnormal calcification of the styloid process (Eagle syndrome).
10. The diameter of the tracheal and deviation down to the carina and assessment for tracheomalacia or invasion of the tracheal tree if any.
11. Laryngeal skeleton and abnormal position of vocal cords.
12. Masses (soft tissue or hard tissues that may be displacing/invading the airway).
13. Correlation with Mallampati score and suggestion of the oral versus nasal route for intubation.

Below, you can find an example of 3 cases that clearly demonstrate the use of 3-D reconstruction and VE of upper airway and how these techniques solved the mystery of the diagnosis:

Case 1: Circular hyoid bone.

CT scan with 3D reconstruction demonstrated a thick hyoid bone with abnormal circular configuration extending posteriorly forming an incomplete ring that caused narrowing of the airway lumen at the supraglottic level. Moreover, the thyroid cartilages' superior Cornu also, encroach on the airway column. Virtual reality of the airway from frontal and lateral projections showed stenosis of the airway at the supraglottic region [39] (Fig. 42.6).

Case 2: Preoperative clinical and nasendoscopic assessment in a patient with trauma to upper airway revealed a web formation at the level of the glottis extending from the anterior commissure to the posterior one-third of the glottis. Virtual endoscopic (VE) evaluation showed the web to be at a supraglottic region, while the glottic region was clear. The finding changed the airway management decision from performing an advanced airway technique toward simple topicalization of the airway [40] (Fig. 42.7).

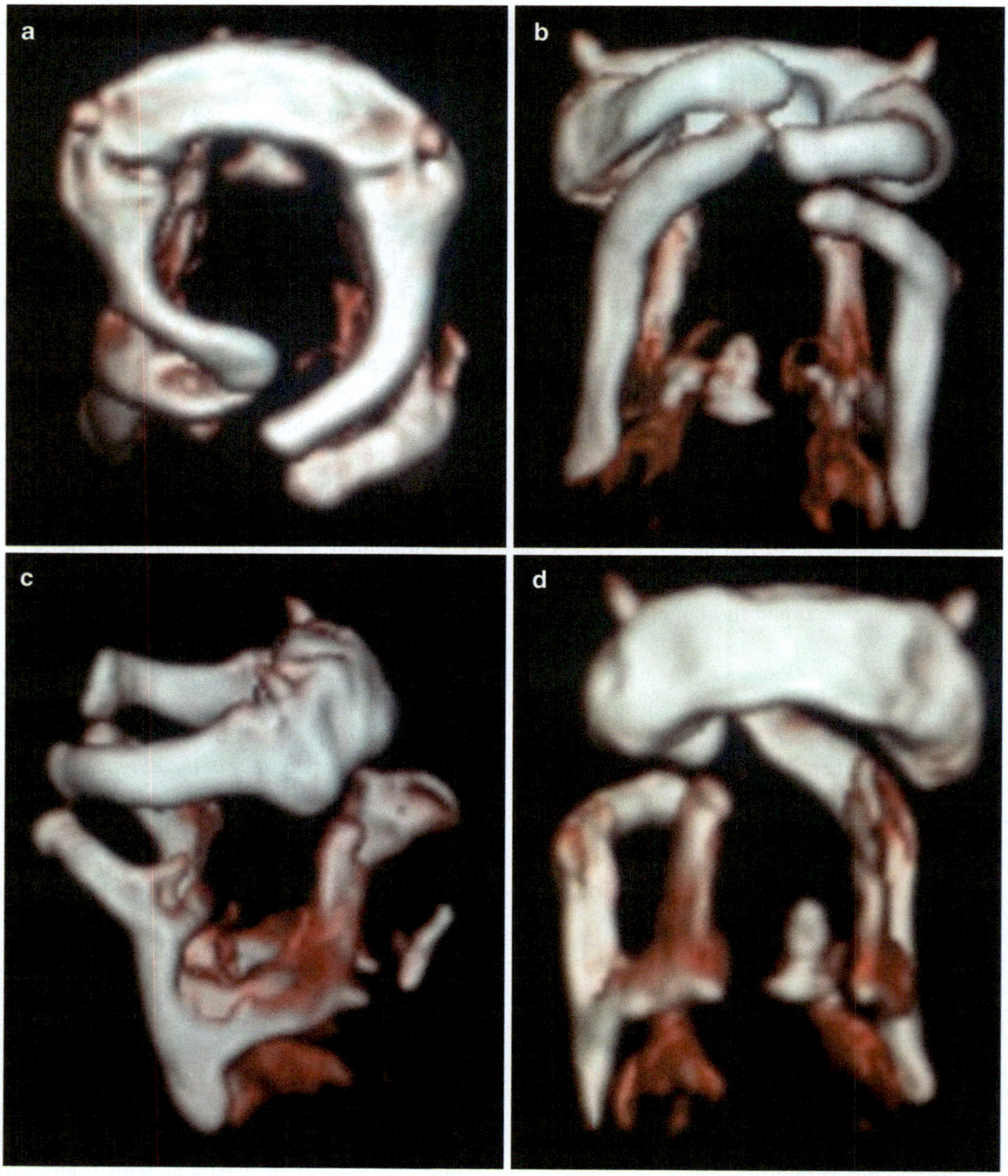

Fig. 42.6 Shows Volume Rendering Technique (VRT) 3-D reconstruction images from different perspectives for the laryngeal cartilaginous framework: (**a**) Craniocaudal projection, (**b**) Right lateral, (**c**) Posterior, (**d**) Anterior projection Showing incomplete ring formation of the hyoid bone forming incomplete ring/circle with overriding of the posterior ends. Similar findings are also noted within the superior Cornu of the thyroid cartilages. (Image courtesy Dr. Nabil Shallik and Dr. Abbas Moustafa).

Case 3: Presented with a hard tissue mass arising from the lateral aspect of airway. Nasendoscopic examination showed a normal vocal cord movement. The nature of the mass couldn't be revealed with either endoscopy or CT scan. The CT 3D reconstruction revealed abnormally configured hyoid bone, leading to mild oropharyngeal airway narrowing. The scan

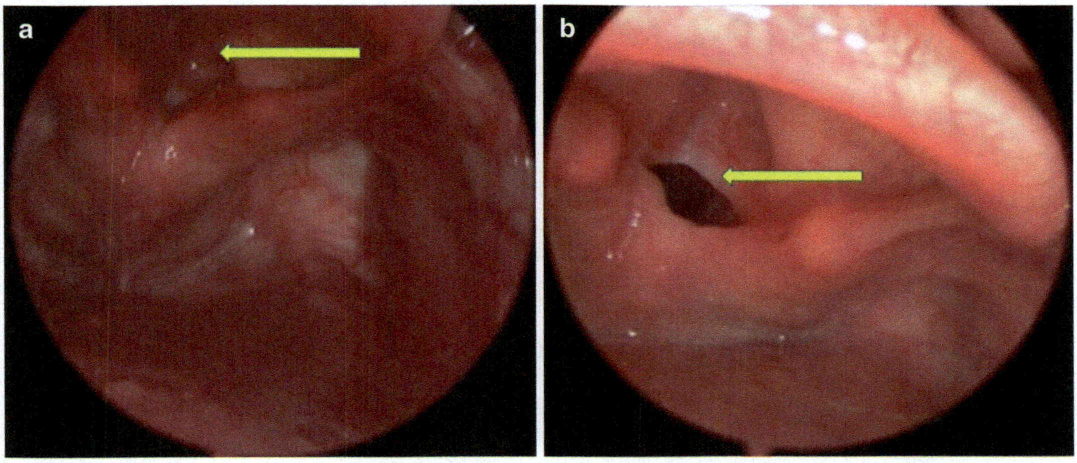

Fig. 42.7 Flexible fibrotic view showing the stenotic glottic opening (Image courtesy Dr. Nabil Shallik)

revealed that the mass is part the hyoid bone, pushed away to one side by the thyroid mass leading to bizarre looking airway. With the use of VE, the diameter of the airway was determined. Surgical, as well as anesthesia plans, were formulated accordingly [41] (Fig. 42.8).

Preoperative Endoscopic Airway Examination (PEAE)

The routine bedside examination of the airway is poorly predictive for difficult tracheal intubation, in part due to the limitation in detecting the presence of pathologies of the upper airway during the inspection. The preoperative use of fiberoptic endoscopic airway examination (PAEA) by ENT surgeons or trained anesthetists in Difficult Airway Clinic (DAC) provides valuable information when assessing patients with supraglottic, the base of the, or vocal cord masses. As well as helps with evaluating the dynamic movement of the vocal cords; hence the examination is usually done as a bedside test under local anesthesia. It is the most reliable method that assess the entirety of the upper airway under dynamic conditions before induction of general anesthesia and is one of the recommendations of NAP4 (Fig. 42.9).

1. Nasopharyngeal endoscopic airway assessment helps the anesthesiologists with formulating a plan to manage patients with a potential difficult airway. A prospective study that investigated whether preoperative endoscopic airway examination (PEAE) would affect airway management decision-making found that the use of PEAE would reduce the use of unnecessary awake intubation by 26% [42].
2. Tracheoscopy also be done also after spraying the vocal cord and tracheal of the patient with local anesthesia by unique technique and need an expert operator to do it without complication. (Fig. 42.10).

42.6 Future Plane in Airway Management

42.6.1 Airway Ventilation Through "Straw"

42.6.1.1 Evone and Tritube in Stenotic Airway

Flow control ventilation (FCV) is a recently developed ventilation strategy which allows keeping the intrapulmonary pressures low while achieving optimal gas exchange [43]. It has been proven in animal models to improve pulmonary function and oxygenation [44] and in cases with acute respiratory distress syndrome (ARDS) [45].

Ventilation through a small endotracheal tube is not uncommon in airway management. It can be used in elective upper airway surgery as well

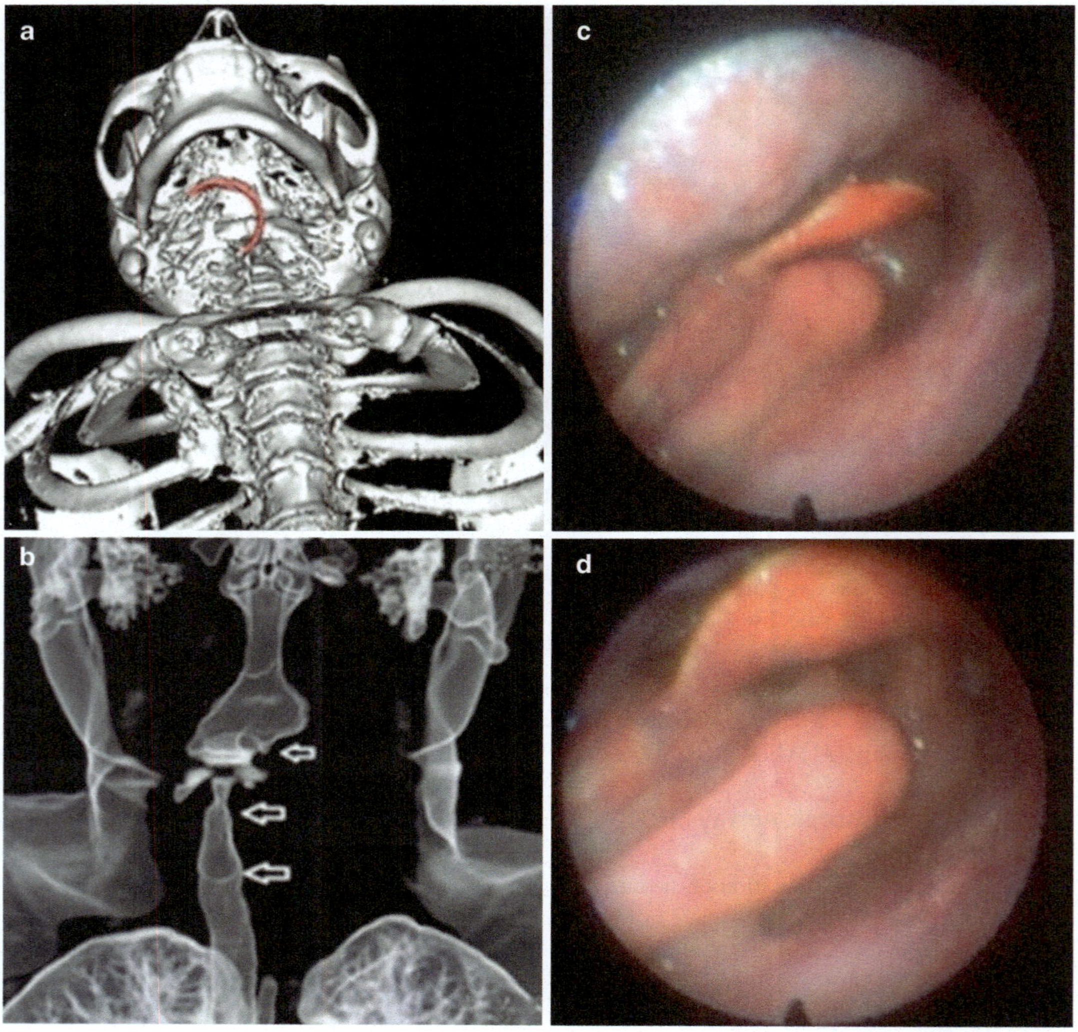

Fig. 42.8 Shows (**a**) 3-D reconstruction images for the laryngeal skeleton and bony framework, (**b**) shaded surface display (SSD) 3-D reconstruction of the airway. Showing axial rotation and right lateral displacement of the hyoid bone as well as the infrahyoid, laryngeal and proximal tracheal airway which is indented and encroached upon with significant reduction of its lumen caliber and appreciable narrowing. but (**c**) and (**d**) show the endoscopic view of nasendoscopic examination of upper airway (Image courtesy Dr. Nabil Shallik and Dr. Abbas Moustafa)

as emergency ventilation through needle cricothyrotomy. The traditional use of jet ventilation by small endotracheal tubes is challenging because of the increased risk of barotrauma and inadequate gas exchange [43]. Keeping in mind that expiration during jet ventilation is a passive process.

Flow Controlled Ventilation (FCV) mode is a unique ventilation technique in which inspiration as well as expiration are controlled processes. This is achieved by generating a continuous flow into the patient's lungs during inspiration and a constant (negative) flow, sucking gasses out of the patient's lungs during expiration. The FCV mode does not allow for ventilation pauses, and this results in linear increases and decreases in intratracheal pressures (Fig. 42.11b). Therefore, the mean airway pressure will be higher compared to conventional large bore Volume Controlled Ventilation

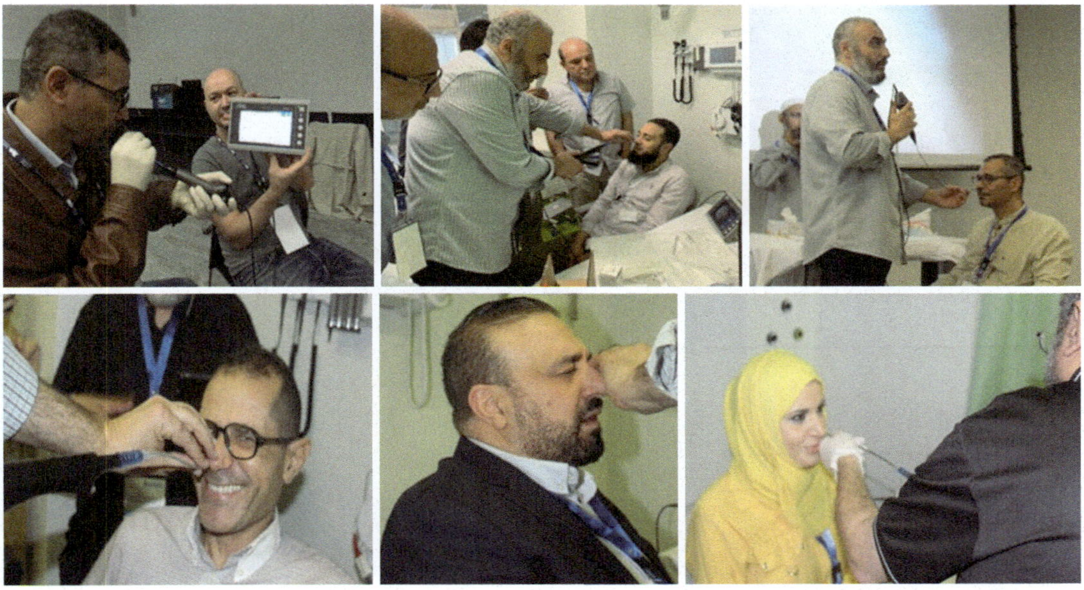

Fig. 42.9 Preoperative Endoscopic Airway Examination (PEAE) of the upper airway. (Image courtesy Dr. Nabil Shallik)

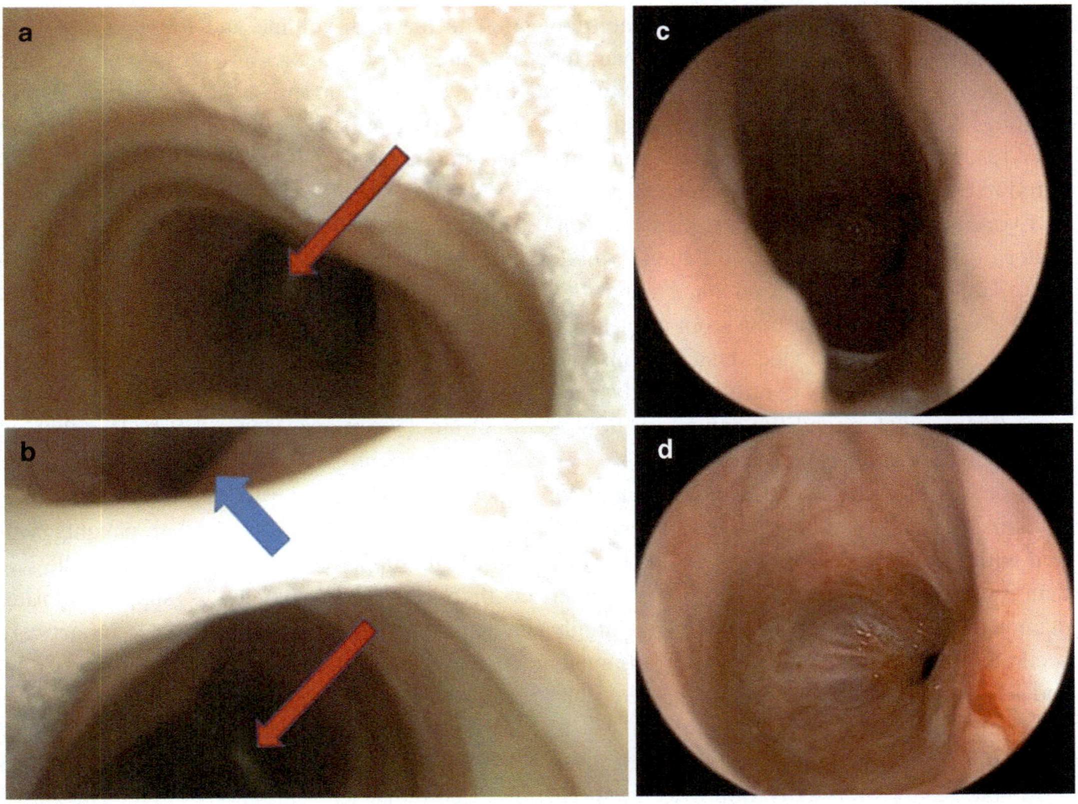

Fig. 42.10 Tracheoesophageal fistula (**a**) and (**b**) red arrow shows carina and blue arrow shows esophagus and (**c**). (**d**) Tracheal stenosis nicely demonstrated by tracheoscopy under local anesthesia. (Image courtesy Dr. Nabil Shallik)

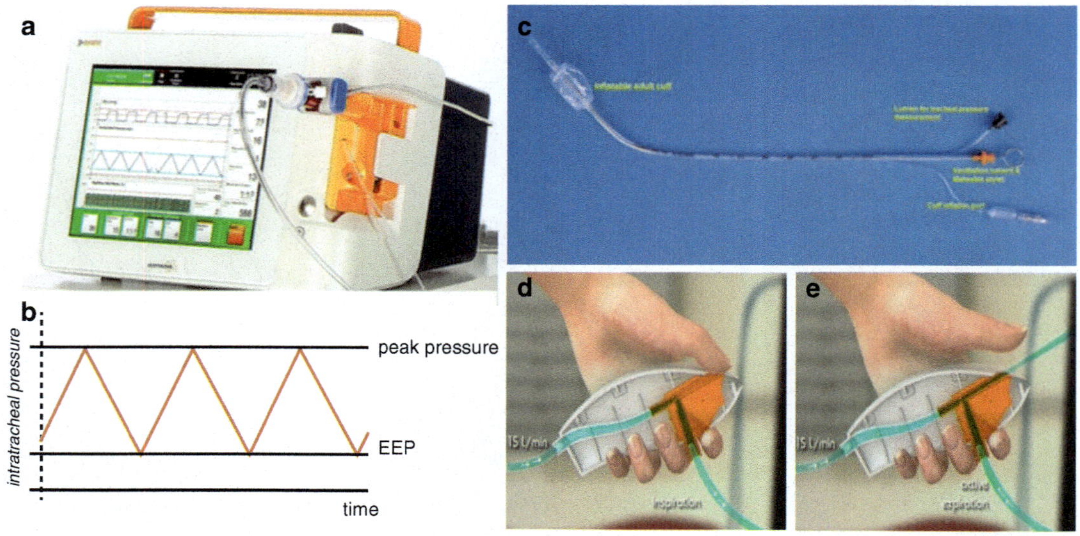

Fig. 42.11 (**a**) Evone ventilator, (**b**) intratracheal pressure waves, (**c**) small diameter tritube and (**d**), (**e**) ventrain during inspiration and expiration

(VCV) or Pressure Controlled Ventilation (PCV). The bronchiole and alveoli will be more opened (stretched) during ventilation facilitating oxygen uptake in the blood. Moreover, the continuous gas flow enhances the gas mixture in the lungs while also improving the gas exchange. FCV results in higher efficient ventilation compared to conventional ventilation techniques.

Evone is the only commercially available ventilator applying FCV ventilation mode (Fig. 42.11a), which is based on a controlled inspiration and expiration flow from a set PEEP to set peak pressure and vice versa. The inspiratory flow is continuously controlled by advanced mass flow regulators and the expiratory flow is controlled by regulated suctioning.

Evone or Ventrain (Ventinova Medical B.V., Eindhoven, The Netherlands) is used in combination with Tritube which has a small caliber (less than 3 mm inner diameter ID and 4.4 mm outer diameter OD) (Fig. 42.11c), enabling highly accurate intratracheal pressure measurements and securing the airway with an inflatable cuff as FCV ventilation requires a sealed airway.

With this small outer diameter (OD), it gives more space in the oral cavity, improves the surgical field, and decreases post-extubation throat pain due to tracheal tube size.

Tritube has three lumens: a ventilation lumen with Murphy's eye; a cuff lumen to inflate and deflate the high-volume and low-pressure cuff; and an intratracheal pressure measurement lumen for continuous intratracheal pressure measurements. Additionally, it has a malleable stylet to facilitate intubation [46, 47].

With this small diameter tube, it carries a risk of aspiration, however, the presence of inflatable cuff decreases this risk without increasing chance for air trapping-induced barotrauma, as in traditional jet ventilation [48–50].

42.6.1.2 Ventrain

Ventrain (Ventinova Medical B.V., Eindhoven, The Netherlands) (Fig. 42.11d, e) is a manually operated small lumen ventilator (manual Evone) that was initially used to ventilate patients with obstructed upper airway following a needle cricothyrotomy [51]. Oxygen is supplied during inspiration and expiration is initiated by actively removing gas from the lungs through jet-flow generated suction based on Bernoulli's principle. This technology has been introduced as expiratory ventilation assistance (EVA) [52]. Compared to the traditional jet ventilation, active removal of gas from the lungs will reduce the risk of intrapulmonary pressure build-up by air trapping, subsequent barotrauma and hemodynamic deterioration, especially in case of a completely obstructed airway. As such, Ventrain has been acknowledged as the lifesaver for CICV situations [53].

Ventrain can ventilate through small lumen such as Tritube, trans-tracheal catheter, intubating catheter, hollow bougie, or airway exchange catheter, via different airway access, either trans-tracheal by puncture or incision, through a tracheostomy, via oral or nasal route. It is used electively in upper airway surgery, improving surgical field, and maintaining adequate ventilation. It also has a side port allowing side stream capnography or measuring airway pressure [53].

42.6.2 Alternative Oxygenation Techniques (THRIVE/HFNO)

42.6.2.1 Introduction

High-flow nasal cannula (HFNC) or transnasal humidified rapid insufflation ventilatory exchange (THRIVE) is a new emerging device for the delivery of oxygen in acute adult medical practice. In this system, humidified oxygen is delivered at a flow rate that reaches up to 80 L/min and an inspired concentration of oxygen up to 100%, making it a good option in hypoxic or oxygen-dependant patients. The system is also able to provide benefits that are more inclusive than other devices, which includes humidification and warming of inspired gases, patient comfort, increased compliance, effective nasopharyngeal dead space washout, and delivery of low-level PEEP during use (Fig. 42.12) [54]. These features allow for the support of various types of patient breathing difficulties, especially those at risk of respiratory deterioration [55].

Initially, this therapy has been used successfully for the management of respiratory failure in neonatal populations. However, it is now being utilized more frequently in adult populations where it has been used to treat patients with hypoxemic respiratory failure, post-extubation in critical care units, and following major surgery to prevent pulmonary complications [56].

It has also been used as an aid for preoxygenation of patients; by improving dead space washout and prolonging the "apneic ventilation" period through enhancing oxygen reserve following induction of anesthesia. This concept may be useful in patients in whom hypoxia is present prior to induction of anesthesia or highly likely following induction, such as critically ill and obese patients, or in those with anticipated difficult airway whom a prolonged apneic window may result due to difficulties in intubation.

Currently, HFNC therapy has a role in critical care units by improving oxygenation and reducing the incidence of desaturation in patients with mild to moderate hypoxia during the period of intubation. A case series of 25

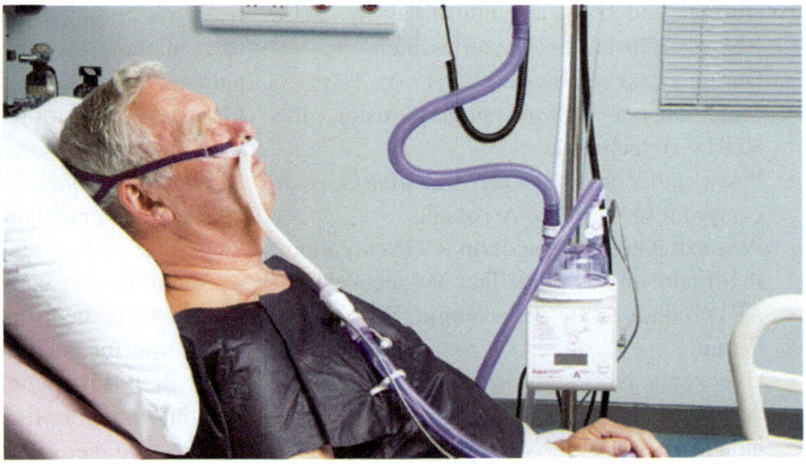

Fig. 42.12 The setup and application of HFNC

patients in which preoxygenation was done for 10 min prior to the induction of anesthesia, showed that the apnea period was significantly prolonged in patients undergoing complex airway and tracheal surgery [56]. However, there is currently no evidence available pertaining to the use of HFNC as a supportive tool in moderate risk elective intubations, such as those that may be encountered in a major head and neck surgical procedures.

These populations often have difficult airways due to previous surgery, radiotherapy or obstructing tumors and have a higher chance of failed intubation and difficulty in securing the airway than other patients. As such, any intervention that may prolong the apneic time and reduce the risk of significant desaturation would be helpful for this patient group [57].

42.6.2.2 Final Outcome After HFNC Application [55]

- It increases FiO_2 and maintains constant FiO_2.
- It improves CO_2 clearance.
- It decreases the work of breathing.
- It creates positive airway pressure.
- It helps in the washout of anatomical dead space.
- It improves pulmonary mechanics.
- It decreases upper airway resistance.
- It helps the mucus clearance.

42.6.2.3 General Indications of HFNC

- Preoxygenation: in all patient especially, difficult airway.
- During endotracheal intubation in ICU, Bariatric, Obstetrics, Pediatrics, etc.
- During awake intubation.
- Minor upper airway surgery using the STRIV-Hi technique.
- Post-extubation in difficult extubation cases or compromised respiratory patients.
- Post-extubation in long-term ICU ventilation.
- In difficult airway guidelines and algorithms.
- ARDS and Acute Hypoxemic Respiratory Failure.
- Hypoxemia induced by severe heart failure.
- Airway instrumentation during rapid sequence induction.
- Hypoxemic and hypercapnic respiratory failure.
- Postoperative in OSA patients.
- Claustrophobia from NIPPV.
- Stridor or end-of-life care.

42.6.3 Tubeless Anesthesia or Tube Free of Upper Airway Surgery

The *Spon**T**aneous **R**espiration using **I**ntra**VE**nous* and *Hi*gh-flow nasal oxygen (*STRIVE Hi*) approach to minor upper airway surgery, which is an open airway technique, and has recently been developed to facilitate micro-laryngoscopy and endoscopic airway surgery in adults without endotracheal tube.

The use of high-flow nasal oxygen (HFNO) is gaining popularity in anesthesia, especially in critical care, as it improves oxygenation and ventilation in both apneic or spontaneously breathing patients [58]. In apneic patients, the Transnasal Humidified Rapid Insufflation Ventilatory Exchange (THRIVE) technique has been associated with a prolonged apnea time and a reduced rate of rising of end tidal carbon dioxide ($ETCO_2$). In spontaneously breathing patients, multiple physiological benefits of HFNO have been described, which include (1) an increased FiO_2, (2) generation of positive airway pressure, (3) improved respiratory mechanics, and (4) reduced upper airway resistance. To date, these clinical benefits during spontaneous ventilation have been limited to awake patients (respiratory supportive care, preoperative preoxygenation, postoperative support), sedated patients [procedural bronchoscopy, or awake fiber-optic intubation (AFOI) or asleep patients with obstructive sleep apnea (OSA). The use of HFNO in spontaneously breathing patients undergoing general anesthesia has not been previously described.

Spontaneous respiration using intravenous anesthesia is the primary technique used at our institution for tubeless airway surgery. We did more than 150 patients using this technique without any complications. Although we have found spontaneous ventilation to be associated with numerous benefits, general anesthesia can have detrimental effects on respiratory mechanics, which may limit the application of the technique in certain patient subgroups, particularly those with severe respiratory comorbidity.

Propofol associated with reduced tidal and minute ventilation, decreases respiratory frequency and an upper airway prone to collapse. We hypothesized that the clinical benefits of HFNO to oxygenation, ventilation and upper airway patency described in awake and sedated patients would be ideally suited to spontaneously breathing patients undergoing general anesthesia. We report our initial experience combining HFNO with our previously described spontaneous respiration technique using intravenous anesthesia in patients undergoing micro-laryngoscopic surgery [59].

Take Home Messages

- Airway management is challenging, being able to recognize and anticipate the difficulty makes the whole process efficient and safe. Difficult airway can be due to difficulty with mask ventilation, use of supraglottic device, tracheal intubation or extubation.
- The familiarity with airway equipment is of paramount important, including the different types of supraglottic devices, direct and indirect laryngoscopes. Providers who deal with airway should be familiar with the recent equipment and recent techniques including the use of apneic oxygenation techniques.
- It is worth mentioning that difficult airway management is a vast chapter with much extensive topics requiring a separate textbook for full discussion. Due to editing limitations in this chapter, we summarize the basic ideas and managements relevant to the ENT surgeon's day-to-day practice focusing on the common problems and providing a very basic guidance for a practical and safe management of difficult scenarios.

References

1. Kheterpal S, Han R, Tremper K, Shanks A, Tait A, O'reilly M, Ludwig T. Incidence and predictors of difficult and impossible mask ventilation. Anesthesiology. 2006;105:885–91. https://doi.org/10.1097/00000542-200611000-00007.
2. Langeron O, Masso E, Huraux C, Guggiari M, Bianchi A, Coriat P, Riou B. Prediction of difficult mask ventilation. Anesthesiology. 2000;92(5):1229–36. https://doi.org/10.1097/00000542-200005000-00009.
3. Cattano D, Katsiampoura A, Corso RM, Killoran PV, Cai C, Hagberg CA. Predictive factors for difficult mask ventilation in the obese surgical population. F1000Research. 2014;3:239. https://doi.org/10.12688/f1000research.5471.1.
4. Brimacombe J. A proposed classification system for extraglottic airway devices. Anesthesiology. 2004;101(2):559.
5. Hernandez MR, Klock PA Jr, Ovassapian A. Evolution of the extraglottic airway: a review of its history, applications, and practical tips for success. Anesth Analg. 2012;114:349–68.
6. Miller DM. A proposed classification and scoring system for supraglottic sealing airways: a brief review. Anesth Analg. 2004;99:1553–9.
7. Ramachandran SK, Mathis MR, Tremper KK, Shanks AM, Kheterpal S. Predictors and clinical outcomes from failed laryngeal mask airway Unique™. Anesthesiology. 2012;116(6):1217–26. https://doi.org/10.1097/aln.0b013e318255e6ab.
8. Apfelbaum JL, Hagberg CA, Caplan RA, Blitt CD, Connis RT, Nickinovich DG, et al. Practice guidelines for management of the difficult airway. Anesthesiology. 2013;118(2):251–70. https://doi.org/10.1097/aln.0b013e31827773b2.
9. Frerk C, Mitchell VS, McNarry AF, Mendonca C, Bhagrath R, Patel A, O'Sullivan EP, Woodall NM, Ahmad I. Difficult Airway Society intubation guidelines working group, Difficult Airway Society 2015 guidelines for management of unanticipated difficult intubation in adults. Br J Anaesth. 2015;115(6):827–48. https://doi.org/10.1093/bja/aev371.
10. Janssens M, Hartstein G. Management of difficult intubation. Eur J Anaesthesiol. 2001;18(1):3–12. https://doi.org/10.1046/j.0265-0215.2000.00777.x.
11. Shallik N, Almustafa M, Zaghw A, Moustafa A. Airway management in ICU setting in Intensive care book. In Intensive care. ISBN: 978-953-51-3360-5. https://doi.org/10.5772/intechopen.69166.
12. Paix AD, Williamson JA, Runciman WB. Crisis management during anaesthesia: difficult intubation. Qual Saf Health Care. 2005;14:e5.
13. Langeron O, et al. Difficult intubation and extubation in adult anaesthesia. Anaesth Crit Care Pain Med. 2018;37(6):639–51. https://doi.org/10.1016/j.accpm.2018.03.013.
14. Belani K, Richtsfeld M. Anesthesiology and the difficult airway – where do we currently stand? Ann Card Anaesth. 2017;20(1):4. https://doi.org/10.4103/0971-9784.197814.

15. Shott SR. Down syndrome: analysis of airway size and a guide for appropriate intubation. Laryngoscope. 2000;110(4):585–92. https://doi.org/10.1097/00005537-200004000-00010.
16. Raj D, Luginbuehl I. Managing the difficult airway in the syndromic child. Contin Educ Anaesth Crit Care Pain. 2015;15(1):7–13. https://doi.org/10.1093/BJACEACCP/MKU004.
17. Meyer AC, Lidsky ME, Sampson DE, Lander TA, Liu M, Sidman JD. Airway interventions in children with Pierre Robin Sequence. Otolaryngol Head Neck Surg. 2008;138(6):782–7. https://doi.org/10.1016/j.otohns.2008.03.002.
18. Major Complications of Airway Management in the United Kingdom. 2011. www.rcoa.ac.uk. Accessed 6 Apr 2020.
19. Chang K, Uitto J, Rowold EA, Grant GA, Kilo C, Williamson JR. Increased collagen cross-linkages in experimental diabetes. Reversal by β-aminopropionitrile and D-penicillamine. Diabetes. 1980;29(10):778–81. https://doi.org/10.2337/diacare.20.10.778.
20. Jurik A. Radiology UP-C, 1984 undefined. Rheumatoid arthritis of the crico-arytenoid and crico-thyroid joints: a radiological and clinical study. Amsterdam: Elsevier. https://www.sciencedirect.com/science/article/pii/S0009926084801464. Accessed 9 Apr 2020.
21. Dargin JM, Emlet LL, Guyette FX. The effect of body mass index on intubation success rates and complications during emergency airway management. Intern Emerg Med. 2013;8(1):75–82. https://doi.org/10.1007/s11739-012-0874-x.
22. Juvin P, Lavaut E, Dupont H, et al. Difficult tracheal intubation is more common in obese than in lean patients. Anesth Analg. 2003;97(2):595–600. https://doi.org/10.1213/01.ANE.0000072547.75928.B0.
23. Riad W, Vaez MN, Raveendran R, et al. Neck circumference as a predictor of difficult intubation and difficult mask ventilation in morbidly obese patients. In: European journal of anaesthesiology, vol. 33. Philadelphia, PA: Lippincott Williams & Wilkins; 2016. p. 244–9. https://doi.org/10.1097/EJA.0000000000000324.
24. Kim JA, Lee JJ. Preoperative predictors of difficult intubation in patients with obstructive sleep apnea syndrome. Can J Anesth. 2006;53(4):393–7. https://doi.org/10.1007/BF03022506.
25. Melissant CF, Smith SJ, Perlberger R, Verschakelen J, Lammers JWJ, Demedts M. Lung function, CT-scan and X-ray in upper airway obstruction due to thyroid goitre. Eur Respir J. 1994;7(10):1782–7. https://doi.org/10.1183/09031936.94.07101782.
26. Ovassapian A, Glassenberg R, Randel GI, Klock A, Mesnick PS, Klafta JM. The unexpected difficult airway and lingual tonsil hyperplasia. Anesthesiology. 2002;97(1):124–32. https://doi.org/10.1097/00000542-200207000-00018.
27. Marple BF, Ludwig WV. Ludwig angina: a review of current airway management. Arch Otolaryngol Head Neck Surg. 1999;125(May):596–9.
28. Galeiras R, Seoane-Quiroga L, Pértega-Diáz S. Prevalence and prognostic impact of inhalation injury among burn patients: a systematic review and meta-analysis. J Trauma Acute Care Surg. 2020;88(2):330–44. https://doi.org/10.1097/TA.0000000000002523.
29. Rönnberg L, Nilsson U, Hellzén O, Melin-Johansson C. The art is to extubate, not to intubate—Swedish registered nurse anesthetists experiences of the process of extubation after general anesthesia. J Perianesth Nurs. 2019;34(4):789–800. https://doi.org/10.1016/j.jopan.2018.11.007.
30. Cavallone LF, Vannucci A. Extubation of the difficult airway and extubation failure. Surv Anesthesiol. 2013;57(6):312–3. https://doi.org/10.1097/01.sa.0000435464.98907.2dnn.
31. Tan J. Extubating techniques for the difficult airway. Int J Anesthetic Anesthesiol. 2017;4(1) https://doi.org/10.23937/2377-4630/1410058.
32. Phillips OC, Duerksen RL. Endotracheal intubation: a new blade for direct laryngoscopy. Anesth Analg. 1973;52:691–8.
33. Bradley P, Chapman G, Crooke B. Airway assessment. Australian and New Zealand College of Anaesthetists (Anzca), Aug 2016.
34. Khan ZH, Arbabi S. Diagnostic value of the upper lip bite test in predicting difficulty in intubation with head and neck landmarks obtained from lateral neck X-ray. Indian J Anaesth. 2013;57(4):381–6. https://doi.org/10.4103/0019-5049.118567.
35. Krage R, Rijn CV, Groeningen DV, Loer S, Schwarte L, Schober P. Cormack–Lehane classification revisited. Br J Anaesth. 2010;105(2):220–7. https://doi.org/10.1093/bja/aeq136.
36. Koh LKD, Kong CF, Ip-Yam PC. The modified Cormack-Lehane score for the grading of direct laryngoscopy: evaluation in the Asian population. Anaesth Intensive Care. 2002;30(1):48–51. https://doi.org/10.1177/0310057x0203000109.
37. Shallik NA, Moustafa AH, Hammad Y. Evaluation of the normal airway using virtual endoscopy and three-dimensional reconstruction. In: Shallik N, Moustafa A, Marcus M, editors. Virtual endoscopy and 3D reconstruction in the airways. Cham: Springer; 2019. https://doi.org/10.1007/978-3-030-23253-5_4.
38. Radiological evaluation of the airway: one-stop shop Abbas H. Moustafa, Nabil A. Shallik. Shallik N., Moustafa A., Marcus M. Virtual endoscopy and 3D reconstruction in the airways. (2019) Springer, Cham. https://doi.org/10.1007/978-3-030-23253-5_3.
39. Shallik N, Haidar H, Dogan Z, Enezi H, Rahman W, Arun N, Ishac N, Moustafa A. Circular hyoid bone: the first reported case in literature. Trends Anaesth Crit Care. 2017;16:27–8. https://doi.org/10.1016/j.tacc.2017.10.040.

40. Shallik N, Zaghw A, Dogan Z, Rahman A. The use of virtual endoscopy for diagnosis of traumatic supraglottic airway stenosis. JCAO. 2017;2(1):103.
41. Shallik N, Dardeer A, Hammad Y, Kumar N, Shaikh N, Ganaw A, Lance M, Moustafa A. Pushed away: how did 3D reconstruction solve this airway problem? Trends Anesth Crit Care. 2020;30:36–7. https://doi.org/10.1016/j.tacc.2019.12.094.
42. Rosenblatt W, Ianus AI, Sukhupragarn W, Fickenscher A, Sasaki C. Preoperative Endoscopic Airway Examination (PEAE) provides superior airway information and may reduce the use of unnecessary awake intubation. Anesth Analg. 2011;112(3):602–7. https://doi.org/10.1213/ANE.0b013e3181fdfc1c.
43. Schmidt J, et al. Flow-controlled ventilation during ear, nose and throat surgery: a prospective observational study. Eur J Anaesthesiol. 2019 Feb 5;36(5):327–34.
44. Schmidt J, et al. Flow-controlled ventilation attenuates lung injury in a porcine model of acute respiratory distress syndrome: a preclinical randomized controlled study. Crit Care Med. 2020;48:e241–8. https://doi.org/10.1097/CCM.0000000000004209.
45. Bergold et al. Flow-controlled ventilation—a novel approach to treating severe acute respiratory distress syndrome. Poster WAMM. 2019.
46. Barnes, Enk. Ventilation for low dissipated energy achieved using flow control during both inspiration and expiration. Trends Anaesth Crit Care. 2019;24:5–12.
47. Schmidt, et al. Improved lung recruitment and oxygenation during mandatory ventilation with a new expiratory ventilation assistance device. Eur J Anaesthesiol. 2018;35(10):736–44.
48. Hagberg C. Benumof & Hagberg's airway management. 3rd ed. Amsterdam: Elsevier; 2013. p. 595–6.
49. Borg PAJ, Hamaekers AEW, Lacko M, Jansen J, Enk D. Ventrain® for ventilation of the lungs. Br J Anaesth. 2012;109:833–4.
50. Shallik N, Zaghw A, Lance M, Hammad Y, Shaikh N, Ganaw A. Clinical feasibility of the tritube with EVA devices in ventilating patients with restricted airway diameter. Trends Anesth Crit Care. 2020;30:51–2. https://doi.org/10.1016/j.tacc.2019.12.130.
51. Paxian M, Preussler NP, Reinz T, Schlueter A, Gottschall R. Transtracheal ventilation with a novel ejector-based device (Ventrain) in open, partly obstructed, or totally closed upper airways in pigs. Br J Anaesth. 2015;115:308–16.
52. Hamaekers AEW, Borg PA, Enk D. Ventrain: an ejector ventilator for emergency use. Br J Anaesth. 2012;108:1017–21.
53. Fearnley RA, Badiger S, Oakley R, Ahmad I. Elective use of the Ventrain for upper airway obstruction during high frequency jet ventilation. J Clin Anesth. 2016;33:233–5.
54. Ward JJ. High-flow oxygen administration by nasal cannula for adult and perinatal patients. Respir Care. 2013;58:98–122.
55. Nishimura M. High-flow nasal cannula oxygen therapy in adults. J Intensive Care. 2016;3:15.
56. Frizzola M, Miller TL, Rodriguez ME, et al. High-flow nasal cannula: impact on oxygenation and ventilation in an acute lung injury model. Pediatr Pulmonol. 2011;46:67–74.
57. Corley A, Caruana LR, Barnett AG, et al. Oxygen delivery through high-flow nasal cannulae increase end-expiratory lung volume and reduce respiratory rate in post-cardiac surgical patients. Br J Anaesth. 2011;107:998–1004.
58. Booth AWG, Vidhani K. Spontaneous ventilation using target-controlled propofol infusion for microlaryngoscopy in adults: a retrospective audit. Anaesth Intensive Care. 2016;44:286–94.
59. Allsop P, Taylor MB, Grounds RM, Morgan M. Ventilatory effect of a propofol infusion using a method to rapidly achieve steady-state equilibrium. Eur J Anaesthesiol. 1988;5:193–303.

Part V

Laryngology and Esophagology

Physiology of the Voice and Clinical Voice Assessment

43

Mayed Radi Alkhafaji and Dina Emam

43.1 Introduction

SPEECH & LANGUAGE is the way of communication used by people. Speech is an expression of ideas and thoughts by means of articulate vocal sounds. Speech requires movement of *sound waves* through the air. Speech itself is air that is moved from the lungs through a series of anatomic structures that *mold* sound waves into intelligible speech. This capacity can be accomplished in any volume from a soft whisper to a loud shout by varying the *force* and volume of air expelled from the lungs.

43.2 Voice Physiology

- Voice = Voiced Sound + Resonance + Articul ation

Voiced sound: The basic sound produced by vocal fold vibration is called "voiced sound." This is frequently described as a "buzzy" sound.

Resonance: Voiced sound is amplified and modified by the vocal tract resonators (the throat, mouth cavity, and nasal passages). The resonators produce a person's recognizable voice.

Articulation: The vocal tract articulators (the tongue, soft palate, and lips) modify the voiced sound. The articulators produce recognizable words.

In humans, there are four main body systems involved in the production of speech.

1. The respiratory system
2. Laryngeal system
3. Articulation
4. The nervous system

The first three systems are responsible for the physical manifestations of speech, and the nervous system is responsible for regulates these systems on both the conscious level.

The rhythmicity center of the medulla: The respiratory center is gray matter in the pons and the upper Medulla, controls automatic breathing consists of interacting neurons that fire either during inspiration (I neurons) or expiration (E neurons)

- *I neurons*—stimulate neurons that innervate respiratory muscles (to bring about inspiration)
- *E neurons*—inhibit I neurons (to "shut down" the I neurons and bring about expiration)
- *Apneustic* center (located in the pons)—stimulate I neurons (to promote inspiration)
- *Pneumotaxic* center (also located in the pons)—inhibits apneustic center and inhibits inspiration

M. R. Alkhafaji (✉) · D. Emam
ENT Department, Hamad Medical Corporation, Doha, Qatar
e-mail: mradi@hamad.qa; DEmam@hamad.qa

A. Al-Qahtani et al. (eds.), *Textbook of Clinical Otolaryngology*,
https://doi.org/10.1007/978-3-030-54088-3_43

43.2.1 The Respiratory System and Airflow

The respiratory system is also called the power system and it's rule is the development and maintenance of a column of air under pressure, which is presented to the glottis and subglottis, whereas the diaphragm is the important muscle for inspiration and expiration—and in particular controlled expiration—is necessary for vocalization.

The relaxing diaphragm interact with the muscles of expiration along with the natural elastic recoil of the act of expiration, also the abdominal muscles play an important rule especially the inner most layers especially in sustaining a long or powerful sound.

- Contraction of external intercostal muscles > elevation of ribs and sternum > increased front- to-back dimension of thoracic cavity > lowers air pressure in lungs > air moves into lungs.
- Contraction of diaphragm > diaphragm moves downward > increases vertical dimension of thoracic cavity > lowers air pressure in lungs > air moves into lungs.

This increase of volume lowers the air pressure in the alveoli to below atmospheric pressure. Because air always flows from a region of high pressure to a region of lower pressure, it rushes in through the respiratory tract and into the alveoli. This is called negative pressure.

Breathing changing the pressure inside the lungs relative to the pressure of the outside atmosphere. In contrast to inspiration, during expiration the diaphragm and intercostal muscles relax. This returns the thoracic cavity to its original volume, increasing the air pressure in the lungs, and forcing the air out.

- Any pulmonary pathology starting from acute upper respiratory tract infection up to the obstructing and restrictive pulmonary diseases can affect the power of the voice as well as weakness in the abdominal wall muscles, also pathology of the thoracic cage as pectus excavatum and kyphosis along with calcifications of the cartilaginous part of the ribs with age can affect the power of the voice.

43.2.2 Vocal Folds (Also Called Vocal Cords)

The vocal cord length is varied between adults and children and between males and females.

The length in adult female is approximately 15–18 mm while in males it is about 20–22 mm. The vocal cords can vibrate together and create sound if they are present in the midline with the presence of subglottic pressure; the pitch is predominantly determined by the stretch of the vocal cord intrinsic muscles while the power of the voice depends on the subglottic pressure.

During the adduction position which is the position of the vocal cords during vocalization there will be a small opened gap. Naturally, the thing which will make the two cords completely adducted for more clear voice is explained by the Bernolli rule which says if a stream of air passes between two surfaces that will create a negative pressure and tends to pull them together.

- So as a general rule is any factor will affect the elasticity of the vocal cords, musculature, regularity of the surface, the completeness of the closure or the mucus that lubricate the vocal cords will have an impact on the voice quality.

One vibratory cycle of the vocal cords is as follows:

- Column of air pressure opens bottom of vocal folds
- Column of air continues to move upward, now toward the top of vocal folds, and opens the top
- The low pressure created behind the fast-moving air column produces a "Bernoulli effect" which causes the bottom to close, followed by the top
- Closure of the vocal folds cuts off the air column and releases a pulse of air
- New cycle repeats

43.2.2.1 Vocal Tract—Resonators and Articulators

The nose, pharynx, and mouth amplify and modify sound, allowing it to take on the distinctive qualities of voice the way that voice is produced is analogous to the way that sound is produced by a trombone. The trombone player produces sound at the mouthpiece of the instrument with his lips vibrating from air that passes from the mouth. The vibration within the mouthpiece produces sound, which is then altered or "shaped" as it passes throughout the instrument. As the slide of the trombone is changed, the sound of the musical instrument is similarly changed.

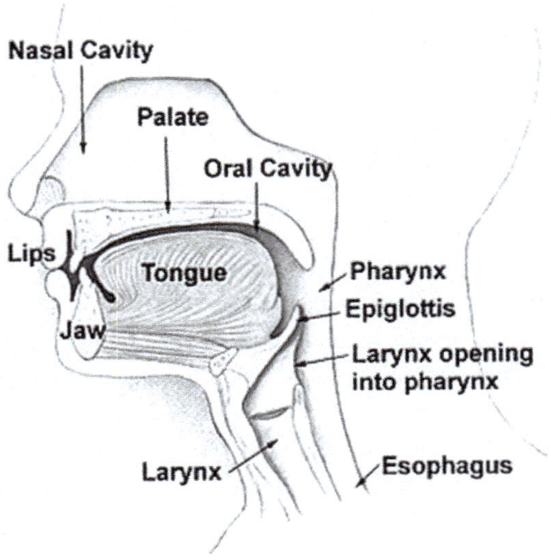

43.2.3 The Nervous System

- The brain typically formed of two cerebral hemispheres connected with nerve fibers called corpus callosum. The speech centers are present mostly in the left hemisphere and in one-third of the people who are left-handed the speech is controlled by the right side of the brain.
- Parts in the brain involved in speech:
  - Cerebrum: The brain is formed of lobes, the speech is controlled by the frontal lobe and temporal lobes.
- Brocas area: an area in the frontal lobe of the dominant hemisphere on the left side of the brain, the function of this area is speech production and it is found to be the most active area immediately before you speak, even if someone has the ability to produce sound the Brocas area is necessary to express the language Brocas area is made up of Brodmann area 44 (pars opercularis) and 45 (pars triangularis).
  - Wernicks area: Works with the angular gyrus, insular cortex, and basal ganglion to process word sequences to determine context and meaning
  - Angular gyrus: Assembles information to help us understand words and concepts
  - Insular cortex: Buried underneath the outer lobes of the cerebral cortex, the insular cortex is important for many functions, including motor control, emotions, and self-awareness, but also important in the processing of language

43.3 Voice Assessment in Outpatient Department

A successful voice assessment determines the cause, the severity, and the prognosis of the problem and enables the planning of the most appropriate treatment program. The voice assessment is complicated and time consuming and it cannot be done in routine ENT clinics; it needs to be done in a specialized voice clinic that is well structured and involves a diagnostic and therapeutic team. The multidisplinary team should include an ENT doctor specialized in laryngology, speech language pathologist, physiotherapist, psychiatrist, and a voice coach and a singing teacher who work together as a team in order to achieve a proper diagnosis and treatment for the different cases of voice disorders.

Voice assessment is multidimensional and it includes history taking, observation, clinical examination, auditory evaluation, and measurement of vocal cords function and physiology.

43.3.1 Voice Case History

A detailed voice history is required in order to do proper assessment and diagnosis for any patient with voice disorder and then to plan your treatment strategies for each case, the history should be detailed regarding the voice change, onset, course and duration, vocal cord demands and stressors, history of reflux, history of special habits as smoking and alcohol consumption.

History should include also medications history as well as the medical and surgical history especially neck surgeries and cardiothoracic surgeries.

43.3.2 Observation (Posture, Breathing, Palpation)

Observation will include general observation for the general appearance of the patient which is a sign of the patient well-being mode and energy, fascial expressions, asymmetry or weakness, tremors, involuntary movements, frequent throat clearance, or coughing.

Position of the neck is important because of the impact on the intrinsic and extrinsic muscles of the larynx, poor posture contributes to many voice disorders and correction of posture has been part of the voice therapy for many years.

Observation should include also observation of breathing, normal breathing will insure a good power for voice production, so observation for any abnormal breathing, use of accessory respiratory muscles, how frequent the patient inhales during conversation and if the patient is running out of air during conversation with excessive shoulder and upper chest movements listing to patient breathing can differentiate between pulmonary and laryngeal disorders.

Palpation for muscles tension is important particularly in the evaluation and treatment of muscle tension dysphonia, and palpation for tension over the temporomandibular, jaw, fascial muscles, and larynx is also important as there is a variety of protocols related to muscles tension and common sites for palpation.

43.3.3 Patient Questionnaire?

Voice disorder is very common and it has its impact on the patient lifestyle and communication especially for the professional voice users and those who depend on their voice in their work as teachers, lecturers, etc.

In most of the specialized voice centers, there will be a questionnaire in order to help the diagnosis and plan the treatment and also to follow up the patient in order to see the improvement and also to facilitate researches.

The questionnaires can be created by each center, but there are well-known questionnaires known worldwide such as Vocal Performance Questionnaire, Voice Handicap Index, and Voice Symptoms Scale.

43.3.4 Endoscopic Evaluation with a Nasopharyngoscopy and Video Stroboscope

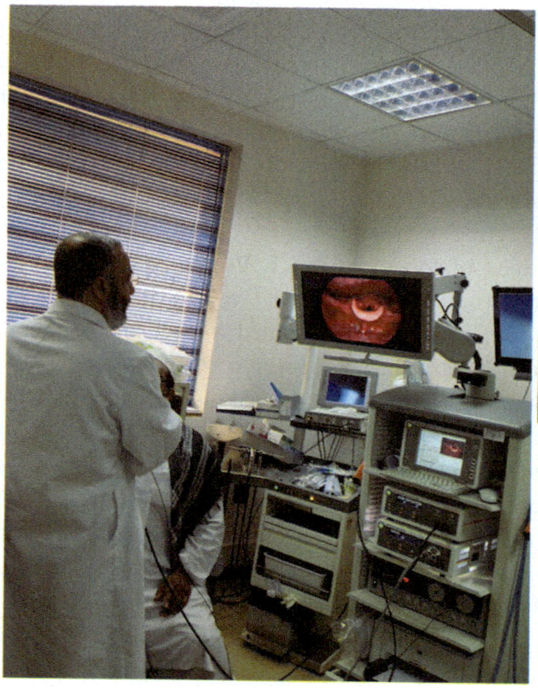
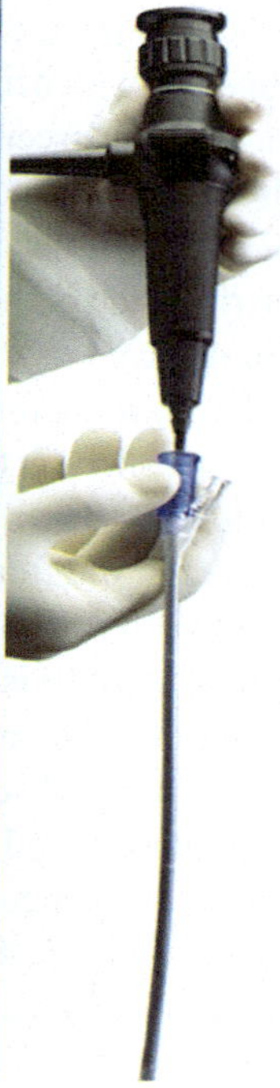

Endoscopic evaluation for the vocal folds and the resonating system considered the most important part in voice assessment because it helps in the diagnosis and in planning the treatment strategy. The endoscopic evaluation can be done through both flexible and rigid endoscopies and also can be done by the video stroboscope (the gold standard test).

43.3.4.1 Flexible Endoscopies

Flexible fiber-optic or what we call it direct laryngoscopy is an important tool in all ENT clinics and in voice clinic in particular for evaluation of both the vibratory and the resonating component of the voice.

The flexible laryngoscope is a well-tolerated test done in ENT-outpatient clinics, it can be done for both adults and pediatric age group, it does not need sedation and the chance of having gage reflex with it is much less in comparison to rigid scopes, and it helps in the evaluation of the upper airway starting from the nose up to the level of the vocal cords. It helps in assessment while the patient is phonating, talking, or singing and it helps the evaluation of the velopharyngeal incompetence and the presence of sings of silent reflux.

The disadvantage of this examination is the magnification so the detailed examination of the mucosa and mucosal wave movements of the vocal cords will not be there and the brightness and clarity of the image for the vocal cords is not as that for the rigid scope or the stroboscope.

43.3.4.2 Rigid Scope

Rigid scope is based on using a rigid metal transoral rode, and this will allow the transmission of a high intensity light and this will give a magnified and much more clear image in comparison to the that of the flexible scope, but still the test needs cooperation from the patient and mostly it will not be tolerated by the patient who are having a strong gage reflex and local xylocaine spray will be required if rigid scope needs to be used, in addition the assessment of full phonatory function is restricted because it interferes with the speech and voice production.

43.3.5 Video Stroboscope

The stroboscopic examination of the vocal cord mobility has the same principle of the rigid scope. The stroboscopic lighting is produced with the same frequency of vocal cords vibration which generated a pseudo slow motion and allows the assessment of the mucosal waves and integrity of the mucosa as well as the closure of the vocal cords.

The stroboscope is done through a rigid scope and it has the same advantage and disadvantage for the rigid scope, so the flexible scope with distal chip camera brought for us the advantage of both the flexible scope and the stroboscope in the same scope and that allowed the laryngologist to go for more detailed voice assessment

43.3.5.1 Simple Aerodynamic Assessment

The maximum phonation time (MPT) is defined as the maximum time in seconds that the patient is able to sustain a vowel letter (ah) in a comfortable pitch and loudness; this test is simple and easy to perform in the clinic and also it has prognostic value in evaluation of patients before and after vocal cords injection. The normal range is between 15–25 s in females and 20–30 s in males.

43.3.5.2 Complex Aerodynamic Assessment

It depend on the measurement of the respiratory function test through a respirometer; this tool is available and easily can be done but the measurement of the subglottic pressure is difficult to be measured directly and can be estimated by intraoral pressure at the time the phonation is stopped.

43.3.6 Electro Laryngography or Electroglottography

The electro laryngography is based on placement of two electrodes on either sides of the larynx and a small current is passing in between, this test is giving evaluation of vibratory cycle behaviors, the output is called Lx, and it gives details about the closing and opening phases of the vibratory cycle.

43.3.7 Electromyography (EMG)

This test is done as an office based test; the test is important to detect the integrity of the laryngeal nerve supple of the larynx through the superior and recurrent laryngeal nerves as well as the muscles supplied by them, for that the test is based on inserting a hooked needle in four pairs of laryngeal muscles, thyroarytenoid, posterior and lateral cricoarytenoids, and the cricothyroid muscles.

This test considered an invasive test and should be avoided in obese patients, patients with bleeding disorders, altered anatomy secondary to infections or previous surgeries or uncooperative patients (children, psychiatric patients, etc.).

For patients on tracheostomy, they require the tube to be removed in order to place the electrodes and to replace it after the test is done.

Take Home Messages

- Voice disorders are a wide range of disorders and the voice assessment in order to have diagnosis and to set up a plan of treatment is not an easy task to be carried out in routine ENT clinics.
- A specialized well-structured and well-equipped voice clinic runner out by ENT doctor specialized in laryngology with his team of SLP and-, singing teachers, etc. is essential to provide the required service for a big sector of patients with voice disorders.

44 Inflammatory, Infectious, and Acquired Conditions of the Larynx

Aisha Larem, Nafil Arimbrathodi, and Rafia Zahid

Key Points

- Steeple sign: funnel-shaped subglottic narrowing on X-ray films, seen in Croup.
- Thumb sign: swollen epiglottis on X-ray, seen in acute epiglottitis.
- Mouse nibbled appearance of vocal cords: seen in TB laryngitis.
- TB has a predilection to posterior larynx whereas syphilis commonly affects anterior larynx.
- Supraglottis: commonly involved in sarcoidosis and amyloidosis.
- Subglottis: commonly involved in Wegerner's granulomatosis and laryngitis sicca.
- C1 esterase inhibitor (Icatibant): used in treating nonallergic angioedema.
- Idiopathic subglottic stenosis: needed work up to rule out autoimmune disorders.

44.1 Introduction

The thorough knowledge of laryngeal anatomy is key in the understanding pathophysiology of laryngeal disorders. It is very important for physician to have a detailed idea about infectious and inflammatory laryngeal pathologies. Early diagnosis and timely management of those conditions are important to secure voice and a patent airway of patients.

44.2 Embryology

Larynx develops from tracheobronchial groove, which starts on fourth week of intrauterine life. Majority of the anatomical features of larynx develop by the third month of intrauterine life. At birth, angle of the thyroid cartilage in males is 110° while in females, 120° [1, 2].

44.3 Anatomy

Larynx is divided by the true vocal cords into three subdivisions

- *Supraglottis* is above the true vocal cords and consists of epiglottis, aryepiglottic folds, arytenoids (laryngeal surface only), false vocal cords, ventricle, vestibule, drain upper deep cervical lymph nodes.

A. Larem (✉) · N. Arimbrathodi · R. Zahid
Hamad Medical Corporation, Doha, Qatar
e-mail: alarem@hamad.qa; NArimbrathodi@hamad.qa; RZahid1@hamad.qa

A. Al-Qahtani et al. (eds.), *Textbook of Clinical Otolaryngology*,
https://doi.org/10.1007/978-3-030-54088-3_44

- *Glottis* is at the level of true vocal cords and contains anterior commissure, posterior commissure, and it has scanty lymph node drainage that is why it rarely shows lymphatic metastasis.
- *Subglottis* is below the true vocal cords up to lower border of cricoid, drain lower deep cervical lymph nodes [3, 4].
- Larynx of infants differs from the adults as it is situated high up (C3–C4) and funnel shaped/conical (adults–cylindrical in shape) with narrow epiglottis.
- Cartilages are soft and collapse easily on forced inspiration.
- The narrowest part of infantile larynx is the junction of subglottic larynx with trachea.
- Cricothyroid is the only intrinsic muscle of the larynx which lies outside the laryngeal framework.
- Posterior cricoarytenoid is the only abductor of vocal cord.
- Vocal cords have no lymphatics except for a small delphian node which lies on cricothyroid membrane.
- Aryepiglottic fold has the richest lymphatic supply in larynx.
- Thyroid cartilage calcifies as a figure of 8 [5, 6].

44.4 Infectious and Inflammatory Conditions of the Larynx

44.4.1 Infectious

- *Viral*
  Croup (influenza and parainfluenza
  Rhinovirus, RSV, adenovirus
- *Bacteria*
  Hemophilus influenza
  Streptococcus spp.
  Epiglottitis
  Diphtheria
  Tuberculosis
  Syphilis
  Leprosy
  Scleroma
- *Fungi*
  Histoplasmosis
  Blastomycosis
  Candidiasis
  Aspergillosis
  Coccidiomycosis

44.4.2 Inflammatory/Autoimmune

- Wegener's granulomatosis
- Relapsing polychondritis
- Systemic lupus erythematosus
- Epidermolysis bullosa
- Cicatricial pemphigoid

44.4.3 Iatrogenic/Trauma

- Radiation laryngitis
- Thermal injury
- Laryngopharyngeal reflux

44.4.4 Idiopathic/Infiltrative

- Amyloidosis
- Sarcoidosis

44.4.5 Allergic

- Angioedema

44.5 Acute Laryngo-Tracheo-Bronchitis (Croup)

Serious infection which affects the entire tracheobronchial tree seen mostly in pediatrics population, viral origin in majority of the time be can be caused by bacteria, common pathogens in pediatric population are Influenza A and Parainfluenza type 1 and 2, while in adults it is caused most of the time by Herpes simplex, Influenza A, CMV, and superimposed bacterial infection caused Hemolytic streptococci.

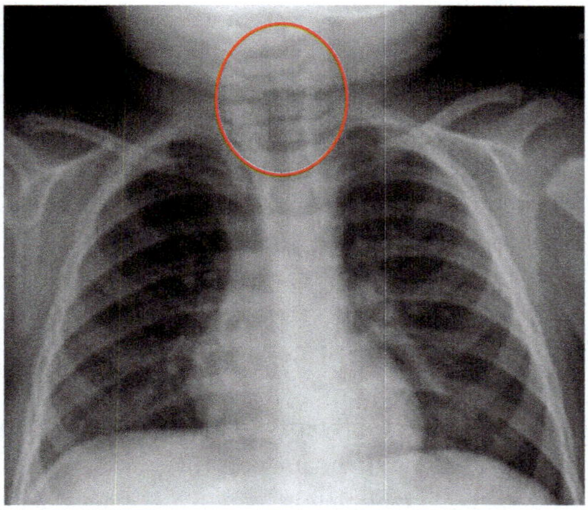

Fig. 44.1 XR Neck AP view showing "steeple" sign

Males are affected more than females, age of presentation is usually 6 months to 3 years, top emergency as airway obstruction issues as a result of mucosal swelling of respiratory tract, subglottic area is the most common involved area causing subglottic edema, and thick mucus is produced with pseudomembrane formation (Fig. 44.1) [7, 8].

44.5.1 Clinical Presentation

Low-grade fever with painful croupy cough (barking cough), the cough is followed by hoarseness of voice and stridor, inspiratory stridor that progress to biphasic, respiratory distress with use of accessory muscle for respiration.

44.5.2 Work Up and Management

44.5.2.1 *"Steeple Sign"* (Steeple or Funnel-Shaped Subglottic Narrowing on X-Ray Films)

Management lines includes supportive measures with, oxygenation, hydration, and nebulization with epinephrine, systemic steroids and broad-spectrum antibiotics for cases with bacterial infection or at high risk of secondary bacterial infections.

If patient deteriorates, intubation needed with reserve option for tracheostomy [7, 8].

44.5.2.2 Acute Epiglottitis (Supraglottic Laryngitis)

Acute inflammation of the supraglottic area, caused most commonly in pediatric population by H. influenza type B, and in adults usually caused by Group A streptococci, *Streptococcus pneumoniae*, *Staphylococcus aureus*, *Klebsiella pneumoniae*, and *Neisseria meningitidis* (cause of fulminant supraglottitis).

44.5.2.3 Clinical Features

Rapidly progressing symptoms commence with URTI and fever, odynophagia and dysphagia are seen in adults, and pediatrics present with drooling, breathing difficulty, and stridor (Inspiratory with worsening on supine position).

Tripod sign: Children sit in position with hyperextended neck relieves the breathing difficulty; adults can present with tachycardia, which is disproportionate to pyrexia which could indicate impending airway obstruction [9, 10].

44.5.3 Work Up and Management

X-ray neck: Swollen epiglottis (*thumb sign*) and absence of well-defined vallecula (*vallecula sign*) can be seen (Figs. 44.2 and 44.3).

Securing airway is the important management step, either by intubation or tracheostomy regardless of the severity of respiratory distress.

Hospitalization required in intensive care unit or under close observation. Mainstay of medical management includes IV antibiotics (preferably third generation cephalosporins, IV corticosteroids, with hydration, oxygenation, and humidified air.

Unvaccinated carriers/contacts should be given prophylactic rifampin for 4 days [10, 11].

44.5.4 Laryngeal Diphtheria

Uncommon after vaccine era, caused by Corynebacterium diphtheria, manifests as exuda-

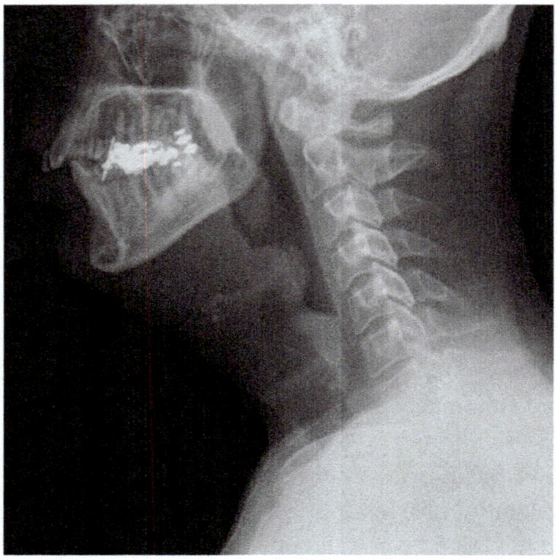

Fig. 44.2 XR neck lateral view showing thumb sign

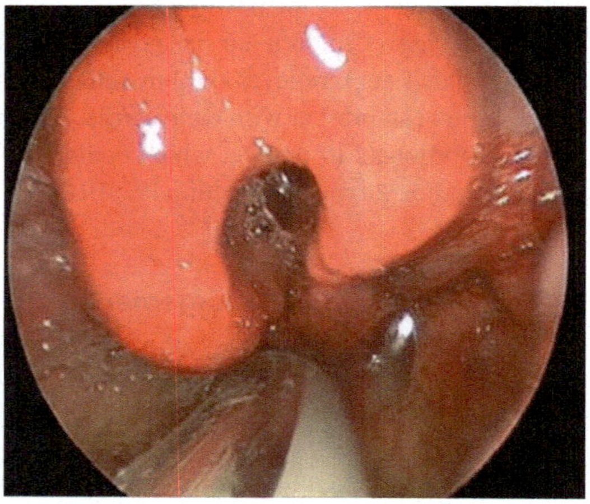

Fig. 44.3 Endoscopic view of inflamed epiglottis. (Image reprinted with permission from Springer Nature: Nature publishing, Infectious disease in pediatric otolaryngology, Laryngeal indections, Tulio Valdez and Jesus Vallejo et al, July 105)

tive inflammation of the mucous membranes, thick, gray plaque-like membranous exudates over tonsils, pharynx, and larynx, complications include nephritis, airway obstruction, death (secondary to neurological toxins).

Treatment lines include diphtheria antitoxin, erythromycin, or penicillin [8, 11].

44.5.5 Tubercular Laryngitis

Seen in association with pulmonary TB, patient may present with hoarseness of voice, cough, dysphagia, odynophagia, voice weakness with periodic aphonia.

Early findings in laryngoscope include hyperemia and ulceration of unilateral vocal cord with impairment of abduction, classically, shallow ulcers with undermined edges are seen in vocal cords (*mouse nibbled appearance*) (Fig. 44.4).

Other findings that may present Turban epiglottis (Pseudo-edema of the epiglottis), Interarytenoid edema and swelling giving a mamillated appearance.

44.5.6 Work Up and Management

Chest X-ray and Sputum for AFB.

Treatment with Anti-TB medications [12, 13].

44.5.7 Lupus of the Larynx

It is an indolent tubercular infection associated with lupus of nose and pharynx, painless condi-

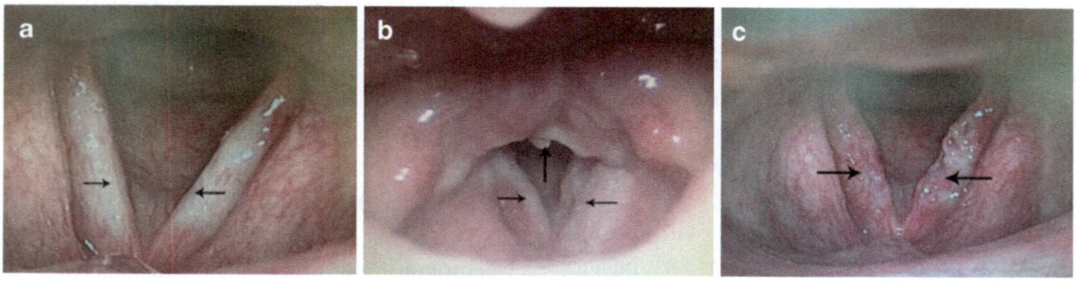

Fig. 44.4 (**a**) True vocal folds fibrinous exudate; (**b**) inter-arytenoid, false vocal folds and true vocal folds ulcer; (**c**) true vocal folds mouse nibbled ulcer. (Image reprinted with permission from Elsevier (Creative Commons Attribution 4.0 International): Otolaryngology case reports, Secondary laryngeal tuberculosis in Tibet China: A report of six cases, HuaidongDu et al, March 2017)

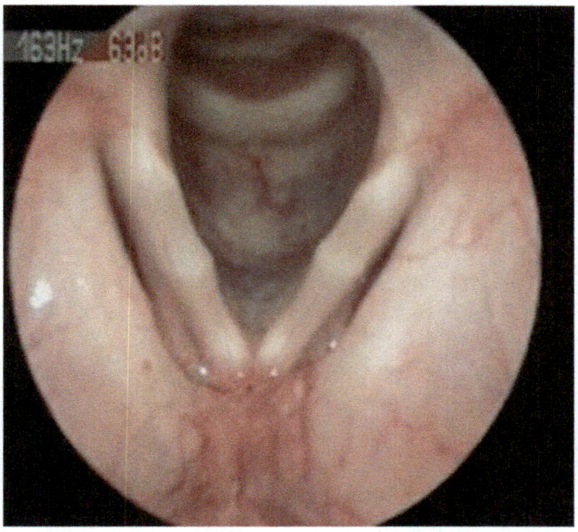

Fig. 44.5 Endoscopic view of bamboo nodules. (Image reprinted with permission from Elsevier: Journal of Voice, Bamboo Nodes on a Series of 15 Patients: Vocal Fold Lesion as a Sign of Autoimmune Disease and Microphonotrauma, Natalie Oker, Aude Julien-Laferrière, Philippe Herman, Gérard Chevaillier, May 2019)

tion with no symptoms, *Bamboo nodules* in vocal cords, carries a good prognosis.

Site affected: Anterior part of the larynx (Epiglottis > Aryepiglottic fold > ventricular bands) (Fig. 44.5) [13, 14].

44.5.8 Syphilis of the Larynx

Can manifest at any stage of the disease,

- *Primary stage*: Mucosal ulceration, primary chancre.
- *Secondary stage*: Multiple vesicles and popular lesions.
- *Tertiary stage*: Gummatous lesion.

Sites affected: Anterior part of the larynx (epiglottis and aryepiglottic fold) [13, 14].

44.5.9 Leprosy

Commonly affects the anterior part of larynx, supraglottic region is first to be affected, gray color lesions and in cases with epiglottis involvement can give an appearance of hook over a buttonhole [13, 14].

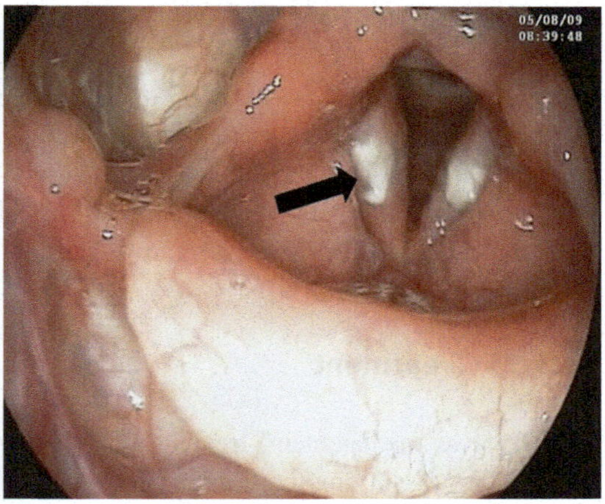

Fig. 44.6 Endoscopic photo of vocal folds of patient with fungal laryngitis. (Image reprinted with permission from Springer Nature: Nature publishing, Indian Journal of Otolaryngology and Head & Neck Surgery volume 66, pages 375–378, A. Ravikumar et al, November 2011)

44.5.10 Histoplasmosis

Systemic fungal disease, caused by Histoplasma capsulatum, nodular superficial granulomas which become painful on ulceration, treatment with amphotericin B [15–17].

44.5.11 Blastomycosis

Fungal infection caused by Blastomyces dermatitidis, multi-organs involvement, histology shows caseous necrosis with acute inflammatory infiltrate, micro-abscesses, giant cells.

Treatment: long-term amphotericin B, ketoconazole, itraconazole.

Complications: Pharyngo-cutaneous fistula if left untreated (Fig. 44.6) [15–17].

44.5.12 Laryngitis Sicca

Also known as atrophic laryngitis, features include atrophy of laryngeal mucosa and crust formation, can be associated with atrophic rhinitis, caused by Klebsiella ozaenae, histology shows metaplasia of respiratory epithelium to squamous type with loss of cilia and glands which leads to dryness and crust formation, affects ventricular folds, posterior region, and subglottic area.

44.5.13 Clinical Features

Females are affected more than males, voice change which improves on crust removal, crusts can cause irritant cough and rarely breathing difficulty (obstruction due to crusts). Mucosal bleeding can happen with crust removal [12].

44.5.14 Treatment

Conservative management, treat the underlying cause, crust dissolving/loosening with laryngeal sprays (glucose in glycerin or oil of pine). Surgical management options include microlaryngoscopy and removal of crust [13].

44.6 Noninfectious Laryngitis in Adults

44.6.1 Chronic Laryngitis

Chronic inflammation of laryngeal mucosa, can be caused by smoking, repeated attacks of acute laryngitis, reflux laryngitis, postnasal drip in chronic sinusitis, allergic rhinitis and chronic allergic cough (Fig. 44.7).

Two types

(a) Hyperemic
(b) Hypertrophic

Metaplasia of pseudostratified epithelium to squamous type associated with hyperplasia and keratinization, implicated in development of granulomas, stenosis, recurrent laryngospasm, globus pharyngeus, cervical dysphagia, asthma, laryngeal carcinoma, and chronic cough, patients often deny heartburn.

Possible findings include

- Red arytenoids with inter-arytenoid mucosal hypertrophy
- Subglottic edema forming "pseudosulcus vocalis"
- Diffuse edema, Reinke edema, or mucosal thickening w/o significant erythema

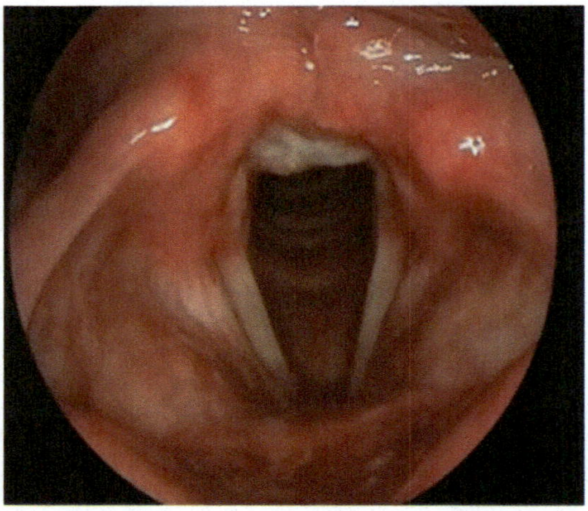

Fig. 44.7 Endoscopic photo of vocal folds in patient with reflux laryngitis showing inflamed mucosa and arytenoid erythema. (Image reprinted with permission from Elsevier: Journal of Voice, Detection of Chronic Laryngitis due to Laryngopharyngeal Reflux Using Color and Texture Analysis of Laryngoscopic Images, Daniel R. Witt, Huijun Chen, Jason D. Mielens, Kieran E. McAvoy, Fan Zhang, Matthew R. Hoffman, Jack J. Jiang, Jan 2014)

Gold standard for diagnosis: 24 h pH double probe monitoring [12, 18].

44.6.2 Traumatic Laryngitis

Vocal abuse, manifests as persistent coughing, muscle tension dysphonia, direct laryngeal injury, treatment: voice conservation and humidification [19].

44.6.3 Angioedema

Vascular dilation and increased vascular permeability, causes include, medications, as ACE inhibitors, insect bites, blood product transfusion, and infections, hereditary angioedema caused by deficiency of C1 esterase inhibitor.

Recurrent attacks of mucocutaneous edema.

44.6.4 Treatment

- O_2, epinephrine, corticosteroids, antihistamines, and minophylline (Fig. 44.8) [18, 20].

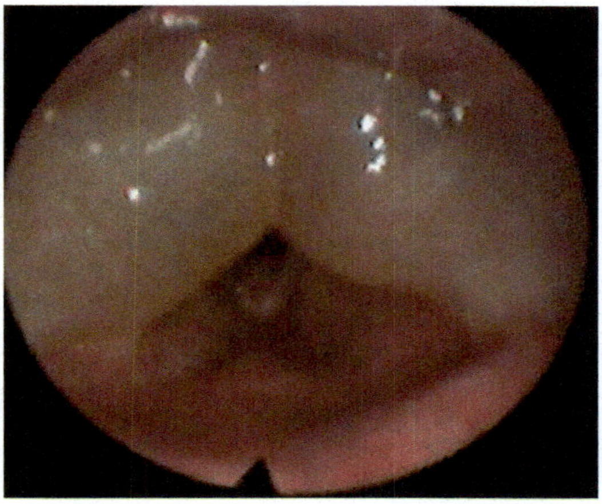

Fig. 44.8 Endoscopic view of edematous larynx. (Image reprinted with permission from Creative Commons Attribution 4.0 International: GMS Current Topics in Otorhinolaryngology - Head and Neck Surgery, Vol. 15, Evidence and evidence gaps of medical treatment of non-tumerous disease of head and neck, Murat Bas, Dec 2016)

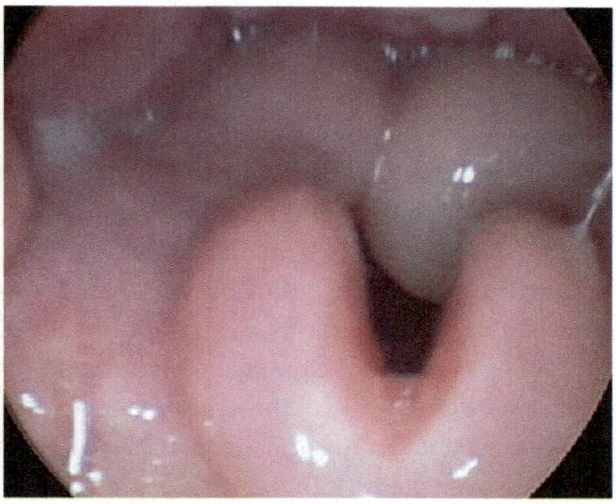

Fig. 44.9 Endoscopic view showing pale, edematous swellings of the epiglottis and arytenoid regions. (Image reprinted with permission from Springer: European Archives of otolaryngology, Clinically isolated laryngeal sarcoidosis, Christina Caroline Plaschke et al., Dec 4, 2010)

44.6.5 Amyloidosis

Manifests as diffuse mucosal thickening, submucosal nodules or polyploid lesion, usually involves supraglottic area, biopsy shows amorphous Congo red-staining material [21].

44.6.6 Sarcoidosis

Noncaseating granulomas and pale diffuse oedema of supraglottic area, diagnosis of exclusion, treatment with steroids (Fig. 44.9) [21, 22].

44.6.7 Wegener Granulomatosis

Necrotizing granulomas with vasculitis involving respiratory tract and kidneys.

Usually affects subglottic area, treatment with cyclophosphamide, corticosteroids, and optional TMP-SMX [21, 23].

44.6.8 Radiation Laryngitis

Erythematous, swollen larynx with exudate and crusting, treatment with hydration, humidification and acid suppression, steroids and antibiotics occasionally in certain circumstances.

Differential diagnosis includes, recurrent cancer, LPR, radio-necrosis, hypothyroidism [24].

44.6.9 Subglottic Stenosis

Subglottic stenosis is a narrowing of the airway below the vocal cords (sub glottis). It could be congenital or acquired. Congenital subglottic stenosis is discussed in pediatric section, subglottis is surrounded from all sides by the cricoid ring, which itself forms the only completely enclosed ring in the complete airway and is a very important contributor to the development of obstructive lesions. The tracheal and thyroid cartilages do not form complete rings and therefore have potential for physiological expansion [25].

44.6.9.1 Etiologies

- Trauma—blunt or penetrating, burns
- Iatrogenic—prolonged intubation, tracheostomy, radiation, surgical trauma
- Inflammatory disease/collagen vascular disease
  Granulomatosis with polyangiitis (Wegener's)
  Sarcoidosis

Amyloidosis
Relapsing polychondritis
Idiopathic

Post-intubation injury is the most frequent cause. It depends upon duration of intubation, endotracheal tube size, number of intubations, traumatic intubations, movement of endotracheal tube and infections. At subglottic level, following mucosal ischemia and ulceration produced by rigid wall of the endotracheal tube, healing occurs with the formation of firm fibrous scar resulting in varying degree of stenosis [25].

44.6.10 Factors Affect Subglottic Stenosis

44.6.10.1 Systemic

- Gastric acid reflux
- Immunocompromised patient
- Anemia
- Neutropenia
- Toxicity
- Poor perfusion
- Radiation therapy

44.6.10.2 Local Factors

- External trauma, penetrating and blunt
- Tracheotomy, especially a high tracheotomy or cricothyroidotomy
- Percutaneous tracheotomy (This has an emerging role as a cause.)
- Chondro-radionecrosis after radiation therapy; may occur up to 20 years later

44.6.10.3 Endotracheal Tube Factors

- Size of ETT, <20 cm H_2O pressure air leak is appropriate
- ETT material, silicone or polyvinyl chloride tube safest
- Duration of intubation, Adults <7–10 days, longer for premature infants
- Shearing motion of ETT, increased trauma to mucosa, increase traumatic changes
- Maintenance and care of ETT and patient, aggressive suctioning, endoscopy, reintubation

44.6.10.4 Infection and Chronic Inflammatory Diseases

Rare causes are tracheal infections including bacterial tracheitis, histoplasmosis and diphtheria and collagen vascular diseases including Wegener's granulomatosis, relapsing polychondritis, polyarteritis and scleroderma.

44.6.10.5 Laryngopharyngeal Reflux/Reflux Laryngitis

In 1983, Brain et al. suggest laryngopharyngeal reflux as a cause of subglottic stenosis. In 1991, Koufman did study on 32 patients, 73% of 32 patients had abnormal lower probe pH and 67% patients had upper probe pH abnormality. In 1998, Walner performed study which concludes that 74 pediatric patients with subglottic stenosis had three times greater incidence of LPR than general pediatric population. Cotton and O'Conner recommend GERD work up in all pediatric patient perioperatively and 3 months in postoperative asymptomatic patients [26, 27].

44.6.10.6 Idiopathic

The peculiar group of patients with subglottic stenosis is represented by those with idiopathic stenosis. This disease is characterized by an inflammatory cicatricle stenosis that occurs almost exclusively in women between third and fifth decade without other identifiable cause of airway stenosis (Fig. 44.10) [25].

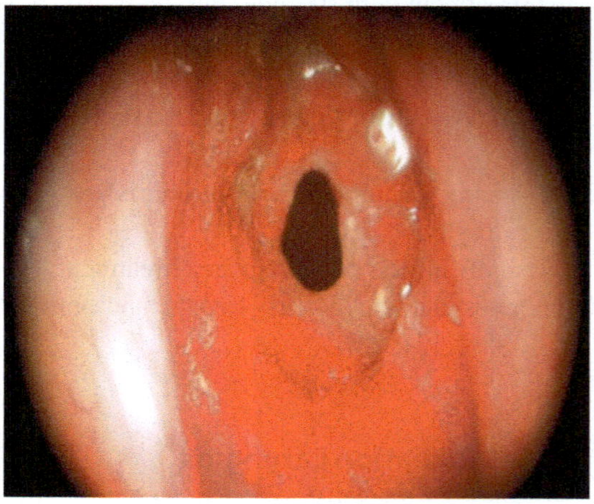

Fig. 44.10 Endoscopic image showing Subglottic stenosis. (Image reprinted with permission from Springer Nature: Springer eBook, Subglottic/Tracheal Stenosis: Laser/Endoscopic Management, Jan 1, 2008)

44.7 Clinical Presentation

Patients with acquired stenosis are diagnosed from a few days to 10 years or more following initial injury. The majority of cases are diagnosed within a year.

Patient presents with clinical symptoms as

Dyspnea, stridor, hoarseness, brassy cough, recurrent pneumonitis, cyanosis.

Many patients would have been diagnosed with asthma and recurrent bronchitis prior to discovery of stenosis. High suspicion is warranted with the onset of respiratory symptoms following intubation, regardless of the duration of intubation [25].

44.7.1 Grading System of Subglottic Stenosis

Grading system is proposed by Cotton Meyer. According to grades, surgical management varies.

Cotton-Meyers Classification

- Grade I: 0–50% obstruction
- Grade II: 51–70% obstruction
- Grade III: 71–99% obstruction
- Grade IV: 100% obstruction

44.7.2 Work Up

Flexible laryngotracheobronchoscopy to assess the stenosis diameter and length and to rule out any other airway problems.

CT neck and Thorax with 3D reconstruction of airway: study but it is not diagnostic.

MRI is useful in evaluating length and width of the stenotic region by coronal and sagittal views.

Laboratory studies: If no past history of trauma: rule out Wegener granulomatosis, relapsing polychondritis, syphilis, tuberculosis, sarcoidosis, leprosy, diphtheria, scleroma [25, 26].

44.7.3 Management

Nonsurgical treatment: for grade 1 and 2 stenosis, corticosteroids injections, dilatation, laser vaporization and stents can be used prior to definitive intervention. The endoscopic dilatation can be good in webs, but stenosis is more than 1–1.4 cm has high failure rates. Mitomycin-c local injection after dilatation can be tried to prevent recurrence, but results are not satisfactory [25].

Surgical treatment: Different interventions vary on length of resection, need for cartilage, and need for mucosal coverage.

- Anterior cricoid division with interposition graft (e.g., hyoid-sternohyoid muscle split clavicle muscle)
- Anterior an posterior cricoid split with stenting
- Resection of stenotic segment with end-to-end repair
- Staged free graft repair [25].

Acknowledgment Authors of the chapter would like to appreciate the help of Dr. Adham Aljariri, an ENT resident in Hamad medical corporation of his help and effort in editing the chapter.

References

1. Bansal M. Textbook of diseases of ear, nose and throat. 1st ed. New Delhi: Jaypee Brothers Medical Publishers Pvt. Ltd. p. 67.
2. Dhingra PL. Diseases of ear, nose and throat, head and neck surgery. 6th ed. Amsterdam: Elsevier. p. 285.
3. Bansal M. Textbook of diseases of ear, nose and throat. 1st ed. New Delhi: Jaypee Brothers Medical Publishers Pvt. Ltd. p. 63–4.
4. Dhingra PL. Diseases of ear, nose and throat, head and neck surgery. 6th ed. Amsterdam: Elsevier. p. 284.
5. Bansal M. Textbook of diseases of ear, nose and throat. 1st ed. New Delhi: Jaypee Brothers Medical Publishers Pvt. Ltd. p. 62–70.
6. Dhingra PL. Diseases of ear, nose and throat, head and neck surgery. 6th ed. Amsterdam: Elsevier. p. 282–5.
7. Bansal M. Textbook of diseases of ear, nose and throat. 1st ed. New Delhi: Jaypee Brothers Medical Publishers Pvt. Ltd. p. 478.

8. Dhingra PL. Diseases of ear, nose and throat, head and neck surgery. 6th ed. Amsterdam: Elsevier. p. 290.
9. Bansal M. Textbook of diseases of ear, nose and throat. 1st ed. New Delhi: Jaypee Brothers Medical Publishers Pvt. Ltd. p. 479.
10. Dhingra PL. Diseases of ear, nose and throat, head and neck surgery. 6th ed. Amsterdam: Elsevier. p. 289.
11. Bansal M. Textbook of diseases of ear, nose and throat. 1st ed. New Delhi: Jaypee Brothers Medical Publishers Pvt. Ltd. p. 480.
12. Bansal M. Textbook of diseases of ear, nose and throat. 1st ed. New Delhi: Jaypee Brothers Medical Publishers Pvt. Ltd. p. 481.
13. Dhingra PL. Diseases of ear, nose and throat, head and neck surgery. 6th ed. Amsterdam: Elsevier. p. 293.
14. Bansal M. Textbook of diseases of ear, nose and throat. 1st ed. New Delhi: Jaypee Brothers Medical Publishers Pvt. Ltd. p. 482.
15. Pasha R, Golub J. Otolaryngology & head and neck surgery clinical reference guide. 6th ed. San Diego: Plural Publishing. p. 112.
16. Mehanna HM, Kuo T, Chaplin J, Taylor G, Morton RP. Fungal laryngitis in immunocompetent patients. J Laryngol Otol. 2004;118:379–81.
17. Scheid SC, Anderson TD, Sataloff RT. Ulcerative fungal laryngitis. Ear Nose Throat J. 2003;82:168–9.
18. Dhingra PL. Diseases of ear, nose and throat, head and neck surgery. 6th ed. Amsterdam: Elsevier. p. 291.
19. Jaworek AJ, Earasi K, Lyons KM, Daggumati S, Hu A, Sataloff RT. Acute infectious laryngitis: a case series. Ear Nose Throat J. 2018;97(9):306–13.
20. Pasha R, Golub J. Otolaryngology & head and neck surgery clinical reference guide. 6th ed. San Diego: Plural Publishing. p. 115.
21. Pasha R, Golub J. Otolaryngology & head and neck surgery clinical reference guide. 6th ed. San Diego: Plural Publishing. p. 114.
22. Schwartzbauer HR, Tami TA. Ear, nose and throat manifestations of sarcoidosis. Otolaryngol Clin North Am. 2003;36:673–84.
23. Gluth MB, Shinners PA, Kasperbauer JL. Subglottic stenosis associated with Wegener's granulomatosis. Laryngoscope. 2003;113(8):1304–7.
24. Villari CR, Courey MS. Management of dysphonia after radiation. Otolaryngol Clin North Am. 2015;48(4):601–9. https://doi.org/10.1016/j.otc.2015.04.006.
25. Medscape: https://emedicine.medscape.com/article/865437-overview.
26. Elumalai G. "Subglottic stenosis" embryological basis and its clinical importance. Int J Insect Morphol Embryol. 2016;100:43458–61.
27. Up to date: https://www.uptodate.com/contents/clinical-presentation-diagnostic-evaluation-and-management-of-central-airway-obstruction-in-adults.

Benign Lesions of the Vocal Folds

45

Mayed Radi

45.1 Introduction

Hoarseness (dysphonia) is a change in the quality of the voice. Hoarseness that lasts more than 4 weeks, especially if patient smokes need to be investigated with an endoscopic evaluation. Also hoarseness of voice can cause a severe change in voice lasting more than a few days. Change in quality of voice can be raspy, strained, breathy, weak, higher or lower in pitch, inconsistent, fatigued, or shaky, with or without difficulty breathing and pain when speaking.

45.2 Types of Office-Based Procedures

In order to have a good evaluation of the patient complaint, any case with hoarseness of voice, we need to have a specialized clinic for voice and swallowing fully equipped with excellent staff to run the clinic. We can do too many procedures in this clinic whether for diagnosis or treatment such us:

1. Trans nasal Flexible Laryngoscopy w/w out Biopsy
2. Injection Laryngoplasty (vocal cord Augmentation)
3. KTP Laser procedures
4. Trans Nasal Tracheoscopy (TNT)
5. Trans Nasal Esophagoscopy (TNE)
6. FEES & FEEST tests
7. Laryngeal EMG

M. Radi (✉)
Laryngology, Hamad Medical Corporation, Doha, Qatar
e-mail: mradi@hamad.qa

45.3 Types of Laryngeal Lesions

Polyp (most common): mucoid/angiomatous, nodules, cyst: mucus retention and dermoid, vocal process granuloma, scar, sulcus vocalis, recurrent respiratory papilloma, polypoid cordites (Reinke's edema), leukoplakia/keratosis. Also there are other lesions but they are rare.

Acute Laryngitis

- Phono trauma—vocal fold edema and possibly hemorrhage due to vocal misuse, overuse, or abuse
- Viral—most common cause of acute laryngitis. Supportive care—rehydration, voice rest, +/− steroids. Croup—children <3 year, most commonly parainfluenza virus
- Bacterial—epiglottitis due to Hemophilus influenzae, decreased incidence with H.I vaccine

  Intubation in controlled setting or awake tracheostomy if respiratory distress

A. Al-Qahtani et al. (eds.), *Textbook of Clinical Otolaryngology*,
https://doi.org/10.1007/978-3-030-54088-3_45

- Fungal—most commonly Candida albicans, dysphonia with white plaques and erythema on the TVFs
- Immunocompromised patients/immunocompetent patients with use of recent use of broad-spectrum antibiotics or inhaled corticosteroids
- Angioedema—inflammatory reaction with vascular dilation and increased vascular permeability

  Causes: 1—Hereditary: C1 esterase inhibitor deficiency. 2—Nonhereditary causes: medications (ACE-I most commonly), food, insect bites, transfusions, infections
- Treatment: oxygenation, epinephrine, steroids, antihistamines

Chronic Laryngitis

- Bacterial—superinfection of injured larynx; commonly Staphylococcus aureus
- Fungal—Blastomycosis—Coccidioidomycosis
- Mycobacterial—Tuberculosis (TB)—Highly associated with active pulmonary TB
- Granulomatous or ulcerative lesions—leprosy (Hansen's Disease)—Mycobacterium leprae
- Laryngopharyngeal reflux (LPR): Symptoms: hoarseness (92%), throat clearing (50%), cough (44%), globus (33%), dysphagia (27%). Over 50% deny heartburn. Laryngeal findings: diffuse laryngeal edema, VF edema, subglottic edema, erythema or hyperemia, ventricular obliteration, posterior commissure hypertrophy (pachydermia), granuloma, thick endolaryngeal secretions

  Diagnosis: gold standard is 24-h dual-probe pH-metry and impedance, Reflux Finding Score (RFS) > 8 suggestive, Reflux Symptom Index (RSI) > 13 suggestive

  Treatment: (PPI) + Change of life style eating habits , Referral to GIT in refractory cases
- Other chronic diseases: Sarcoid—Amyloidosis non-Wegener's granulomatosis

45.4 Vocal Cord Nodules

It is a bilateral, symmetric epithelial swelling of the anterior/mid third of the true vocal folds. It can affect children, adolescents, women, professionals with high voice demands (teachers). Usually arise at the junction of (anterior/middle third) with maximal shearing and repeated collision forces resulting in congestion and edema lead to epithelial hyperplasia. Also, chronic hoarseness and repeated episodes of progressively severe voice loss. Professional singers have inability to sing high notes softly.

Diagnosis: fiber-optic examination/video stroboscope.

Treatment: voice rest, speech therapy, microsurgery in longstanding nodules and speech therapy failure.

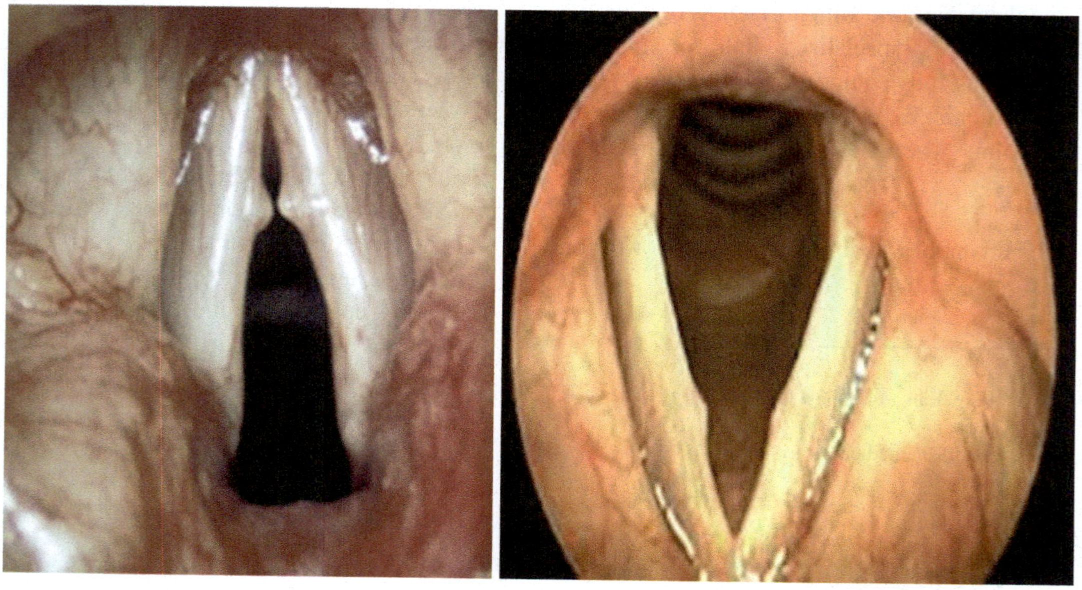

45.5 Vocal Cord Cysts

It is either

1. Mucus retention—(most common) obstructed mucous gland duct (usually during URI or voice overuse)
2. Epidermoid—congenital cell rests in subepithelium from fourth or sixth branchial arch

The cyst can also irritate the contralateral vocal cord, producing a reactive lesion on the opposite vocal cord.

Diagnosis: with video stroboscope, vocal fold asymmetry, significantly decreased or absent mucosal wave which is the most important parameter in differentiating cysts from polyps (diminished or absent in cysts compared to present in 80% of polyps).

Treatment: microsurgery. Keep in mind that cyst recurs if epithelium left behind during surgical excision.

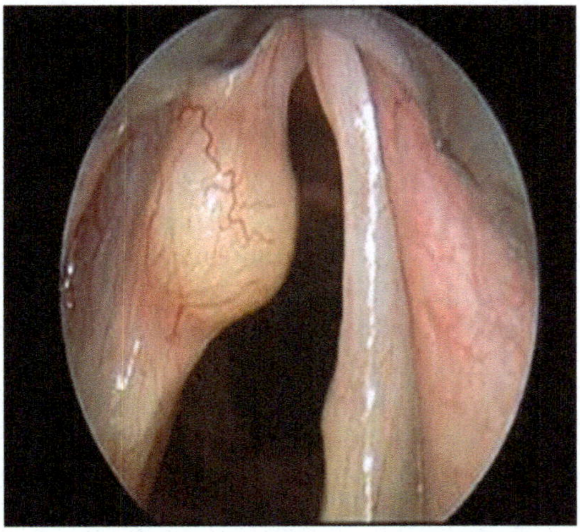

45.6 Vocal Process Granulomas

Pathological lesion informs of inflammatory tissue arising from the perichondrium of the arytenoid cartilage in response to trauma of the arytenoid perichondrium. It occurs at vocal process of the arytenoid, not on the membranous vocal fold. May or may not cause dysphonia. Prolonged or repetitive contact trauma leads to mucosal ulceration, cartilage exposure and inflammation. Mostly unilateral but it can be bilateral.

Risk factors: repeated trauma from hyper adduction of the arytenoid cartilage from excessive clearance of the throat habit, laryngopharyngeal reflux (LPR), chronic cough, throat clearing, post Endo tracheal intubation (contact ulceration).

Diagnosis: fiber-optic examination / video stroboscope.

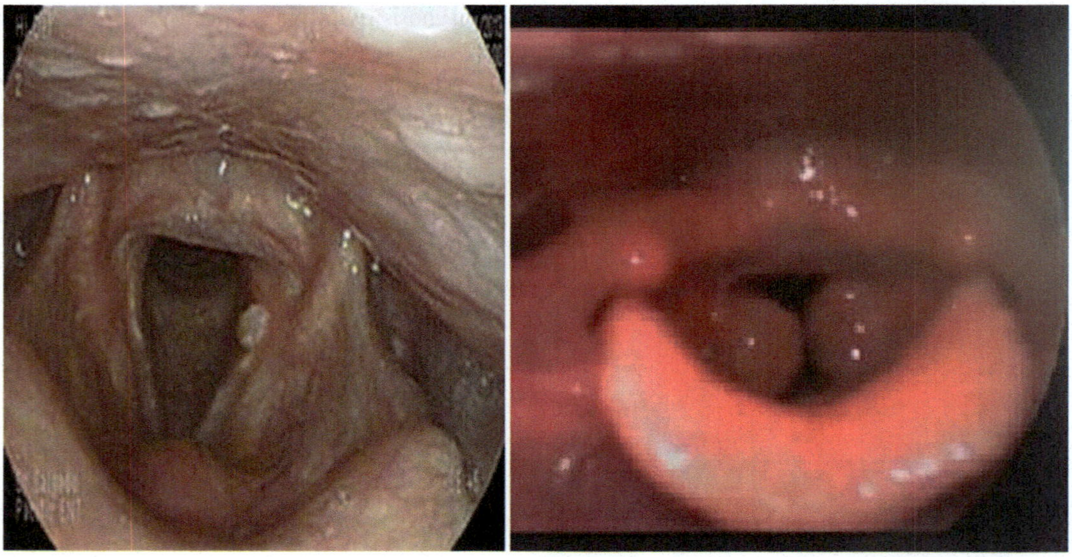

45.6.1 Treatment

1. Conservative: treat LPR (laryngo pharyngo reflux), cough, underlying condition, speech therapy, will often spontaneously resolve over several months. Botox to thyroarytenoid muscle, intralesional corticosteroids
2. Indications for surgery (CO_2 laser or cold knife): enlarging granuloma, compromised voice, breathing or swallowing difficulty or to rule out malignancy

45.7 Sulcus Vocals

The term sulcus vocalis is used specifically to describe a groove or in folding of mucosa along the surface of the vocal fold. In the area of the sulcus, the mucosa is scarred down to the underlying vocal ligament, giving it a retracted appearance, which leads to epithelial scar with loss of superficial lamina propria.

Etiology: unknown but either congenital or acquired by vocal trauma.

Vocal impairment usually due to stiffness of vocal fold and glottic insufficiency.

Symptoms: hoarseness with strained, breathy voice.

Diagnosis: video stroboscope restriction of mucosal wave.

Treatment: difficult to treat with unreliable outcomes.

Options include: speech therapy, excision, collagen or steroid injection, mucosal "slicing" technique, elevation with submucosal grafting, endoscopic fat injection.

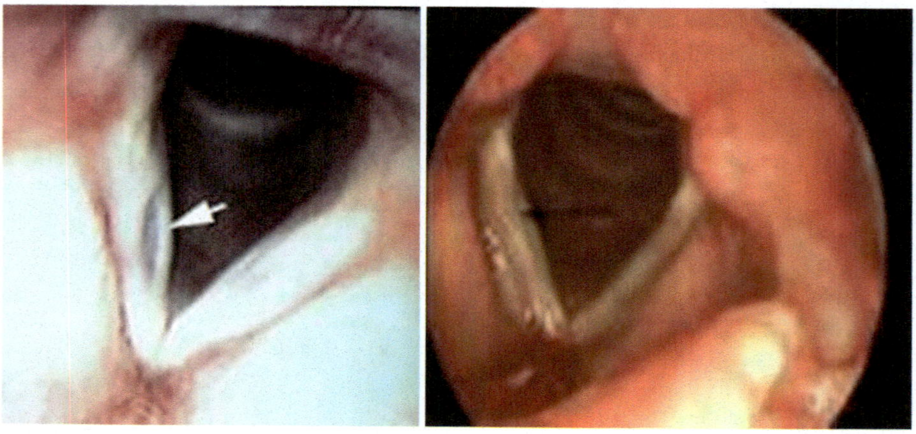

45.8 Recurrent Respiratory Papilloma (RRP)

Most commonly arise at transition between columnar and squamous epithelium. It is the second most common cause of hoarseness in children. Human papilloma virus (HPV) infection (subtypes 6 and 11); 2% likelihood of malignant degeneration (subtypes 16 and 18). Juvenile—onset—Adult-onset.

Symptoms: hoarseness, stridor (inspiratory or biphasic), dyspnea, dysphagia.

Diagnosis: fiber optic examination/video stroboscope.

Treatment: surgical—laryngeal micro-derider, laser CO_2/KTP.

Keep in mind to: avoid tracheostomy.

Adjuvant therapy—HPV vaccine (preventative).

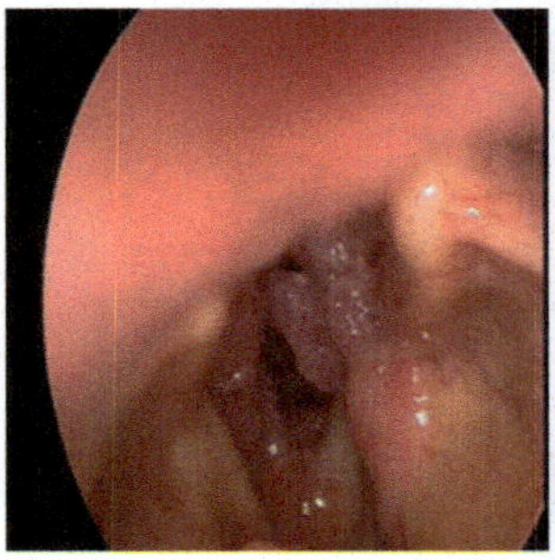

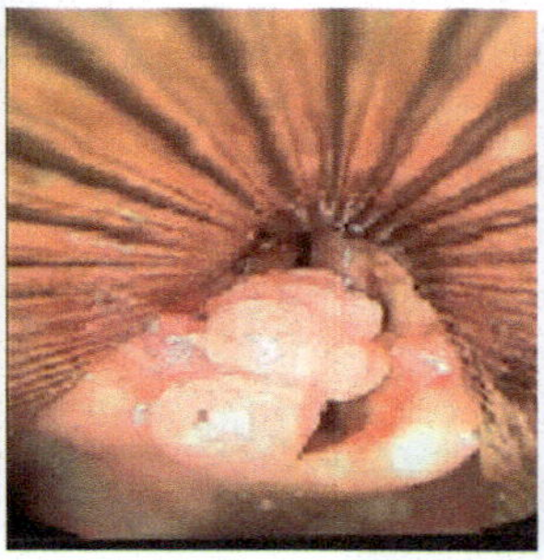

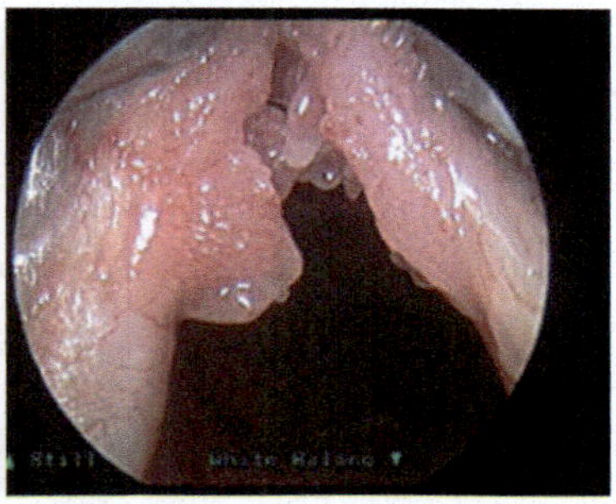

45.9 Leukoplakia

It is a spectrum of diseases affecting vocal fold epithelium (hyperkeratosis, dysplasia, early verrucous changes). 8–14% likelihood of malignant degeneration. Caused by chronic irritation like smoking and genetic predisposition.

Symptoms: hoarseness of voice, breathy voice.

Diagnosis: video stroboscope restriction of mucosal wave.

Treatment: surgical—eradicate disease but preserve surrounding normal anatomy and voice quality.

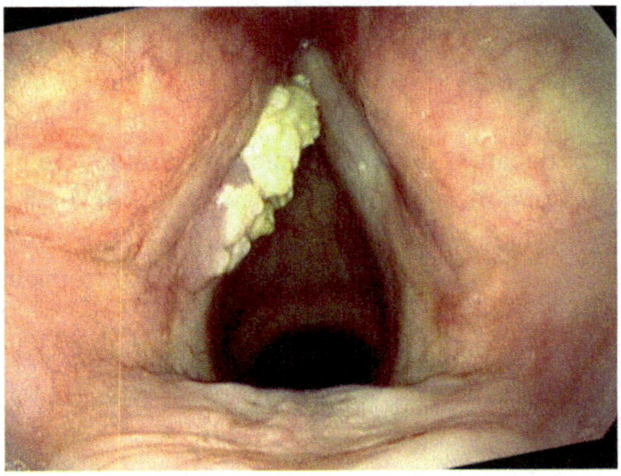

45.10 Ectasias

Vascular lesion of the true vocal fold distinguished by a coalescent hemangiomatous appearance.

Seen in voice professionals, post-radiotherapy. It presented with hoarseness of voice.

Etiology: vocal abuse, trauma. Repeated trauma leads to new blood vessel formation and weakened blood vessel walls.

Diagnosis: video stroboscope.

Treatment: treat underlying trauma-LPR, cough. Stop anticoagulation if possible. Speech therapy.

Surgical indications: enlarging lesion, recurrent hemorrhage, development of a mass. Use pulse dye laser or KTP laser, or surgical excision.

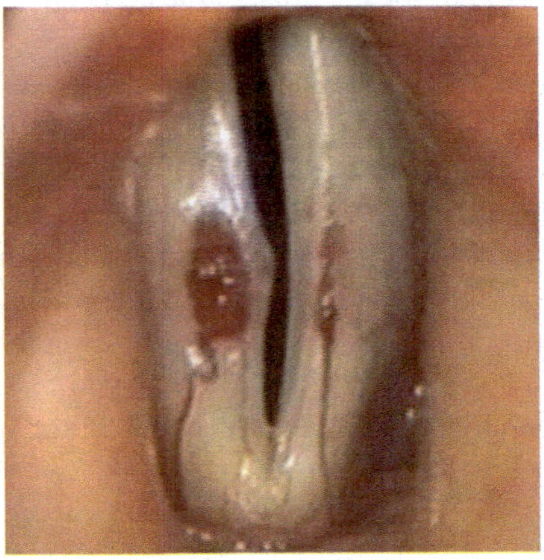

45.11 Polypoid Cordites (Reinke's Edema)

Is an accumulation of a gelatinous type of fluid throughout the superficial aspect of the lamina propria.

Usually, it is bilateral seen in chronic irritant exposure (smoking 95%, LPR, occupational exposures). It is out pouching of membranous vocal folds with edematous appearance. It leads to hoarseness and some time with shortness of breath if it is severe.

Medical treatment involves smoking cessation and control of the LPR. Surgical treatment used to reduce the airway obstruction. Preservation of the epithelium and some of the lamina properia to preserve mucosal wave.

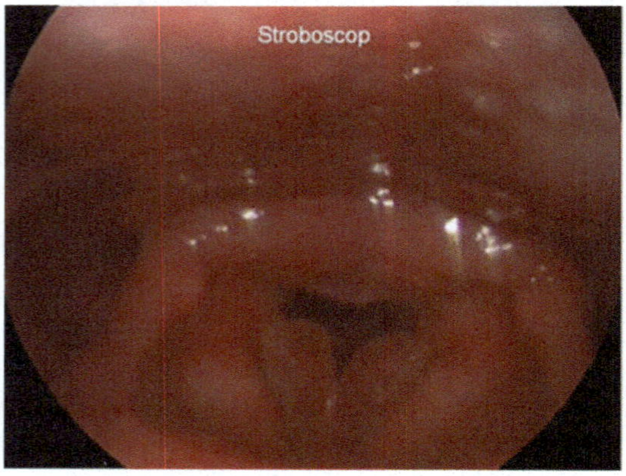

45.12 Rheumatoid Nodules

A rare condition. RA can cause inflammatory fixation of cricoarytenoid joint or inflammatory nodules on vocal fold. It is a bilateral disease which leads to dysphonia and/or stridor.

Symptoms: hoarseness, pain, globus, referred otalgia.

Serology: elevated ESR, RF, decreased complement level, abnormal lupus panel.

Diagnosis: video stroboscope shows immobile arytenoid with erythema and edema (CA joint fixation). RA nodules have "bamboo larynx" appearance with bilateral white stripes perpendicular to the free edge of the vocal fold.

Treatment: medical—steroids, anti-inflammatory medication; surgical—excision of nodule.

In case of severe airway obstruction may necessitate tracheotomy.

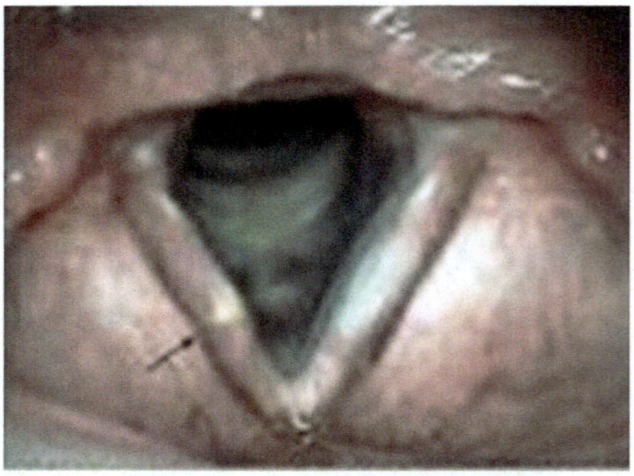

45.13 Vocal Cord Scar

Repeated inflammation, vocal trauma, vocal hemorrhage, presence of intracordal cyst (ruptured epidermoid) leads to intracordal scar. Also it may occur after vocal surgery involving lamina propria, use of CO_2 laser, repeated epithelial procedures.

Diagnosis: video stroboscope: markedly reduced or absent mucosal wave (asymmetric).

Treatment: difficult to treat either excision vs. steroid injections.

45.14 Vocal Hygiene

There is some evidence that vocal hygiene education may be effective in the management of hoarseness. The vocal hygiene programs evaluated included:

- Education in environmental changes (e.g., humidification of the air; avoidance of smoke, dust, and other inhaled irritants)
- Behavior changes (e.g., avoidance of frequent coughing or throat clearing)
- Vocal habit changes (e.g., avoidance of shouting or speaking loudly for prolonged periods)

- Dietary changes (e.g., increased fluid intake; avoidance of large meals, excessive caffeine and alcohol use, and spicy foods). Although the overall education programs were shown to be beneficial, the value of any of the specific components (e.g., individual dietary recommendations or behavior changes) has not been demonstrated

Take Home Messages

- Since many voice disorders are caused by problems in the voice box and/or throat, a careful and detailed examination of the voice box and throat is key to the identification of the cause or causes of voice disorders.
- Video stroboscope is a technique designed to allow the examiner to get information on the vibratory nature of the vocal cords. The technique involves the use of a strobe light which is linked to the frequency of the patient's voice.
- By using the information from the stroboscope exam, the examiner can gather information such as the depth of cancer invasion, the presence of scar or stiffness in a vocal cord, or the relative tone of the vocal cords.
- These technologies provide valuable images to be recorded on video or other media formats, permitting examiners to review the images of the voice box frame by frame, capture still and close-up images, and re-review images with members of the voice care team. Patients can also view the recorded images and see the reason(s) for their voice problems.

Bibliography

1. Rosen CA, et al.. Benign mid-membranous vocal fold lesion nomenclature paradigm. In AAO-HNS annual meeting, Orlando, FL, 23 Sept 2003.
2. Derkay CS, Hester RP, Burke B, Carron J, Lawson L. Analysis of a staging assessment system for prediction of surgical interval in recurrent respiratory papillomatosis. Int J Pediatr Otorhinolaryngol. 2004;68:1493–8.
3. Schweinfurth JM, Powitzky E, Ossoff RH. Regression of laryngeal dysplasia after serial micro-flap excision. Ann Otol Rhinol Laryngol. 2001;110:811–4.
4. Thekdi AA, Rosen CA. Surgical treatment of benign vocal fold lesions. Curr Opin Otolaryngol Head Neck Surg. 2003;10:492–6.
5. Zeitels SM, Hillman RE, Bunting GW, Vaughn T. Reinke's edema: phonatory mechanisms and management strategies. Ann Otol Rhinol Laryngol. 1997;106:533–43.
6. Hochman I, Sataloff RT, Hillman RE, Zeitels SM. Ectasias and varices of the vocal fold: clearing the striking zone. Ann Otol Rhinol Laryngol. 1999;108:10–6.
7. Welham NV, Rousseau B, Ford CN, Bless DM. Tracking outcomes after phono surgery for sulcus vocals: a case report. J Voice. 2003;17:571–8.
8. Rosen CA. Vocal fold scar: evaluation and treatment. Otolaryngol Clin North Am. 2000;33:1081–6.
9. Verdolini K, Rosen CA, Branski R. Classification manual of voice disorders. Mahwah, NJ: Lawrence Erlbaum Associates; 2005.

46 Vocal Cord Paralysis

Rashid Al-Abri and Suresh Pillai

Key Points
By the end of the chapter, the student should be able to:

- Understand the anatomy and nerve supply of the laryngeal musculature.
- Appreciate the pathophysiology of vocal cord paralysis.
- Recognize clinically the two types of vocal cord paralysis, unilateral and bilateral.
- Outline the various management options for treating this condition.

R. Al-Abri (✉)
ORL Division, Department of Surgery, College of Medicine and Health Sciences, Sultan Qaboos University, Muscat, Oman

Medical Education and Informatics Department, College of Medicine and Health Sciences, Sultan Qaboos University, Muscat, Oman

S. Pillai
ORL Division, Department of Surgery, College of Medicine and Health Sciences, Sultan Qaboos University, Muscat, Oman

Department of Otolaryngology and Head and Neck Surgery, Kasturba Medical College, Manipal Academy of Higher Education (MAHE), Manipal, India

46.1 Introduction

Vocal cord paralysis or vocal fold paralysis, (VFP), refers to decreased or absence of movement of one or both vocal cords. There is usually a neurological basis for this, and it can severely affect the quality of life for the patient.

Paralysis of one or both cords can affect laryngeal function in terms of breathing, phonation, and swallowing and the symptoms will, in turn, depend on whether one cord or both are paralyzed. This variability in symptoms between unilateral and bilateral paralysis is related to the actions of the vocal cords which include abduction for respiration and adduction for phonation and prevention of aspiration.

46.2 Pathophysiology

In a majority of cases, vocal cord impairment is due to damage to the peripheral nerves supplying the larynx. In a minority of cases, it can result from central nervous system damage or from cricoarytenoid joint instability or fixation due to laryngeal trauma following procedures such as intubation.

Mild injury to the recurrent laryngeal nerve produces demyelination which is proportional to the extent of the injury. Remyelination over the axon restores nerve conduction and function. If the injury is more severe, as in crush injury or

A. Al-Qahtani et al. (eds.), *Textbook of Clinical Otolaryngology*,
https://doi.org/10.1007/978-3-030-54088-3_46

nerve section, then Wallerian degeneration sets in within 24 h distally, and recovery will depend on the number of viable fibers present and the gap between the distal and proximal segments.

Regeneration of the recurrent laryngeal nerve and the final functional outcome of the vocal cord will depend on the proportion of viable adductor and adductor fibers.

The human larynx has a strong tendency for reinnervation [1]. In fact, reinnervation seems to be the rule rather than the exception [2]. But denervation and reinnervation do not follow the all or none phenomenon. The final state of vocal cord paralysis probably results from partial denervation or complete denervation with variable patterns of reinnervation. This has two important clinical implications.

First, different degrees of reinnervation is responsible for the different positions of the vocal cord after paralysis.

Second, the clinical implication is that the natural tendency for reinnervation maybe responsible for the gradual improvement in the voice over time in unilateral paralysis of vocal cords. A reinnervated vocal cord will retain the muscle bulk and tone rather than undergo atrophy which results in poor quality voice [3].

46.3 Unilateral Vocal Cord Paralysis

Unilateral vocal cord paralysis involves a lesion either at the brainstem, along the course of the vagus nerve or in the recurrent laryngeal nerve. The vagus arises from the nucleus ambiguous within the brainstem (medulla), exits the skull base through the jugular foramen and descends through the neck in the carotid sheath, giving off three branches, the pharyngeal branch, superior laryngeal nerve, and the recurrent laryngeal nerve. The internal branch of the superior laryngeal nerve provides sensation to the larynx down to the level of the vocal cords. The external branch of the superior laryngeal nerve supplies the cricothyroid muscle which adjusts the length of the vocal cord and thereby controls the pitch of the voice.

The recurrent laryngeal nerve arises from the vagus in the upper part of the thorax. On the left side it winds around the aortic arch and on the right, around the subclavian artery and travels back up toward the larynx in the tracheoesophageal groove. The recurrent laryngeal nerve innervates the ipsilateral posterior cricoarytenoid, lateral cricoarytenoid, thyroarytenoid, and interarytenoid (unpaired), muscles. All the intrinsic muscles of the larynx are supplied by the recurrent laryngeal nerve except the cricothyroid which is supplied by the external branch of the superior laryngeal nerve. So, injury to the ipsilateral recurrent laryngeal nerve leads to complete paralysis of the vocal cord. However, the interarytenoid muscle is unpaired and has bilateral innervation which can lead to adduction of the vocal cord during ipsilateral recurrent laryngeal nerve (RLN) paralysis. The cricothyroid muscle does not contribute to adduction or abduction (Fig. 46.1).

46.3.1 Etiology

There are a number of causes for unilateral vocal cord palsy. Surgical iatrogenic causes are one of the most important etiological factors. These include thyroid surgery, esophagectomy with RLN injury in the tracheoesophageal groove and anterior cervical procedures (Table 46.1)

46.3.2 History

46.3.2.1 Voice Quality

The main symptom caused by the paralyzed vocal cord is hoarseness of voice or dysphonia. The range of voice disturbance can vary from mild hoarseness to complete aphonia in poorly compensated cases. The factors affecting the final voice quality are muscle tone and the position of the paralyzed cord. Some develop a high pitched voice due to compensatory contraction of the ipsilateral cricothyroid muscle. This is known as a "paralytic falsetto" [2].

Some patients may complain of swallowing difficulty along with aspiration, if the main trunk

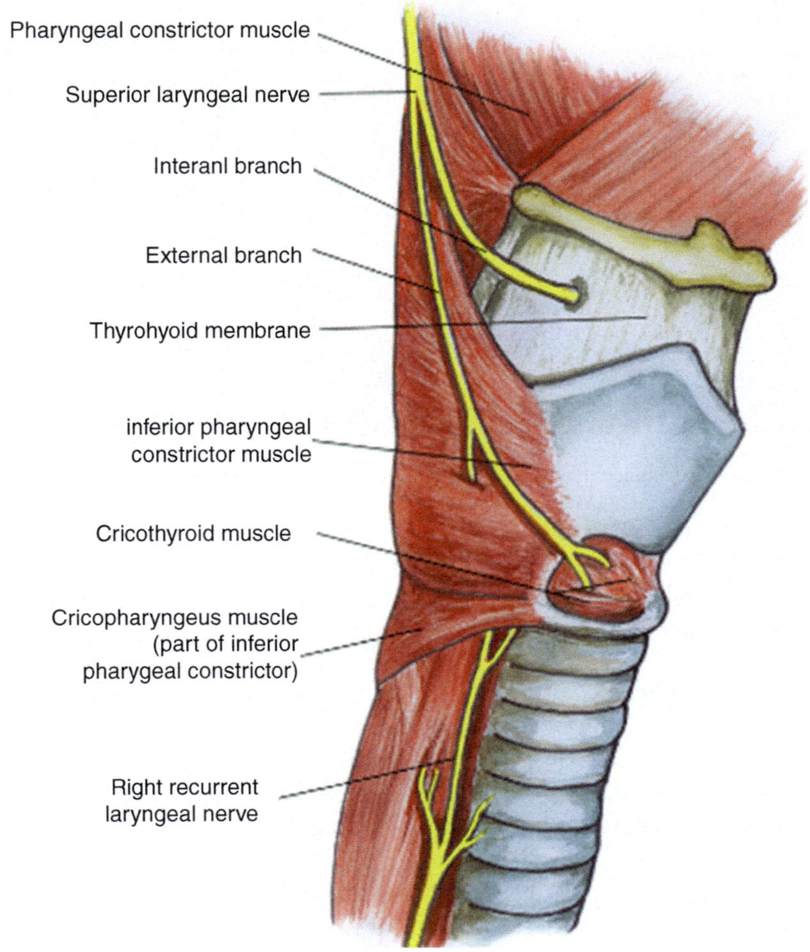

Fig. 46.1 Shows laryngeal muscles and innervation

Table 46.1 Illustrates etiology of unilateral RLN palsy

Iatrogenic causes or surgical trauma
Thyroid surgery
Esophagectomy
Anterior cervical procedures
Carotid endarterectomy
Carotid artery bypass grafting
Pulmonary resection
Malignancy of lung
Idiopathic (?Herpes simplex infection)
Neurological—stroke (brainstem)
Intubation—arytenoid cartilage dislocation

of the vagus is involved, due to denervation of the pharyngeal constrictors and loss of sensation because of involvement of the superior laryngeal nerve.

There may be complaints regarding shortness of breath due to air leak while talking because of poor closure of the glottic airway with a unilateral paralyzed vocal cord.

46.3.3 Clinical Examination

46.3.3.1 Neck

Neck examination must be performed to rule out neck nodes or thyroid enlargement or any other mass leading to RLN palsy. Movement of the soft palate should be observed. If vagus is affected, the palate will move toward the uninvolved side.

Cranial nerve exam should be performed, especially that of the lower four cranial nerves to

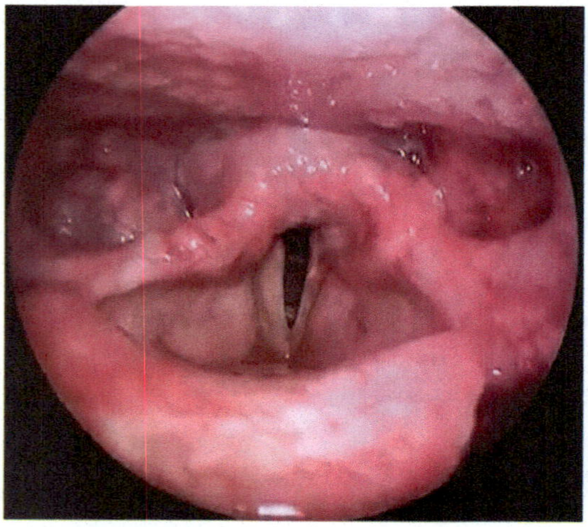

Fig. 46.2 A flexible laryngoscopic examination demonstrates right vocal cord paralysis and left vocal cord abduction

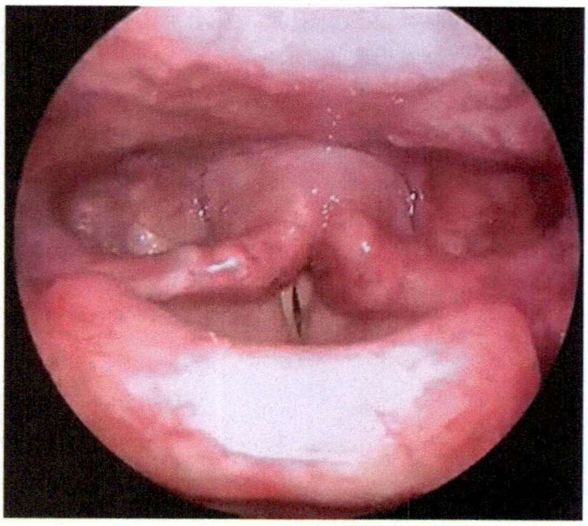

Fig. 46.3 A flexible laryngoscopic examination demonstrates right vocal cord paralysis and left cord adduction

determine whether paralysis is part of a generalized neuropathy.

46.3.3.2 Larynx

Clinical examination of the larynx should start with the help of a flexible laryngoscopic examination to view vocal cord mobility. Rigid endoscopic examination of the larynx with the tongue protruded and grasped with a gauze can alter the natural movements of the cords. The patient should be asked to say "eee" to adduct the vocal cords. A paralyzed vocal cord can be in a variety of positions including median, paramedian, and cadaveric. The final vocal cord position is dependent on the degree of reinnervation and synkinesis (Figs. 46.2 and 46.3).

Another clinical sign that maybe obtained is the anterior displacement or an overhanging arytenoid cartilage on the side of the paralysis. This maybe due to complete denervation or poor reinnervation of the thyroarytenoid muscle.

The degree of air leak and therefore of glottic incompetence can be obtained through the maximal phonation time (MPT). The patient is asked to take a deep breath and say "eee" for as long as possible. In a normal individual, MPT is 25 s. But with a paralyzed vocal cord, the duration can be reduced to 10 or 5 s, depending on the degree of glottic air leak.

46.3.3.3 Investigation

Imaging studies are useful in cases where no cause can be determined for the vocal cord palsy. A CT scan with contrast or magnetic resonance imaging (MRI), extending from the skull base to upper thorax will help in pinpointing lesions affecting the RLN. In case a high vagal lesion is suspected because of palatal paralysis and vocal cord paralysis, the brainstem can also be included in the radiological investigation [4].

Laryngeal electromyography is useful for determining prognosis and identifying suspected case of vocal cord paresis. It is useful if done between 1 and 6 months after the onset of paralysis. It is also able to detect synkinesis due to misdirected reinnervation following injury.

46.3.3.4 Treatment

There are three treatment plans to be considered in cases of unilateral RLN paralysis [2].

1. Observation for 6–12 months in the hope that there will be reinnervation.
2. Patient referred for speech and if required, swallowing therapy.
3. Surgery:
   (a) Temporary—Injection augmentation with filler substance into the vocal cords.
   (b) Permanent—Medialization thyroplasty with or without arytenoid adduction.

The usual waiting time recommended before surgical intervention with permanent methods is 6–9 months.

46.3.4 Surgical Treatment

46.3.4.1 Temporary—Injection Augmentation

Temporary materials can be used as a stop gap arrangement while waiting for the return of function. Gelfoam is short acting (4–6 weeks), therefore rarely used. Other materials that can be tried include carboxymethylcellulose whose duration of action is 1–3 months, calcium hydroxyapatite (18 months), and hyaluronic acid (2–4 months). The injection into the vocal cord is at the posterior aspect of the vocal cord lateral to the vocal process, deep into the thyroarytenoid muscle avoiding Reinke's space. Injection into Reinke's space can lead to loss of vibration of the vocal cord.

This technique of injection laryngoplasty can be done under local anesthesia using a flexible or rigid endoscope either through an oral route or external cutaneous route [5]. Local anesthesia allows for vocal feedback during injection. This can be done under general anesthesia also with the aid of a microscope.

46.3.4.2 Permanent-Framework Surgery

Framework surgery includes medialization thyroplasty or type 1 thyroplasty described by Isshiki and arytenoid adduction.

Type 1 thyroplasty is a reversible technique that can be performed under local anesthesia. Medialization materials that can be used include Gore-Tex strips, silastic blocks, hydroxyapatite and titanium implants. The choice of material depends on the surgeon's preference as there is not much advantage of one material over another. Complications of this procedure include postoperative dysphonia due to edema or submucosal hemorrhage and airway compromise. Postoperative steroids (dexamethasone) given 8 and 16 h postoperatively will reduce airway edema (Fig. 46.4). Both Gore-Tex and Silastic are reversible implants.

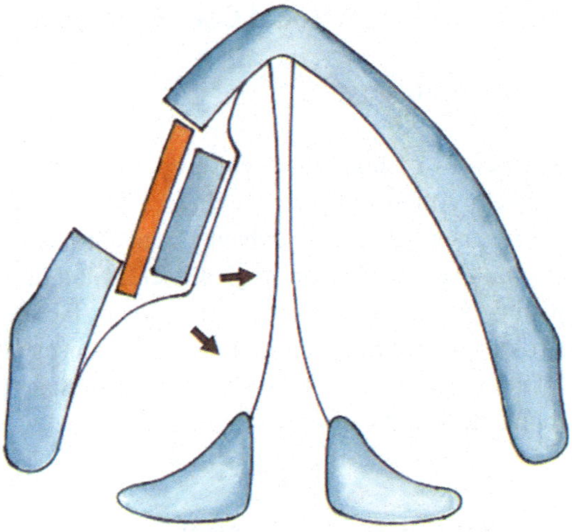

Fig. 46.4 Drawing illustrates medialization thyroplasty with a silastic block (orange) to push vocal cord medially

46.3.4.3 Arytenoid Adduction

This can be combined with medialization thyroplasty. In this procedure, the arytenoid is adducted by taking a suture through the muscular process of the arytenoid and stitching it anteriorly to the thyroid cartilage. This has the effect of medializing the vocal cord.

Laryngeal Reinnervation

Reinnervation procedures are done to establish neural continuity when the RLN is traumatized. This includes end to end anastomosis, hypoglossal to RLN anastomosis, and ansa cervicalis to RLN anastomosis.

> Unilateral vocal cord paralysis is usually caused by thyroid surgery. The cord can be in the median, paramedian or even cadaveric position depending on the degree of reinnervation. A CT scan with MRI will help in ruling out a neck pathology. If there is no movement seen, even after waiting for 12 months, treatment is surgery.

46.4 Bilateral Vocal Cord Paralysis

46.4.1 Etiology

Most cases of bilateral vocal cord paralysis are caused by thyroid surgery. Other causes include malignancy of the esophagus and bronchus, trauma to the neck, neurological factors and idiopathic causes. Among the neurologic factors, stroke is a leading cause. Idiopathic causes of bilateral vocal cord paralysis are rare compared to the unilateral causes.

46.4.2 Clinical Presentation

In bilateral RNL palsy, the clinical presentation is more dramatic than in unilateral RLN palsy. The symptoms can vary from difficulty in breathing on exertion to mild to severe stridor depending on the position of the vocal cords. These symptoms can appear immediately or after a few days or weeks. The glottic airway can range from 1 to 3 mm. The voice of the patient will be normal.

Most patients will give a clinical history of having undergone a surgical procedure in the neck, often a thyroidectomy. It is important to rule out a history of rheumatoid arthritis and intubation when evaluating a patient with bilateral paralysis (Fig. 46.5).

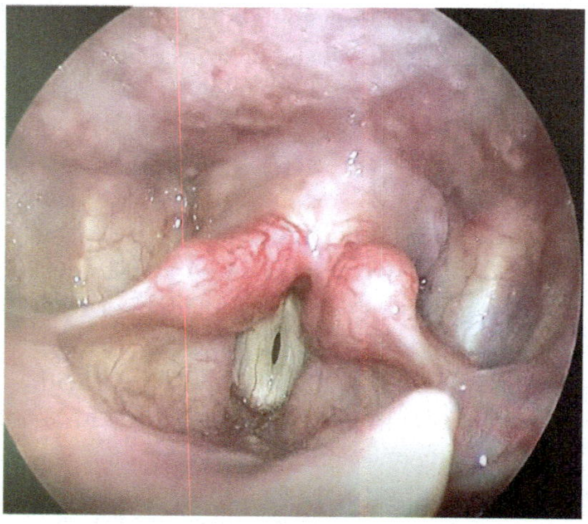

Fig. 46.5 A flexible laryngoscopic examination demonstrates bilateral vocal cord palsy

46.4.3 Clinical Examination

This includes a detailed examination of the head and neck and neurological exam which includes the cranial nerves.

46.4.4 Investigations

Major workup is not required in straight forward cases of surgical trauma. Radiology plays a role in children because the most common causes are neurological like hydrocephalus and Arnold–Chiari malformation in 40% of cases, so an MRI would be useful [6].

46.4.5 Laryngoscopy

This can be carried out under local anesthesia for assessment of vocal cord mobility, and general anesthesia for arytenoid joint fixation and interarytenoid scarring. This examination should be performed without an endotracheal tube in place.

46.4.6 Management

46.4.6.1 Immediate Airway Management

Since most patients will have some degree of airway distress due to the adducted position of the vocal cords, the immediate treatment is to secure the airway. Endotracheal intubation is the preferred method followed by shifting the patient to the intensive care unit, especially after thyroidectomy. If bilateral vocal cord paralysis is still present after 5–10 days, a tracheostomy should be considered.

46.4.7 Reversible Treatments

46.4.7.1 Tracheostomy

This allows for relief of airway obstruction and gives adequate time to see if there is spontaneous recovery of vocal cord mobility within 6–12 months. If within this time the cords are still paralyzed, permanent surgery may have to be undertaken.

46.4.7.2 Extralaryngeal Suture Lateralization [7]

This is performed using a non -absorbable suture taken through the skin of the neck so that it comes out above the vocal process with in the endolarynx and then taken below the cord till it comes out from the neck where it is tied over a button externally.

46.4.7.3 Laryngeal Botox Injection

If injected into the thyroarytenoid—lateral crico-arytenoid muscular complex, will result in some airway improvement that lasts for 2–4 months.

46.4.8 Permanent Surgical Methods

46.4.8.1 Laser Cordotomy

Endoscopic carbon dioxide [8] or KTP 532 laser cordotomy will provide adequate airway. The voice will worsen but is adequate enough to allow for normal conversation to take place. Laser beam is used to vaporize part of the vocal cord and ventricular bands, anterior to the vocal process. This detaches the thyroarytenoid muscle from the arytenoid (Figs. 46.6 and 46.7).

46.4.8.2 Laryngeal Pacing [9]

This is an implant which is placed beneath the skin. It provides electrical stimulation to the posterior cricoarytenoid muscle during inspiration leading to abduction of the vocal cord. This is activated by an electrode on the diaphragm which detects inspiration.

> Bilateral vocal cord palsy is commonly due to thyroid surgery. They symptom of breathing difficulty can be observed after surgery. If after a few days of intubation, stridor persists, tracheostomy has to be considered. Permanent surgical treatment is laser cordotomy. Laryngeal pacing is a recent, promising development.

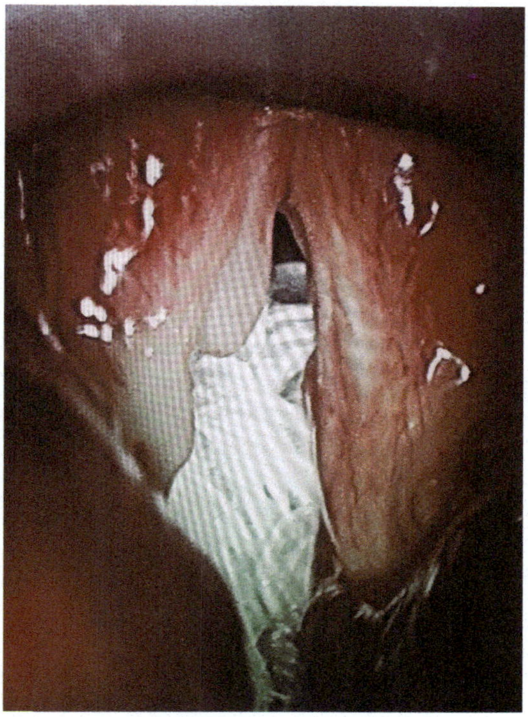

Fig. 46.6 A flexible laryngoscopic examination shows laser cordotomy of left vocal cord using KTP laser

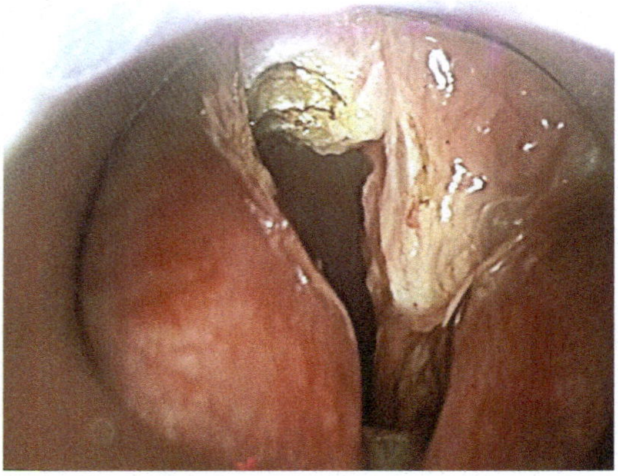

Fig. 46.7 A flexible laryngoscopic examination shows laser cordotomy of left vocal cord with cut thyroarytenoid muscle

> **Take Home Messages**
> - Vocal cord paralysis cannot only affect the quality of life of a patient but can turn into a medical emergency if it is bilateral.

Most of the incidence of paralysis are due to iatrogenic surgical trauma, mainly thyroid surgery. Unilateral vocal cord paralysis can result in hoarseness of voice and treatment consist of temporary or permanent surgical methods.

- Bilateral vocal cord paralysis can result in stridor and requires aggressive management including, intubation. Persisting airway obstruction should be dealt with by tracheostomy. Permanent solution is laser cordotomy. Newer techniques like laryngeal pacing seems promising.

References

1. Woodson GE. Spontaneous laryngeal reinnervation after recurrent nerve or vagus nerve injury. Ann Otol Rhinol Laryngol. 2007;116:66–8.
2. Sulica L. Laryngeal paralysis. In: Snow JB, Wackym PA, editors. Ballenger's otorhinolaryngology head and neck surgery, vol. 2. Shelton, CT: PMPH; 2009. p. 923–30.
3. Bielamowicz S, Stager SV. Diagnosis of unilateral recurrent laryngeal nerve paralysis: laryngeal electromyography, subjective rating scales, acoustic and aerodynamic measures. Laryngoscope. 2006;116:359–64.
4. Koufman JA, Postma GN, Whang SC, et al. Diagnostic laryngeal electromyography: the Wake Forest experience: 1995–1999. Otolaryngol Head Neck Surg. 1992;124:603–6.
5. Simpson CB, Amin MR. Office-based procedures for the voice. Ear Nose Throat J. 2004;83(Suppl 2):10–2.
6. Holinger LD, Holinger PC, Holinger PH. Etiology of bilateral abductor vocal cord paralysis: a review of 389 cases. Ann Otol Rhinol Laryngol. 1976;85:428–36.
7. Lichtenberger G, Toohill RJ. Technique of endo-extralaryngeal suture lateralization for bilateral abductor vocal cord paralysis. Laryngoscope. 1997;107:1281–3.
8. Kashima HK. Bilateral vocal fold motion impairment: pathophysiology and management by transverse cordotomy. Ann Otol Rhinol Laryngol. 1991;100:717–21.
9. Billante CR, Zealear DL, Courey MS, et al. Effect of chronic electrical stimulation of laryngeal muscle on voice. Ann Otol Rhinol Laryngol. 2002;111:328–32.

Dysphagia Disorders Evaluation and Management

47

Mayed Radi Alkhafaji and Olfa Almannai

47.1 Introduction

Dysphagia, difficulty to swallow normally and its sequel, is an extremely common clinical condition that affects millions of people annually in all ages. By examining incidence of dysphagia following stroke, one can begin to grasp the enormity of dysphagia problem.

Approximately 500,000 people per year in the United States have a stroke with up to 65% of those patients experiencing some type of swallowing difficulty. The incidence show up that 10–13% of the hospitalized patients experience some forms of swallowing difficulty.

It is not the acute neurological injury after stroke that usually causes patient demise rather, the pulmonary complications after stroke, in particular aspiration pneumonia, are deadly. Early diagnosis of swallowing disorder will help to avoid aspiration pneumonia, the third cause of killing in elderly patients.

It has found that around 50% of patients with dysphagia are silent aspirators, as a result, some of what one eats or drinks or secretes may enter the lungs, which in turn precipitates severe pulmonary infections.

47.2 The Structure of a Swallowing Clinic?

- Otolaryngologist (chairperson)
- Speech and language pathologist
- Trained registered nurse
- Clark
- Occupational therapist
- Dietician

M. R. Alkhafaji (✉)
Laryngology, Hamad Medical Corporation, Doha, Qatar
e-mail: mradi@hamad.qa

O. Almannai
ENT Department, Hamad Medical Corporation, Doha, Qatar
e-mail: OALMANNAI@hamad.qa

A. Al-Qahtani et al. (eds.), *Textbook of Clinical Otolaryngology*,
https://doi.org/10.1007/978-3-030-54088-3_47

47.3 Neural Control of Swallowing

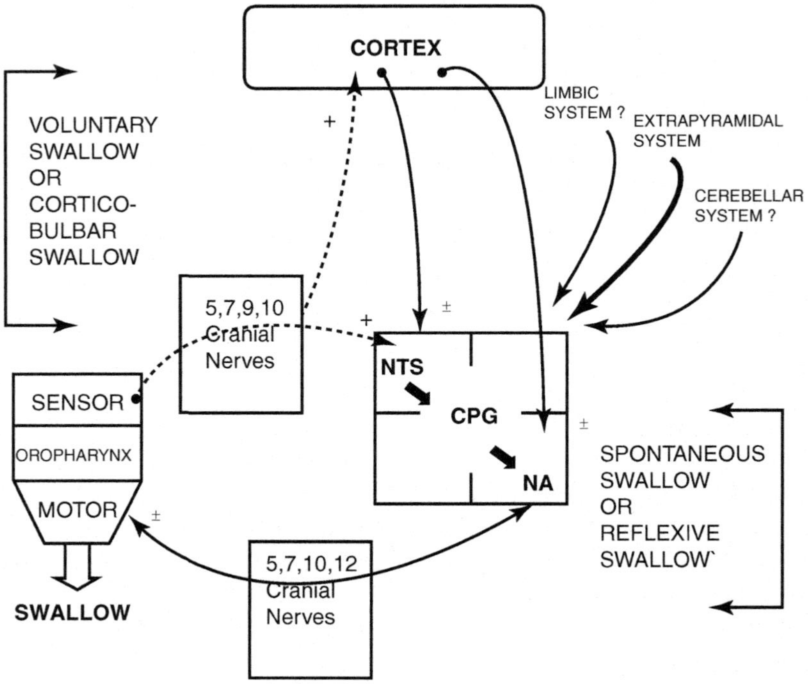

Swallowing is a centrally mediated phenomenon that can be divided into supratentorial and infratentorial regions of control. The supratentorial area of control is located in the frontal cortex anterior to the sensorimotor cortex. The infratentorial or brainstem areas involved in control of swallowing are located in the dorsal region within and subjacent to the nucleus of the tractus solitarius as well as in the ventral region around the nucleus ambiguus. The brainstem is responsible for the involuntary (pharyngeal and oesophageal) phases of swallowing. The dorsal and ventral medullary regions controlling swallowing are represented on both sides of the brainstem and are interconnected.

Either side can coordinate the pharyngeal and oesophageal stages of deglutition, however because they are interconnected, normal motor and sensory functioning on each side of the laryngopharynx depends on intactness on both sides of the medulla.

The clinical implication is that a unilateral medullary lesion, say after an embolic stroke, can result in bilateral pharyngeal motor and sensory dysfunction.

47.4 Stages of Swallowing in Both Adults and Pediatrics

- Pediatric have four stages, they are:
  - Oral preparatory phase
  - Oral transport phase
  - Pharyngeal phase
  - Oesophageal phase
- Adult have three stages, they are:
  - Oral preparatory phase
  - Pharyngeal phase
  - Oesophageal phase

47.5 Signs and Symptoms of Swallowing Disorders

1. Patients with laryngopharyngeal reflux disease (sore throat, phlegm in throat, change in voice.
2. Coughing during or immediately after eating or drinking.
3. Gurgling sound during or after eating or drinking.
4. Recurrent pneumonia or chest infection.

5. Weight loss or dehydration from not being able to eat.
6. Food or drink leaking from mouth or getting stuck in the mouth.
7. Increased congestion in the chest after eating or drinking.
8. Multiple swallows on a single mouthful of food.
9. Obvious extra effort or difficulty while chewing or swallowing.
10. Fatigue or shortness of breath while eating.
11. Temperature rise 30 minutes to an hour after eating.
12. Patients with refractory chronic cough.

47.6 Causes of Swallowing Disorders

1. Neurological: Stroke, parkinsonism, Guillain-Barre syndrome, cases of CP in pediatric age group
2. Infectious: Bacterial, fungal, and viral infections
3. Medications: Anticholinergics, antihypertensives, diuretics, opiates, antipsychotics, antidepressants, antihistamines
4. Psychogenic: Patients with globus hystericus
5. Neoplastic
6. Trauma

47.7 Diagnostic Procedures for the Swallowing Disorders

1. Transnasal flexible laryngoscope
2. Fixable endoscopic evaluation of swallowing safely (FEESS)
3. Fixable endoscopic evaluation of swallowing safely with sensory testing (FEESST)
4. Transnasal esophagoscopy
5. Transnasal tracheoscopy

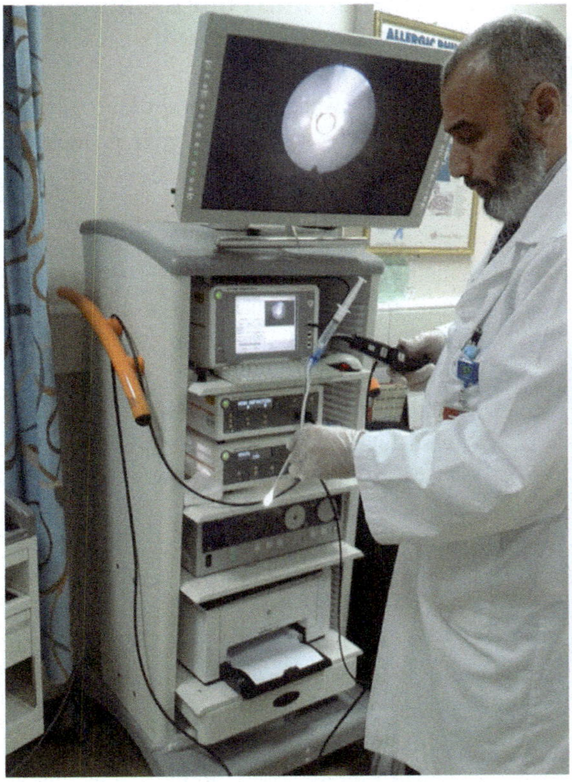

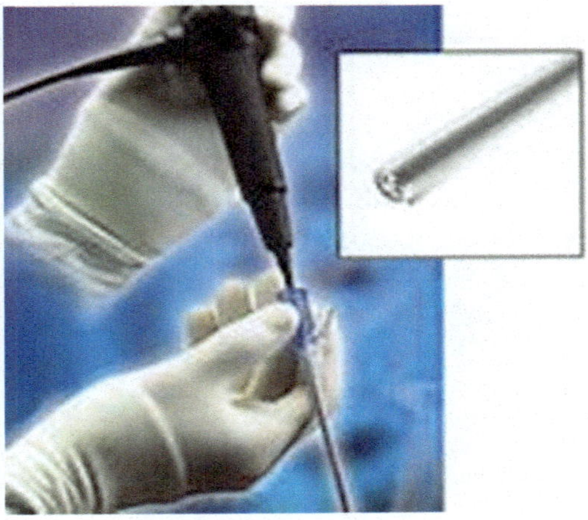

47.8 Transnasal Flexible Laryngoscopy (TFL)

TFL is a way of examining the larynx and throat with a thin, flexible endoscope that is passed via the nose which permits a magnified view of the laryngeal structures and functions. The finding can be show on a monitor and can be recorded and the pictures can be printed out as well.

47.9 Flexible Endoscopic Evaluation of Swallowing Safely (FEESS)

FEES allow for the direct viewing of the swallow function as food passes from the mouth into the throat. It is able to identify functional abnormalities that may occur and is used in "practice swallows" to help determine the safest position and food texture to maximize nutritional status and eliminate the risk of aspiration and unsafe swallowing. The results of the evaluation are photographed and recorded on videotape or CD ROM for later viewing or use for patient and family education and instruction.

Velopharyngeal closure, anatomy of the base of the tongue and hypopharynx, abduction of the vocal folds, pharyngeal musculature and the patient's ability to handle his/her own secretions are assessed. This procedure is painless and well tolerated by most individuals.

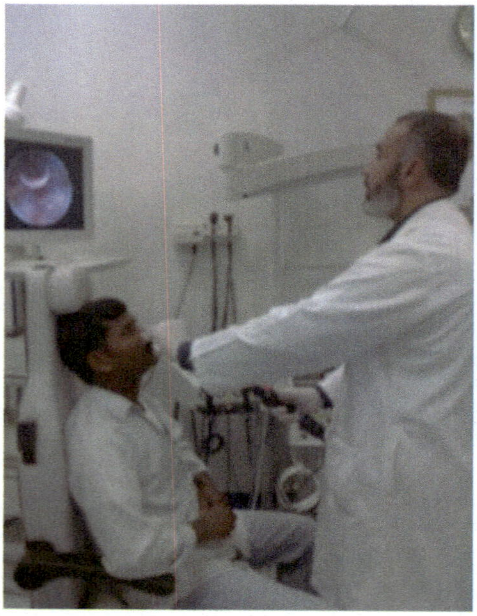

47.10 Fibreoptic Endoscopic Evaluation of Swallowing with Sensory Testing (FEESST)

It is the state of the art nonradioactive alternative to modified barium swallow studies. This exam will allow for direct assessment of the motor and sensory aspects of the swallow in order to precisely guide the dietary and behavioral management of patients with swallowing problems to decrease the probability of aspiration pneumonia.

FEESST is a two-part test. The first part of the test assesses sensation in the larynx in order to illicit an airway protective reflex. The second part of the test involves giving food to the patient (with green food colourings mixed in) and watching/ tracking where the food travels in the throat.

47.11 Swallowing Treatment, or Swallowing Therapy, Is Divided into Four Broad Categories

The purpose of swallowing therapy is to assure a safe swallow. By safe swallow, it is meant a swallow where the chance of choking is very small.

1. Behavioral therapy
2. Dietary therapy
3. Pharmacotherapy
4. Surgery
   1. Behavioral therapy: includes head turn, chin tuck, effortful swallow, shaker exercises, supraglottic swallow, Mendelsohn maneuver, thermal and chemical stimulation.
   2. Food therapy during the FEEST test it may become evident that certain types of food cause the patient to cough or choke, but other foods do not. During the FEESST exam, the various food volumes and consistencies are used until it is determined which combinations allow the patient to swallow easily and safely.

3. Pharmacological therapy:
   (a) Mucolytic agents: medications that thin-out thick secretions.
   (b) Anti-acid medications: swallowing problems are sometimes due to untreated, or insufficiently treated, acid reflux disease. The acid causes swelling in the throat which can contribute to swallowing difficulties.
4. Surgery:
   (a) Zenker's diverticulum cricopharyngeal myotomy diverticulopexy, and (Dolman procedure) peroral end endoscopic division of the party wall between the diverticulum and the esophagus.
   (b) Cricopharyngeal myotomy pharmacologic (botulinum toxin).

Cricopharyngeal myotomy is primarily useful for true cricopharyngeal achalasia such as after vagus nerve injury at the base of the skull where pharyngeal motor function remains otherwise intact. Cricopharyngeal myotomy is contraindicated in conditions when there is impaired pharyngeal peristalsis or when significant reflux disease exists.

47.12 Tube Feeding

Percutaneous endoscopic gastrostomy (PEG) or percutaneous endoscopic jejunostomy (PEJ) are excellent ways to aliment patients who are at high risk for aspiration as a result of severe dysphagia.

Patients who are aspirating regularly frequently become malnourished, which only exacerbates their underlying condition.

47.13 Effect of Tracheostomy on Swallowing

(a) Mechanical impact: (1) prevents proper laryngeal elevation. (2) Direct pressure from the tracheotomy tube → extrinsic oesophageal pressure. (3) Change of the laryngeal function.

(b) Physiological impact: (1) ↓ pharyngeal sensation leads to ↓ sensitivity of the glotticclosure reflex. (2) Loss of subglottic pressure. (3) Impaired cough (cuffed tracheotomy).

***Also consider effect of underlying disease that led to insertion of tracheostomy.

47.14 Management of Swallowing in Patients on Tracheostomy

1. Oro-motor exercise.
2. Tube manipulation (downsizing, light occlusion during swallowing).
3. Diet change.
4. Positioning.

47.15 Benefit of Using the Speaking Valve

1. Provide the facility to produce voice.
2. Eliminate the use digital occlusion.
3. Normalize the pathway of expired air.
4. Restore the subglottic pressure.

***The speaking valve should be used only with use with deflated cuff, fenestrated tube or uncuffed tube.

Take Home Messages

- Dysphagia is a relatively common complaint; it is considered an alarming symptom that needs further evaluation and a diagnosis.
- Flexible endoscopic evaluation of swallowing is helpful in the identification of penetration, aspiration, residue, and the effectiveness of swallowing compensatory strategies.
- The purpose of swallowing therapy is to assure a safe swallow and minimize the chance of choking by behavioral therapy, dietary therapy, pharmacotherapy, and/or surgery.

Further Reading

Abou-Nader L, Wilson JA, Paleri V. Transnasal oesophagoscopy: diagnostic and management outcomes in a prospective cohort of 257 consecutive cases and practice implications. Clin Otolaryngol. 2014;39(2):108–13.

Aviv JE. Transnasal esophagoscopy: state of the art. Otolaryngol Head Neck Surg. 2006;135(4):616–9.

Aviv JE, Martin JH, Kim T, et al. Laryngopharyngeal sensory discrimination testing and the laryngeal adductor reflex. Ann Otol Rhinol Laryngol. 1999;108(8):725–30.

Bennett AM, Sharma A, Price T, et al. The management of foreign bodies in the pharynx and oesophagus using transnasal flexible laryngo-oesophagoscopy (TNFLO). Ann R Coll Surg Engl. 2008;90(1):13–6.

Groher M, Crary M. Dysphagia clinical management in adults and children. Maryland Heights, MO: Mosby; 2015.

Ekberg O, editor. Dysphagia diagnosis and treatment editors. New York: Springer; 2019.

Dhyanesh A, Robert T, Michael F. Evaluation and Management of Dysphagia An Evidence-Based Approach. New York: Springer; 2020.

Herrmann IF, Recio SA. Functional pharyngoesophagoscopy: a new technique for diagnostics and analyzing deglutition. Oper Tech Otolayngol Head Neck Surg. 1997;8(3):163–7.

Johnson CM, Postma NG. Transnasal esophagoscopy. In: Flint PW, Haughey BH, Robbins KT, et al., editors. Cummings otolaryngology-head and neck surgery. Amsterdam: Elsevier Health Sciences; 2014. p. 1020–4.

Langmore SE, Schatz K, Olsen N. Fiberoptic endoscopic evaluation of swallowing safety: a new procedure. Dysphagia. 1988;2:216–9.

Leder SB, Murray JT. Fiberoptic endoscopic evaluation of swallowing. Phys Med Rehabil Clin N Am. 2008;19(4):787–801.

Merati AL. In-office evaluation of swallowing: FEES, pharyngeal squeeze maneuver, and FEESST. Otolaryngol Clin North Am. 2013;46(1):31–9.

Desuter G, editor. Oropharyngeal dysphagia videoendoscopy-guided work-up and management editors. New York: Springer; 2019.

Shaker R. Unsedated trans-nasal pharyngoesophagogastroduodenoscopy (T-EGD): technique. Gastrointest Endosc. 1994;40(3):346–8.

Shih CW, Hao CY, Wang YJ, et al. A new trend in the management of esophageal foreign body: transnasal esophagoscopy. Otolaryngol Head Neck Surg. 2015;153(2):189–92.

Esophageal Diseases

48

Aisha Larem, Ma'in Ali Al Shawabkeh,
and Khalil Sultan

48.1 Introduction

The esophagus can be affected by a wide range of different benign and malignant conditions. Knowledge of these conditions is important as patients can present first to ENT surgeons. Esophagology, which is the study of the esophagus, has developed recently due to the advancements in different technologies like rigid and flexible esophagoscopy.

Esophageal Anatomy [1]

- It measures about 25 cm.
- It extends from C4 till T11.
- Divided into three parts:
  - Cervical (from cricopharyngeus till the suprasternal notch).
  - The thoracic (from suprasternal notch till the diaphragm).
  - Abdominal part (till the gastric entry).
- The narrowest area of the esophagus is at the cricopharyngeus about 15 cm from teeth incisor.
- After that, there are three anatomical constrictions:
  - Aortic arch, about 22 cm from teeth incisors.
  - Left main bronchus, about 27 cm from upper teeth incisors.
  - At the level of the esophageal entry though the diaphragm, about 38 cm from teeth incisors.
- Arterial supply, venous drainage, and lymphatic drainage: see table

	Arterial blood supply	Venous drainage	Lymphatic drainage
Cervical	Inferior thyroid artery	Inferior thyroid via brachiocephalic	Lower deep cervical, paratracheal, and upper mediastinum nodes
Thoracic	Descending aorta or by bronchial and esophageal arteries	Azygos vein and less commonly to hemiazygos and intercostal veins	Posterior mediastinum and tracheobronchial nodes
Abdominal	Left gastric and left inferior phrenic artery	Left gastric vein	Left gastric and celiac nodes

A. Larem (✉) · M. A. Al Shawabkeh · K. Sultan
Hamad Medical Corporation, Doha, Qatar
e-mail: alarem@hamad.qa; MAIGhshoum@hamad.qa; Ksultan@hamad.qa

A. Al-Qahtani et al. (eds.), *Textbook of Clinical Otolaryngology*,
https://doi.org/10.1007/978-3-030-54088-3_48

Histology [1]

- It has four layers:
- Mucosa: keratinizing stratified squamous epithelium till the gastroesophageal junction where the lining changes to columnar epithelium
- Submucosa
- Muscular propria: the proximal is skeletal muscle, the middle is mixed, and the distal is smooth muscle
- Adventitia. There is no serosa layer
- There are two nerve plexuses:
  - Myenteric plexus found between the two muscle layers
  - Meissner's plexus found in the submucosa

Esophageal Disease

Motility disorder	Anatomical causes	Esophagitis/ reflux/caustic	Neoplasia
Achalasia	Strictures	Pill-induced esophagitis	Benign tumor
Diffuse esophageal spasm	Rings and Webs	Infectious esophagitis	Malignant tumor: SCC, and adenocarcinoma
Nutcracker esophagus	Eosinophilic esophagitis	Caustic injury/foreign body/ perforation	
Ineffective esophageal motility	Diverticulum	Reflux	
Systematic diseases affecting the esophagus	Dysphagia lusoria		

48.2 Motility Disorder

Achalasia

- Annual incidence: 1 in 100,000 [2].
- Pathophysiology:
  - Increase in the lower esophageal sphincter (LES) tone due to loss of inhibitory ganglionic cells at Auerbach plexus, leading to unopposed action of myenteric cholinergic stimulation [2–4]
- Symptoms:
  - Dysphagia: to solid, or both solid and liquid
  - Regurgitation
  - Chest pain (vigorous achalasia is a specific type of achalasia with retrosternal chest pain)
  - Weight loss [3]
- Diagnosis:
  - Barium esophagoscopy with fluoroscopy:
    The best study to start with.
    Shows loss of distal two-third primary peristalsis.
    The lower esophagus can appear as a bird beak (Figs. 48.1 and 48.2).
  - Esophageal manometry:
    Abnormality in the relaxation of LES.
  - Upper endoscopy:
    Cancer can resemble achalasia, so endoscopy should be done to rule it out [2, 3].
- Treatment:
  - Graded pneumatic dilation (has a risk of esophageal perforation)
  - Heller myotomy (esphagomyotomy)
  - For nonsurgical candidate consider Botox injection, calcium channel blocker or nitrates [5].

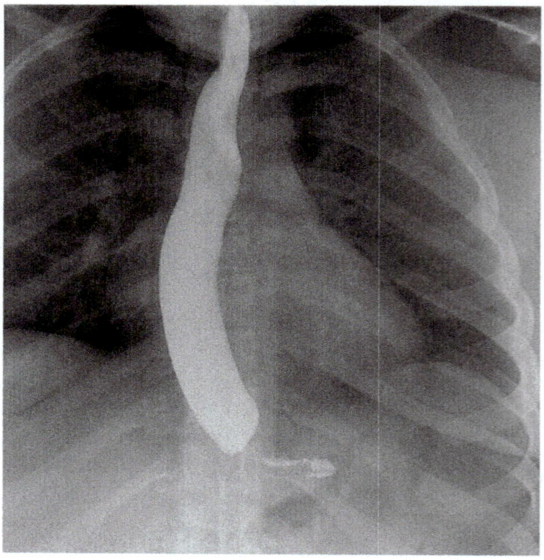

Fig. 48.1 Barium swallow in patient with achalasia showing

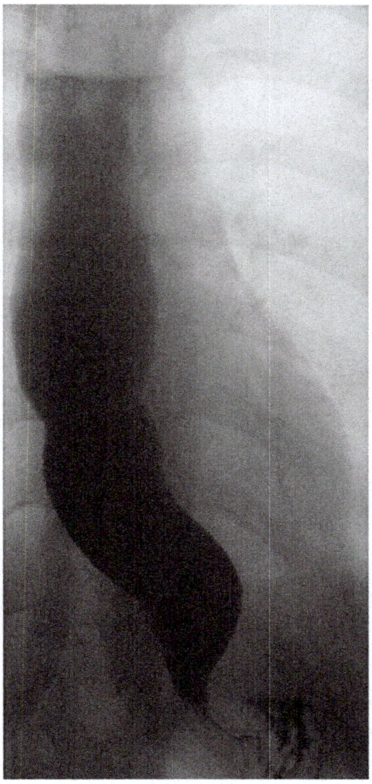

Fig. 48.2 Fluoroscopic image of bird's peak image

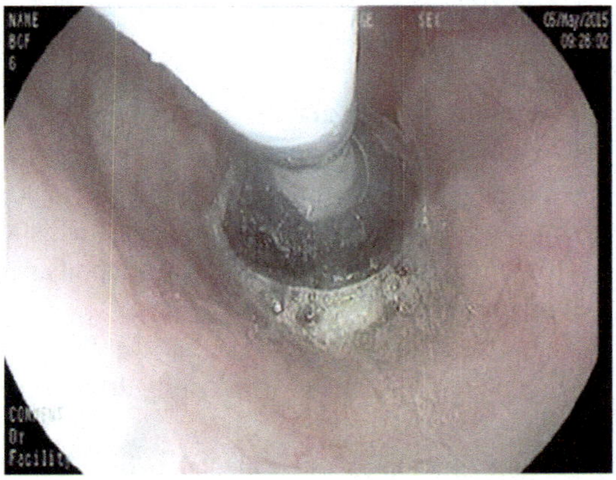

Fig. 48.3 Endoscopic image in patient with achalasia undergoing balloon dilatation

- Patients will have an increased risk of adenocarcinoma or squamous cell carcinoma, so they should have endoscopic surveillance [2] (Fig. 48.3).

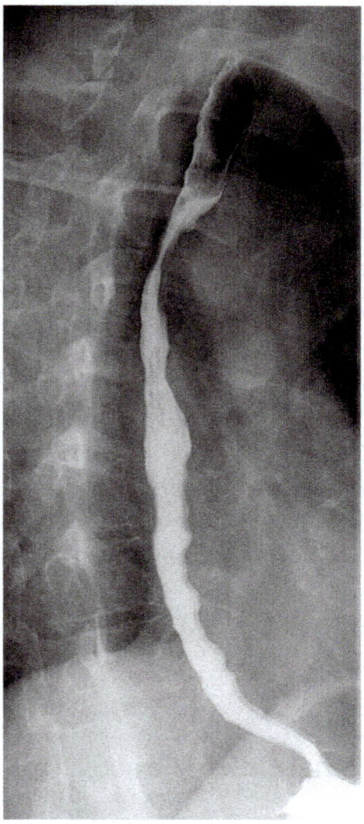

Fig. 48.4 Abnormal esophageal peristalsis is seen in the form of poorly propulsive tertiary contractions, which was better appreciated in the supine position. Contrast is eventually passing into the stomach

Diffuse Esophageal Spasm

- Pathophysiology: high pressure, *non-peristaltic* contraction of the esophagus.
- Symptoms: chest pain, dysphagia to solid and liquid.
- Diagnosis: manometry can show high-pressure simultaneous contraction. Esophagogram appearance is corkscrew.
- Treatment: mainly medical by calcium channel blockers, anticholinergics, nitrates, Botox injection [2, 6] (Fig. 48.4).

Nutcracker Esophagus

- Symptoms: noncardiac retrosternal chest pain.
- Diagnosis: high-amplitude *peristalsis* (the pressure of the contraction more than normal) [1].

Ineffective Esophageal Motility

- It is found in some people with GERD and can result in dysphagia in some cases.
- Diagnosis: decreased in the amplitude of the peristalsis in the distal esophagus to less than 30 mmHg.
- Secondary esophageal motility disorder can be seen in scleroderma, DM, and hypothyroidism [2, 3, 7, 8].

Systematic Disease Affecting the Esophagus

- Scleroderma: affects the smooth muscle of the esophagus, causing an incompetent LES that manifests with GERD.
- Dermatomyositis and other myopathies: affect the skeletal muscle, so mainly it affects the UES.
- Others like SLE, DM, amyloidosis, and hypothyroidism [1].

48.3 Anatomical Causes

Strictures

- Causes: reflux (acid), medication, chemical ingestion, infectious causes, radiation.
- The symptoms can be manifested if the diameter of the lumen is less than 15 mm.
- Treatment: dilatation (consider to dilate to make the diameter more than 15 mm, and do not dilate more than three sequential dilators per session) [1–3].

Rings and Webs

- *Rings*: is circumferential, consists of *mucosa or muscle* and occurs in the *distal* esophagus.
- *Webs*: consists of *mucosa* and occurs in the *proximal* esophagus.
- Symptoms: dysphagia to solid food (symptoms start if the esophageal lumen narrowed from 20 mm to below than 13 mm).
- Diagnosis: barium swallow.
- Treatment: dilation [1–3].
- Note:
  - Plummer–Vinson or Paterson–Kelly syndrome: a triad of proximal esophageal *webs*, iron deficiency anemia, and dysphagia. It occurs in young to middle age female patients, more in Scandinavians. It increases the risk of post cricoid hypopharyngeal tumors. Treatment with iron can alleviate most of the symptoms.
  - Schatzki ring: B-ring is the ring that occurs in the gastroesophageal junction at the distal part of LES, and it is the most common cause of intermittent dysphagia to solid food (Fig. 48.5).
  - A-ring: is the ring that occurs at the proximal part of LES [1–3].

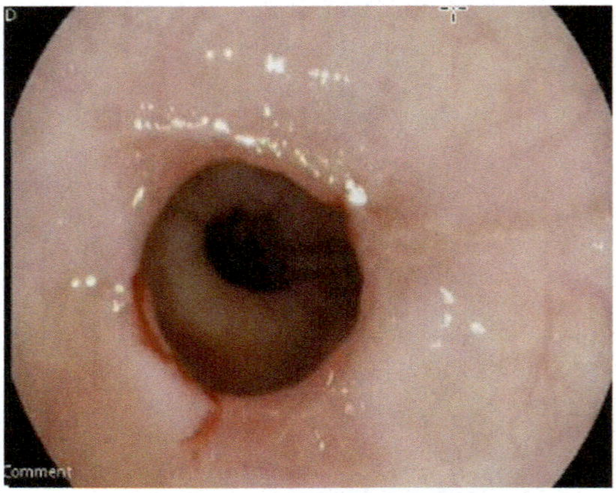

Fig. 48.5 Endoscopic image of Schatzki ring in lower esophagus

Eosinophilic Esophagitis

- Probably caused by an allergy.
- Endoscopy shows multiple esophageal rings.
- Esophageal biopsies at the proximal and distal esophagus show more than 15 eosinophils per high power field.
- Often associated with other atopic diseases and patients often have a family history of atopy.
- Treatment: topical steroid and avoidance of food allergen [9, 10] (Fig. 48.6).

Diverticulum

- The true diverticulum is the one that contains all esophageal layers.
- The false diverticulum is the one that contains mucosa and submucosa [3].
- Types:
  - Zenker's diverticulum (hypopharyngeal diverticulum):

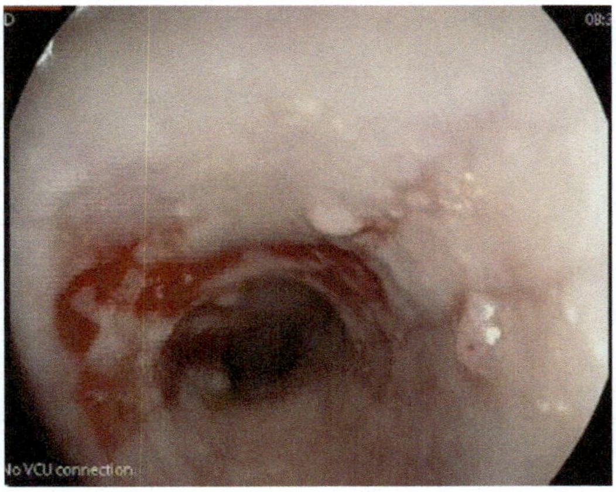

Fig. 48.6 Endoscopic image of eosinophilic esophagitis, multiple features of EoE including exudates, rings, linear furrows, edema, and friability. No strictures

It is considered a false diverticulum.

It occurs more on the left side.

It occurs more in elderly age group patients.

Pathophysiology: it is a pulsion diverticulum resulted from incomplete relaxation of UES, leading to herniation of the mucosa and submucosa through Kilian dehiscence which is found between cricopharyngeus and inferior constrictor muscles.

Symptoms: Regurgitation (most common), dysphagia, halitosis, weight loss, aspiration.

Complication: perforation, fistula, diverticulitis.

Diagnosis: barium swallow and endoscopy.

Treatment:

- Observe for the asymptomatic and small one.
- If symptomatic, then consider the surgical excision of the diverticulum either by external or internal approach. The endoscopic esophago-diverticulostomy is considered now the mainstay of treatment.
- If large in size, then consider trans-cervical diverticulectomy and crico-pharyngeal myotomy.
- The suspension of the diverticulum can be considered as well in inoperable cases [3, 11–13] (Figs. 48.7 and 48.8).

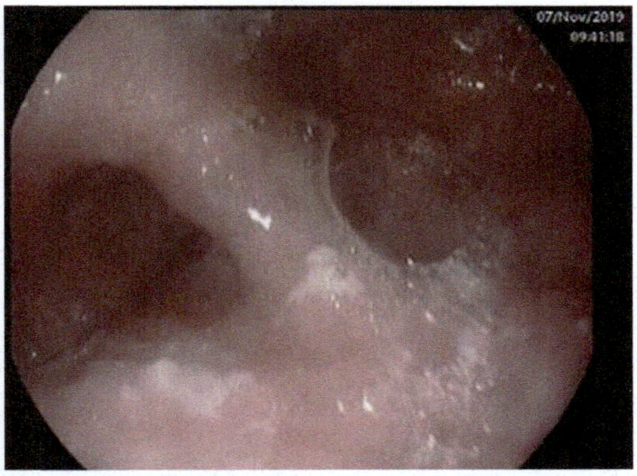

Fig. 48.7 Esophageal diverticulum

- Traction midesophageal diverticulum:

  It is the only true diverticulum in the esophagus.

  It occurs in the middle third of the esophagus.

  It is caused by traction of the esophageal wall by fibrotic tissue (for example TB).

  Usually asymptomatic.

  Treatment: right thoracotomy and diverticulectomy if symptomatic [3, 14].
- Epiphrenic diverticulum:

  Occurs near LES in the distal esophagus.

  It is a pulsion diverticulum.

  Caused by motility disorders like achalasia and esophageal spasm, it can also be associated with carcinoma in some instances.

  Once seen, rule out esophageal motility disorder by doing a manometric study [1, 3].

Dysphagia Lusoria

- It is dysphagia secondary to vascular anomalies.
- Example of these anomalies:
  - Aberrant right subclavian artery (retro esophageal), which is usually associated with right nonrecurrent laryngeal nerve
  - Double aortic arch
  - Right aortic arch

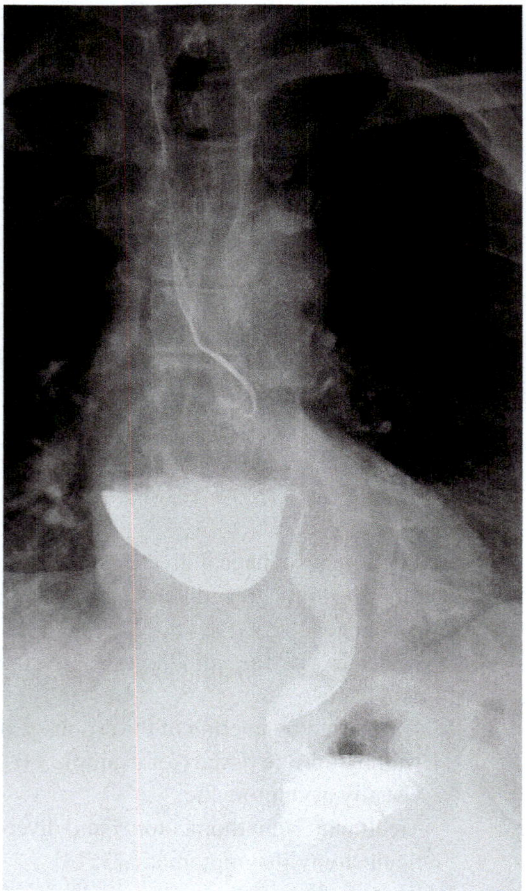

Fig. 48.8 A large esophageal diverticulum measuring 5.5 × 3.6 cm with an air-contrast level is seen at the right side of posterior mediastinum connecting with the esophagus at level of T7/T8 vertebra. There is another 8.5 mm air locule seen on the right side in-between the trachea and esophagus at level of T3 vertebra with no clear communication; this could represent esophagus/tracheal diverticulum with hidden communication. No mediastinal free air to suggest perforation

  - Left ligamentum arteriosum
  - Left subclavian artery
- Diagnosis: endoscopy, arteriography, CT [1, 15].

48.4 Esophagitis

Pill-induced Esophagitis

- Examples are alendronate, tetracycline, quinidine, NSAID, clindamycin, potassium-containing medication.

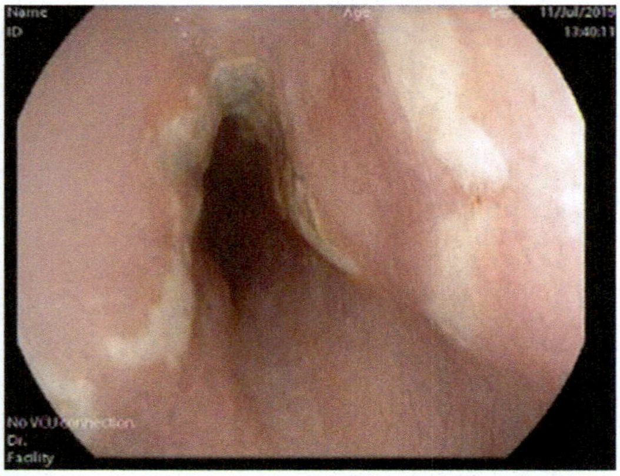

Fig. 48.9 Esophagus shows large clean based superficial ulcers at 26 and 27 cm from esophagus in patient on tetracycline

- Symptoms: chest pain, odynophagia. If the patient has dysphagia consider that stricture has formed.
- Diagnosis: endoscopy might show mucosal changes or strictures.
- Treatment: stop using the medication, always take the medication with fluid in an upright position. Do dilation if strictures happened [3, 16] (Fig. 48.9).

48.4.1 Infectious Esophagitis

Usually, patients present with odynophagia.

Causes

1. Candida:
   - Seen in immunocompromised patients (HIV, DM).
   - Diagnosis: endoscopy can show white patches (not pathognomonic for candida esophagitis). Biopsy should be taken to confirm the diagnosis.
   - Treatment with topical antifungal. Oral antifungal can be used, especially in disseminated cases [1, 3] (Fig. 48.10).
2. CMV:
   - It causes subepithelial infection affecting the fibroblast and endothelial cells.
   - Symptoms: abdominal pain, nausea, and vomiting, along with dysphagia.

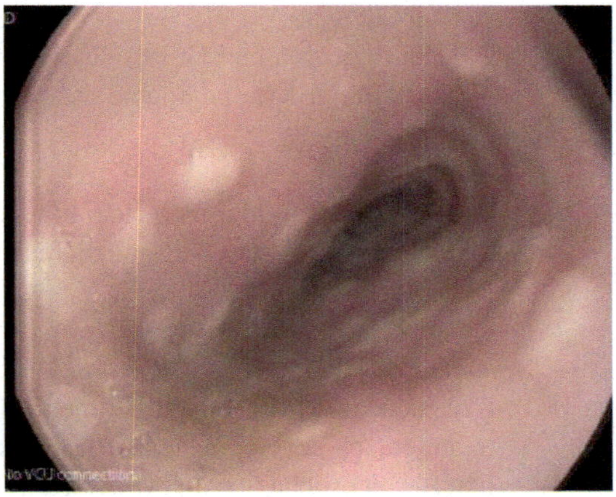

Fig. 48.10 Candidal esophagitis

- Diagnosis: endoscopy shows erosion and ulceration. To confirm biopsy should be taken from the base of the ulcer, and viral culture of the biopsy.
- Treatment: ganciclovir and foscarnet [1, 3].

3. Others: like HSV, HIV, VZV, EBV [1, 3].

Caustic Injury

- Caused by alkali (like those in household cleaning products) or acid.
- Alkali: causes liquefaction necrosis, which causes more severe damage. Stomach acidity can limit injury.
- Acid: causes coagulation necrosis, which limits the damage [1, 17].
- Symptoms: dysphagia, odynophagia, or hypersalivation [1].
- Diagnosis: Endoscopy should be done in the first 24–48 h, grading system as seen in table [18]:

Grade	Feature
0	Normal
1	Mucosal edema
2	2A superficial ulceration 2B deep ulceration
3	3A focal necrosis 3B extensive necrosis
4	Perforation

- Treatment depends on the clinical picture.
  - For stage 1 and 2A, liquid diet can be started and after 24–48 h, to start a regular diet.
  - For grade 2B and 3A, it needs in-hospital observation, to keep patient NPO and if the patient can swallow without pain, then a liquid diet can be started after 48 h.
  - Patients with grade 3 should be observed for symptoms of perforation for one to two weeks after ingestion.
  - Lavage and emetic are contraindicated in cases of caustic ingestion [18].
- Complication:
  - Stricture: mainly at cricopharyngeus, level of aortic arch and LES
  - Esophageal perforation
  - Airway compromise
  - SCC [18]

Foreign Body in Esophagus

- It can present with respiratory distress due to compression on the trachea.
- Examples are coins, food bolus, batteries (which are considered emergency cases as it is an alkaline material that can lead to liquification).
- Diagnosis: obtain both lateral X-ray and Chest X-ray.
- Treatment: rigid esophagoscopy (better than fiberoptic one) can be used for removal under GA.
- Complication: perforation, stricture, and fistula formation [1].

Esophageal Perforation

- Causes: Iatrogenic (most common), spontaneous (due to an increase in the pressure of the abdomen called *Boerhaave syndrome*), trauma, tumor, foreign body.
- Symptoms: chest pain, dysphagia, fever, tachycardia.
- Diagnosis: CXR (can show widening of the mediastinum), water-soluble esophagogram.
- Treatment: in cases of cervical esophageal perforation, usually conservative measures are taken like keeping the patient NPO, starting NG feeding, IV fluid, PPI, and IV antibiotics. Surgical repair can be considered in some instances.
- Complications: mediastinitis, sepsis, and death [2].

Gastroesophageal Reflux Disease (GERD)

- Symptoms:

  We should distinguish between GERD and laryngopharyngeal reflux (LPR) disease, as the former usually presents with heartburn and supine reflux, but the later can manifest with hoarseness, throat clearing, globus sensation, and upright reflux [1].
- Diagnosis:
  - Nasopharyngoscopy shows interarytenoid edema, and pharyngeal and laryngeal erythema [1].
  - Barium swallow: look for stricture or another abnormal esophageal anatomy [19].
  - Endoscopy to identify the severity of esophagitis, to look for Barret's esophagus, and to take biopsies [19].
  - 24-h dual PH monitoring: is considered the gold standard in the diagnosis. In which a probe near the UES and another LES are placed [19].
  - Complication: esophagitis, Barret esophagitis, strictures, vocal cord granuloma (Fig. 48.11).
- Treatment:
  - Behavioral modification: stop smoking, avoid eating before sleep, sleep with head elevation, avoid wearing tight clothes, and avoid eating or drinking caffeine, chocolate, spicy food, and alcohol [19].

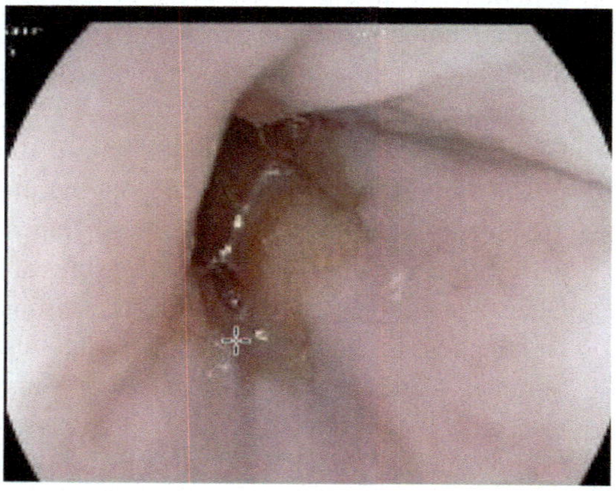

Fig. 48.11 Endoscopic image of lower esophagus in patient with chronic GERD with stricture

  - Medical treatment:

    PPI: first-line treatment. Consider a single dose for GERD and double dose for LPR.

    H2 blocker.

    Prokinetic agents like metoclopramide, it helps in gastric emptying and increase LES pressure.

    Antacids [19].
  - Surgical treatment:

    Indicated in cases of failed medical treatment or developing complications like Barret esophagitis and structure.

    Laparoscopic fundoplication can treat the symptoms in 92 % of cases [19].
- *Note: Barret esophagitis*
  - It is the metaplasia of the squamous epithelial lining of the esophagus to the columnar intestinal one.
  - It increases the risk of adenocarcinoma.
  - Diagnosis: by endoscopy and biopsy (biopsy is important to look for dysplasia).
  - Treatment: close follow up for low-grade dysplasia. While high-grade dysplasia should be treated as adenocarcinoma [1] (Fig. 48.12).

48.5 Neoplasia

Benign Tumor

- It is less common than a malignant one.
- It can present with dysphagia and weight loss.
- Leiomyoma is the most common benign tumor.
- Diagnosis: barium, endoscopy, and CT/MRI [20].

Malignant Tumor

- Mainly SCC and adenocarcinoma. (See Fig. 48.13).
- Incidence increase after the age of 40. It is more common in males.
- Risk factors:
  - SCC: smoking, alcohol, achalasia, low socioeconomic status, diets low in fruit and vegetables, Plummer–Vinson syndrome, HPV infection

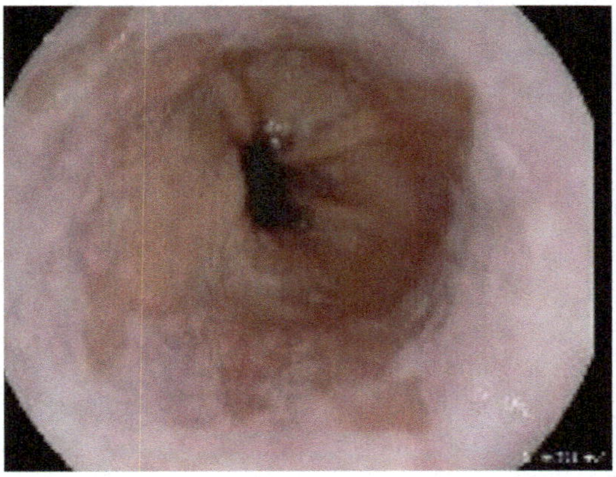

Fig. 48.12 Endoscopic image in patient with Barret esophagus

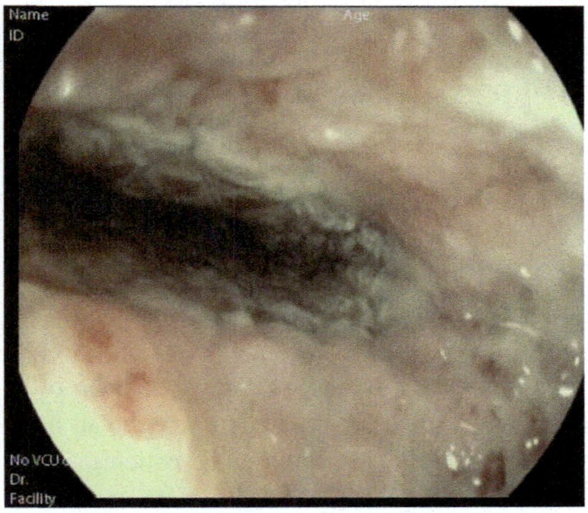

Fig. 48.13 Endoscopic image showing features of malignancy, biopsy of the patient later showed adenocarcinoma

   – Adenocarcinoma: GERD and Barret esophagus [21].
- Symptoms: rapidly progressive dysphagia to solid food due to mechanical obstruction, odynophagia, hoarseness due to recurrent laryngeal nerve injury, weight loss, loss of appetite, early satiety [22].
- Diagnosis: endoscopy and biopsy. Staging CT and the endoscopic US are needed to stage the disease. Endoscopic US is better than CT for assessment depth of invasion [22].
- Distant metastasis to lung, liver, brain, and bone.
- Staging [22]:

Tx: tumor cannot be assessed T0: no primary tumor T1a: invades lamina propria or muscularis mucosa T1b: invades submucosa T2: invades muscularis propria T3: invades adventitia T4: invades adjacent structures
NX: LN cannot be assessed N0: No LN mets N1: LN mets
Mx: distant mets cannot be assessed M0: No distant mets M1: Distant mets

- Treatment: for early-stage surgery can be considered. Patients in late stages will benefit from chemoradiotherapy [22].
- Prognosis: poor prognosis due to lack of serosa in the esophagus that can lead to the early spread of the tumor [22].

Take Home Messages
- Different conditions can affect the esophagus. ENT surgeons have to be aware of them as some patients can present first to ENT.
- Achalasia is caused by an increase in the LES secondary to the loss of ganglionic cells at Auerbach plexus. Barium esophagoscopy with fluoroscopy is the best initial study for diagnosis, and manometry can be beneficial. Endoscopy is essential to rule out malignancies as they can resemble this disease. Treatment can be by graded pneumatic dilatation or Heller myotomy.
- Diffuse esophageal spasm, nutcracker esophagus, and ineffective esophageal motility are other esophageal motility disorders. Scleroderma and dermatomyositis are examples of systemic diseases affecting the esophagus.
- Strictures, rings, and webs can cause dysphagia. They are treated by dilatation. Plummer–Vinson or Paterson–Kelly syndrome is a triad of proximal esophageal webs, iron deficiency anemia, and dysphagia. It usually presents in Scandinavian females.

- Eosinophilic esophagitis can cause multiple esophageal rings. Taking biopsies is essential for diagnosis, which can show more than 15 eosinophils per high power field.
- Zenker's diverticulum is a false pulsion diverticulum resulted from incomplete relaxation of UES, allowing the mucosa and submucosa to herniate through Kilian dehiscence. Surgical excision by an external or internal approach can be considered in symptomatic patients.
- Certain pills (like alendronate, tetracycline, NSAID, clindamycin, quinidine, and potassium-containing medication) and infections (like Candida and CMV) can cause esophagitis, which presents with dysphagia and odynophagia.
- Alkaline caustic injury is more severe than the acidic one. Complications like stricture, perforation, or airway compromise can happen.
- Iatrogenic trauma is the most common cause of esophageal perforation. A chest X-ray can show a widening of the mediastinum. Treatment is by conservative measurement (like keeping patient NPO, NG feeding, IV fluid, PPI, IV antibiotics). Surgical repair can be considered in certain conditions.
- LRP presents with hoarsens, throat clearing, globus sensation, and upright reflux. 24-h pH monitoring is the gold standard for diagnosis. Esophagitis, Barret esophagitis, strictures, and vocal cord granuloma are possible complications secondary to GERD and/or LRP.
- Barret esophagitis, which is the metaplasia of the squamous epithelial lining of the esophagus to a columnar one, can increase the risk of adenocarcinoma.
- Leiomyoma is the most common benign tumor affecting the esophagus.
- Malignancy of the esophagus has a poor prognosis because the esophagus lacks serosa, and that can permit the early spread of the tumor. The most common types are SCC and adenocarcinoma. Smoking and alcohol consumption are the major risk factors for SCC, while GERD and Barret esophagus are the main risk factors for adenocarcinoma. Staging CT and endoscopic US are essential components in management and staging. Distant metastasis can occur in the lung, liver, brain, and bone.

Acknowledgment Authors would like to thank and appreciate the help of Dr. Moutaz Derbala and Dr. Mustafa Tarabolsi from gastroenterology department in Hamad Medical Corporation, and Dr. Adham Aljariri an ENT resident for their effort in finalizing this chapter.

References

1. Snow JB, Ashley Wackym P. Ballenger's otorhinolaryngology and head and neck surgery. 17th ed. Connecticut: People's Medical Publishing House; 2008.
2. Watkinson JC, Clarke RW. Scott-Brown's otorhinolaryngology and head and neck surgery. 8th ed. FL: CRC Press; 2018.
3. Flint P, Haughey B, Lund V, Niparko J, Robbins K, Regan J, Lesperance TM. Cummings otolaryngology. 6th ed. Philadelphia: Elsevier; 2014.
4. O'Neill OM, Johnston BT, Coleman HG. Achalasia: a review of clinical diagnosis, epidemiology, treatment and outcomes. World J Gastroenterol. 2013;19(35):5806–12. https://doi.org/10.3748/wjg.v19.i35.5806.
5. Lopushinksy SR, Urbach DR. Pneumatic dilation and surgical myotomy for achalasia. JAMA. 2006;296:2227–33.
6. Tutuian R, Castell DO. Esophageal motility disorders (distal esophageal spasm, nutcracker esophagus, and hypertensive lower esophageal sphincter): modern management. Curr Treat Options Gastroenterol. 2006;9:283–94.
7. Ergün M, Doğan İ, Ünal S. Ineffective esophageal motility and gastroesophageal reflux disease: a close relationship? Turk J Gastroenterol. 2012;23(6):627–33.
8. Shetler KP, Bikhtii S, Triadafilopoulos G. Ineffective esophageal motility: clinical, manometric, and outcome characteristics in patients with and without abnormal esophageal acid exposure. Dis Esophagus. 2017;30(6):1–8. https://doi.org/10.1093/dote/dox012.

9. Cianferoni A, Spergel J. Eosinophilic esophagitis: a comprehensive review. Clin Rev Allergy Immunol. 2016;50(2):159–74. https://doi.org/10.1007/s12016-015-8501-z. Review.
10. Dellon ES. Diagnosis and management of eosinophilic esophagitis. Clin Gastroenterol Hepatol. 2012;10(10):1066–78.
11. Sasaki CT, Ross DA, Hundal J. Association between Zenker's diverticulum and gastroesophageal reflux disease: development of a working hypothesis. Am J Med. 2003;115(Suppl 3A):169S–71S.
12. Tabola R, Lewandowski A, Cirocchi R, Augoff K, Kozminska U, Strzelec B, Grabowski K. Zenker diverticulum: experience in surgical treatment of large diverticula. Medicine (Baltimore). 2018;97(19):e0557.
13. Bizzotto A, Iacopini F, Landi R, Costamagna G. Zenker's diverticulum: exploring treatment options. Acta Otorhinolaryngol Ital. 2013;33(4):219–29.
14. Ballehaninna UK, Shaw JP, Brichkov I. Traction esophageal diverticulum: a rare cause of gastrointestinal bleeding. Springerplus. 2012;1(1):50.
15. Janssen M, Baggen MG, Veen HF, Smout AJ, Bekkers JA, Jonkman JG, Ouwendijk RJ. Dysphagia lusoria: clinical aspects, manometric findings, diagnosis, and therapy. Am J Gastroenterol. 2000;95(6):1411–6.
16. Kikendall JW. Pill-induced esophageal injury. Gastroenterol Clin North Am. 1991;20:835–46.
17. Poley JW, Steyerberg EW, Kuipers EJ, et al. Ingestion of acid and alkaline agents: outcome and prognostic value of early upper endoscopy. Gastroinest Endosc. 2004;60:372–7.
18. Park KS. Evaluation and management of caustic injuries from ingestion of Acid or alkaline substances. Clin Endosc. 2014;47(4):301–7. https://doi.org/10.5946/ce.2014.47.4.301.
19. Badillo R, Francis D. Diagnosis and treatment of gastroesophageal reflux disease. World J Gastrointest Pharmacol Ther. 2014;5(3):105–12. https://doi.org/10.4292/wjgpt.v5.i3.105.
20. Ha C, Regan J, Cetindag IB, Ali A, Mellinger JD. Benign esophageal tumors. Surg Clin North Am. 2015;95(3):491–514. https://doi.org/10.1016/j.suc.2015.02.005. Review.
21. Domper Arnal MJ, Ferrández Arenas Á, Lanas AÁ. Esophageal cancer: risk factors, screening and endoscopic treatment in Western and Eastern countries. World J Gastroenterol. 2015;21(26):7933–43. https://doi.org/10.3748/wjg.v21.i26.7933.
22. Rubenstein JH, Shaheen NJ. Epidemiology, diagnosis, and management of esophageal adenocarcinoma. Gastroenterology. 2015;149(2):302–17.e1. https://doi.org/10.1053/j.gastro.2015.04.053.

Part VI

General Otolaryngology

Pharyngitis

49

Abdulsalam Al-Qahtani and Zaid Altamimi

49.1 Introduction

Pharyngitis is inflammation of pharyngeal tissue, which mainly affects the oropharyngeal part. Tissues of pharynx prone to frequent inflammation because of the prominent presence of lymphoid tissue and the communication with the external environment during breathing [1]. Sore throat which is one of the most commonly encountered complaints to physicians [2]. Pharyngitis can be classified into infectious and noninfectious or to acute and chronic pharyngitis. A viral infection is the most common cause of pharyngitis in both children and adults. Bacterial infection represents only 30–40% of pediatric pharyngitis, while it is even less in adults with a rate of 5–15% [3]. The deferential diagnosis of pharyngitis is summarized in Table 49.1.

Knowledge of the pharyngeal anatomy and the deep neck spaces is important for a successful diagnosis and understanding the clinical manifestations of the pharyngitis. The pharynx is a 12–14 cm musculo-membranous tube. It has three interior sections: the nasopharynx, oropharynx, and hypopharynx. The nasopharynx extends from the base of the skull superiorly to the pharyngeal isthmus (back of the soft palate and posterior pharyngeal wall) inferiorly, bounded by the nasal cavity and choanae anteriorly, and clivus posteriorly. The oropharynx extends from undersurface of the soft palate to the upper border of the epiglottis bounded by the circumvallate

Table 49.1 Differential diagnosis of pharyngitis

	Bacterial: GABHS (*S. pyogenes*), *Staphylococcus aureus*, *C. diphtheriae*, *N. gonorrhea*, *A. haemolyticum*, *T. pallidum* (*Syphilis*), others
Infectious	*Viral*: Rhinovirus, coronavirus, adenovirus, parainfluenza virus, measles, respiratory syncytial virus, Coxsackie virus, EBV, CMV, HSV, HIV
	Fungal: *C. albicans*, other organisms—*C. glabrata*, *C. tropicalis*, *C. dubliniensis*, *C. rugosa*, and *C. krusei*
Noninfectious	*Inflammatory/autoimmune acute pharyngitis*: PFAPA, Kawasaki disease, PTLD, Oral mucocutaneous diseases
	Inflammatory chronic pharyngitis: Reflux pharyngitis, postnasal drip, granulomatous disease
	Membranous Pharyngitis: Agranulocytosis, aphthous ulcers, traumatic ulcer
	Malignancy: Tonsillar malignancy, leukemia, lymphoma
	Radiation pharyngitis
	Keratosis pharyngitis

A. Al-Qahtani (✉) · Z. Altamimi
Hamad Medical Corporation, Doha, Qatar
e-mail: aalqahtani@hamad.qa; Zaltamimi@hamad.qa

A. Al-Qahtani et al. (eds.), *Textbook of Clinical Otolaryngology*,
https://doi.org/10.1007/978-3-030-54088-3_49

papillae anteriorly, and by the palatopharyngeal arch and palatine tonsils laterally. The hypopharynx extends from the superior border of epiglottis to the inferior border of the cricoid cartilage, contains the pyriform sinuses, post-cricoid region, and posterior pharyngeal wall.

The pharynx contains the Waldeyer's tonsillar ring (pharyngeal lymphoid ring), which consists of the pharyngeal tonsil (adenoids), tubal tonsils (Gerlach tonsil), palatine tonsils (commonly called "the tonsils"), and lingual tonsil. The superior, middle, and inferior constrictor muscles from the external open-tubed structure of the pharynx, and fuse in the posterior midline at the pharyngeal raphe. The pharyngeal wall is surrounded via fascial layers and deep neck spaces. From anterior to posterior these are the bucco-pharyngeal fascia, retropharyngeal space, alar fascia, danger space, and the prevertebral fascia.

49.2 Infectious Pharyngitis

49.2.1 Bacterial Infection

In children, bacterial pharyngitis accounts for 30–40% of cases while in adults it accounts for only 5–15% [3]. Most cases of bacterial pharyngitis are caused by *group A beta-hemolytic streptococcal* (GABHS) *pyogenes* [4].

49.2.1.1 Streptococcal Infection

Group A beta-hemolytic streptococcal (GABHS), also known as Streptococcus pyogenes is the most common cause of acute bacterial tonsillitis pharyngitis. GABHS are Gram-positive cocci. Spread mainly through aerosolized microdroplets. It is a precursor of two serious conditions acute rheumatic fever and poststreptococcal glomerulonephritis.

Clinical Features

- The disease often affects age group of 5–15 years, especially the early school years, but it can affect any age. The incubation period is 1–4 days. Considered contagious during the acute illness and one week after, it becomes noncontagious after 24 h of antibiotics use [1].

Symptoms	Signs
Sore throat	Acute membranous tonsillitis: erythematous swollen tonsils with yellowish spots hyperemia of pillars, soft palate and uvula, that can be easily removed with a swab
Dysphagia, odynophagia	Halitosis
Fever	Tender enlarged jugulodigastric lymph nodes
Earache (referred or due to acute otitis media)	
Other symptoms: headache, myalgia, fatigue and abdominal symptoms, such as vomiting	

- Note that cough, coryza, and nasal congestion are not suggestive of bacterial pharyngitis [5].

Diagnosis

- Diagnosis of GABHS depends on clinical judgment and laboratory testing.
- *Rapid strep test (rapid antigen detection test, RADI): detects* antigen (group-A streptococcal) from a swab. It is highly specific but less sensitive than culture and allows for immediate antibiotic treatment of a positive result. Carriers of GABHS, are around 5–10%, and they will have positive strep testing without acute symptoms [6].
- *Throat culture*: The gold standard laboratory test with the sensitivity of 90–95% [6].

Treatment

- Supportive treatment including analgesics, antipyretics, bed rest, and hydration. Noting that GABHS is usually self-limited and resolved within 3–10 days.
- Antibiotics: avoid the overuse of antibiotics in case of other pathogens, especially in the case of viral pharyngitis. Penicillin or amoxicillin is the drug of choice for 7–10 days. If suspect resistance uses amoxicillin + clavulanic acid or clindamycin. Corticosteroids have not been proven to have benefit in acute streptococcal pharyngitis. The major aim of antibiotic use is

to reduce the rate of rheumatic fever, rheumatic heart disease, suppurative complications, and abscess formation. Noting that antibiotic therapy does not prevent poststreptococcal glomerulonephritis [7].
- Tonsillectomy in case of recurrent infections, despite appropriate antimicrobial therapy.

Complications
- Suppurative complications such as peritonsillar, retro or parapharyngeal abscess, lymphadenopathy with abscess, bacteremia, and sepsis.
- Scarlet fever.
- Rheumatic fever: occur in 3% of untreated GABHS patients, risk can be reduced to 0.3% with the use of antibiotics [1].
- Rheumatic heart disease.
- Poststreptococcal glomerulonephritis.
- Pediatric Autoimmune Neuropsychiatric Disorders Associated with Streptococcal (PANDAS) infections: tonsillectomy in these patients can resolute the neuropsychiatric symptoms [8].

49.2.1.2 Corynebacterium Diphtheriae

This condition caused by gram-positive rod-shaped *Corynebacterium diphtheriae*. A significant reduction in the incidence happened after the introduction of the Diphtheria vaccine [9]. The incubation period for diphtheria pharyngitis is 2–6 days. Spread mainly through infected secretions from the nose, throat, eyes, or skin lesions.

Clinical Features
- The disease often affects children. The patients usually appear ill and toxemic.
- Exotoxin leads to systemic cardiotoxicity and neurotoxicity which account for many of the infection consequences.

Symptoms	Signs
Sore throat	Pseudomembrane tonsillitis*:* adherent greyish-white membrane extends to the uvula, soft palate and can reach the larynx causing asphyxia, it bleeds on removal
Dysphagia, odynophagia	Cervical lymphadenitis (bull-neck) which can cause external compression on the larynx
Fever	*Others*: Nasal cavity can also be affected
Other symptoms: headache, myalgia	

Diagnosis
- Diagnosis is usually based on the clinical picture.
- It is confirmed with the culture of the pseudomembrane on Loeffler or tellurite medium. The growth shows “Chinese character” appearance. Treatment should be starting without wasting of time [1].
- Note that identifying GABHS does not rule out the possibility of diphtheria, as 30% of Diphtheria cases shows positive GABHS [10].
- Serial electrocardiograms: for early detection of cardiac complications.

Treatment
- Treatment consists of antitoxin and antibiotics; penicillin or erythromycin are the recommended antibiotics [1].
- Early administration of medication specially antitoxin significantly affect the outcome.
- In rare cases, with extended pseudomembrane to upper airway intubation or tracheostomy is needed to secure the airway and avoid aspiration.
- Confirm eradication of the disease by having two negative cultures after completion of the treatment.
- Diphtheria toxoid booster injection is recommended every 10 years in adults.

Complications
- Diphtheria exotoxin is toxic to heart and nerves that can occur up to the second or third week of infection.
- Heart involvement includes; myocarditis, arrhythmia, and acute heart failure. It can improve at 2 weeks after onset [7].

- Neurological involvement affects mainly the motor nerves. Commonly affects the soft palate and pharyngeal muscles, other muscles like the diaphragm and ocular muscles can be affected. It can improve from 3 to 7 weeks later [7].
- Other organs can be involved; the larynx with airway obstruction, the kidney can lead to acute tubular necrosis.
- Death can occur due to cardiac or neurological involvement, or from asphyxiation from membranous pharyngitis.

49.2.1.3 Other Bacterial Pharyngitis

- *Vincent's Angina*: ulcerative lesion on the tonsils, mainly unilateral. covered by a slough which may extend to beyond pharyngeal tissues. Came with a characteristic fishy odor. On microbiology, it shows a fusiform bacillus and spirochete. Treatment: penicillin or erythromycin.
- *Others*: *Mycoplasma pneumoniae*, *Neisseria gonorrhoeae*, *Treponema pallidum*, *Chlamydia pneumoniae*, *Mycobacterium tuberculosis*, *Yersinia enterocolitica*.

49.2.2 Viral Infection

A viral infection is the most common cause of infectious pharyngitis in both pediatrics and adults [3]. The most common viruses causing the infection are rhinovirus followed by coronavirus and parainfluenza [4]. It comes with gradual onset, as part of the common cold, symptoms typically include rhinorrhea, cough, and diarrhea, and usually, it is self-limited. Presence of pharyngitis with conjunctivitis, coryza, hoarseness, and cough suggest a viral etiology. Spread is by direct contact and inhalation/ingestion of respiratory secretions. Determining the virologic agent is unnecessary as it does not affect the management. Different viral pharyngitis has been described including the following:

49.2.2.1 Infectious Mononucleosis (Glandular Fever)

Epstein-Barr virus (EBV) is a common cause of acute sore throat in adolescents and young adults. 80–90% of adults are seropositive for EBV [11]. EBV has been associated with nasopharyngeal undifferentiated carcinoma, Burkitt lymphoma, and posttransplant lymphoproliferative disease (PTLD) [7]. It has an incubation period of 3–7 weeks.

Clinical Features

- Affects mainly older children and young adults. The classic triad of sore throat, fever, and lymphadenopathy.

Symptoms	Signs
Sore throat	Exudative pharyngitis enlarged congested membranous tonsils
Severe odynophagia	Lymphadenopathy with enlarged Lymph nodes mainly in the posterior triangle of neck
Fever	*Others*: nasal cavity can also be affected
Myalgia	Hepatosplenomegaly

- Splenomegaly can be found in (50%), while hepatomegaly (10–15%) [11].
- Characteristic feature: Petechiae at the junction of hard and soft palate typically 1–2 mm in diameter, although these are not diagnostic.

Diagnosis

- Diagnosis is usually based on the clinical picture.
- Blood test showed near normal white cell count with increment in lymphocytes, of which 10% are atypical on the blood smear.
- Serological tests: Monospot and Paul Bunnell or Ox-cell. Hemolysis test shows high titers of heterophil antibody. When the Monospot test is negative, but still infectious mononucleosis is highly suspected, EBV-specific antibody studies (to viral capsid antigen) can confirm the diagnosis [11].

Treatment

- Symptomatic treatment including rest, analgesics, antipyretics, and hydration.
- A single dose of dexamethasone during acute symptoms can relieve the symptoms. The steroid also is recommended for complicated infections with upper airway obstruction,

severe hemolytic anemia, severe thrombocytopenia, or persistent severe disease [1, 12].

- Antibiotics: has no role except in secondary bacterial infection. Amoxicillin or ampicillin should be avoided as they can cause a maculopapular rash (salmon-colored rash) in 95% of the patients [12].
- Management of upper airway obstruction: nasopharyngeal airway, high dose steroids, tonsillectomy, endotracheal intubation or a tracheostomy (rarely necessary).
- Recovery from acute phase may take 2–3 weeks. While feelings of malaise may persist for weeks or months. Avoid contact sports to decrease the risk of splenic rupture and hemorrhage until ultrasound examination confirms the resolution of splenomegaly.

Complications

- Secondary bacterial infection up to 30% [7].
- Hemolytic anemia, thrombocytopenia (25–50%).
- Hyperplasia and severe tonsillitis which may cause upper airway obstruction occurs in fewer than 5% [7].
- Splenic rupture, elevated hepatic enzymes.
- Severe neurologic complications occur in 1–5% [7].

49.2.2.2 Coxsackie virus infections (Herpangina)

Mostly it affects children 3–10 years of age. Characterized by a painful vesicular eruption (enanthem) in the palatal and anterior tonsillar pillars area. Treatment is symptomatic, spontaneously resolve in 1 week.

49.2.2.3 Cytomegalovirus

Most infections are asymptomatic, except in immunosuppressed patients, especially post-transplant patients. Infectious mononucleosis-like illnesses but heterophil antibody test is negative. Monoclonal antibodies against CMV is diagnostic. Treatment is symptomatic.

49.2.2.4 Others

Adenovirus (pharyngoconjunctival fever), measles, Herpes simplex virus (HSV).

49.2.3 Fungal Infection

49.2.3.1 Oropharyngeal Candidiasis (Thrush)

Mainly occur in immunosuppressed and chronically debilitated patients as an opportunistic infection [7]. Different Candida species are isolated in oropharyngeal fungal infection. *Candida albicans* is the most common isolated organism [13].

Clinical Features

- It can occur in any age group with immunocompromised status. It is more common in adults, but neonates can be affected as well in 2–5%, which is typically self-limited [1].
- Isolated patches on the pharyngeal mucosa and larynx may be due to inhaled steroids from asthma treatment.

Symptoms	Signs
Sore throat	Mucosal pseudomembranous: characteristic white, cheesy, which can be scraped off to expose an erythematous underlying mucosa
Odynophagia	
Change in taste and burning sensation	
Myalgia	

Diagnosis

- The diagnosis of oral candidiasis is essentially clinical and is based on the recognition of the lesions.
- KOH preparation and microscopic examination. Staining (10% KOH) and culture (Sabouraud dextrose agar).

Treatment

- Topical fluconazole or nystatin are the first line drugs.
- Itraconazole is used for fluconazole-resistant strains, which should be suspected for patients without a clinical resolution after 14 days course of fluconazole.

- Recurrent infections and those with a high risk of systemic infection treated with systemic antifungal therapy [14].
- Prophylactic fluconazole is generally not recommended due to the risk of resistance. May be used with high risk patients for invasive fungal infections.

49.3 Noninfectious Pharyngitis

- *Inflammatory/autoimmune acute pharyngitis*:

Disease	
PFAPA (Periodic Fever, Aphthous Stomatitis, Pharyngitis and Adenitis) syndrome	• Unknown etiology • Affect children <5 years of age • PFAPA is a diagnosis of exclusion (described as regular (clockwork) episodes of high fevers (>39 °C) and oral/neck manifestations every 2–8 weeks and last for 2–7 days with no symptoms between episodes) • Steroids can be used during acute episodes and it mainly reduces the fever episodes • For prevention cimetidine and colchicine can be used • Spontaneous resolution is expected in such pathology, but tonsillectomy has been described to decrease the episodes and possible resolution of PFAPA
Kawasaki disease	• Systemic medium-sized vasculitis of unknown etiology • Treatment focus on Gamma globulin infusion and aspirin to avoid the long-term complications of coronary artery aneurysms and sudden death
Caustic ingestion	• Leads to inflammation or necrosis of the pharynx and upper GI tract
Posttransplant Lymphoproliferative Disorder (PTLD)	• Can present with non-Hodgkin lymphoma • Diagnosis requires a biopsy from Waldeyer's tonsillar ring • Treatment includes a reduction in immunosuppressive therapy, antivirals, and rituximab if EBV titers are high

Disease	
Oral Mucocutaneous *Diseases Epidermolysis Bullosa/Pemphigoid/ Pemphigus/Stevens-Johnson Syndrome*:	• Characterized by blistering and poorly healing ulcers associated with severe pain and dysphagia • Diagnosis is clinical and can be confirmed with a biopsy of an oral or oropharyngeal lesion

- *Membranous Pharyngitis-Tonsillitis*: pharyngitis with exudative membrane can also occur in cases of *agranulocytosis* appears as ulcerative necrotic lesions in the oropharynx, *leukemia*, *aphthous ulcers*, *tonsillar malignancy*, *traumatic ulcer.*
- *Radiation Pharyngitis*: head and neck radiation therapy are known to cause unavoidable acute and long-term pharyngeal inflammation and changes. Starting at an exposure of 20 Gy, and the severity is dose dependent. The acute stage presents with edema, erythema, odynophagia, ulceration, and mucositis. Note that mucositis is worsened in patients with concomitant chemoradiation therapy. Management focuses on symptomatic and superinfection treatments including oral hygiene, topical (analgesia, mouth wash, and antifungals) with or without systemic (analgesia, antibiotics, and antifungal). Healing of acute stage can take around 3–4 weeks or even more [1, 15].

- Inflammatory chronic pharyngitis:
  - *Reflux pharyngitis (laryngopharyngitis)*: presents with gastroesophageal reflux disease (GERD), laryngopharyngeal reflux (LPR), and hiatal hernia. Manifestations include chronic throat pain, burning sensation, sour taste, halitosis, chronic dry cough, hoarseness, globus sensation, and habitual throat clearing. Note that many patients with LPR do not show typical symptoms of GERD of heartburn or indigestion. Clinical exam findings include oropharyngeal erythema, posterior pharyngeal wall cobblestoning, laryngeal edema, contact ulcers and pachydermia on the interarytenoid. The diagnosis is confirmed by a pH probe monitoring study. Treatment using empiric therapy via lifestyle modifi-

cations and proton pump inhibitors or H2-blockers [1].
- *Postnasal drip*: most commonly from allergic rhinitis. Manifestations include globus pharyngeus, chronic cough, and sore throat (irritative pharyngitis). The associate nasal obstruction leads to a habit of mouth breathing which is an important predisposing cause of chronic pharyngitis. Treatment for rhinitis with nasal saline, nasal steroids, and humidification [1].
- *Granulomatous disease*: includes pathologies that induce granulomas, such as tuberculosis (TB), Grahn's disease, foreign body granulomas, iatrogenic (e.g., suture), or as a reaction to hair or keratin debris [1].

- *Malignancy*: Chronic inflammation of the pharynx may hide underlying malignancy in the oral cavity or pharynx.
- *Keratosis Pharyngis*: It is a benign condition, characterized with white/yellow horny keratin outgrowths on the surface of tonsils, pharyngeal wall or lingual tonsils, which is firmly adherent and cannot be removed easily. No accompanying inflammation. No specific treatment is required as usually, it goes into spontaneous regression, the patient needs only reassurance.

Take Home Messages
- Viral infection is the most common cause of pharyngitis in children and adults. Rhinovirus is the most common etiologic agent.
- Bacterial pharyngitis in adults (~10%) is less common than in children (~40%).
- Group A beta-hemolytic streptococci: It is the most common cause of bacterial pharyngitis and can be complicated with deep neck abscess, rheumatic fever, and poststreptococcal glomerulonephritis.
- Poststreptococcal glomerulonephritis risk does not decrease with the use of antibiotics.
- Candidal pharyngitis is common in immunocompromised patients and post-radiotherapy patients.

References

1. Jonas J. Bailey's head and neck surgery: otolaryngology. 5th ed. Philadelphia, PA: Lippincott Williams & Wilkins; 2013.
2. Ebell MH, Smith MA, Barry HC, et al. Does this patient have strep throat? JAMA. 2000;284:2912–8.
3. Pichichero ME. Group A streptococcal tonsillopharyngitis: cost effective diagnosis and treatment. Ann Emerg Med. 1995;25:390–403.
4. Bisno AL. Primary care: acute pharyngitis. N Engl J Med. 2001;344:205–11.
5. Shulman ST, Bisno AL, Clegg HW, et al. Clinical practice guideline for the diagnosis and management of group A streptococcal pharyngitis: 2012 update by the Infectious Disease Society of America. Clin Infect Dis. 2012;55:e86–e101.
6. Choby B. Diagnosis and treatment of streptococcal pharyngitis. Am Pam Physician. 2009;79(5):383–90.
7. Nussenbaum B, Bradford CR. Pharyngitis in adults. In: Flint PW, Haughey BH, Lund V, et al, eds. Cummings Otolaryngology: Head and Neck Surgery. 6th ed. Philadelphia, PA: Elsevier Saunders; 2015:chap 9.
8. Alexander A, Patel N, Southammakosane C, et al. Pediatric autoimmune neuropsychiatric disorders associated with streptococcal infections (PANDAS): an indication for tonsillectomy. Int J Pediatr Otorhinolaryngol. 2011;75(6):872–3.
9. Bimo A, Gerber M, Gwaltney J, et al. Practice guidelines for the diagnosis and management of group A streptococcal pharyngitis. Clin Infect Dis. 2002;35(2):113–25. National Center fur Immunization and Respiratory Diseases: Division of Bacterial Diseases, CDC, Feb 2011.
10. Hodges H. Diphtheria. Pediatric Clin NA. 1979;26:445–59.
11. Papesch M, Watkins R. Epstein-Barr virus infectious mononucleosis. Clin Otolaryngol. 2001;26:3–8.
12. Jenson H. Acute complications of Epstein-Barr virus infectious mononucleosis. Curr Opin Pediatr. 2000;12(3):263–8.
13. Akpan A, Morgan R. Oral candidiasis. Postgrad Med J. 2002;78:455–9.
14. Castagnola E, Macheni M, Bucci B, et al. Antifungal prophylaxis with azole derivatives. Oin Microbiol Infect. 2004;10(Suppl 1):86–95.
15. Scully C, Epstein J, Sonis S. Oral mucositis: a challenging complication of radiotherapy, chemotherapy, and radiochemotherapy: Part 1. Pathogenesis and prophylaxis of mucositis. Head Neck. 2003;25(12):1057–70.

Deep Neck Space Infections

50

Aisha Larem and Adham Aljariri

50.1 Introduction

Deep neck space infection usually arises from the infection of the cervical lymph nodes, the parotid, the mandibular tooth, the sinuses, or the middle ear. With the advancing era of antibiotics, the incidence of deep neck space infection become relatively uncommon, and with immunosuppression, classic signs and symptoms of high-grade fever, systemic toxicity, and local signs of erythema and fluctuant may be absent [1, 2].

50.2 Anatomy

The neck contains different vital structures. Fascial neck space encases these structures and divides them into compartments; this helps to protect vital organs and helps to prevent the direct spread of the infection.

Neck fascial planes are divided into:

(a) *The superficial cervical fascia*: It consists of subcutaneous tissue of the neck that completely encloses and encases head and neck and is continuous with the platysma.

(b) *Deep cervical fascia*: It is subdivided into the superficial, the middle, and the deep cervical fascia. The confluent of all of these three layers of the deep cervical fascia contributes to the carotid sheath. The neurovascular compartment of this sheath contains the carotid artery, the internal jugular vein, and the vagus nerve [1, 3].

Fascial planes are the spaces between the different layers of the cervical fascia: Look at Fig. 50.1

- *Submandibular space*: It lies within submandibular and submental triangles, between mucosa of the floor of the mouth and the superficial (investing) layer of the deep cervical fascia. It is subdivided by the mylohyoid into the sublingual and the submylohyoid spaces. These two spaces communicate posteriorly around the mylohyoid. The infection of the submandibular space can give a condition called Ludwig's angina, where infection of the sublingual space causes gross swelling of the tongue and acute airway obstruction. Infection of the submylohyoid space may spread posteriorly to the parapharyngeal, the retropharyngeal, and may spread to the superior mediastinum [1, 3].
- *Parapharyngeal space*: It is an inverted cone-shaped space at the lateral aspect of the neck with the base at the skull base and the apex

A. Larem (✉) · A. Aljariri
Hamad Medical Corporation, Doha, Qatar
e-mail: alarem@hamad.qa; AAljariri@hamad.qa

A. Al-Qahtani et al. (eds.), *Textbook of Clinical Otolaryngology*,
https://doi.org/10.1007/978-3-030-54088-3_50

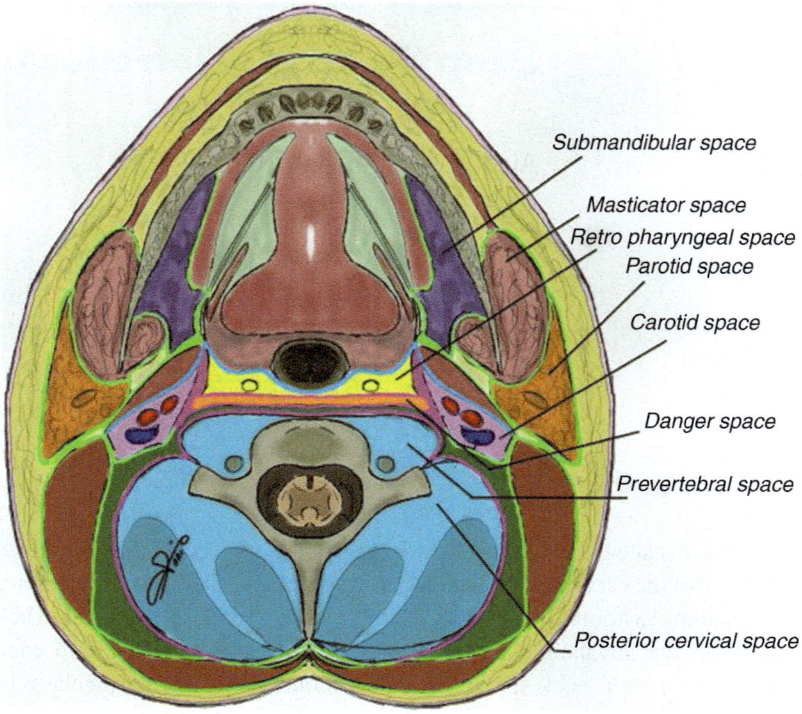

Fig. 50.1 Schematic drawing (axial) demonstrating different deep neck spaces

near the hyoid bone. It lies deep to the pharyngeal constrictor muscle and is continuous with the pretracheal fascia medially and the superficial fascia investing the parotid gland laterally. It is divided by the styloid process into:

Anterior compartment (pre-styloid (muscular)): It contains no vital structures.

Posterior compartment (retro-styloid (Neurovascular)): It contains ninth to twelfth cranial nerves, carotid sheath and its contents, and cervical sympathetic trunk.

Infection of this space may arise from pharyngitis, tonsillitis, otitis, parotitis, mastoiditis, and odontogenic infections [1, 3].

- *Retropharyngeal space*: It is bounded anteriorly by the buccopharyngeal fascia and closely surrounds the constrictor muscles of the neck and bounded posteriorly by the alar layer of the deep layer of the deep cervical fascia. It is situated behind the hypopharynx and the esophagus and communicates with the parapharyngeal fascia laterally [1, 3].
- *Danger space*: It lies behind the retropharyngeal space. It is bounded anteriorly by the alar fascia and posteriorly by the prevertebral fascia. It extends from the base of the skull freely to the entire posterior mediastinum to the level of the diaphragm [1, 3].
- *Prevertebral space*: It is bounded by the prevertebral fascia, which originates from the spinous process and divided into alar fascia anteriorly and prevertebral fascia posteriorly. The prevertebral space extends from the base of the skull to coccyx [1, 3].
- *Pretracheal space*: It compromises the anterior portion of the visceral compartment and completely encircles the trachea and the esophagus. It communicates laterally with the carotid sheath and with the superior mediastinum inferiorly [1, 3].
- *Peritonsillar space*: It lies between the capsule of the palatine tonsils medially and the superior constrictor laterally. Peritonsillar abscess may rupture through the superior constrictor muscle and extend to the parapharyngeal space [1, 3].
- *Parotid space*: It is formed by splitting the investing fascia at the stylomandibular ligament level to enclose the parotid with superfi-

cial capsule and deep capsule. Infection in this space can spread through the deep capsule to the stylomandibular tunnel into the parapharyngeal space [1, 3].

– *Masticator space*: Anterior and lateral to parapharyngeal space. Infection in this space usually ascends from upper odontogenic infection [1, 3].

50.3 Lymphatic Drainage of Head and Neck

Head and neck lymph nodes can be divided into ten groups. Six of them are distributed in a belt-like at the head and neck junction (Sublingual, Submandibular, Maxillary, Parotid, Mastoid, and Occipital). The lateral cervical chain of the neck serves as a common pathway of drainage. The final pathway of head and neck lymphatics is a large lymphatic chain along the carotid sheath, when inflamed cervical lymph nodes become adherent to the cervical fascia, and infection can spread to the bloodstream.

Nasopharynx and oropharynx have mucosal-associated lymphoid tissue as in the gut and the bronchus; in nasopharynx, it is called Waldeyer's ring (Palatine, Lingual, Adenoid, and Tonsillar lymphoid tissue). Acute inflammation of this area may compromise the airway.

Deep cervical fascia is connected with loose connective tissue; the potential spread of infection through this space is possible [4, 5].

50.4 Microbiology for the Deep Neck Space Infections

Deep neck space infections are likely to be polymicrobial. Infections there tend to have five or six bacteria on average with anaerobes outnumbers aerobes [6]. Look at Table 50.1.

The most common isolated organism from deep neck space infections is *viridans Streptococci*, and *Streptococcus anginosus* [17].

Prevertebral space infections usually originate from vertebral abscesses, vertebral osteomyelitis, or local instrumentation of trachea and esophagus, so microbiology is different from other deep neck space infection, IV drug users have increased risk of MRSA [18, 19].

Table 50.1 Microbials in deep neck space infections according to the source of infection

Oral cavity and odontogenic [7–9]	*Viridans Streptococci* *Streptococcus anginosus* *Parvimonas micra* *Peptostreptococcus* species *Fusobacterium nucleatum* *Prevotella melaninogenica*
Pharynx [10, 11]	*Streptococcus pyogens* *Fusobacterium necrophorum* *Haemophilus influenzae*
Ear [12, 13]	*Staphylococcus aureus* *Pseudomonas aeruginosa*
Sinus [7, 14]	*Streptococcus pneumoniae* *H. influenzae* *Moraxella catarrhalis* *S. aureus* *Chronic sinus infections (anaerobes)*
Immunocompromised [15, 16]	*P. aeruginosa and other ESBL*

50.5 Clinical Presentation

Presentation of the deep neck space infections depends on the primary source of the infection (oropharyngeal, sinogenic, otogenic, or odontogenic). However, they share some clinical features like trismus, which is caused by the compression of masticatory muscles by the abscess or caused by the involvement of the motor branch of the trigeminal nerve.

Other signs and symptoms are:

(a) Unilateral sore throat
(b) Neck pain
(c) Neck stiffness
(d) Dysphagia and Odynophagia (may be secondary to the involvement of the cricoarytenoid joint)
(e) Dysphonia or hoarseness of voice (they are late presentations which indicate cranial nerve X involvement)
(f) Bulging of the pharyngeal wall or the floor of the mouth

(g) Oropharyngeal midline shift
(h) Neck swelling
(i) Crepitus
(j) Sign of airway compromise (stridor, muffled voice, or saliva drooling): Stridor and dyspnea signify airway obstruction or an infection spreading to the superior mediastinum
(k) Unilateral tongue paralysis or paresis indicates XII cranial nerve involvement

In patients who are exposed to radiotherapy or had radical neck surgeries, cellulitis, and lymphedema may be the prominent clinical signs. Patients with prolonged tracheostomy or mechanical ventilation may present differently because tracheoesophageal fistula may ease the infection to spread to the mediastinum. Intensive care unit patients with prolonged jugular central line may develop suppurative thrombophlebitis of the internal jugular vein [20, 21].

50.6 Imaging

Clinical features suggesting deep neck space infections should raise the suspicion of this condition and prompt urgent radiologic evaluation. If airway compromise is suspected, the airway should be secured before any image's modality or surgical intervention.

50.6.1 CT Scan

It is the most common imaging modality for evaluation of deep neck space infections, with an excellent evaluation window of the soft tissue and bone. Axial cuts are beneficial in defining the extent of the disease to the mediastinum and cranial vault. Also, a CT scan can be used in diagnostic and therapeutic-guided aspiration or drainage.

50.6.2 MRI

It is useful for soft tissue delineation and assessment of vascular complications. It is superior to CT in soft tissue evaluation and anatomic discrimination, and it is helpful to discriminate between the mass lesion and the surrounding soft tissue when the CT scan is poor. Drawbacks of MRI use are: long study time, minor artifacts caused by breathing, motion and swallowing, cost, discomfort, claustrophobia, and patients with certain implanted devices cannot undergo MRI. These drawbacks limit its use as a standard modality for the evaluation of deep neck space infections.

Plain radiography is of limited use in deep neck space infection. However, dynamic contrast studies still used in the evaluation of the swallowing or detecting foreign bodies [22, 23]

Look at Table 50.2 which shows a comparison between CT scan and MRI.

Table 50.2 Comparison between CT scan and MRI

CT scan	MRI
Short duration study	Long duration study
Good for soft tissue and bone from a single exposure	Poor for bone, very good in visualizing and differentiation of soft tissue
Shows the extent in axial cuts	Expensive
	Cannot be done in certain people (implantable devices, claustrophobic)

50.7 Treatment of Deep Neck Space Infections

Antibiotics, along with drainage of the loculated infections, are the treatment of deep neck space infections. However, in early stages when the infection is confined to the soft tissue of the neck where is no frank abscess or minimal abscess formation, antibiotics alone is sufficient, drainage at these cases may disturb the natural immunity and the defense mechanism in preventing the spread of the infection, and that may exacerbate the condition.

The choice of the antibiotics should be based on the clinical suspicion of the most likely organism depending on the origin of infection before culture result (if sent) is out. A maximum dose of the antibiotic should be given in order to optimize tissue penetration.

The airway should be assessed in every patient with deep neck space infections.

Glucocorticoids can be used to relieve the symptoms of acute airway obstruction, but the data to support this trend remains insufficient [1].

50.8 Peritonsillar Abscess (Quinsy)

It is a suppurative complication of acute tonsillitis. Pus, in this case, accumulates between the capsule of the palatine tonsil and the pharyngeal muscle. At an early stage, cellulitis may be present with no frank abscess or pus collection. Patient with peritonsillar abscess presents with throat pain localized on one side, fever, muffled voice, saliva drooling, and trismus. Physical examination shows bulging of the affected tonsillar side, uvular deviation to the normal side, soft palate swelling, neck swelling, and tender cervical lymphadenopathy.

The presence of trismus may limit throat examination, and the presence of saliva drooling may warn for the possibility of concomitant epiglottitis, so care must be taken. Images and examination in the operating theater with a secured airway may be warranted in some patients.

The diagnosis of a peritonsillar abscess is a clinical one. Images are not necessary unless there is a suspension of another concomitant abscess. Look at Fig. 50.2.

Differential diagnoses of the peritonsillar abscess are epiglottitis, retropharyngeal abscess or cellulitis, parapharyngeal abscess, and severe tonsillopharyngitis.

Differentiation between peritonsillar abscess and peritonsillar cellulitis may be done by intraoral or submandibular ultrasonography, though no sufficient evidence to support this practice.

Management includes surgical drainage with proper antimicrobial coverage and supportive measures as analgesia, hydration, and close observation for complications development [1].

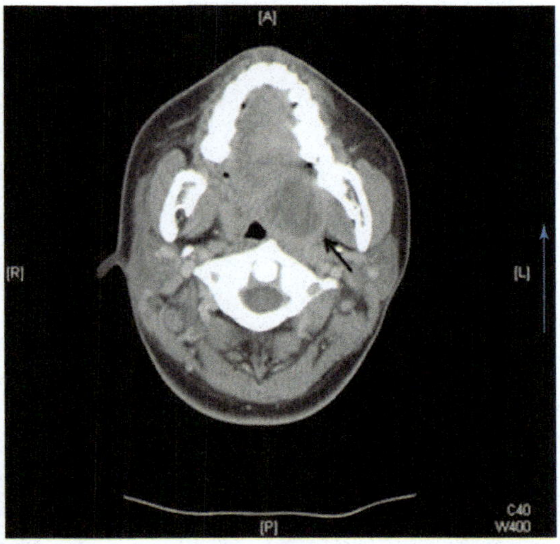

Fig. 50.2 Axial Neck CT scan with contrast showing left peritonsillar abscess (arrow). (Image Reprinted with permission from Elsevier: Pediatrics & Neonatology, Clinical Features of Peritonsillar Abscess in Children, THsiang-Ju Hsiao,Yhu-Chering Huang et al, December 1,2012)

50.9 Parapharyngeal Space Infections

Symptoms of the parapharyngeal space infection are dominated by the primary source of infection, with dental infections being the most common, followed by a peritonsillar abscess, otitis, parotitis, and mastoiditis which are very rare though could still happen.

Patients present with systemic symptoms of fever and rigors, besides to signs and symptoms related to deep neck space infections like trismus, swelling below the mandible, bulging of the medial pharyngeal wall, lymphadenopathy, pooling of saliva, and purulent oral discharge. Dyspnea can occur if epiglottis or larynx is involved. Look at Fig. 50.3.

These signs and symptoms predominate an infection of the anterior compartment of the parapharyngeal space. Infection of the posterior neurovascular compartment, on the other hand, may present with mild trismus and neck pain, systemic signs of sepsis being more prominent, and cranial nerve palsies [24, 25].

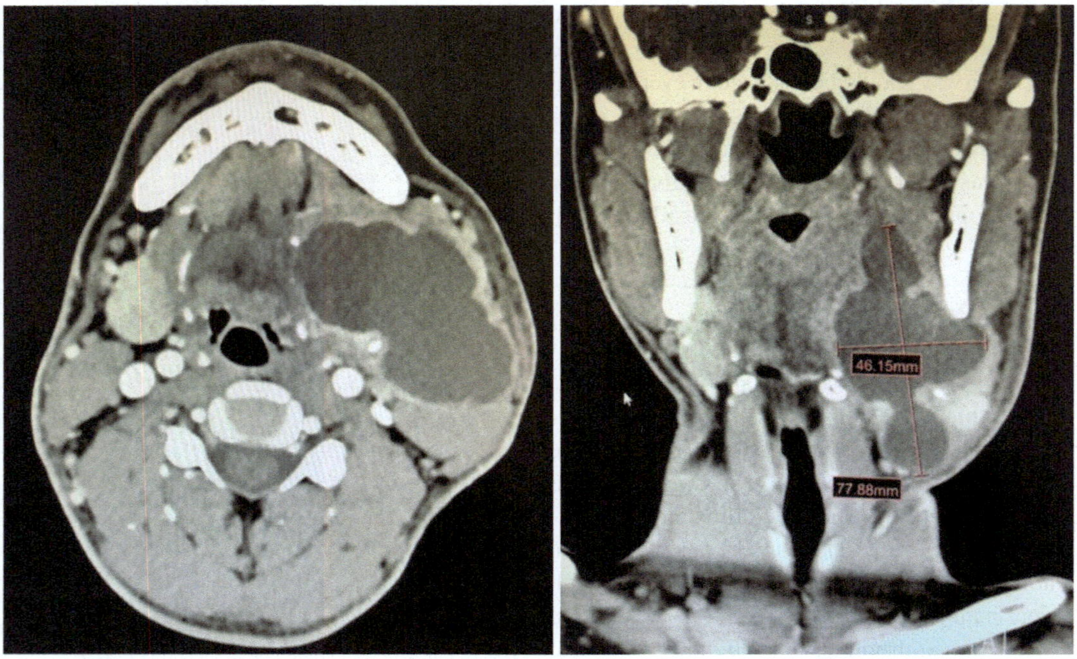

Fig. 50.3 Axial and coronal neck CT scan with contrast in a patient with multiloculated parapharyngeal abscess

Complications:

1. Carotid sheath involvement with subsequent mycotic carotid aneurysm
2. Suppurative jugular thrombophlebitis (Lemierre's syndrome or post-anginal sepsis)

50.10 Retropharyngeal Space Infections

Retropharyngeal abscess is usually secondary to penetrating trauma, foreign body (fishbone), or instrumentation (esophagoscopy, bronchoscopy).

In retropharyngeal infections, signs and symptoms also will depend on the primary source of the infection. Patients may present with sore throat and pressure symptoms like dysphagia and breathing difficulties. Systemic symptoms may be present, depending on the clinical stage of the patient.

Physical examination may show unilateral pharyngeal wall swelling or posterior wall bulging. In the case of retropharyngeal lymph node involvement, the patient will have trismus that will limit the oropharyngeal examination.

Retropharyngeal infections are serious as infection may spread directly to the anterior and posterior areas of the superior mediastinum or into the danger space.

Acute necrotizing mediastinitis is the most serious complication of retropharyngeal infections, as infection may drain via gravity into the posterior mediastinum resulting in mediastinitis and empyema. [1]

A high clinical suspension is needed to diagnose retropharyngeal abscess. Contrast-enhanced neck CT scan and blood cultures should be obtained to all patients with parapharyngeal or retropharyngeal abscess to identify the offending pathogens. Look at Figs. 50.4, 50.5, and 50.6.

Note that necrotic lymph nodes from a metastatic malignant disease may have a similar appearance to an abscess in CT scan, MRI is more helpful in differentiating between them.

Plain radiographs—if done—may have findings that may suggest retropharyngeal space infections as the thickness of prevertebral soft tissue, air-fluid level, the presence of foreign bod-

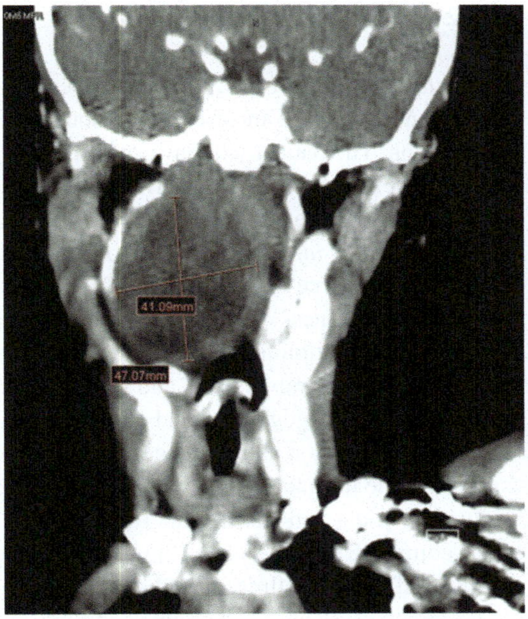

Fig. 50.4 Coronal CT scan with contrast showing retropharyngeal extending to right parapharyngeal space

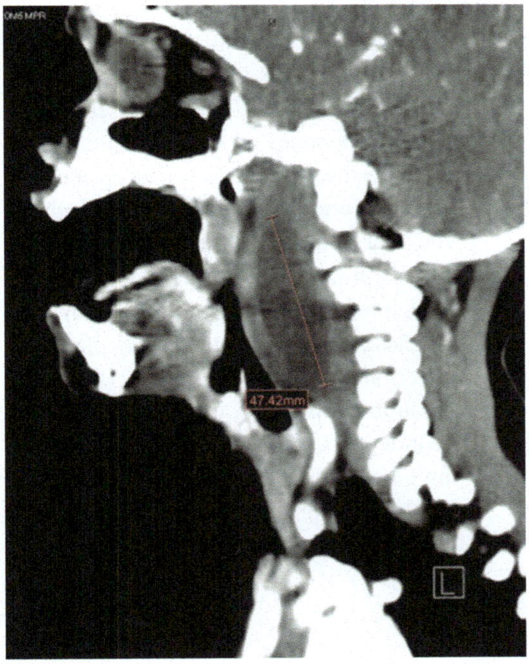

Fig. 50.5 Sagittal CT scan with contrast showing retropharyngeal abscess

ies, cervical lordosis, gas collection, and displacement of the larynx and trachea anteriorly.

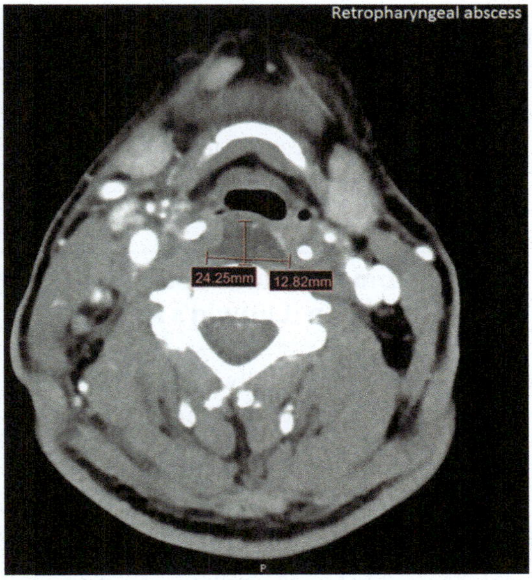

Fig. 50.6 Neck axial CT scan with contrast—retropharyngeal abscess

Treatment:

1. Elimination of the primary source of the infection, whether it is a dental or a foreign body, is recommended.
2. Surgical management is depending on the stage of the infection; localized abscess needs to be drained, while at an early stage cellulitis drainage needs to be delayed. Differentiation between localized abscess and cellulitis is difficult clinically but can be easily identified on images.

The surgical drainage approach depends on: the site of the abscess, whether there is an airway compromise or not, and whether there is a spread to the danger space or not. In general, it is indicated if there is an air-fluid level (gas-producing organism), airway compromise, or failure of improvement after 48–72 h of medical treatment. Ultrasound-guided aspiration is effective if there is no airway compromise. If complicated by necrotizing mediastinitis, surgical drainage through the cervical approach or thoracotomy may be indicted [26, 27].

Surgical drainage will offer a sample for culture to direct the antimicrobial therapy, and establishing an external drainage pathway and a port for irrigation [28].

Prevertebral space infection: It has the same clinical features of the retropharyngeal space infection. Potts' abscess is the osteomyelitis of the spine caused by tuberculosis.

50.11 Submandibular Space Infection (Ludwig's Angina)

It is aggressive and rapidly progressive cellulitis without lymphatic involvement or abscess formation. It usually involves submandibular space on both sides, with both sublingual and submylohyoid space, are affected. The submylohyoid space is affected first as the tooth roots located below the mylohyoid attachment to the mandible. The infection usually arises from the second or the third molar tooth. It may spread from suppurative parotitis or a peritonsillar abscess [29]. Without treatment, Ludwig's angina may lead to airway obstruction. Look at Fig. 50.7.

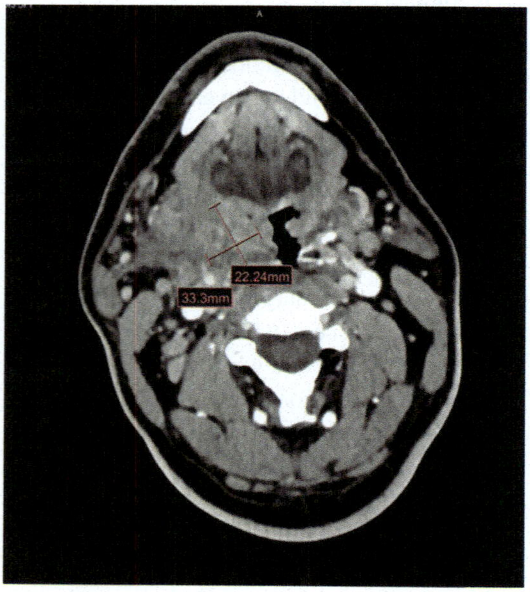

Fig. 50.7 Axial CT scan of a patient with right submandibular space cellulitis (phlegmon)

50.12 Other Space Infections

Masticator space infection: Molars (especially the third molar) is the most common source of the infection. The patient will have swelling over the posterior ramus and trismus. Treatment is by incision and drainage and antibiotics.

Parotid space infection: The parotid is the most common source of the infection. The patient will have tenderness over the parotid area. Treatment is by antibiotics, along with maintaining hydration and oral hygiene and using warm compresses, sialagogues, and massaging. Aspiration or incision and drainage may be necessary in some instances.

Buccal space infection: The teeth are the most common source of the infection. The patient will have swelling over the buccal area extending up till the eyelids. In this condition, it should be treated by aggressive antibiotics and doing incision and drainage urgently to prevent the feared complication of cavernous sinus thrombosis.

Take Home Messages

- Though the incidence of deep neck space infections decreased dramatically, you still could face them during your clinical practice.
- A high index of suspicion is your key to diagnose and treat deep neck space infections.
- Treatment options vary from medical treatment to surgical drainage depending on each patient's situation.
- While treating deep neck space infections, always consider securing the airway.

Acknowledgment Authors of the chapter would like to appreciate the help of Dr. Ma'in Al Shawabkeh, a Clinical fellow at Hamad Medical Corporation, of his help and effort in editing this chapter.

References

1. Chow AW. Deep neck space infections in adults. Up to date.
2. Chow AW. Life-threatening infections of the head, neck, and upper respiratory tract. In: Hall JB, Schmidt GA, Kress JP, editors. Principles of critical care. 4th ed. New York: McGraw-Hill; 2015. p. 676.
3. Grodinsky M. Ludwig's angina, retropharyngeal abscess, and other deep abscesses of the head and neck. JAMA. 1940;114:18.
4. Timon CI, Cafferkey M, Walsh M. Infection of Waldeyer's ring: value of pernasal retropharyngeal swabs. J Otolaryngol. 1991;20:279.
5. Bernstein JM. Waldeyer's ring and otitis media: the nasopharyngeal tonsil and otitis media. Int J Pediatr Otorhinolaryngol. 1999;49(Suppl 1):S127.
6. Todd JK. Bacteriology and clinical relevance of nasopharyngeal and oropharyngeal cultures. Pediatr Infect Dis. 1984;3:159.
7. Brook I. Current management of upper respiratory tract and head and neck infections. Eur Arch Otorhinolaryngol. 2009;266:315.
8. Heim N, Faron A, Wiedemeyer V, et al. Microbiology and antibiotic sensitivity of head and neck space infections of odontogenic origin. Differences in inpatient and outpatient management. J Craniomaxillofac Surg. 2017;45:1731.
9. Cordesmeyer R, Kauffmann P, Markus T, et al. Bacterial and histopathological findings in deep head and neck infections: a retrospective analysis. Oral Surg Oral Med Oral Pathol Oral Radiol. 2017;124:11.
10. Ehlers Klug T, Rusan M, Fuursted K, Ovesen T. Fusobacterium necrophorum: most prevalent pathogen in peritonsillar abscess in Denmark. Clin Infect Dis. 2009;49:1467.
11. Brook I. Microbiology and management of peritonsillar, retropharyngeal, and parapharyngeal abscesses. J Oral Maxillofac Surg. 2004;62:1545.
12. Hull MW, Chow AW. An approach to oral infections and their management. Curr Infect Dis Rep. 2005;7:17.
13. Laulajainen Hongisto A, Aarnisalo AA, Lempinen L, et al. Otogenic intracranial abscesses, our experience over the last four decades. J Int Adv Otol. 2017;13:40.
14. Stephenson MF, Mfuna L, Dowd SE, et al. Molecular characterization of the polymicrobial flora in chronic rhinosinusitis. J Otolaryngol Head Neck Surg. 2010;39:182.
15. Huang TT, Liu TC, Chen PR, et al. Deep neck infection: analysis of 185 cases. Head Neck. 2004;26:854.
16. Lin HT, Tsai CS, Chen YL, Liang JG. Influence of diabetes mellitus on deep neck infection. J Laryngol Otol. 2006;120:650.
17. Rega AJ, Aziz SR, Ziccardi VB. Microbiology and antibiotic sensitivities of head and neck space infections of odontogenic origin. J Oral Maxillofac Surg. 2006;64:1377.
18. Endress C, Guyot DR, Fata J, Salciccioli G. Cervical osteomyelitis due to i.v. heroin use: radiologic findings in 14 patients. AJR Am J Roentgenol. 1990;155:333.
19. Jackson KA, Bohm MK, Brooks JT, et al. Invasive methicillin-resistant *Staphylococcus aureus* infections among persons who inject drugs—six sites, 2005–2016. MMWR Morb Mortal Wkly Rep. 2018;67:625.
20. Jalisi S, Sakai O, Jamal BT, Mardirossian V. Features of prevertebral disease in patients presenting to a head and neck surgery clinic with neck pain. Ann Maxillofac Surg. 2017;7:228.
21. Reihsaus E, Waldbaur H, Seeling W. Spinal epidural abscess: a meta-analysis of 915 patients. Neurosurg Rev. 2000;23:175.
22. Dunnebier EA. Imaging for otolaryngologist. New York: Thieme; 2011.
23. Hurley MC, Heran MK. Imaging studies for head and neck infections. Infect Dis Clin North Am. 2007;21:305.
24. Laupland KB. Vascular and parameningeal infections of the head and neck. Infect Dis Clin North Am. 2007;21:577.
25. Alexander DW, Leonard JR, Trail ML. Vascular complications of deep neck abscesses. A report of four cases. Laryngoscope. 1968;78:361.
26. Brook I, Frazier EH. Microbiology of mediastinitis. Arch Intern Med. 1996;156:333.
27. Daya H, Lo S, Papsin BC, et al. Retropharyngeal and parapharyngeal infections in children: the Toronto experience. Int J Pediatr Otorhinolaryngol. 2005;69:81.
28. Flint PW, et al., editors. Cummings otolaryngology, head and neck surgery. 5th ed. Philadelphia, PA: Mosby Elsevier; 2010.
29. Brook I. Microbiology and principles of antimicrobial therapy for head and neck infections. Infect Dis Clin North Am. 2007;21:355.

51 Obstructive Sleep Apnea

Medhat Shams and Hayam AlTaweel

51.1 Introduction

Sleep is a state with which we are all familiar but is poorly understood. Beginning with the advent of the EEG, investigators began studying the electrical activity of the brain during sleep. Also, it was recognized early on that there are two distinct sleep states: a peaceful, physiologically restive state (NREM sleep), and a different state characterized by muscle atonia and autonomic activity (increased heart rate and blood pressure) and rapid eye movements (REM sleep) when your eyes move quickly in different direction and dreams typically happen.

Using the EEG investigators has divided NREM sleep into four stages. Stage I is the lightest and stage IV is the deepest. Through the night a person cycles up and down through these stages, with REM sleep occurring intermittently between stage II and I. As the night goes on more time is spent in REM sleep. This is important to realize, as the obstructive sleep apnea syndrome is more likely to occur during REM sleep, and thus a partial night sleep study may miss clinically important sleep apnea if done in the first portion of the night [1].

Electronic Supplementary Material The online version of this chapter (https://doi.org/10.1007/978-3-030-54088-3_51) contains supplementary material, which is available to authorized users.

M. Shams (✉) · H. AlTaweel
ENT Department, Hamad Medical Corporation, Doha, Qatar
e-mail: mshafik@hamad.qa; haltaweel@hamad.qa

51.2 Definition

To understand specific disorders one must know some definitions; an apnea is defined as cessation of airflow for 10 s which results in arousal. If the chest wall continues to mechanically move during this time, then it is obstructive apnea, if the chest wall dose not attempt to ventilate then it is presumably due to neurologic etiology and is termed a central apnea, sometimes there is obstructive and central apnea and this is termed mixed apnea. The number of apnea per hour is termed apnea index.

A hypopnea is a diminution of airflow which result in hypoxemia and arousal, the number of apnea and hypopnea is termed apnea-hypopnea index (AHI). The respiratory disturbance index (RDI) is AHI plus the number of arousals per hour.

Generally obstructive sleep apnea syndrome (OSAS) is considered mild when AHI is 5–15, considered moderate if between 15 and 30, and severe if >30. As the field of sleep medicine progressed, there arose an awareness of certain patients who report excessive daytime sleepiness but do not have OSAS (e.g., RDI <5) known to have increased negative thoracic pres-

A. Al-Qahtani et al. (eds.), *Textbook of Clinical Otolaryngology*,
https://doi.org/10.1007/978-3-030-54088-3_51

sure inspiration, thus their increased work of breathing is thought to be responsible for their symptom. This syndrome has been termed upper airway resistance syndrome (UARS). Together with OSAS these are jointly referred to as sleep-disorder breathing (SDB).Those patients who snore but have an RDI <5 and do not have increased intrathoracic pressure upon inspiration simply are primary snorer. One hypothesis is that these disorders represent a spectrum of disease with primary snoring being the mildest, followed by UARS, and ends finally with OSAS as the full manifestation of the disease [2].

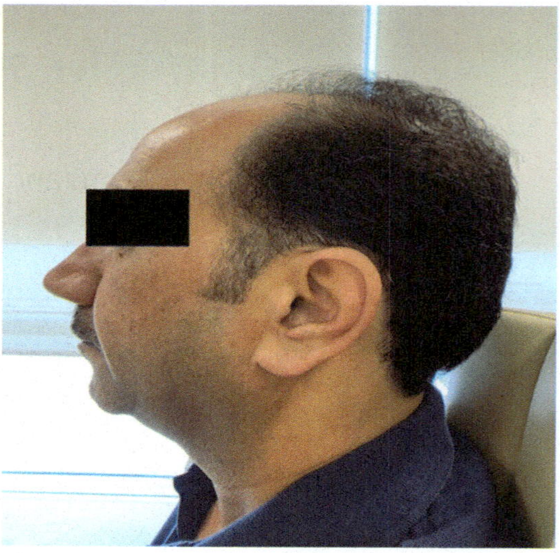

Fig. 51.1 Patient with retrognathia

51.3 Pathophysiology of OSAS

Although incompletely understood, the pathophysiology of OSAS relates to an anatomical small or collapsible pharyngeal airway. During wakefulness, neuromuscular compensatory systems function to increase the activity of the pharyngeal dilator muscles thus preserving airway patency. However, this reflex driven augmented muscle activity is lost at sleep onset, and collapse of the pharyngeal airway occurs.

Nasal obstruction appears to facilitate or exacerbate the syndrome although it does not appear to be primarily responsible. Tonsillar hypertrophy may be a cause for OSAS particularly in the pediatric population. Obesity increases the prevalence of OSAS, as the lateral pharyngeal fat pads may narrow the airway in the lateral dimension. The associated hypoxemia and hypercapnia drive increasing respiratory efforts, and ultimately arousal from sleep occurs, thus reestablishing airway patency and ventilation. Once the patient returns to sleep the cycle begin again. The patient thus suffers the consequences of repeated sleep disruption as well as recurrent hypoxemia and hypercapnia [3].

Unfavorable anatomy appears to be the most important cause. This can be due to a narrow palate, an elongated uvula, redundant tissue at the base of tongue, micro/retrognathia (Fig. 51.1). Additionally, extrinsic factors such as sedating medications may exacerbate the physiologic defects.

51.4 Diagnosis

51.4.1 History

Patients with sleep apnea often present when their bed partner can no longer stand loud snoring. These patients complain of excessive daytime sleepiness, and feeling like they did not sleep the night before. They may complain of awakening multiple times during the night because of apneas or because of the loudness of their own snoring. In the morning, they may have headache or dry mouth. Sometimes these patients are prone to accidents at work or while driving because they fall asleep at inappropriate times. Other symptoms that may be accompanied are memory lapses, poor concentration, gastroesophageal refluxes (GERD), and personality changes [4].

The Epworth sleepiness scale is an invaluable tool for initial assessment of obstructive sleep apnea. This survey asks the likelihood of falling asleep in eight common situations (Fig. 51.2).

Fig. 51.2 Scaled from 0 (never) to 3 (always), and a score greater than 11 is correlated with OSA

Epworth Sleepiness Scale	
How likely are you to doze off or fall asleep in the following situation? **Use the following scale to choose the most appropriate number?**	
0 (No chance) **1** (Slight chance) **2** (Moderate chance) **3** (High chance)	
Sitting and reading	0 1 2 3
Watching television	0 1 2 3
Sitting inactive, in public space	0 1 2 3
Lying down to rest in the afternoon when circumstances permit	0 1 2 3
Sitting and talking to someone	0 1 2 3
Sitting quietly after a lunch without alcohol	0 1 2 3
As a passenger in car for an hour without a break	0 1 2 3
In a car, while stopped for a few minutes in traffic	0 1 2 3

51.4.2 ENT Examination

The nose can be obstructed by nasal valve collapse, septal deviation, turbinate hypertrophy, or nasal masses. Allergic rhinitis, acute rhinosinusitis, nasal polyposis, nasal tumors, and acquired nasal and facial deformities.

Examination of the nasopharynx may reveal adenoid hypertrophy, or other occluding mass. Evaluation of the oral cavity should be done with the tongue inside the mouth in a relaxed position. The tonsils should be graded from 0 to 4, with zero being absent and four being kissing. Examination of the palate and uvula should also be noted. Many patients with OSA will have a long, thick uvula (Fig. 51.3), or redundant soft palate. They may also have macroglossia.

The Muller's maneuver can be performed while occluding the nose and mouth and having the patient take an inspiration. This will allow the examiner to visualize pharyngeal collapse and objectively identify anterior-posterior collapse or lateral wall collapse [5].

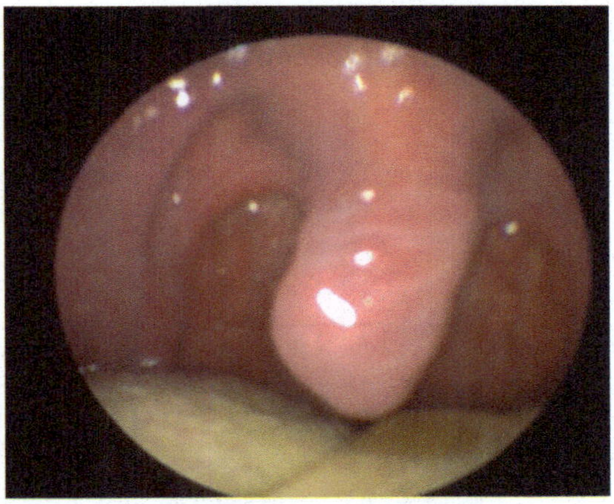

Fig. 51.3 Patient with OSA showing a long and thick uvula

By doing this one can get an idea of the relative collapsibility of the palate as compared to the base of tongue or the hypopharynx. Although not very sensitive or specific, it still can be a helpful examination.

51.4.3 Polysomnography (PSG)

This is the gold standard for diagnosis obstructive sleep apnea this is generally and overnight, attended study performed in a sleep laboratory. EEG, pulse oximetry, EKG, nasal and oral airflow, respiratory effort, and leg movements are all measured during testing (Fig. 51.4).

An apnea is recorded when there is cessation of nasal airflow for at least 10 s. Hypopnea is recorded when airflow decreases by 30% and there is an associated 4% drop in oxygen saturation. The apnea/hypopnea index and respiratory disturbance index as well as the minimum oxygen saturation are the important numbers to review in the report. An AHI or RDI greater than five is considered mild obstructive sleep apnea. When this number is greater than 15, it is moderate, and when it is greater than 30 is severe. Minimum oxygen saturation less than 90% is considered abnormal. After a positive PSG, the patient should be fitted with a CPAP mask and a titration study is performed.

51.4.4 Sleep Endoscopy (DISE)

Drug-induced sedation endoscopy (DISE) has been used in the last two decades in order to determine under fiber optic visualization the exact sites of upper airway collapse in OSA patients.

By directing the surgical procedures towards the obstruction-specific structure, surgical outcome improve (Videos 51.1–51.5).

Additionally, with the help of passive maneuvers, the potential efficacy drug-induced sleep endoscopy has been performed by infusing a sedation administered by an anesthesiologist in the operating room until the patient start to snore and have some blockage of their breathing. We pass a flexible telescope through one side of the nose in order to evaluate the throat and observe the potential blockage of breathing in the palate, lateral pharyngeal wall, and the tongue base.

An assessment of the patient's airway is then performed to determine the sites of obstruction, the use of VOTE classification for the assessment of DISE can facilitate the scientific evaluation in individual centers and also the collection of data across multiple centers. Head rotation during DISE improves upper airway collapse; this improvement is seen in positional obstructive sleep apnea.

Although DISE represents the most widespread diagnostic tool for upper airway endoscopic evaluation of snoring and obstructive sleep apnea-hypopnea syndrome (OSAHS), many controversies exist about how to perform the sedation, the indications for DISE [6].

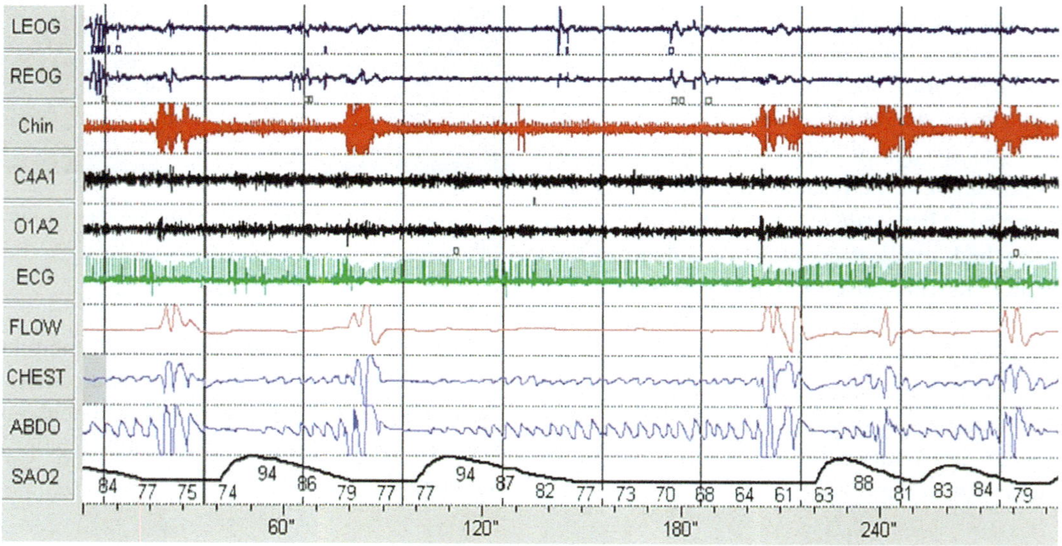

Fig. 51.4 EEG, pulse oximetry, EKG, nasal and oral airflow, respiratory effort, and leg movements are all measured during polysomnography

51.5 Management

Numerous treatment options for obstructive sleep apnea (OSA) presently exist. This treatment ranges from noninvasive behavioral modifications to nightly use of positive airway pressure (PAP) devices to surgical treatments that alter airway anatomy. Selection of patients for these treatments is a complex given the range of variability in patients' anatomy and physiology, patient preference, disease severity, and controversy with regard to the effectiveness of available treatment.

51.5.1 Standard Treatment for Obstructive Sleep Apnea

51.5.1.1 Nonsurgical

In obese patients, one should consider ***weight loss***. It is felt that there is a threshold level of weight for most individuals above which they experience symptoms and below which they do not. Also investigational tools such as computed tomography have demonstrated the increase in the airway with weight loss. Additionally, obese patients have many other medical benefits to gain from weight loss.

Sleep hygiene should be reviewed. Alcohol and sedating medicines may exacerbate OSAS. Patients with insomnia should be counseled to avoid nighttime caffeine and avoid activities such as reading or watching television in bed. Lastly, since OSAS is usually worse when supine, some patients may benefits from relatively simple measures such as sewing a tennis ball into the back of a T-shirt to promote sleeping on the side.

CPAP: Continuous positive airway pressure by passes all of the levels of obstructive sleep apnea and is first-line therapy. The optimal pressure must be achieved and the patient must wear the mask for 5 h/night and 5 nights/week to be considered compliant. Despite all of the benefits of CPAP, some patients cannot tolerate it. The reasons for noncompliance include excessive pressures, noise, air leakage, discomfort, and claustrophobia. They concluded that patients with side effects or noncompliant with CPAP therapy, will benefit from evaluation by an otolaryngologist for possible surgical intervention.

Many patients seen by sleep specialists are never informed of surgical options. They are told that CPAP therapy is their only option. Although CPAP therapy is clearly safer and more effective than any surgical therapy, there is a huge number of patients who cannot or will not use CPAP [7].

Oral appliances: Are also effective in relieving OSAS. These work by mechanically moving the jaw or tongue forward and opening the airway. They have been shown to be more effective for mild or moderate OSAS. Although some find them difficult to use, in general compliance is superior to CPAP.

Individual patient selection in its application remains very crucial. No single appliance has been shown to be superior to another [8].

51.5.1.2 Surgical Treatment

Successful surgical treatment for OSA (Obstructive sleep apnea) is a big challenge. With different surgical techniques to address the upper airway in patients suffering from sleep disordered breathing (SDB), there is no consensus regarding the ideal procedure to improve the success rate with least morbidity. Previous surgical techniques for OSA were mainly focused on excision of tissues and shortening the soft palate.

In the past, surgical therapies focused on treatment of the soft palate. This included snare uvulectomy, uvulopalatoplasty, uvulopalatopharyngoplasty, laser-assisted uvuloplasty, and more recently radiofrequency ablation and soft palate pillar implantation.

The most well-known and popular of these treatments is the uvulopalatopharyngoplasty (UP3). This procedure was developed to address the most probable site of obstruction (the palate) and redundant tissue around. It involves tonsillectomy, followed by trimming the soft palate and repositioning of the anterior and posterior tonsillar pillar, then excision of the uvula with creation of a smaller new uvula. The long-term results of UPPP were rather disappointing and many surgeons said it is not effective and started adapting new techniques [9].

Obstructive sleep apnea is caused by obstruction at multiple sites within the upper airway, thus addressing the site or sites of obstruction should be the goal of any therapy. While CPAP addresses all sites of obstruction, many patients require excessive pressures, or have leaks around the apparatus that preclude its use. Some patients may not obtain a cure with upper airway surgery, but their tolerance and compliance may improve after airway surgery and this was the cause to develop surgeries that address all of the sites of upper airway obstruction [10].

Pharyngoplasty

The recent evolutions regarding techniques of pharyngoplasty aimed to obtain the expansion and stabilization of the pharyngeal airspace through the conservative treatment of LPW and preservation of the pharyngeal soft tissue.

The lateral pharyngeal wall (LPW) collapse plays a significant role in the pathogenesis of OSAHS. The first surgical technique aimed at stabilizing the lateral wall was lateral pharyngoplasty, described by Cahali in 2003; this procedure was not widely used, as it involves a marked modification of the lateral wall with sectioning of the superior pharyngeal constrictor muscle and a significant risk of complications, including postoperative dysphagia [11].

On the other hand, expansion sphincter pharyngoplasty (ESP), described by Pang and Woodson in 2007, had greater agreement. It originated from the technique of sphincter pharyngoplasty, described for the correction of palatal incompetence with the medial rotation of the palatopharyngeal muscle, restricting the velopharyngeal isthmus [12].

This technique was improved by Sorrenti by giving tension on the lateral wall and fixing the palatopharyngeal muscle to the palatine musculature, close to the pterygoid hamulus, allowing advancement of the soft palate more effectively and less invasively than the previous techniques of lateral pharyngoplasty [13].

Among non-resective pharyngoplasty, barbed reposition pharyngoplasty (BRP) have recently been described in the literature. These procedures allow surgeons to achieve widening and stiffening of the nasopharyngeal inlet without any tissue sacrifice using a bidirectional-barbed suture that is inserted through the fibro-muscular tissues of the soft palate and posterior tonsillar pillars, and tightened around the pterygomandibular raphe [14].

Maxillo-mandibular Advancement (MMA)

The jaw advancement surgery of the maxilla and mandible Maxillomandibular advancement may cure the obstructive sleep apnea forever; however, there is a significant difference in the approach.

This procedure requires extensive preoperative measurements and planning in order to achieve surgical success. It is usually performed after the above surgeries have failed to improve obstructive sleep apnea. Cephalometrics can assist in evaluating the hypopharyngeal airway. This is an X-ray taken with the patient in profile, sagittal orientation. The important landmarks are the sella (S), nasion (N), anterior nasal spine (ANS), posterior airway space (PAS), and the hyoid (H). Advancement is performed by at least 10 mm for optimal results. A Lefort I osteotomy is performed with plating of the fractured segment after appropriate advancement. Bone grafts may need to be placed. The bilateral sagittal split osteotomy is then performed. The patient is then kept in maxillomandibular fixation [15].

Trans Oral Robotic Surgery (TORS)

Starting from 2010 TORS as a treatment of OSA has shown to be an effective treatment option for OSA patients.

Transoral robotic surgery (TORS) addresses the tongue base. It permits greater dexterity, precision, and surgical access to the BOT. The robot system used provides improved visualization using high technology and three-dimensional (3D) and HD depth perception and robotic instrumentation, in addition to tremor filtration and. Patient assessment for TORS is paramount in order to improve the possibility of surgical cure and avoid unnecessary operations. Patients eligible for TORS are those who have polysomnographic evidence of moderate-severe OSA with daytime somnolence documented by the Epworth Sleepiness Scale (ESS) and a body mass index (BMI) of less than 35 kg/cm^2.

Only patients that have tried and previously failed or refused treatment with CPAP are deemed suitable. Airway endoscopy, both awake and under drug-induced sedation, allows obstruction at the level of the BOT and/or epiglottis to be diagnosed.

TORS allows the surgeon to address BOT obstruction with excellent visualization and an easier approach that is well tolerated by the patient.

TORS for OSA may be a stand-alone procedure addressing obstruction at the level of BOT and/or epiglottis or can be carried out as part of multilevel surgery that may include either palatal and/or nasal surgery. Furthermore, recent studies demonstrate that TORS can be feasibly performed without the need for tracheostomy [16].

In less than 10 years, TORS for OSA has spread all around the world, and the diffusion of this technique maybe traced through the increasing number of published papers in the literature.

Hypoglossal Nerve Stimulation (HNS)

The American Academy of Otolaryngology-Head and Neck Surgery considers upper airway stimulation (UAS) via the hypoglossal nerve for the treatment of adult obstructive sleep apnea syndrome to be a safe and effective second-line treatment of moderate to severe obstructive sleep apnea in patients who are intolerant or unable to achieve benefit with positive pressure therapy.

Functional surgery of the upper airways is a new technique and aims to increase the caliber of this area without changing the anatomy by the insertion of a neurostimulator which acts selectively on the fibers of the hypoglossal nerve responsible for lingual protrusion. These impulses are synchronized with ventilation, detected using an intercostal sensor [17]. This technique was first described in 2001 by Schwartz and has been approved by the Food and Drug Administration[3] since 2014.

Take Home Messages

- OSA is more common in elderly and obese patients.
- Obese patients with disturbed sleep and daytime sleepiness are high risk for OSAS and must see a sleep physician. To diagnose OSAS we need to do sleep study.
- Polysomnography (PSG) monitors the heart, sleep pattern, blood oxygen, and brain activity.
- Drug-induced sedation endoscopy (DISE) is very important to localize the exact site of obstruction.
- Treatment of mild and moderate cases of OSAS is weight reduction with lifestyle change and some sleep hygiene instructions.
- Severe cases of OSAS patients need to use CPAP which is considered the best treatment if they tolerate it.
- There is no consensus regarding surgical treatment of OSAS as the main idea is to address the specific site responsible for the obstruction.

References

1. Andreasen NC, Black DW. Introductory textbook of psychiatry. Washington, DC: American Psychiatric; 2006. ISBN 978-1-58562-272-6.
2. Simmons J, Barlow. Requiring 4% oxygen desaturation to score hypopnea misses OSA pathology and leaves many patients untreated. An outcome study, treating OSA patients who don't demonstrate 4% desaturation. S. Sleep. 2012;35S:135.
3. Remmers JE, de Groot WJ, Sauerland EK, et al. Pathogenesis of upperairway occlusion during sleep. J Appl Physiol. 1978;44:931–8.
4. Guilleminault C, Brooks SN. Excessive daytime sleepiness: a challenge for the practicing neurologist. Brain. 2001;125(Pt 8):1482–91.
5. Friedman M, et al. Clinical staging for sleep-disordered breathing. Otolaryngol Head Neck Surg. 2002;127(1):13–21.
6. Kakkar RK, et al. Interpretation of adult polysomnogram. Otolaryngol Clin N Am. 2007;40:713–43.
7. Werman HA, Karren K, Mistovich J. Continuous positive airway pressure (CPAP). In: Werman HA,

Mistovich J, Karren K, editors. Prehospital emergency care. 10th ed. Hoboken: Pearson Education Inc; 2014. p. 242.
8. Millman RP, Rosenberg CL, Kramer NR. Oral appliances in the treatment of snoring and sleep apnea. Otolaryngol Clin N Am. 1998;31(6):1039–48.
9. Kahn A, et al. Uvulopalatopharyngoplasty in the management of obstructive sleep apnea: the Mayo experience. Mayo Clin Proc. 2009;84(9):795–800.
10. Chabolle F, Wagner I, Blumen MB, et al. Tongue base reduction with hyoepiglottoplasty: a treatment for severe obstructive sleep apnea. Laryngoscope. 1999;109(8):1273–80.
11. Cahali MB. Lateral pharyngoplasty: a new treatment for obstructive sleep apnea hypopnea syndrome. Laryngoscope. 2003;113(11):1961–8.
12. Pang KP, Woodson BT. Expansion sphincter pharyngoplasty: a new technique for the treatment of obstructive sleep apnea. Otolaryngol Head Neck Surg. 2007;137(1):110–4.
13. Sorrenti G, Piccin O. Functional expansion pharyngoplasty in the treatment of obstructive sleep apnea. Laryngoscope. 2013;123(11):2905–8. https://doi.org/10.1002/lary.23911.
14. Vicini C, Hendawy E, Campanini A, Eesa M, Bahgat A, AlGhamdi S, Meccariello G, DeVito A, Montevecchi F, Mantovani M. Barbed reposition pharyngoplasty (BRP) for OSAHS: a feasibility, safety, efficacy and teachability pilot study. "We are on the giant's shoulders". Eur Arch Otorhinolaryngol. 2015;272(10):3065–70.
15. Yu CC, et al. Computational fluid dynamic study on obstructive sleep apnea syndrome treated with maxillomandibular advancement. J Craniofac Surg. 2009;20(2):426–30.
16. Vicini C, Dallan I, Canzi P, et al. Transoral robotic tongue base resection in obstructive sleep apnoea-hypopnoea syndrome: a preliminary report. ORL J Otorhinolaryngol Relat Spec. 2010;72(1):22.
17. Lurie A. Obstructive sleep apnea in adults. Adv Cardiol. 2011;46:1–42. https://doi.org/10.1159/000327660.

ENT Pharmacotherapy

52

Aisha Larem, Adham Aljariri, Mouna Ghannam, Ahmed Aly, Shaban Mohammed, and Sara Shabana

52.1 Antibiotics in ENT

52.1.1 Introduction

Antibiotics are widely used in otolaryngology to treat infections; prescribing antibiotics rationally is crucial to balance between treating the infections and avoiding the emergence of antimicrobial resistance. This balance can be achieved by a good understanding of the microbiology of the diseases and the antibiotics themselves.

A. Larem (✉)
Hamad Medical Corporation, Doha, Qatar

ENT (ORL-HNS)—HMC, Doha, Qatar
e-mail: alarem@hamad.qa

A. Aljariri
ENT (ORL-HNS)—HMC, Doha, Qatar
e-mail: AAljariri@hamad.qa

M. Ghannam
Karolinska Institute, Solna, Sweden
e-mail: mouna.ghannam@stud.ki.se

A. Aly · S. Mohammed
Pharmacy Department, HMC, Doha, Qatar
e-mail: AALY1@hamad.qa; shaban@hamad.qa

S. Shabana
HMC, Doha, Qatar
e-mail: Sshabana@hamad.qa

52.1.2 Common Organisms in ENT Infections

Most of the infections in otolaryngology can be classified depending on causative organisms, and we have mainly five groups of infections in otolaryngology summarized in (Table 52.1).

Some of those organisms can be responsible for different diseases in many cases, one organism can cause multiple infections, or infections can be caused by multiple organisms.

Table 52.1 Common microbials in ENT

Pneumococcal infections	Acute otitis media, acute rhinosinusitis, mastoiditis
Streptococcal infections	Pharyngitis, tonsillitis
Haemophilus influenzae, Moraxella catarrhalis	Acute otitis media, acute rhinosinusitis, supraglottitis, uvulitis, meningitis, cellulitis, conjunctivitis, acute otitis media, acute rhinosinusitis
Staphylococcal infections	Deep-neck abscesses, chronic tonsillitis, chronic sinusitis, otitis externa
Pseudomonas infections	Malignant otitis externa, perichondritis, nosocomial infections
Anaerobic infections	Sialadenitis, peritonsillar and parapharyngeal, and retropharyngeal spaces abscess wound infections post-surgical

A. Al-Qahtani et al. (eds.), *Textbook of Clinical Otolaryngology*,
https://doi.org/10.1007/978-3-030-54088-3_52

52.1.3 Classification of Antibiotics

Antibiotics are classified according to their chemical structure, their mechanisms of action, or according to their antimicrobial activities.

The following classification of antibiotics depends on their chemical structure.

52.1.3.1 Beta-Lactams

Penicillins

- Considered among the most effective and least novice antibiotics; the main problem is their resistance that altered their use.

  Penicillin members differ from one another in the nature of the side chain, which affects the antimicrobial spectrum, stability to stomach acid, cross hypersensitivity, and susceptibility to bacterial degradative enzymes (β-lactamases).

  There are five categories divided according to the spectrum of activity (Table 52.2).

Natural Penicillin G and V

They are active against pneumococcal and streptococcal infections, actinomycosis, and half of the usual anaerobic organisms of the oral and upper respiratory tract; given orally and intramuscular.

Inactivated by beta-lactamase, renders them noneffective against *Haemophilus influenzae*, *Moraxella catarrhalis*, anaerobes, gram-negative organisms, and *Staphylococcus aureus*. Another issue is that the pneumococcal resistance is increasing by "Alteration of Penicillin-binding protein."

Anti-staphylococcal Penicillin

This group includes: methicillin, oxacillin IV/IM, cloxacillin oral, dicloxacillin oral, nafcillin IV, only cloxacillin and dicloxacillin are given orally. Methicillin used only in vitro to test for resistance, they are active against penicillinase-producing staphylococci (MSSA), but not against MRSA.

Table 52.2 Penicillin's classification

Natural penicillin G and V
Anti-staphylococcal penicillin
Aminopenicillin
Augmented amino penicillin
Antipseudomonal penicillin

Aminopenicillin

This group includes ampicillin and amoxicillin; they are active against pneumococcal and streptococcal infections, except high-level penicillin-resistant strains, and active against gram-negative (*Haemophilus influenza*, *Escherichia coli*, and *Proteus mirabilis*).

Amino penicillin is associated with more rash type reaction (7%) other than penicillin, and if they are given for a patient with infectious mononucleosis, the rash appearance increases to 65–90%; that is why they are not preferred for exudative tonsillitis (the first sign of infectious mononucleosis).

They are inactivated by beta-lactamase.

Augmented Amino Penicillin

By adding beta-lactamase inhibitors like potassium clavulanate to amoxicillin and sulbactam to ampicillin, the spectrum of activity will be extended against *Haemophilus influenzae*, *Moraxella catarrhalis*, *Staphylococcus aureus* except for methicillin-resistant *Staphylococcus aureus* (MRSA), *Bacteroides fragilis,* and other anaerobes.

Extending the spectrum makes this combination very effective in the treatment of acute otitis media and sinusitis, and a broad spectrum of head and neck infections.

While for the pneumococcal, reduced susceptibility to penicillin is not resolved by adding the beta-lactamase, but enhancing the doses improves their susceptibility.

Antipseudomonal Penicillin

This group includes ticarcillin and piperacillin, which are inactivated by beta-lactamase, which is why they are available in combination with beta-lactamase inhibitors, so we have ticarcillin potassium clavulanate and piperacillin tazobactam. They are administered via the parenteral route.

They are active against *Pseudomonas aeruginosa, Proteus mirabilis, Escherichia coli, Klebsiella, Enterobacter, Serratia,* and *Bacteroides fragilis, Staphylococcus* (except MRSA) and anaerobes.

They have a valuable role in treating malignant otitis externa and invasive pseudomonal infections.

Cephalosporins

They belong to beta-lactams, and they are classified into five groups according to their spectrum of activity summarized in (Table 52.3). Because of structural similarity with penicillin cross allergy are present and should be avoided in severe allergic reactions.

Diarrhea and overgrowth of other infections are serious side effects of the broad-spectrum action of cephalosporins.

52.1.3.2 Other B-Lactams

Carbapenem

They are broad-spectrum antibiotics active against *Streptococcus pneumoniae, Staphylococcus aureus* (not MRSA), *Haemophilus influenzae, Bacteroides fragilis* and most anaerobic organism and gram-negative bacteria including *Pseudomonas aeruginosa*, used in serious hospital-acquired or mixed infections, given parenterally only, they have cross allergy with penicillin, and we have to be cautious in patients having seizure with the use of imipenem.

Monobactam

Active against gram-negative bacteria, including *Pseudomonas aeruginosa*, they are safe in patients with a history of penicillin anaphylaxis; they increase the risk of superinfections because they are highly selective for gram-negative bacteria.

52.1.3.3 Macrolides

They are useful as an alternative to beta-lactam and cephalosporin in case of allergy, main issue is increasing resistance.

- Erythromycin

  Effective against streptococci, pneumococci, staphylococci, atypical organisms (*Mycoplasma pneumoniae, Chlamydia pneumoniae, Legionella pneumophila*) and *Moraxella catarrhalis*, but *Haemophilus influenza* is resistant.
- Azithromycin and Clarithromycin

  Have extended antimicrobial activity that includes *Haemophilus influenzae*, azithromycin has a long-acting activity (it is once-daily dosing with a course of only 5 days to accomplish 10 days of therapy), macrolides also have anti-inflammatory and immunomodulatory action.

52.1.3.4 Quinolones

They are broad-spectrum antibiotics that have an important role in the treatment of multidrug-resistant infections. Moreover, they are a good alternative in case of allergy to other classes of antibiotics.

They can be divided into

- Anti-pseudomonal quinolones, ciprofloxacin, and levofloxacin
- Respiratory quinolones, levofloxacin, and moxifloxacin

Ciprofloxacin is effective as an oral treatment for *Pseudomonas aeruginosa* infections of the skin, bone, and respiratory mucosa. Usually, the anti-pseudomonal doses are higher than regular doses (IV:400 mg q8h/ PO: 750 mg BID).

They are used in *Pseudomonal sinusitis* (polyposis) and necrotizing otitis externa, topically they achieve high drug level in the middle ear, with no ototoxic risk if administered through tympanostomy tube or a tympanic membrane perforation, they are used against other gram-negative bacteria like (*Haemophilus influenzae* and *Moraxella catarrhalis*), but they are not effective against streptococci and pneumococci.

Levofloxacin and moxifloxacin are effective against gram-positive bacteria and, gram-negative bacteria; while levofloxacin is active against pseudomonas and moxifloxacin being active against atypical pathogens and anaerobes.

Table 52.3 Cephalosporins classification

Class	Spectrum	Disadvantages	Clinical practice
First generation			
Cefazolin (IV) Cephalexin (Oral)	Gram-positive cocci as streptococcal and pneumococcal (except the penicillin-resistant strains), Staphylococcal infection (except MRSA) Some gram-negative bacilli as *Escherichia coli*, *Proteus mirabilis*, and *Klebsiella*	Poor activity against gram-negative organisms Not effective against *Pseudomonas aeruginosa*, *Bacteroides*, *Haemophilus influenzae* or *Moraxella catarrhalis*	Treatment and prevention of staphylococcal infection Prophylaxis against surgical infections in head and neck infections
Second generation			
Cefuroxime (IV, Oral)	*H. influenzae* infections *Streptococcus pyogenes* Staphylococcal and pneumococcal bacteria	Less active than amoxicillin against pneumococci (reduced susceptibility) Less active than first-generation cephalosporin against *Staphylococcus* Side effect is diarrhea	*Haemophilus influenzae* infections (AOM, sinusitis, epiglottitis) Best absorbed when taken with meals
Third generation			
Cefixime (Oral)	Gram-negative bacilli and cocci (*Haemophilus influenzae*, *Moraxella catarrhalis*, *Neisseria gonorrhea*, and *Neisseria meningitidis*) Gram-positive pneumococci but less effective than other generations	Less active against gram-positive cocci (staphylococci, streptococci, pneumococci) and anaerobes	Treatment of AOM or sinusitis when pneumococci are absent or treated (highly active against *Haemophilus influenzae* and *Moraxella catarrhalis* even Ampicillin- resistant strains) Second generation is more active against pneumococcus
Ceftriaxone (IV, IM)	*Haemophilus influenzae*, *Moraxella catarrhalis*, pneumococci (including penicillin-resistant strains), *Neisseria gonorrhea*, and *Neisseria meningitidis*	Less active against gram-positive bacteria such as staphylococci and anaerobic bacteria such as *Bacteroides fragilis*	Penetrates cerebrospinal fluid (CSF), Broad-spectrum activity against organisms that cause URIT Used to treat patient with intracranial and orbital complications of AO and acute sinusitis
Ceftazidime (IV)	Highly active against *Pseudomonas aeruginosa* Active against gram-negative such as *Haemophilus influenzae* and *Neisseria gonorrhea*	Inactive against *Bacteroides fragilis* and poor activity against staphylococcal	Penetrates well CSF
Fourth generation			
Cefepime (IV)	Very active against *Pseudomonas aeruginosa*, Gram-negative bacteria Active against *Staphylococcus aureus* (not MRSA), *Streptococcus pneumoniae*, *Streptococcus pyogenes*		High CSF penetration
Fifth generation			
Ceftaroline (IV)	The only cephalosporin active against MRSA, poor activity against gram negative if compared to third- and fourth-generation cephalosporin		

Respiratory quinolones are the most effective oral antibiotic available to treat multidrug and highly resistant pneumococcal infections (equivalent to IV ceftriaxone). It is very important to consider drug interactions with this group of medications and their interactions with food and supplements as they can cause tendon toxicity and prolongation of QT interval, and they are not FDA approved for children, because of reports of bone growth impairment in animals. However, they are used with **no risk** in children of cystic fibrosis.

52.1.3.5 Clindamycin

It is effective against all streptococci, most pneumococci, and most penicillin-resistant staphylococci and anaerobes (*Bacteroides fragilis*). However, it has no gram-negative activities, it has a poor CSF penetration, but excellent distribution in bones and oropharyngeal secretion levels indicated in the treatment of infections caused by gram-positive organisms, including MRSA (community-acquired), streptococcus, and anaerobic bacteria.

Also indicated in polymicrobial infections: chronic tonsillitis and deep neck abscess of dental or oral origin, and it is used for prophylaxis against infections in surgery.

The most common side effect being diarrhea, which can be presented in the worst manifestation, which is *Clostridium difficile* colitis overgrowth.

52.1.3.6 Vancomycin

It is highly active against gram-positive cocci (MSSA, MRSA, penicillin-resistant strains of pneumococci, enterococci, and gonococci), so they are mainly indicated in severe infections with resistant gram-positive organisms.

Vancomycin can cause Redman syndrome, a condition that is infusion-related, ototoxicity, especially in patients with renal impairment and nephrotoxicity.

It is important to do vancomycin level monitoring and renal function assessment when taking this antibiotic.

Linezolid and Daptomycin are alternatives for vancomycin.

52.1.3.7 Metronidazole

It has good activity against gram-negative and gram-positive anaerobes, including *Bacteroides*, *Fusobacterium*, and *Clostridium* species, but their activity is poor against aerobic gram-negative and gram-positive organisms.

It is well distributed in nearly all tissues, including CSF, saliva, bone, abscesses.

It has excellent oral bioavailability.

It is indicated as:

- Treatment of mixed infections (combined with other antibiotics)
- It is the primary therapy for antibiotic-induced diarrhea
- Pretreatment of patients who will be using clindamycin.

It is essential to inform the patient to avoid alcohol consumption while taking the medication and 48 h after because of antabuse-like interaction.

52.1.4 Surgical Antimicrobial Prophylaxis

Antimicrobial prophylaxis decreases the incidence of surgical site infection, it is important to weigh benefit against risks when deciding to give antibiotics (allergic reactions, resistance, adverse drug interactions, super-infection, and cost).

Antimicrobial prophylaxis is usually justified for

- Procedures with high infection rates (wound classification)
- Procedure involving implantation of prosthetic material
- Procedures in which the consequences of infection are serious.

Timing is very important in the effectiveness of surgical prophylaxis and usually it should be given "on-call" to the operating room or shortly **BEFORE** anesthetic induction, so that the antibiotic will be present at therapeutic levels at the site and at the time of contamination (incision) and the therapeutic levels should be maintained for the duration of the procedure. So, if the surgery is longer than double the half-life time of the antibiotic re-dosing is justified, giving antibiotics postoperatively has little effect on wound infections and it was proved that it doesn't have protective effect after 24 h.
References [1–4].

52.2 Steroids in ENT

52.2.1 Pharmacology

Corticosteroids are commonly used in a varied range of ear-nose-throat (ENT) disease due to their anti-inflammatory properties. Corticosteroids are small lipophilic molecules that can readily diffuse across cell membrane into the cytoplasm. Where they form steroid-receptor complex, this complex leads to a cascade that decreases the number of inflammatory cytokines secreted by the cell.

Corticosteroids can be administered orally, intravenously, or intranasally/topically (Table 52.4). Moreover, relative potencies of corticosteroids differ and can affect the drug therapy selection (Table 52.5).

52.2.2 Indications

Corticosteroid therapy has been proved to be effective in the treatment of idiopathic facial nerve palsy, allergic rhinitis, acute sinusitis, sinonasal inflammatory polyposis, and croup. The therapeutic efficacy of steroids in the management of Meniere's disease, sudden idiopathic sensorineural hearing loss, chronic otitis media, and vestibular neuronitis remain controversial.

Corticosteroids are usually used in the treatment of Bell's palsy; this is due to their anti-inflammatory effect in decreasing neural edema within the facial canal and/or possible immune modulating effect on the presumed viral etiological agent. A randomized control trial (RCT) reported that compared to placebo, corticosteroids use improved facial nerve recovery in Bell's palsy patients. Another meta-analysis showed that steroid therapy improves complete facial recovery by 17%, which was clinically and statistically significant. In 2007, a Cochrane review of 500 patients showed that early therapy with prednisolone alone significantly increases the chance of complete facial nerve recovery at 3 and 9 months.

Table 52.4 Routes for steroids administration

Steroids route	Preferred medications	Comments
Intravenous steroids	• Methylprednisolone/dexamethasone • Drugs with minimal mineralocorticoid effect is preferred	• Useful during emergencies • One hour is gained when the drug is administered intravenously
Oral steroids	• Prednisolone • Prednisone • Dexamethasone	• Patients need long-term treatment course
Intranasal steroids	• Fluticasone • Beclamethasone dipropionate/ budesonide • Mometasone	• Intranasally administered steroid should be lipophilic • First pass metabolism is avoided • Most glucocorticoid nasal sprays have an onset of action of a few hours • Maximal effect may require several days or weeks in patients with longstanding untreated symptoms

Table 52.5 Commonly used corticosteroids

Oral/IV corticosteroids	Relative anti-inflammatory potency	Equivalent dose (mg)
Short acting (8–12 H) cortisol (hydrocortisone)	1	20
Intermediate acting (18–36 H) Prednisone (inactive precursor of prednisolone)	4	5
Long acting (36–72 H)		
Dexamethasone	25	0.75
Methylprednisolone	5	4
Topical intranasal corticosteroids	**Binding affinity to glucocorticoid receptor**	**Oral-bioavailability (%)** [a]
Beclomethasone	2	26
Budesonide	1	6–11
Mometasone furoate	2.8	<1
Fluticasone	1.8	<1

a = 1

For otitis media with effusion (OME) a Cochrane review assessed the efficacy of systemic and intranasal corticosteroids use. This review showed an improved resolution of OME in the short term with the use of oral steroids alone or in combination with antibiotics. Likewise, topical intranasal steroids combined with oral antibiotic also demonstrated favorable effect.

Vestibular neuritis is believed to have a viral etiology and has an increased rate of spontaneous recovery. In 2011, a meta-analysis assessed the efficacy of corticosteroids in four RCTs (149 patients). There was an overall significant effect of corticosteroid therapy on complete recovery at 1 month.

Nasal topical steroids are well established as first-line therapy in allergic rhinitis, which affects up to 25% of the general population. There is strong benefit in using intranasal corticosteroids over antihistamines in allergic rhinitis. There is no consensus regarding the optimal duration of treatment with published studies reporting efficacy using 4–26 weeks of intranasal steroid therapy.

52.2.3 Complications

Steroids are increasingly being used to treat a wide spectrum of otolaryngologic disorders, it is important for ENT surgeons to understand short- and long-term complications associated with steroid use.

Short-Term Use Complications

- Hypothalamic-pituitary-adrenal axis suppression
- Hyperglycemia
- Gastrointestinal effects
- Psychiatric effects

Long-Term Complications

- Avascular necrosis (AVN)
- Osteoporosis
- Cushingoid appearance
- Accelerated atherosclerosis
- Early cataracts

52.3 Decongestant and Antihistamines in ENT

52.3.1 Pharmacology

Dilation or expansion of blood vessels membranes in the air passages and nose can lead to congestion of the sinuses, nose, and chest. These membranes are stimulated to expand by the release of histamine causing congestion and swelling.

Decongestants are remedies that function by causing constriction or tightening of these membranes blood vessels, which leads to opening up the air passages by pushing the blood out of the

Table 52.6 Decongestants side effects (route)

- Hypertension (IV)
- Headache, insomnia, nervousness, restlessness (oral and IV)
- Blurred vision (IV)
- Decreased urine output (IV)
- Dyspnea, respiratory distress (IV)
- Neck pain, tremor, weakness (IV)
- Rebound nasal congestion-rhinitis medicamentosa (topical/nasal)

Table 52.7 Combination remedies rational

Medication class	Symptoms relieved	Side effects
Antihistamines	Sneezing	Drowsiness
	Runny nose	Dry mouth and nose
	Stuffy nose	
	Itchy eyes	
	Congestion	
Decongestants	Stuffy nose	Stimulation
	Congestion	Insomnia
		Rapid heart beat

membranes and causing them to shrink. Decongestants can trigger numerous side effects, as they are chemically related to adrenaline, a natural stimulant (Table 52.6).

Therefore, combination remedies of decongestants and antihistamines aimed to balance their side effects are produced. For example, the somnolence/drowsiness triggered by antihistamines could be reduced by the stimulation effect of decongestants (Table 52.7). Moreover, to avoid excessively stimulating effects, decongestants should be prescribed with caution for patients with uncontrolled hypertension, cardiovascular diseases, closed angle glaucoma, receiving monoamine oxidase inhibitor therapy, and hyperthyroidism.

In ear-nose-throat (ENT) diseases, oral and topical/nasal decongestants are commonly used in management of allergic rhinitis and common cold (Table 52.8). However, due to side effects the use of topical decongestant should be limited to 2 or 3 days because rebound rhinitis can occur. This disorder is called rhinitis medicamentosa and it develops as downregulation of the alpha-adrenergic receptor starts after 3–7 days. Limiting use to a maximum of approximately 5 days can reduce the risk of developing this condition from nasal decongestants.

Table 52.8 Decongestants

Decongestants rout	Example
Oral	Pseudoephedrine Phenylephrine
Topical/nasal	Phenylephrine Oxymetazoline Xylometazoline Naphazoline

Combination of oral decongestant and antihistamine are part of the management of allergic rhinitis. As a double blind, placebo-controlled, multicenter study showed that oral non-sedating antihistamines (loratadine) combined with the decongestant (pseudoephedrine) offered a better symptomatic relief than antihistamines or decongestant use alone [5]. According to published systematic review and meta-analysis, compared to placebo phenylephrine (10 mg) is less effective for the treatment of rhinitis symptoms [6]. Moreover, recent guidelines indicated that compared with first-generation antihistamines/decongestant combination, second-generation antihistamines/decongestant combination have a better adverse effect profile, including less sedation (with the exception of cetirizine) [7]. Nasal decongestant sprays, which provides a local vasoconstriction, are not recommended as monotherapy in the chronic management of allergic rhinitis [7]. However, the combination of a topical nasal decongestant with topical corticosteroid may effectively treat symptoms without causing rhinitis medicamentosa [8].

In common cold management topical and oral decongestants may lead to moderate relief of nasal congestion compared to no combination [8]. Moreover, a meta-analysis concluded that nasal decongestants produce a very small statistical benefit of 4% and probably clinically insignificant benefit over 3–5 days use in the treatment of common cold [9].

References [5–9].

52.4 Drugs for Vertigo and Motion Sickness

52.4.1 Betahistine

Betahistine facilitate central vestibular compensation by acting like a weak histamine H1 agonist and a potent H3 receptor antagonist. Histamine H1 receptors are pinpointed in the inner ear blood vessels and direct stimulation leads to pressure reduction in the endolymphatic space. Moreover, the strong antagonistic effects of betahistine at H3 receptors cause a potent vasodilatory effect in the inner ear by increasing the amounts of histamine released from nerve endings. All of these mechanisms explain the efficacy of betahistine in the treatment of vertigo [10].

Betahistine uses is preferred over diuretics due to its tolerability and safety (monitoring is not indicated).

52.4.2 Diuretics

Studies indicated that low sodium diet (like Low sodium hypertension-directed diets) could help in the management of Ménière's disease (MD). The use of dietary sodium retractions in combination with diuretics was advocated because it was thought to lower pressure in the hydropic ear, reducing the risk of membrane rupture. Current evidence indicated that diuretics use could slow progression of hearing loss in patient with MD by relieving the inner ear fluid build-up. The thiazide group diuretics can be a part of MD medical treatment; however, loop diuretics are less favored because of their ototoxic effects [10].

When diuretics are used regularly, safety-monitoring parameters are indicated due to its metabolic effects (electrolytes, kidney function test, and blood pressure). Still, if betahistine medication is not available, chronic diuretic therapy is indicated [2] (Table 52.9).

52.4.3 Antihistamines and Anticholinergics

Scopolamine and antihistamines can be used in the treatment of motion sickness (Table 52.10). In 2011, a meta-analysis involving 14 trials (n = 1025) assessing the effectiveness of scopolamine in preventing motion sickness, concluded that it was more effective than placebo, but less effective than antihistamines [4]. Although, antihistamines are effective in the prevention of motion sickness they may cause more sedation than scopolamine [12].

Anticholinergics which affect muscarinic receptors, such as scopolamine, increase motion tolerance. The action looks to be central, while there are receptors in both the periphery and centrally. Moreover, Anticholinergics affect compensation, by producing a reversible overcompensation when administered after compensation has been reached to a vestibular imbalance. Agents with central anticholinergic effects are most important in treating vertigo, since anticholinergic drugs that do not cross the blood–brain barrier are ineffective in controlling motion sickness [13].

Table 52.9 Medication used to treat and prevent vertigo attacks [2]

Medication class	Medication	Dosing
Vasodilator • Act by improving microvascular circulation in the stria vascularis of the cochlea or by inhibiting vestibular nuclei activity	• Betahistine	• Betahistine 8–16 mg orally three times daily
Diuretics • Improve endolymph resorption and also maintain a balanced fluid dynamic in the endolymphatic system	• Hydrochlorothiazide • Furosemide • Acetazolamide	• Hydrochlorothiazide 25 mg/triamterene 37.5 mg orally once daily • Furosemide 20 mg orally once daily • Acetazolamide 250–500 mg orally twice daily

Table 52.10 Medications used in the management of motion sickness [11]

Medication	Dosing	Side effects
Scopolamine (transdermal) • Blocks the action of acetylcholine at parasympathetic sites in smooth muscle, secretory glands, and the CNS • Increases cardiac output, dries secretions, antagonizes histamine and serotonin • At usual recommended doses, causes blockade of muscarinic receptors at the cardiac SA-node and is parasympatholytic (i.e., blocks vagal activity increasing heart rate)	Dose: 1 mg transdermal patch, applied behind the ear at least 4 h (preferably 12 h) before exposure to motion • Patches should be replaced every 72 h if needed	Due to motion sickness ability to cause gastric hypomotility, the transdermal route is advantageous **Potential side effects**: • Sedation, blurred vision, dry mouth and, in older adults, confusion and urinary retention • Dermatitis from the scopolamine patch • Scopolamine is contraindicated in people at risk for angle-closure glaucoma
Antihistamines • Dimenhydrinate, meclizine • Others: diphenhydramine, chlorpheniramine, cyclizine, cinnarizine • Non-sedating antihistamines: cetirizine, loratadine, fexofenadine do not appear to be effective for the treatment of motion sickness [4, 5]	Dimenhydrinate or meclizine Dose: 25 mg orally every 6–8 h as needed • First dose taken 30–60 min prior to anticipated travel • If sedation is excessive, the dose may be reduced to 12.5 mg or even 6.25 mg Dimenhydrinate • Dose: Oral 50–100 mg every 4–6 h (maximum: 400 mg/day) Cinnarizine • Dose: oral 25–75 mg 3 time's daily. (maximum: 225 mg/day) • Is not available in the United States but is widely used in other countries Cyclizine • Dose: Oral: 50 mg up to 3 times daily as needed • Is not available in the United States or Canada	**Potential side effects**: Mainly related to anticholinergic effects • Sedation, blurred vision, dry mouth and, in older adults, confusion and urinary retention Data suggested that cyclizine may be less sedating than dimenhydrinate

Although the detailed role of histamine in central vestibular processing is undefined, there are data signifying that centrally acting antihistamines prevent motion sickness and reduce the severity of its symptoms even if taken after the onset of symptoms besides all antihistamines used for control of vertigo also have anticholinergic activity. The most common side effects of anticholinergics are dry mouth, dilated pupils, and sedation. Scopolamine and atropine are nonspecific muscarinic receptor antagonists [12–15].

Take Home Messages

- Good antimicrobial prescribing practice starts with good understanding of the microbiology and the antibiotics in combination with the adherence to guidelines.
- Corticosteroids are widely used in otolaryngology, using them with the right doses for the right duration with monitoring their side effects and taking precaution with high risk patients will help

to get benefit from their use and reduce their risks.

- Antihistamines and decongestants are widely used to relieve symptoms of allergic rhinitis and common cold. It is important to use the decongestant for the shortest duration to avoid the rebound rhinitis.
- A wide variety of medications is used to treat vertigo and motion sickness; it is always important to remember the right dosing for the indication and the side effects and the precaution related to the different patients.

Acknowledgment Authors would like to thank and appreciate the help of Professor Moza Al Hail Executive Director of Pharmacy in HMC.

References

1. Fairbanks DNF. Pocket guide to antimicrobial therapy in otolaryngology—head and neck surgery. 13th ed: American Academy of Otolaryngology—Head & Neck Surgery Foundation; 2007.
2. Whalen K, Finkel R, Panavelil TA. Pharmacology. 6th ed. Philadelphia, PA: Wolters Kluwer; 2015.
3. Bailey BJ, Johnson JT, Newlands SD, editors. Head & neck surgery—otolaryngology, vol. 1: Lippincott Williams & Wilkins.
4. Abramowicz M. The Medical Letter: Handbook of antimicrobial therapy. The medical letter on drugs and therapeutics. New York. 2000:72–86.
5. Bronsky E, Boggs P, Findlay S, et al. Comparative efficacy and safety of a once-daily loratadine-pseudoephedrine combination versus its components alone and placebo in the management of seasonal allergic rhinitis. J Allergy Clin Immunol. 1995;96(2):139–47. https://doi.org/10.1016/S0091-6749(95)70001-3.
6. Hatton RC, Winterstein AG, McKelvey RP, Shuster J, Hendeles L. Efficacy and safety of oral phenylephrine: systematic review and meta-analysis. Ann Pharmacother. 2007;41(3):381–90. https://doi.org/10.1345/aph.1H679.
7. Treatment of allergic rhinitis. American Family Physician. https://www.aafp.org/afp/2010/0615/p1440.html. Accessed 24 Dec 2019.
8. Berger WE, Meltzer EO. Intranasal spray medications for maintenance therapy of allergic rhinitis. Am J Rhinol Allergy. 2015;29(4):273–82. https://doi.org/10.2500/ajra.2015.29.4215.
9. Taverner D, Latte J. Nasal decongestants for the common cold. Cochrane Database Syst Rev. 2007;1:CD001953. https://doi.org/10.1002/14651858.CD001953.pub3.
10. Lacour M, van de Heyning PH, Novotny M, et al. Betahistine in the treatment of Ménière's disease. Neuropsychiatr Dis Treat. 2007;3(4):429–40.
11. Magnan J, Özgirgin ON, Trabalzini F, et al. European position statement on diagnosis, and treatment of Meniere's disease. J Int Adv Otol. 2018;14(2):317–21. https://doi.org/10.5152/iao.2018.140818.
12. Kohl RL, Homick JL, Cintron N, Calkins DS. Lack of effects of astemizole on vestibular ocular reflex, motion sickness, and cognitive performance in man. Aviat Space Environ Med. 1987;58(12):1171–4. http://www.ncbi.nlm.nih.gov/pubmed/3122717. Accessed 5 Jan 2020.
13. Spinks A, Wasiak J. Scopolamine (hyoscine) for preventing and treating motion sickness. Cochrane Database Syst Rev. 2011;3:CD002851. https://doi.org/10.1002/14651858.cd002851.pub4.
14. Cheung BS, Heskin R, Hofer KD. Failure of cetirizine and fexofenadine to prevent motion sickness. Ann Pharmacother. 2003;37(2):173–7. https://doi.org/10.1177/106002800303700201.
15. Brainard A, Gresham C. Prevention and treatment of motion sickness. Am Fam Physician. 2014;90(1):41–6.

Neck Trauma

53

Furat Abbas and Hossam Makki

53.1 Introduction

Neck trauma occurs in 5–10% of serious trauma [1]. It can be challenging in diagnosis and therapeutic approach for trauma care providers. However, that injury to vital structures in the neck may cause life-threatening situations or functional impairments. These structures, the airway, vascular system, neurological system, and gastrointestinal tract can all be involved in neck injury. Additionally, spinal injuries must always be considered in patients with multiple injuries [2].

- The internal jugular vein and carotid arteries are the most common vessels injured.
- Injuries to the larynx and trachea are more common than injuries to the esophagus and pharynx because they are located anteriorly, which can lead to significant problems with airway patency, voice production, and swallowing.
- The esophagus and pharynx are more protected since they lie between the airway and the spine. Esophageal injuries represent the most frequently missed injury and may be the leading cause of delayed death [3, 4].

F. Abbas (✉) · H. Makki
Hamad Medical Corporation, Doha, Qatar
e-mail: fabbas@hamad.qa; HMAKKI@hamad.qa

53.2 Zones of the Neck and Anatomical Structures [5, 6]

Understanding of the anatomy of the neck, especially the location of important structures, is essential for providing optimal care.

53.2.1 Vital Structures in the Neck

- Airway: (pharynx, larynx, trachea, and lungs)
- Blood vessels: (carotid arteries, innominate artery, aortic arch vessels, Jugular veins and subclavian veins)
- Nerves (spinal cord, brachial plexus, cranial nerves, and peripheral nerves)
- Gastrointestinal tract (pharynx and esophagus)

53.2.2 Skeletal Anatomy

- Mandible
- Hyoid
- Styloid process
- Cervical spine

53.2.3 Muscular Landmarks

Muscular landmarks are also important:

- *Platysma muscle*—Penetration of the platysma muscle defines a deep injury in contrast to a superficial injury.

A. Al-Qahtani et al. (eds.), *Textbook of Clinical Otolaryngology*,
https://doi.org/10.1007/978-3-030-54088-3_53

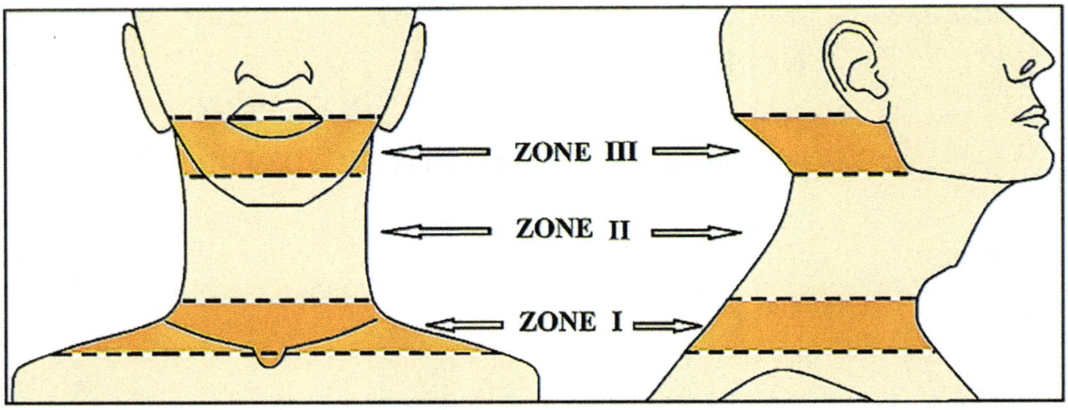

Fig. 53.1 Neck zones

- *Sternocleidomastoid muscle*—the sternocleidomastoid muscle also serves as a valuable landmark, since this large, obliquely oriented muscle divides each side of the neck into anterior and posterior triangles.
- *Anterior triangle*—the anterior triangle contains airway, major vasculature, nerves, and gastrointestinal structures, while the posterior triangle contains the spine and muscle.

The neck is commonly divided into three distinct zones for initial assessment and management, which help in guiding management decisions especially in penetrating trauma [7] (Fig. 53.1 and Table 53.1).

Table 53.1 Content of neck zones [7]

Zone	Area	Contents
I	Between clavicle and cricoid	Proximal carotid and vertebral arteries Subclavian artery and major vessels of upper mediastinum Thyroid gland, trachea, and esophagus Thoracic duct Apices of lungs Spinal cord
II	Between cricoid and angle of mandible	Larynx and trachea Carotid artery and vertebral artery Jugular vein Vagus nerve and recurrent laryngeal nerve Pharynx and esophagus Spinal cord
III	Between angle of mandible and base of skull	Distal carotid and vertebral arteries Distal jugular vein Salivary and parotid glands Cranial nerve IX to XII Spinal cord

53.3 Etiology [3, 7]

53.3.1 Blunt Trauma Include

- *Motor vehicle* crashes, whereby an unrestrained front seat occupant sustains injury to the anterior neck structures striking the steering column or dashboard.
- *Sports-related injuries and clothesline injuries*, the "clothesline" types of blunt trauma to the larynx deserve special attention because of the high impact of the force with the possibility of cricotracheal separation associated with bilateral recurrent laryngeal nerve injury. Injures of this type occur when the anterior part of the neck strikes a stationary objects while bicycling, snowmobiling, or riding. The injury may be caused by a clothesline, chain, or tree branch.
- *Strangulation*

The laryngotracheal airway and cervical spine are the most clinically susceptible to injury. Vascular injuries are potentially devastating but are uncommon overall in blunt trauma; blunt trauma can damage the vessels by the following mechanisms

1. Direct damage
2. Excessive rotation and/or hyperextension: This causes stretching of the arteries and veins resulting in a shear injury

Laryngeal injuries vary by anatomical location, the thyroid cartilage most usually fractured because of its prominence and its thyroid notch. When cricoid fractures are combined with thyroid cartilage fractures, they are usually more extensive and dangerous.

53.3.2 Penetrating Trauma [5, 2]

Penetrating neck injury composes 5–10% of traumatic neck injuries in adults.

Ninety-five percent of penetrating trauma usually results from stabbings or gunshot wounds. It is the violation of the platysma that determines penetrating injury. Wounds which penetrate the platysma have the potential for severe injury. Consequently, it is wise to consider damage to the vital structures if the platysma is violated. Penetrating neck injuries can cause injuries to the aerodigestive and neurovascular systems. Vascular injuries are the most common and occur in up to 40% of patients with penetrating neck trauma and higher in zone I and zone III.

Also, in zone I, the esophagus is at risk for injury.

53.4 History and Physical

The evaluation of a patient with trauma to the neck begins with a detailed history (when possible) that specifically addresses the following items [8]:

1. The development of symptoms,
2. The mechanism of injury,
3. Identify the cause of injury.

The most important part of the evaluation is a careful and thorough *physical examination*. It is important to determine the *extent* of the injury and identify any *associated injuries* particularly in cases involving blunt trauma. Beware that signs and symptoms may be delayed, so *periodic examination* is required to identify deterioration in clinical status.

Assess for penetration of the Platysma. However, wounds should never be probed blindly, as this may dislodge a clot and provoke uncontrolled bleeding. If the platysma is violated, determine whether the wound lays anterior (anterior triangle) or posterior (posterior triangle) to the sternocleidomastoid muscle, and determine in what zone the injury is found [5].

A full neurologic examination should also be performed.

53.4.1 Signs and Symptoms [9]

Signs of Laryngeal or Tracheal Injury

- Voice alteration
- Hemoptysis
- Stridor
- Drooling
- Sucking, hissing, or air frothing or bubbling through the neck wound
- Subcutaneous emphysema and/or crepitus
- Hoarseness
- Dyspnea
- Distortion of the normal anatomic appearance
- Pain on palpation or with coughing or swallowing
- Pain with tongue movement
- Crepitus: in only one-third of cases

Signs of Esophageal and Pharyngeal Injury

- Dysphagia
- Bloody saliva
- Sucking neck wound
- Bloody nasogastric aspirate
- Pain and tenderness in the neck

- Resistance of neck with passive motion testing
- Crepitus
- Bleeding from the mouth or nasogastric tube
- Perforation of the pharynx or the esophagus following blunt neck trauma occurs infrequently. Because the esophagus lacks a serosa layer, it is more susceptible to iatrogenic injury such as following endoscopy, passage of a nasogastric tube, or inadvertent esophageal intubation.
- Esophageal perforation is the most serious and rapidly fatal.

Signs of Carotid Artery Injury
- Decreased level of consciousness
- Contralateral hemiparesis
- Hemorrhage
- Hematoma
- Dyspnea secondary to compression of the trachea
- Thrill
- Bruit
- Pulse deficit (*The presence of a pulse does not exclude a vascular injury, and absence of a pulse is not diagnostic of vascular damage.)*

Signs of Jugular Vein Injury
- These include hematoma, external hemorrhage, and hypotension.

Signs of Spinal Cord or Brachial Plexus Injury
- Diminished upper arm capacity
- Quadriplegia
- Pathologic reflexes
- Urinary retention, fecal incontinence, and paralytic ileus
- Horner syndrome (occurs with injury to the sympathetic chain, and produces ipsilateral miosis with ptosis of the upper eyelid and anhidrosis of the ipsilateral side of the face. It is seen most commonly with zone I injuries.)
- Hypoxia and hypoventilation (can follow disruption of phrenic innervation to the diaphragm.)

Signs of Cranial Nerve Injury
- Facial nerve (cranial nerve VII): Drooping of the corner of the mouth
- Glossopharyngeal nerve (cranial nerve IX): Dysphagia (altered gag reflex)
- Vagus nerve (cranial nerve X, recurrent laryngeal): Hoarseness (weak voice)
- Spinal accessory nerve (cranial nerve XI): Inability to shrug a shoulder and to laterally rotate the chin to the opposite shoulder
- Hypoglossal nerve (cranial nerve XII): Deviation of the tongue with protrusion

53.5 Evaluation

53.5.1 Neck Trauma Diagnostic Measures [6, 7]

1. Anterior and lateral *neck and chest radiographs* should be obtained in all circumstances (especially if the platysma has been penetrated). Any abnormal air surrounding the trachea, mediastinum, or thorax may be the first sign of impending tension pneumothorax and airway embarrassment. Look for widened mediastinum, mediastinal emphysema, apical pleural hematoma, and foreign bodies. *These should be obtained especially for patients with zone* I.
2. *Cervical spine radiography* is indicated for all trauma patients; review the cervical radiographs for emphysema, fractures, displacement of the trachea, and presence of a foreign body (e.g., missile fragments).
3. High-resolution fine cut *computed tomographic* (CT) imaging may be considered for surgical planning in symptomatic patients or in asymptomatic patients with suspected laryngeal injury. Securing the airway is advocated in the setting of acute airway symptoms, such as stridor or respiratory distress, prior to considering imaging.
4. *Multidetector helical computed tomography* (MDCT) is the imaging modality of choice when looking for laryngotracheal injuries in

stable patients with penetrating injury. No consensus exists as to the best diagnostic approach.

5. *Conventional angiography* remains the "gold standard" for evaluating the vascular injury. A four-vessel angiography with venous-phase imaging has a sensitivity of greater than 99%. Routinely is used to evaluate stable patients sustaining penetrating wounds to zones I and III that pierce the platysma.
   - Indications for an angiogram: a stable patient with persistent hemorrhage or neurologic deficits. The presence of Horner syndrome (sympathetic nerve plexus injury) and hoarseness (recurrent laryngeal nerve injury). This suggests a violation of carotid sheath.
6. Consider an *emergent MRI* and/or magnetic resonance angiography (*MRA*) for evaluation of the patient exhibiting neurological impairment with minimal or absent abnormalities on plain radiographs of the cervical spine.
7. *Esophagography* should be performed if an esophageal perforation is suspected (Fig. 53.2).

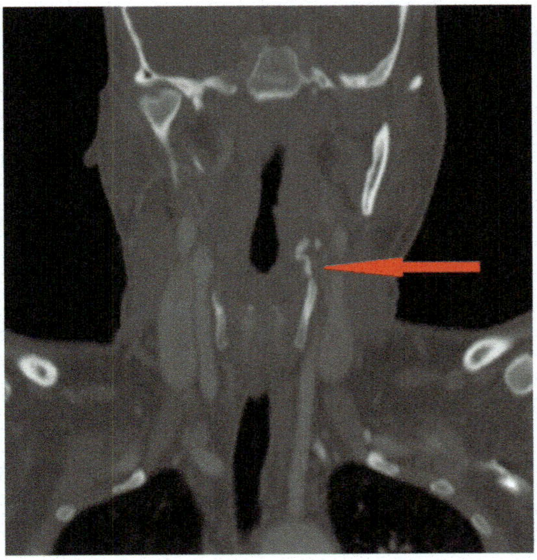

Fig. 53.2 Coronal CT shows fracture of left lamina of thyroid cartilage. (Images courtesy of Dr. Nasser Jassim Al Maslamani, Sr. Consultant & Chief Radiologist, Clinical Imaging Department, Al-Khor Hospital, Hamad Medical Corporation, Qatar)

53.5.2 Other Diagnostic Procedures [10]

Aerodigestive tract injuries, especially those involving the cervical esophagus, should be identified and repaired within 12–24 h after injury to minimize associated morbidity and mortality.

Flexible nasopharyngoscopy allows visualization of the hypo pharynx and supra-laryngeal structures in an awake or sedated patient.

Rigid and flexible esophagoscopy, rigid and flexible bronchoscopy and *rigid direct laryngoscopy* are performed in the operating room under general anesthesia may be useful in the assessment of the aerodigestive tract. Rigid endoscopes are superior to flexible scopes. It may be best to defer examination until the airway is protected and the patient is anesthetized.

53.6 Definitive Management

53.6.1 General Approach [11]

Priorities in the management of patients with neck trauma are like those for any other patient with a life-threatening condition. The primary priorities are securing the airway, breathing, and adequacy of circulation. Cervical spine must be secured and immobilized.

- If the patient is stable, awake flexible fiberoptic examination can be performed.
- If attempts at oral intubation fail or are unsafe due to significant trauma, a surgical airway is required; formal tracheotomy is preferred over cricothyrotomy.
- After securing the airway perform secondary survey; the neck should be methodically examined, searching for clues that indicate damage to vital contents.
- If platysma is violated do not probe.
- Uncontrolled hemorrhage, shock not responding to resuscitation, expanding or pulsatile hematoma, airway compression, bubbling from the wound are all indications for immediate surgical intervention.
- Avoid nasogastric tube placement in patients with penetrating neck injury because of the

risk of hematoma rupture. The agitation of the patient during tube insertion may precipitate bleeding.

Further management of the patient with penetrating neck trauma depends on the anatomic zone of injury, clinical presentation, and hemodynamic stability.

When evaluating a patient with penetrating neck trauma, it is imperative to look for hard and soft signs of injury [4, 12].

Hard signs of vascular injury can include a severe or uncontrolled hemorrhage, rapidly expanding or pulsatile hematoma, thrills and bruits, hypotension unresponsive to aggressive fluid resuscitation, absent or diminished radial pulse, and neurologic deficits consistent with cerebral ischemia (stroke).

Hard signs of aerodigestive injury include air bubbling from a wound, massive hemoptysis, and respiratory distress. Hard signs reflect the presence of a serious injury that generally requires immediate transfer to the operating room.

Soft signs of injury include minor hemorrhage, mild hypotension that responds to fluid resuscitation, minor hemoptysis or hematemesis, subcutaneous or mediastinal air, non-expanding hematoma, dysphonia, and dysphagia. Those patients can be managed non-operatively with serial examination with additional imaging studies and close observation in a monitored setting.

In zone-management approach [2], the most commonly injured area is zone II, which can easily be accessed surgically. The decision for surgical exploration depends on the symptoms. Symptomatic penetrating zone II injuries should undergo neck exploration. Asymptomatic patients with penetrating zone II injuries may be treated with either mandatory exploration or directed evaluation and serial examinations (Fig. 53.1).

However, in zones I and III injuries, exposure and vascular control are more difficult to achieve Therefore, many vascular injuries can be approached by an interventional radiologist.

53.6.2 Specific Injuries [6]

- *Laryngotracheal injury:* A large proportion of patients with traumatic airway injuries require definitive airways, timely repair of certain laryngotracheal injuries is important to prevent long-term complications such as chronic pain, stenosis, or voice change.
- *Pharyngo-esophageal injuries:* Most pharyngo-esophageal injuries are treated surgically, but select patients may be managed non-operatively. Pharyngo-esophageal injuries can cause mediastinitis and abscess or empyema formation from the leakage of gastric contents. Clinicians should begin treatment with broad-spectrum antibiotics in all patients with possible pharyngo-esophageal injuries.
- *Vascular injuries*: Immediate consultation with a vascular surgeon should be obtained if vascular injury is suspected.
- *Neurologic injuries*: Cervical spine injury is uncommon following penetrating trauma to the neck. All patients with cervical spinal cord injury had a neurologic deficit at initial presentation.

For the *management of blunt neck injury* [7] immediate airway protection is needed if any airway compromise is suspected. Subsequent management of blunt aerodigestive injuries depends on the severity of the injury and concomitant injuries.

The laryngotracheal airway and the cervical spine are the two most integral structures that can be damaged in blunt trauma to the neck.

Initial diagnostic airway evaluation with flexible laryngoscopy is helpful in documenting endolaryngeal findings as well as post-injury changes (Tables 53.2 and 53.3).

As described in the penetrating neck trauma hemodynamic instability or signs of vascular injury, such as bruit, expanding/pulsating hematoma, hemorrhage, or loss of pulse, warrant surgical exploration.

Otherwise, stable minimally symptomatic injuries managed conservatively and could undergo initial diagnostic imaging.

All injuries, even those with negative imaging or pan-endoscopy, need observation for at least 24 h, as presentation can be delayed.

Table 53.2 Schaefer Classification System for determining the severity of laryngeal injuries [7, 9]

Group	Severity of injury
1	Minor endolaryngeal hematomas or lacerations without detectable fractures
2	More severe edema, hematoma, minor mucosal disruption without exposed cartilage, or non-displaced fractures
3	Massive edema, large mucosal lacerations, exposed cartilage, displaced fractures or vocal cord immobility
4	Same as group 3, but more severe with disruption of anterior larynx, unstable fractures, two or more fracture lines, or severe mucosal injuries
5	Complete laryngotracheal separations

53.7 Neck Injuries in Children [7]

Children are involved less often in blunt accidents as well as in penetrating. In general, the presentation and management of the pediatric patient with a neck trauma are the same as in adults.

When they are injured, the chances of suffering critical neck injuries are much lower than in the adult population due to more elastic tissue, cartilage instead of bony structures, and mainly because the anterior neck is better protected by the bigger head and chin, and by the shorter neck. In addition, their neck anatomy is often more challenging owing to a high laryngeal position and soft cartilage. Therefore, a pediatric airway is preferably secured with a rigid bronchoscope while maintaining spontaneous respiration before a tracheotomy is performed.

Table 53.3 Evaluation and management based on the Schaefer Classification System [7, 9]

Group	Airway assessment	Evaluation	Management
1	Minimal airway compromise	Flexible fiber-optic laryngoscopy	Generally, medically managed and do not require surgical intervention. Observation and medical supportive care
2	Mild airway compromise	Direct laryngoscopy and esophagoscopy	Serial examinations, since the injuries may worsen over time. These injuries infrequently require a tracheostomy. Observation and medical supportive care
3	Significant airway compromise	Direct laryngoscopy and esophagoscopy performed in the operating room	Tracheostomy and surgical repair are often required. The following injuries of the larynx require surgical repair: disruption of the anterior commissure, major endolaryngeal lacerations, vocal cord tear, immobile vocal cord, cartilage exposure, displaced cartilage fractures
4	Significant airway compromise	Direct laryngoscopy and esophagoscopy performed in the operating room	Tracheostomy is always required Surgical repair requires stent placement to maintain the integrity of the larynx
5	Catastrophic airway obstruction	These patients present in severe respiratory distress and therefore endoscopic evaluation is delayed until an airway is secured	Disruption of the airway usually occurs above or below the cricoid cartilage, either at the cricothyroid membrane or cricotracheal junction. The airway is usually temporarily established using an endotracheal tube inserted through the neck directly into trachea distal to the site of transection. A complex laryngotracheal repair is then performed through a low cervical incision

53.8 Complications [13]

- Airway obstruction
- Aspiration
- Vocal cord paralysis
- Perforated esophagus
- Severe vascular injury
- Necrotizing infection
- Stroke
- Air embolism
- Pneumothorax, hemothorax

53.9 Outcomes [1, 4]

- Overall, injuries to zone I have the highest morbidity and mortality. Death from delayed diagnosis of neck injuries can be from exsanguination, loss of airway, or asphyxiation (in the case of strangulation), and infection due to missed aerodigestive injuries. Carotid artery is the structure most often involved.
- Zone II injuries are the most common in penetrating trauma, but because they can be readily accessible, they also have the best prognosis.
- Due to better diagnostics and management, mortality from neck trauma has improved over the past several decades and now is estimated to be 2–6%. The mortality rate for penetrating neck injuries is as high as 10%.

53.10 Summary and Recommendation [3, 11]

- Injuries that penetrate the platysma are considered penetrating neck injuries.
- Defining anatomical zones is useful in most of penetrating injuries, while in some cases do not guide diagnostic or therapeutic management completely.
- In unstable patients, elective surgical exploration is recommended instead of extensive diagnostic work-up. Unstable patients still need immediate exploration, whereas all stable patients will first be assessed with clinical examination and CT angiography.
- All patients with neck injuries should be monitored in the hospital.
- A high index of suspicion is needed to detect subtle laryngotracheal injuries, especially in the multi-system trauma patient.
- Cervical spine injuries above C6 can result in partial or total loss of respiratory function.
- An inadequate secondary assessment may result in the failure to recognize a spinal cord injury.
- Concentrate on imminent and delayed signs of airway compromise.
- Be prepared to provide a surgical airway immediately if attempts at oral intubation fail.
- Maintain high concern for occult esophageal injuries which can cause life-threatening sequelae (Fig. 53.3).

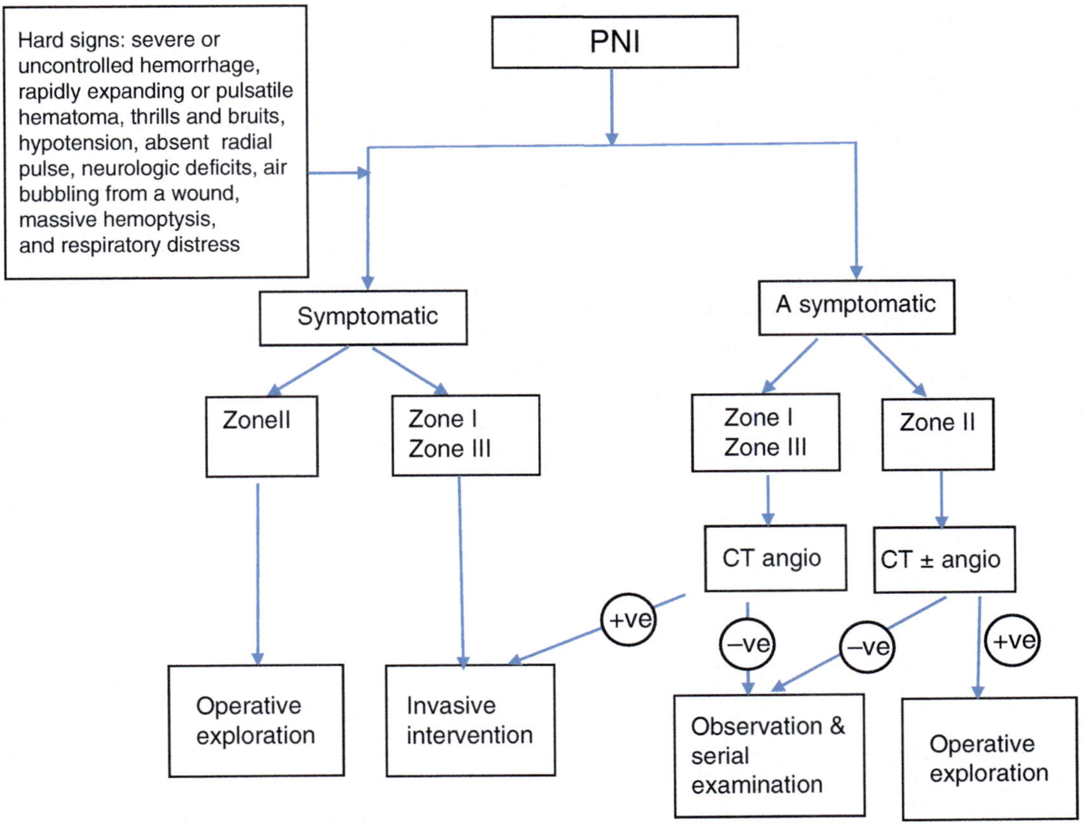

Fig. 53.3 Algorithm for penetrating neck injury (PNI) approach [1, 12]

References

1. Nowicki JL, Stew B, Ooi E. Penetrating neck injuries: a guide to evaluation and management. Ann R Coll Surg Engl. 2018;100(1):6–11. https://doi.org/10.1308/rcsann.2017.0191.
2. Supparerk P et al. "Selective management of penetrating neck injuries using "no zone" approach." Injury. 2015;46(9):1720–1725.
3. Alao T, Waseem M. Neck trauma. Stat Pearls Publishing. 2020. https://www.ncbi.nlm.nih.gov/books/NBK470422/.
4. Swaminathan A. Penetrating neck injuries. REBEL EM blog. 2019. https://rebelem.com/penetrating-neck-injuries/.
5. Newton K. Penetrating neck injuries: initial evaluation and management up to date. 2017.
6. Minerva B et al. "MDCT in the assessment of laryngeal trauma: value of 2D multiplanar and 3D reconstructions." Am J Roentgenol. 2013;201(4):W639–W647.
7. Verdonck, P et al. Penetrating and blunt trauma to the neck: clinical presentation, assessment and emergency management. B-ENT. 2016;12(Suppl. 26/2):69–85.
8. Nathan L. Salinas, MD, Captain, MC. Resident Manual of Trauma to the Face, Head, and Neck First Edition. American Academy of Otolaryngology—Head and Neck Surgery Foundation. 2012. ISBN: 978-0-615-64912-2.
9. Philicia M, Sachdeva UM, and Morse CR. "Management of laryngotracheal trauma." Annals of cardiothoracic surgery. 2018;7(2):210.
10. Park KS. "Evaluation and management of caustic injuries from ingestion of acid or alkaline substances." Clin Endosc. 2014;47(4):301.
11. Poduva JD, Ali IE. Iatrogenic airway trauma: a systematic review. ISSN: 2395-7565. J Med Res. 2016;2(5):166–168.
12. Mahmoodie M, Sanei B, Moazeni-Bistgani M, Namgar M. Penetrating neck trauma: review of 192 cases. Arch Trauma Res. 2012;1(1):14–18. https://doi.org/10.5812/atr.530811.
13. Hussain Zaidi SM, Ahmad R. Penetrating neck trauma: a case for conservative approach. Am J Otolaryngol. 2011;32(6):591–596. https://doi.org/10.1016/j.amjoto.2010.09.001.

54 ENT Manifestations in Systemic and Inflammatory Diseases

Aya Elderee, Ali Al Ansari, Hassan Haidar, and Mazin Al Khabouri

54.1 Introduction

Systemic and Inflammatory Diseases can affect the head and neck regions in a variety of manners. These manifestations may be the initial indications of the systemic disease, or sequela of the established diagnosis. The ENT symptoms and findings may mimic a variety of local illnesses, thus making this distinction an important part of the evaluative process. An awareness of the possible head and neck manifestations of underlying systemic disease is important in a proper diagnosis of the illness with consequent proper management.

A. Elderee (✉) · A. Al Ansari
ENT Department, Hamad Medical Corporation, Doha, Qatar
e-mail: AElderee@hamad.qa; aalansari@hamad.qa

H. Haidar
Hamad Medical Corporation, Doha, Qatar

M. Al Khabouri
ENT Department, Al Nahdha Hospital, Muscat, Sultanate of Oman

54.2 Hereditary Hemorrhagic Telangiectasia HHT (Formerly Osler Weber Rendu)

- It's an autosomal dominant disease.
- Present with multiple telangiectasias of the skin and mucosa.
- **Diagnosis**: Using the Curacao criteria: The HHT diagnosis is Definite if 3 criteria are present, Possible or suspected if 2 criteria are present, and Unlikely if fewer than 2 criteria are present.
  - Epistaxis which is spontaneous and recurrent.
  - Mucosal telangiectasia, multiple, at characteristic sites including lips, oral cavity, fingers, and nose.
  - Visceral lesions such as gastrointestinal telangiectasia (with or w/o bleeding), pulmonary AVM, hepatic AVM, cerebral AVMs, spinal AVM.
  - Family history with a first degree relative with HHT [1].
- **Treatment options showing in** Table 54.1:

54.3 Kawasaki Disease

- Kawasaki disease (KD), also known as mucocutaneous lymph node syndrome. It is an acute febrile disease of childhood and is

A. Al-Qahtani et al. (eds.), *Textbook of Clinical Otolaryngology*,
https://doi.org/10.1007/978-3-030-54088-3_54

Table 54.1 Treatment options for hereditary hemorrhagic telangiectasia (HHT)

Medical management	Surgical management
Topical moisturizers (mupirocin and saline gel)	Cauterization using laser, bipolar, or radiofrequency
Topical or oral estrogen agents	Septodermoplasty
Topical timolol	Young's procedure
Oral tranexamic acid	
Topical or IV bevacizumab (Avastin)	

characterized by medium-sized arteries' vasculitis with predilection for the coronary arteries. This gives a potential for the development of coronary artery aneurysms and sudden death.

- It is the leading cause of acquired heart disease in developed nations [2, 3].
- **Clinical symptoms**:
  - Fever >5 days and have 4–5 of following symptoms:
  - Acute unilateral non purulent cervical lymphadenopathy with size >1.5 cm.
  - Erythematous desquamative rash of palms and soles.
  - Polymorphus rash.
  - Bilateral painless bulbar conjunctivitis.
  - Erythema of tongue (strawberry tongue—protuberance of papillae), lips, oral cavity.
- **Workup**: KD is a clinical diagnosis.
- Labs: could show elevated CRP and ESR, thrombocytopenia.
- Echocardiography to look for CAAs, 7–20% of the patients will develop coronary artery aneurysms.
- Myocardial infarction within 2–12 weeks of disease onset.

Treatment: The main objective is to prevent coronary artery disease. Early administration of IVIG and aspirin within 10 days after the onset of symptoms is the mainstay of treatment to prevent the development of cardiac sequelae [2, 3].

54.4 Giant Cell Arteritis GCA Also Known as (Temporal Arteritis)

- It is a vasculitis of unknown etiology. It is the most common vasculitis in adults and it usually affects the older persons and manifest in a wide variety of systemic, neurologic, and ophthalmologic symptoms.
- Classified as a large-vessel vasculitis but typically also involves medium and small arteries, particularly the superficial temporal arteries hence the term temporal arteritis.
- It most commonly affects the ophthalmic, occipital, vertebral, posterior ciliary, and proximal vertebral arteries.
- More common in females, presents >50 years of age.
- Common signs and symptoms include visual disorder, headache, jaw claudication, cervical pain, and scalp tenderness.

Diagnosis: Temporal artery biopsy remains the criterion standard for diagnosis of this granulomatous vasculitis.

Treatment: Corticosteroids are the mainstay of therapy.

- In steroid-resistant cases, drugs such as tocilizumab, cyclosporine, azathioprine, or methotrexate may be used as steroid-sparing agents.

54.5 Cogan's Syndrome

- **Pathophysiology**: unknown, autoimmune etiology, produce Hydrops similar to Meniere's disease.
- **Symptoms**:
- Non-syphilitic interstitial keratitis (blurriness, rapidly progresses to blindness and labyrinthitis (causing SNHL, vertigo, and tinnitus).
- Most patients have typical syndrome of ocular and sudden true vertigo.

- Hearing loss: initial unilateral, high-frequency loss, followed by bilateral and progressive, can become profound.
- If untreated, may lead to profound sensorineural hearing loss and loss of vestibular function.

Treatment: corticosteroids, cyclophosphamide, Azathioprine.

54.6 Granulomatosis with Polyangiitis (Wegener Granulomatosis)

- Is a rare multisystem autoimmune disease of unknown etiology. Its main features include necrotizing granulomatous inflammation and pauci-immune vasculitis in small- and medium-sized blood vessels.
- Most common granulomatous disease to affect the upper respiratory system.
- Triad of upper/lower airway necrotizing granulomas, systemic vasculitis, glomerulonephritis.
- **ENT manifestations**:
- Chronic sinusitis is the most common initial manifestation; failure to respond to conventional treatment is suggestive for the diagnosis, rhinitis 22%, epistaxis 11%, saddle-nose deformity, serous otitis media and hearing loss and strawberry gingival hyperplasia.
- Stridor, potentially leading to respiratory compromise, from tracheal or subglottic granulomatous masses.
- **Diagnosis**: c-ANCA positive (specificity 90% in systemic vasculitis stage, 65% in granulomatous phase, 30% in remission), and nasal biopsy after thorough removal of nasal crusting.
- **Treatment**:
  - Prednisone 1 mg/kg/day × 4 weeks then taper.
  - Cyclophosphamide 2 mg/kg/day for 6–12 months.
  - IVIG in non-responders.
  - Azathioprine (2 mg/kg/day) for maintenance of remission.

54.7 Sarcoidosis

- Is a systemic noncaseating granulomatous condition of unknown etiology which may affect any part of the body.
- Most frequently involves the lungs and intrathoracic lymph nodes, in over 90% of cases.
- It is 10–20 times more common in African-Americans than Caucasians.
- Is a condition of young adults with a peak onset between the third and fourth decades.
- It is more frequent in women than men.
- **Pathophysiology**: There are abnormalities of both the cell-mediated and humoral immune systems. Macrophages and T-cell activation lead to the release of cytokines, including tumor necrosis factor (TNF), with resultant granuloma formation.
- **ENT manifestation**:
- Sinonasal sarcoid is reported in 1–4%.
- Nasal manifestations are almost always part of chronic multisystem sarcoid.
- Nasal symptoms commonly include obstruction, crusting, bleeding, or facial pain.
- The nasal mucosa: a characteristic granular appearance, 'strawberry skin'.
- The anterior nasal septum is most often affected and may perforate, particularly if traumatized by surgery.
- Patients may present with a soft-tissue mass or expansion of the nasal bridge. This may be associated with thickening and purplish discoloration of the overlying skin known as lupus pernio.
- Salivary gland enlargement is seen in 5–10%.
- Heerfordt's syndrome (enlarged parotid glands, facial nerve palsy, uveitis and fever).
- The larynx is involved in 1–5% of cases, most commonly the supraglottis (85%), with symptoms of cough, hoarseness, dysphagia, and more rarely stridor.
- Unilateral/bilateral facial paralysis.
- Recurrent bilateral parotid swelling.
- **Diagnosis**: Biopsy with the classic histological appearance: noncaseating granuloma with central epithelioid cells surrounded by lymphocytes and fibroblasts.

- Serum angiotensin-converting enzyme (ACE) is elevated in up to 85% during active disease.
- Serum and urinary calcium levels are elevated in approximately 15% of cases.
- Bi-hilar lymphadenopathy on chest X-ray.

Treatment: Include oral corticosteroids, immunosuppressive agents (cyclophosphamide and methotrexate), topical saline rinses and steroids for symptomatic relief and FESS in controlled inflammatory disease.

54.8 Eosinophilic Granulomatosis with Polyangiitis (Churg-Strauss Syndrome)

- It's a small to medium vessel vasculitis, which leads to necrosis, with unknown etiology.
- *American College of Rheumatology criteria for diagnosis*:
  - Asthma.
  - Eosinophilia of more than 10% in peripheral blood.
  - Paranasal sinusitis.
  - Pulmonary infiltrates.
  - Histological proof of vasculitis with extravascular eosinophils.
  - Mononeuritis multiplex or polyneurography.
- *Three clinical phases of disease*:
  - Prodromal Phase with (Asthma and upper respiratory involvement).
  - Peripheral Eosinophilic infiltrative phase with (Pulmonary and GI involvement with eosinophilic tissue infiltration leading to pneumonia/gastroenteritis).
  - Disseminated phase with systemic necrotizing vasculitis affecting (lung, CNS, GI and skin).
- **Diagnosis**: (1) Tissue Biopsy. (2) Labs: p-ANCA positive in 70%.
- **Treatment**: Oral corticosteroids and immunosuppressive agents (such as cyclophosphamide in life-threatening cases or poor prognosis).

54.9 Amyloidosis

- Amyloidosis is an idiopathic clinical disorder caused by extracellular and/or intracellular deposition of insoluble abnormal amyloid fibrils that alter the normal function of tissues.
  - Classification of amyloidosis: historical classification systems for amyloidosis were clinically based.
  - Modern classification systems are biochemically based (Table 54.2).

Table 54.2 Modern classification systems of amyloidosis

1. Based on the cause into:	– Primary: unknown cause; the deposition is in the disease site itself – Secondary: with underlying known disease
2. Based on extent of amyloid deposition:	– Systemic involving multiple organs – Localized amyloidosis involving one or two organs or sites
3. Based on clinical location:	– Pattern I: involves tongue, heart, intestines, skeletal and smooth muscle, skin and nerves – Pattern II: involves liver, spleen, kidney and adrenals – Mixed pattern: involves sites of both pattern I and II
4. Based on tissues in which amyloid is deposited:	– Mesenchymal: organs derived from mesoderm – Parenchymal: organs derived from ectoderm and endoderm
5. Based on the histological basis:	– Peri collagenous: corresponding in distribution to primary amyloidosis – Peri reticulin: corresponding in distribution to secondary amyloidosis
6. Based on precursor biochemical proteins, into a specific type of serum amyloid proteins:	– AL = amyloid light chain – AA = amyloid-associated protein – Aβ2M = amyloid β2-macroglobulin – ATTR = amyloid transthyretin

Biopsy: Using immunocytochemical studies, amyloidosis is diagnosed when Congo red (apple-green birefringence)–binding material is demonstrated in a biopsy specimen.

- **ENT manifestations**:
  - Primary: tongue most commonly involved.
  - localized: larynx most common site of deposition in respiratory tract followed by trachea, can present as subglottic stenosis.

Treatment: Immunotherapy and autologous stem-cell transplantation .

54.10 Relapsing Polychondritis

- Is an episodic and progressive severe inflammatory condition that involves cartilaginous structures, predominantly those of the ears, nose, and laryngotracheobronchial tree. It may also affect the eyes, cardiovascular system, middle and inner ear, and central nervous system.
- **Head and neck manifestation**:
  - Auricular chondritis: 85–95% of the patients develop auricular chondritis, which presents with unilateral or bilateral auricular pain, swelling, and redness develop suddenly but spare the lobules.
  - Nasal chondritis: it is acute and painful and occurs in almost half of patients with relapsing polychondritis. Mild epistaxis may be present. A saddle-nose may develop in longstanding disease.
  - Respiratory tract chondritis: affects 40–56% of patients, weakens the tracheal cartilage rings, resulting in wheezing, dyspnea, cough, and hoarseness.
  - Inflammation and swelling of the laryngeal tissues may require tracheostomy.
  - Audiovestibular derangements are experienced by 46–50% of patients, usually those with concomitant auricular chondritis. Sudden hearing loss is usually permanent, while tinnitus, and vertigo may subside. In some patients, hearing loss is attributed to vasculitic damage to the eighth cranial nerve.
- **Treatment**: the mainstay of treatment is systemic corticosteroid therapy.

54.11 Systemic Lupus Erythematosis

- Is an autoimmune disorder characterized by antibodies to nuclear and cytoplasmic antigens, multisystem inflammation involving (skin, joints, kidneys, blood vessels, nervous system, heart), protean clinical manifestations, and a relapsing and remitting course. More than 90% of cases of SLE occur in women, frequently starting at childbearing age.
- **Head and neck manifestations**:
  - Malar rash (50%)
  - Painful oral mucosal ulcers (25%)
  - Cranial neuropathy (15%)
  - Acute parotid enlargement (10%)
  - Septal ulceration/perforation (3–5)%
  - Telangiectasia
  - Laryngeal/tracheal: vocal cord thickening/paralysis, cricoarytenoid arthritis and subglottic stenosis
  - Chronic xerostomia

54.12 Medications Used to Treat SLE Manifestations Include the Following in Table 54.3

Table 54.3 Medications used to treat systemic lupus erythematosis

Drug class	Examples
Nonsteroidal anti-inflammatory drugs (NSAIDS)	Ibuprofen, naproxen, diclofenac
Corticosteroids	Methylprednisolone, prednisone
Nonbiologic DMARDS (disease-modifying antirheumatic drugs)	Cyclophosphamide, methotrexate, azathioprine, mycophenolate, cyclosporine
Biologic DMARDs (disease-modifying antirheumatic drugs)	Belimumab, rituximab, and/or IV immune globulin
Antimalarials	Hydroxychloroquine sulfate

54.13 Rheumatoid Arthritis (RA)

- Rheumatoid arthritis is a chronic systemic inflammatory disease of unknown cause. An external trigger (e.g., cigarette smoking, infection, or trauma) that triggers an autoimmune reaction, leading to synovial hypertrophy and chronic joint inflammation along with the potential for extra-articular manifestations, is theorized to occur in genetically susceptible individuals.
- HLA DR1 and HLA DR 4 most common serotypes associated with RA.
- HLA-linked RA susceptibility locus accounts for <20% RA in the general population.
- **Head and neck manifestations shown in** Fig. 54.1:
- **Treatment:** analgesics and NSAIDs; anti-rheumatic drugs such as methotrexate.

54.14 Behcet's Syndrome

– Behçet disease is a rare vasculitis disorder with the ability to affect small, medium, and large vessels; it is characterized by a triple-symptom complex of recurrent oral aphthous ulcers, genital ulcers, and uveitis.

54.14.1 Treatment

– For oral and genital ulcerations, topical steroids or sucralfate solution is the first-line therapy.
– For ocular disease, azathioprine is widely accepted as the initial agent [4].

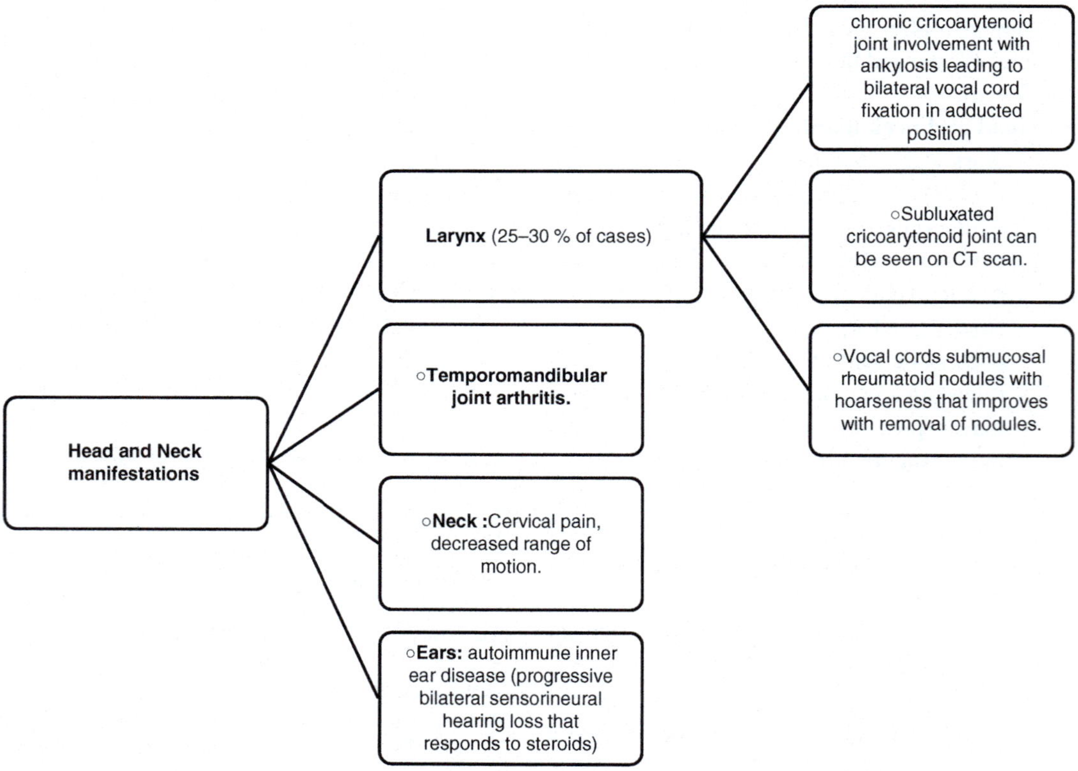

Fig. 54.1 Manifestation of rheumatoid arthritis in head and neck

54.15 Sjogren's Syndrome

- Is the second most common chronic autoimmune connective tissue disorder characterized by xerostomia and xerophthalmia due to profound lymphocytic infiltration into the salivary and lacrimal glands.

54.15.1 Classification

- Primary disease in which there are only symptoms and signs affecting the eye and mouth.
- Secondary Sjogren's syndrome in which there is xerostomia, xerophthalmia and associated connective tissue disorder most frequently rheumatoid arthritis or systemic lupus erythematosus.

54.15.2 ENT Manifestations

- The xerostomia of Sjogren's syndrome can be profound, giving rise to dysarthria and dysphagia. The oral dryness leads to retention of food on the teeth, mucosa, and gingiva and thus increases the frequency of caries and acute gingivitis.
- Affected patients may have intermittent swelling of the major salivary glands—notably the parotid glands, this often reflects non-specific inflammatory change within the glands.
- There is an increased risk of non-Hodgkin's lymphoma of the major salivary gland, mainly MALT tumors.

54.15.3 Diagnosis

1. Biopsy of minor salivary glands (lips, septum, hard palate).
2. Blood tests:
   - Primary: SS-A/Ro (60%), SS-B/La (30%), HLA-DW3, HLA-B8.
   - Secondary: HLA-DW4.
   - Other positive findings: RF, ANA.

54.15.4 Treatment:

1. Local agents, such as salivary substitutes and chewing gum.
2. Systemic agents: as pilocarpine, cevimeline, bethanechol, interferon alpha.
3. Electrostimulation, acupuncture, and dietary supplements.

54.16 Myasthenia Gravis MG

- **Pathophysiology**: is a relatively rare acquired, autoimmune disorder caused by an antibody-mediated blockade of neuromuscular transmission, resulting in skeletal muscle weakness. The autoimmune attack occurs when autoantibodies form against the nicotinic acetylcholine postsynaptic receptors at the neuromuscular junction of skeletal muscles.
- Myasthenic weakness typically affects the extraocular, bulbar, or proximal limb muscles. Droopy eyelids or double vision is the most common symptom at initial presentation of MG, with more than 75% of patients.

ENT Symptoms: Up to 20% of patients with MG may have prominent oropharyngeal symptoms early in the disease course, including dysarthria, dysphagia, and difficulty chewing.

- Slurred Speech (from weakness of the tongue); it worsens with prolonged talking.
- Swallowing may become difficult, and aspiration may occur with fluids which leads to coughing or choking while drinking. Liquids are more difficult to swallow than the solid food. Because of palatal muscle weakness, patients often complain of nasal regurgitation of liquids.

54.16.1 Diagnosis

Following maneuvers are helpful for diagnosis of MG:

- Sustained up gaze (1–3 min); results in fatigable ptosis in one or both eyes.

- Counting loud (from 1 to 50): Enhances dysarthria (nasal, lingual, or labial) and results in dyspnea. Patient may sound relatively clear on speaking initially but will become increasingly dysarthric to the point of becoming unintelligible.
- Weakness of the laryngeal muscles results in dysphonia. This can be evoked by asking the patient to say ("eeee") sound for a several seconds.
- Blood test:
  – The anti–acetylcholine receptor (AChR) antibody (Ab) test is highly specific (about 85%)
- **Electrodiagnostic studies** such as repetitive stimulation of a muscle at 2–3 Hz, also known as repetitive nerve stimulation (RNS) and single-fiber electromyography (SFEMG)
- Treatment:
  – **Medial**: Anticholinesterase (AchE) inhibitors such as (pyridostigmine and neostigmine), intravenous immune globulin (IVIg), plasmapheresis and long-term immunosuppression
  – **Surgical**: Thymectomy

54.17 Pemphigus Vulgaris

- Pemphigus vulgaris is an autoimmune, intraepithelial, blistering disease affecting the skin and mucous membranes. It is mediated by circulating autoantibodies directed against keratinocyte cell surfaces. A potentially life-threatening disease; it has a mortality rate of approximately 5–15%.

54.17.1 ENT Symptoms

- Mucous membranes of the oral cavity are involved in almost all patients (ill-defined, irregularly shaped, gingival, buccal, or palatine erosions, which are painful and slow to heal).
- Erosions may be seen on any part of the oral cavity, and they may spread to involve the larynx, with subsequent hoarseness.

54.17.2 Diagnosis

- Histopathology from the edge of a blister.
- Direct immunofluorescence (DIF) demonstrates in vivo deposits of antibodies and other immunoreactants, such as complement. DIF usually shows immunoglobulin G (IgG) deposited on the surface of the keratinocytes in and around lesions.

54.17.3 Treatment

- Corticosteroids and immunosuppressants to reduce the inflammatory response and autoantibody production.

54.17.4 Scleroderma

- Is a disease characterized by progressive skin hardening and induration.
- Scleroderma is an aspect of systemic sclerosis, which is a systemic autoimmune connective tissue disease that also involves subcutaneous tissue, muscles, and internal organs.
- The risk of systemic sclerosis is much higher in women than in men.
- The peak onset occurs in individuals aged 30–50 years.
- Can be associated with Sjogren's syndrome or **CREST**, which is a limited form of the disease with (calcinosis, Raynaud's phenomenon, esophageal stenosis, sclerodactyly and telangiectasias).
- **Head and neck manifestations**:
  – Difficulty opening mouth secondary to fibrosis of masticatory muscles
  – Nasal cavity telangiectasias leading to epistaxis
  – Esophagus: aperistalsis of lower two-third and esophageal dilation; absent lower esophageal sphincter contraction allowing reflux

Treatment: Symptomatic treatment, immunosuppressants (methotrexate, cyclophosphamide) and phototherapy using ultraviolet A (UVA) light.

Take Home Messages

- ENT symptoms may represent an early sign of an undiagnosed systemic disorder that often requires immediate and aggressive treatment.
- An otolaryngologist should maintain a high index of suspicion to identify the underlying disease as these may be the only manifestations of the systemic disease in early stages.
- Early and accurate diagnosis with prompt treatment or referral to specialists may prevent morbidity and mortality related to these diseases.

References

1. Flint PW, Hughey BH, Lund VJ, et al. Cummings otolaryngology: head and neck surgery. 5th ed. Philadelphia, PA: Mosby Elsevier; 2010.
2. Umezawa T, Saji T, Matsuo N, Odagiri K. Chest x-ray findings in the acute phase of Kawasaki disease. Pediatr Radiol. 1989;20(1–2):48–51.
3. Satou GM, Giamelli J, Gewitz MH. Kawasaki disease: diagnosis, management, and long-term implications. Cardiol Rev. 2007;15(4):163–9. [Medline].
4. Davatchi F, Chams-Davatchi C, Shams H, Shahram F, Nadji A, Akhlaghi M, et al. Behcet's disease: epidemiology, clinical manifestations, and diagnosis. Expert Rev Clin Immunol. 2017;13(1):57–65. [Medline].

Part VII

Pediatrics

Anesthetic Considerations for Pediatric ENT Surgeries for Non-anesthesiologists

55

Nabil A. Shallik, Ahmed Zaghw, Al Moataz Adham, and Sahar Mahadik

55.1 Introduction

Pediatric anesthesia is a rapidly emerging subspecialty requiring a fellowship training. The evolution in anesthesiologists training especially via simulation programs has strived to elevate the safety of children during the perioperative period. The development of pediatric equipment especially the airway tools, monitors and pharmacological agents have, as well contributed in improving the quality and outcome of the anesthesia for the pediatric population. General anesthesia for ear, nose, and throat (ENT) surgeries carries more hazards of perioperative morbidity given the risks related either to the patient such as OSA and/or to the procedure itself such as airway surgeries. The small and narrow pediatric airway is more liable to getting rapidly obstructed from the effects of edema and bleeding.

N. A. Shallik (✉) · S. Mahadik
Weill Cornell Medical College in Qatar, Doha, Qatar
e-mail: Smahadik@hamad.qa

A. Zaghw
Hamad Medical Corporation, Doha, Qatar
e-mail: azaghw@hamad.qa

A. M. Adham
Sidra Medicine, Doha, Qatar
e-mail: madham@sidra.org

55.2 Preoperative Assessment

The preoperative assessment should focus on airway, respiratory and cardiac evaluation, as well as any specific comorbidity for any patient. Preoperative investigations may be ordered depending on the patient and type of surgery. Planning the anesthetic, the post-operative disposal and the analgesia are essential parts of the pre-operative assessment.

55.2.1 Airway Assessment

Any previous anesthetic or airway management records should be obtained. Ideally, these will include details about the feasibility of previous mask or supraglottic device ventilation, and tracheal intubation. Details about earlier devices for the airway as direct or video laryngoscopy, as well as the number of attempts required. Table 55.1 shows the assessment of anatomical features that would predict a difficult airway. Airway assessment in children is difficult to undertake in the smaller uncooperative population. In these cases, the airway assessment is limited to general observation of any facial dysmorphism and more importantly to have a lateral look of the face and mandible inspecting for any retrognathia which might be obscured via the frontal look.

A. Al-Qahtani et al. (eds.), *Textbook of Clinical Otolaryngology*,
https://doi.org/10.1007/978-3-030-54088-3_55

Table 55.1 Summarizes assessment of the anatomical features that predict a difficult airway

Neck	• Limited neck motion • Short neck • Anterior/proximal larynx
Mouth	• Small mouth opening • Presence of loose teeth
Palate	• Deformed midline airway anatomy
Jaw—mandible	• Retro/micrognathia
Facial features	• Craniofacial asymmetry • Soft tissue masses around the airway (tumor, abscesses, burns, scarring)
Tongue	• Macroglossia
Miscellaneous clinical signs of airway obstruction	• Stridor • Known OSA • Intercostal/subcostal/tracheal retraction

55.2.2 Assessment for Comorbidities

Assessment must include a detailed history of allergies, past medical problems including congenital anomalies, recent respiratory illnesses, current medications, recent immunizations, past anesthetic history, or previous problems with anesthetics, including allergies and family history. Extra information about the perinatal course are of considerable importance for neonatal anesthesia. Instructions about the fasting times and discussion of the planned perioperative approach must include anesthetic induction, maintenance, postoperative course and pain management, consequently addressing parental expectations, are important steps of the preoperative assessment. A physical examination is mandatory and should focus on the cardiorespiratory systems. Queries and fears of the child as well as those of the parents need to be addressed. Preoperative investigations may be necessary depending on the complexity of the surgery and the sickness of the patient. Complete blood count (CBC), electrolytes, metabolic profile baseline tests and chest X-ray (CXR) are required on the background of any comorbidity or major surgery such as premature infants, systemic disease, congenital heart disease, renal or metabolic disease, expected blood loss, underlying dehydration, active respiratory disease, and scoliosis.

Table 55.2 International multidisciplinary consensus for preoperative fasting in the pediatric population [6]

Preoperative fasting guidelines for patients with a moderate risk of aspiration • 8 h—solid food or more fried or fatty food or meat • 6 h—solid light meal, nonhuman formula milk if greater than 12 months of age • 4 h—breast milk if less than 12 months of age • 2 h—unlimited clear fluids

Upper respiratory tract infection up to 4 weeks from its onset, is a risk factor for perioperative respiratory adverse events [1]. Decision to proceed versus postponement of the surgery is based on patient, surgical, and anesthetic factors (Kindly refer to Sect. 55.5 for more details) [2].

55.2.3 Preoperative Fasting

Fasting is the restriction of food and fluid intake before general anesthesia or sedation in order to minimize the risk of pulmonary aspiration. Fasting in the perioperative setting is the cornerstone of the patient safety with double-sided effects, as prolonged fasting can result in dehydration, hypoglycemia, hypovolemia, hypotension, and other metabolic complications [3]. It has been shown that children who drank fluids up to 2 h before surgery were less thirsty, hungry, more cooperative, and more comfortable compared to those who were fasted for over 6 h [4]. On the other hand, the less optimal fasting could result in aspiration-induced lung injury [5]. It's noteworthy to mention that most of the fasting guidelines rely on the physiology of gastric emptying and expert opinion, with no compelling evidence that adhering to fasting guidelines may improve clinical outcomes. More extended fasting periods is linked with an increased incidence of nausea and vomiting (Table 55.2).

55.2.4 Preoperative Investigations

The preoperative investigations should be guided based on the underlying comorbidities and the expected surgical complications. Preoperative blood coagulation studies (prothrombin time, activated partial thromboplastin time, international normalized ratio, platelet count, and occasionally a bleeding time) could be done to identify children at risk for perioperative hemorrhage. Other test such as complete blood count (CBC) is useful for anemic cases.

55.3 Airway Management

Airway management is accomplished with mask ventilation, supraglottic device ventilation (SGAD), and tracheal intubation. Mask ventilation is the most fundamental basic skill and most life-saving procedure for all patients who require assisted ventilation either during induction of anesthesia, post-extubation, or during other critical conditions when the ventilatory support is required as in cardiac arrest. Supraglottic airway devices (SGAD) can be used as the primary airway strategy for maintenance of anesthesia, avoiding tracheal intubation if clinically indicated [7]. The tracheal intubation is the only definitive airway management, and it could be done through the nose, the mouth, or the trachea directly as in tracheostomy. The tracheal intubation may be performed by the **Direct Laryngoscopy, Video-laryngoscopy, Flexible Bronchoscopy, and Rigid Bronchoscopy.**

55.3.1 Difference Between the Pediatric and the Adult Airway

The main anatomical differences between the pediatric and the adult are the following:

Infants are obligate nasal breathers, with a relatively large tongue and large occiput. The larynx and trachea are funnel shaped and the vocal cords are slanting anteriorly. In children the larynx is located higher in the neck at the cervical C4 vertebra versus the cervical C6 vertebra in adults. The narrowest part of the pediatric airway is at the cricoid subglottic cartilage. However, the narrowest part in adults is the glottic opening [8]. These differences render the pediatric airway management unique and rather challenging in comparison to the adult's one. For instance, a larger tongue makes the bag-mask ventilation more difficult as it may obstruct the airway after induction. A higher larynx makes laryngoscopy view more anterior, and the narrow subglottic area along with the slanting of the vocal cords in smaller children might impose difficulties in advancing the tube past the vocal cords (Table 55.3).

Table 55.3 Shows difference between the pediatric and the adult airway

Anatomy	Pediatric	Adult
Head	Large occiput-sniffing position	Flat occiput
Tongue	Relatively large	Small
Larynx	Opposite C2–3 (cephalic position) Funnel shaped	Opposite C4–5 Cylindrical
Epiglottis	Omega shaped, soft	Flat, flexible
Vocal cords	Short, concave	Horizontal
Smallest diameter	Cricoid ring	Vocal cord
Cartilage	Soft, non-calcified	Firm, calcified

55.3.2 Pediatric Bag-Mask Ventilation

Pediatric bag-mask ventilation is an essential skill to master in the management of the pediatric airway. Due to different sizes of the pediatric patients, an appropriately sized mask should be selected in order to have a good fit. The mask size selection should cover the area extending from the nasal bridge to the chin with a good seal around the mouth and nose. As in adults, two techniques are described for bag-mask ventilation in children using the C&E maneuver: The two hands technique (with one hand on the mask and chin, and the other hand squeezing the bag, and the three hands technique (where the operator has both hands on the mask and jaw while an assistant is squeezing the bag) (Fig. 55.1).

In contrast to adults, in small children care must be taken not to compress the soft submandibular soft tissues. This may result in total air-

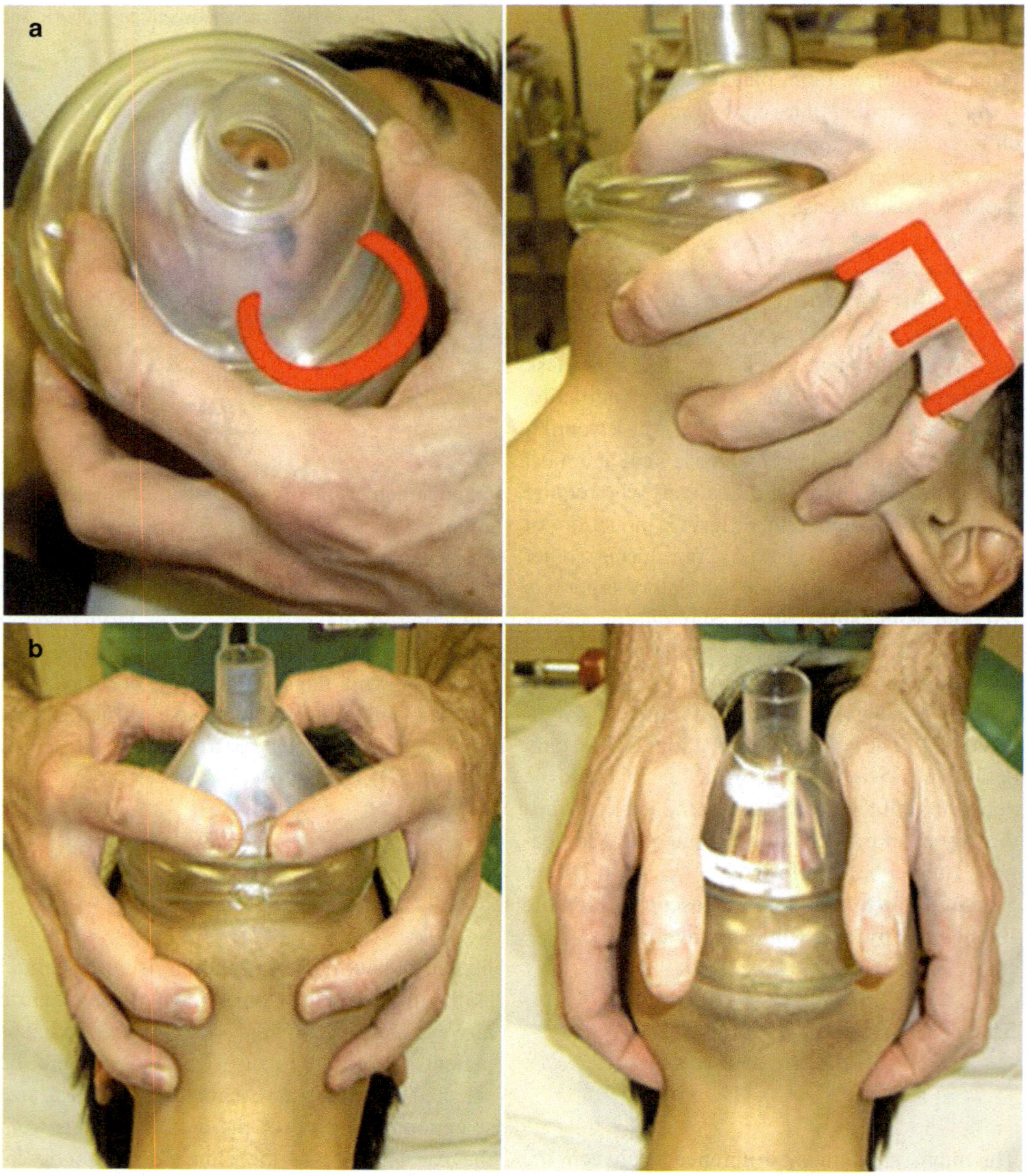

Fig. 55.1 Pediatric mask ventilation (**a**): Two hands bag-mask ventilation technique (C&E). (**b**) Three hands bag-mask ventilation technique

way obstruction, hence the "C & E" maneuver needs to get modified to "C" (with thumb and index on the mask) along with the third finger positioned on the bony part of the chin.

Bag-mask ventilation might be difficult sometimes despite using optimal "jaw thrust" and three hands technique; in such cases an oropharyngeal airway (or nasal) might be necessary for keeping the patient's airway patent.

Selecting an appropriately sized oropharyngeal airway is of a great importance as a small or a large one relatively to the patient's size may worsen the airway obstruction instead of helping its patency.

Selecting the appropriately sized oropharyngeal airway in children is done by externally measuring its length versus the distance between the mouth and the angle of the mandible of the child.

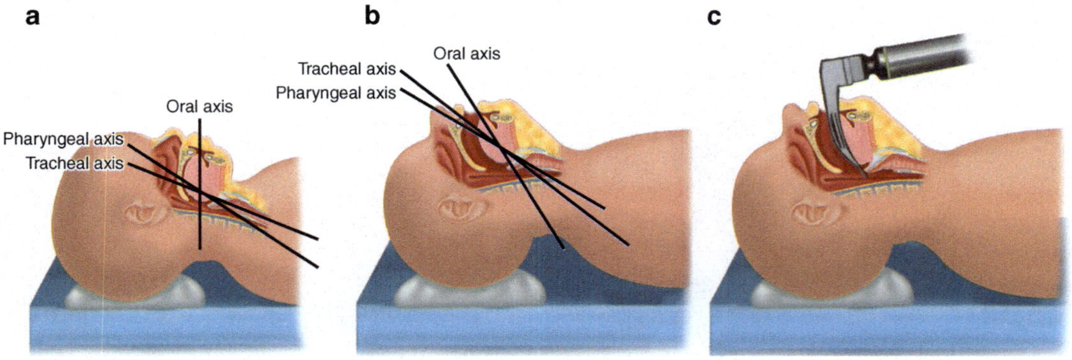

Fig. 55.2 Shows (**a**) axes (oral, pharyngeal, and tracheal); (**b**) alignment of these axes with correct positioning; (**c**) viewing the glottic fold with straight blade

A matching length indicates a proper size of the oropharyngeal airway.

55.3.3 Direct Laryngoscopy (DL)

Direct laryngoscopy (DL) is the most popular intubation technique in nowadays practice [9]. The purpose of the direct laryngoscope is to align the oral, pharyngeal, and laryngeal axis together until the operator obtains only one axis of view (Fig. 55.2). This is achieved by lifting the tongue and the jaw forward using the direct laryngoscopy blades thus exposing the laryngeal inlet. It is a simple and easy technique using an age-appropriate blade size and type.

The most important step in direct laryngoscopy of pediatric patients is to adequately sweep the relatively large tongue to the left out of the field of vision, otherwise an improperly swept tongue might result in a blocked view.

Direct laryngoscopy techniques may be aided by an external laryngeal pressure maneuver ("BURP" backward, upward, and posterior external compression of the larynx) applied by the fingers of an assistant or the operator in order to achieve a better exposure of the glottis.

DL attempts should not exceed a number of two or three trials, with a prompt switch to a further advanced intubation technique if the latter are unsuccessful.

55.3.4 Video-Laryngoscopy (VL)

Video-laryngoscopy is an indirect way of laryngeal visualization and intubation, by which the images are displayed, magnified, and recorded on a screen display. Different devices have shown variable performance in pediatric airway management (See Fig. 55.3 and Table 55.4). Video-assisted visualization is promoted as a first choice in anticipated difficult airway situations as proven by clinical outcome. Intubation with the Glidescope VL has shown a similar success rate at intubation on first attempt, comparable with the fiber-optic bronchoscope intubation, with a significantly higher success rate than the direct laryngoscopy technique [10].

Video-assisted DL (VADL), such as the C-MAC Storz Videoscope, is a technique that allows both DL and indirect laryngoscopy at the same time by combining a videoscope with the traditional laryngoscopy blade that can be used to perform direct laryngoscopy (DL) with the video monitor available to the laryngoscopy operator as well as to the supervisor. While displaying the image on a screen the combined technique a better view than the conventional DL. It also allows, in contrast to DL, a trainee to get adequately coached by an instructor during intubation. It was found that the hyper-angulated blades of Glidescopes and D-Blade of C-Mac have similar success rates of intubations compared to fiber-optic intubation with similar rates of airway trauma [9].

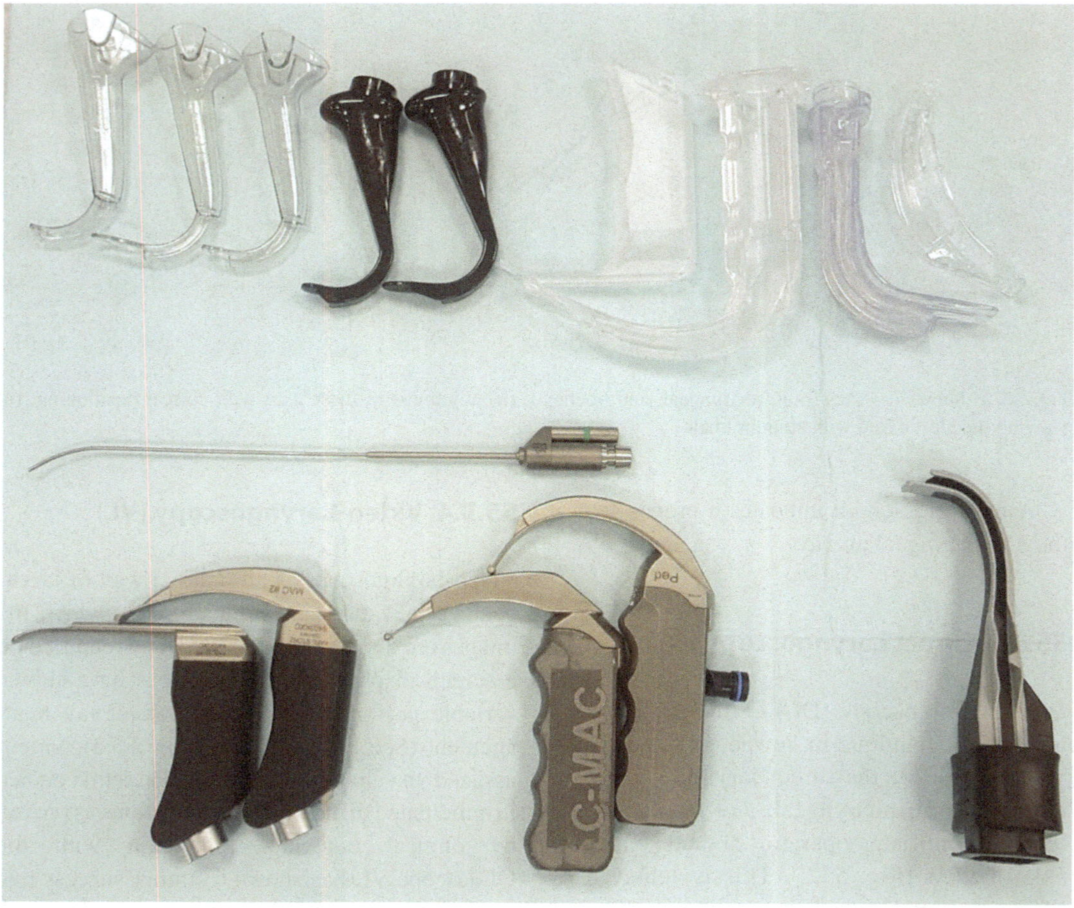

Fig. 55.3 Different video-laryngoscopy tools

Table 55.4 Classification of different video-laryngoscopes (VL) from different manufactures

Rigid blades		Guided channels	Video stylets	
Standard blade	Angled blade	Channeled blade	Rigid stylet	Rigid stylet + Flexing tip
– Storz C-Mac	– Glidescope – Storz D-Blade	– AirTraq	– Bonfils	– Rigid Intubating Fiber-optic Laryngoscope (RIFL)

55.3.5 Fiber-Optic Bronchoscopic Intubation (FOB)

Historically the bronchoscope was made of fiber-optic fibers, but recently it has only a flexible camera scope with CEMOS (Complementary metal oxide semiconductor) technology. It is the gold standard in adult airway management. Awake fiber-optic intubation is one of the most popular techniques in anticipated difficult airway in adults. However, the "Awake" option is almost impossible in the pediatric population. FOB is of great help in pediatric cases with cervical instability or limited mouth opening. It is as successful as intubating with a Glidescope in difficult pediatric airway and could be used as well as an adjuvant combination with video-laryngoscopy or Laryngeal mask airway (LMA).

55.3.6 Complications of Airway Management

According to the Pediatric Difficult Airway Registry (PeDIR), the episodes of severe hypoxia occurred in nearly 9% of cases. Temporary hypoxemia was the most frequent non-severe complication. Among other complications were frequent attempts, airway soft tissue trauma, failure to intubate, and the severest prevailed to be the airway-related cardiac arrest occurring in 2% of cases [9]. Another common complication was inflation of the stomach due to mask ventilation. The inflated stomach can splint the diaphragm of children, leading to lung collapse thus affecting the intraoperative ventilation, it can also lead to postoperative discomfort.

55.3.7 Goals of Anesthetists in-Hospital Course

General Anesthesia goals include preoperative sedation, preoxygenation, a patent airway, adequate ventilation, hemodynamic stability, normal temperature, proper hypnosis, and analgesia. The goals extend postoperatively to the management of postoperative nausea and vomiting (PONV) and postoperative pain (Kindly refer to Sects. 55.7 and 55.8).

55.3.7.1 Preoperative Sedation

In general, preoperative sedation is not mandated for all children. A clinical judgment by the anesthetist based on risk/benefits assessment must be done. Preoperative sedation should be selective for the anxious children who are not at risk of apnea, upper airway obstruction, or aspiration. The most popular medications in the perioperative period are Midazolam, Ketamine, and Dexmedetomidine. Midazolam is water soluble and can be given by parenteral (intravenous IV or intramuscular IM), rectal (PR), intranasal (IN), sublingual (SL), or oral (PO) routes. Intranasal midazolam is faster acting among other routes. Midazolam dose is 0.05–0.1 mg/kg IV with a maximum single dose of 2 mg, but the oral dose is 0.5 mg/kg. Intranasal delivery of 1.5–2 μg/kg dexmedetomidine has been shown to produce preoperative sedation like oral midazolam at 0.5 mg/kg and is associated with lower post-procedural pain scores. Ketamine must be administered in a monitored area, and parents should be informed about its side effects including nystagmus and hallucinations. Several devices can be used for intranasal (IN) administration of sedative drugs such as the mucosal atomization device (MAD), the nasal (aspirator) dropper, or a syringe tip without needle.

55.3.7.2 Preoxygenation

It's a preinduction step by which a 100% oxygen is administered with patient spontaneously breathing through a sealed mask to extend the safe apnea time or duration of apnea without desaturation, the time needed until airway is secured. Infants tolerate shorter periods of apnea and can desaturate in less than 100 seconds of apnea despite adequate preoxygenation. The younger the age, the faster the onset of desaturation. The rate of decline of SPO_2 during apnea in a 1-month old term baby is three times more rapid than in an adult. This makes the airway management in children more difficult for the inexperienced anesthesiologist.

A passive oxygenation technique or "apneic oxygenation" may be useful in prolonging the time of safe apnea without significant desaturation during the intubation process. It is done by passively insufflating oxygen at a low flow via a nasal cannula or a nasopharyngeal tube.

Apneic oxygenation time may be more effectively extended by utilizing a high flow nasal cannula oxygenation (HFNO) during intubation as amounts to providing a much higher flow (>20 L/min) of heated and humidified oxygen at a higher inspired fraction compared to conventional oxygen insufflation. HFNO is gaining great popularity particularly in difficult airway management.

55.3.7.3 Induction

Inhalation induction has been the classical anesthesia induction method in children who don't have a pre-existing intravenous line until the latter is being accessed. Sevoflurane is the most modern and most commonly used inhalation gas for anesthesia induction. It is relatively non-irritant and has a more rapid onset and offset of action as it is less soluble. A concentration of 8% can be used initially and then decreased gradually. Nitrous oxide used concomitantly with sevoflurane may accelerate the induction via its second gas effect property. Minimum alveolar concentration (MAC) values are 3.3% in infants and 2.5% in children.

Intravenous induction is the method of choice for induction in children with an already secured intravenous line. In contrast to inhalation induction, it has the advantage of a quicker onset of action bypassing the "light plane" of anesthesia during which the risk of laryngospasm is high.

Commonly used drugs in intravenous induction in children are: propofol (2–3 mg/kg IV), ketamine (1–2 mg/kg IV), opioids such as fentanyl or morphine should be carefully titrated especially in the smaller children due to their oversensitivity to narcotics. IV lidocaine (1–1.5 mg/kg) could be used as an adjunct to the induction medications in order to blunt the sympathetic reflex response associated with intubation. Muscle relaxants, such as rocuronium, (0.6 mg/kg) are used to facilitate the intubation, however some practices prefer to use a higher dose of propofol and sevoflurane without the use of muscle relaxants for tracheal intubation. Rocuronium with a higher dose (0.9–1.2 mg/kg) can be used for a faster onset of action in rapid sequence induction (RSI).

Choice of Equipment Sizes

Pediatric airway equipment sizes choice should be guided by tables and formulas (See Table 55.5). However, those are just used for guidance and are not accurate estimates. Henceforth, it is recommended that the operator always prepares two more sizes of each equipment (the corresponding size and one size smaller/bigger) before the airway management of any child.

55.3.7.4 Airway Equipment Sizes

Table 55.5 Shows different airway equipment and its suitable pediatric sizes

- **Laryngoscopy blades**:
  - Straight laryngoscope blades (Miller/Wisconsin) are recommended for use in neonates and infants (<2 years)
  - A size 0 blade is preferred in the babies less than 4 kg
  - A curved blade (Macintosh) can be used for children >2 years
- **Endotracheal tubes: "Only a clinical guide—always check clinically"**
  - ETT size = age/4 + 3.5 for cuffed ETT in patients above 1 year of age
  - ETT size = age/4 + 4 for uncuffed ETT in patients above 1 year of age
  - ETT length in cm (at the lip) = age/2 + 12
- **LMA sizes**:
  - 1 up to 5 kg.
  - 1.5 up to 5–10 kg
  - 2 up to 10–20 kg
  - 2.5 up to 20–30 kg
  - 3 for over 30 kg
- **Face masks** and **Oropharyngeal airways are selected visually (see** Sect. 55.3.2)

55.3.7.5 Temperature Management

Temperature management is one of the essential goals in pediatric anesthesia practice.

Intraoperative hypothermia can lead to serious consequences such as coagulopathy, blood loss, increased myocardial stress, acidosis, reduced tissue perfusion, slower drugs metabolism, delayed anesthetic recovery, and wound infection. Infants and smaller children are at a particularly high risk to develop hypothermia in the cold operating room environment due to: high skin surface/ body mass ratio increasing the heat dissipation, little subcutaneous fat with less insulation effect, low muscle mass with inability to shiver for heat production, and immature thermoregulatory center with impaired vasoconstriction leading to increased heat loss from the vasodilated vessels (Table 55.6) [11]. Common sites of core body temperature measurement include the nasopharynx, the esophagus, the rectum, and sometimes the bladder. Less accurate "non-core" peripheral temperature measurement is often done via skin probes [11].

Table 55.6 Temperature control methods

Passive warming techniques:
- Warming the operating room
- Limiting exposure of large areas of skin surface (covering blankets)
- Preservation of heat and moisture by heat and moisture exchanger (HME) filter

Active warming methods
- Use of heated and humidified gases for ventilation
- Forced air warming device
- Underbody conductive heat mattress
- Circulating water mattress
- Radiant warmer
- Fluid warming devices

55.4 Common Challenges in Pediatric Anesthesia for ENT Procedures

55.4.1 Perioperative Management of Children with Obstructive Sleep Apnea

55.4.1.1 Introduction

Obstructive sleep apnea (OSA) has an incidence of 1–3% in the pediatric population. The most common cause of OSA is adenotonsillar hypertrophy [12]. Comorbidities such as childhood obesity, craniofacial anomalies, and neuromuscular diseases are other causes of childhood OSA.

A thorough perioperative management of children with OSA is key for avoidance of complications [13].

55.4.1.2 Diagnosis

The diagnosis of OSA in children might be challenging as patients usually present with very unspecific symptoms such as poor school performance and daytime somnolence. It is also difficult to differentiate those children who have primary snoring from those with a "real" OSA. Other symptoms may include nocturnal enuresis, and mouth breathing. Those with severe long standing OSA might present with secondary pulmonary hypertension as a complication [14].

55.4.1.3 Polysomnography

Polysomnography is the "Gold Standard" for the diagnosis of OSA. It consists of measuring the airflow of breathing, oxygen saturation, and EEG in a sleeping patient. The most important measurement is the apnea to hypopnea index (AHI) (hypopnea being the decrease in airflow for more than 50%, apnea being a complete cessation of airflow) [14] AHI is also very useful to classify the severity of OSA (See Table 55.7) [14].

Table 55.7 Practice guidelines for the perioperative management of patients with obstructive sleep (OSA) Apnea by the American Society of Anesthesiologists (ASA) [15]

OSA severity	AHI children	AHI adults
None	0	0–5
Mild	1–5	6–20
Moderate	6–10	21–40
Severe	>10	>40

55.4.1.4 Preoperative Assessment

The most important aspect in the preoperative assessment of patients with OSA is to identify the symptomatic patient, classify the severity, and anticipate any cardiac involvement such as pulmonary hypertension. This is mainly undertaken via a thorough history and physical examination, followed by selected laboratory investigations and related imaging. Preoperative assessment should be completed by an anesthetic plan addressing all the perioperative precautions mandated to be taken [12] (Fig. 55.4).

55.4.1.5 History

A focused anesthetic history for patients with OSA should aim at reviewing charts for previous established diagnosis and treatment, followed by the inquiry about the symptoms of OSA including snoring during sleep, presence of witnessed apneas along with their duration and frequency, daytime sleepiness, presence of mouth breathing, restless sleep, nighttime sweating, "paradoxical" breathing, sleeping in abnormal positions, nocturnal enuresis, daytime sleepiness, and lack of concentration [14]. A video recording of the child's sleeping pattern and/or respiratory events recorded by the parents, if available, might be very helpful in the assessment.

Additional questions in patients with suspected/confirmed OSA should include other con-

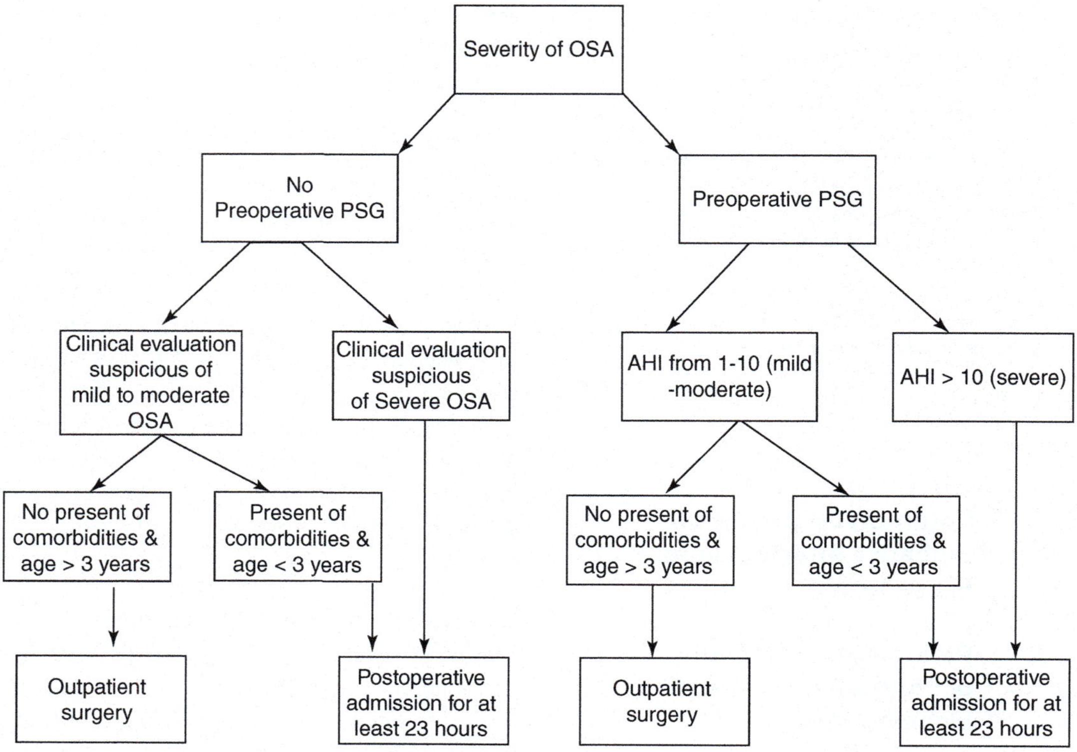

Fig. 55.4 Algorithm of Preoperative evaluation of OSA and postoperative plan [14]

tributing risk factors such as adenotonsillar hypertrophy, craniofacial malformations, some syndromes, obesity, midface hypoplasia, macroglossia, retrognathia, and gloss ptosis.

If the patient is already diagnosed, the latest sleep study should be reviewed in order to categorize severity (Table 55.7):

OSA is classified as mild, moderate, and severe depending on the apnea/hypopnea index (AHI). An AHI below 5 indicates a mild OSA and hence no need for postoperative monitoring. An AHI between 5 and 10 indicates a moderate OSA which may or may not require postoperative apnea monitoring. An AHI above 10 indicates a severe OSA, henceforth the need for a postoperative apnea-monitoring [14].

55.4.1.6 Physical Exam

Important findings during the physical examination may include the presence of mouth breathing, elongated facies, failure to thrive, obesity, tonsillar hypertrophy, presence of any airway abnormality (such as micrognathia, macroglossia, midface hypoplasia) and any craniofacial syndrome such as Pierre-Robin, Goldenhar, Treacher-Collins, and Mucopolysaccharidosis.

55.4.1.7 Investigations

Preoperative evaluation of children for OSA is mainly a clinical assessment done via history and physical exam, thus symptomatic children presenting for a conventional adenotonsillectomy are rarely having a polysomnography study. Polysomnography is kept for patients who have chronic and severe symptoms. Children with severe OSA must undertake a preoperative electrocardiogram (ECG) in addition to referral to cardiology for echocardiography to assess for any secondary pulmonary hypertension. Other investigations for children with OSA may include a complete blood count showing a reactive polycythemia secondary to hypoxia, and an arterial blood gas which may show a metabolic alkalotic compensation for hypercapnic acidosis, a sign of chronic CO_2 retention [14].

55.4.1.8 Intraoperative Considerations

Exposure to general anesthetic in children with OSA can result in airway collapse, hence a vigilant airway management technique and choice of appropriate pharmacological drugs and dose are keys for a safe anesthetic. There is no clear-cut consensus about the anesthetic management of children with OSA. Children with severe OSA and craniofacial anomalies are at higher risk of difficult ventilation/intubation, henceforth a proper plan for a difficult airway should be anticipated with all necessary drugs and equipment (DSAD, Bougies, Video-laryngoscope, Fiber-optic bronchoscope, Difficult Airway Cart…).

A careful inhalation induction is acceptable in patients with mild to moderate OSA, especially those undergoing adenotonsillectomies. However, an intravenous induction with a pre-inserted intravenous line is indicated for severe OSA cases especially those with suspected difficult airway.

As in adults, children with OSA have an increased sensitivity to opioid analgesics [16]. That is mainly explained by the m-opioid receptors; m-opioid upregulation due to chronic hypoxia, which renders them opioids "Naive" and very prone to respiratory depression even with small doses [17]. An "Opioid-sparing" technique, either via decreasing the dose of opioids or avoiding it, is recommended. The choice of opioids, in case used, must favor the short-acting medications (fentanyl, remifentanil…) and avoid the longer-acting drugs such as morphine, which might have an extended postoperative effect. "Non-opioid" analgesics such as nonsteroidal anti-inflammatory drugs and acetaminophen, as well as anesthetic adjuncts with analgesic properties such as ketamine and dexmedetomidine, possess a favorable "opioids-sparing" effect, thus reducing the risk of respiratory depression.

Emergence from anesthesia for children with OSA might be challenging and may take longer than the normal child.

Extubation of such patients must be in a fully awake condition, with full recovery from muscle relaxants effect, a spontaneously breathing child with regular ventilator pattern, and, most importantly, the ability to maintain a relatively patent airway without significant obstruction.

55.4.1.9 Postoperative Care

Children with OSA are at a higher risk of respiratory complications than normal kids. These can range from mild airway obstruction, up to hypopneas, apneas, oxyhemoglobin desaturations, and hypercarbia. For that reason, children with risk factors for postoperative complications must be monitored postoperatively with an apnea monitor consisting of a pulse oximeter and frequent intervals checking of the respiratory rate by a dedicated nurse, preferably in a high dependency unit (HDU) (Table 55.8) [18]. Children who are dependent on BiPAP, a noninvasive ventilation will be required in the postoperative area. Patients with severe forms of OSA may require a postoperative observation in the Pediatric Intensive Care Unit (PICU).

Postoperative pain management in patients with OSA undergoing tonsillectomies is better managed with "opioids-sparing" around the clock drugs such as acetaminophen (IV or PO 15 mg/kg Q6hours) and nonsteroidal anti-inflammatory drugs such as ibuprofen (PO 4–10 mg/kg Q 8 h). "Opioids-sparing" is required to avoid the risks of respiratory depression which are high in such population. If pain is not well controlled with "non-opioids analgesics," a smaller dose of opioids (usually morphine 0.01–

Table 55.8 Risk factors for postoperative respiratory complications after adenotonsillectomy [18]

Children less than 3 years old
Severe OSA
Failure to thrive
Obese patients
Secondary pulmonary hypertension
Down's syndrome
Ex-premature patients
Children with neuromuscular diseases
Craniofacial anomalies
Chronic lung diseases
Sickle cell

0.05 mg/kg) may be given judiciously and under close monitoring with more interval spacing between the doses.

55.4.2 Anesthesia for Children with Upper Respiratory Tract Infection

55.4.2.1 Introduction

Anesthetic management for the patient with upper respiratory tract infection (URI) imposes challenges to the anesthesiologist and the surgeon. Children with recent URTI who undergo anesthesia and surgery are at an increased risk of Perioperative Adverse Respiratory Events (PRAE). On the other hand, most children experience six to eight URI per year, which renders the scheduling of surgical procedures practically difficult [19]. Hence, a careful preoperative risk to benefits assessment of each patient, with specific considerations to surgical, anesthetic, and social factors, is crucial for safe and effective management.

55.4.2.2 Pathophysiology

Pathophysiology of URI is characterized by peripheral airway changes and increased airway reactivity. Peripheral airway changes may lead to decreased diffusion capacity of oxygen as well as increased closing volumes and atelectasis subsequently causing hypoxemia.

Patients with URTI also exhibit an increase in airway reactivity and bronchoconstriction due to over activity of the vagal response secondary to released mediators associated with infection (histamine, bradykinin, and leukotrienes) and viral neurosamidases which in turn inhibit the muscarinic M2 receptors and increasing the release of acetylcholine.

55.4.2.3 Perioperative Respiratory Adverse Events (PRAE)

Children with recent URI are at higher risk of perioperative adverse respiratory events including coughing, breath-holding, laryngospasm, bronchospasm, airway obstruction, oxygen desaturation less than 90% (for 10 s or more), atelectasis, post-extubation stridor, pneumonia, unanticipated tracheal intubation, or re-intubation [2, 3].

The risk of perioperative complications is most significant in the presence of acute infection but remains increased for 2–6 weeks after URI. Realistically, postponing the surgery for 2 weeks may be sufficient for a child with no other comorbidities.

55.4.2.4 Risk Factors for Perioperative Adverse Risk Events (PRAE)

Independent risk factors for PRAE in children with active URIs include the use of an endotracheal tube, children below 5 years of age, a history of prematurity (<37 weeks), a history of reactive airway disease, paternal smoking, a surgery involving the airway, the presence of copious secretions and presence of nasal congestion [20]. The use of an endotracheal tube (<5 years of age). Other than the patient factors, risks include surgical and anesthetic determinants [21], (See Table 55.9).

55.4.2.5 Perioperative Management of Children with URI

Preoperative Management

It was found that the children with current and recent URI (<2 weeks) had more PRAE (25% and 29%, respectively) than did children without URI or with URI between 2 and 4 weeks (12% and 8%, respectively) [22]. Whether the surgery should be cancelled should be a decision, should balances risks and benefits for each individual child, including patient, surgical risk factors of developing PRAE, waste of public healthcare resources, previous surgery cancellation, operation wait time, distance to travel for parents, and difficulties for parents to organize time off work [23]. A good history and clinical examination are sufficient in most children presenting with URI. There's no need to undergo any further testing to assess fitness in the context of URI (Fig. 55.5).

Table 55.9 Risk factors for the occurrence of a perioperative respiratory adverse event in children with upper respiratory tract infection

Patient	• Copious secretions/presence of sputum nasal congestion • Parenteral smoking/passive smoking • History of reactive airway disease, younger age • Prematurity (less than 37 weeks) • Parental belief "the child is sick/has a cold"
Surgery	• Surgery of the airway • Ear nose throat (ENT) surgery • Eye surgery • Upper abdominal surgery • Cardiac surgery
Anesthetic management	• Invasive airway (endotracheal intubation) • Anesthetic agent (desflurane) • Experience and competence of the anesthesiologists in pediatric anesthesia

Reasons to Consider Postponing an Elective Case in the Presence of a URI (Fig. 55.5)

Reasons to consider postponement of surgery in children with URTI include an elective nature of surgery in the presence of severe URTI symptoms such as productive cough, tachypnea, abnormal breath sounds, fever, and lethargy. They also include presence comorbidities such as asthma and parental smoking. A surgery involving the airway is an important reason not to proceed as well. Parental preference not to undertake risks must be taken into consideration.

Reasons to Proceed with Surgery (Fig. 55.5)

Reasons to go ahead with surgery in children with URTI include an urgent surgery, a clear nasal discharge, a mild dry cough with a clear chest exam and the absence of fever. A surgery not involving the airway is also a factor to be considered in favor of proceeding.

Intraoperative Management of Children with URTI

If a decision to proceed with surgery was taken for children with URI, several clinical steps have been shown to decrease the perioperative adverse respiratory events. (See Table 55.10).

- Most importantly, a preoperative inhaled bronchodilator such as albuterol administered 10–30 min prior to surgery has been shown to significantly decrease the risk of perioperative adverse respiratory events. Preoperative premedication with benzodiazepines such as midazolam must be avoided in such patients. Induction of anesthesia would be less hazardous with propofol intravenous induction if feasible compared with inhalation induction (as it bypasses light stage of anesthesia observed with inhalation induction). The airway management must be managed by an experienced anesthetist (preferably pediatric anesthetist) to minimize airway manipulation. Evidence suggests less incidence of PRAE with less invasive airway device whenever possible. Intravenous lidocaine given prophylactically may decrease the risk of laryngospasm if given at the time of intubation or extubation; however it has a very short living effect [24].

55.4.3 Anesthetic Management for a Child with Post-tonsillectomy Bleeding

55.4.3.1 Introduction

Post-tonsillectomy bleeding is infrequent yet a life-threatening complication of tonsillectomy surgeries. It is an emergency requiring imminent medical resuscitation and surgical intervention, which mandates a solid teamwork between the anesthesiologist and the ENT surgeon.

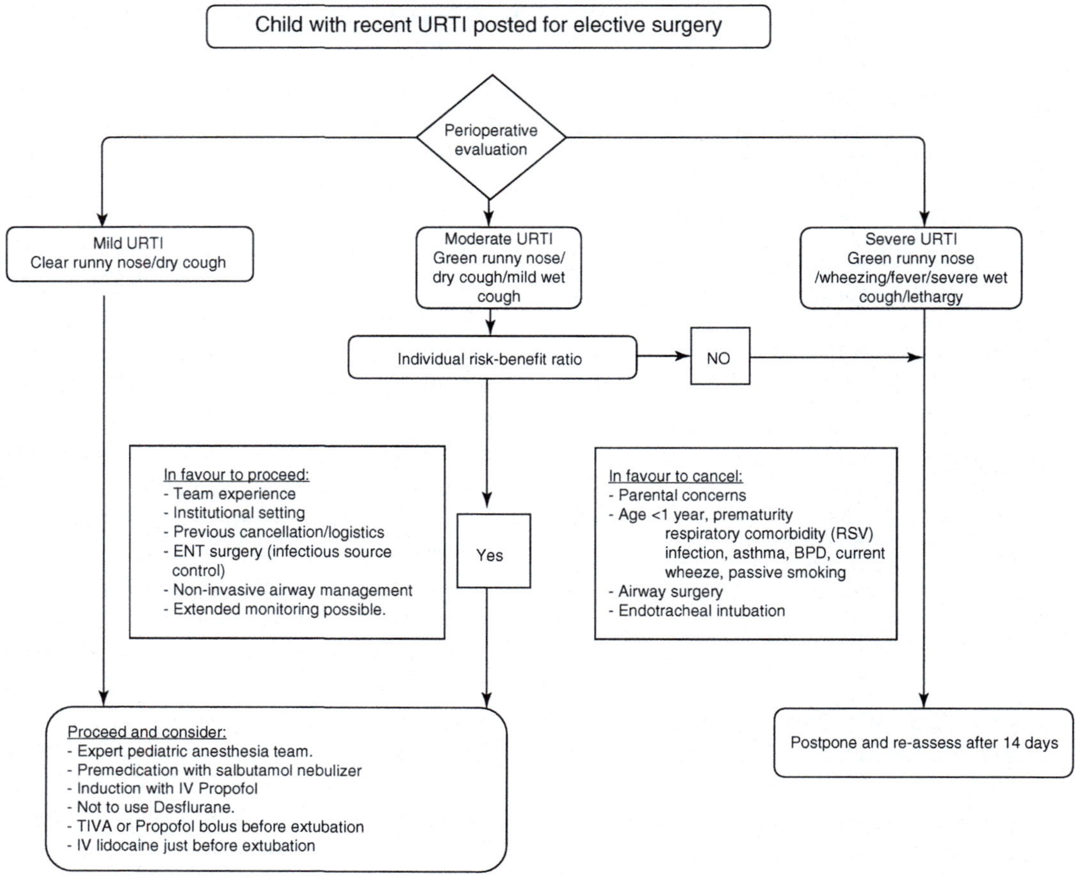

Fig. 55.5 Algorithm to guide perioperative management in children with URTI scheduled for elective surgery [23]

Table 55.10 Evidence-based perioperative management of children with recent URTI

Premedication	– Avoid use of benzodiazepines for premedication – Use clonidine if premedication is required
Lidocaine	– Consider IV lidocaine to suppress laryngospasm in higher-risk patient/higher-risk procedure – Avoid topical lidocaine to the vocal cord – Lidocaine gel on SGAD might be beneficial to decrease postoperative coughing
Bronchodilators	– Preoperative albuterol inhalation 10–30 min before induction, 2.5 mg if WT <20 kg and 5 mg if WT >20 kg) in children with current or recent <14 days [25]
Airway management	– Face mask over SGAD over endotracheal intubation ETT – With ETT preferred the use of uncuffed over cuffed ETT

The incidence of bleeding following tonsillectomy is 0.5–2% depending on the surgical technique [26].

Post-tonsillectomy bleeding can be:

- Primary bleeding occurring within 24 h of surgery, with an incidence of <1% [27].
- Secondary bleeding occurring in up to 28 days after surgery, usually 5–8 days following tonsillectomy, and has an incidence of up to 4% [26] and is usually due to dislodgement of an old blood clot.

The anesthetic management of post-tonsillectomy bleeding brings great challenges even to the experienced anesthetist as he/she has to deal concomitantly with the risks of hypovolemia/acute anemia, pulmonary aspiration of blood, and hypoxemia (due to inability to secure the airway because of bleeding or due to aspiration). Post-tonsillectomy bleeding is usually venous in origin.

55.4.3.2 Risk Factors

Risk factors contributing to post-tonsillectomy bleeding include a history of surgical procedure, children more than 5 years of age, a chronic tonsillar infection, and preoperative use of anti-inflammatory agents [28, 29].

55.4.3.3 Anesthetic Management

The primary anesthetic considerations in the management of a child with post-tonsillectomy bleeding are:

1. Resuscitation and correction of hypovolemia/ blood loss
2. Aspiration precautions from the swallowed blood and full stomach
3. Securing the airway and prevention of hypoxemia which might be challenging in the presence of a bleeding airway and edema (from the swollen tonsils and associated laryngeal edema from previous intubation)

55.4.3.4 Preoperative Preparation

Post-tonsillectomy bleeding is a surgical emergency where the patient must undergo timely surgical hemostasis however, that should not get priority over a quick resuscitation and correction of hypovolemia to prevent the risk of hemodynamic collapse during the anesthetic induction. Preinduction resuscitation must be done imminently in a monitored area or the operating room. Communication between the surgical and anesthetic team in such a situation is of crucial importance to ensure a timely resuscitation without delaying the surgery. Assessment of blood loss may be difficult as the venous bleeding is usually insidious in onset, and a large amount of it is swallowed, in contrast to arterial bleeding where the child is spitting fresh blood. Tachycardia, tachypnea, delayed capillary refill (>2 s), and decreased urine output (<2 mL/kg/h) are early indicators of hypovolemic shock, whereas hypotension and altered mental status are late signs of hypovolemia, with decompensated hypovolemic shock.

Preoperative resuscitation should be guided by the clinical signs and hemodynamic monitors. Laboratory investigations should at least include hemoglobin (CBC), coagulation studies. Blood and other blood products need to be available. The patient should get transfused as necessary. Transfusion with uncrossed matched blood (O negative) should be started if the clinical condition of the patient does not allow waiting for the crossmatch (such as in profuse arterial bleeding).

Fluid resuscitation must be done through a wide-bore intravenous cannula, with a colloid (albumin) or crystalloid solution (lactated ringer or 0.9% normal saline) at boluses of 20 mL/kg repeated as guided by the clinical signs and the monitors. Large volumes, up to 40–60 mL/kg may be required. An assessment of the airway for any potential difficulty (blood clots), as well as the previous anesthetic chart, would be a sensible measure to tailor the anesthetic plan.

55.4.3.5 Anesthesia Set Up

- Proper anesthesia equipment and drug preparation (including emergency medications) before induction are of utmost importance in bleeding post-tonsillectomy management as the anesthetist needs to be extremely vigilant for any life-threatening complication.
- An experienced anesthetist presence is a must and should be called early on.
- Two wide-bore suction devices must be connected and ready to go.
- A wide-bore intravenous cannula suitable for large volumes of fluids and blood administration
- Laryngoscopes with properly sized blades should get checked, cuffed endotracheal tubes of appropriate size with one size smaller ETT

must be available. Intravenous fluid and warming devices at hand and ready.

55.4.3.6 Anesthesia Conduct

Induction

Two anesthesia induction techniques have been described in the literature [30], with each having its advantages and drawbacks:

Inhalation Induction

Its main advantage is that it allows the patient to preserve his spontaneous ventilation, which is favorable in case of difficulty or failure to secure the airway [30], and hence avoiding the risk of hypoxemia. It is also possible to intubate without the use of muscle relaxation and therefore avoid its associated risks [30]. However, this technique is not very popular in practice as it carries the inherent risks of aspiration and laryngeal spasm as well as the unwanted hypotensive effect of inhalation anesthetics.

Intravenous "Rapid Sequence" Induction with Cricoid Pressure

Its main advantage over inhalation induction is that it has a much quicker onset of action and provides optimal intubating conditions for the anesthesiologist to expeditiously secure the airway. It is also done in the supine position which is much comfortable ergonomically for the anesthesiologist to manage his airway.

Intraoperative Management

During the surgery, further fluid and blood administration can be guided by hemodynamic parameters (heart rate, blood pressure), and by arterial blood gas (ABG) displaying the hemoglobin and the acid-base balance.

The child may become cold during surgery due to volume loss and transfusion, hence thermoregulation with a temperature monitor and a forced air warming blanket are mandated. In the case of large intravenous fluids/blood volume administration, it is better to use a fluid warming device.

Once hemostasis is achieved, a large-bore gastric tube should be passed under direct vision to empty the stomach. The neuromuscular blockade should be reversed. The trachea should be extubated after the child is fully awake. Extubation in the left lateral position is favorable in the context of continuing the aspiration precaution [30].

Postoperative Management

Postoperatively, the child is better monitored in a high dependency unit (HDU) for 24 h as the risk of rebleeding is always present. Transfusion management should continue postoperatively if needed.

Nonsteroidal anti-inflammatory drugs are better avoided for pain management in the postoperative period due to the risk of operative site bleeding after tonsillectomy [31]. Postoperative pain can be managed instead with acetaminophen, and judicious doses of opioids. IV Ketamine can also be used if needed in the direct postoperative period while the patient is in the post-anesthesia care unit.

55.4.4 Postoperative Nausea and Vomiting in Children (PONV)

Postoperative nausea and vomiting (PONV) are common in children. It is more likely to happen in children rather than in adults [32]. Some factors influence the incidence of PONV in children including age (PONV is uncommon in children of less than 3 years of age) and nature of surgery (tonsillectomy, strabismus surgeries). PONV prophylaxis is indicated in patients with risk factors such as age >3 years, surgery >30 min, nature of surgery (Strabismus surgery and adenotonsillectomy) and a previous history of PONV [33].

55.4.4.1 Drugs Used for Prophylaxis and Treatment [34]

1. Ondansetron (Dose of 0.1–0.15 mg/kg).
2. Dexamethasone (Dose of 0.05–0.15 mg/kg).

3. Droperidol has fallen out of favor after the FDA warning.
4. Propofol in small doses has been proven to decrease the incidence of PONV [34].

Double therapy for PONV prophylaxis has been proven to be more effective than single therapy.

It is recommended to give a prophylactic double therapy with ondansetron/dexamethasone to children with moderate to high risks. Baseline risk factors play a role in PONV in children. Diminishing baseline risk factors is achieved by utilizing regional anesthesia, avoiding nitrous oxide and inhalational gases, proper hydration and sparing narcotics if possible [35].

55.4.5 Postoperative Pain Management in Children

Analgesia is one of the pillars of perioperative anesthetic management in children. Pain assessment has been evolving to the extent that it is labeled as the sixth vital sign that must get checked regularly.

55.4.5.1 Pain Assessment

Pain assessment in children is challenging and more difficult than in adults as younger children and infants lag the capability to "self-report" any soreness. However, in the last decade, and with the progress of scientific research a wide variety of "non-self-reporting" tools have been validated for the pain assessment in different age groups [36].

Out of those it is worth mentioning the Neonatal Infant Pain "NIPS" scale utilized for neonates, the "Face, Leg, Activity, Cry, Consolability" FLACC scale tool used for young children, and the Modified FLACC scale mainly utilized for children with developmental delay and which incorporates a baseline individual behavior for each element. Adult self-reporting scales such as the numerical pain rating scale or the "Wong Baker" Faces rating scale may be used for older kids with cognitive and communicative ability.

55.4.5.2 Postoperative Analgesia

One of the most popular pain approaches in children is the "WHO" Ladder stepwise guidelines, which utilizes a dynamic scale "ascending" and "descending" relevant to the pain level of the patient.

- **Step 1**: It starts with paracetamol IV or PO (10–15 mg/kg) in addition to nonsteroidal anti-inflammatory drugs such as ibuprofen oral or IV (4–10 mg/kg Q 8 hourly) or IV ketorolac (0.5 mg/kg) for step1 for the mild pain.
- **Step 2**: Escalating to Step 2 for the moderate pain which requires weak opioids.
- **Step 3**: Is a further step up when the pain score is moderate to severe and necessitates strong opioids such as morphine (IV 10–50 μg/kg q 2 h) or Fentanyl (1–2 μg/kg).
- **Step 4**: For the severe pain which includes IV patient-controlled analgesia (PCA), regional/neuro-axial/local analgesia such as epidural analgesia but not for ENT cases [37, 38].

Take Home Messages

- Expected difficult intubation in pediatric practice is common. Potential identifiers include mandibular hypoplasia, facial asymmetry, limited mouth opening, and a history of stridor or sleep apnea. Before proceeding with general anesthesia, the anesthesiologist must ensure that adequate assistance and advanced airway tools as videoscope and fiber-optic devices are available. Induction of anesthesia must not be started unless the proper equipment is available. Maintenance of spontaneous ventilation must be the key when encountering a difficult airway. More than three laryngoscopy attempts are associated increased risk for airway related morbidity or mortality.

- Obstructive sleep apnea is common in children and imposes challenges on the anesthesiologist. Children with OSA are at a higher risk of potentially life-threatening respiratory complications during and after surgery. A coordinated approach between the anesthesiologist, pediatrician, and surgeon is crucial for successful perioperative care. Components of optimal anesthetic care require a proper preoperative clinical assessment of the severity of OSA, an opioid-sparing technique, an adequate analgesia, and postoperative respiratory monitoring for selected cases.
- Children with a recent URI (within 4 weeks) have an increased risk of incidence of perioperative adverse respiratory events such as laryngospasm, bronchospasm, desaturation, breath-holding…).
- The anesthetic management must aim at reducing the incidence of PRAE in children with recent URI (preoperative-inhaled salbutamol, an experienced anesthesiologist manipulating the airway, an intravenous induction with propofol whenever possible, and intravenous lidocaine prior to airway manipulation). Most children can be safely anesthetized even in the presence of an upper respiratory tract infection (URI) if the perioperative anesthetic management is optimized.
- Post-tonsillectomy bleeding is a life-threatening surgical emergency which is challenging to the anesthesiologist and the surgeon. Adequate timely preinduction volume resuscitation with intravenous fluids and blood, a careful well-planned induction, a fully awake extubation and postoperative monitoring are essential components of a safe anesthetic management.
- It is worth mentioning that anesthetic considerations for pediatric ENT surgeries is a vast chapter with much extensive topics requiring a separate textbook for full discussion. Due to editing limitations in this chapter, we summarize the basic principles of pediatric anesthesia relevant to the ENT surgeon's day-to-day practice focusing on the common problems and providing a very basic guidance for a practical and safe management.

References

1. von Ungern-Sternberg BS, Boda K, Chambers NA, Rebmann C, Johnson C, Sly PD, et al. Risk assessment for respiratory complications in paediatric anaesthesia: a prospective cohort study. Lancet. 2010;376:773–83.
2. Lee BJ, August DA. COLDS: a heuristic preanesthetic risk score for children with upper respiratory tract infection. Paediatr Anaesth. 2014;24:349–50.
3. Perioperative fasting in adults and children | Royal College of Nursing. https://www.rcn.org.uk/professional-development/publications/pub-002779. Accessed 27 Feb 2020.
4. Warner MA, Caplan RA, Epstein BS, Gibbs CP, Keller CE, Leak JA, et al. Practice guidelines for preoperative fasting and the use of pharmacologic agents to reduce the risk of pulmonary aspiration: application to healthy patients undergoing elective procedures: a report by the American Society of Anesthesiologists task force on preoperative fasting. Anesthesiology. 1999;90:896–905.
5. Brady M, Kinn S, Ness V, O'Rourke K, Randhawa N, Stuart P. Preoperative fasting for preventing perioperative complications in children. Cochrane Database Syst Rev. 2009:CD005285.
6. Green SM, Leroy PL, Roback MG, Irwin MG, Andolfatto G, Babl FE, et al. An international multidisciplinary consensus statement on fasting before procedural sedation in adults and children. Anaesthesia. 2020;75:374–85.
7. Jagannathan N, Sequera-Ramos L, Sohn L, Wallis B, Shertzer A, Schaldenbrand K. Elective use of supraglottic airway devices for primary airway management in children with difficult airways. Br J Anaesth. 2014;112:742–8.
8. McNiece WL, Dierdorf SF. The pediatric airway. Semin Pediatr Surg. 2004;13:152–65.
9. Fiadjoe JE, Nishisaki A, Jagannathan N, Hunyady AI, Greenberg RS, Reynolds PI, et al. Airway man-

agement complications in children with difficult tracheal intubation from the pediatric difficult intubation (PeDI) registry: a prospective cohort analysis. Lancet Respir Med. 2016;4:37–48.
10. Burjek NE, Nishisaki A, Fiadjoe JE, Adams HD, Peeples KN, Raman VT, et al. Videolaryngoscopy versus fiber-optic intubation through a supraglottic airway in children with a difficult airway: an analysis from the multicenter pediatric difficult intubation registry. Anesthesiology. 2017;127:432–40.
11. Smith CJ. Pediatric thermoregulation: considerations in the face of global climate change. Nutrients. 2019;11(9):2010. https://doi.org/10.3390/nu11092010.
12. Greenfeld M, Tauman R, DeRowe A, Sivan Y. Obstructive sleep apnea syndrome due to adenotonsillar hypertrophy in infants. Int J Pediatr Otorhinolaryngol. 2003;67:1055–60.
13. Katz ES, D'Ambrosio CM. Pathophysiology of pediatric obstructive sleep apnea. Proc Am Thorac Soc. 2008;5:253–62.
14. Patino M, Sadhasivam S, Mahmoud M. Obstructive sleep apnoea in children: perioperative considerations. Br J Anaesth. 2013;111(Suppl 1):i83–95.
15. American Society of Anesthesiologists Task Force on Perioperative Management of patients with obstructive sleep apnea. Practice guidelines for the perioperative management of patients with obstructive sleep apnea: an updated report by the American Society of Anesthesiologists Task Force on Perioperative Management of patients with obstructive sleep apnea. Anesthesiology. 2014;120:268–86.
16. Brown KA, Laferrière A, Lakheeram I, Moss IR. Recurrent hypoxemia in children is associated with increased analgesic sensitivity to opiates. Anesthesiology. 2006;105:665–9.
17. Brown KA. Intermittent hypoxia and the practice of anesthesia. Anesthesiology. 2009;110:922–7.
18. Marcus CL, Chapman D, Ward SD, McColley SA, Herrerias CT, Stillwell PC, et al. Clinical practice guideline: diagnosis and management of childhood obstructive sleep apnea syndrome. Pediatrics. 2002;109:704–12.
19. Bernardo-ocampo MC. Upper respiratory tract infection and paediatric anaesthesia tutorial of the week 246 Assistant Professor/Attending Anesthesiologist University of Washington SOM/Seattle Children ' s Hospital pathophysiology of airway hyper-reactivity. Paediatr Anaesth. 2012; 1–6.
20. Tait AR, Malviya S, Voepel-Lewis T, Munro HM, Siewert M, Pandit UA. Risk factors for perioperative adverse respiratory events in children with upper respiratory tract infections. Anesthesiology. 2001;95:299–306.
21. Regli A, Becke K, Von Ungern-Sternberg BS. An update on the perioperative management of children with upper respiratory tract infections. Curr Opin Anaesthesiol. 2017;30:362–7.
22. Rachel Homer J, Elwood T, Peterson D, Rampersad S. Risk factors for adverse events in children with colds emerging from anesthesia: a logistic regression. Paediatr Anaesth. 2007;17:154–61.
23. Becke K. Anesthesia in children with a cold. Curr Opin Anaesthesiol. 2012;25:333–9.
24. Schebesta K, Güloglu E, Chiari A, Mayer N, Kimberger O. Topical lidocaine reduces the risk of perioperative airway complications in children with upper respiratory tract infections. Can J Anesth. 2010;57:745–50.
25. von Ungern-Sternberg BS, Habre W, Erb TO, Heaney M. Salbutamol premedication in children with a recent respiratory tract infection. Paediatr Anaesth. 2009;19:1064–9.
26. National Prospective Tonsillectomy Audit 2003. London: The Royal College of Surgeons of England; 2005. http://www.rcseng.ac.uk.
27. Handler SD, Miller L, Richmond KH, et al. Post-tonsillectomy hemorrhage: incidence, prevention and management. Laryngoscope. 1986;96:1243–7.
28. Van Der Meulen J. Tonsillectomy technique as a risk factor for postoperative haemorrhage. Lancet. 2004;364:697–702.
29. Lee MS, Montague ML, Hussain SS. Post-tonsillectomy hemorrhage: cold versus hot dissection. Otolaryngol Head Neck Surg. 2004;131:833–6.
30. Pushpanathan E, Sultan N, Sultan P. Anaesthesia for the bleeding tonsil. Br J Hosp Med. 2010;71(2):117.
31. Moiniche S, Romsing J, Dahl JB, et al. Nonsteroidal antiinflammatory drugs and the risk of operative site bleeding after tonsillectomy: a quantitative systematic review. Anesth Analg. 2003;96:68–77, table.
32. Höhne C. Postoperative nausea and vomiting in pediatric anesthesia. Curr Opin Anaesthesiol. 2014;27(3):303–8.
33. Eberhart LH, Högel J, Seeling W, Staack AM, Geldner G, Georgieff M. Evaluation of three risk scores to predict postoperative nausea and vomiting. Acta Anaesthesiol Scand. 2000;44(4):480–8.
34. Kovac AL. Management of postoperative nausea and vomiting in children. Paediatr Drugs. 2007;9(1):47–6.
35. Gan TJ, et al. Consensus guidelines for the management of postoperative nausea and vomiting. Anesth Analg. 2014;118(1):85–113.
36. Verghese ST, Hannallah RS. Acute pain management in children. J Pain Res. 2010;3:105–23.
37. O'Donnell FT, Rosen KR. Pediatric pain management: a review. Mo Med. 2014;111(3):231–7.
38. Vittinghoff M, et al. Postoperative pain management in children: guidance from the pain committee of the European Society for Paediatric Anaesthesiology (ESPA Pain Management Ladder Initiative). Pediatr Anesth. 2018;28:493–506.

Adenoid and Tonsils

56

Amr A. Elhakeem

56.1 Introduction

They are part of the Waldeyer's ring of lymphoid tissues which have no afferent lymphatic.

Their lymphoid follicles are similar to that of other lymph nodes but they also have specialised endothelium covered channels that facilitate antigen uptake directly into the tissues which in turn maximise the development of immunological memory.

They contain T, B lymphocyte and few mature plasma cells.

In addition to their role in antigen processing and immune surveillance, they play part in mucociliary clearance (adenoid).

Removal of either or both has not been found to be clinically or epidemiologically significant in reduction of immunity against polio or increase in incidence of Hodgkin's disease.

56.2 Waldeyer's Ring of Lymphoid Tissues (Fig. 56.1)

Waldeyer's tonsillar ring (pharyngeal lymphoid ring) is a ringed arrangement of lymphoid tissue in the pharynx. Waldeyer's ring surrounds the naso- and oropharynx, with some of its tissue located above and some below the soft palate.

The ring consists of: the adenoid, the tubal tonsils around the openings of Eustachian tubes, the palatine tonsils and the lingual tonsils.

Waldeyer's ring grows throughout childhood until the age of 11 years and after that decreases spontaneously.

Waldeyer's ring tissue serves as a defence against infection and plays an important role in the development of the immune system, comprising the first organs in the lymphatic system that analyse and react to airborne and alimentary antigenic stimulation.

56.3 Adenoids (Nasopharyngeal Tonsils)

They are situated at the junction of roof and posterior aspect of nasopharynx (exit of nose). This anatomic position is important to understand their effects on nasal obstruction and orofacial growth and development (Fig. 56.2).

The frequent question of whether the adenoids are too large for a normal size nasopharynx or the nasopharynx size is smaller in children who develop nasal obstruction remains unresolved.

They are present at birth and reach the maximum period of growth at the age between 3 and 5 years (usually), they then start to regress by the age of 9 years to the age of early adulthood.

A. A. Elhakeem (✉)
Otolaryngology, Head and Neck Surgery, Hamad Medical Corporation, Doha, Qatar
e-mail: aelhakeem@hamad.qa

A. Al-Qahtani et al. (eds.), *Textbook of Clinical Otolaryngology*,
https://doi.org/10.1007/978-3-030-54088-3_56

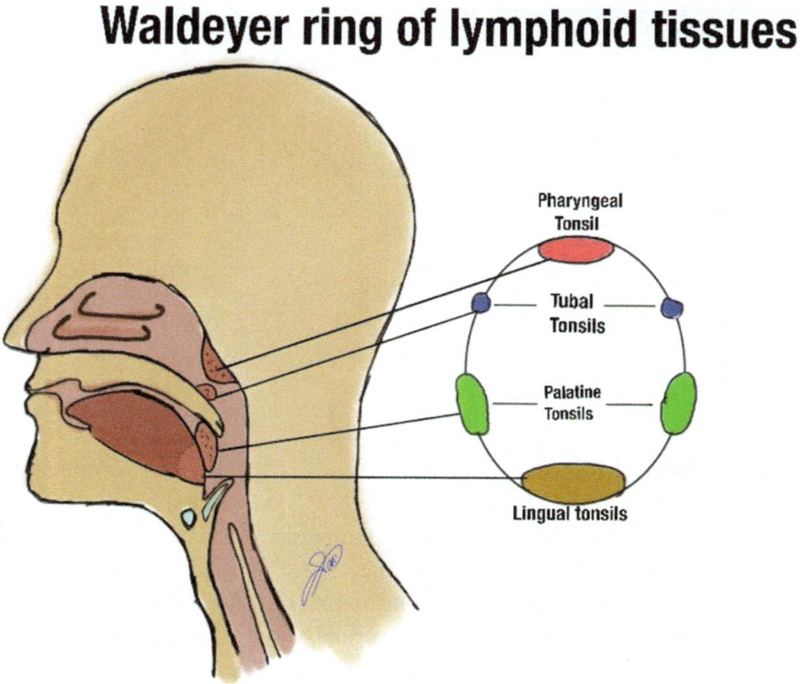

Fig. 56.1 Waldeyer's ring of lymphoid tissues

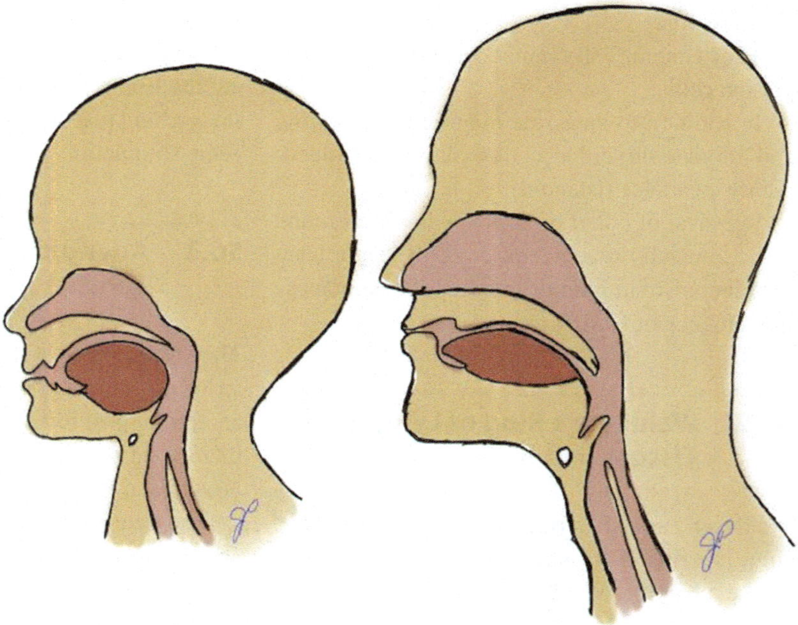

Fig. 56.2 Lateral naso-oropharyngeal airway

56.3.1 Clinical Features and Types

56.3.1.1 Acute Adenoiditis (Table 56.1)

Difficult to differentiate from upper respiratory tract infection (URTI) and are usually associated with it and with rhinosinusitis.

56.3.1.2 Recurrent Acute Adenoiditis (Table 56.2)

The occurrence of four or more episodes of acute adenoiditis in *6 months period*, with complete resolution of symptoms in-between the attacks.

Table 56.1 Acute adenoiditis

Clinical features	Symptoms	Signs
Nose	Obstruction Discharge Mouth breathing	+ + +
Fever	+	+/–
Snoring and sleep disturbance	+ +/– Stop breathing (SDB)	
Ear	+/– Pulling +/– Pain +/– Decrease hearing	Fluid behind TM Tuning Fork Type B Tymp
Voice	+/– Change	Hyponasal
Feeding	+/– Interrupted	
Cough (irritable)	+/–	
Orofacial changes	–	–

Table 56.2 Recurrent acute adenoiditis

Clinical features	Symptoms	Signs
Nose	Obstruction Discharge Mouth breathing	++ ++ ++
Throat	Sore Throat	+/–
Snoring and sleep disturbance	+ +/– Stop breathing (SDB)	
Ear	+ Pulling +/– Pain +/– Decrease hearing	Fluid behind TM Tuning fork Type B Tymp
Voice	+/– Change	+/– Hyponasal
Feeding	+/– Interrupted	
Cough (irritable)	+/–	+
Orofacial changes	+/–	+/–

Table 56.3 Chronic adenoiditis

Clinical features	Symptoms	Signs
Nose	Obstruction Discharge Mouth breathing (Bad)	++++ ++++ ++++
Throat	Recurrent sore throat	
Snoring and Sleep disturbance	+ +/– Stop breathing (SDB)	
Ear	+/– Pulling +/– Pain +/– Decrease hearing	Fluid behind TM Tuning fork Type B Tymp
Voice	Change	Hyponasal
Feeding	Interrupted	Weight not gained
Cough (irritable)	+/–	+
Orofacial changes	++++	Adenoidal faces

56.3.1.3 Chronic Adenoiditis (Table 56.3)

The persistence of one or more symptoms (including nasal discharge, bad breath and ear symptoms) for a minimum of *3 months*.

Chronic adenoiditis is based on chronic inflammation triggered by a persistent bacterial infection. These bacteria, mostly *Staphylococcus aureus*, *Haemophilus* sp. and *Streptococcus* sp., persist predominantly intracellular and within mucosal biofilms. The recurrent or chronic inflammation of the adenoids leads to chronic activation of the cell-mediated and humoral immune response, resulting in hypertrophy of the adenoid lymphoid tissue. This hypertrophic tissue is the cause for the prominent clinical symptoms: obstruction of the upper airways, snoring and sleep apnea.

56.3.2 Adenoidal Facies

Persistence of nasal obstruction during early childhood (from obstructing adenoid and/or tonsils) results in abnormal development of characteristic facial appearance.

Characteristic Facial Appearance:

- Open mouth and dry lips.
- Underdeveloped thin nostrils.
- Short upper lip.
- Prominent upper teeth (incisors).
- Crowded teeth.
- High arched palate.
- Hypoplastic maxilla.

56.3.3 Diagnosis

Is usually based on clinical symptoms (most important), nasopharyngeal endoscopy and radiology (nasopharyngeal X-ray) may be used in addition.

CT or MRI may be useful if other diagnoses are expected or to be excluded (meningeoenchalocoele).

56.3.4 Treatment of Adenoiditis (Table 56.4)

56.3.5 Guidelines and Recommendation for Treatment

Treatment strategies should target the persisting bacteria within their biofilm. Surgical removal of the hypertrophic tissue eliminates not only a mechanical obstacle of the airways, it removes also the basis for the aetiologic cause, the "biofilm carrier".

No good evidence to support curative medical treatment for chronic adenoiditis but surgical removal (Recommendation).

Recommendations are against long-term antibiotic treatment.

The use of local nasal steroid for the treatment to reduce inflammatory changes and the size of the adenoid are optional.

The use of symptomatic treatment is an important tool in the management.

Table 56.4 Treatment of adenoiditis

Options	Acute adenoiditis (Ad)	Recurrent acute Ad	Chronic Ad
Avoidance (allergen, pollution)	+/−	+/−	+/−
Symptomatic Analgesia, Decongestant	++	+	+/−
Antihistamine (If no OSA)	+/−	+/−	+/−
Local nasal steroids	+/−	+	++
Antibiotics	+/−	−	−
Anti reflux	+/−	+/−	+/−
Surgery	−	+	++

56.4 Tonsils

Multiple descriptions have been used to describe the tonsil size, the commonly used is the Brodsky grading.

56.4.1 Brodsky Grading Tonsil Size (Fig. 56.3)

Ratio of the tonsils to the oropharynx in the medial to lateral plane as measured between the anterior pillars (Table 56.5).

56.4.2 Definitions

Tonsillitis is a term used to describe an acute inflammation of the palatine tonsils.

Sore Throat is used to describe any causes of inflammation of the throat.

1. Acute pharyngitis.
2. Laryngitis.
3. Tonsillitis or acute exudative tonsillitis.

56.4.3 Aetiology of Tonsillitis

56.4.3.1 Infectious

- *Bacterial infection*: The most common bacterial cause is Group A beta-haemolytic streptococcus (GABHS) also known as *Streptococcus pyo-*

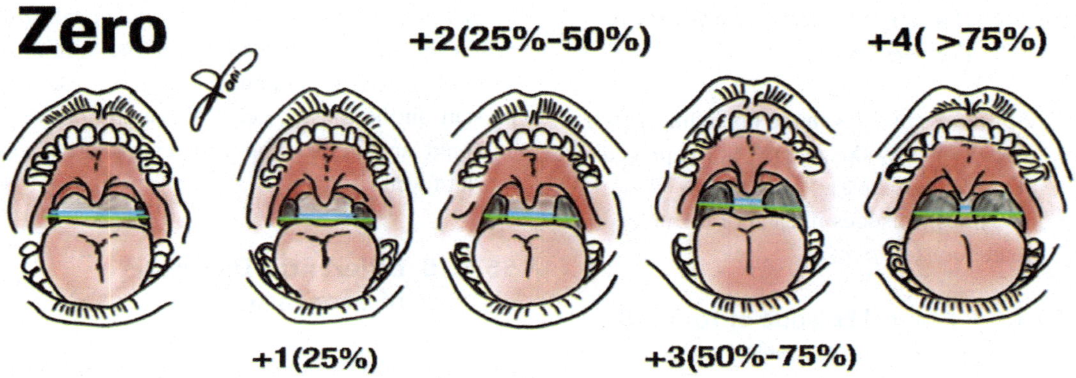

Fig. 56.3 Brodsky grading of tonsil size

Table 56.5 Brodsky grading of tonsil size

Grade	Description
0 Not visible	Tonsils do not reach tonsillar pillars
1+ Less than 25%	Tonsils fill less than 25% of the transverse oropharyngeal space between the anterior tonsillar pillars
2+ 25–49%	Tonsils fill less than 50% of the transverse oropharyngeal space
3+ 50–74%	Tonsils fill less than 75% of the transverse oropharyngeal space
4+ 75% or more	Tonsils fill 75% or more than the transverse oropharyngeal space

genes (*S. pyogenes*) which affect 15–30% of sore throats in children and 10% in adults.

- *Viral infection*: Common viral infectious causes for tonsillitis include: Rhinovirus, Coronavirus, Parainfluenza virus, Influenza types A and B, Adenovirus, Herpes simplex virus type 1 and Epstein–Barr virus.

56.4.3.2 Non-infectious

- Extra-oesophageal or laryngopharyngeal reflux disease.
- Physical or chemical irritation, e.g. from a nasogastric tube, chronic irritation from smoking.
- Others causes like Stevens–Johnson syndrome. Kawasaki disease and oral mucositis secondary to radiotherapy or chemotherapy, which may become secondarily infected.
- Haematological disorders, such as leukaemia and aplastic anaemia.
- Medication side effects, e.g. cytotoxic drugs, carbimazole and sulfasalazine.
- Tonsillar cancer.

Table 56.6 Suppurative complications

Acute otitis media	Mastoiditis
Acute rhinosinusitis	Suppurative cervical adenitis
Peritonsillar abscess (also known as quinsy) presents a risk of airway compromise, aspiration of pus from the abscess, or death due to vascular involvement	Parapharyngeal abscess—may compromise breathing or cause rupture of the carotid artery
Retropharyngeal abscess—common in young children, rare in adults	Metastatic infection, e.g. brain abscess, endocarditis, meningitis or liver abscess
	Streptococcal toxic shock syndrome

56.4.4 Prognosis

For the majority of patients, the following apply:

If caused by a viral or bacterial infection, symptoms resolve within 3 days in 40% of patients and in 1 week in 85% of patients.

Infectious mononucleosis (glandular fever) symptoms usually resolve within 1–2 weeks although mild causes may resolve within days; however, lethargy may continue for months or years in rare cases.

56.4.5 Complications of Tonsillitis Are Either

- *Suppurative* (Table 56.6).
- *Non-suppurative*.
  - Rheumatic fever
  - Post-streptococcal glomerulonephritis

56.4.6 Recurrent Acute Tonsillitis Is Defined as

- *7 or more* episodes in the preceding *1* year.
- *5 or more* episodes in each of the preceding *2* years (*consecutive*).
- *3 or more* episodes in each of the preceding *3* years (*consecutive*).

56.4.6.1 Clinical Episode of Tonsillitis

Sore Throat plus one or more of

1. Temperature >38.3 °C.
2. Cervical lymphadenopathy (tender lymph nodes or >2 cm).
3. Tonsillar exudates.

Others including:

Positive culture for group A beta-hemolytic streptococcus or treatment with antibiotics (conventional dosage for proved or suspected streptococcal episodes).

56.4.7 Chronic Tonsillitis

Persistence of symptoms in-between the attacks of tonsillitis or presence of tonsillolith.

56.4.8 Investigations

56.4.8.1 Full Blood Count

Throat cultures or rapid antigen testing, neither is able to differentiate between carrier states and an invasive infection.

The asymptomatic carrier rate for GABHS is up to 40%, and they have low infectivity and are not at risk of developing complications.

Monospot testing is not routinely recommended.

56.4.9 Viral vs Bacterial

Features indicative of a viral sore throat include malaise, cough, pharynx looks normal or mild erythema and oedema and presence of nasal symptoms or signs.

Features indicative of a streptococcal sore throat include: Odynophagia, nausea, vomiting, abdominal pain (common in children), exudates present on the tonsils, cervical lymph nodes are enlarged and tender and rash characteristic of scarlet fever.

56.4.10 Differential Diagnosis of Sore Throat

Scarlet fever: Caused by streptococcal infection, associated with characteristic erythematous rash which later desquamates with the tongue initially covered with a white coat and enlarged red papillae (strawberry tongue) may be seen.

Acute herpetic pharyngitis: Primary infection with herpes simplex virus may present as acute sore throat. Pain is moderate to severe with possible cervical lymphadenopathy, fever, and exudates and vesicles and shallow ulcers on the palate with gingivostomatitis may be seen.

56.4.11 Treatment of Acute Tonsillitis

The natural history of the illness is self-limiting and most cases last for an average of one week. During this period, patients should be managed through symptom control. Antibiotics should only be used in severe cases.

56.4.11.1 Centor Scoring System

Categorise a patient's risk for Group A beta-haemolytic streptococcus (GABHS) to prescribe antibiotics.

One point is awarded for each of the following:

1. Tonsillar exudates.
2. Tender anterior cervical lymph nodes.
3. Fever.
4. Absence of cough.

Interpretation of scores:

- Score of 3–4 suggests a 40–60% likelihood of GABHS.
- Score <3 indicates infection with GABHS is unlikely.

It is not a diagnostic tool, not valid for children younger than age 3 years with low specificity for bacterial infection.

Antibiotic treatment:

Antibiotics should only be used in severe cases.

Antibiotics *should not* be used for:

1. Patients with a Centor score of <3.
2. Symptomatic relief of sore throat.
3. To prevent suppurative complications.
4. Prophylaxis for recurrent sore throat.
5. Treatment of sore throat specifically to prevent the development of rheumatic fever and acute glomerulonephritis.
6. To prevent cross infection with Group A beta-haemolytic streptococcus (GABHS) in the general community.

56.4.11.2 Choice of Antibiotic

First-line treatment:

- Phenoxymethylpenicillin (penicillin V) for 10 days.
- Ampicillin-based antibiotics, including co-amoxiclav, can be used for 10 days, as alternatives to penicillin V as first line; however, there is a risk of rash when used in the presence of glandular fever.

Second-line treatment:

- Cephalosporin as second-line treatment.

Alternatives to penicillin use:

Clarithromycin for 10 days is recommended.

Close contacts of patients with invasive Group A streptococcal disease should be treated with antibiotics if they have symptoms of localised infection which may include sore throat, fever and skin infection.

56.5 Key Recommendations of the Guideline

- Sore throat including tonsillitis is primarily a condition that should be recognised and managed in primary care.
- Significant complications of sore throat or serious systemic illness should be managed in secondary care.
- Throat swabs and rapid antigen testing are of limited benefit in the diagnosis and management of sore throat.
- Routine treatment of tonsillitis should be symptomatic, with antibiotic use reserved for those most likely to have either:
  - Bacterial infection
  - Complication of tonsillitis
  - Significant risk factors for developing a complication
- Watchful waiting rather than tonsillectomy is a reasonable management approach where the severity of symptoms or frequency of episodes is unclear.
- Recurrent acute tonsillitis and chronic tonsillitis are an indication for tonsillectomy.

Take Home Messages

- Waldeyer's ring grows throughout childhood until the age of 11 years and after that decreases spontaneously.
- Waldeyer's ring tissue serves as a defence against infection and plays an important role in the development of the immune system.
- Removal of either or both doesn't reduce immunity or increase incidence of Hodgkin's disease.
- Treatment of chronic adenoiditis is surgical removal.
- Acute tonsillitis in children is most commonly viral and self-limiting.
- Acute bacterial tonsillitis is most commonly the result of beta-haemolytic streptococcus and is best treated with oral penicillin V.

Further Reading

Glenis K, Scadding Peter D, Bull John M, editors. Pediatric ENT. Graham: Springer-Verlag; 2007.

Mitchell RB, Pereira KD, editors. Pediatric otolaryngology for the clinician. New York: Springer; 2009.

Shapiro NL. Handbook of pediatric otolaryngology: a practical guide for evaluation and management of pediatric ear, nose, and throat disorders. Singapore: World Scientific; 2011.

Wetmore RF, Muntz HR, McGill TJ, editors. Pediatric otolaryngology: principles and practice pathways. Stuttgart: Thieme; 2012.

57 Branchial Arch: Anatomy and Anomalies

Faisal Abdulkader, Francis J. Lannigan, and Mahmoud Taha

Key Points

- Anomalies of the branchial arches usually present as cysts, sinuses, or fistulae.
- Second branchial arch anomalies account for approximately 95% of cases.
- There are no pathognomonic imaging features, so diagnosis depends on a high index of suspicion and knowledge of typical locations.
- Persistent cysts, fistulae, or recurrent localized infection may be due to branchial arch anomalies.
- Surgical excision of the cyst or tract is the most common curative option.
- •The most common is a second branchial system anomaly with persistence of both cleft and pouch.

57.1 Introduction

The branchial arches represent the embryological precursors of the face, neck, and pharynx. Anomalies of the branchial arches are the second most common congenital lesions of the head and neck in children. They may present as cysts, sinus tracts, fistulae, or cartilaginous remnants and present with typical clinical and radiological patterns dependent on which arch is involved. The embryological development of the branchial arches is reviewed and the radiological appearance of branchial arch abnormalities is presented, primarily focusing on branchial cleft anomalies.

57.2 Presentation

- The male:female ratio is 3:2.
- The peak age is the third decade.
- 2/3 are left-sided.
- 2/3 lie anterior to upper sternocleidomastoid.
- 80% present as persistent swelling, 20% are fluctuant.
- FNA—straw-colored fluid containing cholesterol.
- 30% present with pain.
- 15% present with infection.
- 70% are clinically cystic; 30% feel solid.

F. Abdulkader (✉)
Weill Cornell Medical College in Qatar, Doha, Qatar
e-mail: Fabdulkader@sidra.org

F. J. Lannigan
Sidra Medicine, Doha, Qatar

M. Taha
Pediatric Otolaryngology Head and Neck Surgery Department, Sidra Medicine, Doha, Qatar

A. Al-Qahtani et al. (eds.), *Textbook of Clinical Otolaryngology*,
https://doi.org/10.1007/978-3-030-54088-3_57

57.3 Investigations

- FNA.
- U/S, MRI, or CT—can delineate extent of mass but cannot easily differentiate from a metastatic squamous cell carcinoma lymph node that has undergone cystic degeneration.

57.4 Differential Diagnosis

- Benign lymph node.
- Metastatic lymph node.
- Branchiogenic carcinoma.

57.5 Classification

- A cyst is an epithelium-lined structure without an external opening.
- A sinus is a blind tract with an opening either externally through the skin (representing persistence of a branchial cleft) or internally into the foregut (representing persistence of a branchial pouch).
- A fistula is a tract that communicates between the skin externally and the foregut internally and therefore represents persistence of a connection between a branchial cleft and its corresponding pouch.

57.6 Developmental Anatomy

- The most typical feature of the head and neck in an early embryo is the series of branchial arches that begin to develop during the fourth week of gestation and give the embryo its characteristic external appearance.
- Four well-defined pairs of arches appear, while the fifth and sixth are believed to be rudimentary.
- The arches are separated from each other on the external surface of the embryo by ectodermal clefts, and internally within the pharynx by endodermal pouches.
- Each arch contains a cartilaginous rod (which forms the skeleton of the arch), a muscular component, a nerve, and an artery (Fig. 57.1).
- During the fifth week of gestation, the ventral aspect of the second arch grows caudally to overlap the third and fourth arches resulting in the formation of the cervical sinus. This sinus then usually disappears by the 7th week, giving the neck a smooth contour.
- The first pouch and cleft become closely related and ultimately form much of the middle ear, mastoid, and eustachian tube.
- The second pouch remains in part as the tonsillar fossa.

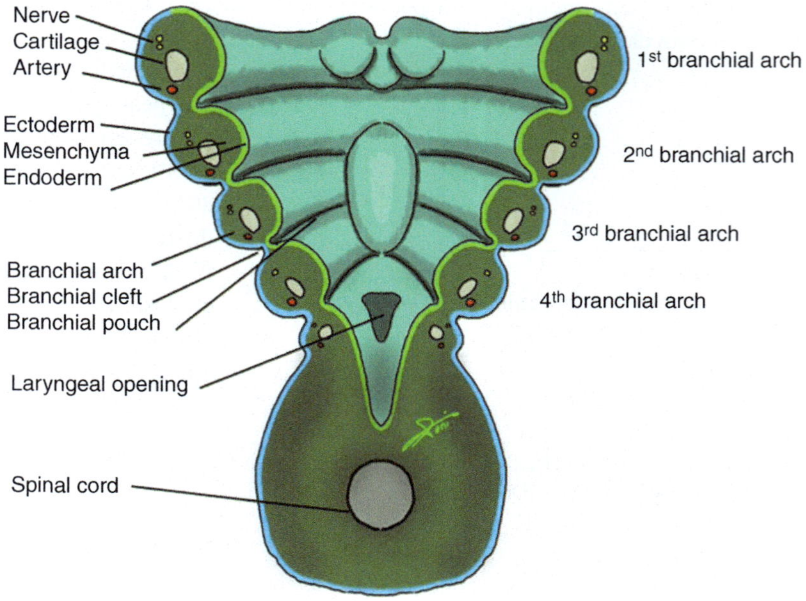

Fig. 57.1 Pharyngeal arches, pouches, and clefts (craniofacial development)

- The third pouch contributes to the thyroid gland and inferior parathyroid, and the fourth to the superior parathyroid gland.
- The external ear begins to develop at week 6 of gestation in the form of three otic folds or hillocks on the first arch and three on the second arch. These ultimately fuse to form the developing auricle.
- The thyroid gland appears as an epithelial proliferation in the floor of the pharynx at a point later indicated by the foramen caecum. The thyroid gland then descends down in front of the pharyngeal gut as a bi-lobed diverticulum. During this migration, the gland remains connected to the tongue by a narrow canal called the thyroglossal duct. By the end of the 7th week, the thyroid has reached its final destination anterior to the trachea; the duct involutes and disappears with time. The thyroid gland begins to function at approximately the end of the 3rd month.

57.7 The Branchial Arches and Their Derivatives

There are six pharyngeal arches, the fifth does not contribute any useful structures and often fuses with the sixth arch.

57.8 Derivatives of the Pouches

- Each pouch has a ventral and a dorsal wing. The fourth pouch has an additional accessory wing. The endodermal lining of the pouches proliferates into glandular organs (Table 57.1).
- *First pouch*: Dorsal and ventral: Middle ear cavity.

Table 57.1 Derivatives of the branchial clefts and pouches

Pharyngeal arch	Muscular contributions	Skeletal contributions	Endocrine	Artery	Nerve
First	Muscles of mastication Anterior belly of digastric Mylohyoid Tensor tympanic Tensor veli palatini	Maxilla Meckel's cartilage Incus Malleus	n/a	Maxillary External carotid	Mandibular
Second	Buccinator Platysma Muscles of facial expression Stylohyoid Posterior belly of digastric Stapedius	Stapes Styloid process Lesser horn and upper body of hyoid	n/a	Inferior branch of superior thyroid artery Stapedial artery	Facial
Third	Stylopharyngeus	Greater horn and lower part of hyoid	ThymusInferior parathyroids	Common and internal carotid	Glossopharyngeal
Fourth	Cricothyroid All intrinsic muscles of the soft palate	Thyroid and epiglottic cartilages	Superior parathyroids	Right—subclavian artery, Left—aortic arch	Vagus
Sixth	All intrinsic muscles of the larynx (except cricothyroid)	Cricoid, arytenoid and corniculate cartilages	n/a	Right—Pulmonary artery, left—Pulmonary artery and ductus arteriosus	Vagus and recurrent laryngeal nerve

- *Second pouch*: Dorsal: Middle ear cavity. Ventral: Tonsillar fossa and palatine tonsil.
- *Third pouch*: Dorsal: Parathyroid. Ventral: Thymus.
- *Fourth pouch*: Dorsal: Parathyroid. Ventral: Accessory: Ultimobranchial body.

57.9 Classification

- Branchial cleft cysts fall into three categories: first, second, and third branchial cleft anomalies (Fig. 57.2).

57.9.1 First Branchial Cleft Anomalies

- First branchial cleft anomalies make up less than 1% of all branchiogenic anomalies and usually appear on the face or near the auricle. There are two types of first branchial anomalies, Type I and Type II.
  - *Type I*—Type I first branchial cleft cysts are duplication anomalies of the external canal and are composed of ectodermally derived tissue. They may pass into the parotid gland and close to the facial nerve.
  - *Type II*—Type II anomalies may comprise ectodermally and mesodermally derived tissues. These lesions typically present below the angle of the mandible, pass through the parotid gland in close proximity to the facial nerve, and end either inferior to the external auditory canal or into the canal at the bony cartilaginous junction (Figs. 57.3 and 57.4).

57.9.2 Second Branchial Cleft Anomalies

- Second branchial cleft anomalies are the most common of the three types.
- They present as discrete, rounded masses below the angle of the mandible and at the anterior border of the sternocleidomastoid muscle.
- The potential tract of an associated sinus passes deep to the second arch structures (e.g., the external carotid artery and the stylohyoid and digastric muscles) and superficial to the third arch derivatives (e.g., the internal carotid artery), opening into the tonsillar fossa (Figs. 57.5 and 57.6).
- Operative Notes Take an ellipse of skin around the tract and start dissecting in a cephalad

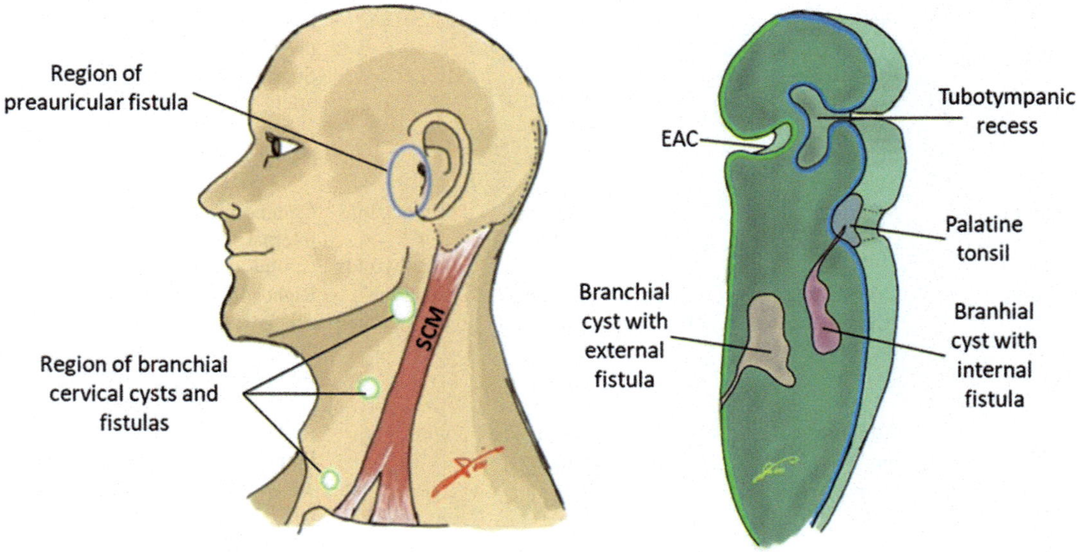

Fig. 57.2 Different types of branchial clefts and pouches anomalies

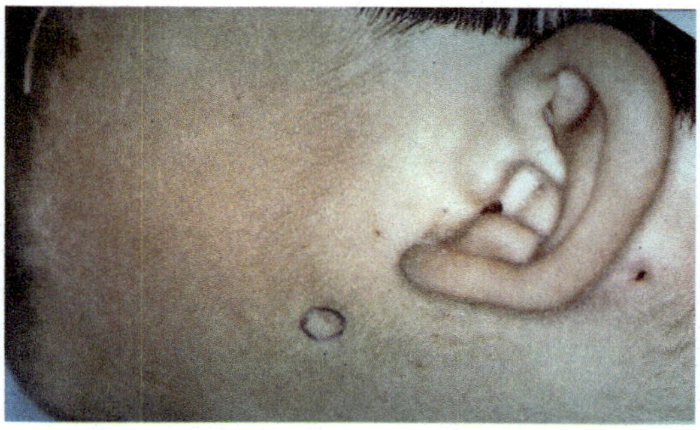

Fig. 57.3 Fistula at anterior border of sternomastoid muscle

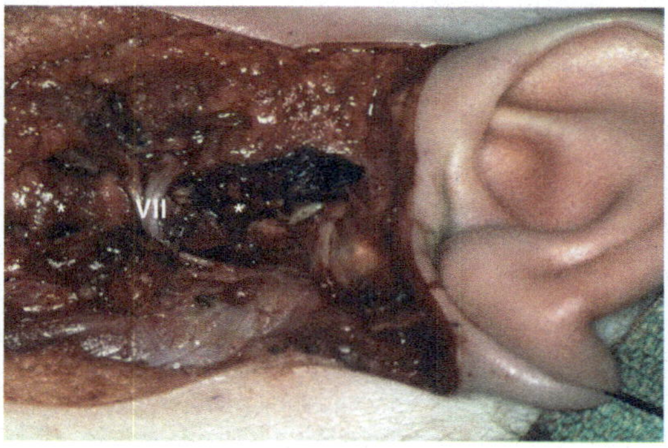

Fig. 57.4 Resection of branchial cyst and its tract (*) by superficial parotidectomy, Notice the tract passing under the trunk of facial nerve (VII) and going towards the ear canal

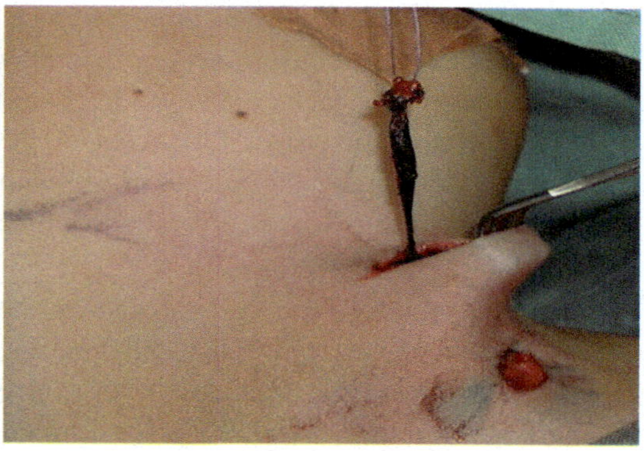

Fig. 57.5 Second branchial arch anomaly tract tracking deep into neck

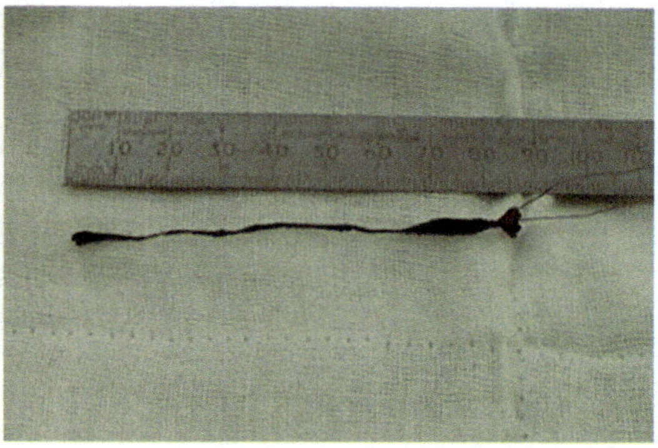

Fig. 57.6 Second branchial anomaly tract totally excised

direction. Then perform further stepladder incisions to follow the tract, taking care that it may course over the hypoglossal and glossopharyngeal nerves, and between the internal and external carotid vessels. Tonsillectomy may be required for internal tract closure.

57.9.3 Third Branchial Cleft Anomalies

- Third branchial cleft cysts present anterior to the sternocleidomastoid muscle and lower in the neck than either first or second branchial cleft anomalies.
- Third branchial cleft cysts are deep to the third arch derivatives (e.g., the glossopharyngeal nerve and the internal carotid artery) and superficial to fourth arch derivatives (e.g., the vagus nerve).
- These anomalies end in the pharynx at the thyrohyoid membrane or pyriform sinus.

57.10 Thymic Cysts/Ectopic Thymic Tissue

- These represent third branchial pouch anomalies.
- They tend to present in first decade of life as a mass in the left paramedian position.
- Treatment is surgical excision in similar fashion as third/fourth branchial system anomalies.

57.10.1 Treatment

- The management of branchial cleft anomalies is initial control of the infection followed by surgical excision of the cyst and tract.

- As a general rule, incision and drainage procedures should be avoided; however, they may be necessary for acute abscess treatment before definitive excision. Placement of the drainage incision should be determined with the need to excise the scar with definitive surgery.
- Needle aspiration and decompression can be beneficial in preventing incision and drainage, which increases the difficulty of definitive excision.

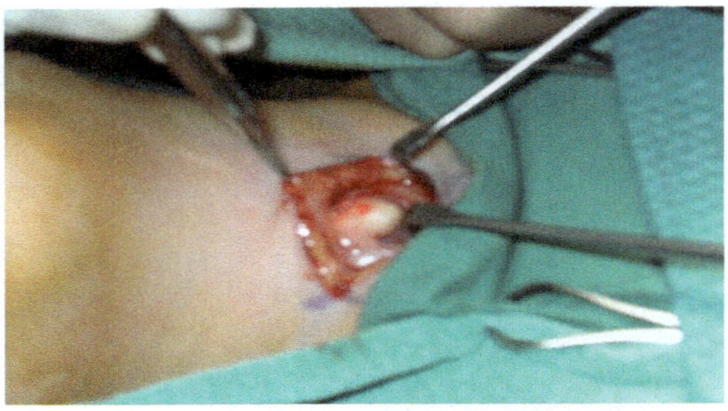

Fig. 57.7 Intraoperative view of thryroglossal duct cyst

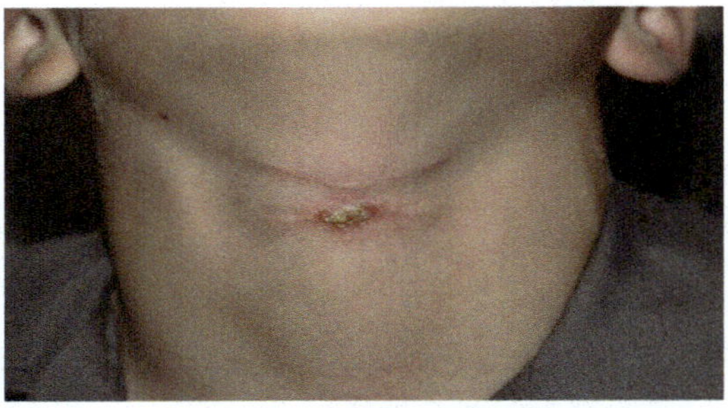

Fig. 57.8 External opening of thyroglossal duct cyst fistula that presented with recurrent neck abscesses

57.11 Thyroglossal Duct Cyst

- Thyroglossal duct cysts account for around 70% of congenital abnormalities in the head and neck region.
- Persistent ducts and cysts occur because of a failure of the thyroglossal duct to involute between the 8th and 10th week of gestation and a cyst can therefore occur anywhere along the duct's natural course from the foramen caecum to the thyroid gland.
- The duct assumes an intimate anatomical association with the hyoid bone, and in approximately 30% of cases, a tract has been found posterior to this structure.

57.11.1 Presentation

- They most commonly present in the first two decades of life.
- Cysts usually appear as a midline cervical mass and lie in close proximity to the hyoid bone.
- Patients can present with a smooth, cystic swelling in the midline of the neck, which moves on swallowing and tongue protrusion.
- Thyroglossal duct cysts can become infected, resulting in a red, painful midline swelling, which can discharge (Figs. 57.7 and 57.8).

57.11.2 Investigations

- An ultrasound examination should be performed to establish the presence of a cystic structure in the neck and to confirm that there is a separate and normal-looking thyroid gland.
- This will prevent the rare possibility of inadvertent removal of an ectopic thyroid gland resulting in post-operative hypothyroidism.

57.11.3 Treatment

- A Sistrunk's procedure is the treatment of choice.
- This is performed through a horizontal skin crease incision at the approximate level of the hyoid bone, taking a skin ellipse around any discharging sinus.

- The cyst and its associated tract are then dissected out in continuity with the middle portion of the hyoid bone and a wedge of muscle superior to the hyoid bone extending up to the foramen caecum.

57.11.4 Complications

- Hypoglossal nerve injury is unlikely, but conceivable.
- This can be prevented by transecting the hyoid at the level of the lesser cornu and maintaining all subsequent dissection medial to the anterior belly of digastric.
- Insertion of a drain will also prevent accumulation of a hematoma.
- Recurrence rates are low when a Sistrunk's procedure is performed (0–3%), but can be as high as 50% if an inadequate surgical procedure is performed initially.

Key point: If there is a midline cyst in the neck and an ultrasound examination confirms a normal thyroid gland, then a Sistrunk's procedure should be performed to avoid recurrence (5% will subsequently turn out to be dermoid cysts).

57.12 Lingual Thyroid

- If the primitive thyroid gland fails to descend during development, it can enlarge and function within the tongue base.

57.12.1 Presentation

- The thyroid mass usually increases in size as the child develops and may manifest as a mass lesion in the tongue base causing dysphagia, dysphonia, and airway compromise.

57.12.2 Investigations

- A radioisotope scan is required to confirm the diagnosis and to determine the amount of functioning thyroid tissue present.
- Thyroid function tests also.

57.12.3 Management

- In an euthyroid and asymptomatic child, no treatment is required.
- If the child has functional symptoms, then thyroid replacement therapy should be commenced to see if regression of the mass occurs.
- If this results in an acceptable improvement in symptoms, then medical therapy can continue.
- An inadequate response requires surgical excision of the mass followed by thyroid replacement.
- Surgery carries no risk to the parathyroid glands, which are derived from the third and fourth arches.

Take Home Messages

- Beware of "simple" skin pits/dimples around the face and neck—they may relate to an underlying branchial anomaly.
- Thyroglossal duct cysts. If there is a midline cyst in the neck and an ultrasound scan confirms a normal thyroid gland, then a Sistrunk's procedure should be performed to avoid recurrence (5% will subsequently turn out to be dermoid cysts).

Further Readings

1. Ang AH, Pang KP, Tan LK. Complete branchial fistula: case report and review of the literature. Ann Otol Rhinol Laryngol. 2001;110(11):1077. [PMID: 11713922] (Discusses the diagnosis and management of branchial cleft cysts).
2. Paczona R, Jori J, Czigner J. Pharyngeal localizations of branchial cysts. Eur Arch Otorhinolaryngol. 1998;255(7):379. [PMID: 9783138] (Reviews the location and development of branchial cysts).
3. Mandell DL. Head and neck anomalies related to the branchial apparatus. Otolaryngol Clin North Am. 2000;33:1309–32.
4. Al-Khateeb TH, Al Zoubi F. Congenital neck masses: a descriptive retrospective study of 252 cases. J Oral Maxillofac Surg. 2007;65(11):2242–7.
5. Al-Dajani N, Wootton SH. Cervical lymphadenitis, suppurative parotitis, thyroiditis, and infected cysts. Infect Dis Clin North Am. 2007;21(2):523–41.
6. Shrime M, et al. Fourth branchial complex anomalies: a case series. Int J Pediatr Otorhinolaryngol. 2003;67(11):1227–33.
7. Verret DJ, et al. Endoscopic cauterization of fourth branchial cleft sinus tracts. Arch Otolaryngol Head Neck Surg. 2004;130(4):465–8.
8. Papadogeorgakis N, et al. Branchial cleft cysts in adults. Diagnostic procedures and treatment in a series of 18 cases. Oral Maxillofac Surg. 2009;13(2):79–85.
9. White WM, et al. Recurrent laryngeal nerve monitoring during thyroidectomy and related cervical procedures in the pediatric population. Arch Otolaryngol Head Neck Surg. 2009;135(1):88–94.
10. Prasad SC, et al. Branchial anomalies: diagnosis and management. Int J Otolaryngol. 2014;2014:237015.

Evaluation of Pediatric Head and Neck Masses

58

Faisal Abdulkader
and Niveen Eltigani Elmusharaf Mukhtar

58.1 Introduction

- Pediatric head and neck masses are common.
- The majority are benign in nature.
- Etiology can be generally divided into inflammatory/infectious, congenital, and neoplastic.
- Inflammatory etiology accounts for the majority (reactive lymphadenopathy secondary to upper respiratory tract infections and tonsillitis) [1].
- A congenital mass may be present at birth or appear in older children. These are best considered in two groups: midline neck abnormalities (most commonly thyroglossal duct cyst and dermoid cyst), and lateral branchial anomalies.
- A very small minority of neck masses are secondary to malignancy: lymphomas and rhabdomyosarcomas are the most common. Squamous cell carcinoma is rare in children [2].
- A thorough history and physical examination are essential in accurately diagnosing neck masses.

The important aspects in the evaluation of a neck masses, the differential diagnosis of neck triangles, investigations, and management will be outlined [3].

58.2 Clinical History

A thorough history will assist in narrowing the differential diagnosis:

- Age at onset:
  - Swelling presents at birth or shortly after are most likely congenital.
  - Reactive lymphadenopathy usually presents in children over 6 months old.
- Duration:
  - Short duration: <3 weeks: acute inflammation
  - Long duration: >6 weeks: chronic inflammation/malignancy
- Progression:
  - Rapid : acute inflammation/malignancy
  - Slow growing: chronic inflammation
- Size:
  - Large swellings (>3 cm) or swellings that do not respond to antibiotics should be investigated.
- Tenderness: Usually indicates inflammatory process
- Other masses: Enlarged masses in the axilla, or groin could indicate lymphoma
- Systemic symptoms:
  - Fever, sore throat, and rhinorrhea generally indicative of upper respiratory tract infection.

F. Abdulkader (✉)
Weill Cornell Medical College in Qatar, Doha, Qatar
e-mail: Fabdulkader@sidra.org

N. E. E. Mukhtar
Sidra Medicine and Research Center, Doha, Qatar
e-mail: nmukhtar@sidra.org

A. Al-Qahtani et al. (eds.), *Textbook of Clinical Otolaryngology*,
https://doi.org/10.1007/978-3-030-54088-3_58

   - Failure to thrive, loss of appetite, loss of weight, or night sweats should be investigated to rule out chronic infections or malignancy
- Past medical history:
   - Birth and pregnancy history
   - Chronic illnesses (e.g., asthma, DM)
   - Any previous surgeries
   - Any previous hospital admissions
- History of contact: Enquire about TB, exposure to farm animals, cats, and ticks
- Medication history
- Family history of malignancies or bleeding conditions

58.3 Physical Examination

- Vital signs (check for fever and tachycardia).
- A careful examination for a source of primary infection should be made. This should include examination of the pharynx, oral cavity, teeth, nose, and ears as well as looking for any cutaneous lesion.
- Search for any associated lymphadenopathy and hepatosplenomegaly.

58.4 Examination of Swelling

The following should be noted:

- Site of mass (anterior triangle/posterior triangle/midline)
- Size
- Consistency (soft/rubbery/hard)
- Tenderness
- Temperature (warmth suggests acute inflammation)
- Fluctuance (suggests abscess or cyst)
- Transillumination (e.g., lymphatic malformation)
- Pulsation (carotid body tumor/aneurysm)
- Overlying skin (erythema/ulceration/punctum/discharging sinus)
- Relation to underlying structure: (tethering/mobility)
- Auscultate for bruit [4]

58.5 Investigation

- The investigation of neck swellings in children is dependent on the clinical assessment.
- In many cases, no investigation is required. Simple observation of presumed viral infection or antibiotic treatment of bacterial infection, with careful clinical follow-up, will often result in resolution [5].
- *Laboratory Tests*
   - Full blood count
   - Monospot test (infectious mononucleosis)
   - Mantoux or IGRAs test (TB)
   - Serology tests (toxoplasmosis, Bartonella (cat scratch), CMV, and HIV)
   - Thyroid function tests
- *Radiology*
   - Plain films: Not routinely performed but occasionally helpful for TB (chest X-ray) or retropharyngeal abscess (soft-tissue neck X-ray).
   - Ultrasound: Non-invasive, distinguishes cystic versus solid masses and provides information regarding lymph node architecture and size [6].
   - CT: Gives information regarding architecture of mass, anatomical, and bony relationships [7].
   - MRI: Consider in diagnosing soft-tissue masses.
- *Biopsy versus Fine Needle Aspiration for Cytology (FNAC)*
   - Persistent or rapidly enlarging masses raise the possibility of malignancy and a tissue diagnosis is required.
   - Lymphomas and sarcomas are less likely to be diagnosed by FNAC, and biopsy remains the gold standard for the diagnosis and treatment.
   - FNAC can be useful in the diagnosis of salivary and thyroid masses [8].

58.6 Differential Diagnosis

- The differential diagnosis for cervical swellings in pediatric patients is broad, but the most common cause is usually infection.
- Mass location assists in the differential diagnosis.

58.7 Anatomy and Differential Diagnosis of Neck Triangles

Site of swelling	Differential diagnosis
Submental triangle	
• Situated underneath the chin • Contains submental lymph nodes, draining the floor of the mouth and parts of the tongue Boundaries: • Inferiorly: hyoid bone • Medially: midline of the neck • Laterally: anterior belly of the digastric • The base is formed by the mylohyoid muscle	• Dermoid • Plunging ranula • Salivary gland pathology • Thyroglossal cyst
Submandibular triangle	
• Located underneath the body of the mandible • Contains the submandibular gland, and lymph nodes • The facial artery and vein pass through it Boundaries: • Superiorly: body of the mandible • Anteriorly: anterior belly of the digastric muscle • Posteriorly: posterior belly of the digastric muscle	• Lymphadenopathy/lymphadenitis • Ludwig's angina • Vascular malformations • Sialadenitis/sialolithiasis • Benign and malignant neoplasia of salivary glands
Posterior/lateral triangle Boundaries:	
• Anteriorly: posterior border of sternocleidomastoid • Posteriorly: anterior border of trapezius muscle • Inferiorly: middle 1/3 of the clavicle • Covered by the investing layer of fascia • Floor is formed by the prevertebral fascia • The omohyoid muscle splits the posterior into two: superiorly the occipital triangle and inferiorly the subclavian triangle	• Lymphadenopathy/lymphadenitis. Most commonly along superficial and deep cervical chains • Branchial cysts • Fibromatosis coli (sternocleidomastoid tumor of infancy) • Carotid body tumors • Mycobacterial infections, including atypical mycobacterium
Supraclavicular triangle	
Boundaries:	
• Above: inferior belly of omohyoid • Below: clavicle • Base: posterior border of sternocleidomastoid • Floor: first rib	• Virchow node • Cervical rib • Subclavian aneurysm
Muscular triangle	
• Contains the infrahyoid muscles, the pharynx, the thyroid, and parathyroid glands Boundaries: • Superiorly: hyoid bone • Medially: imaginary midline of the neck • Superolateral: superior belly of the omohyoid muscle • Inferolateral: inferior portion of the sternocleidomastoid muscle	• Thyroglossal cyst • Dermoid cyst • Thyroid swelling • Laryngocele
Occipital triangle	
Boundaries:	
• In front: sternocleidomastoid muscle • Behind: trapezius muscle • Below: omohyoid muscle • Floor: from above downward: splenius capitis muscle, levator scapulae muscle, and scalenus medius muscle • It is covered by the skin, superficial and deep fasciae, and platysma below	• Lymphadenopathy/lymphadenitis • Vascular malformation • Metastatic lesion • Retropharyngeal abscess
Parotid	
• Lies between the superficial and deep capsules of parotid gland • Formed by splitting of the superficial layer of deep cervical fascia • The superficial capsule is thick and adherent to the underlying parotid gland • Multiple septa run from the superficial capsule into the gland forming numerous intraglandular compartments	• Lymphadenitis • Mumps • Bacterial parotitis • Vascular malformations and hemangiomas • Benign and malignant neoplasia

58.8 Head and Neck Infections in Pediatrics

58.8.1 Bacterial Lymphadenitis

- Most commonly caused by *Staph aureus* and *Group B Streptococci* organisms in neonates.
- Children up to 4 years of age are commonly affected by *Group A Beta Hemolytic Streptococci*.
- *Staph aureus* remains the most common isolated organism in all age groups.
- Anaerobes are common with older children and adolescents, especially those with poor dental hygiene.

58.8.1.1 Treatment

- Antibiotics and surgical drainage for abscess [9].

58.8.2 Mycobacterial Infections

- Tuberculous lymphadenitis is the most common extrapulmonary manifestation of tuberculosis.
- Early-phase lymphadenitis is characterized by a nontender, firm lymph node, which develops caseous necrosis and softens into an abscess.

58.8.2.1 Diagnosis

- Diagnosis is difficult and most commonly require excision biopsy.
- Staining for acid-fast bacilli.
- FNAC and PCR.

58.8.2.2 Treatment

- Tuberculous adenitis is best treated as a systemic disease with antituberculosis medication.
- Atypical mycobacterium requires surgical excision. Macrolides antibiotics may have a role in treatment [10].

58.8.3 Deep Neck Space Infections [11, 12]

Retropharyngeal space: Anatomical boundaries: • Superiorly: lies between the deep layer of the deep cervical fascia (prevertebral fascia) and the buccopharyngeal fascia • Inferiorly: fascia covering the esophagus • Two potential spaces in the retropharyngeal space: – Retropharyngeal/retrovisceral space: lies between fascia covering the pharynx and esophagus, and alar layer of deep cervical fascia. It ends at the level of T2 vertebra – Danger space known as the prevertebral or Grodinsky space: posterior to the alar fascia but anterior to the prevertebral fascia. It allows wider spread of infections into the mediastinum and is commonly involved by rupture of retropharyngeal space abscesses	Retropharyngeal abscess: • Symptoms include difficulty and pain on swallowing, fever, lymphadenopathy, muffled voice, and drooling • Usually caused by a bacterial infection that has spread from the tonsils, throat, sinuses, adenoids, or nose • HIV infection and tuberculosis are becoming more frequent causes in children • Complications: abscess rupture into the airway, laryngeal spasm, pneumonia, and jugular venous thrombosis • Infection may spread to the mediastinum, or to bloodstream causing septic shock • Can compromise the airway Diagnosis and treatment: • Diagnosed primarily clinically and radiologically • Treatment with parenteral broad-spectrum antibiotics and surgical drainage • In severe cases, endotracheal intubation to prevent aspiration of the pus may be needed

Parapharyngeal space: • Situated lateral to the fascia covering the constrictor muscles of the pharynx (buccopharyngeal fascia) • Laterally: pterygoid muscle, mandible, and carotid sheath • Superiorly: it extends up to the skull base • Inferiorly: ends at the level of hyoid bone • The carotid sheath lies close to the posterolateral wall • Posteromedially it communicates with the retropharyngeal space • Anteroinferiorly it communicates with the floor of the mouth • Infections can easily spread to the carotid and retropharyngeal spaces	Parapharyngeal abscess: • Due to infection from tonsils, pharynx or local spread from odontogenic sources. • Can compromise the airway • Can lead to Lemierre's syndrome Clinical features: • Fever, sore throat, odynophagia, neck swelling, and trismus • Medial bulging of tonsil and lateral pharyngeal wall • Posterior abscesses may involve structures within the carotid sheath, possibly causing bacteremia, neurologic deficits, and rarely carotid artery rupture Treatment: • Parenteral broad-spectrum antibiotics and surgical drainage • Airway control
Submandibular area:	Ludwig's angina: • It is a severe diffuse cellulitis that has an acute onset and spreads rapidly • Airway control is mandatory • Affecting the submandibular, sublingual, and submental spaces bilaterally • Caused most commonly by Streptococcus and Staphylococcus organisms • Often follows a mouth injury or infection, such as a tooth abscess • Early diagnosis and immediate treatment planning could be a life-saving procedure

58.8.4 Viral Lymphadenitis

- Commonest viruses: rhinovirus, adenovirus, enterovirus, herpes simplex virus, influenza virus and the Epstein–Barr virus (EBV).
- Usually a self-limited disease.
- HIV can present as cervical lymphadenopathy.

58.8.5 Infectious Mononucleosis (Glandular Fever)

- Caused by the Epstein–Barr virus (EBV).
- Affects adolescence mostly.
- Transmission is via saliva by contact with infected person, or exposure to cough or sneezing.
- Symptoms usually show up about 4–7 weeks after infection.

58.8.5.1 Clinical Features

- Fatigue, fever, sore throat, swollen tonsils that may have white patches, loss of appetite, generalized lymphadenopathy, headaches, sore muscles, hepatosplenomegaly, and abdominal pain.

58.8.5.2 Diagnosis

- Monospot or Paul Bunnell usually confirms the diagnosis.

58.8.5.3 Treatment

- Antibiotics for co-existent bacterial infection.
- Steroids to reduce inflammation in some cases.
- In severe infection with breathing difficulty, endotracheal intubation may be needed [13].

58.8.6 Lemierre's Syndrome

- Characterized by thrombophlebitis of the internal jugular vein and bacteremia.
- Caused by anaerobic organisms, following a recent oropharyngeal infection.
- Should be suspected in young healthy patients with prolonged symptoms of pharyngitis

followed by symptoms of septicemia or pneumonia, or an atypical lateral neck pain.

58.8.6.1 Diagnosis
- Confirmed by identification of thrombophlebitis of the internal jugular vein and growth of anaerobic bacteria on blood culture.

58.8.6.2 Treatment
- Prolonged antibiotic therapy occasionally combined with anticoagulation [13].

58.8.7 Cat Scratch Disease

- Bacterial infection caused by Bartonella Henselae
- One of the most common causes of chronic lymphadenopathy in children and adolescents
- History of sustaining a scratch or bite from a cat

58.8.7.1 Clinical Features
- Papule at the inoculation site, followed by solitary or regional lymphadenopathy within 1–2 weeks.

58.8.7.2 Treatment
- Usually self-limiting disease.
- Analgesics and antibiotics may be needed.
- Applying heat compresses to the affected area may also help.

58.8.8 Actinomycosis

- Subacute-to-chronic bacterial infection caused by *Actinomyces israelii* and other species of *Actinomyces*.
- Exist normally in the lining of the mouth, and throat.
- Can cause suppurative and granulomatous inflammation, formation of multiple abscesses, and sinus tracts that may discharge sulfur granules.
- The most common clinical forms of actinomycosis are cervicofacial (i.e., lumpy jaw), thoracic, and abdominal.

58.8.8.1 Diagnosis
- Culture of sputum, pus, or a biopsy specimen.

58.8.8.2 Treatment
- High dose IV penicillin for four weeks [13].

58.9 Non-infectious Inflammatory Lymphadenopathy

58.9.1 Kawasaki Disease

- Acute multisystem vasculitis.
- Self-limiting disease however in 20% of cases can cause permanent cardiac damage (echocardiogram needed and cardiac follow-up required).
- Unknown etiology.
- Generally, affects children under the age of 5.
- Symptoms usually present in three phases.

58.9.1.1 Clinical Features
- High fever, usually lasting more than 5 days
- Neck lymphadenopathy, usually unilateral
- Erythema, edema, and desquamation of the hands and feet
- Painless bilateral conjunctival infection
- Erythema and injection of the lips and oral cavity
- Joint pain

58.9.1.2 Treatment
- Anti-inflammatory or gamma globulin therapy to reduce inflammatory response [13].

58.9.2 Sinus Histiocytosis (Rosai–Dorfman Disease)

- Present with massive cervical lymphadenopathy
- Unknown cause
- Can be mistaken for infectious mononucleosis or lymphoma

58.9.2.1 Clinical Features
- Fever
- Skin nodules

58.9.2.2 Diagnosis

- Histopathological examination shows dilated sinuses, several plasma cells, and marked proliferation of histiocytes.

58.9.2.3 Treatment

- Observation
- Rarely needed radiation/chemotherapy [13]

58.9.3 Kikuchi-Fujimoto Disease

- Idiopathic disorder.
- Lymphadenopathy can occur anywhere in body but tends to be cervical.
- Young adults affected the most.
- Consider biopsy is to rule out malignancy.
- Self-limiting disease.

58.9.3.1 Clinical Features

- Fever.
- Chills.
- Weight loss is common.

58.9.3.2 Diagnosis

- Histology shows characteristic necrotizing lymphadenitis [13].

Take Home Messages

- Pediatric head and neck masses are common and mostly benign.
- A systemic approach starting from a thorough history and proper examination is required to evaluate masses.
- Mass location assists in the differential diagnosis.
- Biopsy remains the gold standard for the diagnosis and treatment of malignant masses.
- Ultrasound remains the first-line modality of imaging.

References

1. Peters TR, Edwards KM. Cervical lymphadenopathy and adenitis. Pediatr Rev. 2000;21:399–404.
2. Leung AK, Robson WL. Cervical lymphadenopathy in children. Can J Pediatr. 1991;3:10–7.
3. Margileth AM. Sorting out the causes of lymphadenopathy. Contemp Pediatr. 1995;12:23.
4. Peters TR, Edwards KM. Cervical lymphadenopathy andd adenitis. Pediatr Rev. 2000;21:399–405.
5. Torsiglieri AJ Jr, et al. Pediatric neck masses: guidelines for evaluation. Int J Pediatr Otorhinolaryngol. 1988;16:199–210.
6. Ying M, Ahuja A, Metreweli C. Diagnostic accuracy of sonographic criteria for evaluation of cervical lymphadenopathy. J Ultrasound Med. 1998;17:437–45.
7. Elden LM, Grundfast KM, Vezina G. Accuracy and usefulness of radiographic assessment of cervical neck infections in children. J Otolaryngol. 2001;30:82–9.
8. Ramadan HH, Wax MK, Boyd CB. Fine-needle aspiration of head and neck masses in children. Am J Otolaryngol. 1997;18:400–4.
9. De Umapathy R, Donaldson I. Cervical lymphadenopathy in children. Hosp Med. 2003;64:104.
10. Ammari FF, Hani AHB, Ghariebeh KI. Tuberculosis of the lymph glands of the neck: a limited role for surgery. Otolaryngol Head Neck Surg. 2003;128:576.
11. Blomquist I, Bayer A. Life-threatening deep fascial space infections of the head and neck. Infect Dis Clin North Am. 1988;2:237–63.
12. Tom B, Rao V, Guglielmo F. Imaging of the parapharyngeal space: anatomy and pathology. Crit Rev Diagn Imaging. 1991;31:315–6.
13. Graham JM, Scadding GK, Bull P. Pediatric ENT. Berlin: Springer-Verlag; 2008.

Pediatric Head and Neck Vascular Anomalies and Tumors

59

Faisal Abdulkader
and Niveen Eltigani Elmusharaf Mukhtar

59.1 Introduction

The majority of head and neck masses in children are inflammatory in nature, but other etiologies include congenital, inflammatory, and neoplastic lesions.

Vascular anomalies of the head and neck region constitute more than 50% of vascular anomalies diagnosed in children and affect approximately 1 in 20 children. These lesions broadly fall into two categories—vascular tumors and vascular malformations. This is an important distinction because malformations and tumors show different growth characteristics. Infantile hemangioma is the most common and is considered a benign vascular tumor. It will rapidly enlarge, and then slowly regress over time. Vascular malformations are relatively uncommon, rarely regress, and will continue to enlarge and cause increased complications over time.

Neoplasms of the head and neck region account for approximately 5% of all childhood malignancies. The most common pediatric head and neck malignancies include lymphomas (60%), rhabdomyosarcomas (15%), thyroid malignancies (10%), nasopharyngeal carcinomas (NPCs), salivary gland malignancies, and neuroblastomas.

Persistent adenopathy raises more concerns, especially enlarged lymph nodes within the posterior triangle or supraclavicular space, nodes that are painless, firm, and not mobile.

F. Abdulkader (✉)
Weill Cornell Medical College in Qatar, Doha, Qatar
e-mail: Fabdulkader@sidra.org

N. E. E. Mukhtar
Sidra Medicine and Research Center, Doha, Qatar
e-mail: nmukhtar@sidra.org

59.2 Vascular Anomalies-Tumors

- Vascular anomalies occur in the head and neck in approximately 4.5% of children [1].
- They are classified into vascular tumors and vascular malformations (Table 59.1) [2].

Table 59.1 Vascular anomalies based on International Society for the Study of Vascular Anomalies

Vascular tumors	Vascular malformation
Benign: • Infantile hemangioma (IH) • Congenital hemangioma (CH): two types, rapidly involuting and non-involuting • Tufted angioma • Pyogenic granuloma	Low-flow malformations: • Capillary malformations (CM): e.g., Nevus simplex • Lymphatic malformations (LM): macrocytic, microcytotic, and mixed cystic LM • Venous malformations (VM) • Mixed: e.g., VM + LM
Locally aggressive or border line: • Kaposi sarcoma	High-flow malformations: • Arteriovenous malformations (AVM) • Arteriovenous fistula (AVF)
Malignant vascular tumors: • Angiosarcoma	

A. Al-Qahtani et al. (eds.), *Textbook of Clinical Otolaryngology*,
https://doi.org/10.1007/978-3-030-54088-3_59

- The differentiation between the two types is essential as they show different growth characteristics [3].

59.2.1 Infantile Hemangioma

- Has a distinct biologic tumorous entity characterized by rapid endothelial proliferation shortly after birth followed by slow regression over time.
- Most common vascular anomaly seen in approximately 4–10% of infants [1].
- Approximately 60% presents in the head and neck.
- More common in whites, premature babies under 1000 g, and multiple gestations (2–3:1 girl/boy ratio).
- Vascular endothelial growth factor (VEGF) and adrenergic receptor pathway are implicated in its development.
- GLUT-1 has been identified as a specific marker for IH [4].

59.2.1.1 Clinical Features

- Red macule at birth.
- Rapid growth in the first 6 weeks after birth up until the first 8–12 months [5].
- Involution occurs over 3–8 years.
- Subglottic IH presents with stridor.

59.2.1.2 Treatment

- The majority of IH need no treatment due to involution of the hemangioma over time.
- Propranolol (beta blocker) has evolved to become the first-line treatment modality.
- Many protocols for propranolol, most commonly dose is: 1–3 mg/kg/day divided three times a day.
- Propranolol is most effective in the proliferative period. Therefore, mostly given for 6–12 months and then weaned off. If symptoms recur, it can be restarted again [6].
- IH causing functional or cosmetic deformity (covering the eye, nasal tip, subglottic) should be treated early [2].
- High dose steroids (prednisolone) is an effective treatment modality for IH. However, with higher side-effects in comparison to propranolol.
- Prednisolone can be used as primary or adjuvant therapy in non-responders to propranolol [6].
- Other modalities, including interferon and chemotherapy, are rarely used now.
- Surgical interventions are still needed in up to 50% of cases, especially in the proliferating phase, where there is significant damage to surrounding tissues [7].

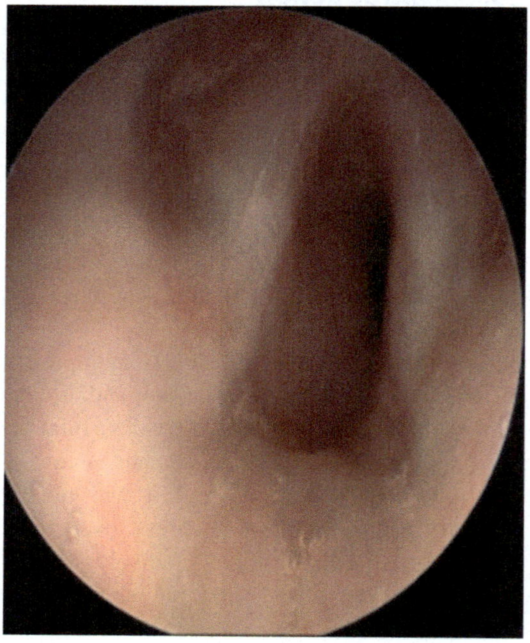

59.3 Vascular Anomalies-Malformations

59.3.1 Capillary Malformation

59.3.1.1 Clinical Features

- Abnormally dilated capillaries in the superficial dermis are present at birth, and eventually change to a deep purple color with age and into adulthood.

- Trigeminal nerve abnormalities lead to a risk of choroidal and intracranial vascular abnormalities called Sturge–Weber Syndrome [8]

59.3.1.2 Treatment
- Pulsed-dye laser achieves significant lightening in 80% of patients.
- Surgical excision in rare cases with skin grafting or advancement flaps [9].

59.3.2 Venous Malformations (VM)

- VMs represent the third most common vascular mass in the head and neck after IH and LM.
- These lesions are structural anomalies that have a normal growth rate (grow with the child) and normal rates of endothelial turnover.
- VMs typically present as compressible masses, often with overlying blue or purplish skin staining. On the mucous membranes, these will be soft purple blebs.
- VMs can present at any site but are more common in the muscle and mucous membranes [10].
- Lesions occur in isolation or part of capillary venous malformation.
- Grow with the child and can expand at puberty, after trauma or subtotal excision.

59.3.2.1 Diagnosis
- Ultrasound: is useful for superficial sites.
- MRI: VM will appear isointense on T1-weighted sequences and hyperintense on T2-weighted sequences

59.3.2.2 Treatment
- Observation: however, most VM will require treatment at some point.
- Treatment modalities: sclerotherapy, surgery, and laser therapy.
- Most VMs will require a multimodality approach to treatment.
- The location, size, and relation to adjacent structures will guide which modality treatment is adopted.
- Sclerotherapy works successfully and results in a significant reduction of the VM.
- Many sclerotherapy agents have been used.
- On average, 1–4 sclerotherapy sessions over a period of 3–12 months is needed.
- Sclerotherapy complications: swelling, ulceration, peripheral nerve palsy, deep vein thrombosis, and muscle contracture.
- Small well-confined VM with clear borders can be cured by simple surgical excision.
- VM with poorly defined borders which can invade normal tissue can be extremely difficult to be excised completely. This type of surgery carries a high risk of bleeding and injury to surrounding structures (e.g., parotid VM).
- Nd:YAG laser has been in the management of VM, typically for airway lesions [11].

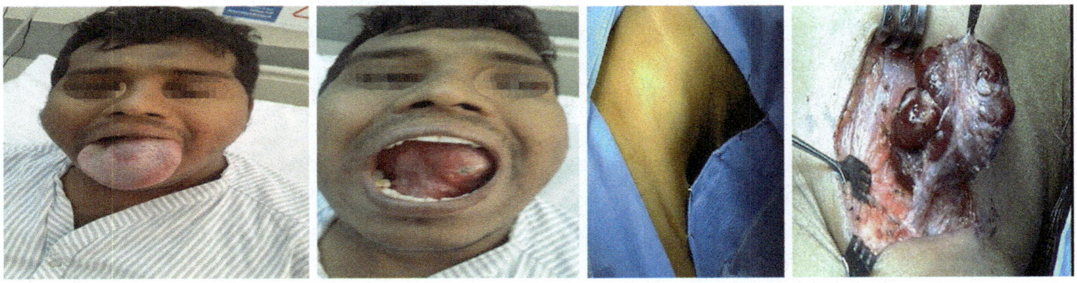

59.3.3 Lymphatic Malformations (LM)

- Known previously as cystic hygroma or lymphangioma.
- Consists of many dilated lymphatic channels lined by single epithelial layer, forming swellings of differing size.
- 75% involves the head and neck due to its abundant lymphatics [12].
- Commonly linked to VM and called venolymphatic malformation (VLM).
- Classified into: macrocystic (>2 cm), microcystic <2 cm), and mixed.
- 4 different types have been described (Serres satging):
  - Type I: Unilateral infrahyoid
  - Type II: Unilateral suprahyoid
  - Type III: Unilateral infra- and suprahyoid
  - Type IV: Bilateral suprahyoid
- Type III and IV are more complex and difficult to treat, requiring frequent treatments.

59.3.3.1 Clinical Features

- Presents at birth or can develop during childhood.
- Sudden swelling can be linked to respiratory infection or minor trauma due to internal hemorrhage.
- On examination: similar to VM, however, less compressible and intertwine with normal tissue leading to cosmetic and functional deformity.
- Macroglossia. Tongue covered in vesicles.
  - Can lead to airway obstruction, a tracheostomy may be necessary.

59.3.3.2 Treatment

- LM treatment is usually complex and depends on the cosmetic and functional deformity.
- The primary goal of treatment is to improve functionality by reducing its size.
- The secondary goal of treatment is the complete eradication of the disease.
- Conservative management mainly with respiratory infections and trauma. This is achieved with antibiotics and steroids.
- Sclerotherapy: ideal for macrocytic type I. However, it may have a role for microcystic lesions.
- Sclerotherapy injections for type I are normally intralesional and done under radiologic guidance leading to an inflammatory response. In microcystic lesion, sclerotic agent is injected submucosally.
- Surgery: total excision of type I and subtotal excision of type II.
- Partial glossectomy may be needed for macroglossia or even surface lasering of tongue vesicles if they are present.
- An immunosuppressant, sirolimus has recently been used for their antilymphangiogenic properties in treating LM [13].
- Psychological support for patients who experience facial disfigurement.

59.3.4 Arteriovenous Malformation (AVM)

- Fast-flow lesions.
- Relatively uncommon in head and neck, except in cranial cavity where they are 20x more common than slow-flow lesions.
- Presents in childhood commonly or adolescence [14].

59.3.4.1 Clinical Features

- Warm and pulsatile swelling.
- If untreated for a long time, skin necrosis and destruction of facial bones can take place.

59.3.4.2 Diagnosis

- Doppler ultrasound used to confirm arteriovenous shunting.
- MRI/ angiography.

59.3.4.3 Treatment

- No treatment for most cases if asymptomatic.
- Selective embolization can be used pre-operatively.
- Subtotal excision means that recurrence is very likely as new vascular channels will develop over time.

- Total excision is the only cure; however, it is a very extensive surgery [11].

59.4 Benign Tumors

59.4.1 Teratoma

- Occurs approximately in 1 in 4000 births.
- Said to be derived from pluripotent cells.
- 7–9% of cases are localized to the head and neck area.

59.4.1.1 Clinical Features

- Most cases occur in sacrococcygeal region, ovaries, testes, anterior mediastinum, and retroperitoneum.
- Malignant transformation is rare in the head and neck.
- Presents as a massive benign neck mass at birth.
- Despite being benign, morbidity and mortality are high.

59.4.1.2 Treatment

- Surgical resection.
- Careful monitoring of tumor markers—alpha fetoprotein and beta human chorionic gonadotrophin—in the blood is highly suggested [11].

59.4.2 Juvenile Nasopharyngeal Angiofibroma

59.5 Malignant Tumors

- 25% of pediatric malignancies will involve the head at some stage.
- Estimated that 5% originate in the head and neck area.
- The most common presentation of a malignancy in the head and neck region in childhood is the asymptomatic mass.
- The best predictors of malignancy in cervical lymphadenopathy are the size of the node, the number of sites involved, and the age of the patient.
- Squamous cell carcinoma is extremely rare in children [14].
- The most common lesions are lymphomas and sarcomas in children, as shown in the following Table 59.2 [15]:

59.5.1 Hodgkin's Lymphoma

- A malignant neoplasm of lymphoreticular system
- Occurs mostly in adolescents

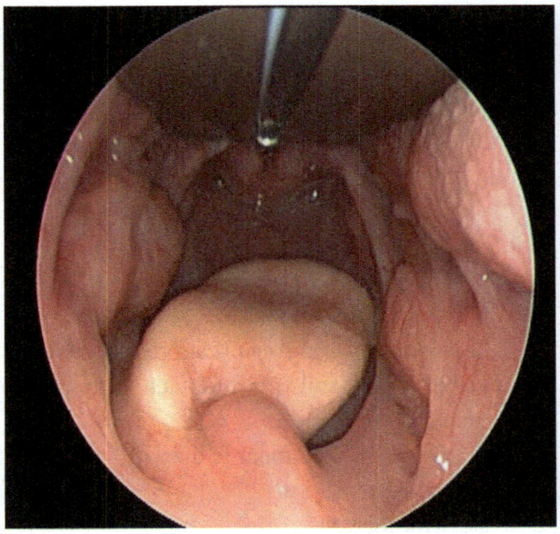

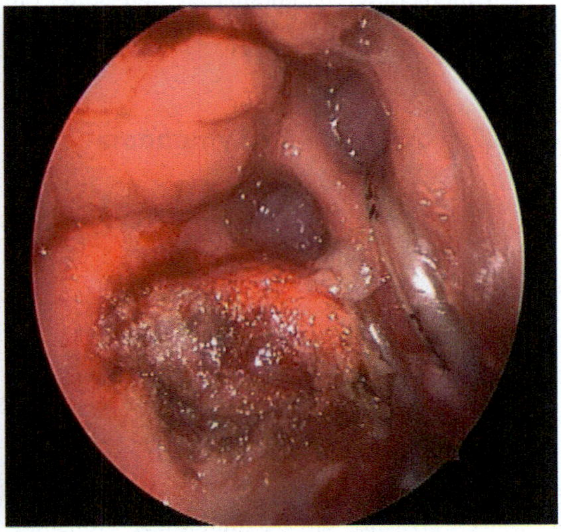

Table 59.2 Histopathology of pediatric head and neck malignancy

Malignancy	Relative incidence
Hodgkin's lymphoma	32%
Non-Hodgkin's lymphoma	29%
Rhabdomyosarcoma	13%
Thyroid carcinoma	9%
Nasopharyngeal carcinoma	4%
Neuroblastoma	5%
Salivary malignancy	2%
Teratoma	1%
Other uncommon tumors	1%

- Distinguished from non-Hodgkin's lymphoma by the presence of Reed–Sternberg cells

59.5.1.1 Clinical Features
- Progressive enlargement of cervical and supraclavicular lymph nodes.
- Enlargement of liver, spleen, and abdominal lymph nodes as the disease spreads.
- Neutropenia, thrombocytopenia, and anemia in peripheral blood film.
- Constitutional symptoms (B symptoms)—fever, night sweats and weight loss in 25–30%.

59.5.1.2 Diagnosis
- FNA has a limited role.
- Excision biopsy is the gold standard.

59.5.1.3 Treatment
- Chemotherapy or radiotherapy depending on stage [16].

59.5.2 Non-Hodgkin's Lymphoma

- A mixed group of solid malignant neoplasms of lymphoreticular system.
- Affects ages 2–12 years mostly.

59.5.2.1 Clinical Features
- Presents commonly as cervical lymphadenopathy but can affect extra-nodal sites.
- Lesions are common in head and neck, nasopharynx, orbit, and skull base.
- May present as asymmetrical tonsillar enlargement.

59.5.2.2 Diagnosis
- FNA has limited role.
- Excision biopsy is the gold standard.

59.5.2.3 Treatment
Chemotherapy or radiotherapy depending on stage [17].

59.5.3 Rhabdomyosarcoma

- Second most common malignancy in pediatric.
- 30–40% of cases occur in head and neck.
- >50% of cases are in <5 years of age.
- Prognosis has improved with multimodality treatments.
- Classified into two types: embryonal and alveolar [18].
- Embryonal affects approximately 80% and has a better prognosis than alveolar type.

59.5.3.1 Clinical Features
- Most common sites are the orbit (most common), nasopharynx, middle ear and mastoid, and sinonasal cavities.
- Typically presents as rapidly enlarging mass in a child under the age of 12 years old.
- Presentation depends on the site involved.
- Nodal involvement is estimated between 3% and 36%.

59.5.3.2 Diagnosis
- Biopsy, MRI, and CT are required.
- Multiple modalities are utilized in staging: chest CT, abdominal ultrasound, bone marrow aspiration, and lumbar puncture [19].

59.5.3.3 Treatment
- Follows guidelines of Inter Group Rhabdomyosarcoma (IRS) (Table 59.3).
- The majority are at stage II at presentation and complete surgical excision is difficult to achieve.
- Multimodality treatment is used:
  - Surgical resection
  - Chemotherapy
  - Radiotherapy

Table 59.3 Staging of rhabdomyosarcoma according to the IRS

Group I
Localized disease completely resected. No regional nodes Confined to muscle or organ origin Contiguous infiltration outside muscle or organ of origin
Group II
Localized disease with microscopic residual disease, or regional disease (lymphnode)
Group III
Incomplete resection or biopsy with gross residual disease
Group IV
Metastatic disease present at onset

59.5.4 Thyroid Malignancy

- More common in adolescents than pediatrics.
- Has a female predominance 4:1.
- Close association with previous radiation history.
- Slow growing tumors and associated with prolonged survival rate.
- 45% are differentiated papillary carcinomas.
- 45% mixed papillary/follicular types.
- 10% follicular lesions.
- Medullary thyroid carcinoma (MTC) is rare (only 10% of thyroid malignancies in children) and must be suspected in children with multiple endocrine neoplasia (MEN) types IIa and IIb.
- Anaplastic and undifferentiated tumors are extremely rare in children and adolescents [20].

59.5.4.1 Clinical Features

- Solitary asymptomatic mass in the anterior or lateral neck is the most common presentation.
- It is estimated that 74% will have nodal metastases and 25% distant metastases at time of presentation.

59.5.4.2 Diagnosis

- Ultrasound scan, usually in conjunction with an ultrasound-guided FNAC.
- Thyroid function tests and plasma thyroglobulin levels.
- Plasma calcitonin when suspecting medullary carcinoma.

59.5.4.3 Treatment

- Complete surgical excision is the ideal approach.
- Possible complications for total thyroidectomy include injury to recurrent laryngeal nerve, hypocalcemia, and airway compromise if both recurrent laryngeal nerves have been injured.
- Following surgery, a whole-body radioiodine scan is performed, and ablative radioiodine treatment is given if necessary [21].
- Plasma thyroglobulin can then be used as a tumor marker and suppressive levothyroxine should be given.
- Radiotherapy is rarely indicated in differentiated thyroid carcinoma in childhood [22].

59.5.5 Neuroblastoma

- Commonest malignancy in children under the age of 1.
- 90% of cases present before 10 years of age.
- Arise from undifferentiated sympathetic nervous system cells of neural crest origin.

59.5.5.1 Clinical Features

- Predominantly found in adrenal gland and sympathetic chain.
- May present as a primary neck mass arising from the cervical sympathetic trunk associated Horner's syndrome.
- Metastases to regional lymph nodes is common (~35%) [23].

59.5.5.2 Treatment

- Surgery can be curative for localized lesions with 90% survival rate in children with resectable disease.
- Radiation and chemotherapy are chosen for metastatic lesions [24].

59.5.6 Nasopharyngeal Carcinoma (NPS)

- 1–2% of pediatric malignancies in the USA and Europe.

- 10–20 % of pediatric malignancies in Africa.
- Originates from epithelium and associated with EBV.
- Undifferentiated NPS is most common in children.
- 5-year survival is similar to adults (30–60%).

59.5.6.1 Clinical Features

- Children will often have metastatic disease in their neck.
- Unilateral otitis media.
- Rhinorrhea.
- Nasal obstruction.
- Cranial nerve palsies and facial pain suggest skull-base involvement.

59.5.6.2 Diagnosis

- Delayed diagnosis is very common.
- Flexible nasopharyngoscopy.
- Biopsy.
- CT and MRI imaging.
- Staging.

59.5.6.3 Treatment

- Dependent on type, location, and extent of spread.
- Chemoradiation.
- Surgery [25].

Take Home Messages

- The pediatric head and neck malignancies differ from adults; hence a different approach is required.
- Squamous cell carcinomas are extremely rare in children.
- Hemangiomas; propranolol have evolved to become the first-line treatment modality in the proliferative period.
- Sirolimus has recently been used for their antilymphangiogenic properties in treating LM.

References

1. Greene AK, Kim S, Rogers GF, Fishman SJ, Olsen BR, Mulliken JB. Risk of vascular anomalies with Down syndrome. Pediatrics. 2008;121(1):e135–40.
2. Mulliken JB, Glowacki J. Hemangiomas and vascular malformations in infants and children: a classification based on endothelial characteristics. Plast Reconstr Surg. 1982;69(3):412–22.
3. Fin MD, Glowacki J, Mulliken JB. Congenital vascular lesions: clinical application of a new classification. J Pediatr Surg. 1983;18:894.
4. North PE, Waner M, Mizeracki A, Mihm MC Jr. GLUT1: a newly discovered immunohistochemical marker for juvenile hemangiomas. Hum Pathol. 2000;31(1):11–22.
5. Mulliken JB, Fishman SJ, Burrows PE. Vascular anomalies. Curr Probl Surg. 2000;37(8):517–84.
6. Frongia G, Byeon J-O, Arnold R, Mehrabi A, Günther P. Cardiac diagnostics before oral propranolol therapy in infantile hemangioma: retrospective evaluation of 234 infants. World J Pediatr. 2018;14(3):254–8. https://doi.org/10.1007/s12519-018-0137-7.
7. Archauer BM, Celikoz B, Vanderkam VM. Intralesional bare fiber laser treatment of hemangioma of infancy. Plast Reconstr Surg. 1998;101:1212–7.
8. Shirley MD, Tang H, Gallione CJ, Baugher JD, Frelin LP, Cohen B, North PE, Marchuk DA, Comi AM, Pevsner J. Sturge-Weber syndrome and port-wine stains caused by somatic mutation in GNAQ. N Engl J Med. 2013;368(21):1971–9.
9. Lee JW, Chung HY. Capillary malformations (Portwine stains) of the head and neck: natural history, investigations, laser, and surgical management. Otolaryngol Clin North Am. 2018;51(1):197–211.
10. Boon LM, Mulliken JB, Enjolras O, Vikkula M. Glomuvenous malformation (glomangioma) and venous malformation: distinct clinicopathologic and genetic entities. Arch Dermatol. 2004;140(8):971–6.
11. Graham JM, Scadding GK, Bull P. Pediatric ENT. Berlin: Springer-Verlag; 2008.
12. Kaur N, Gupta A, Amratash M, Singh N. Giant cystic hygroma of the neck with spontaneous rupture. J Indian Assoc Pediatr Surg. 2007;12:154.
13. Hammill AM, Wentzel MS, Gupta A, Nelson S, Lucky A, Elluru R, Dasgupta R, Azizkhan RG, Adams DM. Sirolimus for the treatment of complicated vascular anomalies in children. Pediatr Blood Cancer. 2011;57:1018–24.
14. Albright JT, Topham AK, Reilly JS. Pediatric head and neck malignancies: US incidence and trends over 2 decades. Arch Otolaryngol Head Neck Surg. 2002;128:655–9.
15. Isaacson PG. The revised European American lymphoma REAL classification. Clin Oncol (R Coll Radiol). 1995;7(6):347–8.

16. Hudson MM, Donaldson SS. Hodgkin's disease. Pediatr Clin North Am. 1997;44:891–906.
17. Patte C. Non-Hodgkin's lymphoma. Eur J Cancer. 1998;34:359–62.
18. Parham DM, Barr FB. Classification of rhabdomyosarcoma and its molecular basis. Anat Pathol. 2013;20(6):387–97.
19. Pappo AS, Shapiro DN, Crist WM. Rhabdomyosarcoma: biology and treatment. Pediatr Clin North Am. 1997;44:953–72.
20. Newman KD, Black T, Heller G, et al. Differentiated thyroid cancer: determinants of disease progression in patients <21 years of age at diagnosis. A report from the Surgical Discipline Committee of the Children's Cancer Group. Ann Surg. 1998;227:533–41.
21. Segal K, Shvero J, Stern Y, et al. Surgery of thyroid cancer in children and adolescents. Head Neck. 1998;20:293–7.
22. Jocham A, Joppich I, Hecker W, et al. Thyroid carcinoma in childhood: management and follow up of 11 cases. Eur J Pediatr. 1994;153:17–22.
23. Haase GM. Head and neck neuroblastoma. Sem Pediatr Surg. 1994;3:194–202.
24. Weinstein JL, Katzenstein HM, Cohn SL. Advances in the diagnosis and treatment of neuroblastoma. Oncologist. 2003;8:278–92.
25. Mertens R, Granzen B, Lassay L, et al. Nasopharyngeal carcinoma in childhood and adolescence. Cancer. 1997;80:951–9.

Evaluation of Stridor and Wheezy Children

60

Amr A. Elhakeem

60.1 Introduction

Normal breathing is quiet.

Partial obstructions to the airway cause turbulence of air flowing, and this in turn produce sounds. The sounds are usually more evident during one or more parts of the respiratory cycle depending on the site of pathology.

On the other hand, if the airway obstruction is becoming severe, sounds quiet down and air flow seriously reduced or stopped.

60.2 Types of Sounds

60.2.1 Stertor

Snoring-type generated at the level of the nasopharynx, oropharynx, and, occasionally, supraglottis.

60.2.2 Stridor

Stridor is a high pitched sound produced at the level of the supraglottis, glottis, subglottis, and/or trachea. It is a symptom, not a diagnosis or disease.

60.2.3 Wheezing

It is an expiratory sound produced in small lower airway (bronchioles).

60.3 Airway in Children

The anatomical differences between adult and pediatric airways make the latter more susceptible for acute airway obstruction.

The recognition of the site, the severity of the airway obstruction, and the impending respiratory distress are essential in the management and avoiding serious consequences.

Multiple causes may produce airway obstruction, which necessitates a proper evaluation (to find the cause and management). Systematic reviews of history and examinations are essential to identify the site, severity, and determine the seriousness of the condition.

60.3.1 Anatomy

- Narrowest at the cricoid, making obstruction with subglottic pathology more likely (Fig. 60.1).
- Ribs and cartilaginous are perpendicular relative to the vertebral column, reducing the effect of the "bucket handle" and pump handle movement of the rib cage (Fig. 60.2).

A. A. Elhakeem (✉)
Otolaryngology, Head and Neck Surgery, Hamad Medical Corporation, Doha, Qatar
e-mail: aelhakeem@hamad.qa

A. Al-Qahtani et al. (eds.), *Textbook of Clinical Otolaryngology*,
https://doi.org/10.1007/978-3-030-54088-3_60

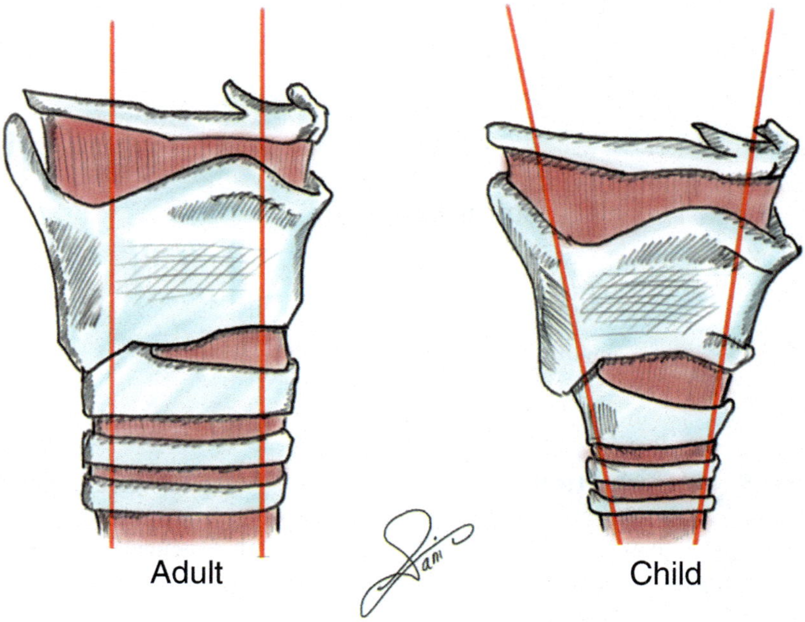

Fig. 60.1 Pediatric larynx anatomy vs. adult showing that the subglottic area is the narrowest area in children

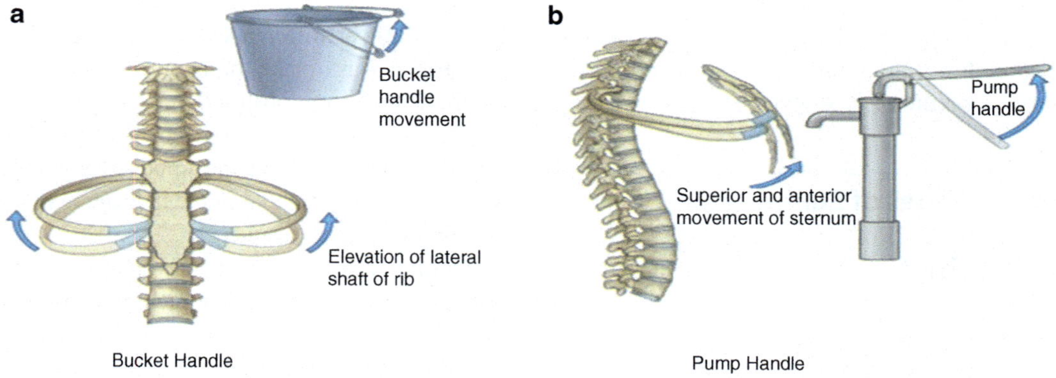

Fig. 60.2 (**a**) and (**b**) show the angular position of the ribs relative to the vertebral column. The elevation of the ribs during breathing results in the effect of the "bucket handle" and "pump handle" movement of the rib cage. (**a**) is the anterior posterior view, while (**b**) is the lateral view

60.3.2 Physiology

1. Higher Basal Metabolism Rate (BMR) and O_2 consumption.
2. Immature CNS: irregular respiration control.
3. Immature intercostal and accessory muscles of ventilation, risk of respiratory muscle fatigue.
4. Smaller and fewer alveoli: less surface area for gas exchange.
5. Increase in O_2 need is maintained by increase in respiratory rate (RR) mainly.

60.3.3 Pathology

1. Congenital diseases.
2. Any decreases in radius lead to big increases in resistance (Fig. 60.3).
3. Susceptible to edema, swelling, and occlusion by secretions.

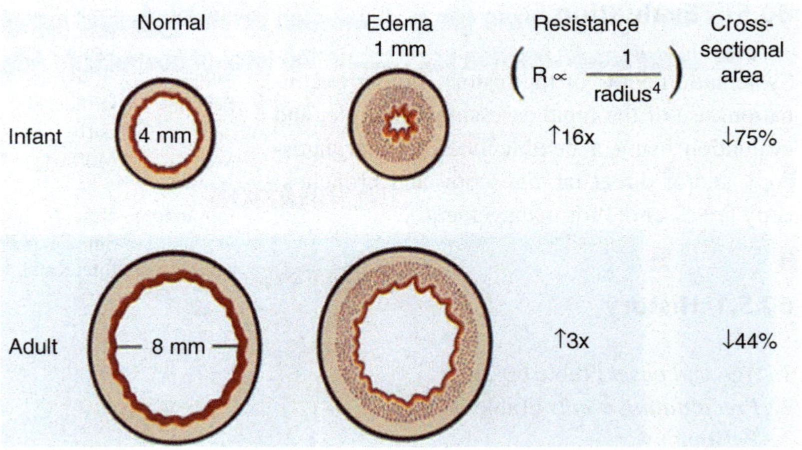

Fig. 60.3 Poiseuille's law states that flow is inversely proportional to the fourth power of the radius. In the already small pediatric airway, tiny impingements on the lumen can create large increases in resistance

Table 60.1 Etiology and site of stridor

	Supraglottis	Subglottic	Trachea
Congenital	Micrognathia Pierre Robin syndrome Macroglossia Down syndrome Storage diseases Choanal atresia Lingual thyroid Thyroglossal cyst	Laryngomalacia (Fig. 60.9) Vocal cord paralysis Laryngeal web Laryngocele Subglottic stenosis (Fig. 60.10)	Tracheomalacia Tracheal stenosis Vascular ring Hemangioma cyst
Acquired	Adenopathy Tonsillar hypertrophy Foreign body Pharyngeal abscess Epiglottitis	Papillomas Foreign body	Croup Bacterial tracheitis Subglottic stenosis Foreign body

60.4 Stridor Causes

60.4.1 Etiology and Site (Table 60.1)

60.4.2 Stridor (Site and Timing) (Fig. 60.4)

60.4.2.1 Sites

1. Nose and mouth
2. Larynx (epiglottis, supraglottis, glottis, and subglottis)
3. Trachea

Timing (during which part of the respiratory cycle the sound is more prominent):

- *Inspiratory phase* = obstruction above glottis.
- *Biphasic (both inspiratory and expiratory)* = glottic/subglottic lesion.
- *Expiratory phase* = lower trachea and bronchi.

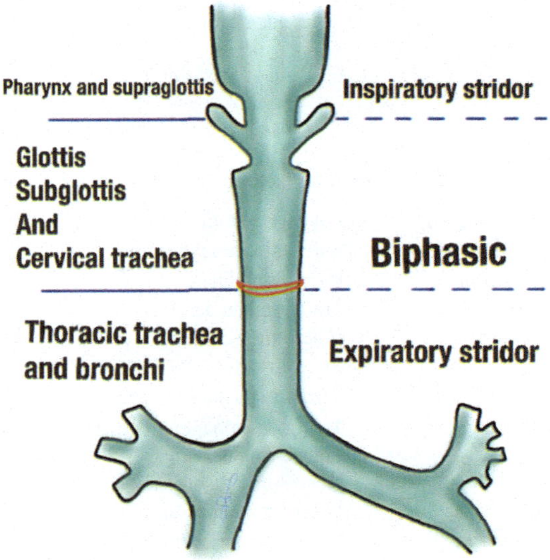

Fig. 60.4 Stridor (site and timing)

60.5 Evaluation

Systematic review of the history, proper examination, use of the rapid assessment triangle, and evaluation using a flexible fiberoptic laryngoscopy and/or direct laryngoscopy and bronchoscopy are essential for management.

60.5.1 History

1. *Age and onset* (Table 60.2).
2. *Precipitating events* (Table 60.3).
3. *Positioning*.
4. *Associated symptoms*. (Table 60.4)
5. *Developmental history*.
6. *Other history including*:

Table 60.2 Age and onset

Neonates	Children	Adults
Laryngomalacia (commonest cause) Chronic	*Infection*— Epiglottitis— Laryngitis Acute	*Infection*— Epiglottitis— Laryngitis Acute
Vocal cord dysfunction Chronic	*Croup: 1–2 days duration* Acute	*Trauma*— acquired stenosis Acute
Congenital tumors Chronic	*Foreign body* Acute	
Choanal atresia Acute or chronic	*Laryngeal dyskinesia* Chronic	
Laryngeal webs Chronic		

Table 60.3 Precipitating factors

Straining or crying	Laryngomalacia Subglottic hemangioma
Position	Laryngomalacia Tracheomalacia Macroglossia Micrognathia
Night	Viral or spasmodic croup
Feeding	Tracheoesophageal fistula Tracheomalacia Neurologic disorder Vascular compression
Upper respiratory tract infection	Croup, bacterial tracheitis
Choking	Foreign body aspiration Tracheoesophageal fistula

Table 60.4 Associated symptoms

Sign	Inspiratory stridor	Biphasic stridor	Expiratory stridor
Feeding	Difficulty Early	Difficulty Late	Difficulty Very Late
Voice	Muffled	Dysphonia	Barking cough
Retractions	Nasal flaring Suprasternal Intercostal	Nasal flaring Suprasternal Intercostal	Nasal flaring Sternal (xiphoid) Subcostal

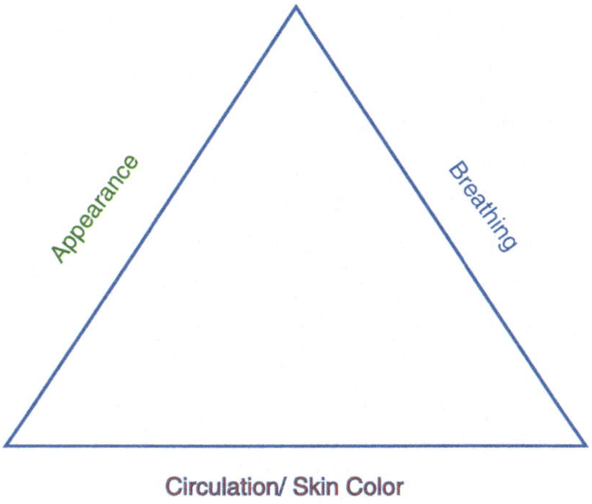

Fig. 60.5 Pediatric assessment triangle

- Endotracheal intubation (size used, duration, and any associated difficulties should be reviewed).
- Presence of congenital anomalies or other craniofacial anomalies.

60.5.2 Examination

Facing a stridulous child, a general impression is formed the first time the physician views the patient, usually within seconds. The pediatric assessment triangle is used as a method of quickly determining the acuity of the child, and can determine whether the child is in respiratory distress or respiratory failure, or shock.

The pediatric assessment triangle consists of three areas of assessment: appearance; work of breathing; and circulation to skin. (Fig. 60.5 and Table 60.5)

Table 60.5 Pediatrics assessment triangle in a stridulous child

Appearance	*Breathing*	*Circulation/Color*
Level of alertness	Respiratory rate	Cyanosis
Interaction	Respiratory effort (retractions, nasal flaring, grunting, abdominal breathing)	Pallor
Response to stimuli		Mottling

Table 60.6 Acceptable range of unwell child

Age (years)	Respiratory rate (per minute)	Heart rate (per minute)
<1	30–40	110–160
1–2	25–35	100–150
2–5	25–30	95–140
5–12	20–25	80–120
>12	15–20	60–100

Suprasternal retractions indicate more severe obstruction than intercosatl and subcostal retractions

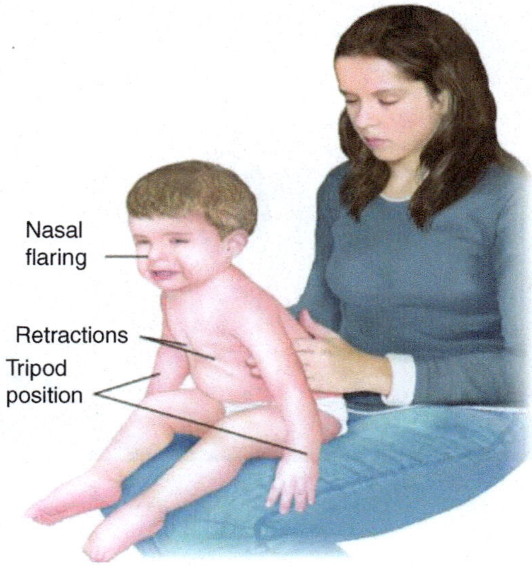

Fig. 60.7 Tripod position

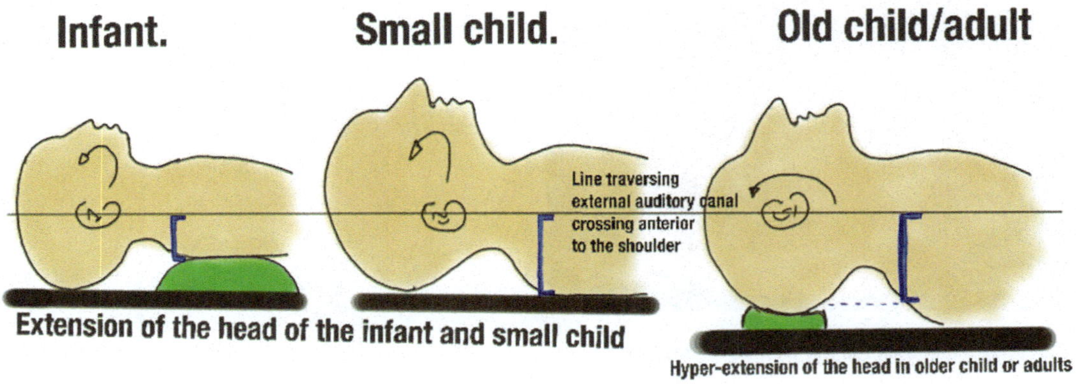

Fig. 60.6 Sniffing position or ear to sternal notch

60.5.2.1 Check the Heart Rate, Respiratory Rate, and Look for Presence of Retraction (Table 60.6)

60.5.2.2 Position of Comfort of the Child

Upper airway obstruction: as the condition worsens, the child assumes an upright posture, leaning forward, self-generating jaw thrust (Sniffing position) (Fig. 60.6).

Lower airway obstruction: as the condition progress, the child tends to assume an upright posture, leaning forward and supporting chest with arms (tripod position) (Fig. 60.7).

60.5.2.3 Flexible Fiberoptic Laryngoscopy and/or Direct Laryngoscopy and Bronchoscopy

Normal Larynx (Fig. 60.8)

See Figs. 60.9 and 60.10.

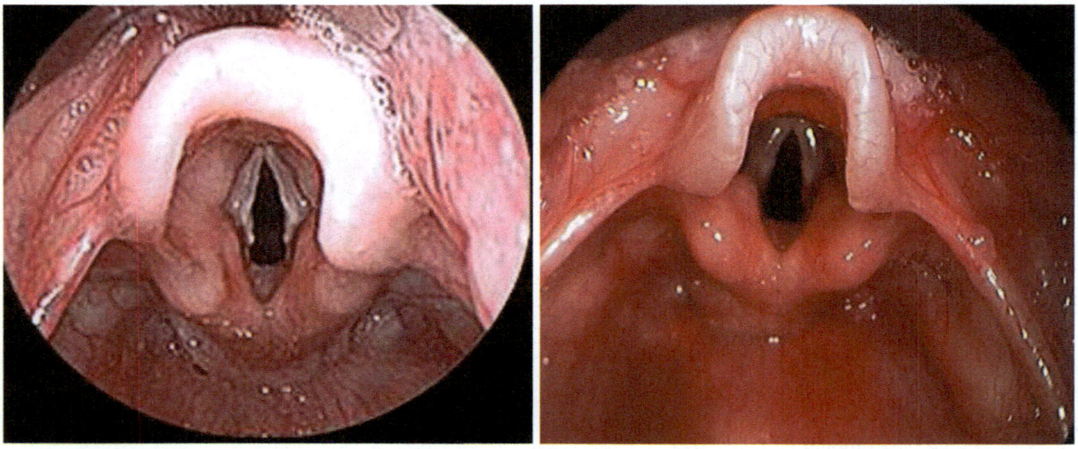

Fig. 60.8 Normal larynx with patent airways

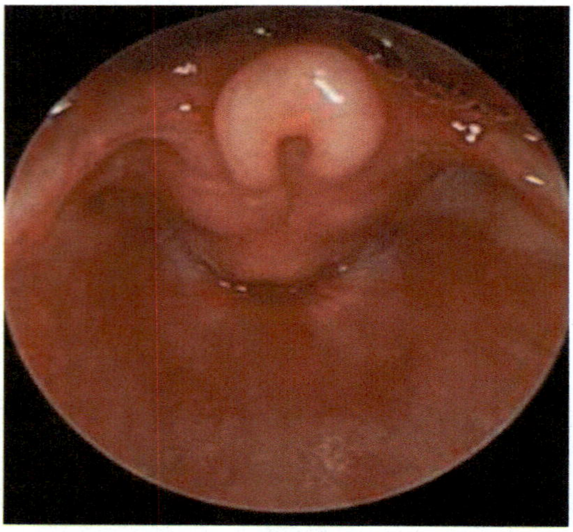

Fig. 60.9 Abnormal Larynx with laryngomalacia

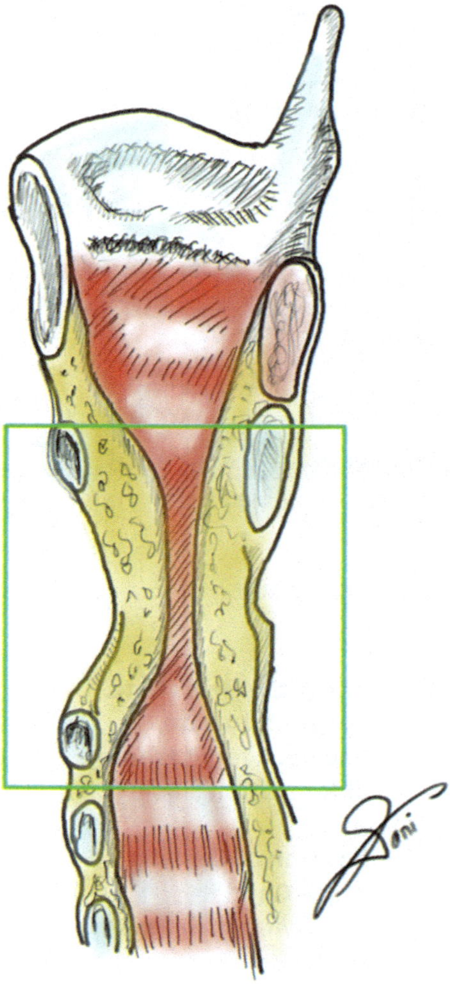

Fig. 60.10 Subglottic stenosis

60.6 Respiratory Distress

(This is the inability to maintain gas exchange.)

Symptoms and signs depend on age and include:

1. Worsening of stridor or wheezing
2. Increase RR and HR.
3. Increase the work of breathing (use of accessory muscles, retraction, nasal flaring, and grunting).

60.6.1 Impending Respiratory Failure

60.6.1.1 Warning Signs

- Retractions.
- Increasing HR.
- Decreasing RR and effort.
- Decreasing stridor or wheezing.
- Unsettled appearance.
- Assuming comfort position (sniffing position or tripod position).

60.6.1.2 Ominous Signs

- Irregular breathing.
- Head-bobbing with each breath.
- Decreased HR.
- Color changes (pallor or cyanosis, which is an extremely late sign in upper airway obstruction).
- Altered level of concentration is essential to determine the need for intervention).

60.6.2 Diagnostic Studies and Monitoring

1. Pulse oximetry (interpretation must be considered carefully if supplemental oxygen has been applied).
2. End-tidal CO_2 monitoring is useful when available, particularly when supplemental oxygen is administered.
3. Arterial blood gas (ABG) can help differentiate between ventilatory and oxygenation failure (a normal $PaCO_2$, in a severely distressed patient, is likely to indicate respiratory fatigue, inability to compensate, and impending respiratory failure).
4. Barium esophagram.
5. CT neck and chest (with airway reconstruction).

Take Home Messages

- Airway obstruction can be life-threatening as it may lead to respiratory failure, which progresses quickly to cardiac arrest.
- Few seconds of observation should make the differentiation between upper and lower airway obstruction easy.
- Failure to manage the airway is the leading cause of preventable deaths in children.

Further Reading

Bruce IA, Rothera MP. Upper airway obstruction in children. Paediatr Anaesth. 2009;19(Suppl 1):88–99.

Croup, Cherry JD. N Engl J Med. 2008;358(4):384–91.

Dobbie AM, White DR. Laryngomalacia. Pediatr Clin North Am. 2013;60(4):893–902.

Mitchell RB, Pereira KD, editors. Pediatric otolaryngology for the clinician. Berlin, Heidelberg: Springer; 2009.

Scadding GK, Bull PD, Graham JM, editors. Pediatric ENT. Berlin, Heidelberg: Springer-Verlag; 2007.

Shapiro NL. Handbook of pediatric otolaryngology: a practical guide for evaluation and management of pediatric ear, nose, and throat disorders. Singapore: World Scientific; 2011.

Wetmore RF, Muntz HR, McGill TJ. Pediatric otolaryngology: principles and practice pathways. Stuttgart: Thieme; 2012.

Zoumalan R, Maddalozzo J, Holinger LD. Etiology of stridor in infants. Ann Otol Rhinol Laryngol. 2007;116(5):329–34.

Managing the Stridulous Child

61

Mai Elhassan

61.1 Introduction

- Stridor: Harsh respiratory sound caused by turbulent airflow through a restricted area.
- Stridor could be: inspiratory sound, expiratory or biphasic stridor; this terminology used to describe intrathoracic and fixed airway obstructions, and usually correlate with the anatomic site of obstruction.
- Stridor mainly originates from the larynx and upper trachea. And should be differentiated from:
  - Stertor: Low pitched snoring sound of breathing during inspiration, originates in the nose or nasopharynx.
  - Wheeze: High pitched whistling sound due to variable intrathoracic obstruction of the tracheobronchial tree, mainly during expiration.
- Stridor is a symptom of underlying airway problem and not a diagnosis [1, 2].

61.2 Anatomy and Pathophysiology of Stridor

Stridor can come from a narrowing of the airway at any point. There are times where the airway involved is at various stages [3, 4].

M. Elhassan (✉)
Pediatric Otolaryngology, Sidra Medicine, Doha, Qatar
e-mail: fabdulkader@sidra.org

61.2.1 Physics of Stridor

- Stridor is mediated by two basic principles of physics:
  - Poiseuille's law of fluid dynamics describes the proportion of flow rate (Q) to the radius of the tube to the fourth power, resulting in an exponential effect on flow rate related to any change in radius. This principle states that as the velocity of airflow increases, the pressure exerted by airflow decreases.
  - Bernoulli principle: Demonstrate that narrowed pediatric airway results in increased airflow velocity that give negative pressure on the walls of the lumen, leading to airway collapse [1].

61.2.2 Evaluation of the Stridulous Patient

Medical History

- Conduct in children with chronic or gradual onset stridor in which the airway is restricted but stable (Box 61.1) [1].
- A thorough history will assist in narrowing the differential diagnosis, and this usually obtains in the absence of severe respiratory distress. Also, it helps in directing the diagnostic evaluation [5].
- Initial observation of the patient's pattern of respiration, assessment of the severity of

A. Al-Qahtani et al. (eds.), *Textbook of Clinical Otolaryngology*,
https://doi.org/10.1007/978-3-030-54088-3_61

airway obstruction, and determination of the potential need for urgent or emergency airway intervention [1].

- Age at onset:
  - Many causes can be predicted from the onset of the symptom.
  - Acute onset of stridor most likely due to infection, inflammation, or foreign body aspiration.
  - A compromised airway manifesting itself immediately at birth, which is commonly due to:
    Bilateral vocal cord paralysis
    Congenital cysts
    Laryngeal webs and atresia
    Choanal atresia
    Vascular mediastinal anomalies
    Severe subglottic stenosis
  - Age: first few weeks of life
    Laryngomalacia
  - Age: 1–4 months
    Moderate subglottic stenosis
    Subglottic hemangioma
  - Age: 1–3 years
    Croup
    Bronchiolitis
  - Age: 3–6 years
    Membranous laryngo-tracheobronchitis
    Epiglottitis
- Aggravating factors
  - Dyspnea and stridor worsen during feeding or agitation, due to increased airway demands.
  - Dyspnea and stertor worsen during sleep in nasopharyngeal or oropharyngeal obstructions, due to loss of muscular tone.
  - In tracheo-esophageal fistulae and clefts: Coughing and choking increase during meals.
- Influence of body position
  - Prone position can reduce noisy breathing resulting from anterior compression of the airway (e.g., glossoptosis, median vallecular cyst, and aberrant innominate artery).
  - Symptoms decrease while the baby lies on the affected side and increase when the baby lies in the contralateral position in: unilateral vocal cord palsy and lateral pharyngeal masses.
- Finally ask about the history of previous intubation, endoscopy, or surgical interventions: in case of obstruction from a vocal cord weakness.
  - In the history of airway obstruction, remember the mnemonic "SPECS" to help in assessing the severity of the condition and in determining the need for diagnostic and therapeutic endoscopy [2].

- S = severity: parents' subjective impression regarding the severity of the obstruction
- *P* = progression: evolution of the obstruction over time
- E = eating: feeding difficulties, aspiration, and failure to thrive
- C = cyanosis: cyanotic episodes, apparent life-threatening events
- S = sleep: disturbed sleep, suprasternal or chest retractions during sleep

61.2.3 Physical Examination

- Careful non-invasive inspection:
  - Evaluation of dysmorphic facial features.
  - Stigmata of a specific syndrome could help in the diagnosis, as many syndromes are linked to congenital airway anomaly, e.g., Down syndrome (congenital subglottic stenosis) and Pallister-Hall (laryngeal cleft).
  - A complete head and neck examination, size and position of the mandible and tongue: helps to locate the source of stridor: e.g., child with micrognathia and stridor may indicate posterior displacement of the tongue and glossoptosis.
  - Signs of increased respiratory effort: nasal flaring, mouth breathing, retraction of suprasternal and intercostal region.
  - Auscultation of the lungs and heart.
  - Careful auscultation for the intensity of the pathological sound and its relation to the phase of respiration; it helps in determining the level of obstruction.
  - Examination of the chest wall and sternum: the presence of a pectus excavatum may suggest significant upper airway obstruction.

  - An accurate diagnosis can be reached when examining infants in various positions and observing the associated changes in the intensity of the pathological sound [2].
- *In-Office Trans-nasal Flexible Laryngoscopy (TNFL)*
  - Is part of the physical examination of the stridulous child.
  - Most effective tool for establishing a diagnosis and for triaging children who need formal bronchoscopic evaluation under general anesthesia.
  - It assesses the patency of the nasal cavities, choanae, nasopharynx, pharyngolarynx and dynamic visualization of the larynx: any abnormalities of the supraglottis and assessing the mobility and lesion within the vocal cords.
  - It's a safe and simple method of diagnosing common pathology inducing stridor.
  - Always provide incomplete information as the subglottis and trachea cannot be visualized [2, 6].

Box 61.1 Stridor history

Timing

- Initiation of symptoms
- Duration of symptoms/episodes
- Episodic versus continuous
- Worsening, steady, or improving

Severity

- Retractions
- Cyanosis
- Fatigue/mental status change
- Weight loss or failure to thrive
- Associated feeding difficulties

Character

- Pitch high versus low
- Phase
- Vibratory
- Positional

Associated symptoms/influence

- Feeding or sleep related
- Strenuous activity
- Spitting up/reflux
- Weight loss
- Dysphagia/aspiration
- Fevers
- Neck mass
- Lymphadenopathy

Medical history

- Intubation history
- Prior surgeries
- Neurologic conditions
- Syndromes/genetics

61.2.3.1 Indication for Endoscopy Under General Anesthesia

- Progression of symptoms.
- Associated abnormalities.
- Atypical clinical presentation.
- Chronic stridor with clinical indications such as: failure to thrive, feeding difficulties, obstructive sleep apneas and cor pulmonale, usually require further assessment and treatment under general anesthesia [2].

61.2.4 Radiological Evaluation

- Lateral and anteroposterior soft tissue X-rays of the neck and chest:
  - Used as the first screening procedure, and can provide useful information of the compromised pediatric airway.
- A helical CT scan using contrast medium:
  - Useful in evaluating extrinsic compressions of the airway by cystic or solid masses.
  - Demonstrate the narrowing of the trachea caused by abnormal mediastinal vessels.
- Computed tomography with three dimensional (3D) reconstructions of the laryngotra-

cheal airway: assist in evaluating airway lesion.

- Useful information as to the location, extent, and severity of the obstruction.
- Virtual endoscopy: It helps in visualizing the distal part of the airway in case of total obstruction of the airway.
- MRI: useful in assessing vascular compressions of the airway secondary to congenital cardiovascular anomalies.
- Ultrasound neck: It helps in differentiating cystic from solid masses, also in assessment and follow-up of vocal cord paralysis.
- Barium esophagram: commonly used in case of unclear dysphagia associated with mild aspiration or recurrent pneumonia, esophagotracheal fistula or cleft, evaluate the function of glottis sphincter and identify vascular compression if it's present [2, 7, 8].

61.2.5 Assessment of the Patient's General Condition

- After conducting a thorough medical history and physical examination, we should be able to differentiate normal infants and children from those with disabilities and visible impairments (e.g., prematurity, severe neurological deficits, and congenital syndromic anomalies).
- Children need to be evaluated and investigated by other specialists. This performed in most tertiary care centers where a child with stridor is evaluated in multidisciplinary fashion:
  - Geneticist evaluation: when congenital anomalies is suspected.
  - Neurological evaluation: when lack of coordinated breathing and swallowing in a mentally retarded child.
  - Cardiac evaluation: If the cause of airway obstruction is intrathoracic, or if cardiac problems are associated with a subglottic stenosis [2].
  - Pulmonary evaluation: provide information about the patient's pulmonary reserve [1, 2].
  - Gastroesophageal investigation: when gastroesophageal reflux (GOR) is suspected [1, 2].
- Similar to acid reflux disease, eosinophilic esophagitis (EoE) can cause inflammation and obstruction of the airways, with similar unfavorable effects on airway healing [9].
- LPR/GERD disorders include laryngomalacia, SGS, and a recurring croup [10].

61.2.6 Resuscitation and Pre-operating Room Management

- Nebulized adrenaline (5 ml of 1:1000 adrenaline) can be administered hourly if indicated: has a drastic impact on the short-term reduction of local mucosal edema, allowing the child to be moved safely.
- Dexamethasone (300 μg/kg) decreases mucosal edema: but slower onset of action, so its main purpose is to avoid late swelling of the mucosa after airway intervention.
- Heliox (a combination of 21% oxygen and 79% helium): a major role in minimizing the breathing function of a child who is fatigued by repeated ventilation into an obstructed airway [11].

61.2.7 Operative Endoscopy

- Definitive diagnosis of an airway problem that causes stridor is often difficult without endoscopic visualization.
- While parts of the airway can or should be examined in the clinic with the patient conscious, other lesions require anesthetics and specialized equipment to fully visualize and examine the airways.
- Age-appropriate laryngoscopes and bronchoscopes are required.
- Excellent communication with anesthesia providers is important if the surgeon is to be given sufficient time to gather information and provide intervention where necessary.
- The ability of the anesthetist to keep the child breathing spontaneously without the endotracheal tube in the airway allows optimal examination and diagnosis of potential causes of stridor.

- Drug-induced sleep endoscopy (DISE) with endoscopy helps to evaluate the stridor and obstruction rates (supraglottic, hypopharynx, or base of the tongue) that occur throughout sleep.
- With advanced endoscopic management, e.g., balloon dilation and endoscopic
- Laryngeal cleft repair, the surgeon can intervene surgically if indicated.
- (Note: Intermittent laryngospasm may sometimes occur when the airway is dilated by a balloon.)
- Suspension laryngoscopy in conjunction with a microscope has the advantages of:
  - Permits accurate diagnosis and endoscopic intervention capability.
  - The surgeon may use both hands, palpate arytenoid for vocal cord mobility, inspect the interarytenoid region for cleavage, and the size of the airway with serial endotracheal tubes to determine the presence or absence of SGS according to Myer–Cotton scale.
  - It also allows intervention such as steroid injection for hemangioma or stenosis, balloon dilation or laser technology for the management of vascular anomalies or stenosis [2].
- *Types of anesthesia*:
- Different types of anesthesia can be performed during examination of the upper airway; these include:
  - Local nasal fossae anesthesia, with or without associated vasoconstriction, for flexible nasal laryngoscopy in ambulatory clinic.
  - Analgesic gas (50% nitrogen monoxide, 50% oxygen) can be used for uncooperative children but has a few side effects.
  - General operating-room anesthesia. During general anesthesia, various techniques of ventilation can be used:
  - Spontaneous ventilation: involve a compromise between spontaneous ventilation and anesthesia that is sufficiently deep to avoid laryngospasm or bronchospasm when entering the endoscope.

- Disadvantage: Clinical and paramedical team inhalation of anesthetic gas
  - Mechanically controlled ventilation after intubation.
  - Intermittent apnea ventilation:
- Advantage: It provides the surgeon with a satisfactory view.
- Disadvantage: short duration.
  - Transglottic or transtracheal jet ventilation:
  - To provide adequate ventilation, a high ventilation frequency of 150–300 breaths/min and 1–3 bar inbreath pressure.
  - Disadvantage: Barotrauma risk can occur with potential pneumothorax or pneumomediastinum [2].

Take Home Messages
- Proper evaluation of the stridulous patient depends on well understanding of the anatomy, physiology, diagnostic tools and potential interventions and complications of the aerodigestive tract.
- Multidisciplinary approach between anesthetists, otolaryngologists, and intensive care specialists are required in the management of pediatric with a difficult airway.

References

1. Ida JB, Thompson DM. Pediatric stridor. Otolaryngol Clin North Am. 2014;47(5):795–819. https://doi.org/10.1016/j.otc.2014.06.
2. Monnier P. Pediatric airway surgery. Berlin, Heidelberg: Springer Verlag; 2011.
3. Rutter MJ, Link DT, Liu JH, et al. Laryngotracheal reconstruction and the hidden airway lesion. Laryngoscope. 2000;110:1871–4.
4. Schroeder JW Jr, Bhandarkar ND, Holinger LD. Synchronous airway lesions and outcomes in infants with severe laryngomalacia requiring supraglottoplasty. Arch Otolaryngol Head Neck Surg. 2009;135:647–51.
5. Michael J. Strider in children. IAPO, 104_116.
6. Vauthy PA, Reddy R. Acute upper airway obstruction in infants and children. Evaluation by the fiberoptic broncho-scope. Ann Otol Rhinol Laryngol. 1980;89:417–8.

7. Singh C, Gupta M, Sharma S. Compression of trachea due to double aortic arch: demonstration by multi-slice CT scan (MSCT). Heart Lung Circ. 2006;15:332–3.
8. Honnef D, Wildberger JE, Das M, et al. Value of virtual tracheobronchoscopy and bronchography from 16-slice multidetector-row spiral computed tomography for assess-ment of suspected tracheobronchial stenosis in children. Eur Radiol. 2006;16:1684–91.
9. Hill CA, Ramakrishna J, Fracchia MS, et al. Prevalence of eosinophilic esophagitis in children with refractory aerodigestive symptoms. JAMA Otolaryngol Head Neck Surg. 2013;139:903–6.
10. Venkatesan NN, Pine HS, Underbrink M. Laryngopharyngeal reflux disease in children. Pediatr Clin North Am. 2013;60:865–78.
11. John M, Gelins K, et al. Pediatric ENT. Belin, Heidelberg: Springer-Verlag; 2007.

62 Congenital and Acquired Disorders of the Larynx

Aisha Larem, Faisal Abdulkader, Zaid Altamimi, and Amr A. Elhakeem

62.1 Introduction

Pediatric airway disorders may be congenital or acquired and may involve the upper, lower, or entire airway. Pediatric laryngeal disorders usually present with airway obstruction, impaired feeding, and abnormal voice production. Pediatric airway disorders can be life-threatening. The laryngeal and upper airway abnormalities described include laryngomalacia, vocal cord paralysis, laryngeal web, cleft, cyst, subglottic stenosis, hemangioma, papillomatosis, foreign body, and laryngeal trauma.

Knowledge of growth, development, and functional anatomy of the upper airways is important to be able to identify the pathology and diagnose it. Larynx develops from the tracheobronchial groove, which starts on fourth week of intrauterine life. The majority of the anatomical features of larynx develop by the third month of intrauterine life. The larynx is divided into three regions: supraglottis, glottis, and subglottis. The supraglottic larynx comprises the epiglottis, aryepiglottic folds, false cords, and ventricles. The glottis consists of the vocal cords; a normal endoscopic view of the infantile glottis is shown in Fig. 62.1. The subglottis extends from the undersurface of the vocal cords to the inferior border of the cricoid cartilage.

The pediatric airway differs from the adult airway, particularly in infancy. Accordingly, clinical presentation and consequences of laryngeal disorders vary by age.

62.2 Difference Between Pediatric and Adult Larynx

Pediatric upper airway has anatomical differences from adult upper airways; Table 62.1 summarize the differences.

Table 62.1 Differences between pediatrics and adult larynx [1]

Pediatric larynx	Adult larynx
Higher in the neck at level of C2 vertebrae	Lies lower at level of C6 vertebrae
Curved epiglottis/omega shaped in contact soft palate	Flat and broad epiglottis, no contact with soft palate
Oblique thyroid cartilage	Longitudinal thyroid cartilage
Shorter vocal folds 4–4.5 mm	Longer vocal folds 14–23 mm
Vocal process 50% in true vocal folds	Vocal process 25–33% of true vocal folds

A. Larem (✉) · Z. Altamimi · A. A. Alhakeem
Hamad Medical Corporation, Doha, Qatar
e-mail: alarem@hamad.qa; ZAITamimi@hamad.qa

F. Abdulkader
Sidra Hospital, Doha, Qatar
e-mail: fabdulkader@sidra.org

A. Al-Qahtani et al. (eds.), *Textbook of Clinical Otolaryngology*,
https://doi.org/10.1007/978-3-030-54088-3_62

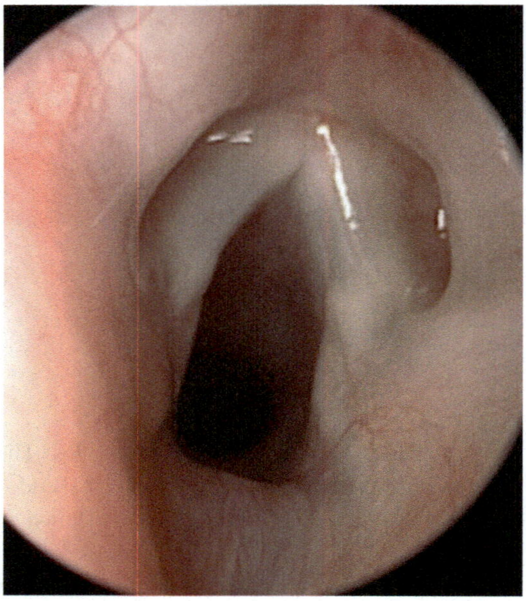

Fig. 62.1 Endoscopic image of normal infantile glottis

Table 62.2 Etiology of laryngeal disorders and upper airway obstruction in pediatrics

Congenital	Acquired
Supraglottic • Laryngomalacia • Saccular cysts and laryngoceles	*Infections* • Laryngotracheo-bronchitis (Croup) • Supraglottitis (Epiglottitis)
Glottis • Vocal cord paralysis • Laryngeal atresia • Laryngeal web	*Reflux disease* • Gastroesophageal reflux disease (GERD) • Laryngopharyngeal reflux (LPR)
Subglottic • Subglottic hemangioma • Congenital subglottic stenosis • Laryngotracheo-esophageal cleft	*Laryngeal trauma* • External • Internal *Others* • Foreign bodies • Papillomatosis

The narrowest part of the infant upper airway is the subglottis (cricoid complete ring); it measures approximately 4.5 by 7 mm in diameter in a full-term infant. Circumferential mucosal edema in infants narrows subglottis by >60% [1]. Figure 62.1 shows an endoscopic view of a normal infantile glottis.

Pediatric upper airway disorders may be congenital affecting different parts of the larynx (supraglottic, glottic, or subglottic) or acquired. The pathophysiology of upper airway obstruction, the clinical presentation, and consequences of airway obstruction vary depend on the underlying pathology. Table 62.2 summarizes the most common etiologies of laryngeal disorders and upper airway obstruction in pediatrics.

62.3 Congenital Anomalies

62.3.1 Supraglottic Anomalies

62.3.1.1 Laryngomalacia

Laryngomalacia is the most common cause of stridor in infants (~60%) [2]. Uncertain pathophysiology thought to be affected by the anatomic factors (floppy supraglottic tissue that leads to a collapse of the supraglottic structures on inspiration), and immature neuromuscular control [3, 4].

Laryngomalacia presents with a high-pitched, fluttering inspiratory stridor, usually present shortly after birth; it is noticeable when the child is lying supine, active or upset, and disappears when lying prone and during sleep. It is more active during the first nine months of life gradually diminishes by 2 years old [2]. Although it is usually considered as non-threatening condition, it can cause complications including severe airway obstruction, cyanosis, difficulty in feeding, failure to thrive, pectus excavatum deformity, and cor pulmonale.

Diagnosis is confirmed by dynamic upper airway study via flexible fiber-optic laryngoscopy or direct laryngoscopy. Figure 62.2 shows an endoscopic view of an infant with laryngomalacia. Examination under general anesthesia is necessary to examine the whole tracheobronchial tree to exclude synchronous airway lesions in patients with severe laryngomalacia or atypical presentation [5].

Management

Most cases will have spontaneous improvement. Medical management can be attained with reflux control, speech-language pathology (SLP) evaluation and feeding strategies. In severe laryngomalacia, surgical intervention

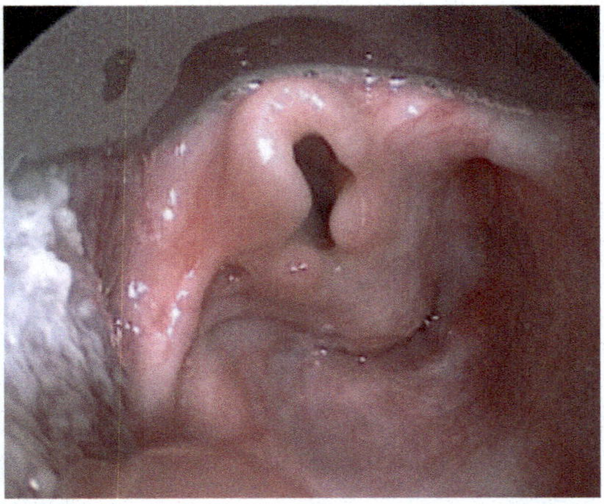

Fig. 62.2 Endoscopic view of an infant with laryngomalacia showing omega-shaped epiglottis and short aryepiglottic fold

might be required. Indications for intervention include severe stridor with failure to thrive, obstructive sleep apnea, weight loss, severe chest deformity, cyanotic attacks, pulmonary hypertension, and cor pulmonale [1]. Surgical intervention is achieved mainly through endoscopic aryepiglottoplasty or supraglottoplasty that include division of aryepiglottic folds, release of epiglottic adhesion, and removal of redundant mucosa, cuneiform, and corniculate cartilages. Tracheostomy might be required in severe cases [2].

62.3.1.2 Saccular Cysts and Laryngoceles

Congenital saccular cysts and laryngoceles are rare (~2%) [6]. The saccular cysts are more common than laryngocele. Saccular cyst is filled with mucus while laryngocele is air-filled, except if it gets obstructed and fill with mucus or become infected, thus becoming like a saccular cyst.

Two types of saccular cyst are identified: the anterior type protrudes into the laryngeal airway between the true and false cords, and the more common lateral type which expands posterosuperiorly into the false cord and aryepiglottic fold [6].

Three types of laryngocele are identified, internal type is confined within the laryngeal framework, the external type when the laryngocele herniates through the thyrohyoid membrane, and the third type is combined [6].

Diagnosis is confirmed by endoscopy, except in the external laryngocele, where no abnormality may be seen except on imaging.

Management

Observation is appropriate in asymptomatic cases. Surgery is indicated if symptomatic by endoscopic marsupialization or lateral cervical approach in case of recurrence [7].

62.3.2 Glottic Anomalies

62.3.2.1 Vocal Cord Paralysis

Vocal cord paralysis is either congenital (second most common congenital anomaly of the larynx after laryngomalacia) or acquired. The. unilateral vocal cord palsy is mainly due to iatrogenic injury to the peripheral nervous system, especially following cardiovascular operations. Bilateral vocal cord palsy is usually the result of a congenital abnormality. Forty five percent of cases are associated with another airway pathology [8].

Etiology vocal cord palsy, unilateral or bilateral include the following:

1. Idiopathic.
2. Iatrogenic, mainly cardiac surgery (esp. patent ductus arteriosus (PDA) ligation with left cord paresis).
3. Trauma; birth trauma is the most common traumatic cause.
4. Neurologic disease as Arnold–Chiari malformation (most common neurological cause), hydrocephalus, cerebral palsy, and hypoxic encephalopathy.
5. Others: malignant disease, familial, brainstem lesions.
6. Drug-related, vinca alkaloids (neurotoxic).

Diagnosis is made through flexible fiber-optic laryngoscopy and other imaging modality as MRI brain, modified barium swallow, speech, and language evaluation.

Management

- Unilateral—rarely any airway/respiratory issues, primarily voice and swallowing. Observation and speech therapy is the usual first step, injection laryngoplasty can be used, and other advanced modalities include reinnervation procedures such as recurrent laryngeal nerve-ansa cervicalis anastomosis [8].

- Bilateral—almost all present with some component of respiratory problems. Observation in case of a patent airway with a spontaneous recovery up to 64% in 5–7 years of age. Surgical options include lateralization suture, lateral cordotomy, partial arytenoidectomy (to be considered at the age of ≥11 years), and cricoid split (endoscopic vs. open); with possible late failures secondary to synkinesis. Tracheostomy is necessary in approximately half the cases [9].

62.3.2.2 Laryngeal Atresia

Uncommon congenital anomaly arises from an incomplete recanalization of the primitive larynx. Incompatible with life unless emergency tracheostomy is performed post-delivery or tracheoesophageal fistula (TOF) presents. Can be diagnosed antenatally on ultrasound imaging and controlled with ex utero intrapartum treatment procedure (EXIT) tracheostomy [10].

62.3.2.3 Laryngeal Web

Laryngeal webs are either congenital (failure of laryngeal canalization) or acquired (post-trauma). It can be found in supraglottic, glottic, and subglottic regions. Anterior glottis webs comprise more than 95% of the cases. Symptoms may appear at any age, which includes hoarse or weak voice, an unusual cry, frequent upper respiratory infections, and stridor.

It is associated with chromosome 22q11.2 deletion syndrome. Diagnosis made with flexible laryngoscopy, micro-laryngoscopy, and bronchoscopy under general anesthesia is used for proper upper airway assessment to confirm the diagnosis and rule out other associated anomalies; it is noticed that longer webs are always thicker than shorter webs. Figure 62.3 shows an anterior laryngeal web between vocal folds.

Cohen's classified congenital glottic web depending on the degree of glottic narrowing as follows [11]:

- *Type I*: Thin anterior web: <35% of the glottic length. Treatment with watchful waiting or CO_2 laser division with mucosal flap.

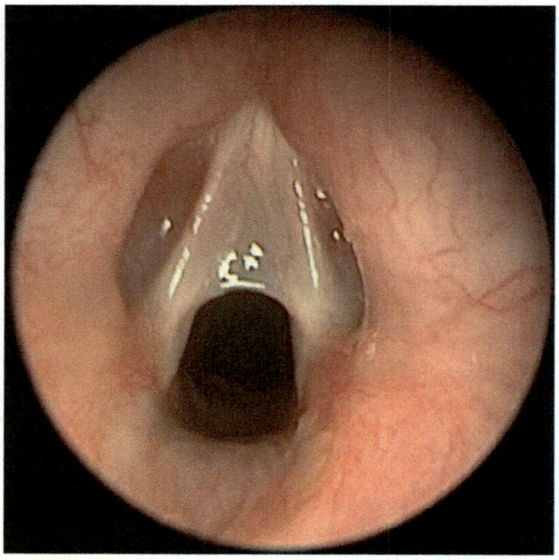

Fig. 62.3 Laryngeal web between vocal folds

- *Type II*: Moderately thick anterior web: 35–50% of the glottic length. Treatment with CO_2 laser division with the endoscopic keel placement to prevent a recurrence.
- *Type III*: Thick anterior web, potentially cartilaginous component 50–75% of the glottic length. Treatment CO_2 laser division with the endoscopic keel or open surgery if a cartilaginous component is present.
- *Type IV*: Uniformly thick web: Cartilaginous segment component 75–90% of the glottic length. Treatment is tracheostomy; two-stage partial cricotracheal resections or laryngotracheal reconstruction with temporary stenting.

62.3.3 Subglottic Anomalies

62.3.3.1 Subglottic Hemangioma

It is a benign vascular tumor. Premature, female and Caucasian newborns are at higher risk of developing a hemangioma. The proliferative phase starts in the 3–4 weeks of life and continues for 4–10 months, then the involuting stage begins around 12 and can talk up to 5–10 years [12].

Subglottic hemangioma is associated with 50% cutaneous lesions, most frequently, with a "beard" distribution. Symptoms include biphasic stridor, croup (barking cough), and failure to

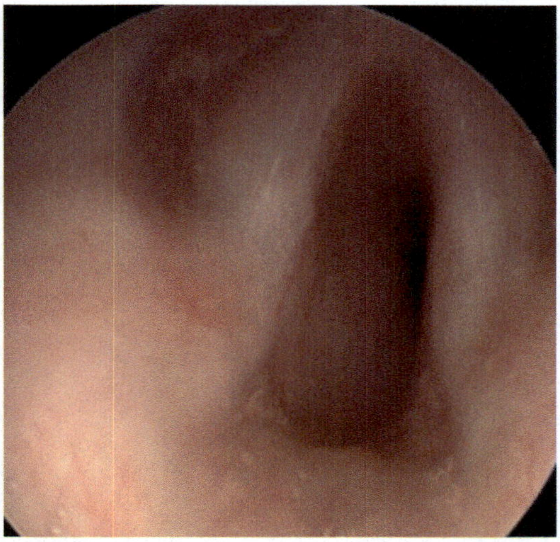

Fig. 62.4 Endoscopic view of subglottic hemangioma

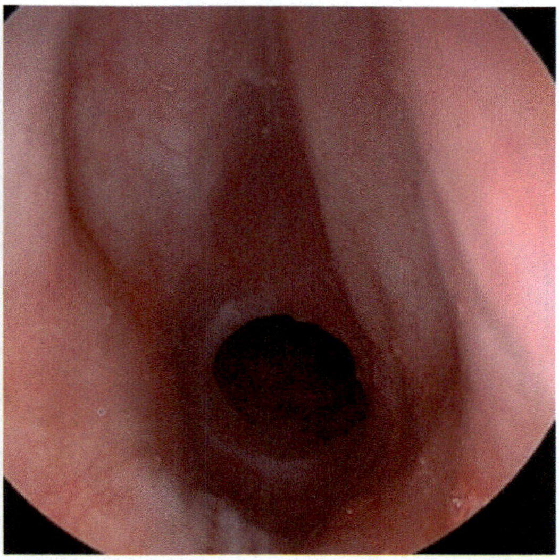

Fig. 62.5 Endoscopic view of a subglottic stenosis

thrive. Diagnosis is made by micro-laryngoscopy and bronchoscopy under general anesthesia. Fig. 62.4 shows an endoscopic view of a subglottic hemangioma. MRI or CT scans can help to identify the severity and site of the lesion.

Management

It depends on the severity of the airway compromised. Observation if the airway is not compromised and asymptomatic. Medical treatment with beta-blockers (propranolol) and high-dose steroids is efficient. Surgical intervention via an endoscopic trial with CO_2 laser or cryotherapy or intralesional injections can be considered. The open laryngofissure approach is an alternative for failure of endoscopic interventions [13].

62.3.3.2 Congenital Subglottic Stenosis

Congenital subglottic stenosis results from defective canalization of the cricoid cartilage and/or conus elasticus. Clinically presents with biphasic stridor and recurrent croup. Diagnosed by micro-laryngoscopy and bronchoscopy under general anesthesia. It is graded by Cotton–Myer to four grades, Fig. 62.5 shows grade III subglottic stenosis. The grading system is described below:

Cotton–Myer grading system of subglottic stenosis [14]:

- *Grade I*: < 50%.
- *Grade II*: 51–70%.
- *Grade III*: 71–99%.
- *Grade IV*: No detectable lumen, complete obliteration.

Management

Surgical intervention is the mainstay treatment, the options depend on the grade and severity and it includes the following:

- Grade I/II endoscopic intervention using a CO_2 laser, Baloon dilation, or cold knife. With/without application of mitomycin C application. Congenital cartilaginous stenosis is a strict contraindication for endoscopic dilation or laser resection.
- Grade III/IV: tracheostomy, laryngotracheoplasty (LTR), or partial cricotracheal resection (PCTR).

62.3.3.3 Laryngeal Cleft

A result from a failure of the posterior cricoid lamina to fuse with or without incomplete development of the tracheo-esophageal septum leading to the slit-defect of the "party wall" between the laryngotracheal airway and the upper digestive tract. Presents with cyanotic attacks on feeding, recurrent chest infections, stridor, and abnormal cry. Type IV clefts cause severe aspiration, cyanosis, and cardiorespiratory failure.

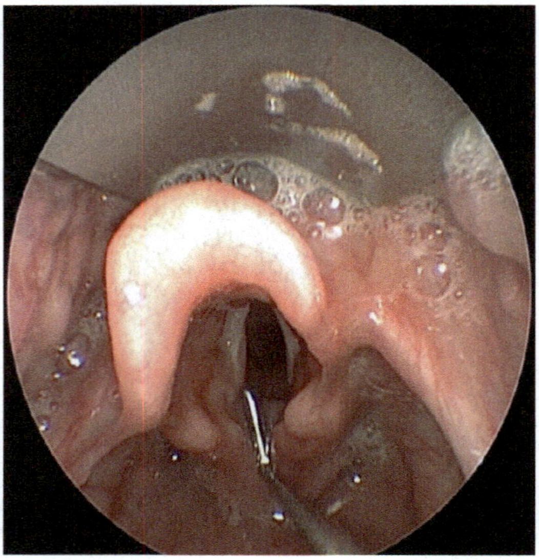

Fig. 62.6 Endoscopic view of laryngeal cleft

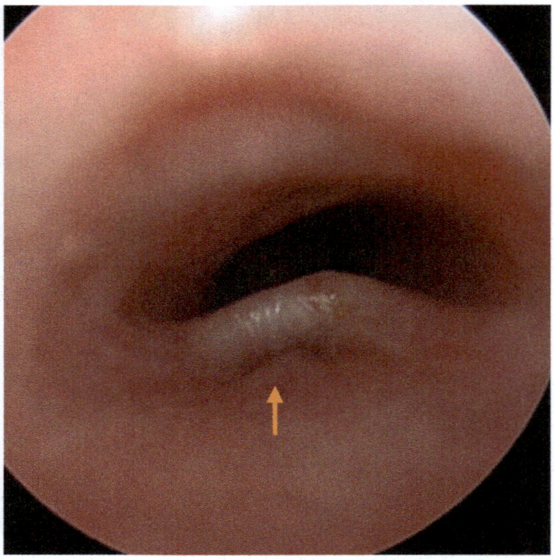

Fig. 62.7 Tracheo-esophageal fistula (red arrow)

Diagnosis is made through esophagram with water-soluble contrast and direct rigid laryngo-tracheo-bronchoscopy with probing of posterior cleft "gold standard." Figure 62.6 shows an endoscopic view of laryngeal cleft with probing.

Benjamin and Inglis classified laryngeal cleft to four types [15]:

- *Type I*: supraglottic interarytenoid cleft to the level of vocal cords. Treatment includes observation, modified diet, injection laryngoplasty, and endoscopic repair.
- *Type II*: partial cricoid cleft extends below the level of vocal cords. Treatment includes observation, diet modification, injection laryngoplasty, and endoscopic or open (extended laryngofissure) repair.
- *Type III*: total cricoid cleft, into the cervical extrathoracic trachea. Treatment includes diet modification, tracheotomy with endoscopic or open (extended laryngofissure) repair.
- *Type IV*: laryngotracheoesophageal cleft (extending into the thoracic trachea). It is challenging to repair and has a poor prognosis.

Management

Laryngeal cleft management depends on the type and severity of the anomaly. The surgical repair of the cleft is undertaken in three layers to optimize healing; the two mucosal layers are reinforced by an interposition graft (tibial periosteum or temporalis fascia).

Type IV cleft presents a more difficult surgical challenge because of the length of the cleft; a tracheostomy is unhelpful, and using a single-stage technique with an anterior cervicothoracic approach via a median sternotomy is recommended. Mortality remains significant, being around 14% overall rising to 66% for type IV laryngotracheoesophageal clefts. The management should be carried with a multidisciplinary team, preferably in a pediatric center.

62.3.3.4 Tracheoesophageal Fistula (TEF)

Presents with immediate feeding problems and aspiration with an inability to pass the feeding tube. Tracheoesophageal fistula has five types, the most common type is esophageal atresia with distal TEF. H-type may present with recurrent pneumonia. The diagnosis is confirmed by fluoroscopy and endoscopy. Figure 62.7 shows an endoscopic view of tracheoesophageal fistula. Surgical correction is required with a considerable risk of postoperative stricture.

Types:

1. Esophageal atresia with distal TEF (85%).
2. Isolated esophageal atresia (10%).
3. H-Type TEF (4%).

4. Esophageal atresia with proximal TEF (0.5–1.0%).
5. Esophageal atresia with proximal and distal TEF (0.5%).

62.4 Acquired

62.4.1 Infections

62.4.1.1 Laryngotracheobronchitis (Croup)

This occurs between the ages of 6 months and 3 years. Parainfluenza virus with types I–III is the most common pathogen. Presents with the classical "croupy" cough ("barking" cough) and stridor. Diagnosed mainly by the clinical presentation, anterior-posterior soft tissue neck X-ray shows "steeple sign" which is demonstrated in Fig. 62.8 [16].

Management

It includes humidification and hydration, aerosolized epinephrine, and high-dose corticosteroids. Tracheostomy is rarely required.

62.4.1.2 Acute supraglottitis (Epiglottitis)

Classically caused by H. influenzae type B. Immunization lead to a dramatic decrease in the incidence of supraglottitis. Peak incidence occurs among 2- to 4-year-old age group. Clinically presents with rapid onset of fever, sore throat, inspiratory stridor, muffled voice, sniffing position, and drooling of saliva [16].

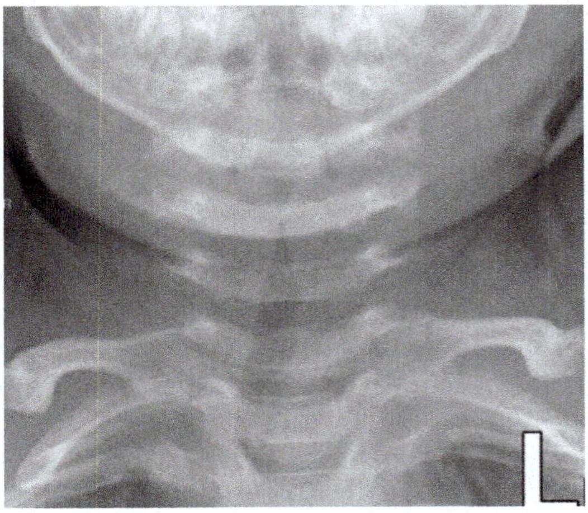

Fig. 62.8 X-ray image shows a steeple sign in cases of croup

Diagnosed mainly by the clinical presentation. Lateral neck X-ray shows the classical "thumbprint sign."

ManagementSecuring the airway should be prioritized in this condition. Avoid procedures (intravenous access, unnecessary physical examination, and diagnostic tests) that might increase the child's anxiety until after the airway is secured. Medical management can be started with aerosolized epinephrine, high-dose corticosteroids. Patients with signs of an advancing upper airway obstruction should be taken to the operative theater immediately to establish the diagnosis and control the airway with intubation with the readiness of a team capable of performing an immediate tracheotomy if needed. Then medical management can be resumed with adding antimicrobial therapy. Extubation is usually possible after 48–72 h.

62.4.2 Gastroesophageal Reflux Disease (GERD)

In pediatric patients, it considered as a causative/aggravating factor for the following disorders:

1. Laryngomalacia.
2. Laryngotracheal stenosis.
3. Laryngitis.
4. Laryngotracheobronchitis.

Diagnosis is made through barium swallow and 24-h esophageal pH monitoring which currently considered as the "gold standard."

Management

Lifestyle modification (lose weight, dietary and behavioral modifications), and a proton-pump inhibitor. Surgical anti-reflux intervention rarely is needed.

62.4.3 Laryngeal Trauma

The pediatric larynx is less prone to injury due to its high position in the neck. Trauma in pediatrics

Table 62.3 Schaefer classification of laryngeal injury

Grade	Findings
Grade 1	Minor endolaryngeal hematomas or lacerations without detectable fractures
Grade 2	More severe edema, hematoma, minor mucosal disruption without exposed cartilage, or non-displaced fractures
Grade 3	Massive edema, large mucosal lacerations, exposed cartilage, displaced fractures, or vocal cord immobility
Grade 4	Same as group 3, but more severe with disruption of anterior larynx, unstable fractures, two or more fracture lines, or severe mucosal injuries
Grade 5	Complete laryngotracheal separation

Source: Schaefer SD. Primary management of laryngeal trauma. Ann Otol Rhinol Laryngol. 1982;91(4 Pt 1):399–402

mainly leads to edema, hematoma, and airway disruption, which can be life-threatening. While true fractures of the pediatric larynx are very rare due its pliable cartilages.

A patient known to have sustained blunt trauma to the neck should be managed with a high index of suspicion for an impending airway problem. Table 62.3 shows the classification of laryngeal injury.

Schaefer Classification System for Determining the Severity of Laryngeal Injuries

Management

Mild injury requires close observation for the airway and medical treatment including steroids, antibiotics, and anti-reflux.

In more severe injuries, secure airway by endotracheal intubation or tracheostomy. When condition becomes stable, complete endoscopic investigation with direct laryngotracheoscopy and bronchoesophagoscopy under general anesthesia. CT scan of the larynx can be useful [17]. In case of disrupted larynx, surgical repair aims to restoring the anatomical and functional integrity of the larynx.

Open surgical exploration by means of laryngofissure with/without stenting. Stenting is required in case of anterior commissure involvement, multiple displaced fractures, or multiple severe lacerations. The condition becomes stable, complete endoscopic investigation with direct laryngotracheoscopy and bronchoesophagoscopy under general anesthesia. CT scan of the larynx can be useful [17]. In a case of a disrupted larynx, surgical repair aims to restoring the anatomical and functional integrity of the larynx.

62.4.4 Corrosive Ingestion

Acidic ingestion leads to coagulative necrosis which is usually superficial. While alkaline ingestion leads to liquefactive necrosis with deeper penetration. Should be treated seriously, as the patient may present with compromised airway [18]. Patients can also present with hot potato voice; drooling, stridor, and dysphonia.

Grading

Grade 1: mucosal erythema

Grade 2: mucosal erythema with non-circumferential exudates

Grade 3: circumferential exudates

Grade 4: circumferential exudates with perforation

Management

Medical management through keeping the patient nil per os (NPO), avoid inducing vomiting, start on IV fluid, steroids, antibiotics, and proton-pump inhibitors. Esophagoscopy and laryngoscopic evaluations at 24/72 h are needed to examine the severity and complications of the injury.

Grade 1–2 injury; Observation, consider steroids [19].

Grade 3–4 injury; more aggressive management, may require laryngeal balloon dilatation or esophagectomy [19]. Figure 62.9 shows balloon dilatation for a patient complicated with tracheal stenosis after corrosive ingestion.

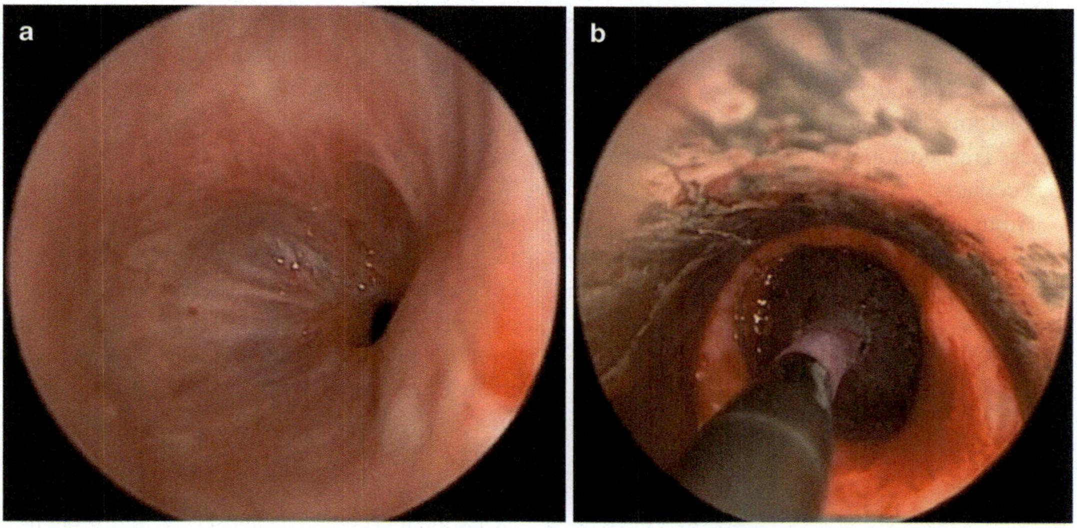

Fig. 62.9 (**a**) Pre-operative endoscopic view of tracheal stenosis post erosive injury. (**b**) Endoscopic view of the undergoing balloon dilatation

62.4.5 Intubation Injury

Endotracheal intubation can traumatize mucosa either directly or indirectly from cuff pressure necrosis. Endotracheal tube cuff pressures >20 mmHg will exceed the capillary filling pressure and cause ischemic damage over time. Intubation injury can lead to mucosal ulceration with chondritis and healing by fibrosis with contracture. The most common site for injury is the cricoid ring [20].

Management

Medical treatment includes systemic steroid, anti-reflex, and antibiotic.

Laryngoscopy at 2- to 3-week intervals is required to assess progress.

62.4.6 Vocal Abuse

Common in screamer children. Presents as fluctuating voice change due to edema of the vocal cords; hoarseness can be due to vocal cord nodules. Diagnosed by awake flexible laryngoscopy.

Management

Speech therapy is the mainstay of management. Vocal cord surgery is not indicated unless there is a specific pathology that needs to be considered.

62.4.7 Recurrent Respiratory Papillomatosis (RRP)

Most common benign tumors of the larynx are caused by HPV 6, 11. Develops at the junction of squamous and respiratory epithelium. High-risk factors include young primigravid mother, vaginal delivery, and firstborn child. Mostly due to vertical maternal transmission. RRP can present with abnormal crying, hoarseness, stridor, respiratory distress, or as a ball-valving glottic lesion [21].

Types:

- Juvenile onset (<12 years old): more common, more aggressive.
- Adult onset.

Diagnosis is made through microlaryngoscopy with bronchotracheoscopy for evaluation of airway and biopsy. Figure 62.10 shows an endoscopic direct laryngoscopy view of laryngeal papillomatosis.

Management

Observation in case the child is asymptomatic and no significant airway obstruction. Surgical interventions should emphasize on function preservation; the surgical debulking is done using a CO_2 laser, microdebrider as shown in Fig. 62.11, or cold knife; it might be required for multiple times. Tracheostomy should be avoided unless it is necessary.

Adjuvant therapies as interferon and cidofovir can be considered. It is indicated in case of more than 4 surgeries/year, need for tracheostomy, distal pulmonary spread, and rapid regrowth of disease with airway compromise.

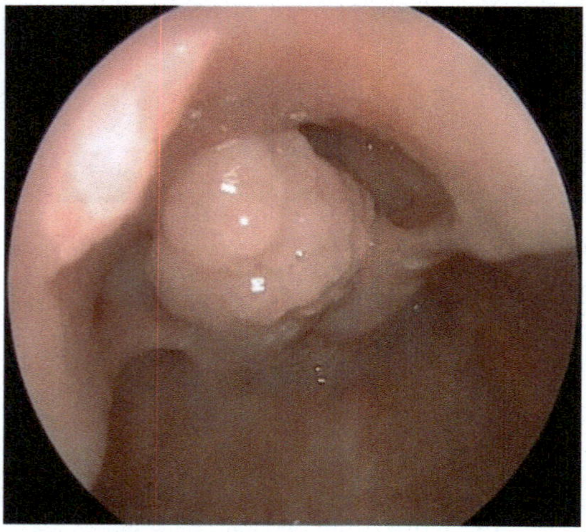

Fig. 62.10 Laryngeal papillomatosis

62.4.8 Foreign Bodies

Large obstructing foreign bodies (FB) may lodge in the laryngeal inlet, causing acute, fatal airway compromise. Esophageal foreign bodies are usually impacted at anatomical points where other structures are compressing the esophagus, it includes cricopharyngeus, aortic arch, left mainstem bronchus, and lower esophageal sphincter.

Management

Esophagoscopy, laryngoscopy, and bronchoscopy under general anesthesia are used to remove the FB. Consider evaluation for esophageal stricture, peristaltic dysfunction, and/ eosinophilic esophagitis.

Some foreign bodies can be followed with serial X-rays to ensure passage with observation for 24 h. Sharp objects and batteries ("double-halo sign") shown in Fig. 62.12 may lead to catastrophic complications and mortality and should be promptly removed [22].

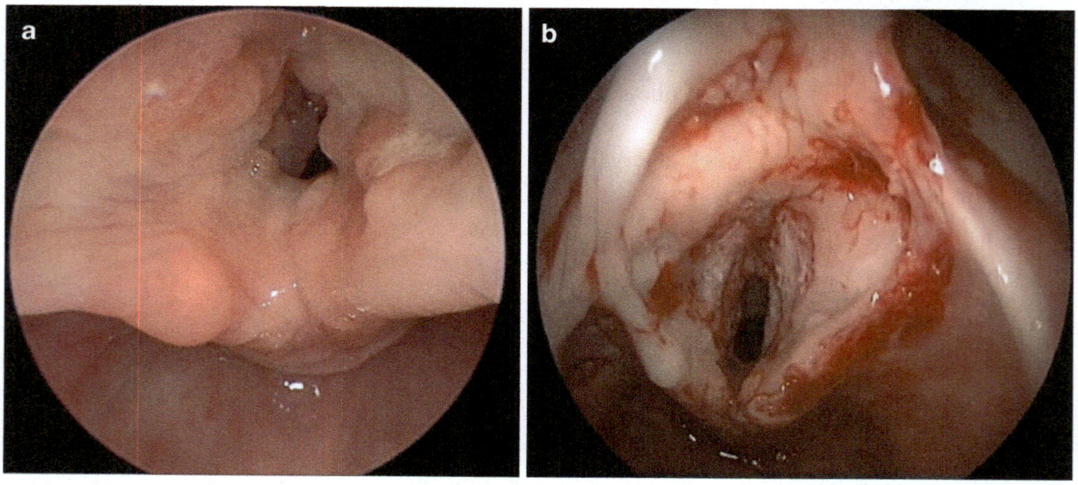

Fig. 62.11 (**a**) Pre-operative endoscopic view of laryngeal papillomatosis. (**b**) Endoscopic view of the larynx after excision of laryngeal papillomatosis with microdebrider

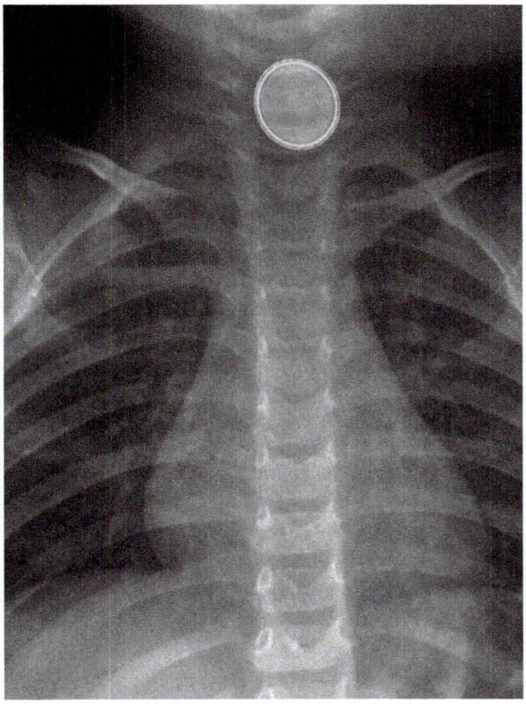

Fig. 62.12 Chest X-ray showing a metallic foreign body (battery) with double hallow sign

Take Home Massages

- Laryngomalacia is the most common cause of stridor in infants. However, surgery is indicated only if there is failure to thrive.
- Direct laryngoscopy should be considered in all cases of bilateral vocal cord palsy as 45% are associated with other upper airway anomalies.
- More severe airway pathology is less likely to respond to endoscopic versus open interventions.
- Endotracheal tube cuff pressures >20 mmHg will exceed the capillary filling pressure and cause ischemic damage over time.
- For any child with stridor and cutaneous lesion, subglottic hemangioma should be ruled out.
- Recurrent croup infections require direct laryngo-bronchoscopy to rule out subglottic stenosis.

Acknowledgement Authors of the chapter would like to appreciate the help of Dr. Adham Aljariri, an ENT resident in Hamad medical corporation of his help and effort in editing the chapter.

References

1. Lin FY, Patel ZM, editors. ENT Board Prep: high yield review for the otolaryngology in-service and board exams. New York: Springer Science Business Media; 2014. p. 19–24. https://doi.org/10.1007/978-1-4614-8354-0_4.
2. Monnier P. Laryngomalacia (LM). Pediatric airway surgery. Berlin, Heidelberg: Springer-Verlag; 2011. p. 100–5. https://doi.org/10.1007/978-3-642-13535-4.
3. Belmont JR, Grundfast K. Congenital laryngeal stridor (laryngomalacia): etiologic factors and associated disorders. Ann Otol Rhinol Laryngol. 1984;93:430–7.
4. Thompson DM. Abnormal sensorimotor integrative function of the larynx in congenital laryngomalacia: a new theory of etiology. Laryngoscope. 2007;117:1–33.
5. Toynton SC, Saunders MW, Bailey CM. Aryepiglottoplasty for laryngomalacia: 100 consecutive cases. J Laryngol Otol. 2001;115:35–8.
6. DeSanto LW, Devine KD, Weiland LH. Cysts of the larynx–classification. Laryngoscope. 1970;80:145–76.
7. Monnier P. Ductal cysts, saccular cysts and laryngoceles. Pediatric airway surgery. Berlin, Heidelberg: Springer-Verlag; 2011. p. 142–5. https://doi.org/10.1007/978-3-642-13535-4.
8. Monnier P. Vocal cord paralysis. Pediatric airway surgery. Berlin, Heidelberg: Springer-Verlag; 2011. p. 108–16. https://doi.org/10.1007/978-3-642-13535-4.
9. Smith ME. Vocal fold paralysis in children. In: Sulica L, Blitzer A, editors. Vocal fold paralysis. Berlin, Heidelberg: Springer; 2006. p. 225–35.
10. Morrison G. Exit-antenatal (pre-natal) diagnoses and management. In: Graham JM, Scadding GK, Bull PD, editors. Pediatric ENT. Berlin, Heidelberg: Springer; 2008. p. 73–81.
11. Cohen SR. Congenital glottic webs in children. A retrospective review of 51 patients. Ann Otol Rhinol Laryngol Suppl. 1985;121:2–16.
12. Bruckner AL, Frieden IJ. Infantile hemangiomas. J Am Acad Dermatol. 2006;55:671–82.
13. Monnier P. Subglottic haemangioma. Pediatric airway surgery. Berlin, Heidelberg: Springer-Verlag; 2011. p. 134–9. https://doi.org/10.1007/978-3-642-13535-4.
14. Myer CM III, O'Connor DM, Cotton RT. Proposed grading system for subglottic stenosis based on endotracheal tube sizes. Ann Otol Rhinol Laryngol. 1994;103:319–23.
15. Benjamin B, Inglis A. Minor congenital laryngeal clefts: diagnosis and classification. Ann Otol Rhinol Laryngol. 1989;98:417–20.

16. Sobol SE, Zapata S. Epiglottitis and croup. Otolaryngol Clin North Am. 2008;41(3):551–66. ix
17. Monnier P. External laryngeal trauma. Pediatric airway surgery. Berlin, Heidelberg: Springer-Verlag; 2011. p. 200–14. https://doi.org/10.1007/978-3-642-13535-4.
18. Holinger LD. Caustic ingestion. In: Cotton RT, Myer CMI, editors. Practical pediatric otolaryngology. Philadelphia, New York: Lippincott-Raven; 1999. p. 595–602.
19. Kay M, Wyllie R. Caustic ingestions in children. Curr Opin Pediatr. 2009;21(5):651–4.
20. Benjamin B. Prolonged intubation injuries of the larynx: endoscopic diagnosis, classification, and treatment. Ann Otol Rhinol Laryngol Suppl. 1993;160:1–15.
21. Monnier P. Recurrent respiratory papillomatosis. Pediatric airway surgery. Berlin, Heidelberg: Springer-Verlag; 2011. p. 220–2. https://doi.org/10.1007/978-3-642-13535-4.
22. Maves MD, Carithers JS, Birck HG. Esophageal burns secondary to disc battery ingestion. Ann Otol Rhinol Laryngol. 1984;93:364–9.

ENT-Related Syndromes

63

Faisal Abdulkader
and Mai Ahmed Mohamed Elhassan Ahmed

Key Points

- Management of ENT-related syndromes are best approached through a multidisciplinary team [1, 2].
- Management of snoring and obstructive sleep apnea in a syndromic child is usually secondary to multiple factors including craniofacial anomalies, hypotonia and hypertrophy and of the tonsils and adenoids [3].
- Hearing impairment is common in a syndromic child. Hearing restoration is an essential component in their management [4].
- A systematic approach to investigation and management of a child with suspected syndrome is of utmost importance [3].

F. Abdulkader (✉)
Clinical Otolaryngology Head & Neck Surgery, Weill Cornell Medical College-Qatar, Doha, Qatar
e-mail: Fabdulkader@sidra.org

M. A. M. E. Ahmed
Sidra Medicine & Research Center, Doha, Qatar
e-mail: melhasenahmed@sidra.org

63.1 Introduction

- A *syndrome* is a group of anomalies that collectively indicate or characterize a disease in which the genetic cause behind it has been identified (e.g., Down syndrome).
- An *association* is a group of anomalies that happen together in which a genetic cause has not yet been identified (e.g., VACTREL association).
- A *sequence* is a descriptive term indicating a single anomaly that leads to other anomalies in the near surrounding structures (e.g., Pierre Robin sequence) [3].
- ENT surgeons most commonly must deal with two distinct presentations:
  – A child who has already been diagnosed with a syndrome: In this presentation, the ENT surgeon must know about the syndrome and its ENT presentations.
  – A child who has not been diagnosed yet and the ENT surgeons suspect a syndrome [1].
- The most common ENT presentations in syndromic child are related to hearing and airway compromise. Other manifestations could include swallowing and feeding difficulties [3].

A. Al-Qahtani et al. (eds.), *Textbook of Clinical Otolaryngology*,
https://doi.org/10.1007/978-3-030-54088-3_63

63.2 General Approach for Evaluation to the Child with Suspected Syndrome

History

History of pregnancy, perinatal and postnatal period is essential in any child with suspected syndrome:

- NICU admission.
- Postnatal infection.
- Exposure to ototoxic medications (e.g., aminoglycosides).
- Co-existing medical conditions (e.g., diabetes, renal disease in the individual and in the family).
- Developmental milestones.
- Family history of hearing loss in first- and second-degree relatives.
- Consanguinity and ethnic origin.
- Hereditary traits within the family.

Examination

A full head and neck examination should be performed to include:

- The overall appearance of the child: normal vs dysmorphic features.
- Shape and position of the external ears (many syndromes).
- Neck examination for cysts, sinuses and scars (branchio-oto-renal syndrome) and swelling of the thyroid gland (may indicate Pendred syndrome).
- Unusual pigmentation of the hair, skin, or eyes (which may indicate an auditory pigmentary disorder).
- Gait and balance should be noted to test the vestibular system.

Investigation

Any child where a syndrome is suspected, the following should be considered:

- Referral to clinical geneticist.
- Referral to cardiology: Echo and ECG, for possible association with Jervell and Lange-Nielsen syndrome or congenital heart conditions.
- Referral to Radiology: CT/ MRI imaging.
- Referral to Ophthalmology: for assessment of visual acuity and dilated fundoscopy as minimum, also for electroretinogram if suspected Usher syndrome.
- Audiology for hearing assessment.
- Thyroid function tests.
- Dipstick of urine: for microscopic hematuria, associated undiagnosed nephritis and nephropathy are rare.

Management of a Child with a Syndrome

- Management of a child with a syndrome is best achieved in a multidisciplinary team (MDT) approach.
- The MDT consists of multiple disciplines; however, most commonly an ENT surgeon is part of a craniofacial head and neck MDT which includes: Craniofacial, ENT, Neurosurgery, Orthodontist, Ophthalmology, Speech and Language therapy, and Audiology. Clinical input from other surgical and medical disciplines is usually required depending on the need of each child [1].

63.3 Syndromes of Particular Relevance to the ENT Surgeon

63.3.1 Pierre Robin Sequence

Characterized by classic triad features (Fig. 63.1):

1. Retrognathia
2. Glossoptosis
3. Cleft palate
    - Pathological *sequence*: Retrognathia prevents descent of the tongue into the oral cavity which prevents secondary palate fusion.

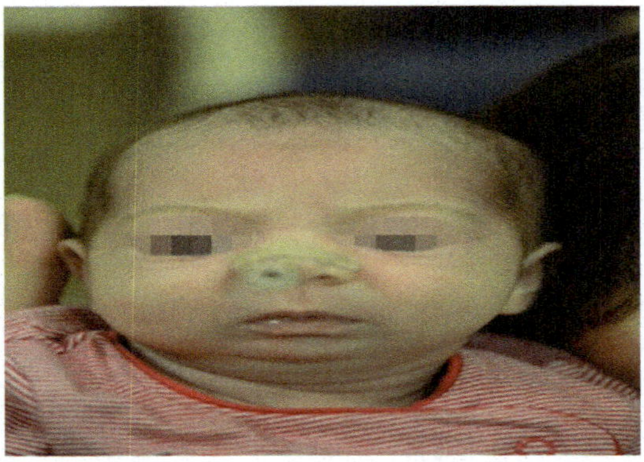

Fig. 63.1 Pierre Robin sequence showing retrognathia, which in this case requires nasopharyngeal airway

- Isolated or syndromic association in 50–80% of cases, most commonly Stickler, and velocardiofacial syndrome.
- Conservative management: in a progressive sequence:
  - Prone positioning
  - Nasopharyngeal airway: most effective management markedly reducing the need for surgical intervention
  - Endotracheal intubation
- Surgical management:
- Tongue–lip adhesion
- Mandibular distraction osteogenesis
- Tracheostomy [4]

63.3.2 Down Syndrome

Genetics

Down syndrome is the most common chromosomal disorder, and ENT sequelae occur frequently [5].

- Most commonly a trisomy of chromosome21, however small proportion could be caused by translocations.
- Incidence is approximately 1 in 700 livebirths.
- Increased risk of trisomy 21 with conceptions and maternal age.
- Antenatal diagnosis is available [1].

ENT Features (Fig. 63.2)

1. Small ears.
2. Narrow external ear canals: can make it difficult to view the tympanic membrane or insert grommets.
3. Increased incidence of glue ear: age related.
4. Otoacoustic emissions often non-reproducible, even in patients with normal hearing ability.
5. Abnormal ossicles.
6. Hearing loss: Mixed (7%) Sensorineural deafness (8%).
7. Airway obstruction from small posterior nasal spine with large tonsils and adenoids.
8. Macroglossia.
9. Subglottis: usually require one anesthetic tube size smaller than expected.
10. Unstable neck, with a risk of atlanto-occipital joint subluxation in 15%, especially during general anesthetic [1].

General Features

1. Typical facial features include:
   - Brachycephaly.
   - Up slanting palpebral fissures.
   - Epicanthic folds and brush field spots (speckling of iris).
   - Flat facial profile.
   - Small nose with depressed nasal bridge.
2. Mental retardation.
3. Hypotonia: contributes to delayed motor milestones, snoring, and OSA.
4. Joint laxity.
5. Congenital heart disease.
6. Single palmar crease.
7. Wide sandal gap (gap between first and second toes).
8. Other medical problems (e.g., hypothyroidism, leukemia).
9. Other congenital problems (e.g., duodenal atresia, Hirschsprung disease) [1].

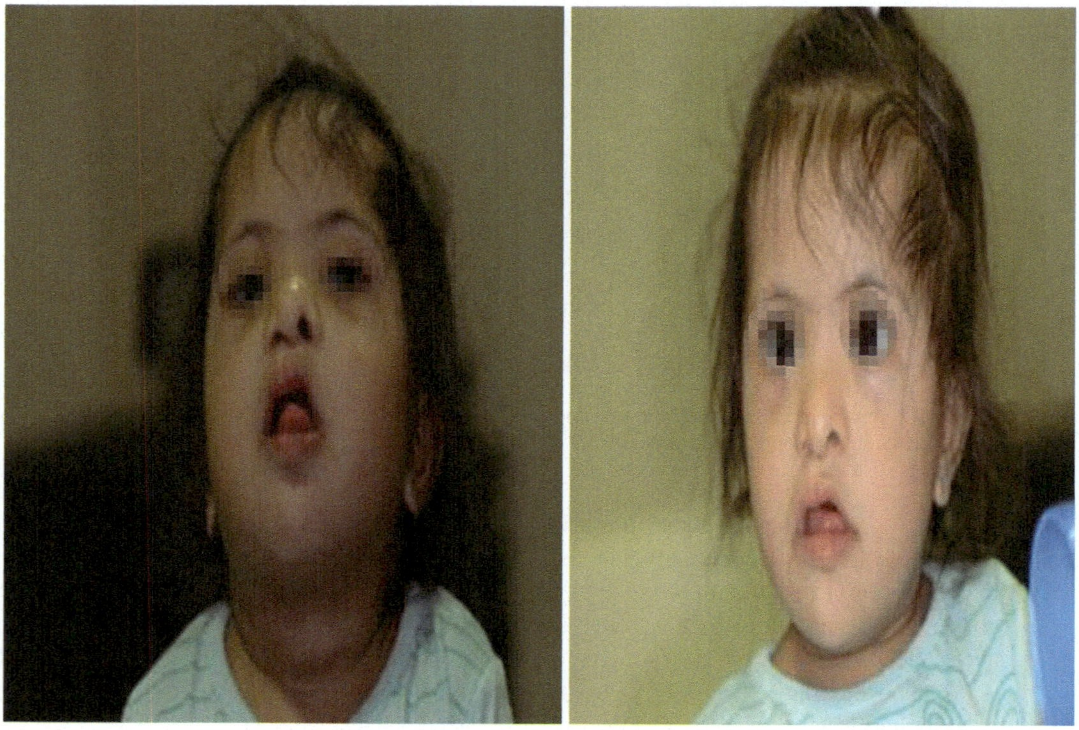

Fig. 63.2 Down syndrome, showing small nose with depressed nasal bridge, and small ears

63.4 Autosomal Dominant Syndromes

63.4.1 Treacher Collins Syndrome

Genetics

- Treacher Collins syndrome (TCS) is a disorder of branchial arch development.
- It is inherited in an autosomal dominant manner and the only gene currently known to be associated is *TCOF1*.
- Classically: features are bilateral, and symmetrical.

ENT Features (Fig. 63.3)

1. Microtia, dysplastic ears (bilateral ear anomalies).
2. Auricular pits/fistula/tags.
3. Deafness: usually conductive due to external auditory canal atresia and malformations of the ossicles.
4. Cleft palate.
5. Micrognathia: cleft palate and micrognathia together may result in significant airway problems in neonates.
6. Mandibular hypoplasia.
7. Flat malar region.
8. Prominent nose.
9. Broad mouth.
10. Narrow nasopharynx.
11. Choanal atresia (rare).

General Features

Typical facial features include:

- downslanting palpebral fissures.
- Coloboma of inferior eyelid.
- Sparse eyelashes [1].

63.4.2 Goldenhar Syndrome (Oculo-Auriculovertebral Spectrum)

Genetics

- First and second branchial arch syndrome [1].

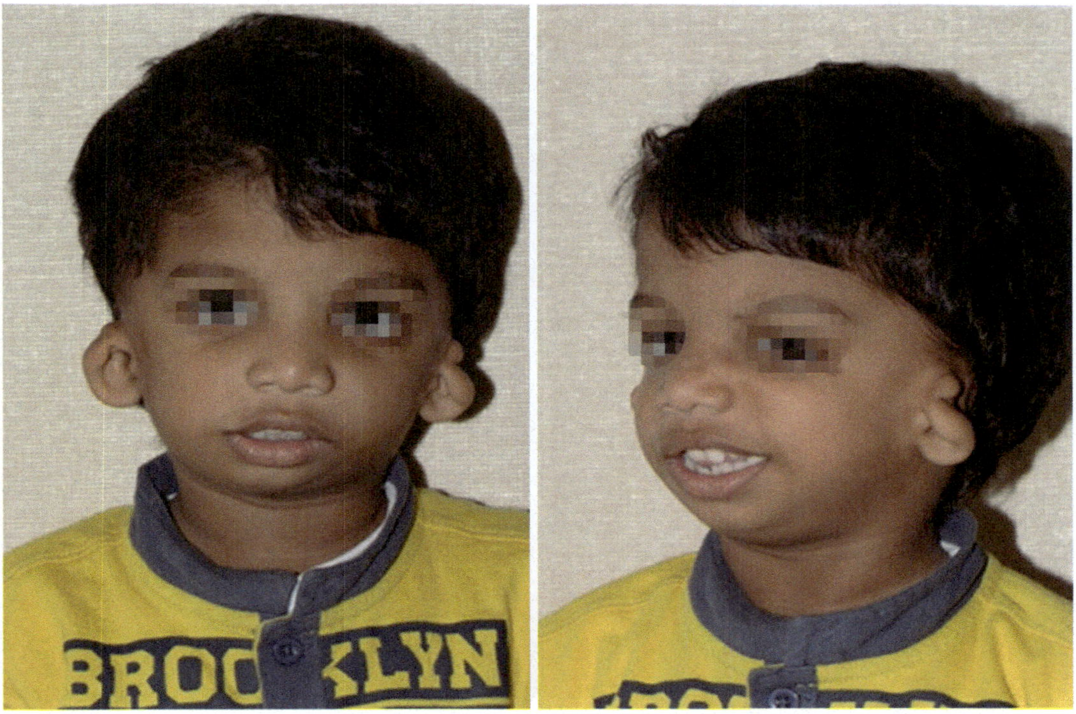

Fig. 63.3 Treacher Collins Syndrome, showing microtia and mandibular hypoplasia

- Most cases sporadic, some autosomal dominant transmission [4].

ENT Features
- Hemifacial macrosomia.
- Unilateral facial asymmetry, unilateral external and middle ear changes.
- Otologic findings: mildly deformed ears to anotia, EAC atresia and ossicular abnormalities [1].

General Features
- Ocular findings: upper lid colobomata.
- Underdevelopment of mandible, orbit, facial muscles, also may have hemivertebrae of vertebral column [3, 4].

63.4.3 CHARGE Syndrome

The term "CHARGE" is taken from its main features:

- Coloboma
- Heart defect
- Atresia choanae
- Retardation of growth and development
- Genital defect and ear anomalies and/or deafness [1]

Genetics
- Mutations in the gene *CHD7* can be identified in approximately 65% of cases.
- Prevalence of approximately 1 in 12,000.
- Diagnosis of CHARGE syndrome is made on the basis of clinical features and temporal bone imaging.
- Unilateral or bilateral, asymmetrical congenital defects involving the first and second branchial arches [1].

ENT Features (Fig. 63.4)
1. Microtia: Usually unilateral or bilateral.
2. Pre-auricular skin tags.
3. Deafness: sensorineural and/or conductive.
4. Middle ear: ossicular malformations.
5. Temporal bone abnormalities: absent or hypoplastic semicircular canals.

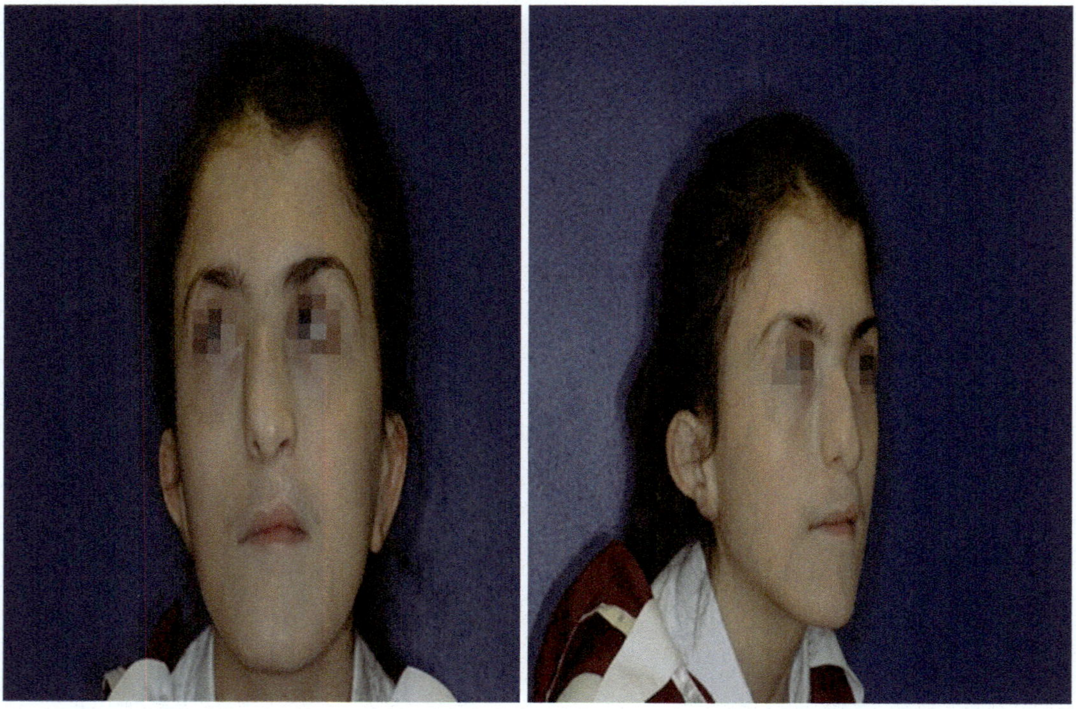

Fig. 63.4 Charge syndrome showing coloboma

6. Macrostomia: occasionally with lateral facial clefting.
7. Choanal atresia/stenosis (unilateral or bilateral) [1].

General Features
1. Facial asymmetry.
2. Epibulbar dermoid.
3. Vertebral defects.
4. Cardiac defects.
5. Renal anomalies.
6. Mental retardation [1].

63.4.4 Branchio-Oto-Renal Syndrome (Melnick–Fraser Syndrome)

Genetics
- This is an autosomal dominant disorder.
- Characterized by external, middle and inner ear anomalies, branchial sinuses and renal dysplasia.
- It is caused by mutations in the *EYA1* gene (less commonly in the *SIX-1* gene) [1].

ENT Features
1. Ear anomalies: pits in the pre-helical region and dysplastic pinnae.
2. Conductive (due to ossicular malformations), sensorineural,or mixed hearing impairment. Inner ear malformations may include Mondini dysplasia of the cochlea, and occasionally, dilated vestibular aqueducts could be found.
3. Branchial fistulae and/or cysts [1].

General Features

Renal malformations: duplex collecting system, hydronephrosis, dysplasia, unilateral or bilateral renal agenesis [1].

63.4.5 22q11.2 Deletion Syndrome

Also known as velocardiofacial syndrome, DiGeorge syndrome, and Shprintzen syndrome.

Genetics

- Inherited in an autosomal dominant pattern.
- The phenotype can be very variable.
- 90% have a de novo deletion of chromosome 22q11.2, but the remaining 10% have inherited it from either parent [1].

ENT Features

Palate

1. Overt or submucous cleft palate.
2. Velopharyngeal incompetence.
3. Hypernasal speech.

Ears

1. Small, low-set ears.
2. Prominent/over folded helices.
3. Absent or hypoplastic ear lobules.
4. Pre-auricular tags.
5. Otitis media.
6. Sensorineural hearing loss.
7. Narrow external auditory canals [1].

63.4.6 Waardenburg Syndrome

Genetics

- Most common type of syndromic autosomal dominant [1].

General and ENT Features

- White forelock (Pigmentary abnormalities).
- Craniofacial anomalies (dystopia canthorum, broad nasal root, synophrys).
- Unilateral or bilateral SNHL [3].

63.4.7 Alport Syndrome

Genetics

- It is caused by mutations in genes that code for collagen IV.
- X-linked Alport syndrome is the most common form.
- Could have autosomal recessive and dominant forms.

ENT Features

- Hearing loss: Progressive SNHL

General Features

- Renal impairment (onset in childhood; progression to end-stage renal failure in 100% of males, 15% of females).
- Ocular lesions: lenticonus (most commonly anterior lenticonus) and macular flecks [1].

63.5 Autosomal Recessive Syndromes

63.5.1 Pendred Syndrome

Genetics

- Autosomal recessive syndrome.
- Discovered in December of 1997 [6].
- Results from two mutations in the SLC26A4 gene: known as PDS gene on chromosome 7.

General and ENT Features

- SNHL associated with iodine metabolism defect leading to euthyroid goiter
- Associated with Mondini's dysplasia and enlarged vestibular aqueduct
- Historically diagnosed with perchlorate discharge test [1]

63.5.2 Usher Syndrome

Genetics

- Autosomal recessive disorder.
- Most common cause of deafness and blindness among pediatrics representing 10% of hereditary deafness.
- The genes associated with USH encode a variety of proteins, including motor and scaffold proteins which regulate hair bundle morphogenesis in the inner ear.

General and ENT Features

- Clinical features: hearing loss, vestibular deficits, ataxia, retinitis pigmentosa (RP) causing progressive visual loss (apparent with electroretinography prior to funduscopic exam)

- Type I: most common (90%), profound deafness, RP by age 10, absent vestibular response
- Type II: moderate/severe deafness, RP by teens/twenties, normal or slightly decreased vestibular response
- Type III: progressive HL, RP begins with puberty
- Type IV: X-linked; clinically similar to type II [4, 7]

63.6 Syndromic Craniosynostosis

This group of disorders contain over 500 syndromes that have craniofacial anomalies.

Genetics

- Crouzon (craniofacial dysostosis), Apert (acrocephalosyndactyly), Muenke, and Pfeiffer syndromes are all part of the *FGFR*-gene-related craniosynostosis syndromes.
- Both Apert and Crouzon are due to mutation of FGFR-2 gene (10q26).
- Muenke is caused by a specific mutation of *FGFR3*, the Pro250Arg mutation.
- They follow an autosomal dominant inheritance pattern, but new mutations are common.
- Saethre-Chotzen is a craniosynostosis syndrome that is caused by mutations in the *TWIST* gene [1].

ENT Features

All craniosynostosis syndrome can share their ENT features:

1. Airway obstruction.
2. Pinna abnormalities: low-set, small or posteriorly rotated ears.
3. External canal atresia.
4. Middle ear abnormalities: both congenital ossicular fixation and Eustachian tube dysfunction that may give rise to a conductive hearing loss.
5. Sensorineural deafness [1].

63.6.1 Crouzon Syndrome

This syndrome affects the face and cranium and occurs in 1: 25,000 live births. Crouzon syndrome is characterized by (Fig. 63.5):

- Craniosynostosis and maxillary hypoplasia
- Congenital enlargement of the sphenoid bone
- Short upper lip
- Shallow orbits causing ocular proptosis
- Bicoronal synostosis (brachycephaly)
- Exorbitism: due to underdeveloped midface which results in prolapse of the globes; main abnormality
- Hypoplasia of the malar bones
- Retromaxillism and a resultant malocclusion [2]

63.6.2 Apert Syndrome

- Occurs in about 1:150,000 live births.
- Craniosynostosis (usually bicoronal).
- Conductive hearing loss secondary to stapes fixation.
- Frontal prominence; exophthalmos (Fig. 63.6).
- Fusion of the digits of the hands and feet (syndactyly).
- Abnormalities of the midface and cranium are evident at birth.
- Brachycephaly and midface retrusion causing an anterior open bite (malocclusion).
- Cleft soft palate or bifid uvula is present in 30% of cases.
- Intellectual ability may vary from normal to significantly impaired [3].

63.6.3 Pfeiffer Syndrome

Similar to Crouzon syndrome and is characterized by:

- Craniosynostosis and midfacial hypoplasia with shallow orbits.

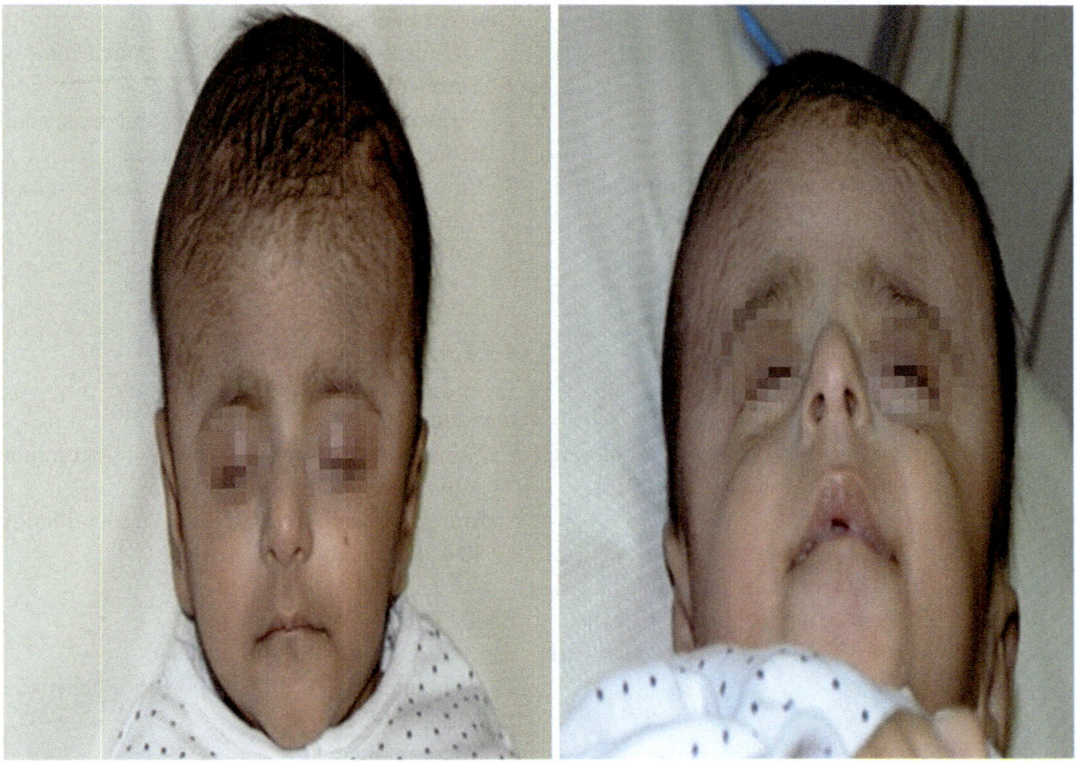

Fig. 63.5 Crouzon syndrome showing craniosynostosis and maxillary hypoplasia

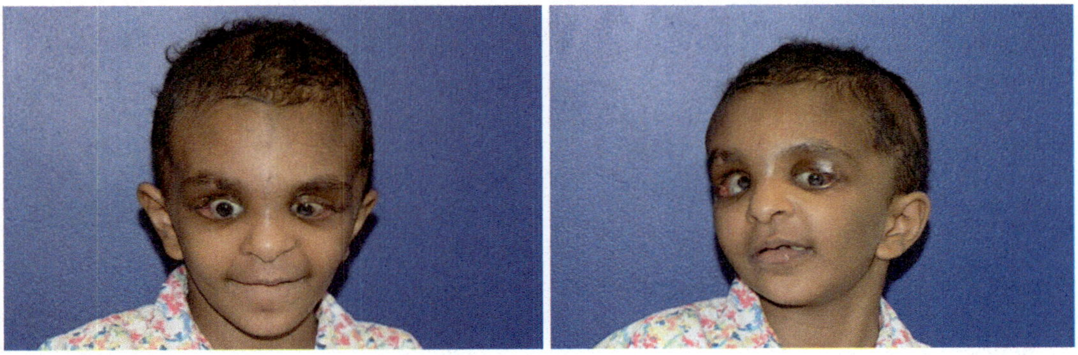

Fig. 63.6 Apert Syndrome showing exophthalmos

- Broad thumbs and broad great toes.
- Severity of craniofacial anomalies can vary from mild midfacial hypoplasia to a cloverleaf skull.
- Skeletal anomalies such as fusion of the elbow joint, solid cartilaginous trachea and choanal stenosis or atresia.
- Central nervous system abnormalities may occur in severe cases [3].

63.7 Other Syndromes That Might Have ENT Involvement

63.7.1 Achondroplasia

Genetics

- An autosomal dominant (*FGFR3*gene).
- Incidence is related to increasing paternal age.
- 80% of patients have de novo mutations [1].

ENT Features
1. Obstructive sleep apnea (OSA) or central apnea.
2. Adenotonsillar hypertrophy.
3. Narrow nasopharynx.
4. Frequent otitis media and glue ear.
5. Sensorineural and conductive hearing loss.
6. Midface hypoplasia [1].

63.7.2 Beckwith–Wiedemann Syndrome

Genetics
- An overgrowth disorder of growth promoting and suppressing genes found at 11p15 [1].

ENT Features
1. Macroglossia: may constitute an anesthetic risk and may occasionally require surgical reduction.
2. Ear lobe creases and/or posterior helical ear pits [1].

General Features
1. Overgrowth: large birth weight, macrosomia, visceromegaly, hemi-hypertrophy. Growth rate slows around age of 7 to 8 years old.
2. Neonatal hypoglycemia.
3. Embryonal tumor risk increased: Wilm's tumor, hepatoblastoma, neuroblastoma, and rhabdomyosarcoma.
4. Renal anomalies [1].

63.7.3 Neurofibromatosis Type 2

Genetics
- Is inherited in an autosomal dominant pattern.
- Is characterized by the presence of vestibular schwannomas.
- New mutations in the *NF2* gene arise in approximately half of cases [1].

ENT Features
- Hearing loss, tinnitus or vertigo caused by schwannoma of the cranial nerves: typically, unilateral or bilateral vestibular (acoustic) neuromas [1].

General Features
1. Meningiomas, ependymomas, spinal tumors, astrocytomas.
2. Peripheral/ subcutaneous schwannomas, cutaneous neurofibromas, NF2 plaques.
3. Cafe au lait patches: these are less common than in NF1.
4. Cataracts, retinal hamartomas [1].

63.7.4 Noonan Syndrome

Genetics
- Noonan syndrome is a relatively common autosomal dominant disorder [8].
- Mutations in *PTPN11* have been identified in 50% of patients [1].

ENT Features
1. Low-set, posteriorly rotated ears.
2. Webbing of the neck, low posterior hairline.
3. Variable hearing loss.
4. Micrognathia [1].

General Features
1. Congenital heart disease.
2. Mild mental retardation.
3. Short stature.
4. Bleeding problems [1].

63.7.5 Prader–Willi Syndrome

Genetics
- Is characterized by poor neonatal feeding and childhood-onset obesity as a result of hyperphagia.
- It is caused by the absence of the paternally derived Prader–Willi syndrome region on chromosome 15 [1].

ENT Features
- Obstructive sleep apnea (OSA): secondary to obesity, a cardinal feature of the disorder.
- Growth hormone (GH) treatment exacerbates OSA in Prader–Willi syndrome [1].

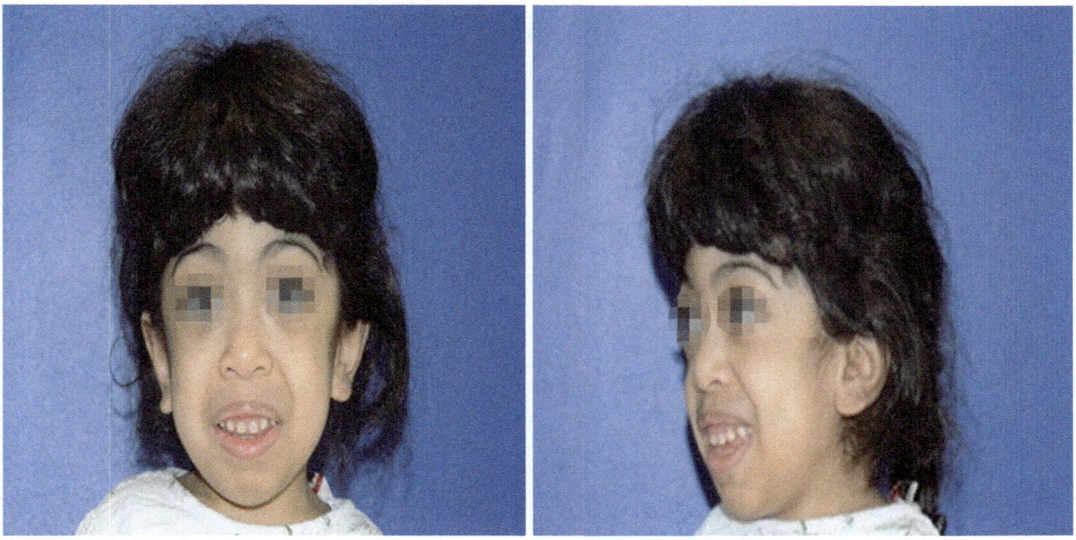

Fig. 63.7 Mucopolysaccaraidoses, showing coarse facial features, thick lips, and short stature

63.7.6 Mucopolysaccharidoses

Genetics

- A group of storage disorders that can affect multiple organs [9].
- Inherited in an autosomal recessive manner with the exception of type II (Hunter syndrome), which is X-linked [1].

ENT Features (Fig. 63.7)

1. Obstructive airway disease and OSA.
2. Diffuse infiltration around the airway.
3. Hearing loss.
4. Atlanto-axial instability in types IV and VI.
5. Coarse or rough facial features with thick lips and enlarged mouth and tongue.
6. Frequent ear infection [1].

General Features

1. Short stature.
2. Skeletal irregularities.
3. Visceromegaly particularly hepatosplenomegaly.
4. Progressive joint stiffness.
5. Heart disease.
6. Corneal involvement in some types.
7. Mental retardation in some types [1].

Take Home Messages

- Whenever a syndromic diagnosis is suspected, the clinician should look for other diagnostic clues and a systematic approach to investigation and management of a child with suspected syndrome is of utmost importance.
- Management of ENT-related syndromes are best approached through a multidisciplinary team and a referral to a geneticist is important for diagnostic purposes, family counselling, and discussion of recurrence risk.

References

1. John M, Glenis K, et al. Pediatric ENT. Belin, Heidelberg: Springer Verlag; 2007.
2. Rosen CL, Storfer-Isser A, Taylor HG, et al. Increased behavioral morbidity in school-aged children with sleep-disordered breathing. Pediatrics. 2004;114:1640.
3. John C, Raymond W. Scott Brown's otorhinolaryngology head and neck surgery. 8th ed. New York: Taylor and Francis Group; 2018.

4. Fred I, Zara M. ENT board prep. New York: Springer Science + Business Media; 2014.
5. Vasudevan PC. Oxford desk reference: clinical genetics. Arch Dis Child. 2006;91(8):717–8. https://doi.org/10.1136/adc.2006.095802.
6. National Center for Biotechnology Information (US). Genes and Disease. Bethesda, MD: National Center for BiotechnologyIn formation (US);1998. Pendred syndrome. https://www.ncbi.nlm.nih.gov/books/NBK22178/.
7. Scott AR, Tibesar RJ, Sidman JD. Pierre Robin sequence: evaluation, management, indications for surgery, and pitfalls. Otolaryngol Clin North Am. 2012;45(3):695–710.
8. El Bouchikhi I, Belhassan K, Moufid FZ, et al. Noonan syndrome-causing genes: molecular update and an assessment of the mutation rate. Int J Pediatr Adolesc Med. 2016;3(4):133–42. https://doi.org/10.1016/j.ijpam.2016.06.003.
9. Tomatsu S, Fujii T, Fukushi M, et al. Newborn screening and diagnosis of mucopolysaccharidoses. Mol Genet Metab. 2013;110(1–2):42–53. https://doi.org/10.1016/j.ymgme.2013.06.007.

Further Reading

1. Marom T, Roth Y, Goldfarb A, Cinamon U. Head and neck manifestations of 22q11.2 deletion syndromes. Eur Arch Otorhinolaryngol. 2012;269(2):381–7.

64 Congenital Anomalies of the Nose

Faisal Abdulkader, Francis J. Lannigan,
and Mahmoud Taha

Key Points
- Congenital nasal anomalies are rare, but will often be associated with other defects.
- CT and MR scanning are essential.
- Decongestion and suction of the nasal cavity immediately prior to scanning improves the quality of the interpretation of the images.
- Intranasal childhood masses should be assumed to be neurogenic and communicate with the cranial cavity until proved otherwise.
- 3D printing of CT scans can facilitate surgical planning in the more challenging anomalies.
- Post-operative stenosis is problematic following choanal atresia surgery despite the use of stents.

F. Abdulkader (✉)
Clinical Otolaryngology Head & Neck Surgery, Weill Cornell Medical College-Qatar, Doha, Qatar
e-mail: Fabdulkader@sidra.org

F. J. Lannigan
Otolaryngology, Sidra Medicine, Doha, Qatar

M. Taha
Pediatric Otolaryngology Head and Neck Surgery Department, Sidra Medicine, Doha, Qatar

64.1 Introduction

Congenital anomalies are the product of errors in embryogenesis (malformations) or the result of intrauterine events that affect embryonic and foetal growth (deformations and disruptions). The more complex the formation of a structure, the more opportunities for malformation.

Development of the Nose
- At about the third week of foetal life, paired thickenings (the olfactory or nasal placodes) appear in the cranial ectoderm, near the embryonic anterior neuropore.
- Invagination of the placodes, consequent on growth of the surrounding mesoderm, results in the formation of the nasal pits which, as they deepen, serve to delineate medial and lateral prominences of the frontonasal process. The medial prominences fuse to form the central portion of the upper lip, the premaxilla, and the primitive nasal septum.
- The floor of the nose is, at first, formed by medial growth of the maxillary processes of the mandibular arch. As the nasal pits deepen, they become slit-like; progressive thinning of the mesoderm, dorsally and caudally, results in the formation of the bucconasal membrane, separating the lumen of the nose from the buccal cavity.
- The bucconasal membrane eventually breaks down, forming the primitive posterior nasal

A. Al-Qahtani et al. (eds.), *Textbook of Clinical Otolaryngology*,
https://doi.org/10.1007/978-3-030-54088-3_64

apertures which, thus, lie horizontally in the roof of the buccal cavity or stomatodaeum.

- The lower, free border of the developing nasal septum, at this stage, lies in contact with the dorsum of the tongue.
- Meanwhile, paired lateral palatal processes are formed, one on each side of the tongue.
- Fusion of these with each other, with an unpaired, ventrally sited, median process and with the caudal border of the septum, gives rise to the definitive palate, finally separating the nasal and nasopharyngeal cavities from the mouth.

Choanal Atresia

- Choana is derived from a Greek word, meaning a funnel. The choanae are, by definition, the posterior apertures of the nose; the use of the term "posterior choanae" is, therefore, a tautology.
- Atresia of the choanae was first described by Roederer in 1775.
- The most consistently quoted figure is one per 8000 live births; bilateral choanal atresia is likely to have been, and may still be, a frequently unrecognized cause of death in the neonatal period.
- Females appear to be affected about twice as often as males and the condition may be unilateral or bilateral in the proportion 3:2.

Embryology

- The anomaly may arise as a result of persistence of the buccopharyngeal membrane.
- It has also been suggested that the aberration is due to a failure of the bucconasal membrane to undergo involution.

Pathology

- Choanal atresia may be bony (90%) or membranous (10%) and is generally sited just in front of the posterior end of the nasal septum.
- Asymmetry of the facial skeleton is common, especially in those with unilateral atresia, and most patients will have a high arched palate.
- Other orthodontic abnormalities, such as transverse maxillary compression, have been described and there may be deformed or absent teeth, especially those of the second dentition.
- Computerized tomography (CT) has demonstrated thickening of the vomer, bowing of the lateral wall of the nasal cavity and fusion of bony elements in the choanal region.
- Various changes have been observed in the cell morphology of the nasal ciliated columnar mucous membrane. They described unevenness of the mucosal surface, thickening of the basal membrane and the presence of ciliary abnormalities including compound cilia, cilia with excessive cytoplasm and ciliary structures with loss of the peripheral membrane.
- Incomplete obstruction of the posterior nasal aperture may also occur, usually taking the form of bony stenosis.
- Congenital atresia of the anterior nares has been described but is excessively rare.

Clinical Features

- Unilateral choanal atresia, unless specifically sought at birth, may not become apparent until later childhood or even adulthood.
- Feeding difficulties may occur, especially during breastfeeding when the non-affected side of the nose is occluded by contact with the breast.
- More commonly, however, it presents as a unilateral nasal discharge.
- Bilateral atresia, on the other hand, almost always presents as a respiratory emergency and is, thus, apparent at birth.
- Newborn infants are, by instinct, nose breathers.
- The reflexes, which in the older child or adult will result in breathing through the mouth in response to nasal obstruction, do not develop until some weeks or months after birth. If, however, the mouth is held open, either by insertion of an artificial airway or during crying, then mouth breathing will occur.
- Thus, neonates with bilateral choanal atresia, or other cause of severe nasal obstruction, will sometimes demonstrate a cyclical change in oxygenation, becoming cyanosed during quiet

periods, normal colour returning when the child cries.

- Choanal atresia has been linked with a limited number of specific defects—the so-called CHARGE association:
  C colobomatous blindness
  H heart disease
  A atresia of the choanae
  R retarded growth or development, including the central nervous system
  G genital hypoplasia in males
  E ear deformities, including deafness

Diagnosis

- The time-honoured method of determining patency of the nose in the newborn infant is the visualized ability to pass a soft red-rubber catheter through each side of the nose into the oropharynx.
- Failure to pass the catheter, however, is not conclusive evidence for the presence of atresia of the posterior nares; the tip may become impacted in the adenoid or may be deflected by minor abnormalities of the turbinates, causing the tube to curl up inside the nasal cavity.
- There are causes of total nasal obstruction in the neonate other than choanal atresia: these include massive congenital hypertrophy of the turbinates or adenoid.
- Radiographic demonstration that contrast medium is blocked at the choanae and doesn't pass beyond (choanography), has been the traditional method of confirming the diagnosis of atresia.
- Computerized tomography gives rather more information, especially with regard to whether the obstruction is membranous or bony and, in the latter case, the actual structures involved and their thickness. The nasal cavity should be decongested and suctioned prior to CT in order to maximize the quality of the study.

Management

- The essential aim of treatment of choanal atresia is the creation of patent nasal airways.
- In the case of unilateral atresia, there is seldom any urgency in the presentation and surgery can be undertaken as a planned or "cold" procedure.
- Bilateral atresia, however, always presents as a respiratory emergency and management must, therefore, be considered under two headings:
  - Primary, or emergency, treatment
  - Secondary, or definitive, surgery

Emergency Management

- In most cases, and especially where it is planned to proceed to definitive surgery within 24 h or so, it will suffice to insert a standard neonatal Waters airway, taping it securely into position.
- The child may, if necessary, be fed through an indwelling orogastric tube.
- In certain circumstances, it is probably wiser to intubate the larynx or, if this is not possible, to perform a tracheostomy (rarely).

Definitive Management

- Four approaches to the posterior end of the nasal cavity have been described:
- trans-nasal
- trans-palatal
- trans-septal
- trans-antral
- Only the first two are in common use today.
- In all surgery of this region, use of the operating microscope not only provides much better illumination but makes the operation easier and safer.
- General anaesthesia with orotracheal intubation is employed. The patient should be in the tonsillectomy position. Operating at the "head end" of the table facilitates directing instruments caudally—away from the cranial cavity.
- The trans-nasal route is valid only in membranous atresia or where the bony plate is thin.
- The simplest procedure is perforation of the atretic lamina followed by dilatation.
- Although Lichtwitz's trocar and cannula is often used to achieve the primary puncture, there is an inherent risk in this method of causing serious damage to the cervical spine and spinal cord. Instead, the author recommends the use of

female urethral dilators which, being curved, direct the perforating force safely downwards, into the lumen of the nasopharynx. An aural suction (Size 5) may also be used. If the atresia is membranous, the tip of the perforator may be palpated with a little finger in the nasopharynx. A 120° rigid telescope enables continuous visualization of the nasopharynx intraoperatively.

- The atretic plate is, almost always, thinnest and weakest at the junction of the floor of the nose and posterior end of the septum. It is, therefore, towards this point that the tip of the instrument should be directed.
- Once puncture has been achieved, the opening may be widened, using progressively larger dilators, up to about 5 mm (14–16 FG). Many surgeons recommend the insertion of Portex or Silastic tubes to prevent restenosis of the choanae.
- Other trans-nasal methods which have been advocated are drilling out the bony atresia with diamond paste burrs or vaporizing the obstruction using the CO2 gas laser.
- In either case, it is imperative that an aural speculum is used to protect the skin of the nasal vestibule as it is very easy, otherwise, to cause circumferential damage, resulting in stenosis of the anterior naris.
- Stenosis can be problematic, despite the use of stents. It is common to require more than one procedure to achieve long-term patency.
- Where the atresia is thick, it may be preferable to employ the trans-palatal approach. The most comfortable operating approach is similar to that used in cleft palate surgery, the child's head overhanging the end of the table and resting on the surgeon's lap. The Denis Browne mouth gag gives rather better exposure of the hard palate and is to be preferred to the more usual Boyle-Davis instrument.
- An incision is made around the summit of the alveolar ridge or at the gingivopalatal margin if teeth are present. The mucous membrane of the hard palate is elevated; using McKenty or Cottle septal elevators and the flap is developed posteriorly, until the edge of the hard palate is reached.
- Care must be taken to avoid damage to the greater and lesser palatine vessels and nerves as they traverse the bony palate on either side, close to its posterior edge.
- The nasopharynx is entered by separation of muscle fibres from the posterior edge of the hard palate and incision of the superior mucosal layer of the soft palate. Using diamond paste or cutting burs of suitable size, the posterior end of the hard palate is removed to expose the bony atresia.
- Continuity of the nasal cavity can now be restored by drilling away the obstructing bone, and the posterior end of the vomer is removed at the same time.
- Care is needed, at this stage, to avoid damage to the vessels and nerves which run in the lateral nasal wall. Before replacing and suturing the palatal flap, soft silastic tubes may be inserted and anchored in position with an anterior septal transfixion suture; the tubes should be removed approximately 6 weeks later.

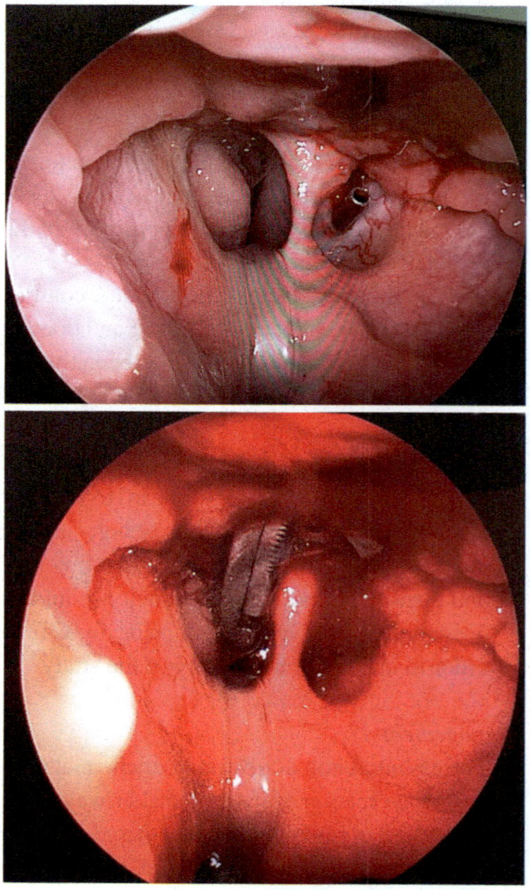

Congenital Nasal Pyriform Aperture Stenosis

- Premature fusion and overgrowth of the medial nasal processes can result in a narrowing of the anterior nasal pyriform aperture.
- The clinical picture is similar to that seen with bilateral choanal atresia.
- Typically, a newborn with congenital nasal pyriform aperture stenosis (CNPAS) presents with nasal airway obstruction that may lead to respiratory distress and failure.
- In its milder form, it may present as feeding difficulties with episodes of cyclical cyanosis that are usually relieved by crying.
- Examination of the nasal cavities may reveal an extremely narrowed nasal vestibule.
- Similar to choanal atresia, it may be difficult to pass a 6-French nasal catheter.
- The pathognomonic sign is the inability to pass a standard-size fibreoptic, flexible nasopharyngoscope (3.5 mm) through the anterior nasal passage.
- Thin-section axial CT with special attention to the pyriform region is the imaging study of choice when CNPAS is suspected. A width less than 11 mm in a term infant is considered to be diagnostic for CNPAS.
- The use of a three-dimensional (3D) CT gives more precise preoperative evaluation of the maxilla.
- CNPAS can occur as an isolated anomaly or in association with other congenital anomalies.
- In a significant number of children, premature fusion of the nasal medial processes may lead to a fusion of the central upper incisors leading to a single, central megaincisor.
- These patients also may have abnormalities of the pituitary-adrenal axis.
- CNPAS might represent a developmental field defect, such as a microform of holoprosencephaly.
- In those patients with a coinciding finding of CNPAS and a central megaincisor on CT or the eruption of teeth, an assumption may be raised that the child may have a microform of holoprosencephaly.
- Chromosomal analysis, evaluation of parents and other relatives, CT and magnetic resonance imaging (MRI) to search for CNS malformations, and an assessment of the hypothalamic-pituitary-adrenal axis may be necessary in these patients.

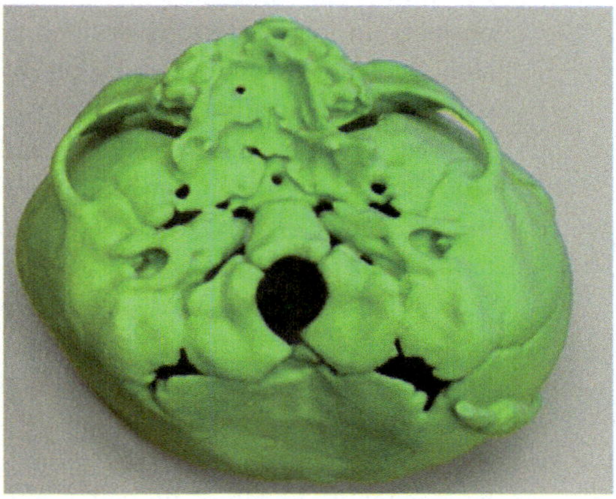

Management

- Strategies for treatment and management of CNPAS include conservative therapy using a McGovern nipple as well as initial gavage feedings until the infant learns to adjust to the nasal obstruction.
- If this fails, surgical enlargement of the nasal pyriform aperture should be performed.
- This surgery typically is approached via a sublabial incision to preserve the nasal mucosa.
- Nasal stenting for 1–2 weeks can be considered to prevent stenosis of the surrounding soft tissues.

Septal Deviation

- Some degree of nasal septal deviation is found in 58% of all newborn babies, and in 4% of births there is also an associated external nasal deformity.
- Two mechanisms explain how deformities may arise:
  - Differences in the rate of growth of the septum as compared to other midfacial structures.
  - Trauma to the nose, either as the result of prolonged contact with the uterine wall or during parturition, especially when this is protracted.

It should be noted that septal deviation is a frequent concomitant of clefting of the upper lip and palate.

The resulting nasal obstruction, which may affect one or both sides, usually presents, in the neonate, as difficult or slow feeding, often accompanied by colic due to air swallowing.

If nasal infection supervenes, the child will become snuffly and in some cases the nasal blockage is so severe as to mimic choanal atresia.

Inspection of the nose may reveal displacement of the quadrilateral cartilage.

Manipulation during the neonatal period is now rarely performed.

By about 6 years of age, the nose is large enough to allow limited septoplasty to be performed.

Congenital Nasal Masses

- Congenital nasal masses are rare, occurring once in every 20,000–40,000 live births.
- All intranasal masses in children, and especially if unilateral should be treated with the gravest suspicion and circumspection.
- Failure to differentiate between a simple nasal polyp and a communicating meningoencephalocele may lead to cerebrospinal fluid rhinorrhoea, with resultant risk of meningitis.
- The differential diagnosis of nasal swellings in a child is given in Table 64.1.

Nasal dermoids

- These are cysts or sinuses occurring anywhere in the midline of the nose from the glabella to the columella, whose walls contain skin adnexae.
- They are formed as the result of sequestration of epithelial elements during fusion of the median nasal processes.
- The diagnosis is often delayed until adolescence or adulthood and may only present if infection occurs.
- Dermoid sinuses, recognized by a dimple or minute opening sometimes containing a single hair, may extend deeply into the nasal septum, occasionally reaching as far as the cribriform plate.
- Contrast sinography will assist in determining both the extent and configuration of the sinus tract.
- Complete excision is often difficult to achieve, but may be facilitated by prior cannulation of the external punctum and instillation of methylene blue.

Nasal Gliomata

- These account for approximately 5% of all congenital nasal swellings.
- More common in males and may occur entirely outside the nasal cavity (60%), entirely within the nasal cavity (30%) or in a combination of both sites (10%).
- Gliomata and meningoencephaloceles share a common origin, resulting from faulty closure of the anterior neuropore. While meningoencephaloceles retain their communication with the subarachnoid space, gliomata become detached from the intracranial cavity by closure of the skull sutures, although in some cases a fibrous tract may remain, connecting the glioma to the skull base.
- Macroscopically, gliomata are smooth and rubbery with a grey, yellow or purple surface.

Table 64.1 Causes of nasal swelling in childhood

Cystic		Solid	
Congenital	Acquired	Congenital	Acquired
Meningoencephalocele	Sebaceous cyst	Glioma	Lipoma
		Haemangioma	Papilloma
Meningocele		Lymphangioma	Lymphoma
		Neurofibroma	Nasopharyngeal carcinoma
Dermoid cyst	Mucocoele	Neuroblastoma	Angiofibroma
		Rhabdomyosarcoma	Ethmoidal polyp
Epidermoid cyst	Lacrimal duct cyst	Chordoma	Antrochoanal polyp
		Craniopharyngioma	Abscess

On histological examination, there are aggregates of mature glial cells, predominantly astrocytes, interspersed with fibrous tissue.

- Most cases are diagnosed at or soon after birth, presenting as either a subcutaneous lump, to one side of the nasal bridge, or as an obstructing intranasal mass. Unlike a meningoencephalocele, a glioma does not increase in size with straining or crying.
- Tomography or CT scanning of the anterior skull base is usually carried out, although it should be noted that absence of a bony defect does not rule out an intracranial communication.
- Generally, the diagnosis is not in doubt but should always be confirmed by biopsy, having first checked for the presence of cerebrospinal fluid by needle aspiration.
- Nasal gliomata tend to enlarge slowly with age although, occasionally, rapid expansion may occur.
- Treatment is by excision. Intranasal masses may require a lateral rhinotomy approach although laser excision is also effective. Incomplete removal may lead to recurrence.
- In those few cases where a dural connection can be demonstrated, anterior craniotomy will be necessary to prevent cerebrospinal fluid leak.

Nasal Meningoencephaloceles

- Meningoencephaloceles are local herniations of glial tissue and meninges, through a defect in the skull.
- They are commonly classified into five main groups, depending upon the size and site of herniation cranioschisis (Table 64.2).
- Most of the meningoencephaloceles seen by otorhinolaryngologists are of the frontoethmoidal or basal types.
- Frontoethmoidal meningoencephalocoeles probably share a common origin with nasal gliomata.
- The sac-like protrusion of meninges contains brain tissue and the subarachnoid space, which is filled with cerebrospinal fluid, communicates freely with the cranial cavity.
- Injury to a meningoencephalocele is, therefore, likely to cause cerebrospinal fluid rhinorrhoea and meningitis.

Table 64.2 Classification of meningoencephalocoeles

Occipital	Basal
Cranial vault	Trans-ethmoidal
Interfrontal	Spheno-ethmoidal
Anterior fontanelle	Trans-sphenoidal
Interparietal	Fronto-sphenoidal or
Posterior fontanelle	Spheno-orbital
Temporal	Cranioschisis
Frontoethmoid	Cranial upper facial cleft
Naso-frontal	Basal lower facial cleft
Naso-ethmoidal	Occipito-cervical cleft
Naso-orbital	Acrania and anencephaly

- A meningoencephalocele usually presents as either a soft cystic mass overlying the root of the nose (frontoethmoidal type) or as a pedunculated intranasal swelling (basal type).
- Crying or straining increases the size and tension of the mass, although, in the case of intranasal swellings, this may not be easy to detect.
- All such swellings must be subject to rigorous radiological examination with CT and MR scanning, to determine the exact site and size of the cranial defect.
- Most cases will require the assistance of a neurosurgeon. Craniotomy is performed, with removal of the herniated brain tissue, followed by closure of the bony defect and repair of the meninges.

64.2 Other Malformations

Haemangioma

- Haemangiomata are common in childhood. Although the majority of these tumours are found in the head and neck region, primary involvement of the nose is relatively rare.
- Histologically, haemangiomata have been identified as capillary, cavernous, mixed or hypertrophic.
- Almost all of these lesions will regress spontaneously, with little or no residual deformity. Those few tumours which do not involute are said to be associated with increasing numbers of arteriovenous fistulae, the development of which can be monitored by serial Doppler examinations.
- In the majority of cases, therefore, masterly inactivity is the treatment of choice, active intervention being restricted to those instances where tumour growth continues.

64.3 Rare Nasal Anomalies

Complete Agenesis of the Nose (Arhinia)

- Complete absence of the nose or nasal cavities is a rare anomaly with less than 40 reported cases.
- Affected infants should be expected to have respiratory distress due to their obligate nasal breathing and some will require a tracheostomy.
- Reconstruction involves establishing both a patent airway and reconstruction of an external nasal skeleton. This reconstruction should be performed in stages with creation of an airway by drilling through the maxilla and lining the nasal cavities with skin grafts. The external nasal skeleton can be created with the use of tissue expanders, bone, cartilage and regional flaps.

Proboscis Lateralis

- This rare anomaly is a 1- to 3-cm long, tubular, rudimentary nasal structure, which usually emanates from the lateral aspect of the nose, typically near the medial canthus.
- Its diameter is 1 cm and it is lined by respiratory and squamous epithelium. The incidence of proboscis lateralis is less than 1 in 100,000 live births.
- It has been classified by Boo-Chai into four groups:
  - *Group I*: proboscis lateralis (PL) with a normal nose (9%).
  - *Group II*: PL with ipsilateral nasal defects (23%).
  - *Group III*: PL with ipsilateral nasal defects and ipsilateral ocular and/or adnexal defects (47%).
  - *Group IV*: group III abnormalities with a cleft lip and/or palate (21%).
- Presenting symptoms and signs of respiratory distress are dependent on the patency of the nasal airway.
- Preoperative evaluation includes CT, MRI, or both to identify both bony and soft tissue abnormalities and exclude any associated CNS abnormalities.
- Depending on the condition of the remaining nose, the PL can be excised or used to reconstruct the external nasal skeleton.

Polyrrhinia (Double Nose)

- This rare anomaly usually is associated with pseudohypertelorism and choanal atresia.
- Surgical reconstruction requires removal of the medial portions of both noses and anastomosis of both lateral halves in addition to the choanal repair.

Pearls

- Congenital nasal anomalies are rare, but will often be associated with other defects.
- CT and MR scanning are essential.
- Decongestion and suction of the nasal cavity immediately prior to scanning improves the quality of the interpretation of the images.
- Intranasal childhood masses should be assumed to be neurogenic and communicate with the cranial cavity until proved otherwise.
- 3D printing of CT scans can facilitate surgical planning in the more challenging anomalies.
- Post-operative stenosis is problematic following choanal atresia surgery despite the use of stents.

Take Home Messages

- Most significant congenital anomalies of the nose are rare.
- Many of these patients have additional congenital abnormalities, especially of the face and central nervous system.

Further Readings

1. Losee JE, et al. Congenital nasal anomalies: a classification scheme. Plast Reconstr Surg. 2004;113(2):676–89.
2. Adelson RT, Karimi K, Herrero N. Isolated congenital absence of the left lower lateral cartilage. Otolaryngol Head Neck Surg. 2008;138(6):793–4.
3. Lewin ML. Congenital absence of the nasal columella. Cleft Palate J. 1988;25(1):58–63.

4. Bilen BT, Kilin H. A congenital isolated alar cleft. J Craniofac Surg. 2006;17(3):602–4.
5. Mazzola RF. Congenital malformation in the frontonasal area: their pathogenesis and classification. Clin Plast Surg. 1976;3:101.
6. De Blecourt R, Roddi R, Berg JP, Bloem JJ. Nasal dysplasia. Ann Plast Surg. 1996;37:633.
7. Nishimura Y. Embryological study of nasal cavity development in human embryos with reference to congenital nasal atresia. Acta Anat (Basel). 1993;147:140.
8. Cohen M. The nose. In: Stevenson RE, Hall JG, Goodman RM, editors. Human malformations and related anomalies. New York: Oxford University Press; 1993.
9. Guerrissi J. Congenital absence of nasal bones. Ann Plast Surg. 1993;30:3.
10. Losken A, Burstein FD, Williams JK. Congenital nasal pyriform aperture stenosis: diagnosis and treatment. Plast Reconstr Surg. 2002;109:1506.

65 Cleft Lip and Palate

Dina Emam, Aya Elderee, and Abdelrahman Alsaleh

65.1 Introduction

Cleft lip and cleft palate are openings or splits in the upper lip, palate, or both (Figs. 65.1 and 65.2). Cleft lip and cleft palate result when facial structures that are developing in fetus don't close completely.

Cleft lip and cleft palate are among the most common birth defects. They most commonly occur as isolated birth defects but are also associated with many inherited genetic conditions or syndromes.

In most babies, a series of surgeries can restore normal function and achieve a more normal appearance with minimal scarring.

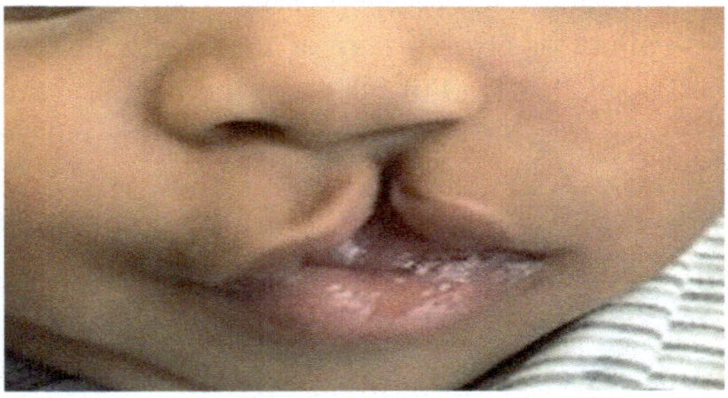

Fig. 65.1 A child with unilateral cleft lip

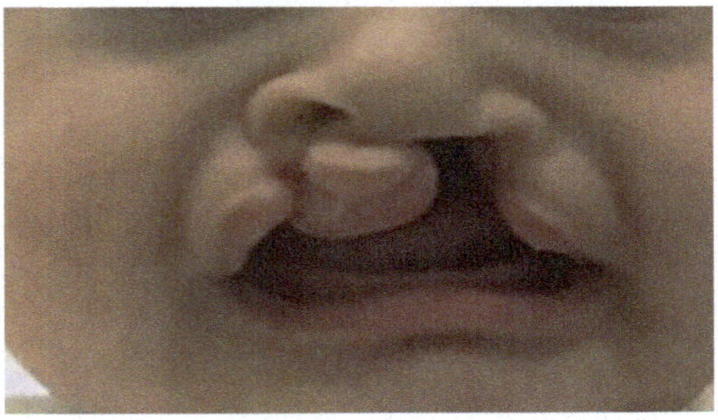

Fig. 65.2 A baby with bilateral cleft lip and palate

65.2 Embryology

- The embryologic development of the face begins at 4 weeks after conception from the neural crest ectomesenchyme that forms five prominences; the frontonasal process, and paired maxillary and mandibular processes surrounding a central depression.
- During the fifth and sixth weeks of embryonic development, bilateral maxillary processes derived from the first brachial arch fuse with the medial nasal process to form the upper lip, alveolus, and the primary palate.
- The formation of the secondary palate begins during the sixth week after conception from the two palatals shelves, which extend from the internal aspect of the maxillary processes.
- During the eighth week, these bilateral maxillary palatal shelves, after ascending to an appropriate position above the tongue, fuse with each other and the primary palate.

D. Emam (✉) · A. Elderee · A. Alsaleh
ENT Department, Hamad Medical Corporation, Doha, Qatar
e-mail: DEmam@hamad.qa

A. Al-Qahtani et al. (eds.), *Textbook of Clinical Otolaryngology*,
https://doi.org/10.1007/978-3-030-54088-3_65

- A disruption in the fusion of these embryonic components can occur due to delay in elevation of the palatal shelves from vertical to horizontal, defective shelf fusion, or post-fusion rupture resulting in a cleft of the secondary palate.
- The lateral nasal process forms the alar structures of the nose.
- The lower lip and jaw are formed by the mandibular processes.
- This process of formation of the face is the consequence of a cascade of processes that involve cell proliferation, cell differentiation, cell adhesion, and apoptosis.
- Failure or error in any of these cellular processes that lead to fusion of the medial nasal process with the lateral nasal and maxillary process can cause orofacial clefts.

65.3 Epidemiology (Fig. 65.3)

- Cleft lip and palate are the second most common congenital malformation after the club foot, which is more common.
- Interracial differences exist in the incidence of cleft lip and palate versus cleft palate.
- The mean incidence of cleft lip and palate is 2.1 cases per 1000 live births among Asians, 1 case per 1000 live births among white people, and 0.41 cases per 1000 live births among black people.
- A high incidence of the cleft lip and palate are seen in North American populations of Asian descent, such as Indians of the southwestern United States and the west coast of Canada.

The incidence of isolated cleft palate is constant among the three racial groups at 0.5 cases per 1000 live births.

- The incidence of cleft lip and palate also rises with increased parental age, and older mothers with additional parity have an increased incidence of having children with cleft palate.
- In relatives of children with cleft lip and palate, the incidence of cleft lip and palate is significantly increased. However, the isolated cleft palate anomaly occurs with the same frequency as that in the general population.
- Relatives of children with isolated cleft palate also have a higher risk of this anomaly, without an increased risk of the cleft lip and palate deformity.
- Overall, 5% of patients with cleft lip and palate and isolated cleft palate have identifiable syndromes.
- Associated syndromes are more common among patients with isolated cleft palate than among others.

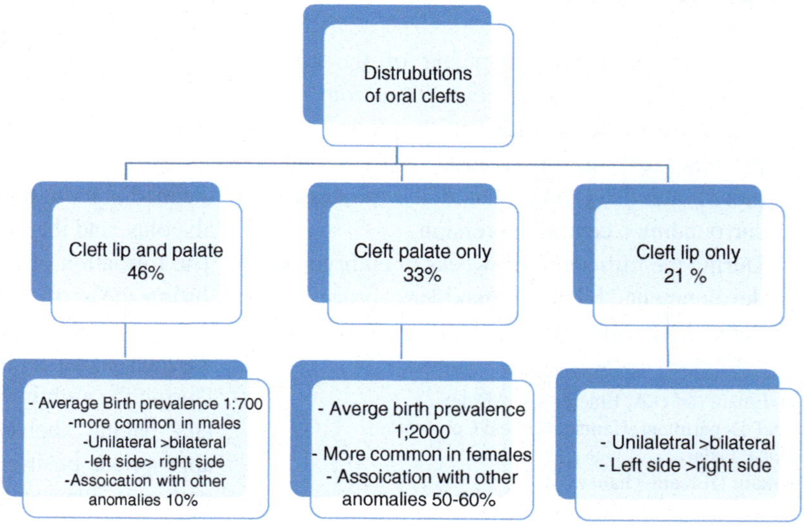

Fig. 65.3 Epidemiology of cleft lip and palate

- Congenital heart diseases are more prevalent in patients with non-syndromic cleft lip and/or palate than in the general population.

65.4 Etiology and Genetics

Non-syndromic CLP is a complex trait with multifactorial etiology resulting from gene–environmental interactions:

- More than ten genes contribute to the development of cleft lip and palate.
- Environmental factors that contribute to the etiology of facial cleft disorders include cigarette smoking; folic acid deficiency during the periconceptional period; and maternal exposure to alcohol and teratogenic medications such as retinoids, corticosteroids, and anticonvulsants (phenytoin and valproic acid).

65.5 Classification of Cleft Lip and Palate

65.5.1 Veau Classification

The Veau classification system divides the cleft lip and palate into four groups, which are as follows and illustrated in Fig. 65.3:

1. Group I—Defects of the soft palate only.
2. Group II—Defects involving the hard palate and soft palate.
3. Group III—Defects involving the soft palate to the alveolus, usually involving the lip.
4. Group IV—Complete bilateral clefts.

65.5.2 International Confederation of Plastic and Reconstructive Surgery Classification

The International Confederation of Plastic and Reconstructive Surgery classification system uses an embryonic framework to divide clefts into 3 groups, with further subdivisions to denote unilateral or bilateral cases:

1. Group I—Defects of the lip or alveolus.
2. Group II—Clefts of the secondary palate (hard palate, soft palate, or both).
3. Group III—Any combination of clefts involving the primary and secondary palates.

65.5.2.1 Submucous Cleft Palate: A Minor Form of Secondary Cleft Palate Defect

Causing a midline diastasis of the levator muscles with the mucosa remaining intact, deficient musculature of the palate causes a blue streak known as zona pellucida, associated with a bifid uvula and loss of posterior nasal spine (notched hard palate).

Risk of velopharyngeal insufficiency is increasing after adenoidectomy.

65.6 Evaluation

A child with a cleft lip and palate present with multiple challenging problems:

- *Airway problems*: Syndromic children, like those with the Robin sequence, for example, present with respiratory distress. Securing the airway is the priority in these patients.
- *Feeding difficulty is the primary problem*, and although these babies have normal sucking and swallowing reflexes, they have difficulty generating enough negative pressure to nurse adequately. As a result, the baby's nutrition must be delivered through bottle-feeding via nipples with large openings to facilitate the delivery of breast milk or formula.
- *Dental and orthodontic problems.*
- *Speech and language difficulties* as hypernasality due to velopharyngeal insufficiency.
- *Hearing impairment* because of Eustachian tube dysfunction leading to recurrent attacks of otitis media secondary to middle ear effusion which will need insertion of auditory tubes to improve the hearing.

Table 65.1 Interdisciplinary care of the cleft patient

Time line	Management
Prenatal	Diagnosis and parental counseling
0–6 months	General assessment for associated anomalies. ENT evaluation—breathing, feeding, swallowing, and hearing. Presurgical orthopedics (0–3 months). Primary lip repair (3–4 months)
6 months–2 years	Speech and oral sensory-motor assessment. Ear tubes (as needed). Primary palate repair (9–12 months)
Preschool: 3–5 years	Dental care. Speech assessment and therapy. Assess the need for lip revision
Childhood: 6–12 years	Correction of velopharyngeal dysfunction. Orthodontic treatment-Phase I. Alveolar cleft repair (8–11 years)
Adolescence: 13–18 years	Orthodontic treatment-Phase II. Orthognathic surgery (if needed) 14–16 years (female), 16–18 years (male). Revision Chielo-rhinoplasty. Replacement of missing teeth (as needed)

- *Social and self-esteem challenges* which lead to psychological and behavioral consequences.

65.7 Management of Cleft Lip and Palate

A multidisciplinary approach is required to assist patients and their families with the comprehensive care of these children. Responsibility for their care is shared by a team of pediatricians, plastic surgeons, otolaryngologists, pedodontists, orthodontists, nurses, speech therapists, audiologists, and social workers (Table 65.1).

Cleft lip and palate surgery should aim to achieve the following:

1. Isolation of the nasal cavity from the mouth.
2. Bone continuity throughout the maxillary alveolus to facilitate the eruption of the permanent dentition.
3. A functional velum that will permit normal speech.
4. An esthetic and functional lip and nose.

65.8 Surgical Repair of Cleft Lip and Palate

65.8.1 Unilateral Cleft Lip

Surgical Anatomy

- The most visible anatomic abnormalities of the complete unilateral cleft lip and nose deformity are due to the abnormal position of the orbicularis oris muscle. Orbicularis oris muscle is directed superiorly in the complete cleft or is hypoplastic in incomplete cleft, the floor of the nose communicate with oral cavity and the maxilla is hypoplastic in the cleft side.
- The nasal deformity is proportionate to the severity of clefting. There is slumping of the alar cartilage on the cleft side, leading to an asymmetric nasal tip.
- The alar base is displaced laterally, inferiorly, and posteriorly leading to a widened nasal aperture.
- There is shortening of the medial crus of the alar cartilage.
- The columella and the caudal edge of the septum and anterior nasal spine are deviated to the non-cleft side.

Repair Timing

- Repair of the unilateral cleft lip is usually performed during the first year of life.
- Follow the "rules of 10": hemoglobin more than 10 g, age older than 10 weeks, and weight more than 10 lb.
- A surgical lip adhesion may be preferred as an initial surgical procedure within 6–8 weeks after birth. Lip adhesion helps to align the maxillary alveolar segments and achieve a tension-free definitive lip repair.

Surgical Techniques

- The most popular technique was introduced by Millard (1955) who described the rotation advancement concept.
- In Millard's technique, the medial flap is rotated downward to achieve length, while the lateral flap is advanced. The advantage of this technique is that the suture line lies on the

recreated philtral column, and incision allows easy access for primary rhinoplasty to reposition the nasal septum, lower lateral cartilage, and alar base. The main disadvantage is that the inexperienced surgeon requires good surgical judgment during the operation as it is not based on exact measurements.

- Other Surgical Techniques include:
  The triangular flap technique, described by Tennison and Randall, is based on exact measurements, can be reproduced well, and used more easily in wide clefts of the lip.
  Millard rotation advancement technique.
  Tennison–Randall (single) triangular flap interdigitation.
  Bardach (double) triangular flap interdigitation.
  Bilateral cleft repair (Millard).

65.8.2 Bilateral Cleft Lip

Complete bilateral clefts of the lip are rare, accounting for only 10% of cleft lips, and therefore, the experience in treating these deformities is limited.

Surgical Anatomy

- The typical anatomical abnormalities that make the bilateral cleft lip deformity so difficult to repair are the absence of muscle in the prolabial segment, resulting in lack of philtral dimple, philtral columns, white roll margin, and the median tubercle; also the central part of the alveolar arch is rotated forward and upward.
- The floor of the nose communicates with the oral cavity bilaterally.
- The nasal columella is short, nasal tip is widened, and cartilaginous nasal septum and nasal spine are deflected forward.

Surgical Techniques

- A number of surgical procedures with many variations for the repair of bilateral cleft lip are well described. Among these are the repairs of Veau, Tennison, Manchester, Millard, and others.
- Bilateral cleft lip repair is much more challenging, and the results are often less satisfactory than those of unilateral cleft lip.

65.8.3 Cleft Palate Repair

Surgical Anatomy

- The muscles of soft palate that help with the function of speech and swallowing include the levator palatini, tensor palatini, palatopharyngeus, palatoglossus, and musculus uvulae.
- The soft palate in a non-cleft individual acts as a muscular valve that can lift superiorly and posteriorly to oppose the pharyngeal wall and achieve velopharyngeal closure during speech.
- In a child with an unrepaired cleft, the soft palate cannot function as a muscular valve leading to velopharyngeal insufficiency.
- The tensor palatini muscle fibers, which control the opening of the Eustachian tube, do not function optimally, often leading to chronic otitis media.

Repair timing: The timing of palate repair to achieve optimal speech with minimal facial growth disturbance has been one of the more debated issues in cleft literature. It is now well accepted, and evidence in the literature shows that speech outcomes are better when soft and hard palate repair is completed before speech development. For most children developing normally, this is around 9–12 months.

Principles and techniques of palate repair:

Surgical repair of the cleft palate falls into two categories. The first is a single-stage repair involving closure with mucoperiosteal flaps. The second involves a multistage approach in which the soft palate is closed initially, followed by delayed closure of the hard palate.

May require orthodontic treatment to move the premaxilla or to realign maxillary segments.

The main principle of cleft palate repair is to detach and retro pose the abnormal insertion of the levator palatini and join the muscles of both halves of the soft palate in the midline at the junction of the middle and posterior third of the soft palate in order to achieve proper elevation of the soft palate.

In the hard palate, the most important principle is to reflect mucoperiosteal flaps posteriorly based on the greater palatine arteries.

At the time of the primary palatoplasty, the ears should be inspected. If there is evidence of serous otitis, a myringotomy is performed, and fluid aspirated with the insertion of ventilating tubes.

1. The two-flap palatoplasty is a commonly used surgical technique for repair of the complete unilateral and bilateral cleft of the palate.
2. The Veau–Wardwill–Kilner (V–Y pushback) technique: is retro position of the mucoperiosteal flap and soft palate, provides additional palate length, used less often for the repair of cleft of the secondary palate.
3. The double reversing Furlow Z-plasty was introduced by Dr. Leonard Furlow Jr. in 1978. This technique uses two reversed Z-plasties of the oral and nasal mucosa to repair the cleft, it yielded excellent speech results for primary cleft palate repair with minimal and acceptable rates of fistula formation, velopharyngeal insufficiency (VPI), and the need for additional corrective surgery.

Take Home Messages

- Clefts of the lip and palate are common congenital birth anomalies.
- Etiology is complex. Known associations are with antenatal anticonvulsants, steroids, maternal smoking, and alcohol. Some of the genes associated with orofacial clefting have now been identified.
- Cleft palate results from failure of bilateral palatine shelves (from maxillary processes) to fuse at midline with developing nasal septum (from frontonasal process and bilateral medial nasal processes).
- Cleft lip results from failure of fusion of maxillary swelling with the medial nasal process.
- Every child born with a CL/P should be thoroughly assessed by complete physical examination and necessary diagnostic tests to check for associated systemic abnormalities, including congenital heart, renal, or airway anomalies.
- Management of patients with cleft lip and palate requires a multidisciplinary approach delivered by a team that includes an otolaryngologist.

Complications of Palatoplasty

- Early complications include bleeding, airway obstruction, and wound dehiscence.
- Late complications include fistula formation, velopharyngeal insufficiency, and maxillary growth disturbance.

Further Reading

Bumsted RM. Management of unilateral cleft lip. In: Smith JD, Bumsted R, editors. Pediatric facial plastic and reconstructive surgery. New York: Raven Press; 1993. p. 131–45.

Cohen MM. Etiology and pathogenesis of orofacial clefting. Oral Maxillofac Surg Clin North Am. 2000;12:379–97.

Cohen MM Jr. Syndromes with cleft lip and cleft palate. Cleft Palate J. 1978;15:306–28.

Cooper ME, Ratay JS, Marazita ML. Asian oral-facial cleft birth prevalence. Cleft Palate Craniofac J. 2006;43:580–9.

Fara M. The importance of physiological reconstruction of the orbicularis oris muscle for esthetic and functional result in operations of unilateral cleft lip. Cesk Stomatol. 1971;71:358.

Forrester MB, Merz RD. Descriptive epidemiology of oral clefts in a multiethnic population, Hawaii, 1986–2000. Cleft Palate Craniofac J. 2004;41:622–8.

Hagberg C, Larson O, Milerad J. Incidence of cleft lip and palate and risks of additional malformations. Cleft Palate Craniofac J. 1998;35:40–5.

Jones MC. The genetics of cleft lip and palate. In: Cleft lip and palate: information for families. Chapel Hill: Cleft Palate Foundation; 2001. p. 4–8.

Marazita ML, Mooney MP. Current concepts in the embryology and genetics of cleft lip and cleft palate. Clin Plast Surg. 2004;31:125–40.

Marazita ML, Field LL, Cooper ME, et al. Nonsyndromic cleft lip with or without cleft palate in China:

assessment of candidate regions. Cleft Palate Craniofac J. 2002;39:149–56.

Melnick M, Bixler D, Fogh-Andersen P, et al. Cleft lip+/– cleft palate: an overview of the literature and an analysis of Danish cases born between 1941 and 1968. Am J Med Genet. 1980;6:83–97.

Mitchell LE, Risch N. Correlates of genetic risk for no syndromic cleft lip with or without cleft palate. Clin Genet. 1993;43:255–60.

Mossey P. Epidemiology underpinning research in the aetiology of orofacial clefts. Orthod Craniofac Res. 2007;10:114–20.

Mossey PA, Little J. Epidemiology of oral clefts. In: Wyszynski DF, editor. Cleft lip and palate: from origin to treatment. Oxford: Oxford University Press; 2002. p. 127–58.

Munabi NCO, Swanson J, Auslander A, Sanchez-Lara PA, Davidson Ward SL, Magee WP 3rd. The prevalence of congenital heart disease in nonsyndromic cleft lip and/ or palate: a systematic review of the literature. Ann Plast Surg. 2017;79(2):214–20.

Randall P, Jackson O. A Short History of Cleft Lip and Cleft Palate. In: Losee, JE; Kirschner, RE - editors. Comprehensive Cleft Care. Columbus: The McGraw-Hill Companies. 2009; p. 194.

Vanderas AP. Incidence of cleft lip, cleft palate, and cleft lip and palate among races: a review. Cleft Palate J. 1987;24:216–25.

Pediatric Audiology

66

Abdulsalam Al-Qahtani, Reni K. Chandran, Khaled Abdulhadi, and Zaid Altamimi

66.1 Introduction

The etiology of childhood hearing impairment can be congenital (at birth) or acquired (after birth). It can affect the child in the pre-lingual or post-lingual stage, depending on whether the child has acquired the ability to speak. Early detection and prevention of childhood hearing impairment play a major role in the management of this condition.

Permanent childhood hearing impairment (PCHI) defined as a confirmed permanent bilateral hearing impairment ≥40 dB HL (hearing level) averaged over the frequencies of 500 Hz, 1 KHz, 2 KHz, and 4 kHz in the better hearing ear. It can result from a structural abnormality in the outer ear, middle ear as well as the inner ear. Hence PCHI can be a conductive, sensorineural, or mixed hearing loss [1].

Congenital hearing loss occurs in approximately 1 to 2 per 1000 live births. Genetic factors account for at least 60% of childhood hearing loss, among children with PCHI, about 70% are non-syndromic, and the remaining 30% are syndromic [2]. The onset of the hearing loss can be prenatal, perinatal, or postnatal in onset. Syndromic or non-syndromic is based on the presence or absence of other clinical abnormalities and the pattern of inheritance (autosomal, X-linked, dominant, recessive, mitochondrial). Eighty percent of cases are autosomal recessive typically of pre-lingual onset or 20% autosomal dominant typically progressive or post-lingual [3]. X-linked or mitochondrial inheritance trait (1%) is passed through the maternal lineage [4]. Table 66.1 shows the most common syndromes with hearing loss.

Table 66.1 Syndromic hearing loss

Autosomal dominant	
1.	Branchio-oto-renal syndrome
2.	Neurofibromatosis
3.	Otosclerosis
4.	Stickler syndrome
5.	Treacher Collins syndrome
6.	Waardenburg syndrome
Autosomal recessive	
7.	Jervell and Lange-Nielsen syndrome
8.	Pendred syndrome
9.	Usher syndrome
X-linked	
11.	Alport syndrome
12.	Norrie syndrome
13.	Otopalatodigital syndrome
14.	Wildervanck syndrome
15.	Mohr-Tranebjaerg syndrome
16.	X-linked Charcot–Marie–Tooth

A. Al-Qahtani · Z. Altamimi
Hamad Medical Corporation, Doha, Qatar
e-mail: aalqahtani@hamad.qa ; Zaltamimi@hamad.qa

R. K. Chandran (✉) · K. Abdulhadi
Audiology Department, Hamad Medical Corporation, Doha, Qatar
e-mail: rchandran1@hamad.qa; Khadi@hamad.qa

A. Al-Qahtani et al. (eds.), *Textbook of Clinical Otolaryngology*,
https://doi.org/10.1007/978-3-030-54088-3_66

For more about congenital hearing loss syndromes, risk factors for permanent congenital, delayed-onset, or progressive childhood hearing loss, please go to the congenital hearing loss chapter.

Acquired causes of childhood hearing loss can be due to: otitis media with effusion (OME), ear infections, meningitis, measles, encephalitis, chickenpox, flu, mumps, ototoxic medications, head injury, and noise exposure.

Otitis media with effusion (OME) is an inflammatory condition, defined by the accumulation of fluid in the middle ear with an intact tympanic membrane without acute infection manifestation. It is the most common cause of pediatric acquired hearing loss and speech delay. Several risk factors associated with an increased incidence of OME include younger age, eustachian tube dysfunction, craniofacial abnormalities, adenoid hypertrophy, recurrent otitis media, daycare attendance, gastroesophageal reflux, and passive smoking. Usually, it resolves spontaneously in >80% of cases; in persistent OME cases with significant hearing loss more than 25 dB, a myringotomy with ventilation tube insertion is indicated.

66.2 Pediatric Hearing Assessment

The goals of a pediatric evaluation are:

1. identify the existence of an auditory disorder.
2. identify the nature of the disorder.
3. identify the extent of the hearing impairment caused by the disorder.

Hearing assessment in infants and young children presents a special challenge in reaching a diagnosis. Infants are usually referred because of a known risk factor for hearing loss or on failing neonatal hearing screening. In contrast, young children are usually referred due to a delay in speech and language or because they have an otologic disease with an effect on hearing. Older children are usually referred because of an otologic problem, failing a school screening, or suspected auditory processing disorder.

66.2.1 Newborn Hearing Screening Program

The newborn hearing screening program aims to identify all children with a moderate–profound PCHI in the better hearing ear [5]. Current screening tests available for newborn hearing screening are automated otoacoustic emissions (AOAEs) using either transient or distortion product otoacoustic emissions or automated auditory brainstem response (AABR) [6]. Most screening programs use a two-stage protocol (either OAE followed by AABR if required or two-stage AABR) [5–7]. A pass in both ears using AOAE, or a pass in both ears on AABR, constitutes an overall screen pass. Though OAE is quick and minimally invasive, the disadvantage is that it can be affected by the presence of fluid/debris in the outer or middle ear. If used alone, it could miss neonates with auditory neuropathy. Babies cared for in NICU for more than 48 hours undergo a transient AOAE screen and an AABR screen. Those that fail the AABR screen in one or both ears are referred for audiological assessment [7].

All cases of bilateral severe to profound sensorineural hearing loss should have a full assessment which includes: *pediatric history* (detailed history of pregnancy, delivery and postnatal period, developmental milestones including speech and language and motor milestones, pre- and postnatal noise exposure, history of ototoxic medications, head injuries, ear disease, meningitis, viral illness, and immunization status), *family history* (deafness or risk factors associated with hearing loss in first- and second-degree relatives), *clinical examination*, *audiological assessment* (age-appropriate tests as mentioned below), *imaging studies* (magnetic resonance imaging and/or computed tomography of inner ears), *referral to clinical geneticist* (connexin 26 and 30 mutations testing with access to clinical genetics service for counseling), *ophthalmic assessment*, *vestibular investigations*, and *other investiga-*

tions (electrocardiograph, viral serology (TORCH), renal ultrasound, thyroid tests).

66.2.2 Pediatric Audiological Test Battery

The 2007 Joint Committee on Infant Hearing 1-3-6 guidelines recommend diagnosis of hearing loss by 3 months of age and intervention by 6 months of age [8]. The Pediatric Hearing Assessment Task Force has delineated the following areas that make up the pediatric audiology assessment test battery:

- History.
- Clinical examination.
- Behavioral observation audiometry (BOA).
- Visual reinforcement audiometry (VRA).
- Conditioned play audiometry (CPA).
  - Frequency-specific stimuli.
  - Speech audiometry.
- Physiologic assessments:
  - Acoustic immittance, including tympanometry and acoustic reflex testing.
  - Otoacoustic Emission (OAE) testing.
- Electrophysiologic audiometry:
  - Auditory Brainstem Response (ABR).
  - At least one electrophysiological measure of threshold prediction should be completed before fitting hearing aids and/or cochlear implant, for any infant under the age of 3 years [8].

Hearing assessment for children can be objective or subjective and it varies according to age. Figure 66.1 shows the hearing tests according to the age group, while Table 66.2 shows the comparison between the subjective and objective hearing tests.

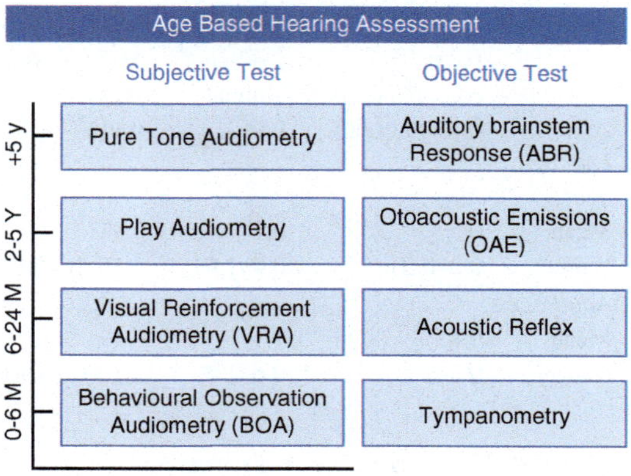

Fig. 66.1 Age-based hearing assessment

Table 66.2 Comparison between subjective and objective hearing

Subjective tests	Objective tests
• Requires reliable and consistent response to sound from the child	• No voluntary response required from the child
• Depends on developmental age	• Can be done on infants, young children, and non-compliant subjects with developmental delay
• Not used in newborn screening	• Used in newborn hearing screening
• Done when the child is awake	• Done mostly in deep sleep/ quiet

66.2.2.1 Immittance Audiometry

Acoustic impedance describes the resistance to energy transmission while acoustic admittance describes the ease of energy transmission through the auditory system. The term "acoustic immittance" has been introduced to express either acoustic condition. Acoustic immittance audiometry serves at least three functions in audiological assessment [9]:

1. Detects middle ear disorder.
2. Differentiates cochlear from retro-cochlear disorder.
3. Cross-checks pure-tone audiometry.

Three immittance measures of middle ear function commonly used are: tympanometry, static immittance, acoustic reflex thresholds. It should be a routine component of the audiological evaluation; the benefit of starting with immittance audiometry is that it provides a useful indication of what to expect from pure-tone audiometry.

The probe tube has three apertures [10, 11]:

1. Transducer which emits a low-frequency probe tone (226 Hz) of approximately 85 dB

Table 66.3 Tympanometry parameters

	Peak compliance (mmho or cc)	Ear canal volume (cm^3)	Middle ear pressure (daPa)
Pediatric age			
Mean	0.5	0.7	
Range	0.2–0.9	0.4–1.0	−50 to +50
Adult age			
Mean	0.8	1.1	
Range	0.3–1.4	0.6–1.5	−100 to +50

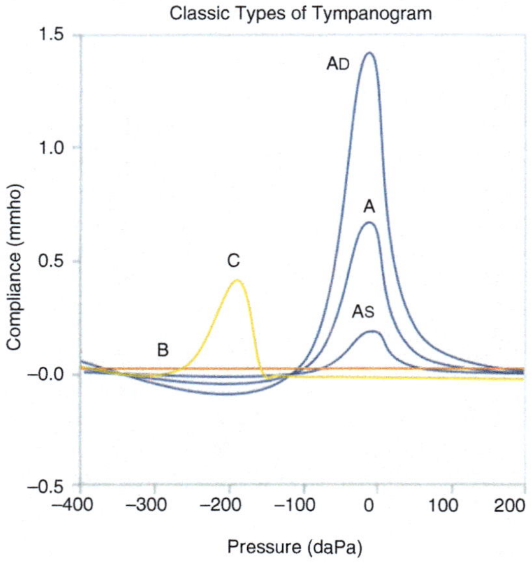

Fig. 66.2 Tympanogram types. *Type A*: normal patients, type AS: otosclerosis, otitis media, type AD: flaccid eardrums, ossicular interruptions. *Type B*: middle ear fluid, eardrum perforations, or impacted cerumen. *Type C*: Eustachian tube disorders, middle ear fluid

sound pressure level (SPL) in adult, but in newborns and infants less than 6 months corrected age 1000 Hz frequency probe tone is recommended.

2. Microphone.
3. Manometer which controls air pressure change within the ear canal.

Parameters in tympanometry include: static compliance, middle ear pressure, and ear canal volume. The values are reviewed in Table 66.3.

Three major types of tympanometry are identified: Type A, Type B, and Type C which are demonstrated in Fig. 66.2.

Table 66.4 Age-based threshold assessment audiometry

Age group	Subjective hearing test
0–6 months	Behavioral observation audiometry (BOA)
6–24 months	Visual reinforcement audiometry (VRA)
2–5 years	Conditioning play audiometry (CPA)
>5 years	Pure-tone audiometry

66.2.2.2 Audiometry

Audiometry can be challenging for the pediatric age especially when it is a subjective test. Table 66.4 shows the age-based audiometry methods.

Behavioral observation audiometry (BOA): used for the age group between 0 and 6 months where it observes the changes in the child's behavior in response to a sound stimulus (eye widening or blink, alteration in sucking response or arousal from sleep, startle or shudder of the body, definite movement of the arms, legs or body). The sound stimulus may be presented for <2 s, in a horizontal plane, 15 cm from the child's ear, out of peripheral vision. The response is observed by the distractor.

Visual reinforcement audiometry (VRA): method of choice for screening children between 6 months and 2 years. Young children are trained by operant conditioning to produce a response to sound. A clear response is a 90° spontaneous head turn within 2–3 s of the sound stimulus reinforced with a visual stimulus, so the child learns to respond to the stimulus to seek a reward. It is considered normal when the response is acquired in the sound field at 25 dB HL.

Conditioned Play Audiometry (CPA): used for the age group between 2 and 5 years. It helps in determining ear-specific and frequency-specific hearing sensitivity. The patient is seated at a child-sized table in an appropriately sized chair. Conditioning is a training session to train the child for the play task test. The transducers can be an insert earphone, supra-aural earphones, bone vibrator, or sound field speakers. Play tasks include placing or tossing a block in a box, stacking blocks in response to an auditory stimulus (speech or frequency-specific).

Pure-tone audiometry (PTA): used for the children above 5 years old. This test provides

Table 66.5 Classification of hearing loss based on hearing threshold (dB HL)

Four commonly used systems of hearing loss classification			
System	WHO	BSA	ASHA
Normal	≤25	<20	−10 to 15
Slight	26–40		16–25
Mild		20–40	26–40
Moderate	41–60	41–70	41–55
Moderately severe			56–70
Severe	61–80	71–95	71–90
Severe to profound	≥81	>95	>90

WHO World Health Organization, *BSA* British Society Audiology, *ASHA* American Speech-Language Hearing Association

quantitative measures of air conduction (AC) and bone conduction (BC) thresholds. AC thresholds assess the entire auditory pathway using headphones or insert phones. BC testing stimulates the cochlea directly, thus bypassing the outer and middle ears. BC thresholds are measured by placing a bone vibrator on the skull (mostly mastoid). AC and BC thresholds are compared to get an idea about the status of conductive and sensory/neural systems. If AC and BC thresholds are elevated equally then the loss is sensorineural, while if AC thresholds are worse than BC thresholds with a gap more than 10 dB, then hearing loss is conductive. The pure-tone average is the mean of thresholds at 500, 1000, and 2000 Hz, which is the same frequencies referred to the speech frequencies. Tables 66.5 and 66.6 show the classification of hearing loss severity and its configuration [12].

Speech audiometry for pediatric age helps to determine the ability to perceive speech and check pure-tone threshold reliability. It includes speech detection threshold (SDT) and speech reception threshold (SRT) using developmentally appropriate spondee words or body-part identification.

66.2.2.3 Otoacoustic Emissions (OAE)

OAE are low-intensity sounds generated by the cochlea either spontaneously or evoked by an auditory stimulus and measured in the ear canal by-product of the active processes of the cochlear outer hair cells, which indicates mechanically active outer hair cells. They are frequency specific

Table 66.6 Criteria for classifying audiometric configurations

Term	Description
Flat	Less than 5 dB rise or fall per octave
Gradually falling	5–12 dB increase per octave
Sharply falling	15–20 dB increase per octave
Precipitously falling	Flat or gradually sloping, then threshold increasing at 25 dB or more per octave
Rising	Less than 5 dB decrease in threshold per octave
Peaked or saucer	20 dB or greater loss at the extreme frequencies, but not at the mid frequencies
Trough	20 dB or greater loss in the mid frequencies (1000–2000 Hz), but not at the extreme frequencies (500 or 4000 Hz)
Notched	20 dB or greater loss at one frequency with complete or near-complete recovery at adjacent octave frequencies

arising from the place on the cochlea's basilar membrane responsible for processing that frequency.

Types of otoacoustic emissions:

- Spontaneous OAEs
  - Sounds emitted spontaneously without an acoustic stimulus.
  - Prevalence estimates vary (found in 40–50% of normal hearing).
  - Not generally used in clinical settings.
- Evoked OAEs
  - *Transient Evoked OAEs (TEOAEs)*: Sounds emitted in response to an acoustic stimulus, usually clicks but also tone bursts can be used.
  - *Distortion Product OAEs (DPOAEs)*: Sounds emitted in response to two simultaneous tones (F1, F2) of different frequencies and the response is a third tone, usually at 2F1–F2.
  - *Sustained Frequency OAEs (SFOAEs)*: Sounds emitted in response to a continuous tone. It is not much used for clinical purposes except for research.

OAEs are primarily analyzed in terms of signal-to-noise ratio (SNR), and the OAE

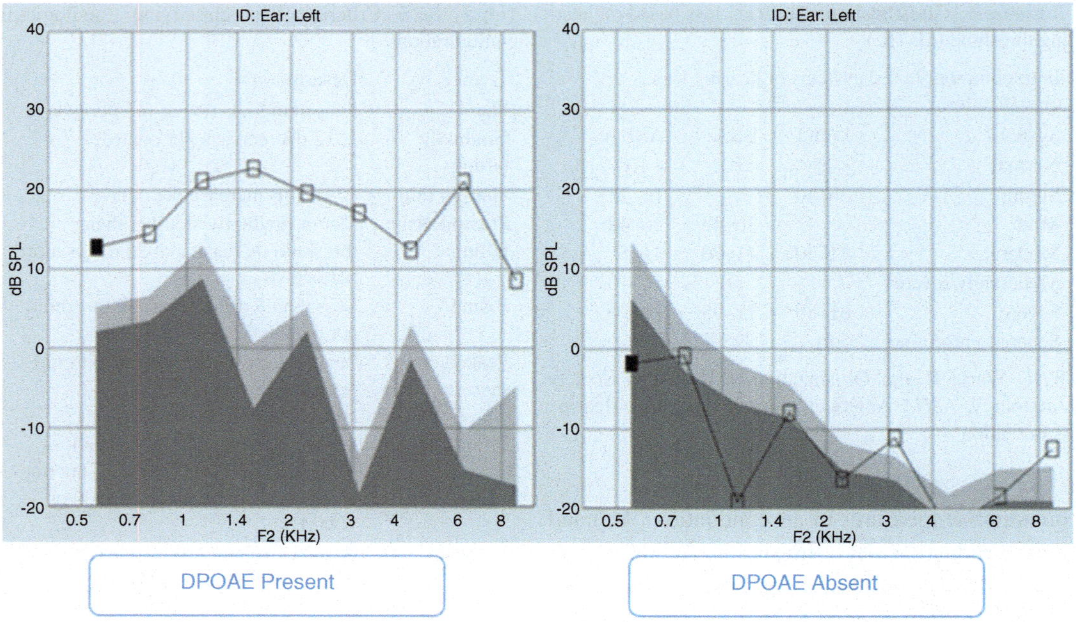

Fig. 66.3 Distortion Product OAEs (DPOAEs) response

response is how many dB above the "noise floor." It is considered present if the response is 3–6 dB above the noise floor (Fig. 66.3). It is also considered present with regard to reproducibility, >70% reproducibility for TEOAEs.

The presence of the response indicates that the outer hair cells function is normal. Normal OAEs generally imply normal hearing, except in cases of auditory neuropathy and give indirect clue about middle ear function, while absent OAE suggests cochlear hearing loss >25–30 dB HL.

The advantages of otoacoustic emission test: It is an objective test, highly sensitive, highly dependent on outer hair cell function, relatively inexpensive; offers immediate response, ear-specific results; and does not require a sound-treated booth. On the other hand, it cannot estimate the type and degree of hearing loss, as OAEs are not a test of hearing.

A *rule of thumb* for comparing OAEs to hearing thresholds is that OAEs are present if thresholds are better than about 30 dB HL and absent if thresholds are poorer than 30 dB HL.

Clinical applications of otoacoustic emission test:

1. Newborns and infant screening.
2. Pediatric assessment.
3. Cochlear function monitoring.
4. Certain cases like ototoxicity and noise-induced hearing loss.

66.2.2.4 Auditory Brainstem Response (ABR)

An auditory evoked potential (AEP) is a waveform that reflects the electrophysiologic function of a certain portion of the central auditory nervous system in response to sound. An ABR is an objective test that elicits brain stem potentials in response to click or tone burst stimuli.

In response to the stimulus onset, the ABR waveform appears as several narrow peaks and troughs within 1–10 ms. The main positive peaks are labeled, in Roman numerals for Waves I, II, III, IV, V, VI, and VII. The following are the neural generators of the waves (Table 66.7).

ABRs can be performed via air conduction or bone conduction. ABRs can be affected by the subjects' gender, age, temperature, and degree of hearing loss but are not acutely affected by the state of arousal or most sedatives anesthesia

Table 66.7 Auditory brainstem response waves

dWave number	Site
I	Distal VIIIth cranial nerve
II	Proximal VIIIth cranial nerve
III	Superior olivary complex
IV	Pons, lateral lemniscus
V	Midbrain, lateral lemniscus, and inferior colliculus
VI and VII	Undetermined (probably medical geniculate body and auditory cortex)

drugs. The ABR should be used in combination with other audiologic procedures.

ABR can be used in different methods:

- *Neurologic ABR*: Evaluates the integrity of the auditory neural pathways, used as a diagnostic and screening tool to indicate auditory nerve and brainstem lesions and to rule out acoustic neuromas/vestibular schwannoma. It requires a high stimulus level of 80–90 dBnHL. A click stimulus generates a response from the 2–4 K Hz region of the basal portion of the cochlea [13]. Click ABR has a specificity of eighty percent for eighth nerve tumor detection [14]. ABRs are not known to be sensitive to small eighth nerve tumors.
- *Stacked ABR*: Enhances small eighth nerve tumor detection up to 95% sensitivity with 88% specificity.
- *Threshold ABR*: Assess the hearing thresholds in children, difficult-to-test patients, and non-organic hearing loss. The wave V peak is identified at each intensity level in a descending method with either a click or tone bursts stimuli until it is no longer identifiable. The click stimuli give an estimated hearing threshold from 1000 Hz through 8000 Hz frequency regions of the cochlea's greatest energy at 3000 Hz [15] while tone burst ABR uses a brief tone stimulus and gives frequency-specific information at 500, 1000, 2000, and 4000 Hz. The thresholds estimated from the ABR are typically higher when compared to behavioral thresholds. They can be as much as 20–30 dB higher, depending on the frequency; this why the corrected ABR is referred to as estimated Hearing Level (eHL) to distinguish it from a typical ABR referenced in normalized Hearing Level (nHL).

A complete ABR test will provide the following information about each ear:

1. Absolute wave and interpeak latencies of all identifiable Waves I–V at different intensities.
2. Wave amplitudes (absolute and relative).
3. Threshold of Wave V if hearing threshold estimation was the purpose of the test.
4. A comparative response with a higher click rate when the ABR was for neurological assessment.

66.2.2.5 The Cochlear Microphonic (CM)

Pre-neural response from the cochlear outer hair cells (OHC) indicating normal OHC function. It follows the characteristics of the external stimulus. The direction of the cochlear microphonic will reverse with changes in the polarity of the stimulus. Responses obtained with positive (condensation) and negative (rarefaction) polarity stimuli show an inversion of the peaks of the cochlear microphonic waveform. CM testing is usually not necessary if OAE is reliably present. However, if OAE may be absent due to a conductive pathology, it is important to consider CM testing to exclude Auditory Neuropathy Spectrum Disorder (ANSD). CM cannot be used to estimate the hearing threshold.

66.3 Management of Hearing Loss

Early detection and prevention is the key to curb the effects of hearing loss. When the results are disclosed to the parents, they may experience a range of emotions, including shock, confusion, depression, anger, and guilt, while parents are still adjusting to being parents. Parents and healthcare professionals are faced with a series of dilemmas and challenges when it is established that a child is deaf.

Medical management consists of

- Developmental assessment
- Identification of coexisting medical conditions
- Extensive investigation to find the underlying cause of deafness

For the best child and family outcomes, an experienced empathic multidisciplinary team should work in a coordinated way with the family. Early intervention should be provided. Exposure to family support groups is very beneficial.

Early intervention services at a very early stage include hearing aids and a cochlear implant in the first 6 months of life, along with audio-verbal therapy with speech and language therapists and teachers of the deaf. Early intervention is a strong predictor of later outcomes, with appropriate early intervention, children with hearing loss can be mainstreamed in regular elementary and secondary education classrooms.

Cochlear implantation: Candidacy for cochlear implantation relies mainly on the audiological assessment. The basic criteria for implanting children include:

- Bilateral severe to profound sensorineural hearing loss (unaided PTA thresholds of ≥90 dB HL)
- Minimal benefit after at least 3–6 months of rehabilitation with well-fitted hearing aids
- No evidence of auditory nerve absence or central auditory lesions
- Have the strong support of his/her family for using oral language with a realistic expectation, and have access to a postoperative rehabilitation program for oral/aural language training [16, 17]

Communication methodologies in these cases include:

1. Auditory-Verbal Approach—based entirely on the use of audition and early amplification with hearing aids/cochlear implant for the development of spoken, receptive and expressive communication skills.
2. American Sign Language (ASL).
3. Aural/Oral Method—child's residual hearing is amplified along with auditory and speech reading training. The child's output is expected to be speech.

66.4 Strategies for Prevention of Hearing Loss

1. Strengthening relevant programs and organizations: Immunization programs to prevent many of the infections and maternal and child health programs.
2. Implementation of screening and intervention programs
   - A newborn hearing screening program
   - Implement school-based hearing screening
3. Training primary-level physicians and healthcare workers about the need for early intervention to address hearing loss
4. Making appropriate technologies accessible
5. Regulation and monitoring of ototoxic medication use
6. Raising awareness via programs targeting children community awareness

Take Home Messages
- Early detection and prevention is the key to curb the effects of hearing loss.
- The newborn hearing screening program aims to identify all children with a moderate–profound PCHI in the better hearing ear.
- Hearing assessment for children can be objective or subjective, and it varies according to age.
- Absent otoacoustic emissions (OAE) suggests cochlear hearing loss >25–30 dB HL.
- Auditory brainstem response (ABR) audiometry is not acutely affected by the state of arousal or most sedatives anesthesia drugs.

References

1. Tharpe AM, Seewald R. Comprehensive handbook of pediatric audiology. 2nd ed. San Diego, CA: Plural Publishing, Inc.; 2016.
2. Shearer AE, Smith RJH. Genetics: advances in genetic testing for deafness. Curr Opin Pediatr. 2012;24(6):679–86.
3. Hilgert N, Smith RJH, Van Camp G. Function and expression pattern of nonsyndromic deafness genes. Curr Mol Med. 2009;9(5):546–64.
4. Saloojee HS, Velaphi Y, Goga N. Congenital syphilis: an overview and recommendations. Bull World Health Organ. 2004;82(6):424–30.
5. Bamford J, Ankjell H, Crockett R et al.. Evaluation of the newborn hearing screening programme in England: studies, results and recommendations. Report to Department of Health and National Screening Committee. 2005.
6. Public Health England. NHS Screening Programmes in England: April 2015 to 31 March 2016. https://www.gov.uk/government/publications/nhs-screening-programmes-annual-report.
7. British Society of Audiology. NHSP audiology protocols and guidance. http://www.thebsa.org.uk/resources/.
8. Joint Committee on Infant Hearing. Year 2007 position statement: principles and guidelines for early hearing detection and intervention programs. Pediatrics. 2007;102:893–921.
9. Martin FN. Introduction to audiology. 11th ed. New York: Pearson; 2017.
10. Hunter LL, Margolis RH. Multifrequency tympanometry. Am J Audiol. 1992;1(3):33–43.
11. Paradise JL. Tympanometry controversy and middle ear effusion: too much concern or too little? Pediatrics. 1976;58(4):626–7.
12. Katz J, Chasin M, English K, Hood LJ, Tillery KL, editors. Handbook of clinical audiology. 7th ed. New York: Wolters Kluwer Health. 2014.
13. Hall JW, Mueller HG. Audiologists' desk reference. Vol. I: Diagnostic audiology principles, procedures, and practices. San Diego, CA: Singular Publishing Group; 1997. p. 395.
14. Burkard RF, Don M, Eggermont JJ, editors. Auditory evoked potentials: basic principles and clinical application. Baltimore, MD: Lippincott Williams & Wilkins; 2007.
15. Hall III. New handbook of auditory evoked responses. New York: Pearson; 2007.
16. Zyfter W, Karlik M, Sekula A, Harris S, Gawęcki W. Current indications for cochlear implantation in adults and children. Otolaryngol Pol. 2019;73(3):1–5.
17. Wackym PA, Tran A. Chapter 15: Cochlear implantation: patient evaluation and device selection. In: Flint PW, Haughey BH, editors. Cummings otolaryngology: head & neck surgery. 6th ed. Philadelphia: Elsevier Inc.; 2015. p. 2428–43.

Part VIII

Facial Plastics

67 Facial Aesthetic Analysis

Rani Hammoud and Hassan Haidar

67.1 Introduction

Human beauty standards, although might vary from culture to another and between times, reflect our evolutionary past and emphasize the role of health assessment in mate choice, where beautiful facial features are indicators of health and fertility.

Aesthetic facial proportions have been used in art since the ancient Egyptians; however, it was the Greek philosophers that made it a formal discipline, where beauty is synonymous to symmetry, harmony, and geometry. In his drawing on the Vitruvian man, Leo da Vinci formulated the ideal human proportion according to Vitruvius, and with this da Vinci formulated the ideal facial proportions by dividing the face into three equal parts. On the other hand, the German printmaker Albrecht Durer divided the face into four equal fourths, and noticed that the length of the nose is equal to that of the ear. From arts to medicine, facial aesthetic analysis plays an important role in the preoperative preparation of patients seeking facial cosmetic and enhancing procedures to get the best result.

R. Hammoud
ENT Department, Hamad Medical Corporation, Doha, Qatar

H. Haidar (✉)
Hamad Medical Corporation, Doha, Qatar

67.2 Skin Classification [1]

Physiologic Changes of the Aging Face

- 1% per year thinning of the papillary dermis
- Decrease of elastin production
- Photodamage
- Increased skin wrinkling and laxity
- Ptosis is of the soft tissue
- Atrophy of the dermis
- Decrease subcutaneous fat and loss of soft tissue volume

Fitzpatrick Skin Classification

- Helps to predict the possible sun damage and the risk of skin cancer (Table 67.1)

The patient fills a questionnaire on genetic disposition, reaction to sun exposure, and tanning habits; a score is formulated that correspond to a fitzpatrick skin phototype.

Dermatone skin analyser is a portable easy to use device that accurately analyzes the skin tone based on the concentration of melanin, Hb, and skin reflection properties of the skin, where the readings have a scale that correspond to various Fitzpatrick skin types.

Glogau Classification of Photoaging

- Photoaging is the premature aging of the skin due to primarily UV light exposure (Table 67.2)

A. Al-Qahtani et al. (eds.), *Textbook of Clinical Otolaryngology*,
https://doi.org/10.1007/978-3-030-54088-3_67

Table 67.1 Fitzpatrick's skin phototypes

Phototype	Sunburn and tanning history (defines the phototype)	Immediate pigment darkening	Delayed tanning	Constitutive color (unexposed buttock skin)
I	Burns easily, never tans	None (−)	None (−)	Ivory white
II	Burns easily, tans minimally with difficulty	Weak (± to +)	Minimal to weak (± to +)	White
III	Burns moderately, tans moderately and uniformly	Definite +	Low +	White
IV	Burns minimally, tans moderately and easily	Moderate ++	Moderate ++	Beige-olive, lightly tanned
V	Rarely burns, tans profusely	Intense (brown) +++	Strong, intense brown +++	Moderate brown or tanned
VI	Never bums, tans profusely	Intense (dark brown) +++	Strong intense brown +++	Dark brown or black

Adapted from Fitzpatrick's Dermatology in General Medicine. McGraw-Hill Professional; fifth edition [2]

Table 67.2 Glogau classification of photoaging

Group	Classification	Typical age	Description	Skin characteristics
I	Mild	28–35	No wrinkles	Early photoaging: mild pigment changes, no keratosis, minimal wrinkles, minimal or no makeup
II	**Moderate**	**35–50**	**Wrinkles in motion**	**Early to moderate photoaging: early brown spots visible, keratosis palpable but not visible, parallel smile lines begin to appear, wears some foundation**
III	**Advanced**	**50–65**	**Wrinkles at rest**	**Advanced photoaging: obvious discolorations, visible capillaries (telangiectasia), visible keratosis, wears heavier foundation always**
IV	**Severe**	**60–75**	**Only wrinkles**	**Severe photoaging: yellow-gray skin color, prior skin malignancies, wrinkles throughout: no normal skin, cannot wear makeup because it cakes and cracks**

Table 67.3 Classification of Facial Wrinkles

Facial wrinkle	Class	Description
Horizontal forehead lines		
Glabellar frown lines		
Periorbital lines		
Preauricular lines	0	No wrinkles
Cheek lines	1	Just perceptible wrinkle
Nasolabial folds	2	Shallow wrinkles
Radial upper lip lines	3	Moderately deep wrinkle
Radial lower lip lines	4	Deep wrinkle, well-defined edges
Corner of the mouth lines	5	Very deep wrinkle, redundant fold
Marionette lines		
Labiomental crease		
Horizontal neck folds		

67.3 Facial Wrinkles [3]

- Superficial wrinkles: texture changes due to photoaging of the typographically defined areas, limited superficial dermal creases
- Mimetic wrinkles: deep dermal creasing, caused by repeated facial movements and dermal elastosis
- Lines (partial thickness)
- Furrows (full thickness) (Fig. 67.1 and Table 67.3)

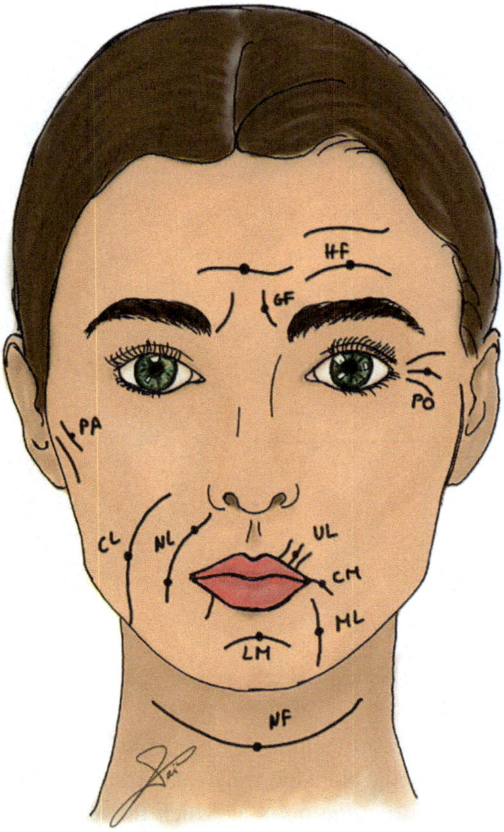

Fig. 67.1 Frontal view showing the facial wrinkles. *HF* horizontal forehead lines, *GF* glabellar frown lines, *PO* periorbital lines, *PA* preauricular lines, *NL* nasalabial lines, *CL* cheek lines, *UL* upper lip lines, *CM* corner of the mouth lines, *LB* labiomental crease, *NF* neck fold, *ML* marionette lines

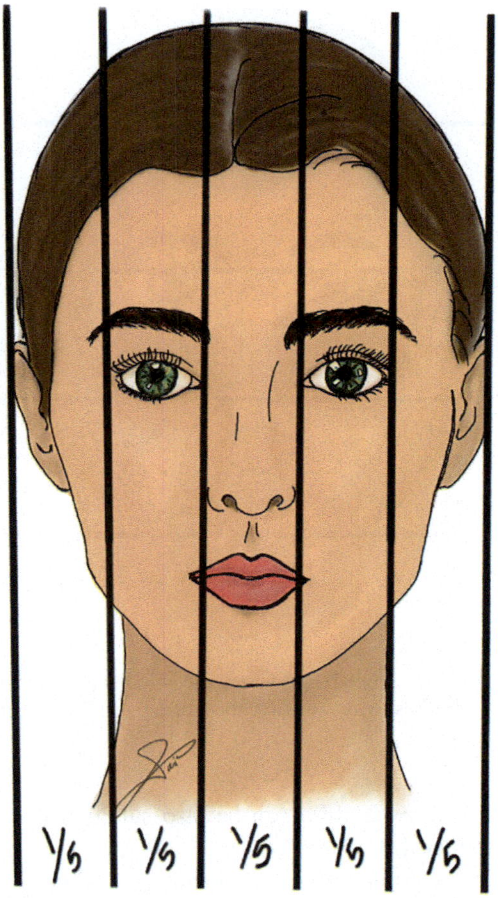

Fig. 67.2 Frontal facial view showing the facial fifths

67.4 Poor Candidates for Cosmetic Facial Plastic Surgeries

The selection of a patient suitable for cosmetic facial surgery is very important to get the best result that meets with the patients expectations; hence a patient with unrealistic expectations is a poor candidate. A patient with multiple physician visits also makes him/her a poor candidate. The physician should always check for any patterns in the patient's personality that shows any signs of psychiatric instabilities such as depression and anxiety. Finally smoking decreases the healing process, hence the patient should stop smoking to allow proper healing and less skin scarring after the surgery, hence a patient unwilling to stop smoking is a poor candidate for any cosmetic facial plastic surgeries.

67.5 Proportions [4]

67.5.1 The Frankfurt Horizontal Plane (FHP)

- Line drawn from superior aspect of external auditory canal to most inferior point of the orbital rim
- This is line used in the preoperative photos

67.5.2 Vertical Fifths (Fig. 67.2)

67.5.3 Horizontal Facial Thirds (Fig. 67.3)

- The lower third can be subdivided into upper 1/3 and lower 2/3

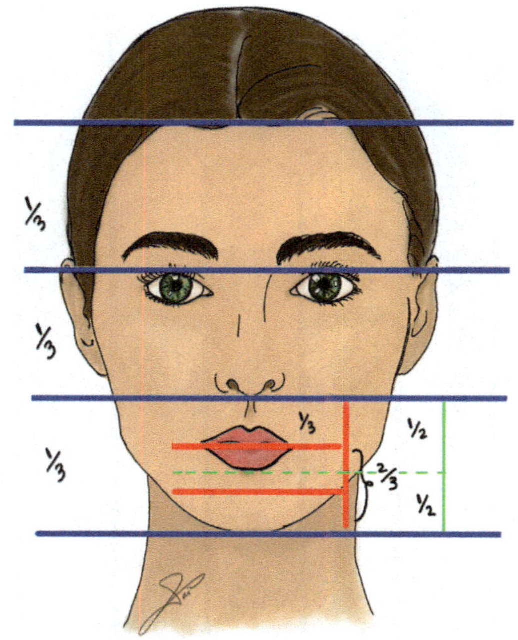

Fig. 67.3 Frontal facial view showing the horizontal facial thirds, with the lower third being also divided into thirds

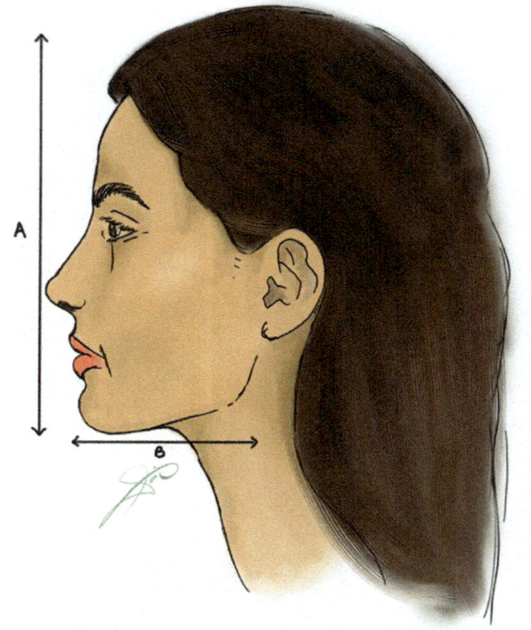

Fig. 67.4 Lateral facial view with A = 2B

- The lower third can be also subdivided into three 1/3
- The lower third can be again subdivided into 2 half

67.5.4 Lateral View (Fig. 67.4)

- The distance from the mentor to mandibular angle is half the distance from mention to hairline

67.6 Soft Tissue Anatomic Reference Points (Fig. 67.5) [5]

- *Trichion*: hairline in the midsagittal plane
- *Glabella*: most prominent portion of forehead in midsagittal plane, above root of the nose
- *Nasion*: deepest point in the nasofrontal angle, corresponds to nasofrontal suture
- *Radix*: root of nose
- *Rhinion*: junction of bony and cartilaginous nasal dorsum; thinnest skin of the nose
- *Tip*: most anterior projection of nasal tip
- *Nasal b*ase: includes the tip in addition to the columella, alar side walls, and nasal sill
- *Subnasale*: the point at which the nasal columella merges with the upper cutaneous lip
- *Pogonion*: most prominent anterior projection of chin
- *Menton*: inferior border of chin
- *Cervical point*: innermost area between the submental region and the neck
- *Sellion*: osseocartilaginous junction on the dorsum of the nose
- *Labrale superius*: vermilion border of upper lip
- *Labrale inferius*: vermilion border of lower lip
- *Mentolabial sulcus*: most posterior point between lower lip and chin

67.7 On Cephalometric Reference Point [6]

Anthropometry: standardized measuring technique that expresses the quantitative dimensions of the human body.

Cephalometry: the discipline of anthropometry that deals with the measurement of the head

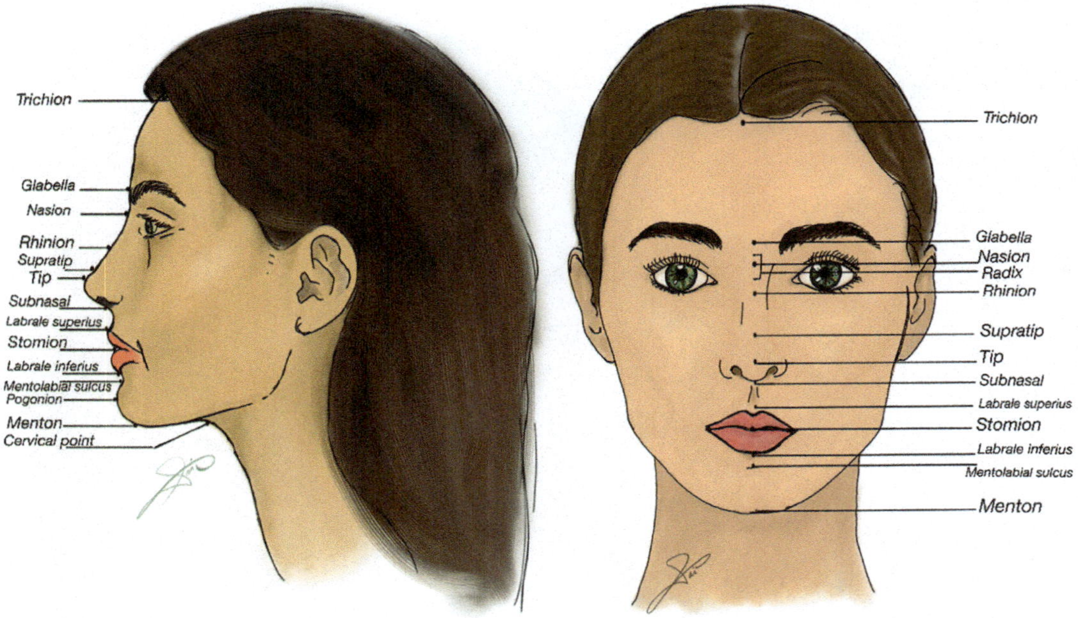

Fig. 67.5 Frontal and lateral facial view showing the major soft tissue anatomic reference points

and face bony landmarks taken directly or by radiograph using specific reference points. Cephalometry is used in forensic studies, orthodontic treatment, orthognathic surgery, and facial/ reconstructive evaluation.

Cephalometric reference points (Fig. 67.6):

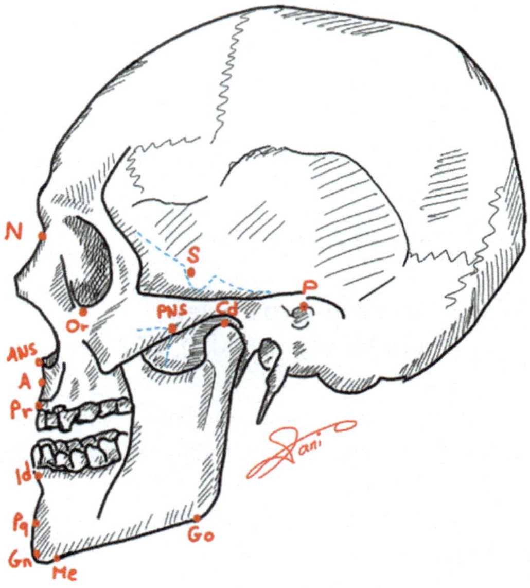

Fig. 67.6 Cephalometric reference points

- (*N*) nasion
- (*S*) Sella: midpoint of the hypophyseal fossa
- (*Or*) Orbitale: most inferior point on the infraorbital rim
- (*P*) Porion: most superior point on the external auditory meatus
- (*Cd*) Condylion: most superior point on the head of the mandibular condyle
- (*ANS*) Anterior nasal spine
- (*PNS*) Posterior nasal spine
- (*A*) Point A, subspinale: deepest point in the concavity of the premaxilla
- (*Pr*) Prosthion: lowest most anterior point on the alveolar portion of the premaxilla
- (*Id*) Infradentale: highest most anterior point on the alveolar portion of the mandible
- (*Pg*) Pogonion: Most anterior point on the bony chin in the midline
- (*Gn*) Gnathion: point between (Pg) and (Me)
- (*Me*) Menton: lowest point on the mandible
- (*Go*) Gonion: midpoint at the angle of the mandible

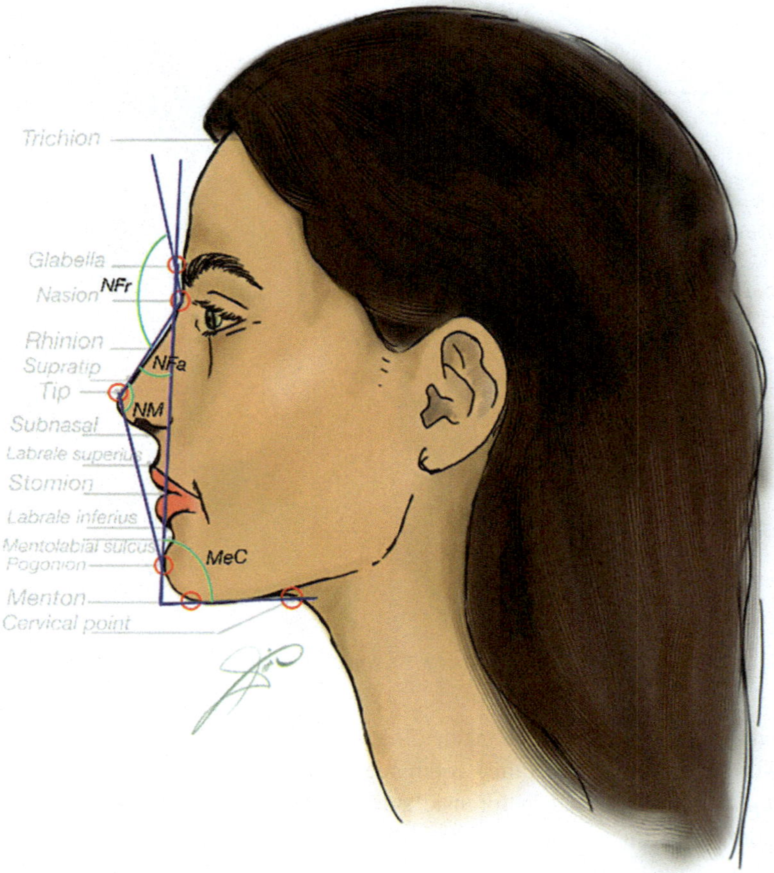

Fig. 67.7 Lateral facial view showing the facial angles according to Powell and Humphrey

67.8 Facial Angles [5]

67.8.1 According to Powell and Humphrey (Fig. 67.7)

Nasofacial angle (*NFa*): angle between the plane of the face (glabella to pogonion) and the nasal dorsum; normally 30–40°.

Nasolabial angle (*NL*): angle between a line from the upper lip mucocutaneous border to the subnasale and a line from the subnasale to the most anterior point on the columella; ideal range is 90–105° in men, and 95–120° in women.

Nasofrontal angle (*NFr*): angle between the nasal dorsum and a tangent passing through the nasion and the glabella; ideal range is 115–130°.

Nasomental angle (*NM*): angle between the nasal dorsum and the nasomental line (nasal tip to pogonion); ideal range is 120–132°.

Cervicomental angle (*MeC*): angle between a line from the glabella to the pogonion and a line from the menton to the cervical point; ideal range is 80–90°.

67.8.2 According to Peck and Peck (Fig. 67.8)

Facial angle (*F*): angle created by intersection of a line drawn from tragion to subnasal and line from nasion to pogonion; the mean angle is 102.5.

Maxillofacial angle (*MF*): angle created by intersection of line drawn from nasion to labium

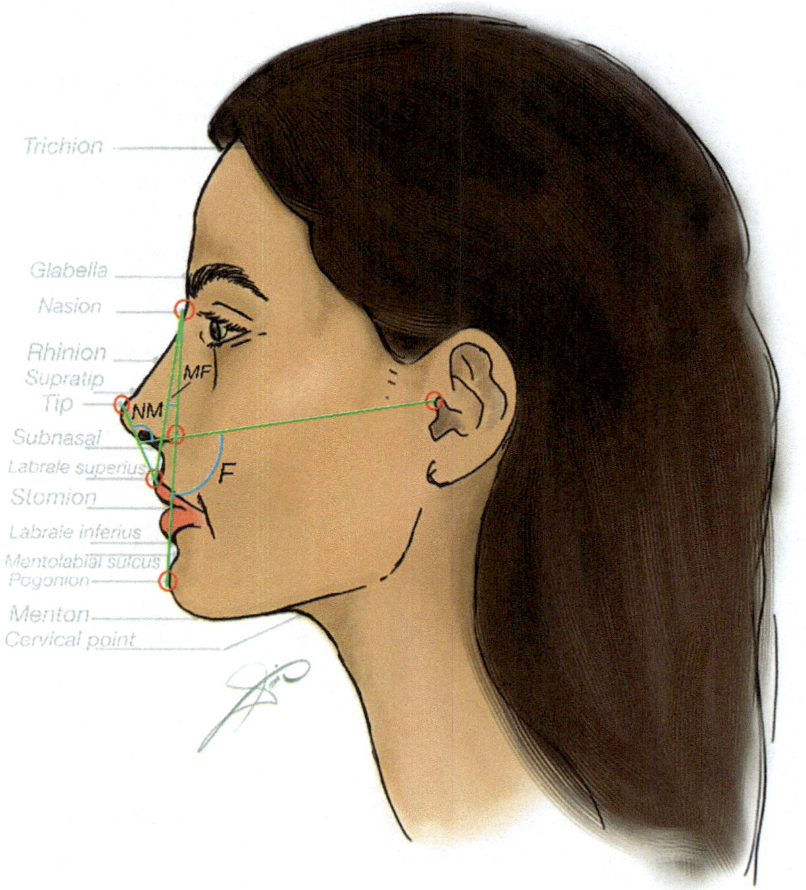

Fig. 67.8 Lateral facial view showing the facial angles according to peck and peck

superior and line from nasion to pogonion; the mean angle is 5.9°.

Nasomaxillary angle (*NM*): angle created by intersection of line drawn from nose tip to superior labium and line from tragion to subnasal; the mean angle is 106.1.

67.9 Forehead [5, 7]

- Height: from the hair line to the glabella
- Nasofrontal angle: 115–130 as described above (Fig. 67.7).
- Position of the eyebrow (Fig. 67.9):
- Medial brow is a clublike shaped start from a point on the vertical line passing from the medial canthus of the eye to the Lateral most of the nasal ala.
- Lateral brow is a point on the line passing from the nasal ala to the lateral canthus of the eye.
- In men: the eyebrow sits on the superior orbital rim with a roughly horizontal shape.
- In women: the eyebrow has a more arc shaped and usually sits above the superior orbital rim with the lateral brow slightly superior to the medial brow.
- The apex which is the highest point of the arc is usually found between the lateral limbus and the lateral canthus of the eye.

67.10 The Eyes

The boundaries of the orbit:

Lower third of the upper face and the upper third of the midface.

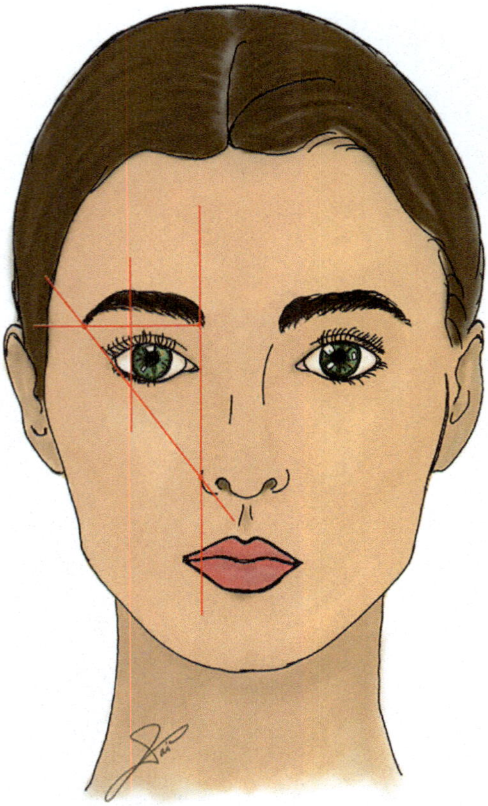

Fig. 67.9 Frontal facial view showing aesthetic analysis of the forehead

Measurements

The intercanthal distance is on average around 31–33 mm and tends to be equivalent to 1/5 the facial width; however, a distance of 33–36 mm is considered attractive.

In men, the intercanthal distance ranges from 26.5 to 38.7 mm while in women it ranges from 25.5 to 37.5 mm.

The intercanthal axis is a bit tilted with the lateral canthus 2° higher.

The upper eyelid crease is usually at the level of the nasion, with the distance from the crease to the lash line being around 8–11 mm.

The average palpebral opening is 10–12 mm, with the upper eyelid covering around 1.5 mm of the limbus while the lower eyelid covers not more than 0.5 mm of it.

The lower eyelid crease should be <5–6 mm from lid margin.

67.11 The Nose [5, 7, 8]

The nose is found in the middle facial third. Starting from the nasion which is usually at the level of the upper eyelid crease down to the subnasale. In the frontal view, a smooth continuous line can be drawn from the eyebrow along the lateral edge of the dorsum up until the nasal tip.

The nose can be divided into thirds:

- Upper third: nasal bone
- Middle third: upper lateral cartilages and septum
- Lower third: lower lateral cartilage and septum

General Measures

- The ideal nasal length from the rhinos to the tip is equal of that from the stomion to the menton, and usually is equal 2/3 of the middle facial third's height
- Dorsal width is equal to the intercanthal distance, which is equal to the 1/5 facial width

General Angles (Fig. 67.7)

- Nasofacial angle: 36°
- Nasofrontal angle: 120°
- Nasomental angle: 120–132°
- Nasolabial angle: male 90–95 female 95–110°
- Columellar-lobular angle: 30–45°
- Formed by the junction of the columella and the infratip lobule, it's usually around 30–45°. In case of prominent caudal septum, there will be increased fullness in this area giving the appearance of increased tip rotation while the nasolabial angle is unchanged

Nasal Symmetry

- An imaginary vertical line passing by the midsagittal plane is used to assess the symmetry of the nose, taking into consideration to assess each nasal third independently in order to correct the underlying cause of the asymmetry according to the deformed structure.

Nasal Tip Projection

- It's the distance of the nasal tip from the coronary plane, and it is determined by the size

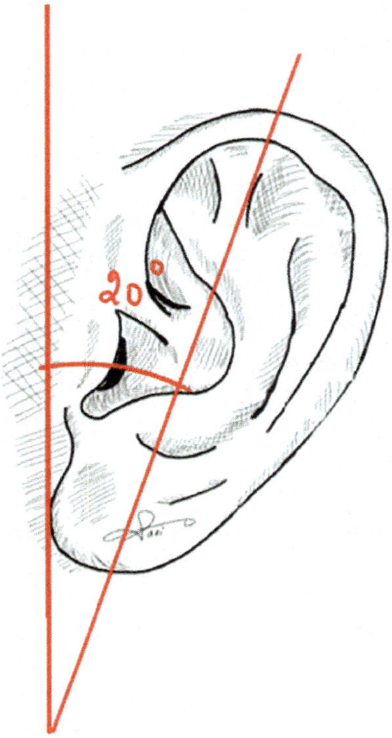

Fig. 67.10 View showing the auriculocephalic angle

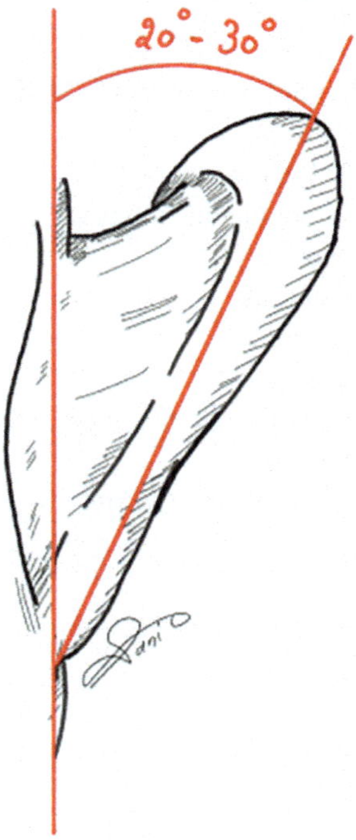

Fig. 67.11 View showing the long axis of the ear

and the shape of the lower lateral cartilages, and the height of the caudal cartilage outs septum

The distance between the tip and a vertical line drawn passing by the upper most projecting portion of the lip is usually 50–60% of the distance from the tip of the nose to the alar-cheek junction

- If >60%, it means that is overprojected
- If <50%, it mean that projection is inadequate

This relationship is only effective if the lip projection is normal

The tip projection is usually equal of the alar base width

Tip Rotation

- The rotation of the nose tip is on long the radius based at the external auditory canal, with increased rotation along the upper operation of the arc while decreased rotation is along the lower portion of the arc

The tip rotation is usually determined by the nasolabial angle (discussed in the angle section)

67.12 The Ears [7]

Angles

- Auriculocephalic angle: angle between the scalp and the anterolateral aspect of the helix, usually around 20–30° (Fig. 67.10).
- Long axis of the ear is inclined posteriorly 15–20° from the vertical line (Fig. 67.11).

Measures

- The vertical height of the ear is equal to the height of the nose from the nasion to the subnasal and it is usually around 6 cm.
- The width is around 50% the ear length.
- The helix is around 15–25 mm away from the mastoid skin.
- The helix projects 2–5 m more laterally from the antihelix.

67.13 The Mouth

The key point and landmarks to be assessed:

- Dental occlusion
- Vermilion-cutaneous junction
- Cupid's bow
- Philtral columns
- Perioral rhytids
- The volume
- The lateral angles of the mouth. Usually it gets down with age
- Upper lip length; at rest the upper lip should expose around half inch of the upper incisor teeth
- The depth of nasolabial groove at rest and during animation

67.14 Chin

- The chin is a pivotal facial unit when analyzing the nose and the neck
- The chin should be at the line perpendicular to the Frankfort and passing by the nasion
- The labiomental groove should be around 4 mm deep to the abovementioned line
- Evaluation of microgenia which is the diminished chin eminence that requires augmentation, versus the retrognathia which is the retrodisplaced mandible that requires sagittal split osteotomies

67.15 The Neck

The neck ideally has to be well defined from the pogonion to the mandibular angle, with the mentocervical angle around between 80° and 90° as discussed previously; the neck should always be assessed along with the chin, Because an obtuse mentocervical angle gives a false perception of a poor projected chin.

Take Home Messages

- The patient's skin quality affects the result of the operations.
- A proper communication between the physician and the patient is needed to insure that the patient expectations are congruent with what the surgeon can do.
- It's important to consider both the facial subunit and the face as whole during the preoperative aesthetic evaluation.
- There are people with aesthetically appealing faces that don't have these ideal facial proportions.
- Facial angles and proportions are adjuvant tools that facilitate the surgeon's work in order to provide the best result for the patients.

References

1. Sachdeva S. Fitzpatrick skin typing: applications in dermatology. Indian J Dermatol Venereol Leprol. 2009;75(1):93. https://doi.org/10.4103/0378-6323.45238.
2. Faghihi G, Fatemi-Tabaei S, Abtahi-Naeini B, Siadat AH, Sadeghian G, Nilforoushzadeh MA, Mohamadian-Shoeili H. The effectiveness of a 5% retinoic acid peel combined with microdermabrasion for facial photoaging: a randomized, double-blind, placebo-controlled clinical trial. Dermatol Res Pract. 2017;2017:1–6. https://doi.org/10.1155/2017/8516527.
3. Lemperle G, Holmes RE, Cohen SR, Lemperle SM. A classification of facial wrinkles. Plast Reconstr Surg. 2001;108(6):1751–2. https://doi.org/10.1097/00006534-200111000-00050.
4. Prendergast PM. Facial proportions. In: Erian A, Shiffman M, editors. Advanced surgical facial rejuvenation. Berlin, Heidelberg: Springer; 2012. p. 15–22. https://doi.org/10.1007/978-3-642-17838-2_2.
5. Flint PW. Cummings otolaryngology—head & neck surgery. Philadelphia, PA: Elsevier/Saunders; 2015.
6. Darkwah WK, Kadri A, Adormaa BB, Aidoo G. Cephalometric study of the relationship between facial morphology and ethnicity: review article. Transl Res Anat. 2018;12:20–4. https://doi.org/10.1016/j.tria.2018.07.001.
7. Chan Y, Goddard JC. K.J. Lees essential otolaryngology: head and neck surgery. New York: McGraw-Hill; 2019.
8. Park SS. Fundamental principles in aesthetic rhinoplasty. Clin Exp Otorhinolaryngol. 2011;4(2):55. https://doi.org/10.3342/ceo.2011.4.2.55.

Rhinoplasty

68

Hassan Haidar and Rani Hammoud

68.1 Introduction

Rhinoplasty is widely performed and is often regarded as one of the more rewarding and challenging surgeries. Many aspects of this operation give rise to the perpetual learning curve. This chapter is designed to cover broad concepts that are fundamental principles in primary rhinoplasty.

68.2 Surgical Anatomy of Rhinoplasty (Figs. 68.1 and 68.2)

Upper lateral cartilage: paired triangular cartilages connected medially to the middle third of the dorsal septum at a 10–15° angle. Bordered superiorly by the nasal bones, laterally by the maxillary pyriform aperture, and inferiorly by the lower lateral cartilage.

Lower lateral cartilage: paired C-shape cartilages with three segments (medial crus, intermediate crus, and lateral crus) that form the domes and nasal tip.

Dome: the junction between the medial and lateral crura that creates the most anterior and angulated segment of the lower lateral cartilages.

Scroll region: attachment of the upper and lower lateral cartilages.

Alae: lateral nostril walls that extend from the nasal tip to the alar crease and nasal base.

Alar crease: crease where the ala meets the cheek.

External nasal valve: the nasal aperture bordered medially by the membranous septum, superiorly and laterally by the nasal ala, and inferiorly by the nasal sill.

Internal nasal valve: the internal nasal aperture bordered medially by the caudal septum, superiorly by the upper lateral cartilage, laterally by the inferior turbinate, and inferiorly by the rim of the pyriform aperture.

Major tip support mechanisms (Fig. 68.3)

- Intrinsic strength of the lower lateral cartilages
- Attachments of medial crura of lower lateral cartilages with the caudal septum
- Attachments of the lower lateral cartilages with the upper lateral cartilages (scroll region)

H. Haidar (✉)
Hamad Medical Corporation, Doha, Qatar

R. Hammoud
ENT Department, Hamad Medical Corporation,
Doha, Qatar

A. Al-Qahtani et al. (eds.), *Textbook of Clinical Otolaryngology*,
https://doi.org/10.1007/978-3-030-54088-3_68

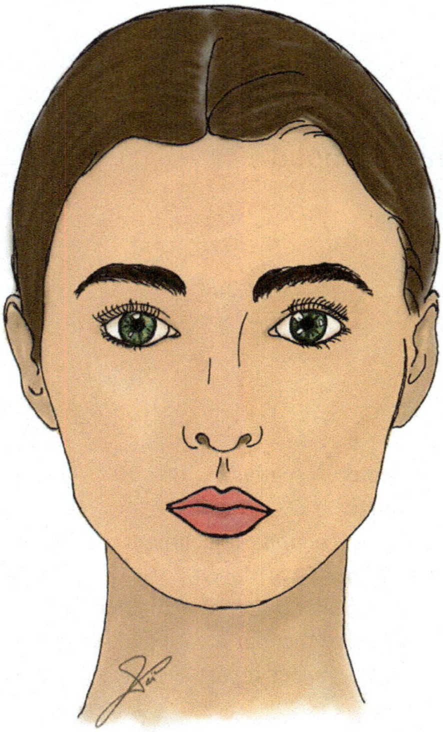

Fig. 68.1 Skeletal anatomy of nose from frontal view

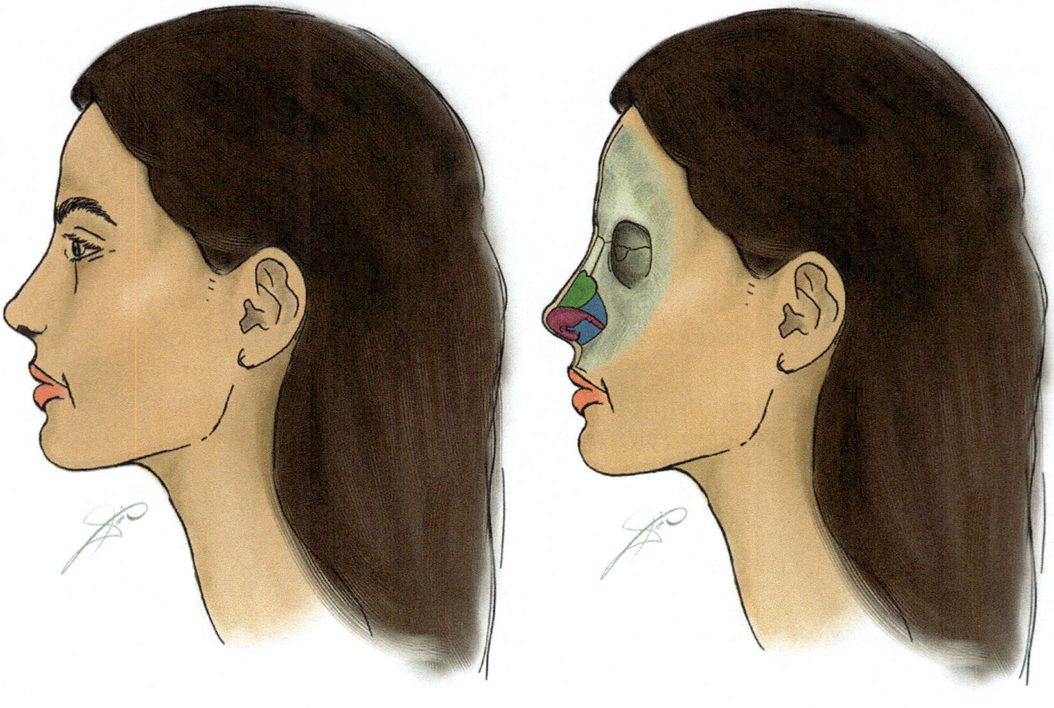

Fig. 68.2 Skeletal anatomy of nose from lateral view

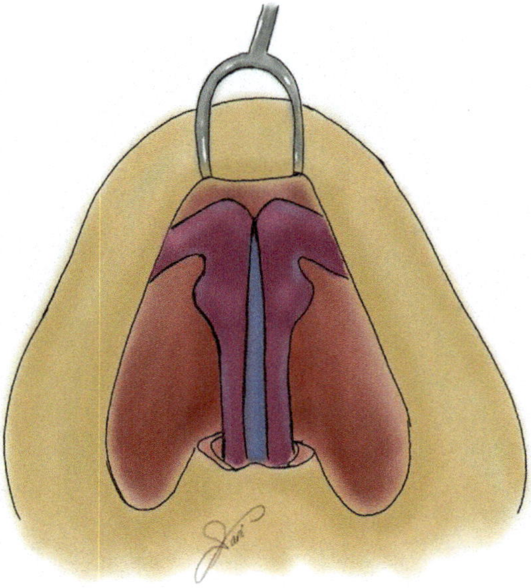

Fig. 68.3 Major tip support mechanism is defined by intrinsic strength of the lower lateral cartilages and attachments of medial crura of lower lateral cartilages with the caudal septum

68.3 Rhinofacial Analysis

68.3.1 Functional Analysis

Septum: cartilaginous and/or bony deviation, dislocation, or spur.

External nasal valve: collapse. Examine from basal view during nasal inspiration.

Internal nasal valve:

- *Cottle Maneuver*: examiner places thumbs on patient's cheeks and retracts the cheek soft tissue and nasal walls laterally during inspiration
- *Modified Cottle Maneuver*: examiner places a Freer (or other blunt instrument) into the nose to push the lateral nasal wall laterally

68.3.2 Aesthetic Analysis (Figs. 68.4, 68.5, and 68.6)

Upper third (Bony pyramid): fractures, deviation, symmetry, narrowing, depth of radix.

Middle third (Cartilaginous dorsum): deflection, "twisted nose," dorsal hump.

Lower third: asymmetry, tip projection, tip rotation, alar collapse, columellar show, alar width.

Nasofrontal angle: angle formed by (1) a line drawn from the nasal tip to the nasion and (2) a line drawn from the glabella to the nasion; "ideal": 115–130°.

Nasofacial angle: angle formed by (1) a vertical line drawn from the glabella to the pogonion and (2) a line drawn from the nasal tip to the nasion; "ideal": 30–40°.

Nasomental angle: angle formed by (1) a line drawn from the nasion to the nasal tip and (2) a line drawn from the nasal tip to the pogonion; "ideal": 120–130°.

Nasolabial angle: angle between the columella and the upper lip; males: 90–95°; females: 95–105°.

Columellar show: amount of columella visualized caudal to the ala on lateral view; "ideal" is 2–4 mm.

Thick skin:

- Advantages: hides imperfections in underlying nasal skeleton framework
- Disadvantages: increased scarring (increased risk of pollybeak deformity)

Thin skin:

- Advantages: allows for improved definition of underlying nasal skeleton
- Disadvantages: contour imperfections and irregularities are easily visible

68.4 Surgical Techniques

68.4.1 Incisions

- Marginal—an incision along the caudal edge of the lower lateral cartilage
- Intercartilaginous—an incision between the caudal edge of the upper lateral cartilage and the cephalic edge of the lower lateral cartilage
- Intracartilaginous (cartilage-splitting)—an incision through the lateral crus of the lower lateral cartel

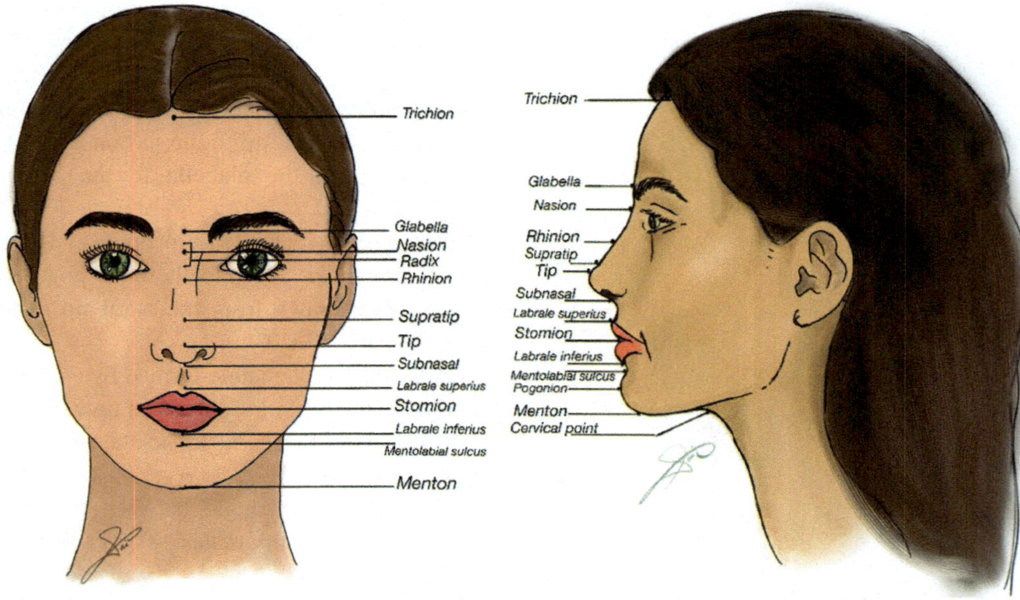

Landmark	Definition
Trichion	Midline of the hairline at the top of forehead
Glabella	Most prominent midline point of forehead
Nasion	The deepest point of the frontonasal angle
Radix	Distance measured from the plane of cornea to the nasion
Rhinion	Midline at the junction of nasal bones and dorsal septum
Supratip	Area just above the tip
Tip	Most projecting point on nasal tip
Subnasale	Point where the columellar base meets the upper lip
Nasolabial Angle	Angle formed by the junction of columella and the upper lip
Pogonion	Most anterior point in the midline of the chin
Menton	Most inferior point in the midline of the chin
Cervical Point	Junction of posterior chin with the neck

Fig. 68.4 Major facial landmarks

- Transcolumellar—a W-shaped or inverted V-shaped incision through the columella that extends to the posterior edges of the medial crura to meet the marginal incisions
- Transfixion:

  Full transfixion—a through-and-through incision made through the membranous septum caudal to the cartilaginous septum, separating the medial crura from the caudal septum

  Hemitransfixion—an incision through one side of the membranous septum just caudal to the cartilaginous septum without separating the medial crus from the septum

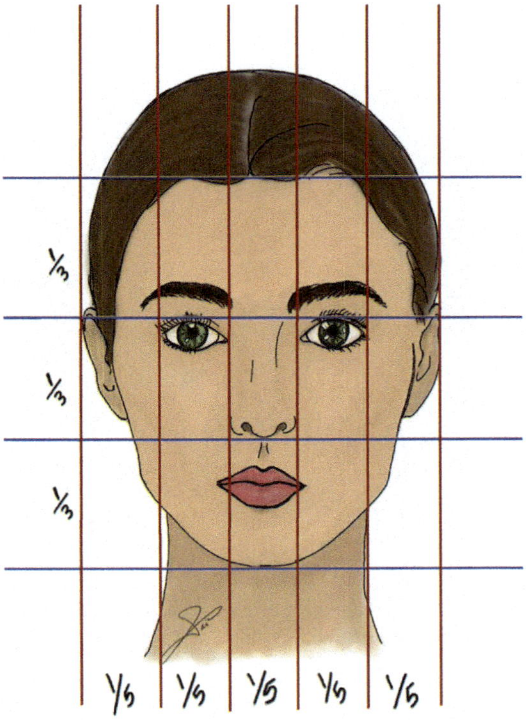

Fig. 68.5 Aesthetic nasal analysis from lateral view

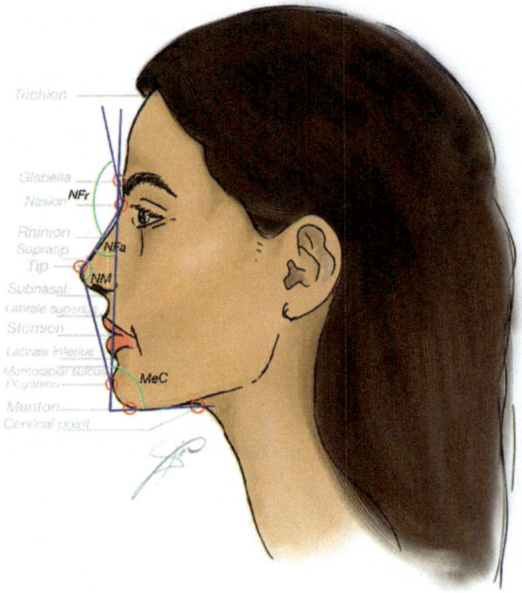

Fig. 68.6 Aesthetic nasal analysis from lateral view

- Alar base—an incision made through the nasal vestibule, nasal sill, and nasal crease to release the ala

68.4.2 Surgical Approach (Closed or Open)

68.4.2.1 Closed

Non-delivery: minor tip work performed through intracartilaginous incision or an intercartilaginous incision with retrograde dissection.

Delivery: extensive tip work performed after delivering the lower lateral cartilages through marginal and intercartilaginous incisions.

- Advantages—provides full access to the lower lateral cartilages to perform extensive tip work, no external scar
- Disadvantages—intercartilaginous incision disrupts a major tip support mechanism

68.4.2.2 Open

Performed through transcolumellar and marginal incisions

- *Advantages*: provides complete access to the lower lateral cartilages, septum, and upper lateral cartilages for extensive tip work, major reconstruction, revision rhinoplasty, dorsal septal deviations, easier placement of sutures/grafts/implants, and academic teaching/learning
- *Disadvantages*: may disrupt major tip support mechanism if medial crura are separated from the caudal septum, external scar, increased post-operative edema, more time-consuming, nasal tip anesthesia

68.4.3 Tip Modifications

68.4.3.1 Tip Narrowing/Refinement

Refinement of the broad nasal tip is one of the more common goals in cosmetic rhinoplasty. Surgical options to achieve this can be categorized as:

- Volume reduction
- Cartilage reorientation
- Augmentation
- Soft tissue debulking

Choosing the appropriate technique is highly dependent on an accurate preoperative diagnosis in terms of the anatomic etiology.

Volume Reduction

- *Complete Strip*: The cephalic border of the lower lateral cartilage is often the culprit in tip bulbosity and its direct excision can have dramatic effects on the nasal tip. The primary effect is to narrow the supratip region and allow the tip lobule to blend in better with the upper nose. The secondary effects of such a maneuver are to create some cephalic tip rotation as well as deprojection. This technique was referred to as the "complete strip" procedure, making reference to the complete strip of cartilage left behind.
- It is important to preserve at least 8 mm of caudal strip of alar cartilages; excessive cephalic trimming of lower lateral cartilage should not be excessive as the "dead space" created by this resection may lead to continued contracture, collapse, and tip deformities. These stigmata include excessive columellar show due to alar retraction and nasal obstruction due to collapse of the nasal side wall.
- *Dome-binding suture*: Single dome-binding suture: one horizontal mattress suture between the two domes used to correct a boxy or bifid tip.
- Double dome-binding suture: three sutures: one suture in each dome and one suture to bring the two domes together. Useful for more severely bifid or boxy tips, results in more narrowing than single dome-binding suture. The combination of a cephalic trim with dome-binding sutures is a useful tandem (Fig. 68.7).
- *Interrupted Strip*: interrupts the continuity of the lower lateral cartilage to obtain major changes in tip projection and narrowing. A bilateral, vertical dome division and resection of the intermediate crura or *Goldman tip technique* is useful for extremely boxy or bulbous tips with resilient intrinsic cartilage strength. Cartilaginous edges are re-approximated with simple stitches and often camouflaged with a tip graft (Fig. 68.8).

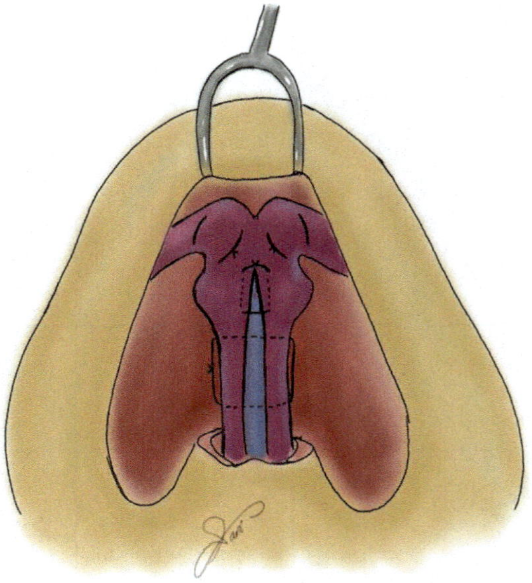

Fig. 68.7 Tip refinement using complete strip technique and double dome binding

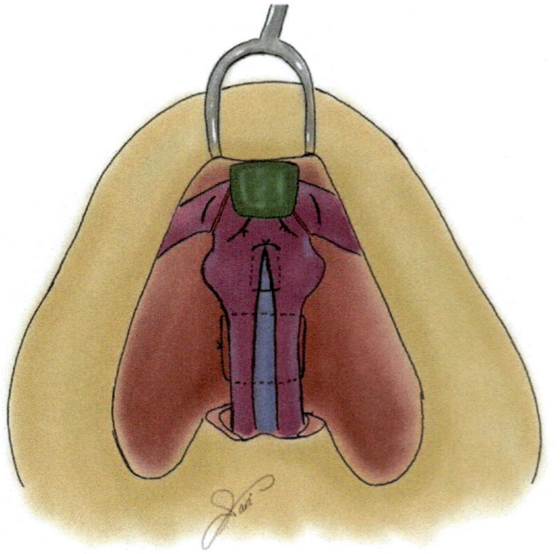

Fig. 68.8 Tip refinement using interrupted strip technique and tip graft

Tip Augmentation

Augmentation can be an effective way of improving tip definition. The amorphous tip may be best served with a strong tip graft that protrudes beyond the existing framework and creates a new

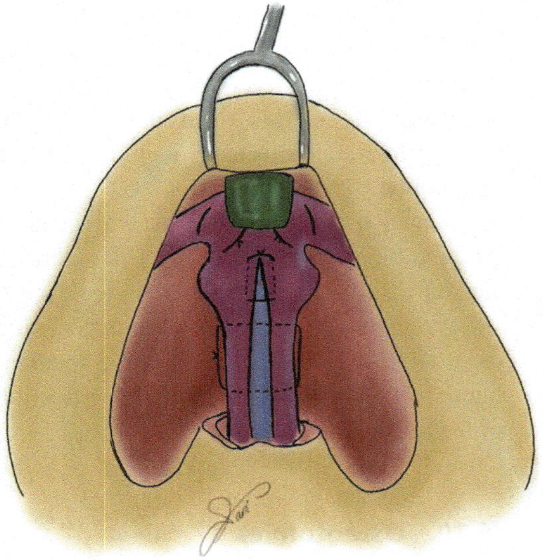

Fig. 68.9 Tip augmentation using tip graft, the outcome is better definition of the tip and more projection

scaffold for tip support. This graft can camouflage pre-existing asymmetries, form new tip defining points, and effectively narrow the tip lobule (Fig. 68.9).

Conventional "shield" tip grafts will support the tip, increase projection and create some derotation.

Soft Tissue Debulking

In individuals with extremely thick skin, who paradoxically often have a poorly developed cartilaginous framework, it may be necessary to debulk some of the overlying soft tissue envelope in order to improve the amorphous nasal tip. This is often done in conjunction with strong augmentation grafts designed to push through the thick overlying skin. This debulking must be done conservatively in order to avoid the subdermal vascular plexus and jeopardizing flap viability.

68.4.4 Techniques to Increase Projection

- *Tripod concept*: lengthen all three legs → increase projection (augment medial and lateral crura)
- *Suture techniques* can create small increases in projection:
- Suturing together the medial crura, septocolumellar sutures, transdomal and/or interdomal sutures
- *Augmentation of tip*
- *Columellar strut*

68.4.5 Techniques to Increase Rotation

- Most techniques that increase tip projection will also increase tip rotation.
- *Complete strip technique* with single dome-binding suture will increase rotation without major changes in projection
- *Reduction of dorsal hump*

68.4.6 Techniques to Decrease Projection

All procedures that destroy tip support mechanisms will reduce projection.

- *Tripod concept*: shorten all three legs → decrease projection
- *Reduction of medial and lateral crura*
- *Complete transfixion incision*
- *Reduction of caudal septum*

68.4.7 Techniques to Decrease Rotation

- The techniques to decrease tip projection typically result in a decrease in rotation
- *Augmentation of nasal dorsum*
- *Augmentation of lateral crura with overlay grafts*

68.4.8 Dorsal Augmentation

- Augmenting the dorsum is a very common goal.

- There are numerous techniques employed, each with their unique merits.
- The anatomic etiology of the low dorsum may be limited to the upper third, namely the nasal bones or it can be isolated to the middle vault, the classic “saddle nose deformity.”
- Augmentation can be done using preferably cartilage allograft harvested from nasal septum, conchal cartilage, or costal cartilage or by using prosthetic implants or even injectable soft tissue fillers.

68.4.9 Dorsal Hump Reduction

- Dorsal hump is composed of caudal anterior nasal bones and superior dorsal septal cartilage.
- Hump removal will create open roof deformity, so osteotomies are performed to medialize the nasal bones and upper lateral cartilages (Fig. 68.10).
- Hump removal may disrupt attachments of upper lateral cartilages with septum, may require spreader grafts to prevent nasal valve collapse.
- Upper lateral cartilages may collapse inferomedially away from the nasal bones causing an inverted-V deformity.
- Leaving too much dorsal septum at the anterior septal angle leaves a pollybeak deformity.
- Overresection, on the other hand, leads to more dire consequences including nasal obstruction.
- A nasion that sits low on the face will create a “pseudo-hump” and resection of this dorsum can be disastrous. Instead, one should consider augmenting the radix area and raising the nasion. This may camouflage the apparent hump and allow a more conservative resection of the dorsum.

68.4.10 Osteotomies

- Osteotomies are necessary to correct cosmetic deformities of bony upper third of nose (open roof, deviated nasal bones, narrow nasal vault, and widened nasal vault).
- *Medial osteotomy*: mobilizes the nasal bones to allow infracturing after the lateral osteotomies.
- *Lateral osteotomy*: the nasal bones along with a small portion of the maxilla are mobilized, allowing infracture of the bones.
- *Intermediate osteotomy*: an osteotomy performed between the medial and lateral osteot-

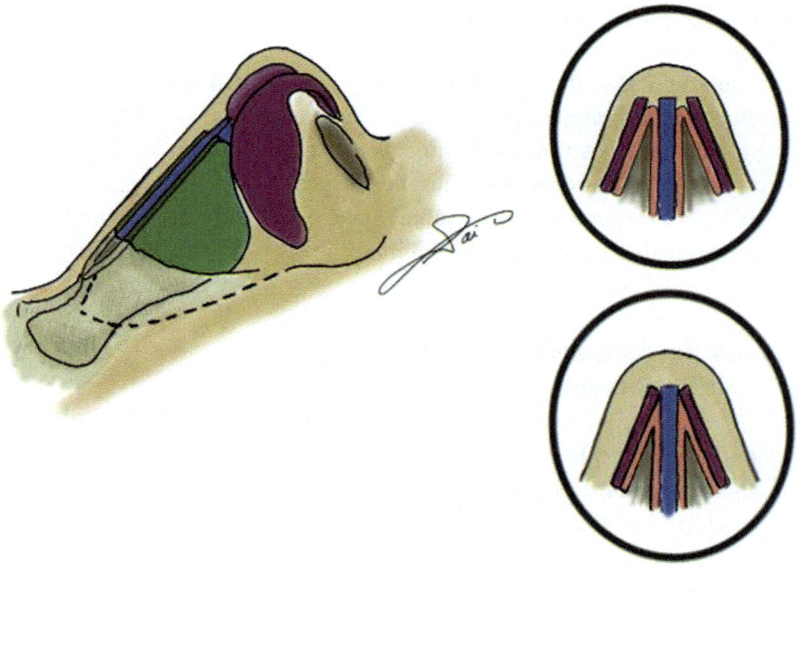

Fig. 68.10 Hump removal will create open roof deformity, so osteotomies are performed to medialize the nasal bones and upper lateral cartilages to close the open roof deformity

omies in conjunction with the other two. It provides additional medialization and infracturing of prominent nasal horns, severely deviated bony vaults, or excessively convex nasal bones.

68.4.11 Twisted Nose

- It is also important to delineate exactly which part of the nose is deviated, and in which direction.
- Deviations of the upper third are generally post-traumatic and are repaired with osteotomies. Traditional medial and lateral osteotomies do not necessarily cut through previous fractures. Because of this, it is often necessary to perform intermediate osteotomies which create smaller pieces of bone that can be better controlled and realigned.
- Middle vault deviations primarily involve the dorsal septum and straightening it can be challenging. This procedure involves release of the dorsal septum from the ULCs and progressive destabilization, realignment, followed by firm fixation and stabilization of the dorsal septum. It is usually necessary to splint the corrected cartilage with a strong piece of spreader graft.
- Significant deviations of the caudal septum may require a complete extracorporeal septoplasty and re-implantation to provide a solid dorsal and caudal "L" strut. Securing the cartilage at the dorsum to the ULCs and to the lower lateral cartilages are essential to establish a solid platform.

68.4.12 Functional Considerations

Alar collapse: place batten grafts caudal to the lateral crura at the point of nasal valve collapse.

Upper lateral cartilage collapse: spreader grafts placed between upper lateral cartilage and septum to widen nasal valve.

68.5 Complications of Rhinoplasty

Asymmetric tip: caused by unequal reduction of tip or asymmetric dome-binding sutures.

Twisted nose: caused by inadequate straightening of septum, bony vault, or asymmetric tip.

Bossing: knuckling of nasal tip caused by contractual scarring of weakened/overresected lower lateral cartilages. Patients with thin skin, bifid tips, strong cartilages, and those who have undergone vertical dome division may be at higher risk of bossing.

Treatment: excise the weakened bossing area, cover with small cartilage graft.

Saddle nose deformity: collapse of nasal dorsum caused by overresection of septum or failure to preserve a dorsocaudal L-strut.

Pollybeak deformity: soft-tissue or cartilage fullness of the supratip

- Inadequate tip support and decreased tip projection
- Excessive reduction of columella
- Inadequate reduction of dorsal hump
- Supratip dead space scar formation from inadequate skin taping

Inverted-V deformity: During dorsal hump removal, ensure preservation of the nasal mucoperichondrium, which supports the upper lateral cartilages. If nasal mucoperichondrium is violated, the upper lateral cartilages may collapse inferomedially away from the nasal bones.

If the nasal bones are inadequately infractured with osteotomies, then the patient will have an inverted-V deformity in which the caudal edges of the nasal bones are overly visible.

Treatment: new osteotomies with infracturing/narrowing of the bony nasal vault, placement of spreader grafts.

Take Home Messages

- Rhinoplasty is considered to be the most challenging, rewarding, and humbling of all otolaryngology procedures.
- No single maneuver can be applied to all rhinoplasty patients; only experience tells us how to pair an aesthetic goal with the appropriate technical maneuver.
- Every rhinoplasty operation presents the surgeon with a diversity of nasal anatomy, contours, and proportions, requiring a series of organized and interrelated surgical maneuvers tailored to each patient's anatomical and functional needs.
- Any single suture or graft can have different outcomes, especially after long-term follow-up.
- Following sound fundamental principles, beginning with analysis, is the cornerstone to a successful rhinoplasty career.

Further Readings

Daniel RK. Mastering rhinoplasty: a comprehensive atlas of surgical techniques with integrated video clips. Berlin, Heidelberg: Springer; 2010.

Daniel RK, Pálházi P. Rhinoplasty: an anatomical and clinical atlas book. Berlin, Heidelberg: Springer; 2018.

Gubisch W. Mastering advanced rhinoplasty. Berlin, Heidelberg: Springer; 2018.

Shiffman MA, Di Giuseppe A, editors. Advanced aesthetic rhinoplasty: art, science, and new clinical techniques. Berlin, Heidelberg: Springer; 2013.

Otoplasty

69

Rani Hammoud and Hassan Haidar

69.1 Introduction

The term otoplasty refers to surgical procedures designed to give the auricle a more natural and anatomic appearance and it is mainly performed for protruding ears (bat ears).

Congenitally prominent ears are a cosmetic deformity that can have a severe emotional and behavioral effect on a child, although they typically do not affect a youngster's self-image until the child is older than age 5 or 6 years; surgery for prominent ears is best performed by age 6–7 years.

69.2 Development of the Auricle

- The auricle starts to develop from the six hillocks of His (first 2 months of gestation) [1]:
  - *First branchial arch*: Anterior three hillocks—contributes the tragus, the root of helix, and superior helix only (upper third of ear)
  - *Second branchial arch*: Posterior three hillocks—contributes the rest (antihelix, antitragus, lobule) (lower two-thirds of the ear)
- Ear begins to protrude from developing face at approximately 3–4 months of gestation.
- The antihelical furl develops later over the subsequent 4 weeks, medializing the helical rim.
- The auricle is fully shaped at birth.
- By the third year of life, the ear has attained 85% of its adult size.
- The transverse auricular growth and the conchal depth growth are fully completed at the age of 6–7; however, the auricular longitudinal length is completed at around the age of 11–12 [2].

69.3 Ear Aesthetics

- The normal auricle measures approximately 6 cm vertically, and its long axis should recline approximately 20° from the vertical plane (Fig. 69.1a).
- Correct placement of the ear: The helix-to-mastoid distance falls in the normal range of 10–12 mm at the top, 16–18 mm in the middle, and 20–22 mm in the lower third.
- The normal auricle protrudes 20–30° from the skull (Fig. 69.1b).
- *A protruded ear also known as apostasis otis is* commonly caused by a combination of two defects:
  - Underdevelopment of antihelical folding (the common and the superior crura only) (Fig. 69.2)
  - Overdevelopment of the conchal wall

R. Hammoud
ENT Department, Hamad Medical Corporation, Doha, Qatar

H. Haidar (✉)
Hamad Medical Corporation, Doha, Qatar

A. Al-Qahtani et al. (eds.), *Textbook of Clinical Otolaryngology*,
https://doi.org/10.1007/978-3-030-54088-3_69

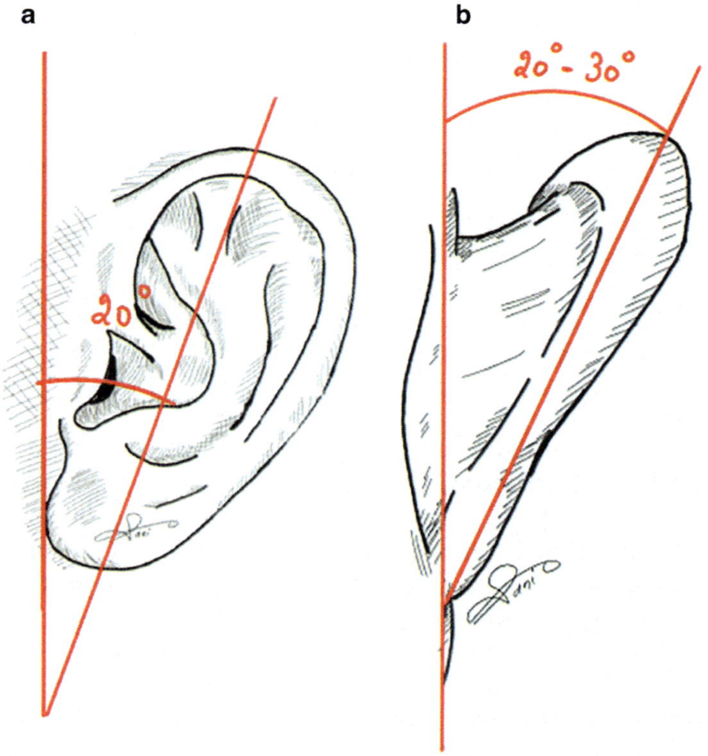

Fig. 69.1 (**a**) The normal auricle long axis should recline approximately 20° from the vertical plane. (**b**) The normal auricle protrudes 20–30° from the skull

69.4 Epidemiology

- Relatively common, with an incidence in whites of about 5%
- Autosomal dominant trait with variable penetrance
- 59% of affected individuals have a family history
- Congenital genitourinary tract deformities may be present

69.5 Nonsurgical Treatment

Nonoperative correction of protruded ear anomalies can be performed by molding if initiated within the first 2 weeks of life.

- Takes advantage of circulating maternal hormones that result in more pliable and malleable cartilage [3].
- Perform continuously for 6–8 weeks.
- May avoid surgical treatment.
- Options: Splinting, taping, and gluing.

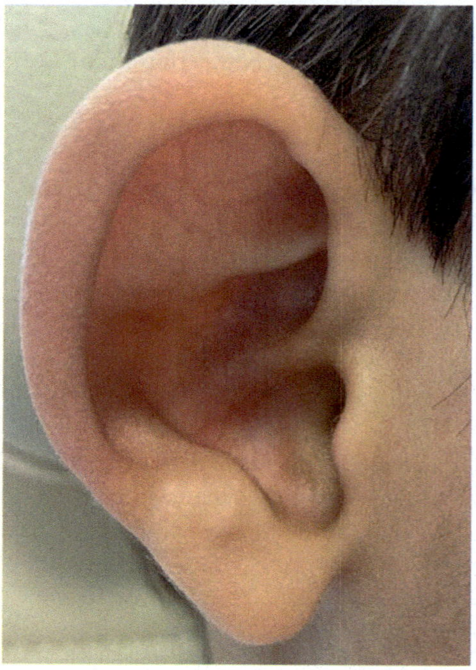

Fig. 69.2 A child with protruded ears exhibits the lack of an antihelical fold. The inferior crus is generally well developed, but the common and the superior crura can be affected. Isolated hypoplasia of the superior crus causes a superior pole deformity; if the common crus is also affected, the entire ear appears lateralized

- Fair-to-excellent results were reported in more than 70% of the cases [4].

69.6 Surgical Treatment

69.6.1 Indications

Despite benign physiologic consequences, numerous studies attest to the psychological distress, emotional trauma, and behavioral problems; this deformity can inflict on children.

Otoplasty is indicated for correction of ears that protrude more than 20 mm and at an angle greater than 35° from the occipital scalp.

Because the ear is nearly fully developed by age 6–7 years, the correction may be performed by this time.

69.6.2 Preoperative Evaluation

- The following should be assessed:
  - Degree of antihelical folding
  - Depth of the conchal bowl
  - Distance between the helical rim and the mastoid bone
  - Elasticity of the auricular cartilage
  - Comparison of both ears
  - The timing of the surgery is an important factor for better results, usually it's advisable to perform the procedure before the age of 6 since at that age the ear size is at 90 % of the adult size, therefore early surgery can reduce bullying and the psychological effects on the child [2].

69.6.3 Goals of Surgical Treatment

- All traces of protrusion in the upper third of the ear must be corrected. (Some remaining protrusion in the middle or lower portions may be acceptable.)
- From the front view, the helix of both ears should extend beyond the antihelix.
- The ear should not be placed too close to the head.
- The positions of the two ears (i.e., the distances from the lateral borders to the head) should match fairly closely—*to within 3 mm at any given point.*

69.6.4 Surgical Techniques

Two philosophies of otoplasty exist, cartilage cutting (splitting) and cartilage sparing.

Cartilage cutting technique includes incision, excision, scoring and/or abrasion. A significant drawback of incisional cartilage techniques is the potential loss of the smooth, undulating surface of the auricle because of the sharp angles at the cartilage cuts. However, it provides long-term stability.

The cartilage sparring techniques including the suture techniques were developed to overcome the disadvantages of the cartilage cutting techniques, hence providing a smooth cartilaginous contour and structural support; however, this technique has lower long-term stability.

Cross-hatching, rasping, or abrading the lateral surface of the auricular cartilage allows for medialization by contracture of the medial side and expansion of the lateral surface of the cartilage.

Modern otoplasty combines when appropriate suture techniques and cartilage cutting techniques to provide the desired result with minimal disadvantages.

Classification of the Otoplasty Surgical Techniques [5]

- Cartilage cutting otoplasty
- Converse and Becker: an incision and suturing technique
- Stenstrom: An incision and scoring technique
- Crikelair and Congchet: anterior scoring with rasp

- Walter: a cartilage incision and excision technique
- Pitanguy: cartilage island flap technique
  - Cartilage sparing techniques:
    Mustarde: a suturing technique
    Furnas: suturing technique

Mustarde Technique

- Used to correct a poorly defined antihelical fold.
- Sutures (scaphaconchal sutures) placed from the scaphoid fossa to the concha to create an antihelical fold (Fig. 69.3).
- Because no cartilage incisions are made, the antihelical contour is smooth.
- Correct placement and incremental tension on the Mustarde sutures creates a conchoscaphoid angle of 90° [6].

Furnas Technique

- Used to correct conchal excess through conchamastoid sutures (several permanent mattress sutures between conchal cartilage and the mastoid periosteum → medial conchal repositioning) (Fig. 69.4).
- Directing the sutures posteriorly is important to avoid advancing the conchal bowl into the external auditory meatus.
- Can be combined with other techniques for correcting an absent antihelical fold [6].

Stenstrom

- Rasping alone of the lateral surface of the antihelix in order to promote medially directed folding of the antihelix [7].
- Cartilage scoring techniques are based on the observation that cartilage curls away from a cut surface, which has been attributed to “interlocked stresses” that are released when the perichondrium is incised [8, 9].
- Narrow rasper can be introduced into subcutaneous pockets on the lateral surface from posterior access via small transcartilage fenestration.

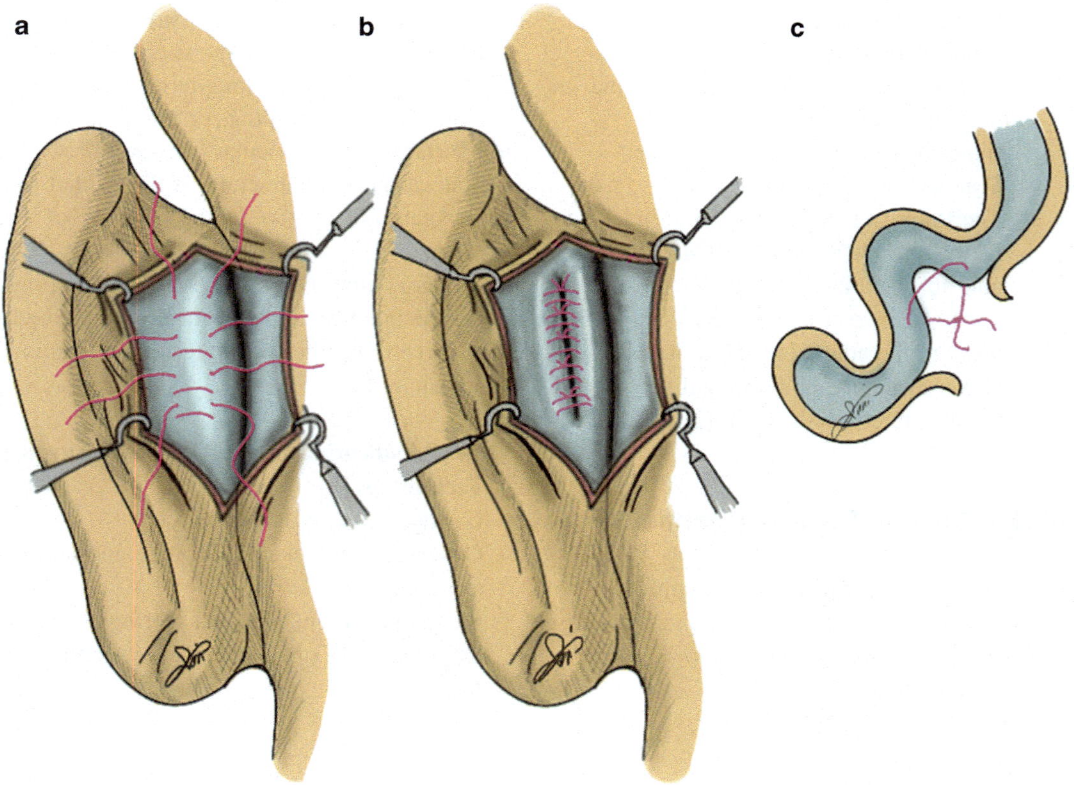

Fig. 69.3 Mustarde suture placement

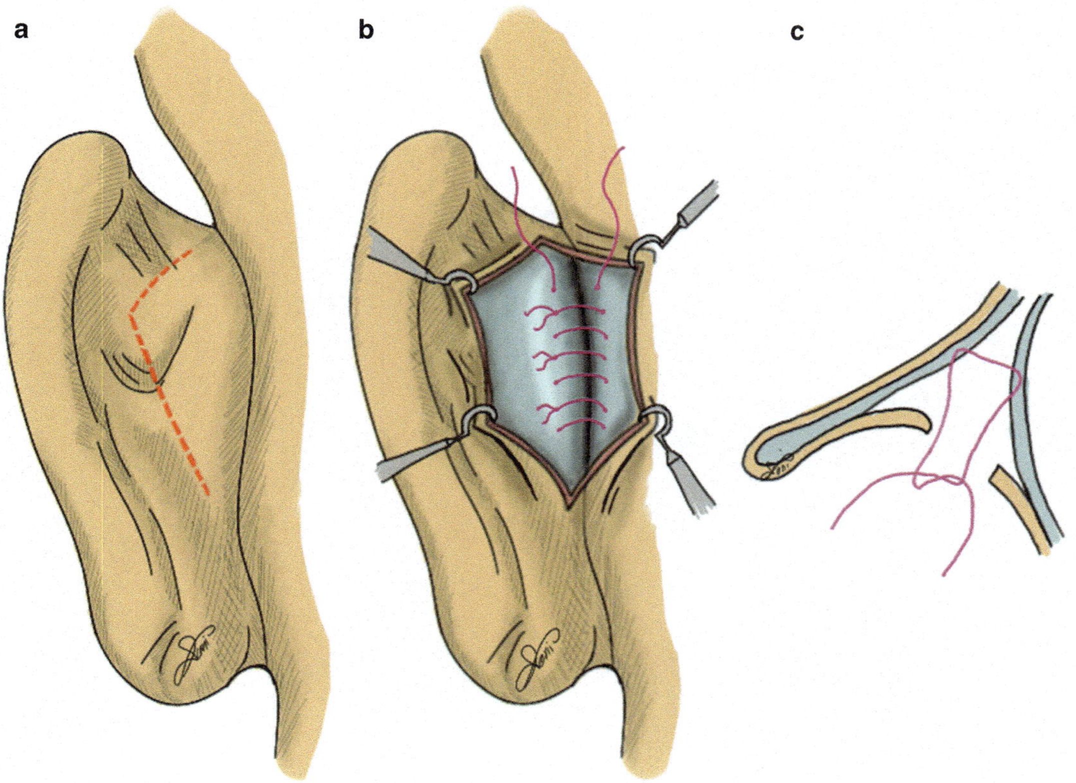

Fig. 69.4 Furnas technique: Conchal setback sutures

"Incisionless" Otoplasty

- Used to correct a poorly defined antihelical fold.
- Uses small stab incisions to pass mattress sutures on both sides of the antihelical curl.
- The suture is passed through these incisions below and out of the skin, then turned and passed through the incision again to exit at the next incision site.

Correction of Lobule Prominence

A prominent lobule can be caused by medial skin excess or an abnormal cauda helicis:

- Medial skin excess: Corrected using the modified fishtail excision (Fig. 69.5)
- Long and abnormally positioned cauda helicis → simple resection of the cauda helicis corrects lobule position

69.7 Complications [10]

Hematoma

- Most immediate and pressing postoperative problem
- If sudden onset of persistent, unilateral pain, then suspect hematoma
- Management: urgent suture removal, and evacuation of clot. Reexploration and hemostasis, if active

Wound Infection

- Rare, usually from s-aureus
- Antibiotics are useful in preventing spread of infection and chondritis

Chondritis

- The most feared complication of otoplasty because it can deform the ear beyond recognition.

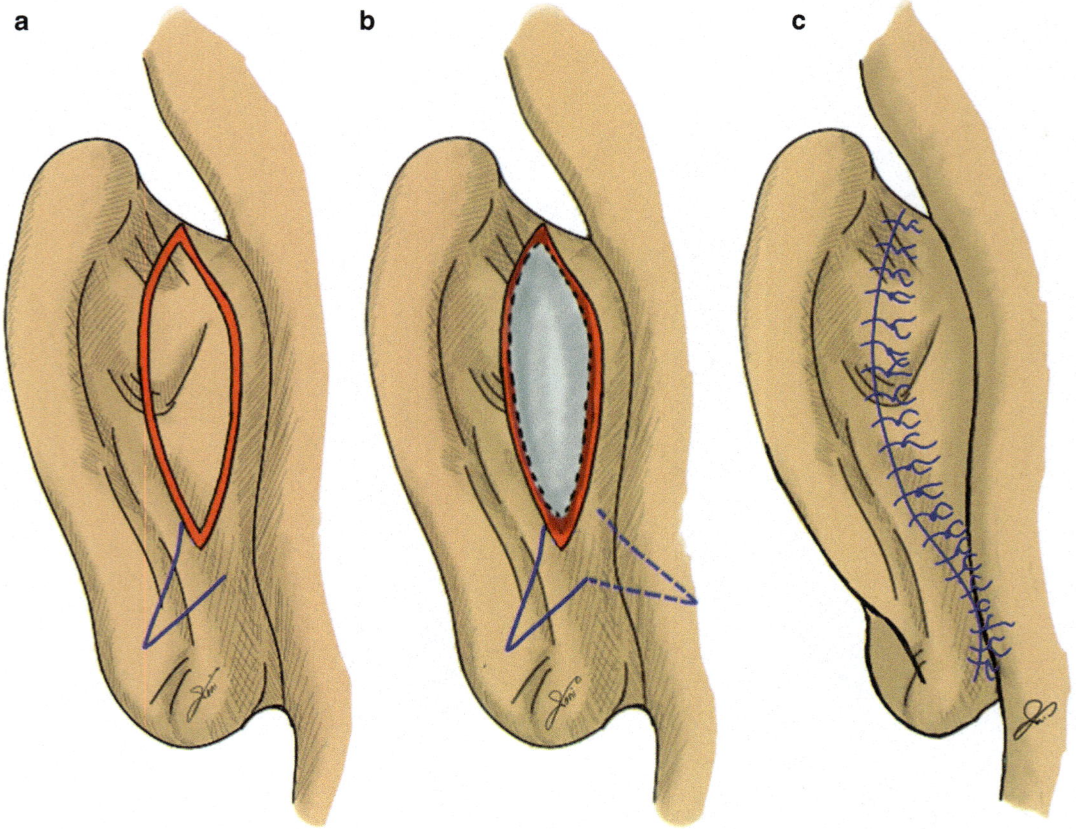

Fig. 69.5 Modified fishtail excision technique: Mark a "V extension" from the inferior aspect of the postauricular incision used for correction of prominent ear deformity (e.g., Mustarde, Furnas). Transpose the marking to the mastoid skin while the ink is still fresh, forming a mirror image pattern in the shape of a fishtail. Excise along the demarcated line

- Appropriate perioperative antibiotics and drainage of any collection of serum or blood can prevent chondritis.
- Chondritis requires prompt exploration and debridement of necrotic cartilage.

Undesirable Outcome

- Incomplete correction of prominent ears is probably the most common undesirable outcome of otoplasty.
- Correction of the mid portion of the auricle greater than the superior and inferior poles leads to a "telephone ear" deformity.
- A reverse telephone ear deformity is a result of inadequate medialization of the central portion of the auricle.
- Overcorrection of a prominent ear can lead to obliteration of the postauricular sulcus.
- Loss of correction after otoplasty can be a frustrating complication. Early loss may be a result of manipulation by the patient, or it may be caused by suture breakage or poor suture placement.
- The most common long-term complication is recurrence of the deformity, which is technique and surgeon dependent.

Hypertrophic scars or keloids may form along the incision line. This is more likely if excess tension is placed on the closure.

Take Home Messages

- Ear cartilage is very malleable immediately after birth, and deformities can sometimes be corrected nonsurgically through molding techniques.
- Otoplasty for prominent ear deformities usually is performed around age 6–7 years.
- Two deformities that make up the prominent ear: poorly defined antihelical fold and/or conchal excess.
- The best surgical approach to treat a prominent ear: combination of cartilage scoring and cartilage molding.
- Hematoma and infection are rare but need to be treated immediately and aggressively.
- The most common long-term complication is recurrence of the deformity, which is technique and surgeon dependent.

References

1. Streeter GL. Development of the auricle in the human embryo. Contrib Embryol. 1922;14:111–3.
2. Naumann A. Otoplasty—techniques, characteristics and risks. GMS current topics in otorhinolaryngology. Head Neck Surg. 2007;6:Doc04.
3. Cottler PS, McLeod MD, Payton JI, Pineros-Fernandez A, Black JS. Plasticity of auricular cartilage in response to hormone therapy. Ann Plast Surg. 2017;78(6S Suppl 5):S311–4.
4. van Wijk MP, Breugem CC, Kon M. Non-surgical correction of congenital deformities of the auricle: a systematic review of the literature. J Plast Reconstr Aesthet Surg. 2009;62(6):727–36.
5. Taş S. Prominent ear correction: a comprehensive review of fascial flaps in otoplasty. Aesthet Surg J. 2018;38(7):695–704. https://doi.org/10.1093/asj/sjx254.
6. Aston SJ, Beasley RW, Throne CH, editors. Grabb and Smith's plastic surgery. 6th ed. Philadelphia: Lippincott Williams & Wilkins; 2007.
7. Stenstroem SJ. A natural technique for correction of congenitally prominent ears. Plast Reconstr Surg. 1963;32:509.
8. Gibson T, Davis W. The distortion of autogenous cartilage grafts: its cause and prevention. Br J Plast Surg. 1958;10:257.
9. Fry HJ. Interlocked stresses in human nasal septal cartilage. Br J Plast Surg. 1966;19:276.
10. Furnas DW. Complications of surgery of the external ear. Clin Plast Surg. 1990;17:305.

Blepharoplasty

70

Maryam Abdulraheem, Rani Hammoud, Shanmugam Ganesan, and Alwyn D'Souza

70.1 Introduction

Blepharoplasty is one of the most common surgical procedures performed for both functional improvements in the aging patient as well as aesthetic rejuvenation of the periocular region and midface [1]. It is a surgical procedure in which the eyelid skin, orbicularis oculi muscle, and orbital fat are excised or sculpted to rejuvenate the aesthetic look of the patient along with the correction of any functional abnormality [2]. Usually, the upper eyelid blepharoplasty is performed for both aesthetic and functional indications, while the lower eyelid blepharoplasty is commonly performed for esthetic reasons [3, 4].

70.2 Eyelid Anatomy

The eyelid is a bilamellar structure comprising an anterior lamella and a posterior lamella separated by the orbital septum (Figs. 70.1 and 70.2).

M. Abdulraheem (✉) · R. Hammoud · S. Ganesan
ENT Department, Hamad Medical Corporation, Doha, Qatar
e-mail: mabdulraheem1@hamad.qa; Rhammoud3@hamad.qa; Sganesan@hamad.qa

A. D'Souza
University Hospital Lewisham, London, UK

70.2.1 The Anterior Lamella

The eyelid has two lamellas, an outer and an inner lamella separated by the orbital septum, which is also known as the palpebral pigment. It is a dense fibrous membrane extending from the periosteum of the orbital rim to the tarsus, and in the upper eyelid, it fuses with the levator aponeurosis. The orbital septum is considered a barrier to both neoplastic and inflammatory invasion.

The outer lamella consists of two parts, the skin measuring around 0.3 mm and the oculi muscle, which is supplied by the facial nerve, and it furtherly subdivided into three parts.

The outermost is the pretarsal fibers found over the tarsal plate responsible for the involuntary blink and the mechanism of lacrimal pumping. The second part is the preseptal fibers that overlie the orbital septum; these fibers assist with blinking. The orbital fibers overlying the orbital rims are responsible for the voluntary and forceful eyelid closure.

The tarsal plate is a dense connective tissue found at the margin of the eyelids approximately 1–2 mm in thickness attached medically to the anterior lacrimal crest by the medial canthal tendon and to the orbital tubercle of the zygomatic bone by the lateral canthal tendon.

The superior tarsus is around 12–15 mm in vertical height and serves as an attachment for the Muller's muscle and the levator aponeurosis superiorly. On the other hand, the inferior tarsus

A. Al-Qahtani et al. (eds.), *Textbook of Clinical Otolaryngology*,
https://doi.org/10.1007/978-3-030-54088-3_70

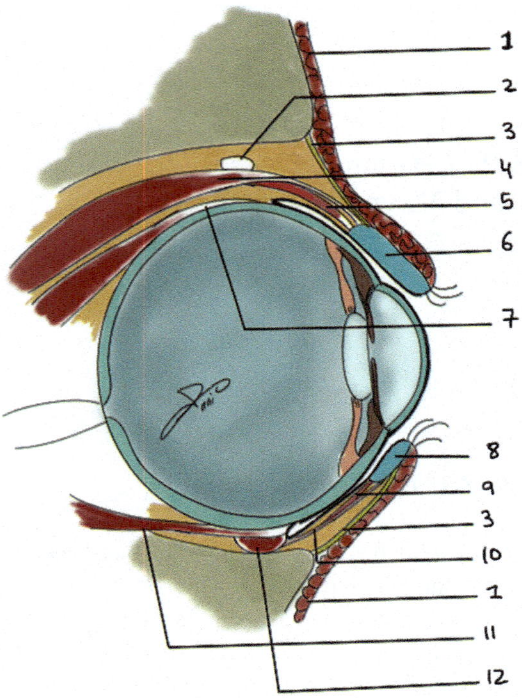

1. orbicularis oris muscle
2. Whitnall's ligament
3. Orbital septum
4. Levator palpebrea superioris muscle
5. Muller's muscle (superior trasal muscle)
6. Superior tarsus
7. Superior rectus muscle
8. Inferior tarsus
9. Inferior tarsus muscle
10. Capsulopalpebral fascia
11. Inferior rectus muscle
12. Inferior oblique muscle

Fig. 70.1 Sagittal view. (1) Orbicularis oris muscle. (2) Whitnall's ligament. (3) Orbital septum. (4) Levator palpebrae superioris muscle. (5) Muller's muscle (superior tarsal muscle). (6) Superior tarsus. (7) Superior rectus muscle. (8) Inferior tarsus. (9) Inferior tarsus muscle. (10) Capsulopalpebral fascia. (11) Inferior rectus muscle. (12) Inferior oblique muscle

is smaller and has a Vatican height of 4–10 mm and is usually continuous with the capsulopalpebral fascia inferiority.

70.2.2 The Eyelid Retractors

The upper lid has two retractors, the Muller's muscle which arises from the inferior part of the levator muscle fibers and inserts into the superior part of the superior tarsus and is innervated by the sympathetic nervous system, and the levator palpebrae superioris that arises from the sphenoid wing and extends to the superior edge of the superior tarsus. The levator is supplied by the superior division of the oculomotor nerve.

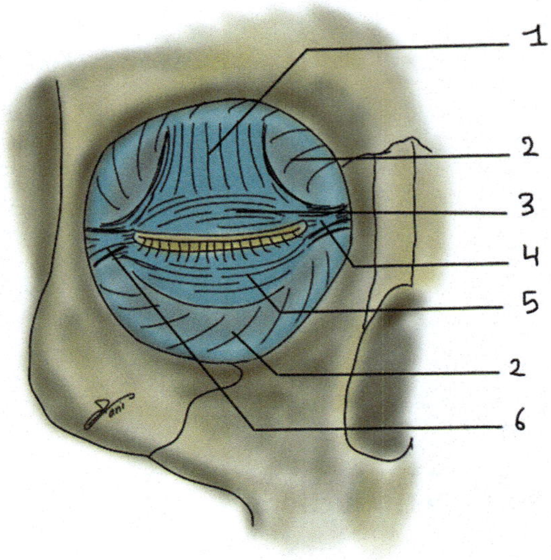

1. Tendon of the levator palpebrea superioris muscle
2. Orbital septum
3. Superior tarsus
4. Medial canthal ligament
5. Inferior tarsus
6. Lateral canthal ligament

Fig. 70.2 Frontal view. (1) Tendon of the levator palpebrae superioris muscle. (2) Orbital septum. (3) Superior tarsus. (4) Medial canthal ligament. (5) Inferior tarsus. (6) Lateral canthal ligament

The Whitnall's ligament is a dense fibrous connective tissue that serves as a fulcrum that redirects the vector of pull from horizontal to vertical for the lid retraction.

The lower lid has one main retractor, the capsulopalpebral fascia, a dense fibroelastic tissue found anterior to the lockwood ligament, and joins the inferior tarsus.

70.2.3 The Layers Found at the Upper Eyelid Crease

1. Skin
2. Orbicularis muscle
3. Orbital septum

4. Orbital fat
5. Levator aponeurosis
6. Muller's muscle
7. Tarsal portion

70.3 Indication

Indications for blepharoplasty include dermatochalasis, which is an acquired draping of excess skin over lids, and blepharochalasis which is characterized by recurrent attacks of lid edema resulting in swelling and edema of the lids, progressive tissue breakdown, prolapse of the orbital fat, and drooping of the lid. Other indications also include pseudoherniation, where orbital fat protrudes through a lax orbital septum behind orbicularis muscle resulting in baggy lids, orbicularis hypertrophy which also results in bagginess, and blepharoptosis in which droopy eyelid caused by levator muscle malfunction [5].

70.4 Preoperative Evaluation [6]

70.4.1 History

Proper selection of patients is crucial to achieve the most satisfying results in blepharoplasty and avoid unhappy patients. It is also essential to discuss the patient's goals and expectations as unrealistic expectations will lead to an unhappy patient. Limitations, the normal healing process, and complications of the surgery should be clearly explained during the preoperative evaluation. When taking history, it is essential to inquire about history of systemic diseases, such as Graves' disease, Sjogren's syndrome, rosacea, myasthenia gravis, and diabetes. Previous eye surgery, especially a history of laser in situ keratomileusis (LASIK) or previous cosmetic surgery, should also be included while taking history. It is also important to query patients preoperatively regarding bleeding disorders, the use of medications that may increase their risk of bleeding (e.g., aspirin, warfarin), and factors associated with poor wound healing, such as smoking and steroid use [1].

70.4.2 Physical Examination

Before surgery, an examination of the forehead, brows, and eyelids should be performed, as abnormalities or asymmetries in these structures may require repair at the same time as blepharoplasty to ensure a satisfactory result. Brow position must be assessed in all patients. Patients with significant brow ptosis, as well as dermatochalasis, should be considered for combined correction of the brow ptosis along with blepharoplasty. Eyelids should be evaluated preoperatively for pre-existing ptosis, asymmetrical lid creases, as well as any scarring that may be indicative of previous surgery or trauma. It is also essential to look for exophthalmos, lid retraction, inferior scleral show, lid laxity, entropion, and ectropion. Evaluation should also include palpebral fissure, marginal reflex distance, amount of lagophthalmos, and lid crease height. Corrected visual acuity, extraocular motility evaluation, and Schirmer's test can be helpful before blepharoplasty. Lastly, clinical photos should be obtained in order to document the patient's preoperative appearance, as well as for postoperative comparison [1, 7].

70.5 Surgical Technique [8, 9]

70.5.1 Upper Eyelid Blepharoplasty

Address the upper lid after the brow and before the lower lid. Mark the estimated upper lid skin to be excised. With the patient in an upright position, pinch the excess skin with forceps. To prevent webbed scar formation, avoid extending the incision beyond the medial canthus. Intraoperatively the lid should leave 1–2 mm lagophthalmos. Address lateral hooding by extending the incision lateral to the orbital rim. For better definition, a strip of orbicularis oculi may be removed with the heavy lid. The orbital septum is opened to access the pseudoherniated fat, which is clamped and excised. Lacrimal gland ptosis may be treated by plication to the periosteum.

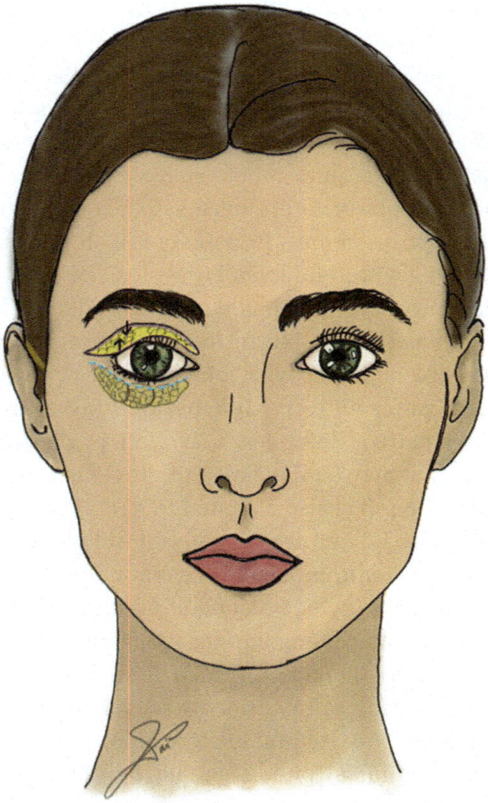

Fig. 70.3 Upper and lower blepharoplasty

70.5.2 Lower Eyelid Blepharoplasty

The two main approaches are subciliary and transconjunctival. Subciliary approach is most common, and it allows easier modification of skin and muscle. The transconjunctival approach avoids lid retraction and has no visible scar. It may be used effectively in patients with excessive fat herniation with little skin redundancy. Depending on the underlying anatomy and the desired result, the skin, muscle, and pseudoherniated fat are excised in a customized fashion. Inferior orbital fat can be repositioned inferiorly with the SOOF by opening the orbital septum for subtle changes (Fig. 70.3).

70.6 Complications

The complication of blepharoplasty include ptosis, lagophthalmos, and upper eyelid overcorrection, ectropion and lower eyelid correction, asymmetries, dry eye syndrome, chemosis, hematomas, diplopia, infection, and wound dehiscence [1, 7]. True ptosis secondary to blepharoplasty is usually temporary and is usually caused by eyelid edema, hematoma, or supratarsal fixation sutures in the perioperative period. It usually resolves during the first several postoperative weeks. Permanent post-blepharoplasty ptosis is usually caused by direct trauma to the levator muscle. When persistent ptosis occurs, it is advised to wait at least 3 months before surgical correction, as it often improves spontaneously. Lagophthalmos is common in the first postoperative week and is most often self-limited. It is managed with aggressive ocular lubrication, with both artificial tears during the day and lubricating ointment at bedtime. Persistent lagophthalmos is usually due to excessive skin resection or traction on the orbital septum. When the surgical site has completely healed, and conservative measures have failed, only then should surgical reconstruction be considered. Ectropion and lower lid malposition is the most common complication of transcutaneous lower lid blepharoplasty; it is usually due to either middle lamellar contracture, excess skin removal or both. Dry eye syndrome is very common in the early postoperative period and is usually managed with ocular surface lubrication with artificial tears during the day time and lubricating ointment at bedtime. Preserving orbicularis oculi and its innervation, avoiding inadvertent resection of the lacrimal gland, especially in patients who may have prolapse of their lacrimal gland, can minimize the risk of persistent dry eye syndrome. Superficial hematomas occur more commonly after lower eyelids blepharoplasty. These are most commonly preseptal and have no impact on visual function. They usually resolve without intervention in several weeks. Orbital or retrobulbar hemorrhages are rare; however, it can lead to significant visual loss if untreated. The following measures should be taken to minimizing the risk of a retrobulbar hemorrhage; the patient is in a relaxed condition with well-controlled blood pressure, meticulous surgical technique with cauterization of any bleeding vessels and avoidance of excess traction on orbital fat, and adequate postoperative pain and nausea control to avoid blood pressure spikes and episodes of emesis.

Symptoms will include significant pain and pressure, double vision, blurred vision, nausea, and vomiting. On examination, patients often have significant eyelid and subconjunctival ecchymosis with a firm periocular area, chemosis, restricted extraocular motility, decreased vision, and an afferent papillary defect. When suspected, prompt surgical intervention is indicated as permanent visual loss can occur in as little as 90 min. Diplopia following blepharoplasty usually results from muscle injury by aggressive dissection or use of thermocautery. Knowledge of the periocular anatomy and careful dissection in the areas of extraocular muscles can minimize the risk of postoperative diplopia. Due to the rich vascular supply of the periorbital soft tissue, infection following blepharoplasty is rare. Infection is most commonly caused by Staphylococcus and b-hemolytic streptococcus and is usually preseptal. Symptoms include swelling, warmth, and erythema along the surgical incision. It can be safely treated with broad-spectrum oral antibiotics. Orbital cellulitis following blepharoplasty is significantly less common than preseptal cellulitis. Symptoms include pain and swelling of the eyelid and may be associated with proptosis, ptosis, restricted eye movement, pupillary defects, impaired color vision, and decreased visual acuity. Orbital cellulitis is a medical emergency as it can progress rapidly, and without proper management can lead to optic nerve compression, blindness, meningitis, panophthalmitis, and brain abscess. Treatment includes appropriate intravenous broad-spectrum antibiotics [1].

Take Home Messages

- Patient selection and thorough preoperative assessment, including clear discussion regarding complications and outcomes, will enhance both patient and surgeon satisfaction.
- While serious blepharoplasty complications are rare, the surgeon needs to be aware of the possible complications and have a thorough understanding of the management of these complications if they do arise.
- Although hemorrhages following blepharoplasty are usually preseptal and resolve without intervention, however, the surgeon should always be mindful of the possibility of retrobulbar hemorrhage and intervene quickly if a retrobulbar hemorrhage is suspected.

References

1. Sniegowski M, Davies B, Hink E, Durairaj VD. Complications following blepharoplasty. Expert Rev Ophthalmol. 2014;9(4):341–9.
2. Bhattacharjee K, Misra DK, Deori N. Updates on upper eyelid blepharoplasty. Indian J Ophthalmol. 2017;65:551–8.
3. McCord CD. Upper blepharoplasty and eyebrow surgery. In: Chen WP, editor. Oculoplastic surgery. New York: Thieme; 2001. p. 125–45.
4. Rees TD. Blepharoplasty. In: Rees TD, Wood Smith D, editors. Cosmetic facial surgery. Philadelphia, PA: Saunders; 1973. p. 44–133.
5. Raza P, Justin SG. Otolaryngology head and neck surgery clinical reference guide. 4th ed. California: Plural Publishing; 2014. p. 487–93.
6. Golan S, Goldberg RA. Time course analysis of upper blepharoplasty complications. Dermatol Surg. 2017;43(2):307–9. https://doi.org/10.1097/DSS.0000000000000919.
7. Oestreicher J, Mehta S. Complications of blepharoplasty: prevention and management. Plast Surg Int. 2012;2012:252368. https://doi.org/10.1155/2012/252368.
8. Charles HT. Blepharoplasty. In: Mark AC, Derek TF, editors. Grabb and smith's plastic surgery. 6th ed. Philadelphia: Lippincott Williams & Wilkins; 2007. p. 486–97.
9. Jeffery EJ. Eyelid reconstruction. In: Jason EL, Smita RR, Jeffery EJ, editors. Essentials of plastic surgery. 2nd ed. Florida: CRC Press; 2014. p. 392–402.

Facelifting

71

Rani Hammoud and Hassan Haidar

Key Points

- To understand the main anatomical consideration during the facelift surgeries.
- To be able to describe the layers of the face.
- To describe the distribution of fat compartments, as well as what makes up the malar fat compartment.
- To be familiarized with the various surgical players technique available for the face life surgeries.
- To be able to identify the common postoperative complications.

71.1 Introduction

Facelifting, also known as a rhytidectomy, technically means the removal of wrinkles by surgery to give a more youthful appearance to the face.

Skin wrinkles typically appear because of the aging processes of skin tissue such as glycation (1). Wrinkles begin to form in the mid-30s. They usually start in the thin skin of the periorbital area. As the body gets older, skin and subcutaneous fat lose its volume and the collagen and elastic fibers lose their elasticity, which results in superficial wrinkles in the remaining face.

Sun exposure is one of the main reasons for wrinkles. The sun makes the skin look older and constant exposure of skin to sun exacerbates this matter. A facelift can rejuvenate patients.

71.2 Facelift Anatomy (Fig. 71.1) [1]

– The first layer in facelift anatomy is the skin. The dermal vascular plexus is responsible for the skin blood supply.
– The next layer is the subcutaneous fat which is in close contact with deeper SMAS and superficial dermis. This layer can be safely undermined without damaging the anatomic structures.
– The third layer is the SMAS layer. This layer separates the subcutaneous fat from the parotidomasseteric fascia and facial nerve branches. The SMAS layer is continuous with the platysma in the neck, the temporoparietal fascia in the temples, and the galea in the scalp. The SMAS layer consists of suspensory ligaments that encase the cheek fat, thereby causing them to remain in their normal position. The SMAS is thicker and more adherent over the parotid, whereas it becomes thinner and

R. Hammoud (✉)
ENT Department, Hamad Medical Corporation, Doha, Qatar

H. Haidar
Hamad Medical Corporation, Doha, Qatar

A. Al-Qahtani et al. (eds.), *Textbook of Clinical Otolaryngology*,
https://doi.org/10.1007/978-3-030-54088-3_71

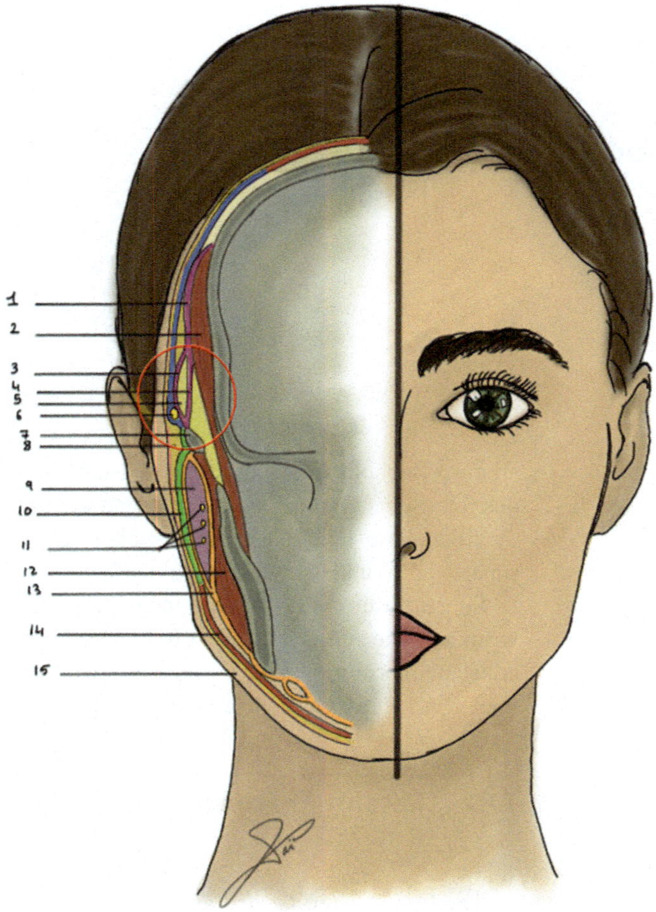

Fig. 71.1 Coronal view showing the face layers, and the red circles represent the temporal region. (1). temporal fascia proper. (2) Temporalis muscle. (3) Superficial layer of deep temporal fascia. (4) Deep layer of the deep temporal fascia. (5) Superficial fat pad. (6) Frontal-temporal branch of facial nerve. (7) Zygomatic arch. (8) Subcutaneous fat. (9) Parotid gland. (10) SMAS. (11) Facial nerve branches within the parotid gland. (12) Masseter muscle. (13) Parotidomasseteric fascia. (14) Platysma muscle. (15) Skin

mobile medially. Resuspension and securing the SMAS anatomical layer can lead to rejuvenation of the face, by counteracting aging and gravity caused laxity. When this layer is stretched or pulled, it moves the entire lateral face in the desired vector. Superficial Musculo-Aponeurotic System (SMAS) layer using one of a multitude of facelift surgeries is vital in achieving natural and long-lasting outcome techniques.

– The fourth surgical plane is the sub-SMAS plane. It contains the parotidomasseteric fascia (investing fascia over the parotid gland and masseter muscle). It is important to know that the facial nerve motor branches and the parotid duct run under this layer. Hence by operating superior to this layer, the facial nerve branches are protected (Fig. 71.1).

71.2.1 Malar Fat Compartment (Fig. 71.2)

The malar fat compartment described by owsley is considered to play a very important part in the youthfulness of the cheek area.

The malar fat compartment is the inverted triangular areas that consist of the nasolabial fat compartment, the medial cheek fat and in some extent the inferior orbital fat compartment.

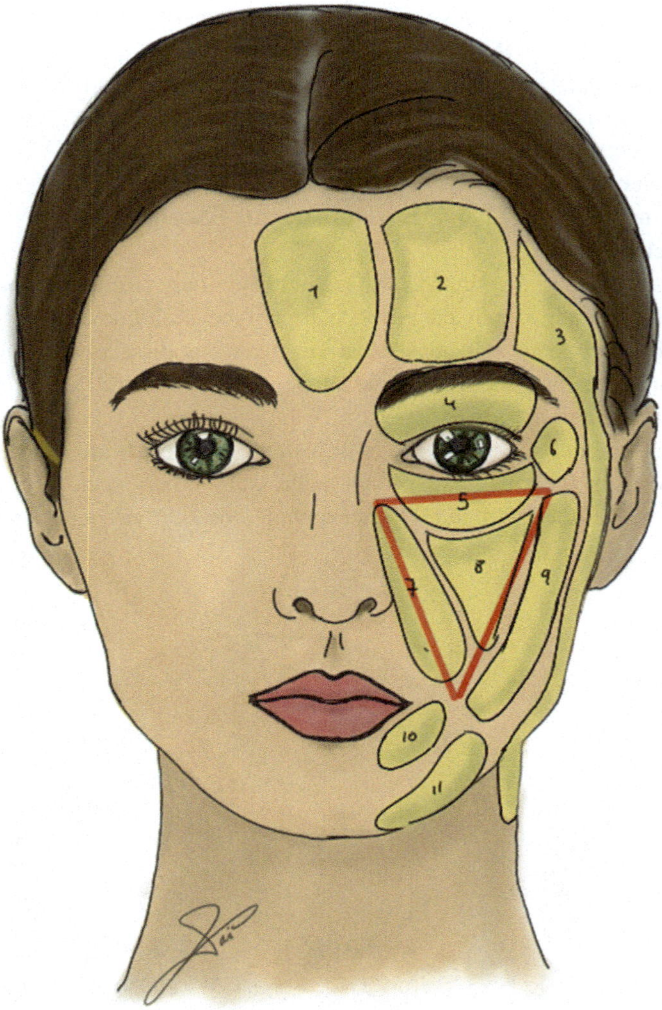

Fig. 71.2 Showing the superficial fat compartment and the malar fat compartment in the red triangle. (1) Central forehead fat compartment. (2) Middle temporal fat compartment. (3) Lateral temporal-cheek fat compartment. (4) Superior orbital fat compartment. (5) Inferior orbital fat compartment. (6) Lateral orbital fat compartment. (7) Nasolabial fat compartment. (8) Medial cheek fat compartment. (9) Middle cheek fat compartment. (10) Superior jowl fat compartment. (11) Inferior jowl fat compartment

71.3 Indications for Facelift Surgery

Ideally, the patient should be around the age of 50 or below.

A facelift is performed to rejuvenate the appearance of the face. Aging of the face is most shown by a change in position of the deep anatomical structures, notably the platysma muscle, cheek fat and the orbicularis oculi muscle. These lead up to three landmarks namely (Fig. 71.3):

- An appearance of the jowl (a broken jaw line by ptosis of the platysma muscle).
- Increased redundancy of the nasolabial fold (caused by a descent of cheek fat).
- Increased distance from the ciliary margin to the inferior-most point of the orbicularis oculi muscle (caused by decreasing tone of the orbicularis oculi muscle).

Evaluation of the psychological aspect of the patient must be done carefully.

71.4 Facelift Techniques

Many different procedures of rhytidectomy exist. The differences are mostly the type of incision and the area of the face that is treated. Expectations of the patient, the age, possible recovery time, and areas to improve are some of the many factors taken in consideration before choosing a technique of rhytidectomy.

In the traditional facelift, an incision is made in front of the ear extending up into the hairline. The incision curves around the bottom of the ear and then behind it, usually ending near the hairline on the back of the neck. After the skin incision is made, the skin is undermined from the deeper tissues with a scalpel or scissors over the cheeks and neck. At this point, the deeper tissue (SMAS) is exposed and can be manipulated.

The excess skin is then removed, and the skin incisions are closed.

71.4.1 Subcutaneous Facelift

Subcutaneous facelift or skin-only facelift was initially the major concept of the facelift procedure.

It consists of subcutaneous dissection above the SMAS and suitable only to reduce the facial skin excess.

The results of a skin-only facelift are limited because of not addressing other senile facial structures. After a while, the skin viscoelasticity

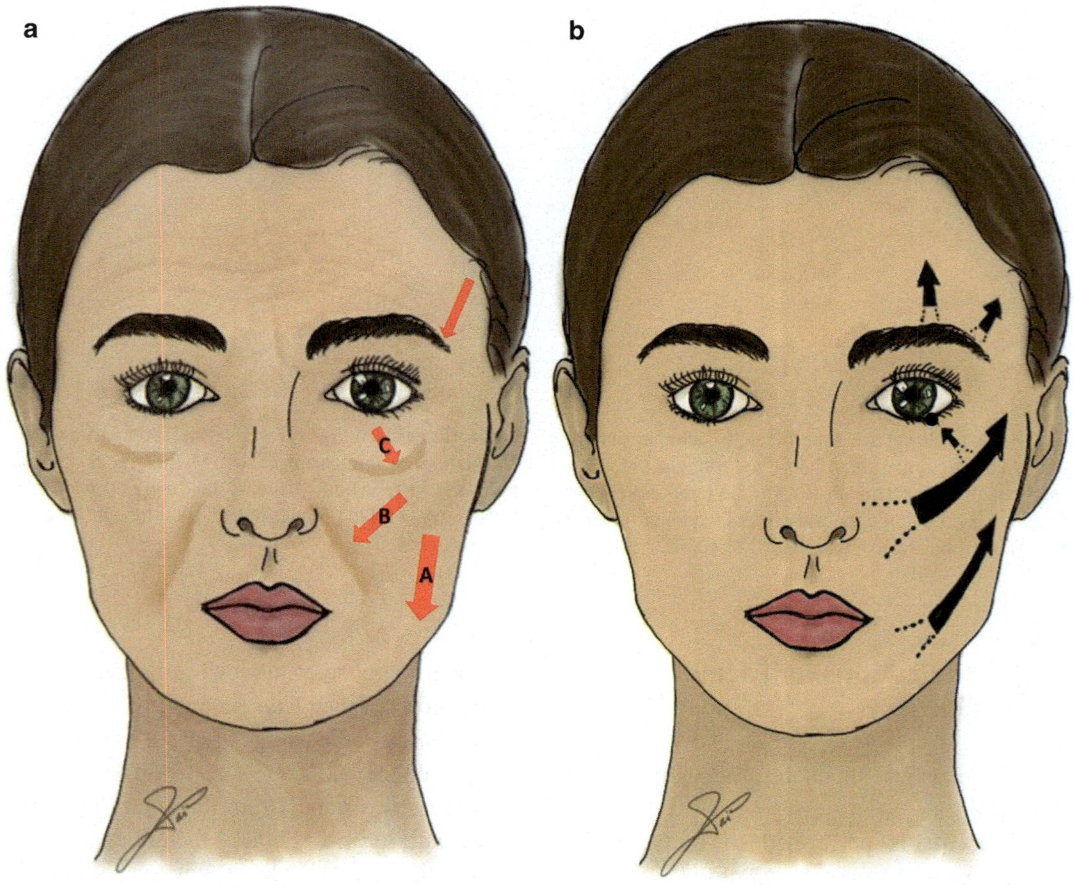

Fig. 71.3 (**A**) Jowl (a broken jaw line by ptosis of the platysma muscle); (**B**) Increased redundancy of the nasolabial fold (caused by a descent of cheek fat). (**C**) Orbital folds in the eye area (caused by decreasing tone of the orbicularis oculi muscle). Black arrows: The intended effect of a facelift

property causes loosening of tightened skin [2]. Intact subcutaneous tissues are susceptible to ptosis after some time because they are not manipulated in this technique.

This skin-based facial rejuvenation and facelift surgeries did not have outcome longevity. Skin by its very nature accommodates stretch and over time, in a matter of months, the effects of the initial surgery had been lost.

71.4.2 SMAS Plication Facelift

Manipulation of the SMAS would yield a more natural and a long-lasting facial rejuvenation and facelift results.

This technique solves the senile changes of the face including skin wrinkles and deep soft tissue sagging simultaneously. The strong fibrous composition of the SMAS layer gives it greater strength against gravity than skin.

The simplest SMAS-based surgery involves widespread skin undermining from in front of the ear, to close to the lips and across the cheek (Fig. 71.4). Skin undermining often extends into the neck as the procedures often need to be combined for a harmonious and good outcome. The dissection plane in this technique is supra-SMAS. After dissecting in the subcutaneous plane, the SMAS layer is exposed. At this point the redundancy in the SMAS is marked out and using permanent sutures, the mobile segment of the SMAS layer is plicated and fixed to the posterior relatively immobile layer (Fig. 71.5). This lifts the lower face and the neck but is unable to address the mid-cheek region. The skin excess is then excised and the skin is closed in layers.

The advantage of this operation is that it is very safe in regard to any possible threats to the facial nerve. The facial nerve traverses in the sub-SMAS plane.

The disadvantage of this surgical technique lies in its inability to address the mid-cheek region. The widespread undermining of the facelift surgery skin flaps leaves them prone to small areas of necrosis at the most distal part near or behind the ear.

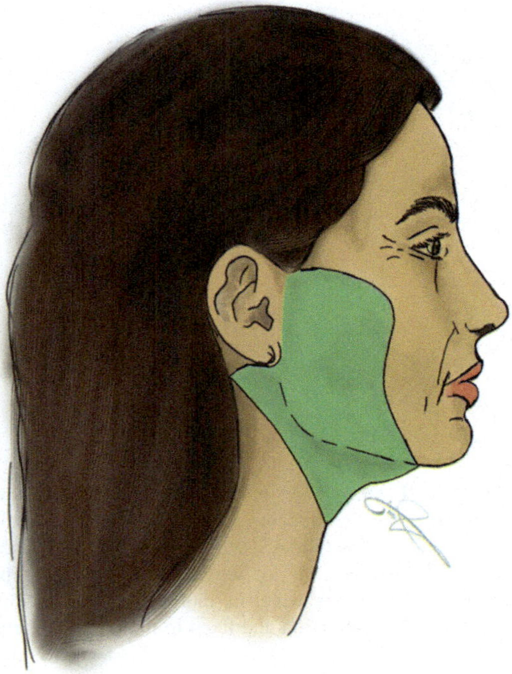

Fig. 71.4 Extent of facelift skin flap undermining in SMAS plication and lateral SMAS-ectomy

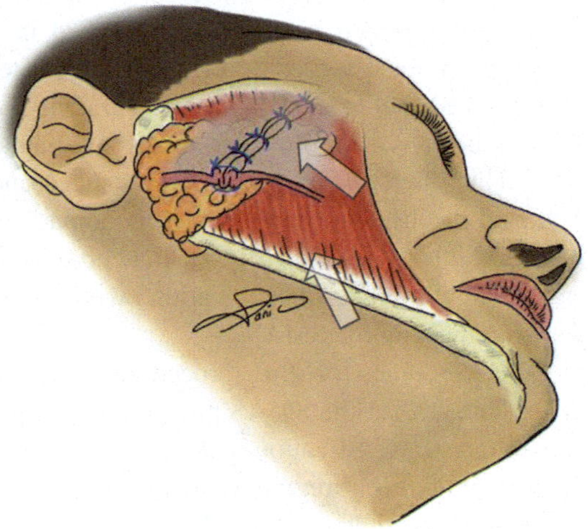

Fig. 71.5 In SMAS plication technique, the mobile segment of the SMAS layer is plicated and fixed to the posterior relatively immobile layer. This lifts the lower face and the neck (arrows)

71.4.3 Lateral SMAS-ectomy

Lateral SMAS-ectomy is a technique that involves the excision of the redundant lateral

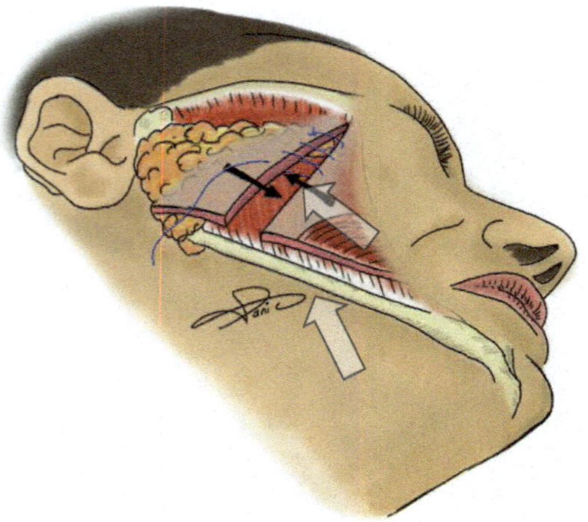

Fig. 71.6 Lateral SMAS-ectomy technique involves the excision of the redundant lateral SMAS between the mobile and the fixed SMAS. With excision of redundancy in the SMAS, tightening of the SMAS is achieved. The anterior SMAS layer which is mobile is stretched in a superoposterior direction and fixed to the posterior fixed SMAS layer. The vector of tracing the SMAS layer is perpendicular to the nasolabial fold

SMAS between the mobile and the fixed SMAS. With excision of redundancy in the SMAS tightening of the SMAS is achieved. The anterior SMAS layer which is mobile is stretched in a superoposterior direction and fixed to the posterior fixed SMAS layer. The vector of tracing the SMAS layer is perpendicular to the nasolabial fold. This often allows for a more nuanced and sculpted facelift surgery outcome in comparison to SMAS plication. The risk of facial nerve damage is slightly higher than plication owing to the incision made in the SMAS.

The outcomes of this procedure continue much longer than the SMAS plication technique due to the stronger fixation of the SMAS layer.

The mid-cheek region remains out of the scope of this technique (Fig. 71.6).

71.4.4 Deep Plane Facelift (DPFL)

Deep plane rhytidectomy was suggested in place of traditional facelifting to correct aging changes of midface (i.e., malar fat pad) and nasolabial grooves more accurately. The SMAS lift is an effective procedure to reposition the platysma muscle; however, the nasolabial fold is better addressed by a deep plane facelift or composite facelift.

The main concept of this technique was based on reversing gravity's effect by manipulating tissues deep to SMAS (example repositioning the malar fat pad and release of facial ligament) to make more satisfying changes in older patients. Dissecting in sub-SMAS layer allows manipulating deep soft tissues of the face gives rise to major changes and improvements of senile faces. By dividing the ligaments that connect the overlying skin and SMAS to the underlying skeleton, the composite unit is advanced as a whole. With permanent retaining sutures put in place, both the amount of skin undermining and skin excision become minimal. The skin is closed without a dead space or tension resulting in better wound healing, less postoperative edema, and faster recovery.

This technique is associated with high risk of facial nerve damage.

Patients with significant aging changes of midface and mentolabial fold are good candidates for this procedure.

71.4.5 Extended SMAS Lift

The main procedure protocol in this method is dissecting and drawing skin and SMAS flaps separately. The vector of stretching the SMAS layer is different from the skin.

After widespread undermining of the skin towards and very close to the nose and the corner of the mouth (Fig. 71.7), the SMAS is accessed on the zygomatic or the cheekbone skeleton and is undermined towards the apple of the cheek (Fig. 71.8). Resuspension of the undermined SMAS against the skeleton or underlying stable tissues then achieves the lift. Finally, the skin is closed over the lifted SMAS.

The vector of retracting the SMAS layer is more vertical than the skin flap. The SMAS and platysma flaps can be rotated in the postauricular area to improve the jowl and cervical contour. The SMAS flap is advanced superolaterally, perpendicular to the nasolabial fold in the malar fat pad area.

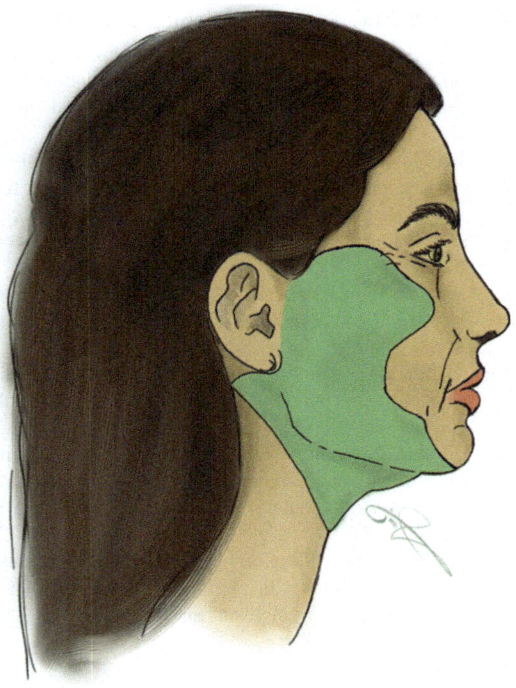

Fig. 71.7 The extent of the skin undermining and the neck incision in an extended or high SMAS facelift technique

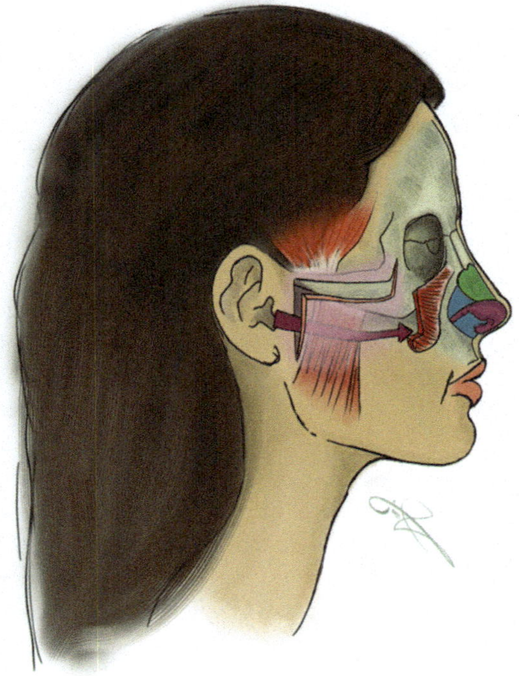

Fig. 71.8 Extended SMAS technique for access to the midface and cheek

The advantage of this technique is that it is a powerful tool in addressing aging and the descent of the mid-cheek.

Maximum effects on lower face and neck can be achieved by creating a continuous SMAS-platysmal flap.

The outcomes of this technique are long-lasting due to releasing the facial ligaments and repositioning of the malar fat pad.

The risk of facial nerve damage is relatively high in this method.

The compromised viability of the skin flap is a major concern in this technique.

71.4.6 Complications of the Facelift Procedure [3–6]

The most feared complications of facelift surgery are facial nerve damage (1%) and flap necrosis (1–2%).

Hematoma (the most common complication, it is dangerous because it may lead to infection and flap necrosis).

Infection.

Venous thromboembolism.

Pre- and postauricular skin necrosis.

Pre- and postauricular scar hypertrophy.

Temporal alopecia.

It has been reported that the complication rate in patients with a high body mass index (BMI) over 25 was 9.5%, compared to 4.7% in normal-weight patients undergoing a facelift [5].

Take Home Messages

- The facial changes during aging are due to the loss of the soft tissue elasticity, volume redistribution, and skin changes.
- There is no single surgical technique that has proven to be superior in the treatment of the different varieties of facial aging; hence the surgeon should

always individualize each case to provide the best outcome for the patient.

- The surgeon should always try to minimize the chances of causing a facial nerve injury, by following the right anatomy and planes during dissection; in addition, the use of the nerve stimulation tool should be always considered.
- Postoperative hematoma can be reduced by good intraoperative hemostasis and blood pressure control.
- It's not advisable to operate on an active smoker, since the risk of skin necrosis is increased.

References

1. Mitz V, Peyronie M. The superficial musculo-aponeurotic system (SMAS) in the parotid and cheek area. Plast Reconstr Surg. 1976;58:80–8.
2. Gamble WB, Manson PN, Smith GE, Hamra ST. Comparison of skin-tissue tensions using the composite and the subcutaneous rhytidectomy techniques. Ann Plast Surg. 1995;35:447–53; discussion 453–4.
3. Gupta V, Winocour J, Shi H, et al. Preoperative risk factors and complication rates in facelift: analysis of 11,300 patients. Aesthet Surg J. 2016;36(1):1–13.
4. Chaffoo RA. Complications in facelift surgery: avoidance and management. Facial Plast Surg Clin North Am. 2013;21:551–8.
5. Abboushi N, Yezhelyev M, Symbas J, Nahai F. Facelift complications and the risk of venous thromboembolism: a single center's experience. Aesthet Surg J. 2012;32:413–20.
6. Moyer JS, Baker SR. Complications of rhytidectomy. Facial Plast Surg Clin North Am. 2005;13:469–78. Facelift: Current Concepts, Techniques, and Principles.

72 Fillers and Neurotoxins

Maryam Abdulraheem, Rani Hammoud, Shanmugam Ganesan, and Alwyn D'Souza

72.1 Neurotoxins

72.1.1 Introduction

Neurotoxins, or botulinum neurotoxins type A (BoNT/A) are the most commonly performed non-surgical aesthetic procedure in the world [1]. It is a protein produced by the anaerobic gram positive bacteria, *Clostridium botulinum* [2]. Botox can be used for aesthetic and functional reasons in various regions of the head and neck. Seven serotypes of BoNT (named types A through G) have been identified so far, with only BoNT types A and B being available for therapeutic use. The therapeutic value of botulinum neurotoxin A (BoNT A) was first recognized in 1989 when the Food and Drug Administration (FDA) approved oculinum for the treatment of strabismus and blepharospasm. It was not until April 2002 that the use of BoNT A (onabotulinumtoxinA) was approved for the treatment of glabellar lines by the FDA. In September 2013 and October 2017, the FDA eventually approved BoNT A for the treatment of lateral canthal lines and forehead lines, respectively [3].

M. Abdulraheem (✉) · R. Hammoud · S. Ganesan
ENT Department, Hamad Medical Corporation, Doha, Qatar
e-mail: mabdulraheem1@hamad.qa; Rhammoud3@hamad.qa; Sganesan@hamad.qa

A. D'Souza
University Hospital Lewisham, London, UK

72.1.2 Neurotoxin Serotypes

There are seven serotypes (A, B, C, D, E, F, and G) of BoNT. Each serotype has multiple subtypes that are based on a ≥2.6% difference in amino acid sequences [4]. Five subtypes of BoNT A have been described previously; three of the five subtypes of BoNT A are currently used for treating rhytides [5]. There are four commercially available botulinum neurotoxin type A (BoNT/A) preparations; they are either lyophilized as in abobotulinumA (Dysport®) and incobotulinumA (Xeomin®), or vacuum-dried powder as in onabotulinumA (Botox®) and prabotulinumtoxinA-xvfs (Jeuveau) [6].

72.1.3 Mechanism of Action

The botulinum toxin heavy chain binds selectively and reversible to the receptor found on the presynaptic cell, then enters the cytoplasm by endocytosis. Once in the cytoplasm, the light chain acts on the SNAP/SNARE (synaptosome-associated protein/soluble N-ethylmaleimide-sensitive factor attachment protein receptor) docking protein complex, thus preventing the binding and the release of the acetylcholine at the neuromuscular junction. This results in what is called chemodenervation of the muscles, which causes reversible relaxation of the local muscle, which in turn results in reduced facial wrinkles/lines. The serotypes A, B, and E target the SNAP-

A. Al-Qahtani et al. (eds.), *Textbook of Clinical Otolaryngology*,
https://doi.org/10.1007/978-3-030-54088-3_72

25 protein within the SNARE complex. The serotype B, D, F, and G targets the synaptobrevin via the VAMP (vesicles-associated membrane protein) within the SNARE complex [7, 8].

72.1.4 Indication (Fig. 72.1)

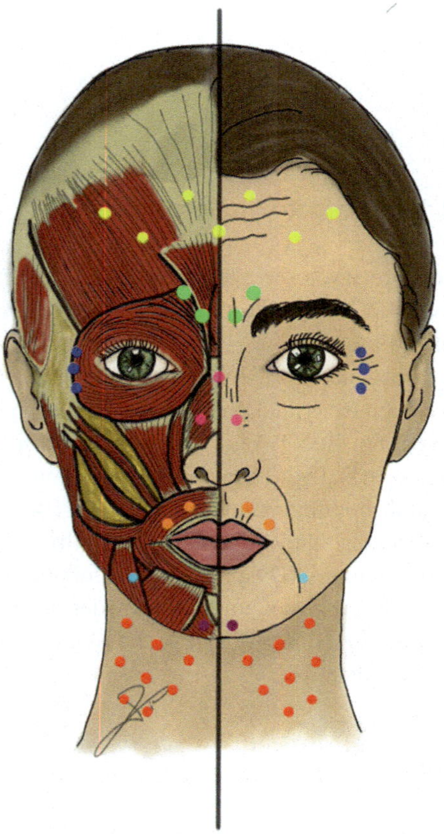

Fig. 72.1 Frontal facial view showing the site of Botox injection: *Yellow*: horizontal forehead lines (frontal is ms); *Green*: glabellar complex and vertical forehead lines (corrugator supercilii, procerus, orbicularis oculi ms); *Blue*: crows feet lines ("lateral orbital wrinkles" lateral portion of orbicularis oculi ms); *Pink*: bunny's lines (nasals and procerus mss); *Orange*: perioral wrinkles (orbicularis oris); *Jad*: marionette lines (depressor anguli oris ms); *Purple*: dimpled chin (mentalis ms); *Red*: platysmal bands (platysma ms)

72.1.4.1 In Upper Face

Glabellar rhytides, horizontal lines on the forehead, lateral canthal lines (crow's feet), depressed brow, hypertrophic orbicularis oculi muscle (small palpebral aperture) [9, 10].

72.1.4.2 In Mid Face

Rhytides from upper nasalis muscle contraction (bunny lines), nasolabial folds (selected patients) [11, 12].

72.1.4.3 In Lower Face

Vertical perioral rhytides, mouth frown, gummy smile, melomental folds (marionette lines), mental crease (horizontal crease on the chin), Peau d'orange chin, masseteric hypertrophy (square jaw) [11, 12].

72.1.4.4 In the Neck

Horizontal neck lines, platysmal bands [11, 12].

72.1.5 Contraindication

72.1.5.1 Absolute Contraindications

It includes infection at the site of injection and known hypersensitivity to any component of the product. Abobotulinumtoxin A is contraindicated in patients with allergies to cow's milk protein [13, 14].

72.1.5.2 Relative Contraindications

It includes neuromuscular disorders that could amplify the effect of the toxin, such as myasthenia gravis, Eaton–Lambert syndrome, myopathies, or amyotrophic lateral sclerosis. It can be used with caution in patients taking drugs that can interfere with neuromuscular transmission (e.g., aminoglycosides, cholinesterase inhibitors, quinidine, magnesium sulfate, succinylcholine, and curare-type nondepolarizing blockers) [13, 14].

72.1.5.3 Pregnancy and Lactation

OnabotulinumtoxinA, abobotulinumtoxinA, incobotulinumtoxinA, and rimabotulinumtoxin-B are pregnancy class C agents (can be used with caution if benefits outweigh risk). As for the risks of maternal-infant transmission of botulinum toxin in lactating women it is unknown [15].

72.1.6 Side Effects

The most common side effects include bruising at the injection site, pain, and swelling. These can be avoided by using thinner needles and diluting Botox with saline [16, 17]. Mild headache may also occur but will usually resolve within 2–4 weeks and can be treated using systemic analgesics [16, 18, 19]. Other side effects may include malaise, nausea, and influenza-like symptoms [16, 17].

Ectropion may also develop due to the local diffusion process of Botox when injected into the lower eyelids. Botox injections used to treat crow's feet or bunny lines (periorbital) may cause strabismus caused by inadvertent injection and local diffusion of Botox [16, 20]. Nevertheless, all of these side effects will gradually resolve after the paralytic effect of the toxin diminishes [16, 21].

72.1.7 Complications

72.1.7.1 In the Upper Face

Diffusion of toxin in the upper face can result in several adverse effects such as brow ptosis. It occurs due to excessive weakening of the frontalis muscle and eyelid ptosis due to the weakening of the upper eyelid levator muscle secondary to diffusion into the orbital septum. Ptosis can remain for several weeks but can be treated with alpha-adrenergic agonist ophthalmic drops [20, 21]. Another possible adverse effect is quizzical or "cockeyed" appearance ("Mr. Spock" eyebrow), which results from weakening the medial frontalis muscles, allowing the unaffected lateral muscle fibers of the frontalis to elevate the lateral brow. The quizzical-appearing brow can be remedied through injection of the lateral frontalis musculature. Other adverse effects that can occur in the upper face include diplopia, ectropion, lower eyelid droop, epiphora, decreased strength of eye closure, and dry eye. These adverse effects usually last for 2–12 weeks and will gradually resolve as the paralytic effect of the toxin diminishes [21].

72.1.7.2 In the Lower Face

Complications in the lower face affect muscle function and facial expression; they are usually due to the use of excessive doses or injection into inappropriate locations. When placing the injection too close to the mouth, injecting in the mental fold, or when Botox interacts with the orbicularis oris muscle, a group of complications can result. These include flaccid cheek, incompetent mouth, asymmetrical smile, and loss of the ability to whistle [21].

72.1.7.3 In the Neck

Dysphagia and weakness of the neck flexors can result if high doses were administered in the neck area [21].

72.2 Fillers

72.2.1 Introduction

Skin wrinkles and loss of tissue volume due to aging, atrophy, and displacement of subcutaneous fat contribute significantly to facial aging. Fillers can be used to restore a youthful appearance by replacing the lost tissue volume and by filling and enhancing coarse wrinkles. Fillers are an option for the treatment of volume deficiency, scars, and rhytides, as well as for facial sculpting. Fillers are also used for facial contouring and augmentation of specific anatomical sites such as the lips. Multiple products are currently Food and Drug Administration (FDA) approved to be used to provide facial volume. The substances most commonly used for facial volumizing are hyaluronic acid (HA), calcium hydroxylapatite (CaHA), poly-L-lactic acid (PLLA), and polymethyl methacrylate (PMMA) [22].

72.2.2 Types of Injectable Filler

They can be permanent; that persist indefinitely or temporary; that are eventually resorbed by the body.

Currently, permanent fillers are less desirable due to the adverse results that required surgical removal.

Permanent fillers: (polymethylmethacrylate microspheres, hydrogel polymers, and silicone).

Temporary fillers: (hyaluronic acid, collagen, calcium hydroxylapatite, and poly-L-lactic acid) [22].

72.2.3 Indications (Fig. 72.2)

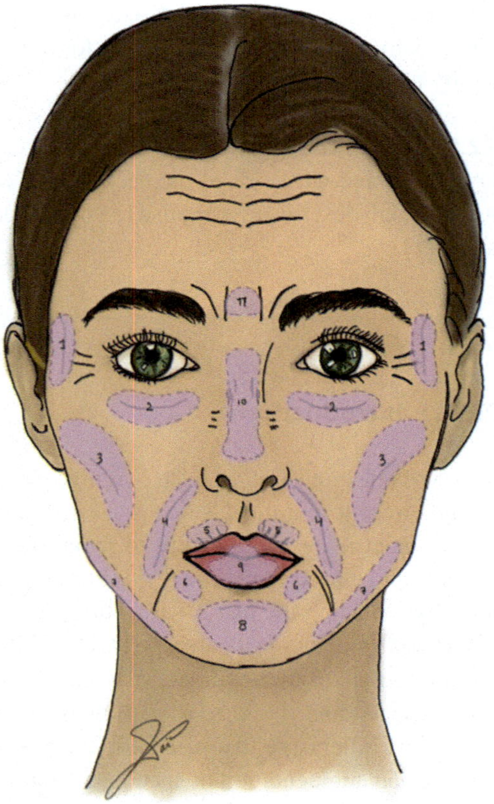

1- temporal hollows
2- submalar area
3- cheeks
4- nasolabial folds
5- perioral vertical lines
6- marionette lines
7- jaw line
8- mental crease and chin
9- lips augmentation
10- nose
11- frown lines

Fig. 72.2 Frontal facial view showing the most common area for filler injection. (1) Temporal hollows. (2) Submalar area. (3) Cheeks. (4) Nasolabial folds. (5) Perioral vertical lines. (6) Marionette lines. (7) Jaw line. (8) Mental crease and chin. (9) Lips augmentation. (10) Nose. (11) Frown lines

72.2.3.1 Cosmetic Indications

In upper face: Deep vertical *glabellar lines*, *horizontal forehead lines*, lateral brow ptosis and reduced lateral brow projection, *and temporal fossa wasting*.

In mid face: *Nasojugal fold (tear trough depression)*, hypoplasia of the zygoma and the descent, and atrophy of midfacial fat.

In lower face: *Nasolabial folds*, vertical perioral wrinkles, mouth frown, lip augmentation, melomental folds (marionette lines), horizontal creases in the chin, chin and mandibular augmentation.

In the neck: to reduce the appearance of wrinkles.

72.2.3.2 Therapeutic Indications

HIV-associated lipoatrophy: sunken cheeks, bitemporal wasting, and deep nasolabial folds.

Scarring: pitted atrophic scars that often result from acne vulgaris and depressed scars that result from the treatment of skin cancer, trauma, or other causes.

Facial asymmetry and soft tissue defects: congenital, postsurgical or posttraumatic [23–26].

72.2.4 Complications

72.2.4.1 Early Injection Site Reactions

Erythema, swelling, pain, and bruising are common injection site reactions. They usually resolve within 1–2 weeks. There are few measures to be taken to avoid or minimize the risk of site reactions and these include using a small gauge needle, blunt cannula, and slowly injecting small volumes [27, 28].

72.2.4.2 Inappropriate Placement

Inappropriate placement of fillers by injecting too superficially can lead to palpable nodules and papules. These are treated simply by local massage or by aspiration or incision and drainage. Superficial injection of hyaluronic acid fillers result in blue-grey discoloration under the skin (Tyndall effect), and this can be treated by injecting hyaluronidase which will dissolve the filler [27].

72.2.4.3 Delayed Nodules

Delayed nodules may result from infections, biofilms, foreign body granulomas, or inflammatory/

immune-mediated causes. In case of infected nodule or abscess treatment measures should include incision and drainage and/or broad-spectrum antibiotics until the culture results are back. As for biofilms, maintaining a sterile technique is key to reduce the risk of acquiring them. Foreign body granulomas are another potential cause of delayed nodules which result from poly-L-lactic acid (PLLA) injection. In order to avoid this reaction, PLLA should not be injected intradermally. Treatments options used for delayed nodules include intralesional hyaluronidase; topical, oral, or intralesional corticosteroids; oral antibiotics and lasers; or a combination of these treatments [28–32].

72.2.4.4 Vascular Occlusion and Necrosis

Interruption of vascular supply by direct injection of the filler into the vessel is considered the most serious complication. Symptoms can include pain, blanching, and reticulated violaceous erythema. It can progress to skin necrosis and scarring or visual complications such as ocular pain and immediate unilateral vision loss. Sites that are at high risk for vascular compromise are glabella, nasal region, nasolabial fold, and forehead. To avoid such complications, firm knowledge of vascular anatomy is crucial. There are some strategies that can be implemented to reduce the risk of vascular occlusion which include using low volumes of product, injecting slowly, and using a small gauge needle or cannula [33, 34].

Take Home Messages

- The demand for non-surgical aesthetic procedures is increasing worldwide due to the advantage of minimal invasion and fewer side effects.
- Complete knowledge of indications and contraindications of the use of neurotoxins and injectable fillers help with better patient selection and hence lead to better result.
- It is important to understand the different types of fillers available in the market and the advantage and disadvantages of each one of them in order to choose the most suitable type for the patient.
- Detailed knowledge of anatomy of the face significantly reduces the risk of complications.

References

1. Haney B. The aging face. In: Aesthetic procedures: nurse practitioner's guide to cosmetic dermatology. Cham: Springer; 2020.
2. Huang W, Foster JA, Rogachefsky AS. Pharmacology of botuli- num toxin. J Am Acad Dermatol. 2000;43(2):249–59.
3. Hanna E, Pon K. Updates on botulinum neurotoxins in dermatology. Am J Clin Dermatol. 2019;21:157. https://doi.org/10.1007/s40257-019-00482-2.
4. Jacobson MJ, Lin G, Tepp W, Dupuy J. Purification, modeling, and analysis of botulinum neurotoxin subtype A5 (BoNT/A5) from *Clostridium botulinum* strain A661222. Appl Environ Microbiol. 2011;77:4217–22.
5. Won CH, Kim HK, Kim BJ, Kang H. Comparative trial of a novel botulinum neurotoxin type A versus onabotulinumtoxinA in the treatment of glabellar lines: a multicenter, randomized, double- blind, active-controlled study. Int J Dermatol. 2015;54(2):227–34.
6. Haney B. Reconstitution and dosing of neurotoxins. In: Aesthetic procedures: nurse practitioner's guide to cosmetic dermatology. Cham: Springer; 2020.
7. Khawaja HA, Hernandez-Perez E. Botox in dermatology. Int J Dermatol. 2001;40(5):311–7.
8. Lowe NJ. Minimally invasive treatments and procedures for aging skin. In: Burns T, Breathnach S, Cox N, Griffiths C, editors. Rook's textbook of dermatology. 8th ed. London: Blackwell Publishing; 2010. p. 80.1–80.14.
9. Carruthers A, Carruthers J. Botulinum toxin type A: history and current cosmetic use in the upper face. Semin Cutan Med Surg. 2001;20:71.
10. Carruthers A, Carruthers J, Cohen JA. Prospective, double-blind, randomized, parallel- group, dose-ranging study of botulinum toxin type a in female subjects with horizontal forehead rhytides. Dermatol Surg. 2003;29(5):461–7.
11. Carruthers J, Carruthers A. Botulinum toxin A in the mid and lower face and neck. Dermatol Clin. 2004;22:151.
12. Lowe NJ, Yamauchi P. Cosmetic uses of botulinum toxins for lower aspects of the face and neck. Clin Dermatol. 2004;22:18.
13. Allergan, Inc. Botox cosmetic (botulinum toxin type A) purified neurotoxin complex (prescribing information). Irvine, CA: Allergan, Inc.; 2005.

14. Feily A, Fallahi H, Zandian D, Kalantar H. A succinct review of botulinum toxin in dermatology; update of cosmetic and noncosmetic use. J Cosmet Dermatol. 2011;10:58.
15. https://www.accessdata.fda.gov/drugsatfda_docs/label/2019/761085s000lbl.pdf. Accessed 11 June 2019.
16. Satriyasa BK. Botulinum toxin (Botox) A for reducing the appearance of facial wrinkles: a literature review of clinical use and pharmacological aspect. Clin Cosmet Investig Dermatol. 2019;12:223–8. https://doi.org/10.2147/CCID.S202919.
17. Cohen JL, Freeman SR. Botulinum toxins. In: Draelos ZD, editor. Cosmetic dermatology products & procedures. United Kingdom: Wiley-Blackwell Publishing Ltd; 2010.
18. Ascher B, Talarico S, Cassuto D, et al. International consen sus recommendations on the aesthetic usage of botulinum toxin type A (Speywood Unit)—Part II: Wrinkles on the middle and lower face, neck and chest. J Eur Acad Dermatol Venereol. 2010;24(11):1285–95. https://doi.org/10.1111/j.1468-3083.2010.03728.x.
19. Maio M, Rzany B. Patient selection. In: Acquilla R, Patel T, Gonzales M, editors. Botulinum toxin in aesthetic medicine. New York: Springer; 2007. p. 11–9.
20. Cox SE, Adigun CG. Complications of injectable fillers and neurotoxins. Dermatol Ther. 2011;24(6):524–36. https://doi.org/10.1111/j.1529-8019.2012.01455.x.
21. Klein AW. Complications, adverse reactions, and insights with the use of botulinum toxin. Dermatol Surg. 2003;29(5):549–56.
22. Ballin AC, Brandt FS, Cazzaniga A. Dermal fillers: an update. Am. J. Clin. Dermatol. 2015;16(4):271–83.
23. Greco TM, Antunes MB, Yellin SA. Injectable fillers for volume replacement in the aging face. Facial Plast Surg. 2012;28:8–20. https://doi.org/10.1055/s-0032-1305786.
24. de Maio M, Swift A, Signorini M, Fagien S. Facial assessment and injection guide for botulinum toxin and injectable hyaluronic acid fillers. Plast Reconstr Surg. 2017;140(2):265e–76e. https://doi.org/10.1097/PRS.0000000000003544.
25. de Maio M, DeBoulle K, Braz A, Rohrich RJ. Facial assessment and injection guide for botulinum toxin and injectable hyaluronic acid fillers. Plast Reconstr Surg. 2017;140(4):540e–50e. https://doi.org/10.1097/PRS.0000000000003716.
26. de Maio M, Wu WL, Goodman GJ, Monheit G. Facial assessment and injection guide for botulinum toxin and injectable hyaluronic acid fillers. Plast Reconstr Surg. 2017;140(3):393e–404e. https://doi.org/10.1097/PRS.0000000000003646.
27. Cohen JL. Understanding, avoiding, and managing dermal filler complications. Dermatol Surg. 2008;34(Suppl 1):S92–9.
28. Rzany B, DeLorenzi C. Understanding, avoiding, and managing severe filler complications. Plast Reconstr Surg. 2015;136(5 Suppl):196S–203S.
29. Glashofer MD, Flynn TC. Complications of temporary fillers. In: Carruthers J, Carruthers A, editors. Soft tissue augmentation. Toronto: Elsevier Saunders; 2013. p. 179–87.
30. Beleznay K, Carruthers JA, Carruthers A, et al. Delayed-onset nodules secondary to a smooth cohesive 20 mg/mL hyaluronic acid filler: cause and management. Dermatol Surg. 2015;41:929–39.
31. Wildemore J, Jones D. Persistent granulomatous inflammatory response induced by poly-L-lactic acid for HIV lipoatrophy. Dermatol Surg. 2006;32:1407–9.
32. Jones D. Treatment of delayed reactions to dermal fillers. J Dermatol Surg. 2014;40(11):1180.
33. Jagdeo J, Hruza G. The Food and Drug Administration Safety Communication on unintentional injection of soft-tissue filler into facial blood vessels: important points and perspectives. Dermatol Surg. 2015;41(12):1372–4.
34. Beleznay K, Carruthers J, Humphrey S, Jones D. Avoiding and treating blindness from fillers: a review of the world literature. Dermatol Surg. 2015;41:1097–117.

The manufacturer's authorised representative in the EU is Springer Nature Customer Service Centre GmbH, Europaplatz 3, 69115 Heidelberg, Germany. If you have any concerns regarding our products, please contact ProductSafety@springernature.com

Printed and bound by CPI Group (UK) Ltd, Croydon, CR0 4YY
30/09/2026
02225594-0009